THE WASHI[…] OF SURGERY

Ninth Edition

Department of Surgery
Washington University in St. Louis
School of Medicine
St. Louis Missouri

Editors

Paul E. Wise, MD

Jeffrey A. Blatnik, MD

Associate Editors

Katharine E. Caldwell, MD

Ina Chen, MD

Bradley S. Kushner, MD

Martha M.O. McGilvray, MD

Jorge G. Zarate Rodriguez, MD

Foreword by:

John A. Olson, Jr., MD, PhD

William K. Bixby Professor
Chair, Department of Surgery

Wolters Kluwer

Philadelphia • Baltimore • New York • London
Buenos Aires • Hong Kong • Sydney • Tokyo

Acquisitions Editor: Keith Donnellan
Development Editor: Barton Dudlick
Editorial Coordinator: Chester Anthony Gonzalez
Editorial Assistant: Kristen Kardoley
Marketing Manager: Kirsten Watrud
Production Project Manager: Justin Wright
Manager, Graphic Arts & Design: Stephen Druding
Manufacturing Coordinator: Lisa Bowling
Prepress Vendor: TNQ Technologies

9th edition

9 8 7 6 5 4 3 2 1

Printed in the United States of America

Library of Congress Cataloging-in-Publication Data

ISBN-13: 978-1-975201-25-8

Cataloging in Publication data available on request from publisher.

shop.lww.com

MPP0923

Contributors

Rami Al-Aref, MD
Assistant Professor of Surgery
Section of Acute and Critical Care Surgery
Department of Surgery

Erin G. Andrade, MD, MPH
Resident
Department of Surgery

Bracken A. Armstrong, MD
Adjunct Assistant Professor of Surgery
Section of Acute and Critical Care Surgery
Department of Surgery

Sandra Garcia Aroz, MD
Resident
Department of Surgery

Michael M. Awad, MD, PhD
Professor of Surgery
Section of Minimally Invasive Surgery
Department of Surgery

Louisa Yun Zhu Bai, MD
Resident
Department of Surgery

Sydney C. Beache, MD, MPHS
Resident
Department of Surgery

Jeffrey A. Blatnik, MD
Associate Professor of Surgery
Section of Minimally Invasive Surgery
Department of Surgery

Tiffany K. Brocke, MD
Resident
Department of Surgery

L. Michael Brunt, MD
Pruett Professor and Section Chief, Minimally Invasive Surgery
Department of Surgery

Sara A. Buckman, MD, PharmD
Assistant Professor of Surgery
Section of Acute and Critical Care Surgery
Department of Surgery

Katharine E. Caldwell, MD, MSCI
Chief Resident
Department of Surgery

Cameron Casson, MD
Resident
Department of Surgery

William C. Chapman, MD
Eugene M. Bricker Professor of Surgery Chief, Section of Abdominal Transplant Surgery
Division of General Surgery
Department of Surgery

Ina Chen, MD
Resident
Department of Surgery

Julie M. Clanahan, MD
Resident
Department of Surgery

Graham A. Colditz, MD, DrPH
Niess-Gain Professor and Chief, Division of Public Health Sciences
Department of Surgery

Leah Conant, MD
Resident
Department of Surgery

Heidy Cos, MD
Resident
Department of Surgery

Cathleen M. Courtney, MD
Resident
Department of Surgery

Francesca Dimou, MD, MS
Assistant Professor
Section of Minimally Invasive Surgery
Department of Surgery

James Doss, MD
Resident
Department of Obstetrics and Gynecology

Maria Bernadette Doyle, MD, MBA
Professor of Surgery
Section of Abdominal Transplant Surgery
Department of Surgery

Shaina Eckhouse, MD
Associate Professor
Section of Minimally Invasive Surgery
Department of Surgery

Nyssa Farrell, MD
Assistant Professor
Department of Otolaryngology

Ryan C. Fields, MD
Kim and Tim Eberlein Distinguished Professor
Chief, Section of Surgical Oncology
Department of Surgery

C. Corbin Frye, MD
Resident
Department of Surgery

Faiz Gani, MBBS
Resident
Department of Surgery

Will D. Gerull, MD
Resident
Department of Surgery

William E. Gillanders, MD
Professor and Vice Chair
Section of Surgical Oncology
Department of Surgery

Sean C. Glasgow, MD
Associate Professor
Section of Colon and Rectal Surgery
Department of Surgery

Andrea R. Hagemann, MD, MSCI
Associate Professor
Department of Obstetrics and Gynecology

Chet Hammill, MD, FACS
Associate Professor of Surgery
Section of Hepatobiliary, Pancreatic and Gastrointestinal Surgery
Department of Surgery

Britta J. Han, MD, MSEd
Resident
Department of Surgery

William Hawkins, MD
Professor of Surgery and Section Chief of Hepatobiliary, Pancreatic and Gastrointestinal Surgery
Department of Surgery

Brendan T. Heiden, MD, MPHS
Resident
Department of Surgery

Sara E. Holden, MD
Assistant Professor of Surgery
Section of Minimally Invasive Surgery
Department of Surgery

Steven R. Hunt, MD
Associate Professor
Section of Colon and Rectal Surgery
Department of Surgery

Obeid N. Ilahi, MD
Associate Professor of Surgery
Section of Acute and Critical Care Surgery
Department of Surgery

Alston James, MD
Resident
Department of Surgery

Momodou L. Jammeh, MD
Vascular Surgery Resident
Department of Surgery

Meghan O. Kelly, MD
Resident
Department of Surgery

Paul Kepper, MD, MS
Resident
Department of Surgery

Adeel S. Khan, MD, MPH
Associate Professor of Surgery
Section of Abdominal Transplant
Department of Surgery

Vipul Khetarpaul, MD
Assistant Professor
Section of Vascular Surgery
Department of Surgery

Eric H. Kim, MD
Associate Professor of Surgery
Division of Urologic Surgery
Department of Urology

John Kirby, MD, MS
Associate Professor of Surgery
Section of Acute and Critical Care Surgery
Department of Surgery

Jordan M. Kirsch, DO
Clinical Instructor
Section of Acute and Critical Care Surgery
Department of Surgery

Jessica Kramer McCool, MD
Assistant Professor of Surgery
Section of Acute and Critical Care Surgery
Department of Surgery

Lindsay Kranker, MD
Assistant Professor of Surgery
Section of Acute and Critical Care Surgery
Department of Surgery

Bradley S. Kushner, MD
Chief Resident
Department of Surgery

Angela Lee Hill, MD
Resident
Department of Surgery

Jessica Lindemann, MD, PhD
Resident
Department of Surgery

Robert M. MacGregor, MD
Resident
Department of Surgery

Julie A. Margenthaler, MD
Professor of Surgery
Section of Surgical Oncology
Department of Surgery

Christopher M. McAndrew, MD, MSc
Associate Professor
Department of Orthopaedic Surgery

Martha M.O. McGilvray, MSt, MD, MPHS
Resident
Department of Surgery

Bryan F. Meyers, MD, MPH
Professor of Surgery and Section Chief of Thoracic Surgery
Department of Surgery

Matthew G. Mutch, MD
Solan and Bettie Gershman Professor of Surgery
Chief, Section of Colon and Rectal Surgery
Department of Surgery

Ken Newcomer, MD
Resident
Department of Surgery

Oluseye Oduyale, MD
Resident
Department of Surgery

J. Westley Ohman, MD
Associate Professor of Surgery
Program Director of Integrated Vascular Surgery Residency
Department of Surgery

Emily J. Onufer, MD, MPH
Resident
Department of Surgery

Hannah M. Phelps, MD
Resident
Department of Surgery

Nicholas A. Pickersgill, MD
Resident
Division of Urologic Surgery
Department of Surgery

Varun Puri, MD, MSCI
Professor of Surgery
Section of Thoracic Surgery
Department of Surgery

Nanette R. Reed, MD, FACS
Assistant Professor
Section of Vascular Surgery
Department of Surgery

Keenan J. Robbins, MBBS, MPHS
Health Policy Research Fellow
Department of Surgery

Sophia H. Roberts, MD
Resident
Department of Surgery

Luis A. Sanchez, MD
Professor of Surgery
Chief, Section of Vascular Surgery
Department of Surgery

María del Pilar Martínez Santos, MD
Resident
Department of Surgery

Matthew R. Schill, MD
Instructor
Section of Cardiac Surgery
Department of Surgery

Douglas J. Schuerer, MD
Professor of Surgery
Section of Acute and Critical Care Surgery
Department of Surgery

Surendra Shenoy, MD, PhD
Professor of Surgery
Section of Abdominal Transplant Surgery
Department of Surgery

Eileen R. Smith, MD
Resident
Department of Surgery

Radhika Smith, MD
Assistant Professor
Section of Colon and Rectal Surgery
Department of Surgery

Jason Snyder, MD
Assistant Professor of Surgery
Section of Acute and Critical Care Surgery
Department of Surgery

Jessica K. Staszak, MD, MS
Assistant Professor of Surgery
Section of Acute and Critical Care Surgery
Department of Surgery

Melissa K. Stewart, MD
Assistant Professor
Section of Acute and Critical Care Surgery
Department of Surgery

Julia Suggs, MD
Vascular Surgery Resident
Department of Surgery

Brian Sullivan, MD, MSc
Vascular Surgery Resident
Department of Surgery

Kerry A. Swanson, MD
Resident
Department of Surgery

Shoichiro Tanaka, MD, MPH
Assistant Professor
Division of Plastic and Reconstructive Surgery
Department of Surgery

Damini Tandon, MD
Resident
Division of Plastic and Reconstructive Surgery
Department of Surgery

Theresa Tharakan, MD
Resident
Department of Otolaryngology: Head and Neck Surgery

Andrea Tian, MD
Resident
Department of Orthopaedic Surgery

Isaiah Turnbull, MD, PhD
Associate Professor
Section of Acute and Critical Care Surgery
Department of Surgery

Brad E. Warner, MD
Surgeon-in-Chief, St. Louis Children's Hospital and Jessie L. Ternberg, MD, PhD
Distinguished Professor of Pediatric Surgery
Department of Surgery

Jason R. Wellen, MD, MBA
Professor of Surgery and Surgical Director of Kidney and Pancreas Transplantation
Department of Surgery

Jorge G. Zarate Rodriguez, MD
Resident
Department of Surgery

Mohamed A. Zayed, MD, PhD, MBA
Associate Professor of Surgery and Radiology
Section of Vascular Surgery
Department of Surgery

Felicia Zhang, MD
Resident
Department of Surgery

Foreword

I am delighted to present the ninth edition of *The Washington Manual™ of Surgery*. For over a quarter century, the manual has provided essential knowledge and guidance to residents, surgeons, and medical students worldwide. It is with great anticipation that I invite you to explore the wealth of information contained within this latest edition.

Since its inception in 1997, *The Washington Manual™ of Surgery* has established itself as an indispensable resource in the field. Our commitment to delivering the most up-to-date and comprehensive content remains unwavering. With each edition, we strive to meet the evolving needs of the surgical community and equip our readers with the necessary tools to provide exceptional patient care.

In this ninth edition, a dedicated team of resident authors, supported by expert faculty coauthors and our esteemed editors, Drs. Jeffrey Blatnik and Paul Wise, has meticulously crafted a manual that addresses the specific needs of surgical trainees, practicing surgeons, and students alike. Building upon evidence-based medicine, advanced surgical techniques, and current research, we have curated a concise reference that embodies the pinnacle of surgical knowledge.

This edition places a strong emphasis on clarity and efficiency. We understand the time constraints faced by busy trainees and surgeons and have organized the content to allow for easy navigation and quick reference. Whether you require guidance in complex surgical decision-making or a concise overview of a particular procedure, this manual serves as a reliable companion in the care of surgical patients.

As we enter this new era at Washington University, I extend my heartfelt appreciation to all those who have contributed to the success of *The Washington Manual™ of Surgery*. Specifically, I would like to recognize all of the residents who have played a pivotal role in shaping the content, and the faculty members who have shared their expertise and guidance to this publication over the years. Likewise, I am grateful to each and every reader whose support and dedication to surgical excellence have sustained this unique and important resource.

May this ninth edition serve as a trusted companion in your pursuit of surgical mastery. Our collective commitment to healing, innovation, and the relentless pursuit of excellence ensures that the art and science of surgery continue to positively impact the lives of patients.

John A. Olson, Jr, MD, PhD
St. Louis, Missouri

Preface

This ninth edition of *The Washington Manual™ of Surgery* is designed to complement *The Washington Manual of Medical Therapeutics*. Written by resident and faculty members of the Department of Surgery at Washington University in St. Louis, we present a brief, rational approach to the assessment and management of surgical conditions and topics relevant to surgeons. The text is directed to the reader at the second- or third-year surgical resident level, although all residents, surgical and nonsurgical attendings, medical students, physician assistants, nurse practitioners, and others who provide care for patients with surgical conditions will find this Manual of interest and assistance. The book provides a succinct discussion of surgical diseases, with algorithms for addressing problems based on the opinions of the authors, as well as key steps to routine and major operative procedures. Although multiple approaches may be reasonable for some clinical situations, this Manual attempts to present a single, effective approach for each. We have limited extensive details on diagnosis and therapy as this is not meant to be an exhaustive, detailed surgical reference. Coverage of pathophysiology, the history of surgery, and extensive reference lists have been excluded from most areas.

The first edition of this Manual was published in 1997, followed by editions in 1999, 2002, 2005, 2007, 2012, 2016, and 2019. As with editions in the past, we have attempted to focus on relevant and timely topics, but we hope to bring this edition into the modern, multimedia age with the edition of podcasts by the authors and associate editors to further delve into important aspects of their chapters. This ninth edition continues to provide review questions at the end of each chapter so that readers can self-assess their knowledge and practice for examinations (but given the litany of multiple choice question resources now available to learners both online and in print, we have focused on short answer questions in this edition). We have added a chapter on "Endovascular Basics" and expanded "Biostatistics" with "Study Design." Some chapters have been consolidated and reorganized (e.g., "Radiology," "Anesthesia," coagulation/transfusion, fluid/electrolyte/nutrition, and subspecialty chapters) to best reflect the nature of today's surgical practice and improve on flow and topic relevancy. All chapters have again been updated with evidence-based medicine, with the latest information and treatment algorithms in each section, including new material and citations. We have added more operative and procedure steps in a brief, succinct format, hopefully helpful for learners and trainees as they prepare for cases or their Board exams. We have also added a "Key References" section to each chapter to allow for those readers who want a deeper understanding of the subject matter to review the landmark trials and important publications that inform each topic.

This continues to be a resident-prepared Manual, and each chapter was updated and revised (or authored) by a resident with assistance from faculty coauthors. Editorial oversight for the Manual was shared by five senior resident associate editors (Katharine Caldwell, Ina Chen, Bradley Kushner, Martha McGilvray, and Jorge Zarate Rodriguez). The tremendous effort of all involved—resident and faculty authors, and particularly the above-noted senior resident associate editors—is reflected in the quality and consistency of the chapters.

We are indebted to the former senior editors of this work, Gerard M. Doherty, MD, who developed and oversaw the first three editions, and then Mary Klingensmith, MD, who oversaw the next five editions of this Manual, continuing this Manual as a perpetually well-organized project as it was handed over to P.E.W. as co-editor of the eighth edition. M.E.K. was instrumental in moving the Manual forward, as she did with surgical education as a whole, and now J.A.B. is joining as co-editor. We are grateful for the continued tremendous support from Wolters Kluwer Health, especially through the complexities of publishing during the pandemic. They have been very supportive of our efforts and have supplied dedicated, knowledgeable assistance. Keith Donnellan remains an incredibly helpful Acquisition Editor, with Anne Malcolm as Associate Director of Content Development, Barton Dudlick and Ariel Winter as Development Editors, and Anthony Gonzalez as Editorial Coordinator, all keeping us on point and on schedule.

Finally, we are grateful to have the support of our new Chair of the Department of Surgery, John A. Olson, MD, PhD, in allowing us to continue the Manual's tradition of excellence. Dr. Olson steps in for Timothy J. Eberlein, MD, our Chair for almost 25 years. Dr. Eberlein's dedication and leadership of the Department of Surgery at Washington University in St. Louis through a quarter of a century has been inspiring, and we are indebted to him for his support for us and this Manual through the years. Most importantly, though, we want to deeply thank our families for their love, support, patience, and encouragement as we wouldn't be who we are and do what we do without them!

We hope you enjoy this latest edition of *The Washington Manual™ of Surgery*!

J.A.B. and P.E.W.

Contents

Contributors iii
Foreword viii
Preface ix

1 Preoperative Assessment and Care of the Surgical Patient 1
Angela Lee Hill, Bradley S. Kushner, and Sara E. Holden

2 Intraoperative Considerations 13
Ina Chen, Felicia Zhang, Jason Snyder, and Lindsay Kranker

3 Management of Common Postoperative Problems 43
Louisa Yun Zhu Bai, Katharine E. Caldwell, Rami Al-Aref, and Isaiah Turnbull

4 Critical Care 85
Robert M. MacGregor and Sara A. Buckman

5 Trauma Resuscitation and Adjuncts 115
Emily J. Onufer and Jessica Kramer McCool

6 Head, Neck, and Spinal Trauma 132
Erin G. Andrade and Jessica K. Staszak

7 Chest Trauma 148
Hannah M. Phelps, Jordan M. Kirsch, and Melissa K. Stewart

8 Abdominal Trauma 163
Kerry A. Swanson and Douglas J. Schuerer

9 Extremity Trauma 176
Andrea Tian and Christopher M. McAndrew

10 Burns 194
Oluseye Oduyale, Bracken A. Armstrong, Jessica Kramer McCool, and John Kirby

11 Wound Care 209
Tiffany K. Brocke and Bracken A. Armstrong

12 Acute Abdomen 233
Sophia H. Roberts and Obeid N. Ilahi

13 Esophagus 250
William D. Gerull and Bryan F. Meyers

14 Stomach 269
Alston James and William Hawkins

15 The Surgical Management of Obesity 285
Ina Chen and Francesca Dimou

16 Small Intestine 301
Cameron Casson and Radhika Smith

17 Surgical Diseases of the Liver 330
Sandra Garcia Aroz and William C. Chapman

18 Surgical Diseases of the Biliary Tree 346
Heidy Cos and Adeel S. Khan

19 Pancreas 362
Katharine E. Caldwell and Chet Hammill

20 Spleen 389
Keenan J. Robbins and Maria Bernadette Doyle

21 Abdominal Transplantation 412
Jessica Lindemann and Jason R. Wellen

22 Appendix 435
Paul Kepper and Sean C. Glasgow

23 Colon and Rectum 444
Jorge G. Zarate Rodriguez and Steven R. Hunt

24 Anorectal Disease 475
Julie M. Clanahan and Matthew G. Mutch

25 Hernias 499
Bradley S. Kushner and Jeffrey A. Blatnik

26 Endoscopic, Laparoscopic, and Robotic Surgery 517
Leah Conant and Michael M. Awad

27 Breast Disease 527
Faiz Gani and Julie A. Margenthaler

28 Skin and Soft Tissue Tumors 551
Ken Newcomer and Ryan C. Fields

29 Adrenal Gland and Hereditary Endocrine Syndromes 573
C. Corbin Frye and L. Michael Brunt

30 Parathyroid and Thyroid Glands 597
Eileen R. Smith and William E. Gillanders

31 Lung and Mediastinal Diseases 620
Louisa Yun Zhu Bai, Brendan T. Heiden, and Varun Puri

32 Cardiac Surgery 650
Meghan O. Kelly and Matthew R. Schill

33 Endovascular Basics 678
Martha M. O. McGilvray and J. Westley Ohman

34 Cerebrovascular Disease 688
Momodou L. Jammeh and Mohamed A. Zayed

35 Thoracoabdominal Vascular Disease 702
Martha M. O. McGilvray, J. Westley Ohman, and Luis A. Sanchez

36 Peripheral Arterial Disease 733
María del Pilar Martínez Santos and Vipul Khetarpaul

37 Venous and Lymphatic Disease 761
Julia Suggs and Nanette R. Reed

38 Dialysis Access 782
Brian Sullivan and Surendra Shenoy

39 Pediatric Surgery 795
Cathleen M. Courtney and Brad W. Warner

40 Subspecialty Surgery for the General Surgeon 822

Obstetrics and Gynecology for the General Surgeon 822
James Doss and Andrea R. Hagemann

Otolaryngology for the General Surgeon 832
Theresa Tharakan and Nyssa Farrell

Plastic and Reconstructive Surgery for General Surgeons 849
Damini Tandon and Shoichiro Tanaka

Urology for the General Surgeon 867
Nicholas A. Pickersgill and Eric H. Kim

41 Biostatistics and Study Design 882
Sydney C. Beache and Graham A. Colditz

42 Patient Safety and Quality Improvement 897
Britta J. Han and Shaina Eckhouse

Answer Key 907
Index 925

1 Preoperative Assessment and Care of the Surgical Patient

Angela Lee Hill, Bradley S. Kushner, and Sara E. Holden

I. INTRODUCTION

A. To provide an introduction and brief overview of important considerations for the preoperative care for surgical patients
   1. Two components are emphasized:
      a. The decision to proceed with surgery
      b. Preoperative optimization

B. A special population highlighted is older adult care: By the year 2050, elderly Americans are projected to make up 20% of the US population[1]
   1. When evaluating surgical risk in an older adult population, several questions emerge:
      a. What is the significance of chronological age?
      b. How do we weigh risks versus benefits?
      c. As such, this chapter focuses on surgical decision-making, how to best evaluate frailty, and options for preoperative optimization.

II. SURGICAL DECISION-MAKING

A. Preoperative planning begins with surgical decision-making including a discussion regarding capacity and realistic goal setting.

B. Identifying patient goals
   1. The first step in any patient's preoperative care is determining the need for surgery.
   2. Prior to deciding on operative management, patients should **determine their health care goals** and determine how the possible risks and benefits of surgery align with those goals.[2]
      a. Especially important in elective surgeries, such as ventral hernia repairs, where postoperative risks vary by patient age and functional health.[3]
      b. Critical in patients for whom surgery may not increase quality or length of life, such as in metastatic oncologic disease.[4]
      c. Discussing patient goals and preferences is not limited to an older and frailer or terminally ill population; rather, this decision is applicable to many common conditions, e.g., appendicitis and diverticulitis.
         i. Trials comparing surgery and comparative management for these two pathologies did not demonstrate one option as being

superior across all measures. For example, patients treated with antibiotics for appendicitis have a higher recurrence rate; however, surgical patients reported worse pain and longer hospitalizations.[5] This suggests the importance of assessing patient goals in even more robust patients.

3. In **emergent situations**, thoughtful goals-of-care conversations can be especially difficult; only 36.7% of patients have completed an advance directive and illness severity can preclude meaningful conversations with patients in these settings.[6]
4. It is important to revisit previously stated patient priorities when patients may not be able to advocate for themselves.
   a. Despite many critically ill patients prioritizing quality of life, nearly 10% of patients over the age of 65 years had an operation in their last week of life.[6]
5. Not only is it more difficult to assess patients' goals but also it can be more challenging to predict perioperative risk in emergent situations.
   a. Patient factors like frailty can compound postoperative risk in the emergent setting.
   b. For surgeries that can be postponed, and prior to which health optimization can be pursued, surgeons and patients may decide to delay surgery in favor of prehabilitation (*see "Prehabilitation" below*).[7]

C. Decision-making capacity

1. For many older adult or critically ill patients who lack decision-making capacity, the decision-making responsibility falls on patients' power of attorney or next of kin.
   a. **Decision-making capacity** can be assessed by the clinician based on the patient's ability to articulate therapeutic options, explain their preference, rationalize this preference, and delineate the consequences of each treatment option.
      i. "Capacity" can be fluid and can change pending the patient's clinical status.[8]
      ii. For example, patients with waxing and waning delirium may have intermittent capacity. Patients can regain capacity when off sedation following a period of mechanical intubation.
   b. A health care power of attorney (HCPOA) should be established prior to any operation.
      i. Unfortunately, only a minority complete this. Being female, widowed or having an increased American Society of Anesthesiology score has been associated with the presence of HCPOA documentation preoperatively.[9]

III. PREOPERATIVE ASSESSMENT

A. Age and frailty

1. While advanced age is often associated with increasing age-related risk factors, termed **geriatric syndromes**, age is often an imperfect measurement for determining postoperative complications.

a. Geriatric syndromes include conditions such as multimorbidity (multiple chronic conditions), polypharmacy (multiple medications concurrently), poor functional status, cognitive impairment, sarcopenia (reduced muscle mass), and malnutrition.[3]

b. Geriatric syndromes do not affect all older adult patients and may affect younger patients, suggesting that chronological age alone is insufficient in screening patients preoperatively.

2. The terms "chronological age" vs. "biological age" have been developed as a means of distinguishing between a patient's age and a more complex measure of a patient's physiologic health, incorporating age, lifestyle, disability, etc.[10]

   a. **Biological, or physiologic, age** is meant to account for functional status, assessed via a patient's activities of daily living. This is measured in metabolic equivalents (METs), with 1 MET equaling the resting oxygen consumption of an average 40-year-old male.[11]

      i. Functional capacity can be classified as excellent (>10 METs), good (7-10 METs), moderate (4-6 METs), or poor (<4 METs).

   b. Across surgical subspecialties, biological age with chronological age is more effective in predicting postoperative outcomes than chronological age alone.

      i. For example, among patients with ventral hernias, increased **chronological age** alone does not increase the risk for postoperative complications or readmission.[12]

      ii. Increased biological age, meanwhile, has shown to be significantly associated with systemic complications following laparoscopic gastrectomy for gastric cancer.[13]

3. **Frailty** is often used as an indicator and measure of biological age.

   a. Frailty has been defined as a depleted physiologic reserve resulting in decreased resistance to stressors, as associated with decreased strength and endurance.[1]

   b. It has been further characterized via a phenotypic versus cumulative deficit model, with the former assessing weight loss, exhaustion, physical activity, speed, and grip strength and the latter incorporating 48 deficits associated with advanced age.[14]

      i. Several tools for measuring frailty exist, ranging from single-item assessment tools, such as a timed walking test and sarcopenia, to scales and survey, including the Clinical Frailty Scale, the FRAIL scale, Vulnerability Elders Survey-13 and The Frailty Index, and the Comprehensive Geriatric Assessment.[13,15]

      ii. No single frailty assessment has demonstrated superior prediction of postoperative outcomes.[16]

   c. Across the surgical literature, frailty is associated with an increased rate of postoperative complications, hospital length of stay, discharge to residential care facility, and mortality.[15,16]

      i. As such, frailty should be assessed preoperatively to assist with perioperative risk assessment and surgical decision-making in all patients.

B. Medical and surgical history

1. In addition to age and functional health, medical comorbidities should be reviewed thoroughly during the preoperative patient assessment.

2. **Cardiovascular disease**

   a. Remains one of the leading causes of death after noncardiac surgery.

   b. **Risk factors**

      i. Factors associated with perioperative cardiac morbidity and mortality include age above 70 years, unstable angina, recent (prior 6 months) myocardial infarction (MI), untreated congestive heart failure (CHF), diabetes mellitus, valvular heart disease, cardiac arrhythmias, peripheral vascular disease, and functional impairment.

      ii. Procedural factors also convey risk. In 2014, the American Heart Association condensed procedures into two risk levels: *Low* risk (major adverse cardiovascular event—MACE—risk <1%) and *elevated* risk (MACE risk >1%). The category of intermediate risk is no longer used, as the management of patients undergoing these and elevated risk procedures is similar.

   c. **Cardiac risk indices/calculators**

      i. Several tools have been created to aid in predicting preoperative risk of a MACE.

      ii. The American College of Surgeons NSQIP Surgical Risk Calculator combines cardiac and noncardiac factors to calculate the risk of overall postoperative complications and can be found at riskcalculator.facs.org.

   d. **Preoperative testing**

      i. Preoperative workup is based on several factors including medical history, urgency of surgery, risk of surgical procedure, patient functional status, and goals of care.

      ii. When it is determined that a patient requires further testing prior to surgery, a multidisciplinary team including a cardiologist is employed to determine which noninvasive or invasive measure should be taken to optimize the patient.

   e. **Preoperative management**

      i. **Patients with pacemakers** should have their pacemakers turned to the uninhibited mode (e.g., DOO) before surgery. In addition, bipolar cautery should be used, when possible, in these patients. If unipolar cautery is necessary, the dispersive electrode should be placed away from the heart.

      ii. **Patients with internal defibrillators** should have these devices turned off during surgery.

      iii. **Perioperative beta-blockade**

         a) Recent studies, including the POISE trial, suggest that β-blockers reduce perioperative ischemia and may reduce the risk of MI and cardiovascular death in high-risk patients.[17]

      iv. **Patients with recent angioplasty or stenting**

         a) Several studies have shown a high incidence of cardiovascular complications when noncardiac surgery is performed shortly after coronary angioplasty or stenting.

b) Current guidelines (ACC/AHA 2016) are to delay noncardiac surgery at least 6 weeks after coronary angioplasty or placement of bare metal stents for stable ischemic disease as these require at least 1 month of dual antiplatelet therapy (DAPT), aspirin 81 mg, and clopidogrel.

c) In contrast, DAPT should be continued for at least 6 to 12 months following placement of newer-generation drug-eluting stent (first generation rarely if ever used clinically), which can affect timing of elective operations.

d) If coronary stents were placed for percutaneous coronary intervention following acute or recent acute coronary syndrome, then DAPT should be continued for 12 months.

e) For all patients, the risk of bleeding and thrombosis need to be considered.

f) Surgery in an open body space, such as the abdomen, is possible on patients taking antiplatelets, albeit with an elevated bleeding risk.

3. **Pulmonary disease**
   a. **History**
      i. Preexisting lung disease confers a dramatically increased risk of perioperative pulmonary complications.
      ii. Risk factors for pulmonary complications include chronic obstructive pulmonary disease, smoking, asthma, obstructive sleep apnea, advanced age, obesity, surgical site located near the diaphragm, and poor functional status.
   b. **Physical examination**
      i. Attention directed toward signs of lung disease (e.g., wheezing, prolonged expiratory–inspiratory ratio, clubbing, or use of accessory muscles of respiration).
   c. **Diagnostic evaluation**
      i. A **CXR** should only be performed for acute symptoms related to pulmonary disease, unless indicated for the specific procedure under consideration.
      ii. An **arterial blood gas** can be considered in patients with a history of lung disease or smoking to provide a baseline for comparison with postoperative studies, but it is not reliable to accurately predict postoperative pulmonary complications.
      iii. **Preoperative pulmonary function testing** is controversial and probably unnecessary in stable patients with previously characterized pulmonary disease undergoing nonthoracic procedures.
   d. **Preoperative prophylaxis and management**
      i. **Pulmonary toilet.** Increasing lung volume by the use of preoperative incentive spirometry is potentially effective in reducing pulmonary complications.
   e. **Antibiotics** do not reduce pulmonary infectious complications in the absence of preoperative infection. Elective operations should be postponed in patients with respiratory infections. If emergent surgery is required, patients with acute pulmonary infections should receive IV antibiotic therapy.

f. **Smoking cessation.** All patients should be encouraged to and assisted in smoking cessation before surgery.
g. **Bronchodilators.** In the patient with obstructive airway disease and evidence of a significant reactive component, bronchodilators may be required in the perioperative period. Elective operation should be postponed in the patient who is actively wheezing.

4. **Renal disease**
   a. **History**
      i. Patients with chronic renal insufficiency (CRI) are at a substantially increased risk of perioperative morbidity and mortality.
      ii. The timing and quality of the patient's last dialysis session, the amount of fluid removed, and preoperative weight provide important information about the patient's volume status.
      iii. In nonanuric patients, the amount of urine made daily should also be documented.
   b. **Physical examination** should be performed to assess the volume status.
      i. Elevated jugular venous pulsations or crackles on lung examination can indicate intravascular volume overload.
   c. **Diagnostic testing**
      i. Serum electrolyte and bicarbonate levels should be measured, as well as blood urea nitrogen (BUN) and creatinine.
      ii. A complete blood cell count should be obtained to evaluate for significant anemia or a low platelet level.
      iii. Normal platelet numbers can mask platelet dysfunction in patients with chronic uremia.
   d. **Perioperative management**
      i. **Timing of dialysis.** Dialysis should be performed within 24 hours of the planned operative procedure.
      ii. **Intravascular volume status.** Cardiac events are the most common cause of death in patients with CRI. Both hypovolemia and volume overload are poorly tolerated, and invasive monitoring in the intra- and postoperative periods may assist in optimizing fluid balance.
   e. **Preventing perioperative renal dysfunction**
      i. **Risk factors**
         a) Patients without preexisting CRI may be at risk of developing postoperative acute renal failure (ARF), depending on certain patient and procedure risk factors.
         b) Incidence of postoperative ARF ranges from 1.5% to 2.5% for cardiac surgical procedures to more than 10% for patients undergoing repair of supraceliac abdominal aortic aneurysms.
         c) Other risk factors for the development of ARF include elevated preoperative BUN or creatinine, CHF, advanced age, intraoperative hypotension, sepsis, aortic cross-clamping, intravascular volume contraction, and use of nephrotoxic and radionuclide agents.

ii. **Prevention**
   a) **Intravascular volume expansion.** Adequate hydration is the most important preventive measure for reducing the incidence of ARF.
   b) **Radiocontrast dye administration.** Patients undergoing radiocontrast dye studies have an increased incidence of postoperative renal failure. Fluid administration (1-2 L of isotonic saline) alone appears to confer protection against ARF. Additional commonly used but unproven measures for reducing the incidence of contrast dye–mediated ARF include the use of low-osmolality contrast agents, a bicarbonate drip, and oral N-acetylcysteine.
   c) **Other nephrotoxins**—including aminoglycoside antibiotics, NSAIDs, and various anesthetic drugs—can predispose to renal failure, as well, and should be avoided in patients at high risk for postoperative renal failure.

5. **Diabetes mellitus**
   a. Diabetic patients are at increased risk of morbidity and mortality.
   b. Vascular disease is common in diabetics, and MI, often with an atypical presentation, is the leading cause of perioperative death among diabetic patients.
   c. **Preoperative evaluation**
      i. All diabetic patients should have their blood glucose measured in preop holding and intraoperatively to prevent unrecognized hyperglycemia or hypoglycemia.
      ii. **Patients with diet-controlled diabetes mellitus** can be maintained safely without food or glucose infusion before surgery.
      iii. **Oral hypoglycemic agents** should be discontinued the evening before scheduled surgery. Long-acting agents such as chlorpropamide or glyburide should be discontinued 2 to 3 days prior.
      iv. **Insulin-dependent diabetic patients** require insulin and glucose preoperatively to prevent ketosis and catabolism. Patients undergoing major surgery should receive half of their morning insulin dose and 5% dextrose IV. Subsequent insulin administration by either SC sliding-scale or insulin infusion is guided by frequent blood glucose determinations. SC insulin pumps should be inactivated the morning of surgery.

6. **Infectious complications**
   a. Infectious complications are a major cause of morbidity and mortality following surgery.
   b. They may arise at the surgical site itself or in other organ systems. It is impossible to overemphasize the importance of frequent handwashing or antiseptic foam use by all health care workers to prevent the spread of infection.
   c. In addition to impacting the patient, rates of postsurgical infections are closely monitored by hospitals and health care providers and are increasingly being used as a metric by which hospitals, departments, and surgeons are measured.

d. **Assessment**
   i. Risk factors for infectious complications after surgery can be grouped into procedure- and patient-specific risk factors.
   ii. **Procedure-specific risk factors** include the type of operation, the degree of wound contamination (whether the case is classified as clean, clean–contaminated, contaminated, or dirty), and the duration and urgency of the operation.
   iii. **Patient-specific risk factors** include age, diabetes, obesity, immunosuppression, malnutrition, preexisting infection, smoking, and other chronic illness.

e. **Prophylaxis**
   i. **Surgical site infection**
      a) Several modifiable factors under control of the surgical team have been identified as preventable contributors to surgical site infections. Updated guidelines addressing strategies for the prevention of surgical site infections were published in *JAMA* and include when prophylactic antimicrobials are appropriate, the importance of glycemic control, etc.[18]
   ii. **Respiratory infections**
      a) Risk factors and measures for preventing pulmonary complications are discussed elsewhere.
   iii. **Genitourinary infections** may be caused by instrumentation of the urinary tract or placement of an indwelling urinary catheter.
      a) Preventive measures include avoiding catheterization for short operations, sterile insertion of the catheter, and removal of the catheter on postoperative day 1. Some operations that include a low pelvic dissection will require longer catheterization because of local trauma.

IV. PREOPERATIVE OPTIMIZATION

A. Individual behavior modification

1. **Smoking:** Across multiple studies, smoking at time of operation has been associated with increased postoperative complications, especially wound and tissue flap necrosis; anastomotic leakage; and surgical site infection. Long-term smokers are more likely to develop hernias and have delayed fistula and bone healing.[19]
   a. Several prospective cohort studies and randomized controlled trials have been developed to examine the efficacy of perioperative smoking cessation programs. The studied programs often utilize counseling in addition to nicotine replacement therapy.[20]
   b. In the majority of studies, this multimodal programming has decreased the prevalence of smoking on the day of surgery, with more intense programs (e.g., those lasting 6-8 weeks) demonstrating improved cessation rates.[21]
   c. When possible and available, longer and more intensive counseling programs, combined with pharmaceutical treatment, such as varenicline, are more likely to benefit patients.

2. **Obesity:** The impact of patient obesity on postoperative surgical outcomes has been varied. In large studies of general surgery patients, obesity has been associated with increased risk of wound infection after open elective surgery.[22]
   a. Furthermore, preoperative weight loss has had a demonstrable benefit in patients with hernia. Obesity has been demonstrated to be a significant predictor of recurrence in incisional hernias and groin hernias following repair.[23,24]
   b. Together, this suggests that preoperative weight loss may be beneficial in general surgery patients, especially those undergoing hernia repair.
3. **Malnutrition:** Malnutrition has consistently been associated with poor postoperative outcomes. Although multiple nutrition criteria have been utilized preoperatively, common components include hypoalbuminemia, low body mass index, recent weight loss, and sarcopenia.
   a. When comparing nutritional assessments, such as the subjective global assessment and nutritional risk index, no significant differences were found in predicting postoperative outcomes.[25]
   b. Among patients with cancer, malnutrition has been associated with increased reoperation, prolonged mechanical ventilation, incidence of pneumonia, postoperative blood product transfusion, and mortality.[26] Furthermore, in patients with lung cancer, malnutrition has been associated with other postoperative complications, such as ARF requiring dialysis and development of arrhythmias.[27] Given the consistently increased surgical risk associated with malnutrition, preoperative nutrition optimization may be beneficial in these patients.

B. Organized programming (prehabilitation)
1. The perioperative period can be a valuable time to optimize a patient's physiologic health, especially for patients at higher risk for postoperative complication.
2. Recently, prehabilitation has gained popularity as a means of preoperative optimization.
   a. To date, exercise frequency, methodology, and intensity, as well as diet recommendations, have not been standardized.
   b. Typically prehabilitation is a several-weeks-long program with physical and mental health components, including[28]:
      i. Physical health: Exercise regimen including resistance training
      ii. Pulmonary: Regular incentive spirometry
      iii. Nutrition-based intervention[29]
3. Although studies of patients undergoing abdominal surgery have not demonstrated differences in hospital length of stay, prehabilitation has been associated with decreased postoperative complications and postoperative morbidity. Unfortunately, these associations are not consistent across randomized control groups.[3,30]
   a. Heterogeneities in programming, adherence quantification, and initial patient physical fitness assessment have made comparing studies' results difficult.[29] However, given the promising early results demonstrated by prehabilitation, further investigation is warranted.

Key References

Citation	Summary
Devereaux PJ, Xavier D, Pogue J, et al. Characteristics and short-term prognosis of perioperative myocardial infarction in patients undergoing noncardiac surgery: a cohort study. *Ann Intern Med*. 2011;154(8):523-528.	• In a cohort study looking at the 8,351 patients undergoing noncardiac surgery, 5% of patients suffered a perioperative MI; 74% of MIs occurred within 48 h of surgery and 65% did not experience ischemic symptoms. The 30-d mortality rate was 11.6% among patients who had a perioperative MI, compared with 2.2% among those who did not.
Fleisher LA, Fleischmann KE, Auerbach AD, et al. 2014 ACC/AHA guideline on perioperative cardiovascular evaluation and management of patients undergoing noncardiac surgery: a report of the American College of Cardiology/American Heart Association Task Force on practice guidelines. *J Am Coll Cardiol*. 2014;64(22):e77-e137.	• Risk stratification for major adverse cardiac events (or MACE, defined as death, Q-wave MI, and need for revascularization) should be done preoperatively, and pending MACE risk, further workup may include 12-lead EKG, left ventricular functional assessment, and exercise testing.
Wijeysundera DN, Duncan D, Nkonde-Price C, et al. Perioperative beta blockade in noncardiac surgery: a systematic review for the 2014 ACC/AHA guideline on perioperative cardiovascular evaluation and management of patients undergoing noncardiac surgery—a report of the American College of Cardiology/American Heart Association Task Force on Practice Guidelines. *Circulation*. 2014;130(24):2246-2264.	• Guidelines following expert review recommend that routine administration of higher perioperative β-blockade started within 1 d of noncardiac surgery prevents nonfatal MI at the cost of increased risk of stroke and death.

CHAPTER 1: PREOPERATIVE ASSESSMENT AND CARE OF THE SURGICAL PATIENT

Review Questions

1. What term is used to describe age-related risk factors, such as multimorbidity, polypharmacy, and sarcopenia?
2. How can frailty be measured?
3. How should pacemakers be managed perioperatively?

4. How long should patients continue dual antiplatelet therapy (e.g., aspirin and clopidogrel) after undergoing drug-eluting stent placement?
5. When should a urinary catheter placed intraoperatively be removed?
6. What postoperative complications are associated with smoking?
7. What can be done in the preoperative period to improve patients' postoperative outcomes?

REFERENCES

1. Hanna K, Ditillo M, Joseph B. The role of frailty and prehabilitation in surgery. *Curr Opin Crit Care*. 2019;25(6):717-722.
2. Dworsky JQ, Russell MM. Surgical decision making for older adults. *JAMA*. 2019;321(7):716.
3. Hamilton J, Kushner B, Holden S, Holden T. Age-related risk factors in ventral hernia repairs: a review and call to action. *J Surg Res*. 2021;266:180-191.
4. A controlled trial to improve care for seriously ill hospitalized patients. The study to understand prognoses and preferences for outcomes and risks of treatments (SUPPORT). The SUPPORT Principal Investigators. *JAMA*. 1995;274(20):1591-1598.
5. Chhabra KR, Sacks GD, Dimick JB. Surgical decision making: challenging dogma and incorporating patient preferences. *JAMA*. 2017;317(4):357-358.
6. Morris RS, Ruck JM, Conca-Cheng AM, Smith TJ, Carver TW, Johnston FM. Shared decision-making in acute surgical illness: the surgeon's perspective. *J Am Coll Surg*. 2018;226(5):784-795.
7. Pache B, Grass F, Hubner M, Kefleyesus A, Mathevet P, Achtari C. Prevalence and consequences of preoperative weight loss in gynecologic surgery. *Nutrients*. 2019;11(5):1094.
8. Ganzini L, Volicer L, Nelson WA, Fox E, Derse AR. Ten myths about decision-making capacity. *J Am Med Dir Assoc*. 2005;6(3 suppl l):S100-S104.
9. Marks S, Wanner JP, Cobb AS, Swetz KM, Lange GM. Surgery without a surrogate: the low prevalence of healthcare power of attorney documents among preoperative patients. *Hosp Pract*. 2019;47(1):28-33.
10. Diebel LWM, Rockwood K. Determination of biological age: geriatric assessment vs biological biomarkers. *Curr Oncol Rep*. 2021;23(9):104.
11. Harb SC, Bhat P, Cremer PC, et al. Prognostic value of functional capacity in different exercise protocols. *J Am Heart Assoc*. 2020;9(13):e015986.
12. Kushner BS, Han B, Otegbeye E, et al. Chronological age does not predict postoperative outcomes following transversus abdominis release (TAR). *Surg Endosc*. 2022;36(6):4570-4579.
13. Tanaka T, Suda K, Uyama I. ASO author reflections: chronological or biological age—which is more important for making clinical decisions in geriatric patients? *Ann Surg Oncol*. 2019;26(suppl 3):810-811.
14. Kulminski AM, Ukraintseva SV, Kulminskaya IV, Arbeev KG, Land K, Yashin AI. Cumulative deficits better characterize susceptibility to death in elderly people than phenotypic frailty: lessons from the Cardiovascular Health Study. *J Am Geriatr Soc*. 2008;56(5):898-903.
15. Ethun CG, Bilen MA, Jani AB, Maithel SK, Ogan K, Master VA. Frailty and cancer: implications for oncology surgery, medical oncology, and radiation oncology. *CA Cancer J Clin*. 2017;67(5):362-377.

16. Lin HS, Watts JN, Peel NM, Hubbard RE. Frailty and post-operative outcomes in older surgical patients: a systematic review. *BMC Geriatr*. 2016;16(1):157.

17. POISE Study Group; Devereaux PJ, Yang H, Yusuf S, Guyatt GH. Effects of extended-release metoprolol succinate in patients undergoing non-cardiac surgery (POISE trial): a randomised controlled trial. *Lancet*. 2008;371(9627):1839-1847.

18. Berrios-Torres SI, Umscheid CA, Bratzler DW, et al. Centers for disease control and prevention guideline for the prevention of surgical site infection, 2017. *JAMA Surg*. 2017;152(8):784-791.

19. Sørensen LT. Wound healing and infection in surgery: the clinical impact of smoking and smoking cessation—a systematic review and meta-analysis. *Arch Surg*. 2012;147(4):373-383.

20. Wong J, Lam DP, Abrishami A, Chan MT, Chung F. Short-term preoperative smoking cessation and postoperative complications: a systematic review and meta-analysis. *Can J Anaesth*. 2012;59(3):268-279.

21. Thomsen T, Villebro N, Moller AM. Interventions for preoperative smoking cessation. *Cochrane Database Syst Rev*. 2014;2014(3):CD002294.

22. Dindo D, Muller MK, Weber M, Clavien PA. Obesity in general elective surgery. *Lancet*. 2003;361(9374):2032-2035.

23. Sauerland S, Korenkov M, Kleinen T, Arndt M, Paul A. Obesity is a risk factor for recurrence after incisional hernia repair. *Hernia*. 2004;8(1):42-46.

24. Rosemar A, Angeras U, Rosengren A, Nordin P. Effect of body mass index on groin hernia surgery. *Ann Surg*. 2010;252(2):397-401.

25. Kuzu MA, Terzioğlu H, Genc V, et al. Preoperative nutritional risk assessment in predicting postoperative outcome in patients undergoing major surgery. *World J Surg*. 2006;30(3):378-390.

26. Hu WH, Chen HH, Lee KC, et al. Assessment of the addition of hypoalbuminemia to ACS-NSQIP surgical risk calculator in colorectal cancer. *Medicine (Baltimore)*. 2016;95(10):e2999.

27. Bagan P, Berna P, De Dominicis F, et al. Nutritional status and postoperative outcome after pneumonectomy for lung cancer. *Ann Thorac Surg*. 2013;95(2):392-396.

28. Shaughness G, Howard R, Englesbe M. Patient-centered surgical prehabilitation. *Am J Surg*. 2018;216(3):636-638.

29. Moran J, Guinan E, McCormick P, et al. The ability of prehabilitation to influence post-operative outcome after intra-abdominal operation: a systematic review and meta-analysis. *Surgery*. 2016;160(5):1189-1201.

30. Hughes MJ, Hackney RJ, Lamb PJ, Wigmore SJ, Christopher Deans DA, Skipworth RJE. Prehabilitation before major abdominal surgery: a systematic review and meta-analysis. *World J Surg*. 2019;43(7):1661-1668.

2 Intraoperative Considerations

Ina Chen, Felicia Zhang, Jason Snyder, and Lindsay Kranker

I. CULTURE OF SAFETY IN THE OPERATING ROOM

It is crucial to promote a culture of safety in the operating room, in which all team members share perceptions, beliefs, and values that prioritize patient safety. All team members should be empowered to communicate concerns and take action if patient safety is compromised. The following principles are key to maintaining a culture of safety among team members.

A. Clear speech
   1. Masks and machine noise are often a hindrance. Adjust your volume accordingly and speak distinctly.
   2. Use precise language with your team members to avoid misunderstandings.

B. Use of names
   1. Using names enhances communication and respect among team members.

C. Closed-loop communication
   1. Each message or question is met with an explicit accuracy check.
   2. Example:
      Surgeon: "Roger, can you set the Bovie to 30/30?"
      Circulator: "Sure, Dr. Cutsalot. Setting the Bovie to 30 'Coag' and 30 'Cut.'"

D. Speak up
   1. Immediately notify your team members if you notice something amiss.
   2. Example:
      Medical student: "Our suction has stopped working."
      Surgeon: "Rhonda, can you check to see if our suction tubing is clogged?"
      Scrub nurse: "Looks like it is clogged, Dr. Cutsalot. I'll fix it."

E. Mutual respect
   1. Acknowledge that each professional and trainee is fulfilling their role in the operating room to care for the patient.

II. TIMEOUT

Timeouts occur before anesthesia induction. The goal is patient safety. Note that the patient is often awake during the timeout.

A. Components of standard surgical timeout. Please see **Table 2.1**.

B. Emergency situations
   1. Often patient identification and consent is foregone in emergent cases.
   2. An abbreviated timeout is performed with confirmation of emergent status, type of operation, and any necessary equipment or blood products.

TABLE 2.1 Components of Surgical Timeout

Component of Timeout	Description
Patient identification	• Patient name, date of birth, and other patient health information stated and confirmed
Identification of team members	• Team members state their names and roles
Procedure verification	• Surgeon states operation, declares laterality, and verifies correct side has been marked on patient
Verify consent has been obtained	• Team verifies stated surgery matches signed consent
Prophylactic antibiotics	• Surgeon states if antibiotics are indicated, and, if so, which ones • Anesthesia confirms delivery within a time frame from incision
Blood products	• Is there an up-to-date type and screen? • Are blood products available? • Surgeon states expected estimated blood loss
Specimens	• Will there be a specimen? • How should the specimen be processed (fresh, frozen, formalin), and who is responsible for the specimen
Special considerations	• Intraoperative tools: ultrasound for liver surgery, nerve monitor for neck surgery • Medications (e.g., immunosuppression for transplant, antiplatelet therapy)

III. ANESTHESIA INDUCTION, MAINTENANCE, AND OXYGEN ADMINISTRATION

A. Types of anesthesia

1. General

Provides full unconsciousness, amnesia, analgesia, and usually neuromuscular blockade. Gives significant physiologic control to the anesthesia provider and requires constant monitoring.

a. Oxygenation/Ventilation: Requires mechanical ventilation via endotracheal tube (ETT) or laryngeal mask airway

b. Monitoring: Full physiologic monitoring, including "twitch" monitoring if neuromuscular blockade is used. See the "Intraoperative monitoring" section in Part VI for a full list of basic monitoring tools and adjuncts.

   c. Example procedure: Any laparoscopic surgery, open chest or abdominal surgery

2. Monitored anesthesia care (MAC)

   Often patients have significant comorbidities that prevent them from undergoing general anesthesia without great risk. MAC consists of a combination of local/regional anesthesia with sedation.

   a. Oxygenation/Ventilation: Oxygenation via nasal cannula or face mask is required. May use nasal/oral airway device to prevent obstructive apnea. Mechanical ventilation is not indicated.
   b. Monitoring: Basic vitals and capnography
   c. Example procedure: Breast surgery, melanoma excision with lymph node dissection

3. Conscious sedation

   Involves light use of sedatives and analgesia in conjunction with local or regional anesthesia.

   a. Oxygenation/Ventilation: Oxygenation via nasal cannula or face mask is necessitated by level of sedation. May use nasal/oral airway device to prevent obstructive apnea. Mechanical ventilation is not indicated.
   b. Monitoring: Basic vitals and capnography
   c. Example procedure: Epidermoid cyst removal, bedside incision and drainage

B. Regional/local anesthetic

Often used in conjunction with general, MAC, or conscious sedation to reduce dose of systemic medications.

1. Peripheral nerve blockade
   a. Upper extremity
      i. Brachial plexus blockade: Interscalene, supraclavicular, infraclavicular, axillary blockade
      ii. Distal upper extremity blockade includes radial, median, ulnar, and digital blocks
      iii. Intravenous regional anesthesia (Bier block): Often used in carpal tunnel surgery. Involves intravenous local anesthetic administration after tourniquet application to isolate analgesia to the distal extremity.
   b. Lower extremity
      i. Includes femoral, popliteal, saphenous, and ankle blocks
   c. Miscellaneous techniques
      i. Thoracic: Intercostal, paravertebral, or erector spinae blocks
      ii. Abdominal: Transversus abdominis plane block—targets the cutaneous branches of the low thoracic and lumbar spinal nerves that travel in the plane between the transversus abdominis and internal oblique muscles. Often used with laparotomy incisions.
2. Common anesthetic agents
   a. Local anesthetics for infiltration. See **Table 2.2**.
      i. Mechanism of action: Blockade of voltage-gated sodium channels

TABLE 2.2 Local Anesthetics for Infiltration

	Maximum Dose (mg/kg)		Length of Action (h)	
Agent	Plain	With Epinephrine	Plain	With Epinephrine
Procaine	7	9	0.5	0.5-1
Lidocaine	4	7	0.5-1	2
Mepivacaine	4	7	0.75-1.5	2
Bupivacaine	2.5	3	2-4	3-4
Ropivacaine	3	4	2-4	3-4
Tetracaine	1.5		24	

ii. Two classes based on chemical structure:
   a) Aminoesters (one i): Tetracaine, procaine, cocaine, chloroprocaine
   b) Aminoamides (two i's): Lidocaine, bupivacaine, ropivacaine, mepivacaine

b. Can be mixed with epinephrine, which prolongs blockade, reduces systemic drug absorption, and allows for higher maximum dose
   i. Contraindicated when arterial spasm would cause tissue necrosis (mnemonic "fingers, toes, penis, nose") as well as in patients with arrhythmias, unstable angina, poorly controlled hypertension, or uteroplacental insufficiency.

3. Local anesthetic systemic toxicity
   a. Central nervous system (CNS) toxicity
      i. Symptoms: Mental status changes, dizziness, perioral numbness, metallic taste, tinnitus, visual disturbances, seizures
   b. Cardiovascular (CV) toxicity
      i. Symptoms: Decreased cardiac output, hypotension, or cardiovascular collapse at worst
      ii. Most anesthetics cause CNS toxicity prior to CV toxicity
      iii. Treatment: Airway and cardiovascular support, seizure suppression, lipid emulsion therapy
         a) Hypersensitivity reactions occur rarely. Symptoms include urticaria, bronchospasm, hypotension, anaphylactic shock.

C. Neuroaxial blockade

Low-dose anesthetic is injected around the nerve roots with the aim of blocking sympathetic and dermatomal sensory fibers.

1. Spinal anesthesia
   a. Injected into the subarachnoid space at the level of the lumbar spine.

2. Epidural anesthesia
   a. Injected into the epidural space without advancement through the dura.
   b. Slower onset of action than spinal anesthesia.
   c. A catheter is often advanced into the epidural space to allow for repeat boluses or continuous infusion.
3. Complications
   a. High spinal blockade: May result in hypotension (blocking dermatomes T1-T4: Preganglionic cardioaccelerator nerves), dyspnea (loss of chest proprioception or intercostal muscle function, diaphragmatic paralysis due to C3-C5 blockade), or apnea (decreased medullary perfusion secondary to hypotension).
      i. Treatment: Ventilatory support and/or intubation, IV fluids, chronotropic and inotropic support.
   b. Hypotension: Occurs as a result of sympatholytic-induced vasodilation. Consider 500 to 1,000 mL of crystalloid prior to spinal block.
      i. Treatment:
         a) IV fluids, decrease epidural infusion rate, vasopressors, positive inotropic and chronotropic drugs
         b) Leg elevation and Trendelenburg positioning increases venous return to the heart.
   c. Headache: Occurs more often in spinal anesthesia but can occur with inadvertent dural puncture in epidural anesthesia. Look for a postural component (i.e., symptoms worsened by sitting up or standing). The use of smaller-caliber needles has reduced the frequency of this complication.
      i. Treatment: Bed rest, abdominal binders, oral or IV fluids, oral analgesics, and caffeinated beverages. Severe refractory headache may require placement of an epidural blood patch to prevent ongoing leakage of cerebrospinal fluid.
   d. Urinary retention: A urinary catheter is advisable to prevent bladder distention.
   e. Rare complications
      i. CNS infection: May result in meningitis, epidural abscess, or arachnoiditis.
      ii. Permanent nerve injury: Seen with the same frequency as in general anesthesia.
      iii. Intravascular catheter placement (usually in epidural veins): Potentially devastating due to the potential for intravascular injection of local anesthetic and risk of systemic toxicity.
      iv. Epidural hematoma: Usually occurs in patients with coexisting coagulopathy. Emergent laminectomy may be required to decompress the spinal cord and avoid permanent neurologic injury.

D. Common anesthetic agents
1. Short-term sedation and analgesia

Often used in minor procedures, including bedside procedures. Below are common agents used with standard adult dosing.

a. Dexmedetomidine (Precedex)
  i. Mechanism of action (MOA): Selective alpha$_2$-adrenoreceptor agonist leading to inhibition of norepinephrine release
  ii. Role: Provides sedation and some analgesia
  iii. Dose: 1 μg/kg over 10 min, then 0.2 to 1 μg/kg/h IV
  iv. Side effects: May cause bradycardia and hypotension, transient hypertension during loading
  v. Reversal: None
b. Fentanyl
  i. MOA: Short-acting synthetic opioid
  ii. Role: Provides analgesia with unpredictable sedative effects
  iii. Dose: 25 to 50 μg q5 to 10 min IV
  iv. Side effects: Respiratory depression
  v. Reversal: Naloxone
c. Midazolam
  i. MOA: Binds postsynaptic GABA receptor
  ii. Role: Provides sedation and anxiolysis, not analgesia
  iii. Dose: 0.5 to 1 mg q15 min IV
  iv. Side effects: Respiratory depression, vomiting
  v. Reversal: Flumazenil
d. Propofol, etomidate, and ketamine are additional common agents used for short-term sedation. These are described in the next section on induction agents.

2. Induction agents for general anesthesia
  a. Propofol
    i. MOA: $GABA_A$ agonist
    ii. Role: Can be used for both induction and maintenance; does not provide analgesia. Advantages include low incidence of postoperative nausea and vomiting and unchanged pharmacokinetics in the setting of chronic hepatic or renal failure.
    iii. Dose: 1 to 3 mg/kg IV
    iv. Side effects: May cause hypotension, especially with bolus dosing
      a) Propofol infusion syndrome: Rare but fatal syndrome observed in critically ill patients sedated with prolonged infusion of propofol, characterized by electrolyte abnormalities, arrhythmia, renal failure, and cardiovascular collapse.
  b. Etomidate
    i. MOA: Imidazole $GABA_A$ modulator
    ii. Role: Use for induction only as it has short duration of action. Advantages include no effect on hemodynamics, favoring its use in hemodynamically unstable patients.
    iii. Dose: 0.3 mg/kg IV
    iv. Side effects: Mild direct hemodynamic depressant effects and high incidence of postoperative nausea and vomiting. Adrenal insufficiency may result from single administration.
  c. Ketamine
    i. MOA: Phencyclidine derivative and N-methyl-D-aspartate receptor antagonist

ii. Role: Provides dissociative anesthesia and excellent analgesia. Favorably, it does not cause respiratory depression and it is often used in pediatrics as it can be given intramuscularly.
iii. Dose: 1 to 2 mg/kg IV
iv. Side effects: Increases heart rate, cardiac output, and blood pressure. Patients can experience hallucinations with emergence.

3. Maintenance agents
 a. Inhalational
  i. Volatile agents include the "-fluranes"
  ii. Dose-dependent respiratory depression
  iii. Advantages include ease of administration, bronchodilation, decrease in cerebral metabolic rate, and increase in cerebral blood flow.
  iv. Increased risk of postoperative nausea and vomiting compared with IV maintenance agents
  v. Nitrous oxide
   a) Never used alone due to low potency and usually used in combination with other inhalational agents
   b) Has analgesic and anxiolytic properties with minimal hemodynamic effects
 b. Intravenous. When used alone, termed TIVA (total IV anesthesia)
  i. Sedative: Propofol
  ii. Analgesia: Opioids
  iii. Adjuvants: Dexmedetomidine, ketamine, lidocaine

4. Paralytics
 a. Neuromuscular blockade is achieved with acetylcholine receptor antagonists that act on postsynaptic receptors in the neuromuscular junction. This produces muscle relaxation, which facilitates endotracheal intubation as well as many surgical procedures. See **Table 2.3** for description of paralytic agents.
 b. Neuromuscular, or "twitch" monitoring, is often used to assess depth.
 c. Considerations before succinylcholine consideration
  i. Malignant hyperthermia
   a) Autosomal dominant mutation of RYR1 gene resulting in a hypermetabolic skeletal muscle disorder characterized by intracellular hypercalcemia and rapid ATP consumption.
   b) Treat with depolarizing agent cessation and dantrolene.
  ii. Hyperkalemia
  iii. Contraindicated in patients with crush or burn injuries as succinylcholine can result in significant potassium release from muscle cells

E. Rapid sequence intubation
 1. Algorithm that guides endotracheal intubation in emergent scenarios OR in patients at increased risk for aspiration (nonfasted, patients with delayed gastric emptying, reflux, pregnancy, bowel obstruction)[1]

F. Venous thromboembolism (VTE) prophylaxis
 1. Multiple risk factors contribute to the perioperative thrombogenic state, including general anesthesia. See **Table 2.4**.

TABLE 2.3 Agents Producing Neuromuscular Blockade

Agent	Initial Dose (mg/kg)	Duration (min)	Elimination	Associated Effects
Depolarizing				
Succinylcholine	1-1.5	3-5	Plasma cholinesterase	Fasciculations, increase or decrease in heart rate, transient hyperkalemia, malignant hyperthermia trigger agent
Nondepolarizing				
Atracurium	0.2-0.4	20-35	Ester hydrolysis	Histamine release
Cisatracurium	0.1-0.2	20-35	Ester hydrolysis	
Vecuronium	0.1-0.2	25-40	Hepatic and renal	Histamine release
Rocuronium	0.6-1.2	30	Hepatic and renal	
Pancuronium	0.04-0.1	45-90	Primarily renal	Increase in heart rate, mean arterial BP, and cardiac output

BP, blood pressure.

2. Commonly mechanical prophylaxis with sequential compression devices is enough intraoperatively.
3. Surgeon/institutional preference varies on chemical prophylaxis.
4. Balance with bleeding risk based on operation and patient's disease profile.
5. See **Table 2.4** for overview of thromboprophylaxis in hospitalized patients.

IV. POSITIONING

A. See **Table 2.5** for standard patient positions

B. Table positioning

TABLE 2.4 Levels of Thromboembolism Risk and Recommended Thromboprophylaxis in Hospital Patients

Risk Level	Type of Patient	Symptomatic DVT Risk w/o Prophylaxis (%)	Suggested Thromboprophylaxis Options
Very low	Most outpatient/ same day surgery	<0.5	Early and aggressive ambulation
Low	Minor surgery in mobile patients Medical patients who are fully mobile	~1.5	Mechanical prophylaxis with IPC Mechanical prophylaxis with IPC
Moderate	Most general, cardiothoracic, nononcologic, gynecologic, or urologic surgery Medical patients who are on bed rest, "sick"	~3	LMWH or LDUH or mechanical prophylaxis with IPC LMWH or LDUH or mechanical prophylaxis with IPC
	Moderate VTE risk plus high bleeding risk		Mechanical prophylaxis with IPC until risk decreases, then chemical prophylaxis
High	Major trauma, bariatric surgery, pneumonectomy, spinal cord injury, TBI, or craniotomy	~6	LMWH or LDUH AND mechanical prophylaxis with IPC or elastic stockings
	High VTE risk plus high bleeding risk High risk plus oncologic, abdominal, or pelvic surgery		Mechanical prophylaxis with IPC until risk decreases, then chemical prophylaxis extended duration LMWH (4 wk) AND mechanical prophylaxis with IPC or elastic stockings while hospitalized

DVT, deep vein thrombosis; IPC, intermittent pneumatic compression; LDUH, low-dose unfractionated heparin; LMWH, low-molecular-weight heparin; TBI, traumatic brain injury; VTE, venous thromboembolism.

Adapted from Gould MK, Garcia DA, Wren SM, et al. Prevention of VTE in nonorthopedic surgical patients. Antithrombotic therapy and prevention of thrombosis, 9th ed: American College of Chest Physicians evidence-based clinical practice guidelines. *Chest*. 2012;141(2):e227S-e277S.Copyright 2012, The American College of Chest Physicians. With permission.

TABLE 2.5 Standard Patient Positions

Position	Description	Common Operation	Comments
Supine	Patient lies flat with extremities in neutral position	Most commonly encountered position	• Arm abduction should not exceed 90° to prevent brachial plexus injury • Arm tucking considerations include line access for the anesthesiologist, space for equipment, and avoiding hindering the surgeon from reaching the operative field of work
Lithotomy	Modified supine position in which the patient's lower extremities, with the use of stirrups, are slightly abducted at the hips and flexed at both hips and knees	Colorectal resection Urology Gynecology	• Allows access to perineum and abdomen at the same time • Pad the fibular head to prevent foot drop due to pressure on the peroneal nerve
Prone/ Prone Jackknife	Patient lies face down on pillows, padded frames, or rolls. Prone jackknife is a modification that involves flexing the table at the patient's hips	Anorectal Spine	• Oxygenation must be carefully monitored as the patient's airway is not easily accessible • Pad-dependent pressure points
Lateral decubitus	Patient lies with the operative side up with slightly flexed lower extremities and supportive padding or bean bag to keep the patient from rolling off the table	Thoracotomy	• Axillary roll used to prevent pressure on brachial pressure • Pad-dependent pressure points • Ensure neutral neck alignment
Beach Chair	Patient lies supine with neck extended. The table is flexed at the hips and slightly flexed at the knees	Head and neck operations	• Neck extension can be enhanced with a shoulder roll. Avoid overextension.

1. Use gravity to enhance visualization of working field
   a. Trendelenburg: Tilt patient head down, when exposure is needed in lower abdomen (i.e., colorectal resection)
   b. Reverse Trendelenburg: Tilt patient feet down, when exposure is needed in upper abdomen (i.e., gastric resection)
2. Must ensure patient is well secured to table with safety strap, footboard, and nonstick pad

V. ERGONOMICS

A. Surgeons and interventionalists are at high risk for work-related musculoskeletal disorders (MSDs), including degenerative cervical and lumbar spine disease, rotator cuff pathology, and carpal tunnel syndrome.
   1. The prevalence of cervical and lumbar spine disease has been estimated to have increased by 18% and 27%, respectively, in recent years. As high as 12% of those with work-related MSD have required a leave of absence, practice restriction/modification, or early retirement.[2]

B. Enhance surgeon comfort and prevent injury
   1. Maintain back, neck, and elbows at neutral position
   2. Avoid working with extended arms
   3. Minimize truncal twisting or sustained bending
   4. Consider microbreaks
   5. Support the ergonomics of other team members

C. Environmental adjustments
   1. Table height
   2. Light, screen, or monitor positioning
   3. Use of step stools, floor mats, or other supportive furniture

VI. PREPARATION AND DRAPING

A. Surgical site infection (SSI) prevention

As high as 20% of all hospital-associated infections are estimated to be SSI.[3] A substantial cause of postoperative morbidity and mortality, SSI has become a key focus of multiple national organizations. The Surgical Care Improvement Project, whose members include, among others, the American College of Surgeons and The Joint Commission, is a national effort garnered toward improving postoperative outcomes. Much of its publicly reported measures are focused on preventing SSI.

   1. Prophylactic antimicrobial choice and timing
      a. Timing
         i. Initial dosing: Administer within 1 hour before incision or within 2 hours for vancomycin or fluoroquinolones.
         ii. Redosing is based on agent half-life OR for every 1,500 mL of blood loss.
         iii. Discontinue prophylactic antibiotics after incision closure.
      b. With some exceptions, there is no evidence that continuing antibiotics post incision closure decreases SSI risk.

c. Antimicrobial choice
   i. Specific antibiotic use is based on institutional antibiograms. See **Table 2.6** for general recommendations.

2. Hair removal
   a. Shaving with a razor is associated with more SSI than clipping.[4]
   b. Current guidelines recommend clipping only when necessary.[5]
   c. Lower rates of SSIs when hair is removed on the day of compared with day before surgery.[6]

TABLE 2.6 General Recommendations for Antibiotic Prophylaxis

Operation	Likely Pathogens	Recommended Antibiotics[a]
Cardiac (including prosthetic valve)	Staphylococci	Cefazolin, cefuroxime
Thoracic	Staphylococci	Cefazolin, ampicillin-sulbactam
Vascular (including prosthetic graft)	Staphylococci, streptococci, enteric gram-negative bacilli, clostridia	Cefazolin, clindamycin
Orthopedic (including total joint replacement)	Staphylococci	Cefazolin
Upper GI and Hepatobiliary	Enteric gram-negative bacilli, enterococci, clostridia	Cefazolin, cefoxitin, cefotetan, ceftriaxone, ampicillin-sulbactam
Colorectal	Enteric gram-negative bacilli, anaerobes, enterococci	Cefazolin + metronidazole, cefoxitin, cefotetan, ceftriaxone + metronidazole, ertapenem
Appendectomy	Enteric gram-negative bacilli, anaerobes, enterococci	Cefoxitin, cefotetan, cefazolin + metronidazole
Obstetrics/gynecology	Enteric gram-negative bacilli, anaerobes, group B streptococci, enterococci	Cefazolin, cefotetan, cefoxitin, ampicillin-sulbactam

GI, gastrointestinal.

[a]Vancomycin can be considered in hospitals that have high methicillin-resistant *Staphylococcus aureus* (MRSA) SSI rates or in patients with a beta-lactam allergy or a history of MRSA. If vancomycin is used in place of cefazolin, additional gram-negative coverage may be required.

3. Antiseptic agents
   a. 4% chlorhexidine gluconate
      i. Most common antiseptic agent
      ii. Alcohol-based solution, thus flammable until completely dry
      iii. Site contraindications: Mucous membranes, meninges, corneas, inner ear
   b. 10% povidone–iodine
      i. Indicated for surgeries with open wounds, higher fire risks (i.e., tracheostomy)
4. Temperature regulation
   a. Hypothermia is theorized to cause tissue hypoxia secondary to vasoconstriction, increasing wound infection susceptibility. Patient warming and normothermia maintenance has been found to be associated with decreased wound infections.[7,8]
5. Blood glucose
   a. Glucose control between 110 and 150 mg/dL is associated with lower SSI risk.[5]
6. Note on evidence behind current SSI prevention guidelines
   a. There are numerous trials, reviews, and other studies with sometimes concurrent and other times contradictory findings in regards to factors and methods of SSI prevention. In addition, there are multiple evidence-based guidelines with evolving recommendations. See Key Reference table for additional reading.
7. **Extent of preparation and draping**
   a. A wide or narrow prep takes into account several variables.
      i. Incision length and field of operation
      ii. Elective or emergent
      iii. Possibility of additional future fields of operation, e.g., distal extremity preparation if a proximal thrombus were to embolize
   b. Occasionally it is appropriate to prep widely but drape narrowly.
   c. When in doubt, discuss preparation and draping with the lead surgeon ahead of time.

VII. THE OPERATION

A. General steps in an operation. See **Figure 2.1**.
   1. Access (see **Figure 2.2** for common open incisions)
   2. Exploration
   3. Dissection
   4. Resection
   5. Reconstruction
   6. Closure
B. Closure considerations
   1. Commonly involves closure of at least two layers, e.g., fascial layer and skin layer
      a. Fascial closure allows less tension on the cutaneous closure, which facilitates wound healing.[9]

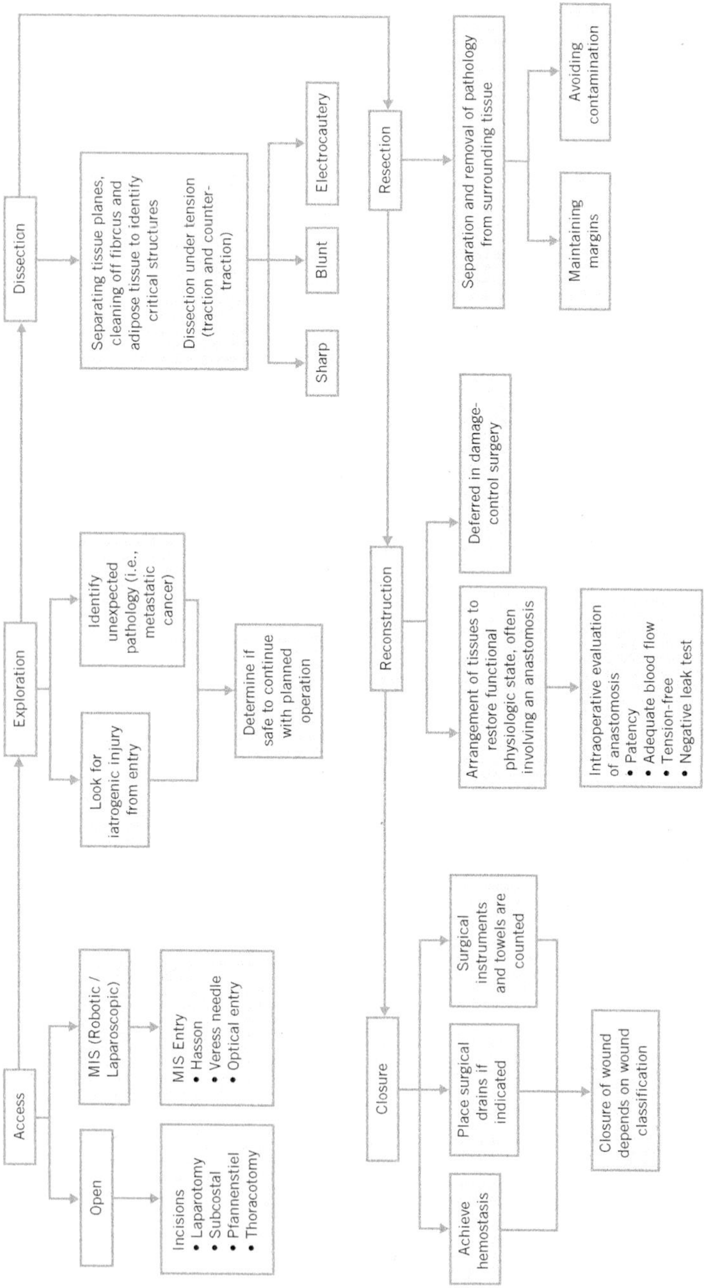

FIGURE 2.1 General steps in an operation.

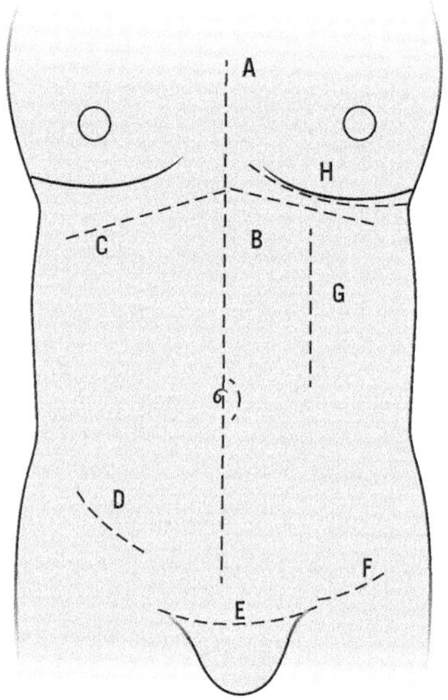

FIGURE 2.2 Common anterior open incisions in general surgery. A, Sternotomy. B, Midline laparotomy. C, Subcostal incision, can be extended superiorly and contralaterally to form a Mercedes incision. D, McBurney incision. E, Pfannenstiel incision. F, Inguinal incision. G, Paramedian incision (now rarely used due to high risk of hernia and loss of rectus nervous supply). H, Anterolateral thoracotomy.

b. Skin closure
  i. Choice of skin closure material (nonabsorbable suture, absorbable suture, staple, closure devices) as well as type of closure (e.g., subcutaneous vs. mattress stitch) depends on a multitude of factors, including wound tension, healing aesthetics, the patient's anticipated healing ability, and surgeon preference.
  ii. Delayed primary closure is often considered in clean contaminated (see **Table 2.7**) cases or contaminated/dirty cases that have since been adequately irrigated and debrided.
  iii. Healing by secondary intention (i.e., granulation) may be considered in persistently dirty or infected wounds. May be assisted by negative pressure wound therapy.

VIII. ELECTROSURGERY

Electrosurgery is an essential tool that utilizes electric current to apply heat with precision to cut, coagulate, and destroy tissue. See Fundamental Use of Surgical Energy modules for additional information.[10]

A. The effects of heat on tissue include
  1. Protein denaturation
  2. Desiccation

TABLE 2.7 Surgical Wound Classification

Wound Classification	Description
Class I—Clean	• Uninfected wound • No break in antiseptic technique • Gastrointestinal, respiratory, or urogenital tracts are not entered • Closed primarily
Class II—Clean-Contaminated	• Gastrointestinal, respiratory, or urogenital tracts are encountered in a controlled fashion
Class III—Contaminated	• Break in aseptic technique • Open wounds with nonpurulent inflammation • Gross spillage from gastrointestinal tract
Class IV—Dirty	• Open wound with foreign body or devitalized tissue • Active infection • Ruptured viscous

3. Cellular vaporization
4. Carbonization

B. The main types of electrosurgery instruments are

1. Monopolar
   - **a.** Electric current transmitted via patient tissue between active electrode (tip of instrument) and dispersive electrode (grounding pad on patient)
   - **b.** Example: Bovie electrocautery
   - **c.** There are two major waveforms of electric current that monopolar instruments can use to achieve specific results.
     - **i.** Cut
       - **a)** Continuous low voltage: Less tissue desiccation/fulguration
     - **ii.** Coagulation (or "Coag" for short)
       - **a)** Intermittent high voltage: More tissue desiccation/fulguration
     - **iii.** Blend: A combination of "cut" and "coag"
2. Bipolar
   - **a.** Both electrodes are positioned on the surgical instrument.
   - **b.** Only a small amount of patient tissue is involved in the circuit, dramatically reducing risk of current diversion inherent in monopolar instruments.

C. Mechanisms of injury

1. Direct coupling
   - **a.** Electrode within circuit touches or arcs to an instrument outside of the circuit.
   - **b.** Ensure no extraneous instruments are in field of operation prior to activation of energy device.

2. Insulation failure (during laparoscopic procedures)
   a. Insulation material around laparoscopic instrument is compromised, thus increasing risk of direct coupling injury.
   b. Inspect all instruments to ensure insulation is intact prior to start of case.
3. Unintentional activation of the active electrode
   a. Store active electrode in holster when not in use.
4. Injury due to direct thermal extension
   a. Heat from active electrode can extend to surrounding structures.
   b. Isolate tissue of interest from surrounding critical structures. If unable to do this, avoid electrosurgery in these sensitive areas.
5. Alternate site–related injury
   a. Patient is in contact with metal objects that may conduct electricity outside of intended circuit.
   b. Remove all metal objects from patient. If unable to remove, apply padding with nonconductive materials to effectively remove from circuit.

IX. INTRAOPERATIVE MONITORING

A. Role of the anesthesia provider
   1. Basic anesthesia monitoring
      a. Oxygenation—pulse oximetry
      b. Ventilation—continuous end-tidal CO_2
      c. Circulation—blood pressure, heart rate, ECG
      d. Temperature—core temperature probes (axilla, bladder, nasopharynx)
      e. Neuromuscular blockade—nerve stimulation or "twitch monitor"
   2. Monitoring adjuncts
      a. Arterial lines are useful for precise, continuous blood pressure monitoring.
      b. Central venous pressure from a central line is an imperfect measure of fluid responsiveness and volume status.
      c. Cerebral oximetry, evoked potentials, and carotid artery stump pressures can monitor cerebral perfusion.
      d. Electroencephalogram can measure brain electrical activity. Bispectral index can be used to monitor depth of anesthesia.
      e. Transesophageal echocardiogram is useful in mainly cardiac cases to assess cardiac structure, function, and volume status.
      f. Urine output is a useful indicator of volume status.
      g. Laboratory values such as blood gas, lactate, and hematocrit are useful physiologic and metabolic indicators, especially during long procedures.
   3. Mutually effective communication between the anesthesia provider, the surgeon, and the rest of the operative team is paramount to patient safety.
B. Common intraoperative problems
   1. Hypotension
      a. Many patients without physiologic reserve can become hypotensive upon induction and may need pressor support briefly or throughout the case.

2. Bleeding
   a. See "Hemostasis" below
3. Failure to ventilate
   a. Can be manifest by hypoxemia or hypercarbia.
   b. Pause operation while the anesthesia provider is checking the system (ETT connection, position, etc.).
   c. Maneuvers to consider include airway suctioning, recruitment, and fiberoptic bronchoscopy.
   d. High peak pressures might indicate high intra-abdominal pressure during laparoscopic surgery or tension pneumothorax.
4. Tachycardia, bradycardia, or arrhythmia
   a. Concomitantly evaluating for hemodynamic instability, oxygenation, and ischemic ECG changes can give context for etiologies and guide treatment.
5. Hypothermia
   a. Occurs due to increased heat loss secondary to peripheral vasodilation.
   b. At-risk populations include pediatric and burn patients.
   c. May lead to prolonged emergence, cardiac arrhythmias, coagulopathy.
   d. Prevent with atmospheric (room) or active (forced warm air) warming and limiting exposure.

C. Less common intraoperative problems
1. Aspiration
   a. Can occur when the patient has a significant amount of stomach contents prior to induction, e.g., emergent settings.
   b. Treatment is often supportive. May require intubation for further airway protection. Antibiotics or steroids are often not indicated.
2. CO_2 embolism
   a. Can occur during laparoscopy
   b. Treat with immediate desufflation, Trendelenburg and left-side-down table positioning, 100% FiO_2
3. Anaphylaxis
   a. Can still occur despite fastidious preoperative allergy reconciliation with the patient
   b. Treat with epinephrine and supportive measures
   c. Often safest to abort case if occurs on induction
4. Tension pneumothorax
   a. Can occur with high positive airway pressure, especially in patients with chronic obstructive pulmonary disease, or when the pleura is accidently violated during surgery
   b. Treat with decompression

X. HEMOSTASIS

A. Normal mechanisms of hemostasis
1. Thrombus formation
   a. Platelet plug formation (primary hemostasis)
      i. Injury to the endothelium → endothelial cells and platelets release vWF → vWF binds exposed collagen → platelets bind vWF via

glycoproteins (i.e., glycoprotein 1B) → platelets undergo a critical shape change and release ADP and thromboxane A2 → ADP induces platelet glycoproteins 2b/3a, which allows formation of fibrinogen bridges between platelets (aggregation)

b. Coagulation and platelet plug stabilization (secondary hemostasis). **See Figure 2.3**.

B. Inherited and acquired disorders of coagulation

Excessive bleeding or clotting may be due to underlying coagulopathy. Knowledge of the patient's comorbidities and perioperative risk factors can help guide diagnosis and etiology.

1. Common inherited disorders

a. Von Willebrand disease (vWD)

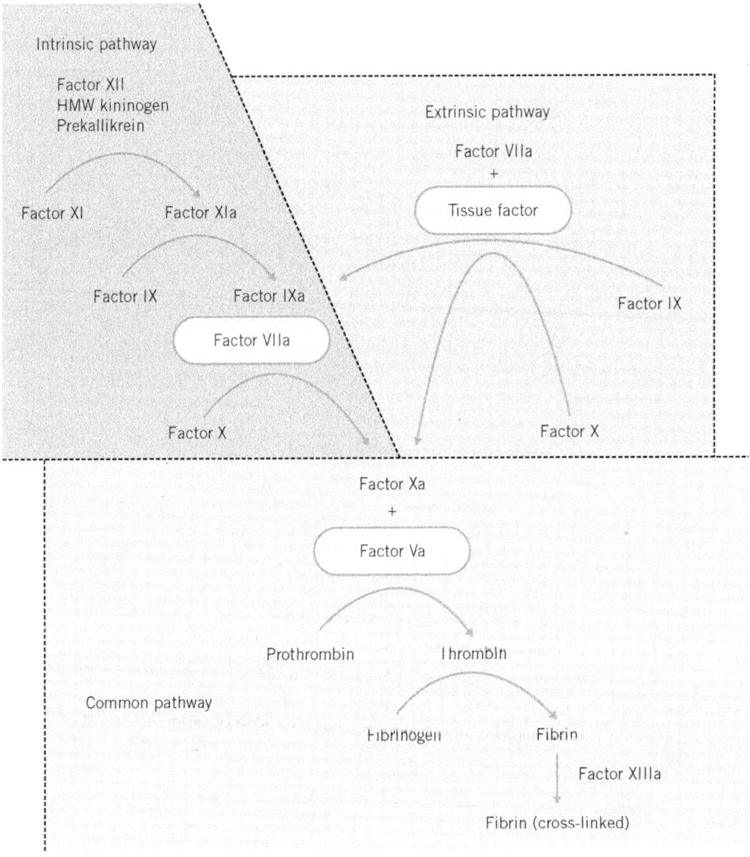

FIGURE 2.3 Coagulation cascade. *(Adapted from Klingensmith ME, Wise P. Washington Manual of Surgery, 8th ed. Wolters Kluwer; 2019.)*

i. Most common inherited bleeding disorder. Prevalence may be as high as 1% of the general population. Characterized by decreased activity of von Willebrand factor (cWF).
ii. Types of vWD
a) Type 1: Decreased concentration and activity of vWF
b) Type 2: Dysfunctional vWF
c) Type 3: Absent or severe reduction in vWF
iii. Screening tests: vWF antigen, functional activity assays, or testing factor VIII activity (vWF is a carrier for factor VIII)
iv. Possible laboratory abnormalities:
a) Mild thrombocytopenia
b) Increase in thrombocytopenia with administration of desmopressin
c) Increased partial thromboplastin time (PTT) if factor VIII activity is significantly reduced

b. Hemophilia
i. X-linked bleeding disorder. Hemophilia A (factor VIII deficiency) at 1 in 5,000 live births is more common than hemophilia B (factor IX deficiency).
ii. May see prolonged activated PTT with moderate to severe disease.
iii. Factor assays confirm diagnosis.

c. Factor V Leiden (FVL) deficiency
i. Most common inherited hypercoagulable disorder. A frequency of 5% of the general white American population for FVL heterozygosity has been reported.
ii. Genetic mutation in factor V, rendering the protein resistant to breakdown by activated protein C.
iii. Genetic testing or functional assays can confirm diagnosis.

2. Common acquired disorders
a. Liver disease
i. Leads to complex coagulopathy, as hepatocytes synthesize both procoagulants (fibrinogen; thrombin; factors V, VII, IX, X, and XI) and anticoagulants (protein C, protein S, and antithrombin)
ii. May have varying degrees of thrombocytopenia

b. Vitamin K deficiency
i. Vitamin K is an essential cofactor in activation of factors VII, IX, X; prothrombin; and proteins C/S.
ii. Can occur in patients without oral intake for 1 week or longer, those with biliary obstruction or malabsorption, or those receiving some antibiotics or warfarin.

c. Uremia
i. Leads to platelet dysfunction, including adhesion and aggregation
ii. Secondary to renal failure

d. Heparin-induced thrombocytopenia (HIT)
i. HIT types
a) Type 1—Nonimmune
1) Begins within 4 days of therapy
2) Prevalence between 5% and 30% of population
3) Heparin cessation may not be needed

b) Type 2—Immune mediated
   1) Caused by heparin-induced antiplatelet antibodies (anti-PF4 heparin complex).
   2) Occurs 5 to 10 days after initial exposure and immediately after reexposure.
   3) Platelet count <100,000 or decreases by >30% of baseline.
   4) Thrombotic events may occur.
   5) Immediately stop heparin administration.

ii. Laboratory testing
   a) HIT is a clinical diagnosis.
      1) 4T score can be used to calculate pretest probability of HIT.
         - Thrombocytopenia
         - Timing of platelet count fall
         - Thrombosis or other sequelae
         - Other causes of thrombocytopenia
   b) A HIT panel is an ELISA that is useful for screening but with low specificity.
   c) A serotonin release assay is gold standard as a confirmatory test.

e. Disseminated intravascular coagulation (DIC)
   i. Inciting events include sepsis, extensive trauma, or burns.
   ii. Pathogenesis involves inappropriate generation of thrombin within the vasculature, leading to platelet activation, formation of fibrin thrombi, and increased fibrinolytic activity.
   iii. Often presents with complications from microvascular thrombi in the vascular beds of the kidney, brain, lung, and skin.
   iv. Consumption of coagulation factors (i.e., fibrinogen) and activation of the fibrinolytic pathway leads to bleeding.
   v. Laboratory findings include thrombocytopenia, hypofibrinogenemia, increased fibrinogen degradation products, and prolonged PTT.
   vi. Therapy is focused on treatment of underlying cause.

f. Malignancy
   i. Production of procoagulants (e.g., tissue factor) leads to a hypercoagulable state.

g. Pregnancy
   i. An increase in coagulation factors, decrease in protein S, increase in resistance to protein C, and increase in fibrinolytic inhibitors in pregnancy all contribute to a hypercoagulable state.

h. Hemolysis
   i. Hemolysis can occur in operations requiring extracorporeal bypass.

C. Hemostasis techniques

When intraoperative bleeding is encountered, there are several ways to achieve hemostasis.

1. Direct pressure
   a. Often one finger placing direct pressure on the source of bleed is the most expedient temporizing measure. This can be replaced with a clamp, sponge, or packing as necessary.

b. Small venous bleeding can often resolve with a period of direct pressure.

2. Energy devices
   a. Refer to the "Electrosurgery" section above
3. Ligation
   a. Ligation refers to using ties, clips, or suture to occlude the offending vessel.
   b. Control of bleeding is highly effective as long as the vessel is visible and in reach.
4. Topical hemostatic agents
   a. Effectively controls mild bleeding. Large-volume, pulsatile bleeding will not respond to topical agents. See **Table 2.8**.

TABLE 2.8 Common Hemostatic Agents

Agent	Mechanism	Notes
Gelatin sponge	Absorbs many times its weight of blood through capillary action, provides matrix for thrombus formation	• Resorbs in 4-6 wk without much inflammatory reaction
Oxidized cellulose	Absorbs blood into a scaffold of knitted cellulose, provides matrix for thrombus formation	• Slow resorption can create a foreign body reaction
Collagen sponge	Bovine tendon collagen promotes platelet adhesion	• Slow resorption can create a foreign body reaction
Microfibrillar collagen	Stimulates platelet adhesion and thrombus formation	• Can be sprayed into areas that are difficult to reach • Should be avoided in procedures that use cell saver as it can pass through autotransfusion filters
Topical thrombin	Promotes formation of a fibrin-rich plug	• Can be applied onto dressings or directly onto wound
Gelatin matrix	Provides matrix for thrombus formation	• Often used in conjunction with topical thrombin
Fibrin sealant	Insoluble, cross-linked fibrin mesh that provides a matrix for thrombus formation	• Thrombin and fibrinogen are mixed prior to application via a dual-syringe system
Evarrest	Human fibrinogen and human thrombin embedded in a flexible composite patch	• Absorbs in approximately 8 wk

D. Lab assessment of ongoing bleeding and coagulation
   1. A combination of visualization of bleeding on the surgical field, quantification of blood loss in suction cannisters and surgical sponges, hemodynamic monitoring, and laboratory values guides transfusion. Many tests are available as point-of-care (POC) tests that are valuable when needed for quick decision making. See **Figure 2.4**.
   2. Note on thromboelastography (TEG) and rotational thromboelastometry (ROTEM)
      a. Available as POC systems, both are viscoelastic hemostatic assays that provide broad functional assessments of the coagulation system in real time.
      b. Both TEG and ROTEM give the same information, but nomenclature differs. **Figure 2.5** is an example of a TEG tracing with its associated nomenclature definitions.

XI. TRANSFUSION

A. Preparation
   1. All nonemergent transfusions require patient consent.
   2. A type and screen is generally good practice to send in advance of possible bleeding.
      a. The patient's serum is screened against a panel of known red blood cell (RBC) antigens.
   3. A type and cross is performed if bleeding is expected.
      a. Each unit of blood is cross-matched against the patient's serum to check for patient preformed antibodies against donor RBC antigens.

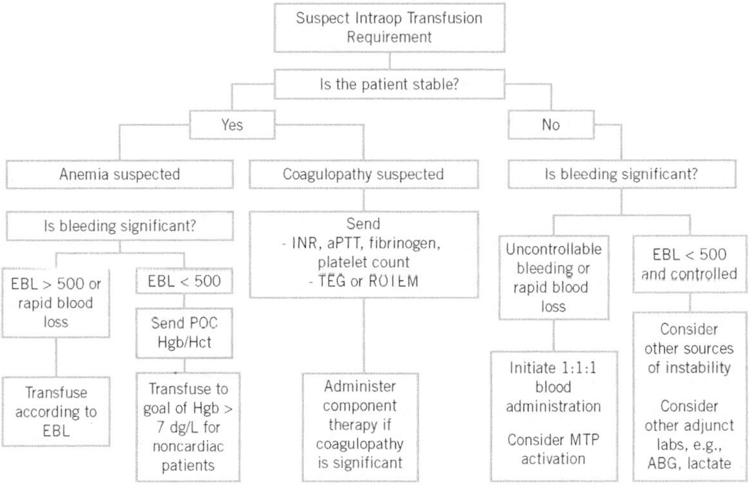

FIGURE 2.4 Laboratory assessment prior to transfusion. Hgb, hemoglobin; Hct, hematocrit; INR, International Normalized Ratio; aPTT, activated partial thromboplastin time; EBL, estimated blood loss; dg/L, decigram per liter; MTP, Massive Transfusion Protocol.

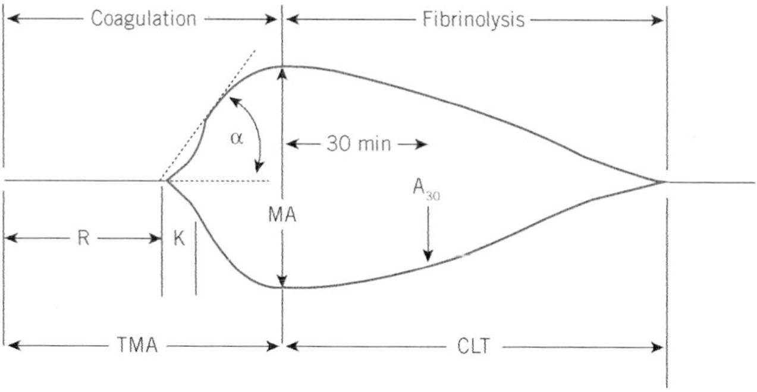

R	Period of latency from when blood is placed into the TEG analyzer until the initial fibrin formation. Represents the enzymatic portion of coagulation.
K	Measures the speed to reach a certain level of clot strength (20 mm above baseline). This represents clot kinetics.
α	Measures the rapidity of fibrin buildup and cross-linking (clot strengthening). This represents fibrinogen level.
MA	Maximum amplitude, is a direct function of the maximum dynamic properties of the fibrin and platelet binding via GPIIb/IIIa and represents the ultimate strength of the fibrin clot. This represents platelet function/aggregation.
LY30	Measures the rate of amplitude reduction 30 min after MA. This represents clot lysis.

FIGURE 2.5 Thromboelastogram.

4. Preoperative autologous blood donation or intraoperative blood salvage may be considered prior to operations with large expected blood loss.

B. Blood components
   1. Generally, in hemorrhagic shock, packed red blood cells (pRBCs), platelets, and fresh frozen plasma are given in a 1:1:1 ratio.[11,12]
   2. TRICC trial. In noncardiac, critically ill patients, we generally reserve RBC transfusion for patients with hemoglobin less than 7 g/dL and aim to maintain hemoglobin levels between 7 and 9 g/dL.[13]
   3. Component therapy and its common uses are detailed in **Table 2.9**.
   4. In trauma resuscitation, where massive transfusion may be indicated, the use of whole blood has been shown to be associated with improved survival.[14]

C. Transfusion risks
   1. Allergic reactions—most common
      a. Reaction against donor plasma proteins
      b. Signs and symptoms: Usually mild, rarely bronchospasm or laryngospasm (i.e., anaphylaxis)
      c. Cessation and anaphylaxis treatment is required if reaction is severe.
   2. Febrile nonhemolytic reactions
      a. Reaction against donor white blood cells

TABLE 2.9 Blood Product Components

Blood Product	Volume (mL)	Additional Factors	Expected Response	Common Use
PRBC 1 unit	200-250	Fibrinogen: 10-75 mg Clotting factors: None	Increase: 1 mg/dL Hgb 3% HCT	ABLA MTP Surgical blood loss
Platelets SDP (apheresis) RDP[a]	300-500; 50 per unit	Fibrinogen: 2-4 mg/mL (360-900 mg) Clotting factors: Equivalent of 200-250 mL of plasma (hemostatic level) "6 pack" of pooled RDP similar to SDP	Increase: 30-60 K/mm^3 Increase: 7-10 K/mm^3/U	Plt count <10 K MTP; Bleeding with known qualitative plt defect
FFP[b] 1 unit	180-300	Fibrinogen: 400 mg Clotting factors: 1 mL contains 1 active unit of each factor (II, V, VII, IX, X, XI)	Decrease: PT/INR PTT	Coagulopathy Warfarin overdose DIC
Cryo 10 pack		Fibrinogen: 1,200-1,500 Clotting factors: VIII, vWF, XII	Decrease: PT/INR PTT Increase: fibrinogen level	vWD DIC Hemophilia A

ABLA, acute blood loss anemia; Cryo, cryoprecipitate; DIC, disseminated intravascular coagulation; FFP, fresh frozen plasma; HCT, hematocrit; Hgb, hemoglobin; INR, international normalized ratio; MTP, massive transfusion protocol; plt, platelet; PRBC, packed red blood cells; PT, prothrombin time; PTT, partial thromboplastin time; RDP, random donor platelets; SDP, single donor platelets; vWD, von Willebrand disease; vWF, von Willebrand factor.

[a]About 4 to 10 RDP units are pooled prior to transfusion.

[b]Duration of FFP effect is approximately 6 h. INR of FFP is 1.6 to 1.7.

b. Symptoms: High fever during or within 24 hours of transfusion, general malaise, chills, nausea, headaches
c. Patients with a history should receive leukoreduced blood products.

3. Acute immune hemolytic reactions
   a. Patient antibodies to donor RBC antigens (usually ABO or Rh incompatibility) leads to intravascular hemolysis.

b. Signs and symptoms: Nausea, chills, anxiety, flushing, chest or back pain, excessive bleeding, or oozing from mucous membranes. May progress to shock or renal failure with hemoglobinuria.
c. Requires immediate transfusion cessation. Perform repeat cross-match
4. Delayed hemolytic reaction
a. Mediated by amnestic patient antibodies to non-ABO antigens.
b. Signs and symptoms: Often nonspecific. May see falling RBC count or elevated bilirubin on laboratory evaluation in 1 to 2 weeks.
c. Therapy is supportive.
5. Transfusion-related acute lung injury
a. Donor antibodies against recipient antigens or another factor in the donor component activates recipient neutrophils in the lung, leading to release of cytokines, reactive oxygen species, etc. that damage the pulmonary capillary endothelium.
b. Signs and symptoms: Sudden-onset hypoxemic respiratory insufficiency within 6 hours of transfusion, often within minutes of initiation.
c. Requires immediate transfusion cessation. Therapy is supportive, ranging from supplemental oxygen to intubation/mechanical ventilation.
6. Graft-vs.-host disease
a. Immunocompetent T cells are transfused into immunocompromised recipients.
b. Signs and symptoms: Rash, elevated liver function tests, pancytopenia. Associated mortality of 80%.
c. Prevent by irradiating donor blood.
7. Transfusion-associated circulatory overload
a. Pulmonary edema develops secondary to circulatory volume overload.
b. Signs and symptoms: Acute respiratory distress, increased blood pressure, tachycardia, positive fluid balance.
c. Therapy is supportive with judicious use of diuretic therapy.
8. Infection
a. Incidence is extremely low, with a reported rate of bacterial, viral, parasitic, and prion infection in the US of 0.2 per million RBC units. Infection rate is slightly higher with platelets theoretically because they are kept at room temperature.
b. Signs and symptoms: Fever, rigors, tachycardia
c. Requires immediate transfusion cessation. Rule out other transfusion reactions and take a blood culture from the opposite arm. Initiate broad-spectrum antibiotics. Immediately notify the blood bank.

XII. EXTUBATION

A. Reversal of neuromuscular blockade

Timing of reversal often requires discussion between the anesthesia provider and surgeon.

1. Common agents
a. Acetylcholinesterase inhibitors (neostigmine, edrophonium).

   b. Sugammadex directly binds rocuronium and vecuronium but does not affect acetylcholine.

B. Sedation is often weaned during skin closure.

C. Delayed emergence

   1. Affected by residual medication effect, hypercarbia, hypoxia, hypoglycemia, hypothermia, electrolyte abnormalities, neurologic complications, or patient metabolism

D. Criteria for successful extubation include adequate oxygenation, spontaneous breathing, hemodynamic stability, and normal acid–base status.

XIII. HANDOFF

A. Documentation

   1. Operative note

      a. At least a brief operative note should be finished in a timely fashion so that postoperative caretakers have a general idea of the operation performed and any potential complications.

   2. Postoperative orders

      a. Placing postoperative orders is an opportunity to communicate with those caretakers beyond the post-anesthesia care unit, such as floor nurses and technicians to whom the operative team does not traditionally give handoff.

B. Handoff to PACU nurse or ICU team

   1. Handoffs to postoperative care providers is often standardized within an institution in order to avoid misinformation or omission of key information that could lead to adverse patient outcomes.

   2. Ideally, the nurse, surgeon, and anesthesia providers involved in the case should each give a handoff.

   3. General handoff components

      a. From the nurse:

         i. Confirmation of patient identifiers

         ii. Review of patient medical history and allergies

      b. From the anesthesia provider

         i. Ease of airway management

         ii. Total dose and timing of opioids, paralytics, muscle relaxants, antiemetics, and antibiotics

         iii. Total fluids administered, including blood products

         iv. Intraoperative complications

         v. Critical laboratory values

         vi. Ongoing physiologic parameters and pressor requirements

         vii. Identification of retained invasive monitors

      c. From the surgeon:

         i. Procedure performed and incisions made

         ii. Identification and management of surgical drains

         iii. Intraoperative complications

         iv. Expected postoperative course and/or complications

         v. Plan for postoperative analgesia

         vi. Disposition

Key References

Citation	Summary
Berríos-Torres SI, Umscheid CA, Bratzler DW, et al. Centers for disease control and prevention guideline for the prevention of surgical site infection, 2017. *JAMA Surg.* 2017;152(8):784-791.	• Updated guidelines based on a systematic review of 170 studies from 1998 to 2014 that categorizes recommendations based on quality of evidence.
Deerenberg EB, Harlaar JJ, Steyerberg EW, et al. Small bites versus large bites for closure of abdominal midline incisions (STITCH): a double-blind, multicentre, randomised controlled trial. *Lancet.* 2015;386(10000):1254-1260.	• Randomized control trial that found that small fascial bites of 0.5 mm spaced 0.5 mm apart was superior to the traditional 1 cm by 1 cm bites in terms of rate of incisional hernia at 1-y follow-up.
Holcomb JB, del Junco DJ, Fox EE, et al. The prospective, observational, multicenter, major trauma transfusion (PROMMTT) study: comparative effectiveness of a time-varying treatment with competing risks. *JAMA Surg.* 2013;148(2):127-136.	• Prospective cohort study that compared higher platelet or plasma to RBC ratios with lower ones within different resuscitative time frames that found that higher ratios (1:1 or higher) were associated with improved in-hospital mortality if given within the first 6 h of active resuscitation.
Holcomb JB, Tilley BC, Baraniuk S, et al. Transfusion of plasma, platelets, and red blood cells in a 1:1:1 vs. a 1:1:2 ratio and mortality in patients with severe trauma: the PROPPR randomized clinical trial. *J Am Med Assoc.* 2015;313(5):471-482.	• Randomized clinical trial that compared blood product ratios of 1:1:1 vs. 1:1:2 during active resuscitation that found that more patients in the 1:1:1 group achieved hemostasis and fewer experienced death due to exsanguination in the first 24 h.
Hébert PC, Wells G, Blajchman MA, et al. A multicenter, randomized, controlled clinical trial of transfusion requirements in critical care. Transfusion requirements in critical care investigators, Canadian critical care trials group. *N Engl J Med.* 1999;340(6):409-417.	• In noncardiac, critically ill patients, we generally reserve RBC transfusion for patients with hemoglobin less than 7 g/dL and aim to maintain hemoglobin levels between 7 and 9 g/dL.

CHAPTER 2: INTRAOPERATIVE CONSIDERATIONS

Review Questions

1. What is the maximum volume of plain lidocaine 1% solution (without epinephrine) that should be locally administered to a 60-kg patient?
2. What pathogens should be covered by antibiotic prophylaxis in an appendectomy case?
3. There was gross spillage of enteric contents into the abdomen during your ileostomy creation. Under which surgical wound classification would this case fall?
4. A patient's systolic blood pressure during an elective case drops to 50 mm Hg after induction of anesthesia. Is blood transfusion indicated?
5. You are using the Bovie to dissect through soft tissue in a breast case when you come across an actively bleeding vessel that immediately fills your field with blood. Multiple attempts at coagulation with electrocautery fails. You can visualize the vessel clearly. What can you do to achieve hemostasis?
6. During liver transplant, the patient's TEG readout shows a decreased alpha angle, which you interpret as indicating a low fibrinogen level. What blood product would you consider giving?
7. What is the ratio of pRBC, platelets, and plasma recommended in patients with hemodynamically significant and severe active hemorrhage?

REFERENCES

1. Reynolds SF, Heffner J. Airway management of the critically ill patient: rapid-sequence intubation. *Chest.* 2005;127(4):1397-1412.
2. Epstein S, Sparer EH, Tran BN, et al. Prevalence of work-related musculoskeletal disorders among surgeons and interventionalists: a systematic review and meta-analysis. *JAMA Surg.* 2018;153(2):e174947.
3. Magill SS, Edwards JR, Bamberg W, et al. Multistate point-prevalence survey of health care-associated infections. *N Engl J Med.* 2014;370(13):1198-1208.
4. Tanner J, Norrie P, Melen K. Preoperative hair removal to reduce surgical site infection. *Cochrane Database Syst Rev.* 2011;11:Cd004122.
5. Ban KA, Minei JP, Laronga C, et al. American College of Surgeons and Surgical Infection Society: Surgical Site Infection Guidelines, 2016 update. *J Am Coll Surg.* 2017;224(1):59-74.
6. Tanner J, Melen K. Preoperative hair removal to reduce surgical site infection. *Cochrane Database Syst Rev.* 2021;8(8):Cd004122.
7. Sobel J, Khan AS, Swerdlow DL. Threat of a biological terrorist attack on the US food supply: the CDC perspective. *Lancet.* 2002;359(9309):874-880.
8. Kurz A, Sessler DI, Lenhardt R. Perioperative normothermia to reduce the incidence of surgical-wound infection and shorten hospitalization. Study of Wound Infection and Temperature Group. *N Engl J Med.* 1996;334(19):1209-1215.
9. Deerenberg EB, Harlaar JJ, Steyerberg EW, et al. Small bites versus large bites for closure of abdominal midline incisions (STITCH): a double-blind, multicentre, randomised controlled trial. *Lancet.* 2015;386(10000):1254-1260.

10. Fundamental Use of Surgical Energy (FUSE). 2022. https://www.fuseprogram.org/

11. Holcomb JB, del Junco DJ, Fox EE, et al. The prospective, observational, multicenter, major trauma transfusion (PROMMTT) study: comparative effectiveness of a time-varying treatment with competing risks. *JAMA Surg.* 2013;148(2):127-136.

12. Holcomb JB, Tilley BC, Baraniuk S, et al. Transfusion of plasma, platelets, and red blood cells in a 1:1:1 vs a 1:1:2 ratio and mortality in patients with severe trauma: the PROPPR randomized clinical trial. *J Am Med Assoc.* 2015;313(5):471-482.

13. Hébert PC, Wells G, Blajchman MA, et al. A multicenter, randomized, controlled clinical trial of transfusion requirements in critical care. Transfusion Requirements in Critical Care Investigators, Canadian Critical Care Trials Group. *N Engl J Med.* 1999;340(6):409-417.

14. Spinella PC, Perkins JG, Grathwohl KW, Beekley AC, Holcomb JB. Warm fresh whole blood is independently associated with improved survival for patients with combat-related traumatic injuries. *J Trauma.* 2009;66(4 suppl I):S69-S76.

3 Management of Common Postoperative Problems

Louisa Yun Zhu Bai, Katharine E. Caldwell, Rami Al-Aref, and Isaiah Turnbull

I. NEUROLOGIC CONSIDERATIONS

A. The physiologic stress of surgery can affect neurologic function. This may be especially true for patients with underlying neurologic disorders or for elderly patients. It is important to differentiate recovery from general anesthesia, delirium, withdrawal, and other neurologic complications due to differences in necessary treatment.

B. Delayed emergence from anesthesia

1. Presentation[1]
   a. Normal emergence from anesthesia is a gradual return to consciousness after administration of general anesthesia.
   b. Most patients should be awake and aware of surroundings 15 minutes post extubation.
   c. All patients should be responsive 60 minutes after last administration of sedative, opiate, or anesthetic agent.
2. Risk factors
   a. Hepatic or renal insufficiency → delayed drug clearance
   b. Hypothermia → slows drug metabolism
   c. Advanced age → slows drug metabolism
   d. Prolonged duration of surgery
   e. Inappropriate dose
   f. Drug interactions
3. Treatment
   a. Airway protection
      i. Evaluate need for reintubation
   b. Consider role of modifiable risk factors
      i. Correction of hypoxemia, hypothermia, or electrolyte abnormalities
   c. Consider specific agents for additional reversal as required[2]
      i. Opiates
         a) Naloxone 40 to 80 μg IV
            1) Can repeat at 40-μg dose at 2- to 5-min intervals until patient is responsive.
            2) May require redosing due to short half-life (1-1.5 h) generally shorter than half-life of many opiates.

- ii. Benzodiazepines
  - a) Flumazenil 0.2 mg IV given over 30 seconds
    - 1) Can repeat 0.2-mg doses up to 1 mg maximum.
- iii. Neuromuscular blockade
  - a) Sugammadex 2 mg/kg IV
- iv. Note: No reversal agents are available for volatile inhalational anesthetics (sevoflurane, desflurane) or sedative-hypnotic agents (propofol).

d. Consider other causes of alterations in level of consciousness (i.e., stroke, seizure).

C. Altered mental status (AMS)

1. Presentation
   - a. AMS is any change in baseline mental status including abnormal thought content, change in level of consciousness, confusion, and agitation.
   - b. Always consider patient's baseline level of cognition and orientation.
   - c. AMS is a symptom and not a diagnosis. Patients should be evaluated with a broad differential regarding the etiology of their neurological discrepancy.
2. Differential diagnosis
   - a. Infections—sepsis, meningitis
   - b. Hypoxia
   - c. Hypoperfusion—hypovolemia, cardiogenic shock
   - d. Trauma—head injury, carbon monoxide exposure
   - e. Toxidromes—alcohol, barbiturates
   - f. Metabolic—acid–base electrolyte or glucose derangements
   - g. Neurologic—stroke, seizure, intracranial bleed
   - h. Psychiatric—depression, bipolar disorder, schizophrenia
   - i. Endocrine—thyroid or adrenal disorders
   - j. Pharmacologic—medication effects or intoxication
   - k. Delirium (see below)
3. Treatment
   - a. Treatment of the precipitating cause should be initiated.
   - b. Patient safety should be considered for patients with significant alterations in mental status who are at risk for falls, accidental removal of lines or drains, or accidental self-injury.

D. Delirium

1. Presentation[3]
   - a. Extremely common in hospitalized patients especially patients with intensive care unit (ICU) stays or the elderly.
   - b. Symptoms
     - i. Waxing and waning symptoms
     - ii. Alterations in memory, orientation, and perception
     - iii. Alterations in level of consciousness and attention
     - iv. Altered sleep patterns
   - c. Patients with hyperactive delirium may experience agitation, restlessness, and aggression.
   - d. Patients with hypoactive delirium may experience slowing of motor function and speech, as well as sedation.

2. Diagnosis
   a. Delirium is a diagnosis of exclusion, and full evaluation of underlying metabolic or physiologic causes should be completed.
   b. Should consider a patient's baseline level of orientation and functioning.
   c. Often precipitated by other medical causes (infectious, toxic, metabolic, etc.).
3. Treatment
   a. Treatment of underlying causes
   b. Frequent reorientation
   c. Minimize sleep disturbance and normalize sleep/wake cycles
   d. Provide access to vision and hearing aids if utilized
   e. Avoidance of physical restraints
   f. Involvement of family members or other patient support network
   g. Use of pharmacologic agents for severe agitation to provide for patient safety may be required.
      i. Haloperidol 0.5 to 1 mg IV or IM is generally the agent of choice.
      ii. Benzodiazepines (lorazepam 0.5-1 mg) have a limited role for extreme agitation and may worsen confusion and sedation.
      iii. Other sedative agents (dexmedetomidine, propofol) may be used in critical care settings to manage delirium; however, they may further contribute to delirium symptoms.

E. Perioperative stroke
1. Presentation
   a. Focal neurologic deficit (unilateral weakness or clumsiness)
   b. Sensory loss
   c. Speech changes
   d. Diplopia
   e. Vertigo
2. Risk factors[4]
   a. Advanced age
   b. History of myocardial infarction (MI) within 6 months
   c. Acute renal failure
   d. End-stage renal disease requiring hemodialysis
   e. History of transient ischemic attack or stroke
   f. Chronic obstructive pulmonary disease (COPD)
   g. Active tobacco use
   h. Surgical type (major intra abdominal procedure, vascular surgery, pulmonary resection, transplant surgery)
3. Diagnosis
   a. Physical examination
      i. FAAST Scale[5]
         a) Face—uneven smile or facial droop
         b) Arm—arm or leg numbness or weakness
         c) Anesthesia—evaluate for residual anesthetic effect
         d) Speech—slurring of speech or difficulty speaking
         e) Time—get help immediately

ii. Emergent head CT
 a) Essential to rule out hemorrhagic stroke
iii. Emergent neurologic evaluation
iv. MRI/electroencephalogram (EEG)
 a) May be helpful adjuncts for evaluating the possibility of stroke.
 b) Must consider patient stability before MRI due to need for prolonged time to complete scan.

4. Treatment
 a. Appropriate resuscitation and supportive care should be provided.
 b. Neurology consult
  i. Rapid consideration of thrombolysis is essential for all patients with ischemic strokes.
   a) Thrombolysis may be contraindicated in patients in the immediate postoperative period due to risk of hemorrhage and consideration for thrombolytics should only be initiated in close consultation with a neurologist and surgeon.

F. Seizures

1. Presentation
 a. Can vary widely based on the region of the brain affected
 b. Symptoms
  i. Motor symptoms
   a) Rhythmic jerking movements (clonic)
   b) Limp or weak muscles (atonic)
   c) Stiffening of muscles (tonic)
   d) Brief muscle twitching (myoclonus)
  ii. Nonmotor symptoms
   a) AMS
   b) Staring spells (absence)
   c) Changes in sensations or emotions
   d) Autonomic dysfunction
 c. Causes
  i. Discontinuation of home seizure medications in the postoperative period
  ii. Anesthesia
  iii. Electrolyte abnormalities (e.g., hyponatremia and hypocalcemia)
  iv. Withdrawal (e.g., alcohol or benzodiazapine)
  v. Hypoglycemia
  vi. Fever
  vii. Mediations (e.g., imipenem)
  viii. Head trauma
  ix. Intracranial bleeding

2. Diagnosis
 a. A thorough investigation for the cause of new-onset seizures in a postoperative patient should be performed.
  i. Electrolyte and glucose evaluation
  ii. Head CT
  iii. EEG
  iv. Arterial blood gas (ABG)

v. Evaluation of potential medication causes
vi. Consideration of lumbar puncture

3. Treatment[6]
   a. Airway—the most important step in the treatment of a patient having a seizure is to assess and, if necessary, secure the airway to prevent aspiration.
   b. Correct hypoglycemia or metabolic derangements.
   c. All patients with new-onset seizures in the postoperative period should be evaluated by a neurologist.
   d. Acute medical management of status epilepticus
      i. Seizures lasting >5 min or a series of multiple continuous seizures without return to baseline is a medical emergency.
      ii. Emergent neurology consultation should be obtained.
      iii. Medication management of convulsive status epilepticus
         a) Lorazepam/diazepam 0.1 mg/kg IV, repeated if necessary
            1) Rectal or intranasal diazepam can be given at 0.2 mg/kg (max 20 mg) for patients without IV access.
         b) Antiseizure medication should be given to prevent recurrence after cessation of seizure activity.
            1) Phenytoin 20 mg/kg loading dose
            2) Keppra 60 mg/kg (maximum dose 4,500 mg)
            3) Valproate 40 mg/kg (maximum dose 3,000 mg)

G. Withdrawal

1. The prevalence of alcohol use disorder is estimated to be approximately 14% in the US, and withdrawal will affect approximately 50% of those patients. Mortality for patients who develop severe alcohol withdrawal symptoms is between 1% and 4%.[7]
2. Presentation
   a. Begins as soon as 8 hours after blood alcohol levels normalize
   b. Peak symptomatology will occur at 72 hours.
   c. Symptoms
      i. Insomnia or restlessness
      ii. Tachypnea
      iii. Fever
      iv. Hypertension
      v. Seizures (between 12 and 48 hours after normalization of blood ethanol level)
      vi. Disorientation
      vii. Hallucinations
      viii. Diaphoresis
3. Diagnosis
   a. Clinical diagnosis made based on history of alcohol use and symptoms
   b. Should be considered a diagnosis of exclusion, and other causes of alterations in mental status and vital signs should be ruled out
4. Treatment
   a. Clinical Institute Withdrawal Assessment (CIWA) protocols
      i. The CIWA Scale for Alcohol is a tool to evaluate symptom severity for patients with alcohol withdrawal and guide symptom-triggered treatment.[8]

a) Evaluates 10 symptoms on a scale from 0 (not present) to 7 (severe)
   1) Nausea/vomiting
   2) Headache
   3) Paroxysmal sweats
   4) Auditory disturbances
   5) Anxiety
   6) Visual disturbances
   7) Agitation
   8) Tactile disturbances
   9) Tremor
   10) Orientation and sensorium clouding—scored on a scale from 0 (fully oriented) to 4 (disoriented)

ii. Scores
   a) <10: None or very mild withdrawal
   b) 10 to 15: Mild withdrawal
   c) 16 to 20: Modest withdrawal
   d) >20: Severe withdrawal

b. Seizure prevention
   i. Long-acting benzodiazepines
      a) For initial management or more severe withdrawal
         1) Diazepam 5 to 10 mg IV q 5 to 10 min as needed
         2) Lorazepam 2 to 4 mg IV q 15 to 20 min as needed
      b) For prolonged management or less severe symptoms
         1) Chlordiazepoxide (Librium) 25 to 100 mg PO q6h
         2) Diazepam 5 to 20 mg PO q6h
      c) Consider lorazepam or oxazepam for patients with advanced cirrhosis due to poor metabolism in these patients.

c. Autonomic hyperactivity
   i. Patients with tachycardia or hypertension should undergo close hemodynamic monitoring and consideration for administration of agents to control autonomic hyperactivity.
      a) Clonidine 0.1 mg PO qid
      b) Atenolol 50 to 100 mg PO once daily

d. Nutritional supplementation
   i. Thiamine 500 mg IV for 3 days followed by 100 mg PO daily should be given to prevent Wernicke encephalopathy.
   ii. Folate 1 mg daily
   iii. Careful electrolyte correction as metabolic derangements (e.g., hypomagnesemia) are common.

II. PAIN CONTROL

A. Opiates (**Table 3.1**)

1. Overdose management
   a. Presentation
      i. Depressed mental status
      ii. Decreased respiratory rate
      iii. Constricted pupils

TABLE 3.1 Dosing and Morphine Equivalents of Commonly Used Opiates

Agent	Morphine Equivalent	Oral Dosing	Parenteral Dosing
Morphine	1:1	10-20 mg q4h	1-5 mg q4h
Codeine	1:0.1	30-60 mg q4h	N/A
Fentanyl	1:100	N/A	50 mg q2h
Hydrocodone	1:1	5-10 mg q4h	N/A
Hydromorphone	1:5	2mg q4h	1mg q4h
Oxycodone	1:1.5	5-10 mg q4h	N/A
Tramadol	1:0.1	25-100 mg q4h	N/A

b. Diagnosis
   i. Evaluate recently given opiate medication
      a) Consider operating room administration of medication
      b) Consider hepatic function
c. Treatment
   i. Supportive treatment for the patient's airway and breathing
      a) Evaluate for supplemental O_2 requirements and possible need for bag-valve respiration until naloxone can be administered.
   ii. Administer naloxone
      a) Spontaneously breathing patients should receive 0.04 mg IV naloxone with up titration every few minutes until respiratory rate is >12.
      b) Apneic patients 0.2 to 1 mg IV naloxone
      c) Patients in cardiac arrest 2 mg naloxone

2. Opioid use disorder
   a. Opioid use and overdose remain a significant problem in the US. Approximately two-thirds of drug overdose deaths are related to opioids. https://pubmed.ncbi.nlm.nih.gov/32191688/
   b. Management of postoperative pain in the patient with opiate use disorder:
      i. For patients in recovery from opiate use disorder, discuss patient's wishes regarding opiate administration.
      ii. For patients currently using pharmacologic treatment for opiate use disorder (buprenorphine or methadone), consider consultation with a pharmacist or pain medicine specialist for recommendations regarding dosing opiates. https://pubmed.ncbi.nlm.nih.gov/30500943/
      iii. For patients with active opiate use disorder, higher doses than typical postoperative doses may be required to achieve pain control due to tolerance. Monitor for respiratory depression.

c. For interested individuals who are seeking treatment, referral for pharmacologic management (buprenorphine or methadone) and psychosocial management should be placed.

B. Nonopiate adjuncts (Tylenol, NSAIDs, gabapentin)

1. Nonopiate adjuncts can be used alone or in combination with narcotic pain medication to control postoperative pain.
2. Choice of specific agents will depend upon surgical type and patient risk factors (see **Table 3.2**).

TABLE 3.2 Doses of Commonly Used Nonopiate Medications

Agent	Typical Dose	Typical Formulation	Mechanism of Action	Adverse Events
Acetaminophen (Tylenol)	325-1000 mg q4-6h (maximum 4 g/d)	PO or IV	Inhibition of COX and action of metabolite AM404 on cannabinoid receptors	Hepatotoxicity in chronic use or acute overdose
Gabapentin	100-900 mg q8h	PO	$\alpha_2\delta$ Ligand reducing calcium channel delivery to the cell membrane preventing neurotransmitter release	Sedation, dizziness, and ataxia. Caution with renal impairment
Cyclobenzaprine (Flexeril)	5-10 mg q8h	PO	5-HT2 receptor antagonist	Sedation, dizziness, tachycardia
Ibuprofen	400 mg q4h	PO	Inhibition of COX enzymes	Can cause or worsen renal insufficiency. Risk of gastropathy
Ketorolac	15-30 mg q6h (maximum 120 mg/d × 5 d)	PO or IV	Inhibition of COX enzymes	Can cause or worsen renal insufficiency. Risk of gastropathy

5-HT, 5-hydroxytryptamine; COX, cyclooxygenase.

C. Regional and local anesthesia
1. Local anesthetics are medications that lead to sensory nerve impulse blockade near the site of their administration.
2. Often infiltrated in or near the surgical site at the time of operation to improve postoperative pain control.
3. Regional anesthesia refers to the injection of a local anesthetic to induce neuraxial or peripheral nerve blockade.
   a. Spinal anesthesia—injection of anesthetic into the subarachnoid space at the level of the lumbar spine
   b. Epidural anesthesia—catheter is inserted into the epidural space and local anesthetic is administered.
   c. Peripheral nerve block—injection of local anesthetic into specific locations to induce anesthesia of a particular area of the body
      i. Upper extremity block—generally brachial plexus nerve blockade
      ii. Lower extremity—generally femoral, popliteal, or saphenous nerve blockade
      iii. Intercostal nerve block
      iv. Transversus abdominis plane block—injection into the plane between the transversus abdominus and internal oblique to induce cutaneous nerve block for the abdomen
4. Grouped as esters (one "i") or amides (two "i's")
   a. Esters: Tetracaine, procaine, cocaine
   b. Amide: Lidocaine, bupivacaine, ropivacaine
5. Can be dosed plain or with epinephrine
   a. Epinephrine leads to vasoconstriction near the site of instillation and decreases vascular absorption, increasing the maximum dose that can be used and total length of action.
6. Local tissue acidosis (often due to infection) decreases the efficacy of local anesthetic medications.
7. General rules for dosing
   a. 1% lidocaine (10 mg/mL)—give up to 0.5 mL/kg
   b. 2% lidocaine (20 mg/mL)—give up to 0.25 mL/kg
   c. 0.25% bupivacaine (2.5 mg/mL)—give up to 1 mL/kg
   d. 0.5% bupivacaine (5 mg/mL)—give up to 0.5 mL/kg
8. Toxicity
   a. Toxic dose administration or accidental intravascular administration of local anesthetics can lead to
      i. Central nervous system symptoms (AMS, perioral numbness, visual disturbances, seizures)
      ii. Cardiovascular symptoms—hypotension, cardiovascular collapse
   b. Treatment is generally supportive with management of arrhythmia, seizure, or hypotension.
      i. Lipid emulsion therapy can be used for severe toxicity with 1.5 mL/kg IV bolus of 20% lipid emulsion followed by continuous infusion at 0.25 mL/kg/min.

Agent	Max Dose Plain (mg/kg)	Max Dose With Epi (mg/kg)	Length of Action Plain	Length of Action With Epi
Procaine	7 mg/kg	N/A	40 min	N/A
Lidocaine	4.5 mg/kg	7 mg/kg	30-60 min	60-240 min
Bupivacaine	2.5 mg/kg	3 mg/kg	120-240 min	180-360 min
0.5% Ropivacaine	3 mg/kg	3.5 mg/kg	15-60 min	

III. CARDIAC CONSIDERATIONS

The physiologic stress of surgery can affect cardiac function for a multitude of reasons including fluid shifts common in the postoperative period. Patients with underlying heart disease are especially at risk.

A. Postoperative hypotension
  1. Presentation
    a. Hypotension (systolic blood pressure <90 mmHg, mean arterial pressure <65 mmHg) postoperatively should raise immediate concern, particularly for postoperative bleeding.
    b. Can be associated with tachycardia, AMS, oliguria.
  2. Diagnosis
    a. Most common postoperative causes
      i. Bleeding
      ii. Underresuscitation/hypovolemia
      iii. Sepsis
      iv. Anesthesia/analgesics (epidural catheters, narcotics)
      v. Premature resumption of home antihypertensive medications
    b. Close patient evaluation
      i. Vitals
      ii. Physical examination, with emphasis on region of recent surgery
      iii. Complete laboratory evaluation (complete blood count [CBC], basic metabolic panel [BMP], coagulation)
      iv. Check surgical drains
      v. Evaluate Ins and out (I&O) including intraoperative fluid administration
      vi. Evaluate medication administration
      vii. Laboratory evaluation (CBC, BMP)
  3. Treatment
    a. Ensure IV access and initiate fluid challenge.
    b. If evidence of bleeding on physical examination or laboratory tests, promptly initiate balanced transfusion.
    c. Ensure there an active type and screen and prepare blood products as appropriate.
    d. If epidural catheter in place, consider slowing or stopping infusion.

e. Stop medications with hemodynamic effects (β-blockers, diuretics, narcotics).
f. Consider Foley catheter placement for monitoring of urine output.
g. Consider transfer to higher level of care if hypotension is persistent despite initial interventions and vasopressors are required.

B. Hypertension
1. Presentation
a. Evaluate in relation to the patient's baseline preoperative blood pressure (BP).
b. Aim to achieve baseline BP as opposed to absolute normotension.
i. Chronic hypertension→ shift in cerebral autoregulatory system that may not allow for adequate cerebral perfusion at normotension
c. Causes
i. Essential hypertension
ii. Pain
iii. Ethanol withdrawal
iv. Hypoxemia
v. Hypertensive urgency
a) Severe hypertension without evidence of end-organ damage
vi. Hypertensive emergency
a) Severe hypertension (usually diastolic BP > 120 mmHg) with evidence of acute end-organ damage, such as stroke, acute heart failure, acute aortic dissection
2. Diagnosis
a. Thorough evaluation and physical examination, including neurological examination
b. Assess for underlying causes (pain, withdrawal, hypoxemia).
3. Treatment
a. Address underlying causes
b. When possible, resume home antihypertensive agents.
c. For acute hypertension
i. Labetalol 10 to 20 mg IV q10 min (maximum dose 300 mg)
ii. Hydralazine 10 to 20 mg IV q6h
iii. Clonidine 0.1 mg PO q6h
d. Patients with hypertensive urgency or emergency should be evaluated for need for transfer to a higher level of care.

C. Postop MI
1. Presentation
a. Dyspnea, hypotension, atypical pain, or asymptomatic
b. Commonly occurs on postoperative day (POD) 2
2. Diagnosis
a. All patients with new-onset chest pain should be evaluated for possible MI.
i. Vital signs
ii. Laboratory evaluation (CBC, BMP, serial troponin levels)
iii. ECG—compare with prior tracings
iv. CXR

b. Role of troponin
   i. Elevated troponin + new ischemic ECG changes (ST-segment or new conduction system changes) is diagnostic for MI.
   ii. Elevated troponins in the absence of ECG changes may indicate other underlying abnormalities (global shock, renal failure) and may be difficult to interpret.

3. Treatment
   a. For patients with ECG findings consistent with ischemia
      i. Emergent cardiology consultation
      ii. Telemetry
      iii. Supplemental O_2
      iv. Morphine for pain control (1-4 mg IV q hour)
      v. Aspirin 325 mg PO
      vi. Nitroglycerin 0.4 mg sublingual until pain resolves in patients without hypotension
      vii. β-Blocker administration (three doses of metoprolol 5 mg IV q5 min) has been demonstrated to improve patient outcomes.
      viii. Heparin infusion
         a) Safety of heparin administration must be discussed between surgical and consulting cardiology teams due to risk of bleeding in postop patients.

D. Postop congestive heart failure exacerbation
1. Presentation
   a. Shortness of breath and hypoxia
   b. Edema
   c. Frequently occurs immediately postop due to intraoperative fluid administration or POD1-2 due to mobilization of sequestered fluids
2. Diagnosis
   a. Physical examination to evaluate for fluid overload
   b. Vital signs
   c. Evaluation of recent I&O and body weights
   d. Laboratory evaluation (troponin, B-type natriuretic peptide, ABG, CBC, BMP)
   e. CXR
   f. ECG
3. Treatment
   a. Supplemental oxygen
   b. Fluid restriction
   c. Diuresis (as tolerated)
      i. Lasix 20 to 40 mg IV up to 200 mg q6h
      ii. Monitor serum potassium and bicarbonate closely.
      iii. If contraction alkalosis occurs, substitute acetazolamide.
   d. Use of vasodilator and inotrope therapy are reserved for patients with refractory end-organ hypoperfusion.

E. Postop atrial fibrillation
1. Presentation
   a. Often asymptomatic
   b. Can present with palpitations, dyspnea, or hypotension

c. Consider personal history of atrial fibrillation
d. More common with advanced age, male sex, colon resections, coagulopathy[9]

2. Diagnosis
   a. ECG
   b. Electrolyte evaluation
3. Treatment
   a. Chronic atrial fibrillation
      i. Resume home β-blocker and anticoagulation therapy when able.
   b. New-onset atrial fibrillation
      i. Initiate rate control with IV metoprolol or diltiazem.
      ii. Majority of patients will convert to sinus rhythm spontaneously within 24 hours.
      iii. If new-onset atrial fibrillation lasts >48 hours and CHA2DS2-VASc score ≥ 2, recommend initiation of therapeutic anticoagulation when able.
      iv. If persistent, consider transesophageal echocardiogram to rule out left atrial thrombus followed by direct current cardioversion.
   c. Atrial fibrillation with rapid ventricular response[10]
      i. Rate control with IV metoprolol
      ii. Pharmacologic rhythm control with amiodarone
   d. For hemodynamic instability, perform urgent cardioversion (120-200 J).

F. Perioperative use of antiplatelet therapy[11]
   1. Aspirin should be continued perioperatively for noncardiac surgery.
   2. For patients with coronary stents placed within 6 to 12 weeks on dual antiplatelet therapy (DAPT) delay elective surgery until completion of DAPT therapy, continuation of both agents when possible for nonelective surgery, or stopping one antiplatelet agent 7 to 10 days prior to surgery.
      a. In patients with coronary stents placed within the last 3 to 12 months undergoing elective surgery, recommend stopping P_2Y_{12} inhibitor prior to surgery.

IV. PULMONARY CONSIDERATIONS

Patients are at risk of pulmonary complications in the postoperative period because of anesthesia, prolonged immobility, pain, and decreased breathing, as well as other causes. These effects are most pronounced for patients with underlying lung disease.

A. Atelectasis[9]
   1. Collapse of alveoli as the result of general anesthesia, recumbent position, and increased intra-abdominal pressure (**Figure 3.1**)
   2. Presentation
      a. Dyspnea
      b. Hypoxia
      c. Pain with deep inhalation
      d. Inability to deep cough
      e. Fever (within 24-48 hours postop)

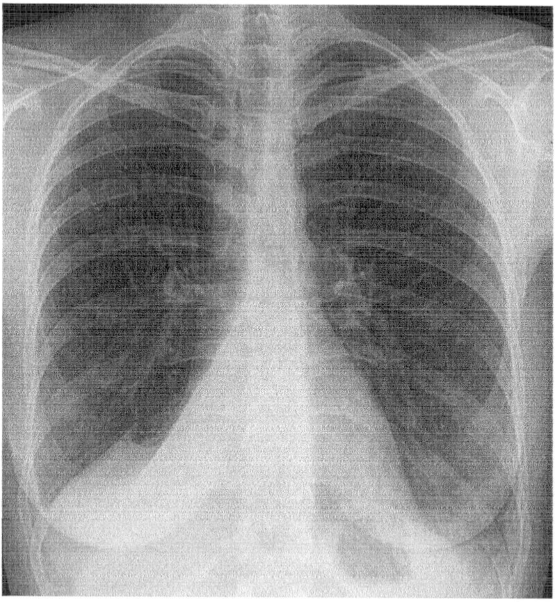

FIGURE 3.1 Right lower lobe atelectasis. (*Reprinted from https://commons.wikimedia.org/wiki/File:Unterlappenatelektase_rechts_pa.jpg; https://creativecommons.org/licenses/by-sa/3.0/deed.en.*)

3. Diagnosis
   a. CXR—low lung volumes, lung opacification especially in lung bases, hilar or hemidiaphragmatic shift toward the affected area
4. Management
   a. Encourage incentive spirometry
   b. Chest physical therapy
   c. Ambulation
   d. Ensure adequate pain control

B. Pneumothorax
   1. See Chapter 7—Chest Trauma

C. Pulmonary effusion
   1. See Chapter 31—Lung and Mediastinal Disease

D. Asthma or COPD exacerbation
   1. Presentation
      a. Dyspnea
      b. Hypoxia or hypercapnia
      c. Wheezing
   2. Diagnosis
      a. CXR, ABG, ECG
   3. Management
      a. Supplemental O_2
      b. Inhaled β-agonist (albuterol)

i. Albuterol inhaler 90 µg/inhalation 2 inhalations q20 min for 3 doses
ii. Albuterol nebulizer 2.5 mg q20 min for 3 doses
c. Anticholinergics (ipratropium bromide)
i. Ipratropium 500 µg q20 min for 3 doses
d. In patients with life-threatening exacerbations refractory to medical therapy, intubation, mechanical ventilation, and transfer to higher level care may be required.

E. Pulmonary embolism
1. See Hematologic Considerations

F. Postoperative pneumonia
1. See Infectious Disease Considerations

G. Acute respiratory distress syndrome
1. See Chapter 4—Critical Care

H. Respiratory support (**Table 3.3**)
1. For additional details, see Chapter 4—Critical Care.
2. In the postoperative period due to emergence from anesthesia, sedating effects of mediation, pain control, etc., patients may require additional supplemental oxygen.
3. Different modalities of oxygen delivery are indicated for patients based on differing O_2 concentration requirements.

V. RENAL CONSIDERATIONS AND FLUIDS/ELECTROLYTES/NUTRITION

A. Overview of renal insufficiency and renal failure (**Table 3.4**)
1. Oliguria—less than 0.5 mL/kg/h of urine output
2. Acute kidney injury—increase in serum creatinine (Cr) by 0.3 mg/dL or 1.5-fold above baseline in the setting of oliguria
a. Prerenal azotemia—hypotension, intravascular volume contract, decreased effective renal perfusion
b. Intrinsic renal causes—drug-induced acute tubular necrosis, radiocontrast dye administration, acute interstitial nephritis, rhabdomyolysis, prolonged ischemia from suprarenal aortic cross-clamping
c. Postrenal causes—obstruction of ureters or bladder from stones, iatrogenic injury, enlarged prostate, obstructed urinary catheter
3. RIFLE criteria
a. Risk, Injury, Failure, Loss of kidney function, and End-stage kidney disease
b. **Figure 3.2**. RIFLE criteria
4. Indications for dialysis
a. Volume overload with respiratory insufficiency
b. Electrolyte abnormalities (i.e., hyperkalemia, hyperphosphatemia)
c. Metabolic acidosis
d. Ingestion of dialyzable toxins
e. Uremia (i.e., encephalopathy, pericarditis)

B. Postoperative urinary retention
1. Presentation
a. Inability to void
b. Suprapubic discomfort/pain

TABLE 3.3 Methods of Oxygen Administration

Modality of Respiratory Support	Mechanism	Indication
Nasal cannula	O_2 concentrations 20%-40% Flow rates 1-6 L/min	Spontaneously breathing patients with low-flow O_2 requirement
High-flow nasal cannula	O_2 concentrations up to 100% Flow rates: 40-60 L/min	Spontaneously breathing patients with severe hypoxemic respiratory failure as an alternative to other noninvasive ventilation methods
Simple mask	O_2 concentrations: 35%-50% Flow rates 6-10 L/min	Spontaneously breathing patients who require moderate oxygen to maintain O_2 saturation
Non-rebreather mask	O_2 concentrations 60%-80% Flow rates 8-10 L/min	Spontaneously breathing patients with high-dose oxygen requirements
Bilevel positive airway pressure	Regulates inspiratory and expiratory positive pressure levels	Patients with acute respiratory failure or those with chronic hypoventilation (e.g., obstructive sleep apnea)
Continuous positive airway pressure	Allows for spontaneous ventilation and provides constant positive airway pressure throughout respiratory cycle	Patients with chronic hypoventilation
Intubation	Direct oxygen delivery into the respiratory tract	Patients with acute respiratory failure, patients who are unable to protect their airway

TABLE 3.4 Laboratory Evaluation of Oliguria and Acute Renal Failure

Category	FE_{Na} (%)	FE_{Ur} (%)	U_{Na}	U_{Osm}	RFI	U_{Cr}/P_{Cr}
Prerenal	<1	≤35	<20	>500	<1	>40
Renal (intrinsic)	>1	>50	>40	<350	>1	<20
Postrenal	>4	NA	>40	<50	>1	<20

FE_{Na}, fractional excretion of sodium; FE_{Ur}, fractional excretion of urea; NA, not applicable; RFI, renal failure index; U_{Cr}/P_{Cr}, urine–plasma creatinine ratio; U_{Na}, urine sodium in mmol/L; U_{Osm}, urine osmolality in mOsm/kg.

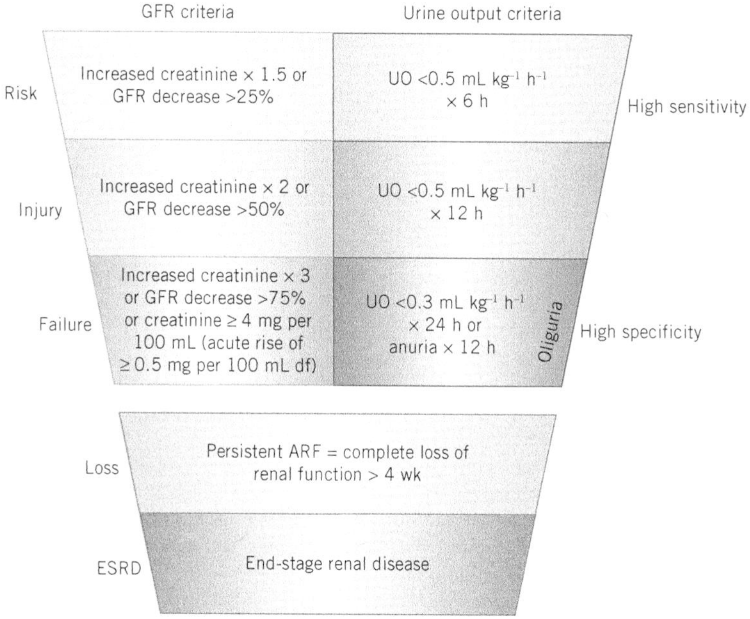

FIGURE 3.2 RIFLE criteria.[12] ARF, acute renal failure; GFR, glomerular filtration rate; UO, urine output. *(Reprinted from Ricci Z, Cruz D, Ronco C. The RIFLE criteria and mortality in acute kidney injury: a systematic review. Kidney Int. 2008;73(5):538-546. Copyright 2008, International Society of Nephrology. With permission.)*

2. Diagnosis
    a. Bladder ultrasound (>500 mL of urine)
    b. History of prostate issues
    c. Review home medications (i.e., tamsulosin)
3. Management
    a. Bladder catheterization with in-and-out catheter or indwelling Foley catheter insertion
    b. Initiation or resumption of α-blockade (tamsulosin)

C. Electrolyte abnormalities—**Table 3.5**

D. Nutrition

1. Evaluation of nutritional status
    a. Two of six criteria[13]
        i. Weight loss
        ii. Insufficient energy intake
        iii. Subcutaneous fat loss
        iv. Muscle mass loss
        v. Localized or general fluid accumulation (may mask weight loss)
        vi. Diminished functional status (measured by hand grip strength)
    b. Laboratory tests
        i. Albumin
        ii. Prealbumin

iii. Transferrin
iv. Specific vitamin and mineral levels
c. Nutric score calculator[14]
i. Quantifies the risk of critically ill patients developing adverse events that may be modified by aggressive nutritional therapy
ii. Validated in ICU patients
iii. Online calculator tool: https://www.criticalcarenutrition.com/resources/nutric-score/nutric-score-calculator
2. Enteral nutrition
a. Oral feeds
i. Requires intact chewing/swallowing mechanism and mental alertness
ii. Those with difficulty swallowing may require modified diets such as mechanical soft or pureed.
b. Assisted enteral feeds
i. Nasogastric tube—temporary, cannot be used for high gastric residuals
ii. Gastrostomy tube—percutaneous, laparoscopic or open, long-term enteral access, cannot be used for high gastric residuals
iii. Nasoduodenal tube—temporary, for gastric outlet obstruction
iv. Jejunostomy tube—percutaneous, laparoscopic or open, for proximal intestinal obstruction
3. Parenteral nutrition
a. Peripheral parenteral nutrition (PPN)
i. Peripheral IV access
ii. Osmolarity of PPN is limited to 900 mOsm to avoid phlebitis.
iii. Volumes are typically too high to meet full nutritional requirements.
b. Total parenteral nutrition (TPN)
i. Central venous access (internal jugular or subclavian)
ii. Can provide complete nutritional support
iii. Complications: Catheter-associated blood stream infection, cholestatic liver disease
4. Important that consideration of intake of vitamins (**Table 3.6**) and trace elements are considered (**Table 3.7**).

VI. GASTROINTESTINAL CONSIDERATIONS

Surgery on the gastrointestinal tract, general anesthesia, and pain medications may lead to a variety of gastrointestinal events that are commonly seen in the postoperative period.

A. Postoperative nausea and vomiting
1. Presentation
a. Occurs on POD 0 to 1
b. Can affect up to 30% of patients
2. Diagnosis
a. Abdominal x-ray
b. Abdominal CT

TABLE 3.5 Electrolyte Abnormalities and Management

Electrolyte	Deficiency	Excess
Sodium (normal 135-145 mmol/L)	Presentation: • Confusion, lethargy, nausea, vomiting, seizures, coma Management: • If severe (Na <110) or neurologic symptoms, then treat with hypertonic (3%) saline and loop diuretics • If hypovolemic, fluid replacement with normal saline • If SIADH, water intoxication, or liver disease, then restrict fluid and consider sodium tablets • If secondary to hyperglycemia, hyperproteinemia, or hyperlipidemia, correct underlying disorder Risk of osmotic demyelination syndrome: • Can occur with rapid correction of chronic hyponatremia • Maximum of 8 mEq/L sodium correction over 24 h	Presentation: • Lethargy, weakness, irritability, fasciculations, seizures, coma Management: • Replace free water deficit • If hypodipsia, encourage fluid intake • If central diabetes insipidus, administer desmopressin and dietary sodium restriction • If nephrogenic diabetes insipidus, dietary sodium restriction and thiazide diuretics Risk of cerebral edema: • Can occur with rapid correction of hypernatremia • Only half of the water deficit should be corrected over the first 24 h, with the remainder being corrected over the following 2-3 d
Potassium (3.3-4.9 mmol/L)	Presentation: • ECG with ectopy, T-wave depression, prominent U-waves, reentry arrhythmias Management: • Oral or parenteral repletion with 40-100 mEq of potassium (administered as chloride, acetate, or phosphate salts) • For every 0.1 mmol/L deficiency, correct with 10 mEq of potassium	Presentation: • ECG with peaked T waves, reduced P-wave voltage, widened QRS complex, sinusoidal pattern Management: • If mild (5-6 mmol/L), then low K diet, loop diuretics, cessation of exacerbating medications • If severe (>6 mmol/L), then temporize with 10% calcium gluconate, dextrose with insulin, inhaled β-agonists, $NaHCO_3$, and treat with Kayexalate, normal saline infusion with loop diuretics, dialysis

(continued)

TABLE 3.5 Electrolyte Abnormalities and Management (*Continued*)

Electrolyte	Deficiency	Excess
Magnesium (1.3-2.2 mEq/L)	Presentation: • Altered mental status, tremors, hyperreflexia, tetany • T waves and QRS complex broadening, PR and QT prolongation, arrhythmias Management: • If severe hypomagnesemia (<1 mEq/L) or life-threatening arrhythmias, administer 1-2 g parenteral $MgSO_4$ over 5 min then continuous infusion • If mild hypomagnesemia and able to tolerate PO, administer 20-80 mEq of Mg daily in divided doses, as magnesium oxide, chloride, or gluconate	Presentation: • Depression of deep tendon reflexes, paralysis, hypotension, sinus bradycardia, prolongation of PR, QT, QRS intervals Management: • If life-threatening arrhythmias, administer 10% calcium gluconate • Administer normal saline infusion with loop diuretics to promote renal elimination
Phosphate (2.5-4.5 mg/dL)	Presentation: • Diffuse weakness, flaccid paralysis, respiratory muscle depression Management: • For average-weight adult (61-80 kg): • If < 1 mg/dL → 40 mmol IV Phos • If 1-1.7 mg/dL → 30 mmol • If 1.8-2.2 mg/dL → 15 mmol • Once serum phosphorus >2, can start oral therapy with sodium-potassium-phosphate salt	Presentation: • Hypocalcemia, tetany, soft tissue calcifications (if chronic) Management: • Limit dietary phosphorus • Fluid hydration and acetazolamide for renal elimination • Phosphate binders (aluminum hydroxide) • Dialysis if refractory

TABLE 3.5 Electrolyte Abnormalities and Management (*Continued*)

Electrolyte	Deficiency	Excess
Calcium (8.9-10.3 mg/dL)	Presentation: • Tetany, Chvostek sign (facial muscle spasms elicited by tapping over branches of facial nerve), perioral numbness and tingling, QT prolongation, ventricular arrhythmias Management: • If symptomatic, IV 10% calcium gluconate or calcium chloride (3× elemental Ca compared with gluconate), followed by infusion • If asymptomatic, oral calcium carbonate or gluconate • Consider supplementation with vitamin D if hypocalcemia is severe	Presentation: • Altered mental status, diffuse weakness, adynamic ileus, severe constipation, nausea, vomiting, QT shortening, arrhythmias Management: • If severe and symptomatic, normal saline infusion with loop diuretics, adjusted to maintain urine output of 100-150 mL/h • Bisphosphonates • Calcitonin • Dialysis if refractory

SIADH, syndrome of inappropriate antidiuretic hormone.

TABLE 3.6 Essential Vitamins

Vitamin	Function	Deficiency State
Fat Soluble		
A (Retinol)	Rhodopsin synthesis	Xerophthalmia, keratomalacia
D (Cholecalciferol)	Intestinal calcium absorption, bone remodeling	Rickets (children), osteomalacia (adults)
E (α-Tocopherol)	Antioxidant	Hemolytic anemia, neurologic damage
K (Naphthoquinone)	τ-Carboxylation of glutamate in clotting factors	Coagulopathy (deficiency in factors II, VII, IX, and X)
**Problems with fat digestion and absorption can result in deficiency of vitamins A, D, E, and K. Vitamin K is also produced by enteric microbiota.*		
Water Soluble		
B_1 (Thiamine)	Decarboxylation and aldehyde transfer reactions	Beriberi, neuropathy, fatigue, heart failure
**Bodily thiamine stores are relatively small, making deficiency common in hospitalized patients, and especially those with a history of alcoholism. As such, early thiamine supplementation, especially in the ICU, can be useful in the prevention of altered mental status and lactic acidosis. Furthermore, since thiamine is needed to breakdown glucose, supplementation should proceed glucose delivery in at-risk patients, to prevent Wernicke–Korsakoff syndrome* (Attaluri P, Castillo A, Edriss H. Nugent K. Thiamine deficiency: an important consideration in critically ill patients. *Am J Med Sci.* 2018:356:382-390).		
B_2 (Riboflavin)	Oxidation–reduction reactions	Dermatitis, glossitis
B_3 (Niacin)	Oxidation–reduction reactions	Pellagra (dermatitis, diarrhea, dementia, death)
B_6 (Pyridoxine)	Transamination and decarboxylation reactions	Neuropathy, glossitis, anemia
B_7 (Biotin)	Carboxylation reactions	Dermatitis, alopecia
B_9 (Folate)	DNA synthesis	Megaloblastic anemia, glossitis

(continued)

TABLE 3.6 Essential Vitamins (*Continued*)

Vitamin	Function	Deficiency State
B_{12} (Cyanocobalamin)	DNA synthesis, myelination	Megaloblastic anemia, neuropathy
**Vitamin B_{12} requires intrinsic factor (produced by gastric parietal cells) for absorption.*		
C (Ascorbic acid)	Hydroxylation of hormones, hydroxylation of proline in collagen synthesis, antioxidant	Scurvy

Modifications and supplementary information from authors are indicated by asterisks and italicized text.

Adapted with permission from Nedeau AE, Unger LD, Rombeau JL. Nutrition, digestion, and absorption. In: Atluri P, Karakouisis GC, Porrett PM, et al., eds. *The Surgical Review: An Integrated Basic Science and Clinical Science Study Guide.* 2nd ed. Lippincott Williams & Wilkins; 2006:252.

TABLE 3.7 Essential Trace Elements

Trace Element	Function	Deficiency
Chromium	Promotes normal glucose utilization in combination with insulin	Glucose intolerance, peripheral neuropathy
Copper	Component of enzymes	Hypochromic microcytic anemia, neutropenia, bone demoralization, diarrhea
Fluorine	Essential for normal structure of bones and teeth	Caries
Iodine	Thyroid hormone production	Endemic goiter, hypothyroidism, myxedema, cretinism
Iron	Hemoglobin synthesis	Hypochromic microcytic anemia, glossitis, stomatitis
Manganese	Component of enzymes, essential for normal bone structure	Dermatitis, weight loss, nausea, vomiting, coagulopathy

(*continued*)

TABLE 3.7 Essential Trace Elements (*Continued*)

Trace Element	Function	Deficiency
Molybdenum	Component of enzymes	Neurologic abnormalities, night blindness
Selenium	Component of enzymes, antioxidant	Cardiomyopathy
Zinc	Component of enzymes involved in metabolism of lipids, proteins, carbohydrates, nucleic acids	Alopecia, hypogonadism, olfactory and gustatory dysfunction, impaired wound healing, acrodermatitis enteropathica, growth arrest

Adapted with permission from Nedeau AE, Unger LD, Rombeau JL. Nutrition, digestion, and absorption. In: Atluri P, Karakouisis GC, Porrett PM, et al., eds. *The Surgical Review: An Integrated Basic Science and Clinical Science Study Guide.* 2nd ed. Lippincott Williams & Wilkins; 2006:253.

3. Management
   a. Aggressive management with antiemetic
      i. Ondansetron
      ii. Promethazine
      iii. Prochlorperazine
      iv. Scopolamine
      v. Dexamethasone
   b. Ondansetron, promethazine, and prochlorperazine may cause QT prolongation
   c. For patients with persistent nausea with single-agent therapy and no evidence of acute intra-abdominal process, consider multimodal treatment

B. Paralytic ileus

1. Presentation
   a. Obstipation and constipation
   b. Nausea
   c. Vomiting
   d. Intolerance of PO diet
   e. Abdominal distension
2. Diagnosis
   a. Upright abdominal radiograph
      i. Dilated stomach and loops of bowel
      ii. Air should be visualized in the colon, helping to differentiate ileus and small bowel obstruction.
   b. Abdominal CT
      i. May be used to rule out obstruction as a possible cause of ileus

c. Upper gastrointestinal (GI) study with small bowel follow through
 i. Used if diagnosis is uncertain from radiographs or CT scans
 ii. Can be diagnostic as well as therapeutic
3. Management
 a. Nothing by mouth
 b. Nasogastric tube (NGT) placement
 c. Intravenous fluid replacement should be started to compensate for enteric loses.
 d. Correction of electrolyte deficiencies
  i. Deficiency of potassium and magnesium may prolong ileus.
 e. Limit use of narcotics as able.
 f. Await return of bowel function.
4. Pitfalls
 a. Ensuring nutritional supplementation with TPN is considered for patients with prolonged ileus (>7 days) or sooner for those with poor nutritional status preoperatively.

C. Postoperative bowel obstruction
1. Presentation
 a. Nausea, vomiting
 b. Abdominal pain and distension
 c. Surgical history
2. Diagnosis
 a. Abdominal examination
 b. Upright abdominal radiograph
 c. Abdominal CT
  i. Evaluate for fascial dehiscence, hernias, bowel incarceration or strangulation, closed loop obstructions, internal hernias, bowel ischemia, or perforation.
3. Management
 a. NPO, bowel rest
 b. NGT placement will not help for closed-loop bowel obstructions
 c. IV fluids, electrolyte repletion.
 d. If there is concern for technical failure or acute postoperative bowel obstruction, consider return to operating room for abdominal exploration.

VII. HEMATOLOGIC CONSIDERATIONS

A. HIT (heparin-induced thrombocytopenia)
1. Presentation
 a. HIT type I (5%-30%)
  i. Nonimmune, heparin-associated thrombocytopenia
  ii. Typically begins within 4 days of initiation of heparin.
 b. HIT type II
  i. Severe immune-mediated syndrome caused by heparin-dependent antiplatelet antibodies (anti-PF4–heparin complex) occurring 5 to 10 days after initial exposure but within hours after re-exposure

ii. In minority of cases, thrombotic events may ensue, including extensive arterial and venous thrombosis, including skin necrosis, limb loss, end-organ infarction.[15]

2. Diagnosis
   a. 4T score (thrombocytopenia, timing, thrombosis, other causes)
   b. HIT antibody testing (ELISA)
   c. Serotonin release assay (confirmatory test)
3. Treatment
   a. HIT type I
      i. Do not need to stop heparin.
      ii. Close monitoring of laboratory values
   b. HIT type II
      i. Stop all heparin products immediately.
      ii. Initiate anticoagulation with nonheparin products, such as direct thrombin inhibitors (e.g., bivalirudin).

B. DIC (disseminated intravascular coagulopathy)

1. Presentation
   a. Common in severe sepsis, extensive trauma, or burns
   b. Complications from microvascular thrombi in kidney, brain, lung, skin
   c. Often intractable bleeding from GI tract, genitourinary tract, surgical incisions
   d. Mechanism: Inappropriate thrombin generation within vasculature → platelet activation → fibrin thrombi formation → increased fibrinolytic activity
2. Diagnosis
   a. Laboratory tests reveal thrombocytopenia, hypofibrinogenemia, increased fibrin degradation products, prolonged partial thromboplastin time (PTT).
3. Treatment
   a. Treatment of underlying cause
   b. Supportive care
   c. High mortality

C. DVT (deep vein thrombosis)

1. Presentation
   a. Pain and swelling of the affected extremity
   b. Fever or leukocytosis
      i. Especially consider in patients with poor functional status or with prolonged ICU stays
   c. Erythema, warmth of the affected extremity
2. Diagnosis
   a. Maintain a high index of suspicion in patients with
      i. Prolonged immobility
      ii. Recent surgical intervention
      iii. Risk for hypercoagulability (pregnancy, inherited coagulation disorders, malignancy, etc.)
   b. Lower extremity venous duplex
      i. Sensitivity 90%
      ii. Can differentiate chronic and acute clots and evaluate the progression of clots

- **iii.** Limitations: Calcified vessels may limit evaluation
- **c.** Contrast venography (gold standard)
  - **i.** Rarely used because invasive

3. DVT prophylaxis—**Table 3.8**

4. Treatment—**Table 3.9**

- **a.** Therapeutic anticoagulation
  - **i.** In patients with venous thromboembolism (VTE), initiation of therapy with direct thrombin inhibitor or direct factor Xa inhibitors is recommended over vitamin K antagonists.
  - **ii.** For cancer-associated thrombosis, direct factor Xa inhibitors are recommended over low-molecular-weight heparin.
- **b.** Duration of treatment
  - **i.** Recommend treatment of VTE for at least 3 months, followed by assessment for need of extended therapy.
  - **ii.** If VTE is diagnosed in the context of a major transient risk factor, 3 months of anticoagulation therapy is recommended.
  - **iii.** If VTE is unprovoked or provoked by a persistent factor (i.e., malignancy), extended therapy over 3 months with a direct oral anticoagulants is recommended.

D. PE (pulmonary embolism)

1. Presentation

- **a.** Shortness of breath
- **b.** Hypoxemia
- **c.** Tachypnea
- **d.** Tachycardia
- **e.** Dysrhythmias
- **f.** EKG changes
  - **i.** S1Q3T3 (highly specific, but rarely seen)
  - **ii.** Nonspecific ST-segment or T-wave changes

2. Diagnosis

- **a.** ABG, ECG, CXR
- **b.** D-dimer not helpful because often elevated after surgery.
- **c.** If patient is unstable for transport, bedside transthoracic echocardiography can evaluate for signs of right-sided heart strain.
- **d.** Spiral CT scan
  - **i.** Sensitivity is 83%, specificity is 96%.[16]
  - **ii.** Preferred over gold standard pulmonary angiography because of availability, speed, and noninvasive nature
- **e.** V/Q scan
  - **i.** Useful if patients are unable to undergo contrasted CT scan
  - **ii.** Limitations: Difficult in patients with underling lung disease

3. Treatment

- **a.** Supportive measures: O_2 administration, hemodynamic monitoring
- **b.** Anticoagulation
  - **i.** IV unfractionated heparin or subcutaneous low-molecular-weight heparin should be started.
  - **ii.** Target PTT 50 to 80 seconds

TABLE 3.8 Levels of Thromboembolism Risk and Recommended Thromboprophylaxis in Hospital Patients

Risk Level	Type of Patient	Symptomatic DVT Risk w/o Prophylaxis (%)	Suggested Thromboprophylaxis Options
Very low	Most outpatient/same day surgery	<0.5	Early and aggressive ambulation
Low	Minor surgery in mobile patients Medical patients who are fully mobile	~1.5	Mechanical prophylaxis with IPC Mechanical prophylaxis with IPC
Moderate	Most general, cardiothoracic, nononcologic, gynecologic, or urologic surgery· Medical patients who are on bed rest, "sick"	~3	LMWH *or* LDUH *or* mechanical prophylaxis with IPC LMWH *or* LDUH *or* mechanical prophylaxis with IPC
	Moderate VTE risk plus high bleeding risk		Mechanical prophylaxis with IPC until risk decreases, *then* chemical prophylaxis
High	Major trauma, bariatric surgery, pneumonectomy, spinal cord injury, TBI, or craniotomy	~6	LMWH *or* LDUH *AND* mechanical prophylaxis with IPC *or* elastic stockings
	High VTE risk plus high bleeding risk. High risk plus oncologic, abdominal, or pelvic surgery		Mechanical prophylaxis with IPC until risk decreases, *then* chemical prophylaxis extended duration LMWH (4 wk) *AND* mechanical prophylaxis with IPC *or* elastic stockings while hospitalized

TBI, traumatic brain injury; IPC, intermittent pneumatic compression; LDUH, low-dose unfractionated heparin; LMWH, low-molecular-weight heparin; VTE, venous thromboembolism.

Adapted from Gould MK, Garcia DA, Wren SM, et al. Prevention of VTE in nonorthopedic surgical patients. Antithrombotic therapy and prevention of thrombosis, 9th ed: American College of Chest Physicians evidence-based clinical practice guidelines. *Chest*. 2012;141(2):e227S-277S. Copyright 2012, The American College of Chest Physicians. With permission.

TABLE 3.9 Anticoagulant Medications

Drug	Mechanism	Metabolism	Dose for DVT Prophylaxis	Dose for Therapeutic Anticoagulation	Therapeutic Target	Reversal Agent
Heparin	Potentiates antithrombin: IIa, Xa, IXa, XIa, XIIa inhibition	Hepatic, RES, and 50% renal excretion	5,000 U SC bid to tid	Bolus = 80 μ/kg Infusion = 18 μ/kg/h; adjust to target PTT	aPTT = 60-80 s	Protamine: Start with 25-50 mg
LMWH (e.g., enoxaparin [Lovenox])	Potentiates antithrombin: Xa inhibition	Mainly renal excretion	40 mg SC once daily	1 mg/kg SC bid	Chromogenic anti-Xa assay: 0.6-1 anti-Xa U/mL	None
Fondaparinux (Arixtra)	Potentiates antithrombin: Xa inhibition	Renal	2.5 mg SC once daily	5 or 7.5 or 10 mg SC once daily	Chromogenic anti-Xa assay 0.6-1 anti-Xa U/mL	None
Rivaroxaban (Xarelto)	Direct Xa inhibition	Likely liver	10 mg PO once daily		Chromogenic anti-Xa assay 0.6-1 anti-Xa U/mL	None
Apixaban (Eliquis)	Direct Xa inhibition	Liver	5 mg PO bid		Chromogenic anti-Xa assay 0.6-1 anti-Xa U/mL	None

(continued)

TABLE 3.9 Anticoagulant Medications (*Continued*)

Drug	Mechanism	Metabolism	Dose for DVT Prophylaxis	Dose for Therapeutic Anticoagulation	Therapeutic Target	Reversal Agent
Warfarin (Coumadin)	Prevents carboxylation of X, IX, VII, II, proteins C and S	Hepatic, marked genetic variability		2-10 mg PO daily; adjust to target INR	INR = 2-4	Vitamin K: 1-10 mg PO or plasma; start with 2-4 U
Lepirudin (Refludan)	Direct thrombin inhibition	Renal		Bolus = 0.4 mg/kg Infusion = 0.15 mg/kg/h; adjust to target PTT	aPTT = 60-80 (1.5-2.5 times control)	None
Bivalirudin (Angiomax)	Direct thrombin inhibition	Proteolytic cleavage and renal (20%)		Bolus = 1 mg/kg Infusion = 0.2 mg/kg/h; adjust to target PTT	aPTT = 60-80 s	None
Desirudin (Iprivask)	Direct thrombin inhibition	Renal	10-15 mg SC id		Prolongs the aPTT	None
Argatroban (Acova)	Direct thrombin inhibition	Hepatic		Infusion = 2 Hg/kg/min; adjust to target PTT	aPTT = 60-80 s; may prolong INR	None
Dabigatran etexilate (Pradaxa)	Direct thrombin inhibition	Renal (unchanged) and some conjugation with glucuronic acid	150 mg PO once daily	150 mg PO bid	Prolongs aPTT	None

iii. See "Treatment" under "DVT" for choice of anticoagulation and duration of treatment.

c. Catheter-directed thrombolytic therapy
   i. May be considered for patients with significant PE with associated shock with imminent threat to life

d. Transvenous or open embolectomy
   i. May be considered for patients with significant PE with associated shock who are not candidates for thrombolytics due to recent surgery or high risk of bleeding

e. Special consideration: inferior vena cava (IVC) filters
   i. IVC filters are not recommended for patients with acute DVT/PE who are able to be treated with therapeutic anticoagulation.

VIII. INFECTIOUS CONSIDERATIONS

A. Postop fever

1. Definition
   a. Elevation in a patient's body temperature >38°C in the postoperative period and is classified as immediate (within hours of surgery), early (POD1-3), or late (>POD3).
2. Differential diagnosis ("wind, water, walking, wound, wonder drug")
   a. Immediate postoperative period (within hours of surgery)
      i. Inflammation due to surgery (release of inflammatory cytokines—IL6, TNFa, IFNy)
      ii. Malignant hyperthermia
      iii. Immune-mediated reaction to medication or blood products
      iv. Infections predating the operation
   b. Early fever (24-72 hours)
      i. Continued stress-mediated response to surgery
      ii. Infections predating the operation
      iii. Urinary tract infection (UTI)
         a) See below
      iv. Early surgical site infection (SSI)
         a) *Clostridium perfringens* or group A strep can cause early SSIs
      v. Pneumonia
         a) See below
      vi. Alcohol withdrawal
      vii. VTE
   c. Late fever (>72 hours from surgery)
      i. Pneumonia
      ii. UTI
      iii. Central line–associated blood stream infections
      iv. Wound infection
      v. Colitis/enteritis
      vi. Abscess
      vii. Febrile drug reaction
   d. Diagnosis
      i. Thorough inspection of all wounds, catheters, lines

ii. CBC, CXR, urinalysis, blood/urine/sputum cultures
iii. Ultrasound or CT of deep space infection in the cavity where the surgery was performed

B. Surgical Site Infections (SSIs)
1. Presentation
a. Fever, erythema, pain, induration, drainage at surgical site
b. Risk factors
i. Patient factors: Age, diabetes, smoking status, nutritional status, obesity, other coexisting infections, colonization, altered immune response, prolonged length of stay
ii. Operation factors: Surgical technique (poor hemostasis, tissue trauma), antimicrobial prophylaxis, preoperative shaving, adequate skin antisepsis, surgical wound class (**Table 3.10**)
iii. Local wound factors: Contaminated wound, proximity to other contaminated sites, edema, local tissue perfusion
c. Definitions
i. Superficial SSI—involvement of the skin
ii. Deep SSI—involvement of the fascia and/or muscle
iii. Organ space infection—involvement below the fascia (intra-abdominal, etc.)
d. Diagnosis
i. Physical examination: Warmth, erythema, drainage
ii. Imaging
a) Cross-sectional imaging is helpful in evaluating for undrained abscesses.
b) Ultrasound may be helpful in identification of subcutaneous abscess but can miss deeper fluid collections.
2. Treatment
a. Superficial infection → open wound to allow drainage, and pack wound
b. Parenteral antibiotics should be given if extensive erythema or deeper infection is present (**Table 3.11**).
c. Most common pathogens are enteric and anaerobic following bowel or perineal surgery.
d. Intra-abdominal abscesses
i. See below
e. Consider the presence of necrotizing infection
i. See below

C. Necrotizing soft tissue infections (NSTI)
1. Presentation
a. Necrotizing infections include fasciitis, myositis, and cellulitis.
b. Significant tissue destruction with associated clinical signs of toxicity.
c. Risk factors
i. Traumatic injury
ii. Skin breach (varicella, insect bite, intravenous drug use)
iii. Recent surgery
iv. Immunosuppression (diabetes, HIV, neutropenia)
v. Malignancy
vi. Obesity

TABLE 3-10 Recommendations for Antibiotic Prophylaxis

Nature of Operation	Specific Procedure	Preferred Antibiotic Regimen	History of Delayed Hypersensitivity to Beta-Lactams
Cardiac Surgery	Median sternotomy, CABG, valve replacement, VAD insertion	Cefazolin[a] + Vancomycin[b]	Vancomycin[b] + Aztreonam[c]
	Pacemaker or ICD insertion	Cefazolin[c]	Vancomycin[b]
	Pacemaker or ICD insertion with MRSA colonization/infection or generator exchange	Cefazolin[a] + Vancomycin[b]	Vancomycin[b]
Colon and Rectal Surgery	**Clean surgeries:** Planned hernia repair, exploratory laparotomy/laparoscopy without colon entry, other planned nonemergent intra-abdominal surgeries that do not involve entry into the GI tract	Cefazolin[a]	Vancomycin[b]
	Clean-contaminated surgeries at or below the duodenum: Planned intestinal resection, bowel obstruction repair without risk of perforation, other colorectal surgery	Cefazolin[a] + Metronidazole[d] OR Cefoxitin[c] OR Ertapenem[e]	Clindamycin[f] + Aztreonam[c] OR Ciprofloxacin[g] + Metronidazole[d]
	Contaminated surgeries: Perforated bowel obstruction repair, perforated diverticulosis repair, repair of colorectal fistulae, or any surgery involving a grossly perforate GI tract or infected viscous	Ertapenem[e] OR Ceftriaxone[h] + Metronidazole[d] OR Piperacillin/tazobactam[i]	Clindamycin[f] + Aztreonam[c] OR Ciprofloxacin[g] + Metronidazole[d]
Thoracic Surgery	Lobectomy, pneumonectomy, lung resection, thoracotomy, VATS, esophageal procedures	Cefazolin[a]	Vancomycin[b]
Vascular Surgery	Carotid and brachiocephalic procedures, upper extremity procedures with prosthetic grafts, lower extremity procedures	Cefazolin[a]	Vancomycin[b]
	Abdominal aorta procedure or procedure with groin incision	Cefazolin[a]	Vancomycin[b] + Aztreonam[c]

(continued)

TABLE 3-10 Recommendations for Antibiotic Prophylaxis (Continued)

Nature of Operation	Specific Procedure	Preferred Antibiotic Regimen	History of Delayed Hypersensitivity to Beta-Lactams
General Surgery	**Clean surgeries:** Splenectomy, gastric banding, planned hernia repair, exploratory laparotomy/laparoscopy without colon entry, other planned nonemergent intra-abdominal surgeries that do not involve entry into the GI tract	Cefazolin[a]	Vancomycin[b]
	Clean-contaminated surgeries above the duodenum: Gastric bypass, sleeve gastrectomy, planned foregut repair, PEG placement	Cefazolin[a]	Vancomycin[b] + Aztreonam[c] OR Vancomycin + Gentamicin[j]
	Clean-contaminated surgeries at or below the duodenum: Planned intestinal resection, bowel obstruction repair without risk of perforation, appendectomy without risk of perforation, or colorectal surgery; Planned cholecystectomy, hepatectomy, pancreatoduodenectomy, pancreatectomy, hepaticojejunostomy, liver resection, bile duct revision, and other biliary procedures	Cefazolin[a] + Metronidazole[d] OR Cefoxitin[c]	Clindamycin[f] + Aztreonam[c] OR Ciprofloxacin[g] + Metronidazole[d]
	Contaminated surgeries: Appendectomy with possible or confirmed perforation, perforated bowel obstruction repair, perforated diverticulosis repair, repair of infected pancreas, repair of colorectal fistulae, or any surgery involving a grossly perforate GI tract or infected viscous	Ceftriaxone[h] + Metronidazole[d] OR Piperacillin/tazobactam[i]	Clindamycin[f] + Aztreonam[c] OR Ciprofloxacin[g] + Metronidazole[d]
Gynecologic Surgery	Cesarean delivery procedures with labor (spontaneous, or induced, with contractions and cervical dilation) or rupture of the membranes	Cefazolin[a] + Azithromycin[k]	Clindamycin[f] + Gentamicin[j]
	Cesarean delivery (elective, no labor)	Cefazolin[a]	Clindamycin[f] + Gentamicin[j]
	Hysterectomy (vaginal or abdominal)	Cefazolin[a]	Clindamycin[f] + Gentamicin[j] OR Clindamycin[f] + Ciprofloxacin[g]
	Hysterectomy with possible colon resection (vaginal or abdominal)	Cefazolin[a] + Metronidazole[d]	Clindamycin[f] + Gentamicin[j] OR Clindamycin[f] + Ciprofloxacin[g]
	Hysterectomy with planned colon resection (vaginal or abdominal)	Ertapenem[e]	Ciprofloxacin[g] + Metronidazole[d]
	Repair of cystocele or rectocele	Cefazolin[a]	Clindamycin[f]

Orthopedic Surgery	Foot/Ankle procedures with hardware, open reduction/internal fixation (Grade 1, 2 fracture), laminectomy	Cefazolin[a]	Vancomycin[b]
	Laminectomy with MRSA risk factors	Cefazolin[a] + Vancomycin[b]	Vancomycin[b]
	Joint preservation, closed reduction hip fracture	Cefazolin[a]	Vancomycin[b] + Aztreonam[c]
	Open reduction/internal fixation (Grade 3 fracture)	Ampicillin/sulbactam[m] + Gentamicin[j]	Vancomycin[b] + Gentamicin[j] + Metronidazole[d]
	Lawn mower injury	Cefazolin[a] + Metronidazole[d] OR Ampicillin/sulbactam[m]	Clindamycin[f] + Ciprofloxacin[g]
	Total joint replacement	Cefazolin[a]	Vancomycin[b] + Aztreonam[c]
	Spinal fusion	Cefazolin[a]	Vancomycin[b] + Aztreonam[c]
	Total joint replacement with MRSA risk factors, spinal fusion with MRSA risk factors	Cefazolin[a] + Vancomycin[b]	Vancomycin[b] + Aztreonam[c]

Krekel T, Neuner E, Portell J. *The Barnes-Jewish Hospital Tool Book: Drug Dosing and Usage Guidelines.* 19th ed. Department of Pharmacy, Barnes-Jewish Hospital; 2023.

[a]Cefazolin pre/intraoperative dosing: 2,000 mg for adult patients <120 kg; 3,000 mg for adult patients ≥120 kg.

[b]Vancomycin pre/intraoperative dosing: 1,000 mg for adult patients <80 kg; 1,500 mg for adult patients 80 to 120 kg; 2,000 mg for adult patients >120 kg.

[c]Aztreonam and Cefoxitin pre/intraoperative dosing: 2,000 mg for all adult patients.

[d]Metronidazole pre/intraoperative dosing: 500 mg for all adult patients.

[e]Ertapenem pre/intraoperative dosing: 1,000 mg for all adult patients.

[f]Clindamycin pre/intraoperative dosing: 900 mg for all adult patients.

[g]Ciprofloxacin pre/intraoperative dosing: 400 mg for all adult patients.

[h]Ceftriaxone pre/intraoperative dosing: 2,000 mg for all adult patients.

[i]Piperacillin/tazobactam pre/intraoperative dosing: 3.375 g for all adult patients.

[j]Gentamicin dosing for nonobstetric surgical prophylaxis:

- Normal renal function: gentamicin 5 mg/kg
- Renal impairment (CrCl < 30 mL/min or SCr > 1.5 mg/dL): gentamicin 1.5 mg/kg
- In obese patients with SCr ≤ 1.5 mg/dL or CrCl ≥ 30 mL/min, use single-dose gentamicin 5 mg/kg based on adjusted body weight (ABW)
  - ABW equation: (ABW= IBW + 0.4[TBW-IBW])
  - ABW: adjusted body weight; IBW: ideal body weight; TBW: total body weight.

[k]Azithromycin pre/intraoperative dosing: 500 mg for all adult patients.

[l]Gentamicin dosing for obstetric surgical prophylaxis: Because the volume of distribution and renal function in the obstetric population are altered, for patients with an SCr of <0.9 mg/dL, a single dose of gentamicin 5 mg/kg (max dose 600 mg) based on TBW is suggested. For patients with known SCr > 0.9 mg/dL, a single dose of gentamicin 1.5 mg/kg TBW is suggested.

[m]Ampicillin/sulbactam pre/intraoperative dosing: 3,000 mg for all adult patients.

TABLE 3.11 Recommendations for Antibiotic Prophylaxis

Nature of Operation	Likely Pathogens	Recommended Antibiotics	Adult Dose Before Surgery[a]
Cardiac: Prosthetic valve and other procedures	Staphylococci, corynebacteria, enteric gram-negative bacilli	Vancomycin and cefazolin Vancomycin and aztreonam[a]	1-1.5 g IV 1-3 g IV 1-1.5 g IV 1-2 g IV
Device insertion		*Cefazolin or vancomycin*	1-3 g IV 1-1.5 g IV
Thoracic	Staphylococci	Cefazolin Vancomycin[a]	1-3 g IV 1-1.5 g IV
Vascular: Peripheral bypass or aortic surgery with prosthetic graft	Staphylococci, streptococci, enteric gram-negative bacilli, clostridia	Cefazolin Vancomycin and aztreonam[a]	1-3 g IV 1-1.5 g IV 1-2 g IV
Abdominal wall hernia	Staphylococci	Cefazolin Clindamycin[a]	1-3 g IV 900 mg IV
Orthopedic: Total joint replacement or internal fixation of fractures	Staphylococci	Cefazolin Vancomycin Vancomycin and aztreonam[a]	1-3 g IV 1-1.5 g IV 1-1.5 g IV 1-2 g IV
Gastrointestinal (GI)			
Upper GI and hepatobiliary	Enteric gram-negative bacilli, enterococci, clostridia	Cefotetan Cefoxitin Clindamycin and gentamicin[a] Ciprofloxacin and metronidazole[a]	1-2 g IV 1-2 g IV 900 mg IV 5 mg/kg IV 400 mg IV 500 mg IV
Colorectal	Enteric gram-negative bacilli, anaerobes, enterococci	Cefoxitin Cefotetan Ertapenem Cefazolin and metronidazole[a]	1-2 g IV 1-2 g IV 1 g IV 1-3 g IV 500 mg IV
Appendectomy (no perforation)	Enteric gram-negative bacilli, anaerobes, enterococci	Cefoxitin Cefotetan Ciprofloxacin and metronidazole[a]	1-2 g IV 1-2 g IV 400 mg IV 500 mg IV

(continued)

TABLE 3.11 Recommendations for Antibiotic Prophylaxis (*Continued*)

Nature of Operation	Likely Pathogens	Recommended Antibiotics	Adult Dose Before Surgery[a]
Obstetrics/ gynecology	Enteric gram-negative bacilli, anaerobes, group B streptococci, enterococci	Cefotetan Cefoxitin Cefazolin Clindamycin and gentamicin[a]	1-2 g IV 1-2 g IV 1-3 g IV 900 mg IV 1.5-5 mg/kg IV

ABW, actual body weight; TBW, total body weight.

For vancomycin, dose of 1 g for patients <80 kg, 1.5 g for ≥80 kg.

For cefazolin, cefotetan, cefoxitin, and aztreonam, pre- and intraoperative dosing of 1 g is suggested for patients <80 kg, 2 g for patients ≥80 kg and <120 kg, and 3 g for patients ≥120 kg.

In obese patients, single-dose gentamicin should be dosed at 5 mg/kg of adjusted body weight (ABW = IBW + 0.4[TBW − IBW]).

[a]Indicated for patients with penicillin/cephalosporin allergy.

Reprinted with permission from Krekel T, Neuner E, Portell J. *The Barnes-Jewish Hospital Tool Book: Drug Dosing and Usage Guidelines.* 19th ed. Department of Pharmacy, Barnes-Jewish Hospital; 2023.

vii. Alcoholism

d. Associated organisms

i. Polymicrobial (type I)

ii. Monomicrobial (type II), generally the result of group A strep or *Staphylococcus aureus*

2. Diagnosis

a. Suggestive laboratory findings include elevations in white blood cells (WBCs), glucose, C-reactive protein, Cr, and anemia.

i. LRINEC score[17]

a) Can be used to calculate likelihood of necrotizing soft tissue infection, based on serum laboratory values including total WBC, hemoglobin, sodium, glucose, Cr, and C-reactive protein

b) Score >= 6 is highly indicative of NSTI.

c) Tool has variable sensitivity, and low scores do not rule out NSTI.[18]

b. Surgical exploration is needed to definitively establish the presence of necrotizing infection.

c. Should *not* delay operative intervention for radiographic, culture, or other diagnostic information

d. Suggestive radiographic findings

i. Soft tissue gas

ii. Fluid collection or abscess

iii. Tissue enhancement

e. Evaluation for clear physical signs of NSTI

i. Crepitus

ii. Severe pain out of proportion

iii. Rapid progressive clinical symptoms

3. Treatment
   a. Rapid broad-spectrum antimicrobial therapy including coverage of gram-positive (e.g., streptococcal species) and anaerobic bacteria (e.g., clostridial species), fluid resuscitation
   b. Urgent surgical exploration to evaluate tissue, debride devitalized tissue, and obtain cultures
   c. Patients may require takeback to the operating room to evaluate for additional spreading infection.

D. Intra-abdominal abscess
1. Presentation
   a. Abdominal pain, fever, ileus, peritonitis
   b. Can develop after anastomotic leak, missed enterotomy that has walled off
2. Diagnosis
   a. CT abdomen and pelvis with IV contrast (may consider PO contrast scan if concern for an anastomotic leak)
3. Treatment
   a. Percutaneous drainage under radiologic guidance, if able
   b. Empiric antibiotics covering enteric pathogens and anaerobes, can be de-escalated based on culture data from drainage procedure
   c. If generalized peritonitis or not amenable to percutaneous drainage refractory to empiric antibiotics → operative exploration and drainage
   d. Duration of antibiotics should be 4 days from adequate source control, assuming improvement in clinical signs and symptoms (STOP-IT Trial).[19]

E. Urinary tract infection (UTI)
1. Presentation
   a. Dysuria, hematuria, fever, leukocytosis
   b. Recent urinary catheterization or indwelling Foley placement
   c. Increased UTI risk with increasing duration of catheter placement
   d. Patients with indwelling Foleys with positive UAs should not be considered to have UTIs without symptoms.[20]
2. Treatment
   a. Empiric antibiotic therapy, tailored to culture data
   b. Start with parenteral therapy if patient is systemically ill, otherwise can move to oral antibiotic therapy.

F. Pneumonia (PNA)
1. Definition
   a. Community acquired
      i. Pneumonia acquired by community exposure
      ii. Lower risk of multidrug-resistant organisms or methicillin-resistant *S. aureus* (MRSA)
   b. Hospital acquired
      i. Pneumonia acquired after >48 hours of hospitalization
   c. Aspiration
      i. Pneumonitis due to aspiration of gastric or oropharyngeal contents
   d. Ventilator acquired
      i. Culture-proven pneumonia that develops at least 72 hours after intubation

2. Presentation
    a. Fever, cough, purulent sputum production, infiltrate on CXR, leukocytosis
3. Diagnosis
    a. Consolidation on CXR
    b. Culture data
        i. Sputum culture, bronchoalveolar lavage, tracheal aspirate, biopsy of lung tissue
4. Treatment
    a. Consider patient risk factors for MRSA/Multidrug resistant organisms (MDRO)
        i. Prolonged hospitalization
        ii. Recent IV antibiotics for other process
        iii. Septic shock at the time of presentation
        iv. MRSA colonization
    b. For patients with Health care-associated pneumonia/Ventilator-associated pneumonia, start empiric antibiotics aimed at nosocomial organisms
        i. Consider need for coverage of MRSA/MDRO
        ii. If no risk factors for MRSA or MRDOs → antimicrobial coverage for gram-negative bacilli, meticillin-sensitive *S. aureus*, and pseudomonas only
            a) Piperacillin–tazobactam, cefepime, levofloxacin, imipenem, meropenem
        iii. At risk for MRSA only but not MRDOS
            a) Add vancomycin or linezolid
        iv. At risk for MRDOs without MRSA
            a) Piperacillin–tazobactam, cefepime, levofloxacin, imipenem, meropenem PLUS
            b) Ciprofloxacin, levofloxacin, gentamicin, tobramycin
        v. At risk for both MRDOs and MRSA
            a) Piperacillin–tazobactam, cefepime, levofloxacin, imipenem, meropenem PLUS
            b) Ciprofloxacin, levofloxacin, gentamicin, tobramycin PLUS
            c) Vancomycin, linezolid
    c. De-escalate based on culture data

G. *Clostridioides difficile* infection (CDI)
1. Presentation
    a. Recent use antibiotics (including preoperative dosing)
    b. Recent hospitalization
    c. Diarrhea, ileus, abdominal pain, blood/mucus in stool, fever, hypotension, peritonitis, perforation, septic shock, toxic megacolon
2. Diagnosis
    a. *C. difficile* A or B toxin assay
    b. Assess disease severity[21]
        i. Nonsevere CDI: WBC <15 K, Cr < 1.5
        ii. Severe CDI: WBC >15 K, Cr > 1.5
        iii. Fulminant colitis: CDI associated with hypotension, shock, ileus, or megacolon

3. Treatment
   a. Fluid resuscitation, cessation of unnecessary antibiotics, contact isolation
   b. Antibiotic therapy[21]
      i. Initial nonfulminant episode → 10 days oral fidaxomicin, or vancomycin (if fidaxomicin is not available).
      ii. First recurrent episode → 10 days oral fidaxomicin or pulse-tapered oral vancomycin or high-dose oral vancomycin
      iii. Second recurrent episode → oral fidaxomicin or pulse-tapered oral vancomycin or high-dose oral vancomycin plus rifaximin
         a) Consideration for fecal microbiota transplantation where available
      iv. Fulminant disease without ileus → oral vancomycin plus IV metronidazole
      v. Fulminant disease with ileus → rectal vancomycin
   c. Fecal microbiota transplant recommended for patients with at least three CDI episodes
4. Complications
   a. See Toxic Megacolon in Chapter 23

H. Catheter-related blood stream infections
1. Presentation
   a. Fever, leukocytosis, systemic bacteremia, localized erythema or purulence around line/catheter/port insertion sites
2. Treatment
   a. Source control with removal of infected catheter[22]
   b. Empiric broad-spectrum IV antibiotics, can de-escalate based on culture data.
      i. Gram-positive organisms → vancomycin
      ii. Gram-negative bacilli → cefepime, piperacillin–tazobactam, imipenem, meropenem
   c. If line needs to be replaced, wait approximately 48 hours before inserting new line[23]

Key References

Citation	Summary
Sawyer RG, Claridge JA, Nathens AB, et al. Trial of short-course antimicrobial therapy for intraabdominal infection [published correction appears in *N Engl J Med.* 2018]. *N Engl J Med.* 2015;372(21):1996-2005.	• This study is a randomized control trial in which 518 patients were randomly assigned to receive either a fixed course of antibiotics for 4 d after source control as compared with standard therapy of antibiotics with duration until 2 d after the resolution of fever and leukocytosis following source control. From this study, it was determined that fixed-duration antibiotic therapy of 4 d after source control was noninferior to longer courses of antibiotic therapy.

Citation	Summary
Wong CH, Khin LW, Heng KS, Tan KC, Low CO. The LRINEC (Laboratory Risk Indicator for Necrotizing Fasciitis) score: a tool for distinguishing necrotizing fasciitis from other soft tissue infections. *Crit Care Med.* 2004;32(7):1535-1541.	• This retrospective observational trial evaluated 145 patients with necrotizing fasciitis and compares them with 309 patients with severe cellulitis or abscesses. From this they created a scoring system that predicts the likelihood that a patient has a necrotizing soft tissue infection based on total white cell count, hemoglobin, sodium, glucose, serum creatinine, and C-reactive protein. Scores ≥6 are highly indicative of necrotizing fasciitis in this cohort.
Stevens SM, Woller SC, Kreuziger LB, et al. Antithrombotic therapy for VTE disease: second update of the CHEST guideline and expert panel report [published correction appears in *Chest.* 2022; 62(1):269]. *Chest.* 2021;160(6):e545-e608.	• This consensus document outlines several essential guidelines for management of VTE including anticoagulants should be stopped after 3 mo for patients with acute DVT provoked by surgery and IVC filters should not be used for patients who can be treated with anticoagulation.

CHAPTER 3: MANAGEMENT OF COMMON POSTOPERATIVE PROBLEMS

Review Questions

1. What medication should be given for an unresponsive patient with concern for acute opioid overdose?
2. What treatment is preferred for a first event of *C. diff*?
3. What diagnosis should be considered for a patient with a LIRNEC score ≥6 and what treatment is recommended for this diagnosis?
4. What is the most common postoperative pulmonary condition and how is it treated?
5. What are the earliest signs of postoperative hemorrhage?
6. What is the next best step for management of postoperative atrial fibrillation with hemodynamic instability?
7. What is the appropriate duration of antibiotic therapy after source control has been obtained?
8. What alternative anticoagulation can be used for HIT type II?

REFERENCES

1. Cascella M, Bimonte S, Di Napoli R. Delayed emergence from anesthesia: what we know and how we act. *Local Reg Anesth.* 2020;13:195-206.
2. Anderson JA. Reversal agents in sedation and anesthesia: a review. *Anesth Prog.* 1988;35(2):43-47.
3. Oh ES, Fong TG, Hshieh TT, Inouye SK. Delirium in older persons: advances in diagnosis and treatment. *J Am Med Assoc.* 2017;318(12):1161-1174.

4. Mashour GA, Shanks AM, Kheterpal S. Perioperative stroke and associated mortality after noncardiac, nonneurologic surgery. *Anesthesiology*. 2011;114(6):1289-1296.
5. Sun Z, Yue Y, Leung CC, Chan MT, Gelb AW; Study Group for Perioperative Stroke in China POSIC. Clinical diagnostic tools for screening of perioperative stroke in general surgery: a systematic review. *Br J Anaesth*. 2016;116(3):328-338.
6. Perks A, Cheema S, Mohanraj R. Anaesthesia and epilepsy. *Br J Anaesth*. 2012;108(4):562-571.
7. Grant BF, Goldstein RB, Saha TD, et al. Epidemiology of DSM-5 alcohol use disorder: results from the national epidemiologic survey on alcohol and related conditions III. *JAMA Psychiatr*. 2015;72(8):757-766.
8. Sullivan JT, Sykora K, Schneiderman J, Naranjo CA, Sellers EM. Assessment of alcohol withdrawal: the revised clinical institute withdrawal assessment for alcohol scale (CIWA-Ar). *Br J Addict*. 1989;84(11):1353-1357.
9. Miskovic A, Lumb AB. Postoperative pulmonary complications. *Br J Anaesth*. 2017;118(3):317-334.
10. Danelich IM, Lose JM, Wright SS, et al. Practical management of postoperative atrial fibrillation after noncardiac surgery. *J Am Coll Surg*. 2014;219(4):831-841.
11. Douketis JD, Spyropoulos AC, Murad MH, et al. Perioperative management of antithrombotic therapy: an American College of Chest Physicians clinical practice guideline. *Chest*. 2022;162(5):e207-e243.
12. Ricci Z, Cruz D, Ronco C. The RIFLE criteria and mortality in acute kidney injury: a systematic review. *Kidney Int*. 2008;73(5):538-546.
13. White JV, Guenter P, Jensen G, et al. Consensus statement of the Academy of Nutrition and Dietetics/American Society for Parenteral and Enteral Nutrition: characteristics recommended for the identification and documentation of adult malnutrition (undernutrition). *J Acad Nutr Diet*. 2012;112(5):730-738.
14. Heyland DK, Dhaliwal R, Jiang X, Day AG. Identifying critically ill patients who benefit the most from nutrition therapy: the development and initial validation of a novel risk assessment tool. *Crit Care*. 2011;15(6):R268.
15. Arepally GM, Ortel TL. Clinical practice. Heparin-induced thrombocytopenia. *N Engl J Med*. 2006;355(8):809-817.
16. Stein PD, Fowler SE, Goodman LR, et al. Multidetector computed tomography for acute pulmonary embolism. *N Engl J Med*. 2006;354(22):2317-2327.
17. Wong CH, Khin LW, Heng KS, Tan KC, Low CO. The LRINEC (Laboratory Risk Indicator for Necrotizing Fasciitis) score: a tool for distinguishing necrotizing fasciitis from other soft tissue infections. *Crit Care Med*. 2004;32(7):1535-1541.
18. Fernando SM, Tran A, Cheng W, et al. Necrotizing soft tissue infection: diagnostic accuracy of physical examination, imaging, and LRINEC score. A systematic review and meta-analysis. *Ann Surg*. 2019;269(1):58-65.
19. Sawyer RG, Claridge JA, Nathens AB, et al. Trial of short-course antimicrobial therapy for intraabdominal infection. *N Engl J Med*. 2015;372(21):1996-2005.
20. Golob JF Jr, Claridge JA, Sando MJ, et al. Fever and leukocytosis in critically ill trauma patients: it's not the urine. *Surg Infect (Larchmt)*. 2008;9(1):49-56.
21. Johnson S, Lavergne V, Skinner AM, et al. Clinical practice guideline by the Infectious Diseases Society of America (IDSA) and Society for Healthcare Epidemiology of America (SHEA): 2021 focused update guidelines on management of *Clostridioides difficile* infection in adults. *Clin Infect Dis*. 2021;73(5):e1029-e1044.
22. Burnham JP, Rojek RP, Kollef MH. Catheter removal and outcomes of multidrug-resistant central-line-associated bloodstream infection. *Medicine (Baltimore)*. 2018;97(42):e12782.
23. Lee YM, Ryu BH, Hong SI, et al. Clinical impact of early reinsertion of a central venous catheter after catheter removal in patients with catheter-related bloodstream infections. *Infect Control Hosp Epidemiol*. 2021;42(2):162-168.

4 Critical Care

Robert M. MacGregor and Sara A. Buckman

I. INTRODUCTION

This chapter provides a general overview of the assessment and management of critically ill patients. A systematic approach is crucial to care of patients in the intensive care unit (ICU) as these patients have multiple concomitant physiologic derangements.

II. MONITORING OF THE CRITICALLY ILL PATIENT

A. Temperature monitoring
   1. Catheter-based probes (i.e., Foley catheter) provide more accurate measurements of core temperature.
   2. The fever cutoff is traditionally ≥38.5 °C.
   3. Antipyretics as a strategy of temperature control should be avoided due to increased mortality.[1]

B. ECG
   1. Continuous ECG monitoring with telemetry allows for rapid detection of dysrhythmias.

C. Arterial pressure monitoring
   1. Indirect—Noninvasive blood pressure cuff
   2. Direct—Intra-arterial catheters allow for continuous arterial pressure measurement and access for frequent laboratory tests and arterial blood gas measurements.
      a. Indicated for patients on vasoactive medications or those with a tenuous respiratory status
      b. The most common site is the radial artery, chosen because of accessibility and collateral blood flow. Alternative sites are the axillary or brachial artery, both of which have a similar incidence of complications.[2,3]
      c. The extremity distal to the catheter should be assessed prior to and after insertion for signs of ischemia.

D. Central venous pressure (CVP) monitoring
   1. Central venous catheters provide access to measure CVP, central venous oxygen saturation ($ScvO_2$)
   2. CVP—assess for volume status and ventricular preload
   3. $ScvO_2$—reflects balance between oxygen delivery and consumption. Can be used as a variable to guide resuscitation in shock.

E. Pulmonary artery (PA) catheters

1. Provides more accurate measurements of cardiac output (CO), PA pressure, and mixed venous oxygen saturation (SvO_2).
2. May be useful in patients with severe cardiogenic shock or pulmonary hypertension.
   a. Not routinely indicated for all critically ill patients—use of PA catheters has not been shown to improve mortality.[4]
3. Complications
   a. Right bundle branch block
   b. Balloon rupture resulting in air or balloon fragment emboli
   c. PA perforation
      i. Presents with hemoptysis, typically after balloon inflation.
      ii. Management—position the patient with the involved side in the dependent position and emergent thoracic surgical consultation.
   d. Other complications include malposition (e.g., coronary sinus), right ventricular rupture, cardiac tamponade, and decreased CO.

F. Noninvasive CO monitoring
1. Esophageal Doppler—measures descending aortic blood velocity to extrapolate patient CO.
2. Pulse contour analysis—uses an arterial pressure waveform to calculate the stroke volume and CO.
3. Devices such as the NICOM Cheetah use four electrodes to measure the bioreactance across the thorax to provide continuous CO measurements.[5]

G. Respiratory monitoring
1. Pulse oximetry—provides continuous assessment of arterial oxygen saturation (SaO_2).
   a. An elevated carboxyhemoglobin falsely raises the measurement, and methemoglobinemia results in a persistent reading of 85%.
2. Capnography provides a quantitative, continuous assessment of expired CO_2 concentrations.
   a. Increased $ETCO_2$ may indicate a decrease in alveolar ventilation or an increase in CO_2 production, as seen with sepsis and fever.
   b. Decreased $ETCO_2$ may indicate an increase in alveolar ventilation or an increase in dead space, as seen with massive pulmonary embolism (PE), endotracheal tube (ET) or mainstem bronchus obstruction.

H. Neurologic monitoring
1. Intracranial pressure (ICP) monitoring requires invasive placement of catheters in intraventricular, intraparenchymal, subarachnoid, or epidural spaces. Indication limited to patients at risk of elevated ICP with reduced Glasgow Coma Scale (i.e., unable to follow neurologic examination accurately).
2. Electroencephalogram (EEG)—measures electrical activity of brain.
   a. Processed EEG monitors (e.g., Bispectral Index and SedLine) use proprietary algorithms to analyze the EEG waveform and provide a number that is intended to indicate sedation or anesthetic depth.

III. NEUROLOGIC

A. Sedation: Provides temporary reduction in consciousness
  1. Sedation often is necessary for ICU patients who are critically ill or require invasive procedures.
  2. Sedating the critically ill patient
    a. Benzodiazepines act through γ-aminobutyric acid-A ($GABA_A$) receptors.
      i. Midazolam is hepatically metabolized and renally cleared, which may result in accumulation of metabolites with prolonged infusions.
      ii. Lorazepam has a slower onset and longer half-life, and its long-term use may cause propylene glycol toxicity.
      iii. Benzodiazepines are associated with higher rates of delirium, especially in older patients.[6]
      iv. Benzodiazepines are also indicated for alcohol or benzodiazepine withdrawal.
    b. Propofol acts through potentiation of $GABA_A$ receptors.
      i. It is short-acting with rapid onset due to its lipophilicity and ability to quickly cross the blood–brain barrier.
      ii. It has no analgesic properties and is typically used with an opioid in postoperative patients.
      iii. Side effects include significant hypotension due to myocardial depression, vasodilation, and increased venous capacitance, respiratory depression, and bradycardia.[7]
        a) Profound hypotension has been described when propofol is administered to patients receiving rifampin.[8]
        b) Prolonged use can lead to an elevation of triglycerides and subsequent pancreatitis, so triglyceride levels should be checked periodically.
        c) Propofol infusion syndrome is a rare but lethal complication, presenting with arrhythmia, rhabdomyolysis, and lactic acidosis.[9]
    c. Dexmedetomidine is a centrally acting α_2-adrenoceptor agonist with sedative and analgesic properties.
      i. Its use has become more widespread, as it is associated with less delirium than other sedative agents, has analgesic properties, and does not depress respiration.
      ii. Dexmedetomidine may be useful during a breathing trial to decrease anxiety while other anxiolytics are discontinued.
      iii. Side effects include hypotension and bradycardia.[7]
    d. Ketamine is a dissociative anesthetic agent that maintains CO and mean arterial pressure by also activating the sympathetic nervous system.
      i. It is used in patients with depressed cardiac function, especially after cardiac surgery.
  3. Richmond Agitation–Sedation Scale—provides clinical score to guide dosing and titration of sedation (**Table 4.1**).

TABLE 4.1 Richmond Agitation–Sedation Scale

Score	Characteristics
+4	Combative: Danger to self or staff
+3	Very agitated: Aggressive, pulling at tubes
+2	Agitated: Frequent nonpurposeful movements
+1	Restless: Anxious, movements vigorous but not aggressive
0	Calm and alert
−1	Drowsy: In response to voice; eye contact sustained >10 s
−2	Light sedation: In response to voice; eye contact sustained <10 s
−3	Moderate sedation: In response to voice; movement but without eye contact
−4	Deep sedation: In response to physical stimulation; any movement
−5	Unarousable: No response to verbal or physical stimulation

4. Protocols that minimize sedation have been shown to decrease the number of days on mechanical ventilation and the ICU length of stay, as well as reduce risk of long-term effects such as posttraumatic stress disorder and sleep disorder.[10,11]
   a. Patients who meet criteria should have a daily interruption of sedation to wakefulness.

B. Delirium. See **Figure 4.1** for overview of management of delirium.
   1. Delirium is a common manifestation of acute illness and is associated with increased mortality.[12]

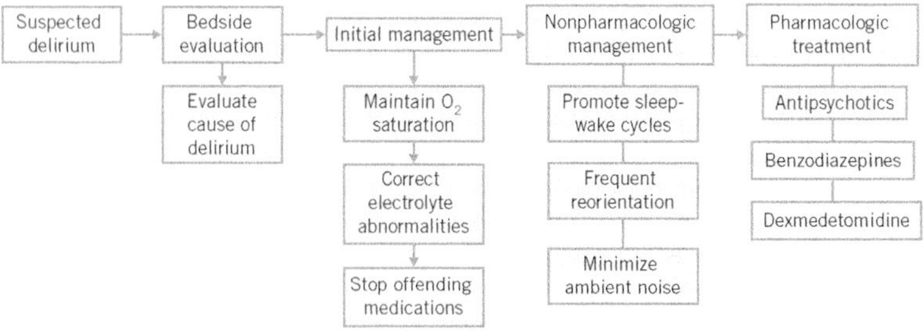

FIGURE 4.1 Management of acute postoperative delirium.

a. Characterized by waxing and waning inattention and disorganized thinking coupled with an acutely altered level of consciousness. Most patients have hypoactive delirium.
b. Often indicates underlying pathology, such as shock or infection.
2. Nonpharmacologic management
a. Mild confusion or agitation may resolve with environmental manipulations, including minimizing night-time interruptions and promoting sleep–wake cycles.
b. Delirium can be exacerbated by polypharmacy. ICU patients should have their medications routinely reviewed and reconciled.
3. Medical therapy
a. Antipsychotics
i. Haloperidol is an antipsychotic used to treat hyperactive delirium. Major toxicities include hypotension, prolongation of the QT interval, and extrapyramidal symptoms.
ii. Quetiapine is a second-generation antipsychotic that might be used as an alternative to haloperidol.[13]
iii. Olanzapine causes less QTc prolongation, so may be used in patients with a longer QTc.
b. Dexmedetomidine may be used in patients with agitated delirium receiving mechanical ventilation and has been shown to increase ventilator-free hours at 7 days.[14]
4. Brain death
a. Definition: Irreversible cessation of all brain function, including brainstem reflexes, legally equivalent to death by cessation of cardiopulmonary function.
b. Diagnosis confirmed after correcting reversible causes of severe neurologic dysfunction.[15]
i. Apnea test—evaluate for spontaneous respirations in response to hypercarbia ($PaCO_2 > 60$ mm Hg)
ii. Interval second physician clinical assessment may be required.
c. Once brain death has been confirmed, organ donation discussions can be initiated with the patient's surrogate decision makers.

IV. RESPIRATORY

A. Respiratory failure
1. Respiratory failure results from inadequate gas exchange caused by
a. Ventilation/perfusion (V/Q) mismatch: Airflow within the lung that does not equilibrate with blood–gas content (i.e., PE).
b. Pulmonary shunt: Perfusion of lung tissue that is poorly ventilated, such as severe pulmonary edema, acute respiratory distress syndrome (ARDS), or pneumonia.
c. Hypoventilation, or impaired systemic delivery/extraction.
2. Diagnosis—Signs or symptoms of respiratory distress should prompt evaluation of patient with physical examination, CXR, ECG, pulse oximetry, arterial blood gas, and possible chest CT with PE protocol pending suspicion of PE.

a. Oxygen saturation (SaO_2) <90% can be reflective of impaired tissue oxygenation.
b. An acute rise in $PaCO_2$ accompanied by a decrease in pH (respiratory acidosis) implies a significant imbalance between carbon dioxide production and elimination.
c. It is important to note that adequate oxygenation does not guarantee adequate ventilation.

3. Treatment—The urgency of the situation may necessitate management prior to a diagnosis.
   a. Oxygen therapy—Supplemental oxygen can be administered to increase the alveolar oxygen concentration. Modalities are presented in **Table 4.2**.
   b. Establishment of airway and mechanical ventilatory support

B. Overview of mechanical ventilation

1. Airway management
   a. **Procedural approach: ET intubation—technique**
      i. Prepare the patient for intubation by providing sedation/analgesia and adequately preoxygenating with bag mask ventilation.
      ii. Position the patient supine in "sniffing position." In trauma patients, if cervical spine injury is suspected, neck alignment should be maintained.
      iii. Insert laryngoscope with blade tip in epiglottic vallecula to directly visualize vocal cords.
      iv. The ET is inserted past the vocal cords into the trachea under direct visualization.
      v. Confirm placement with auscultation, return of end-tidal CO_2, and imaging with CXR.
   b. Tracheostomy
      i. Provides a more secure airway, improves patient comfort and oral hygiene, increases patient mobility, and enhances secretion removal
      ii. Indicated for patients requiring extended ventilatory support, although timing of this is hard to define.[16,17]
      iii. **Procedural approach: Tracheostomy technique**
         a) Incise the skin and subcutaneous tissue to expose the trachea. Be careful of bleeding from anterior jugular veins.
         b) Create defect on the anterior trachea wall and insert tracheostomy under direct visualization. Tracheostomy is ideally placed below the cricoid cartilage at the 2nd or 3rd tracheal ring to reduce the risk of subglottic stenosis.
         c) Confirm placement with detection of end-tidal CO_2 and subsequent CXR.
         d) Secure tracheostomy in place. Allow approximately 2 weeks for tract to mature before attempting tracheostomy exchange.
      iv. Tracheostomies can also be placed percutaneously.
2. Modes of mechanical ventilation (**Table 4.3**)

TABLE 4.2 Oxygen Delivery Systems

Type	FiO_2 Capability (%)	Comments
Nasal cannula	24-48	Flow rates of 1-8 L/min; true FiO_2 uncertain and highly dependent on minute ventilation; simple, comfortable, and can be worn during eating or coughing
Simple face mask	35-55	Flow rates of 6-10 L/min
High-humidity mask	Variable from 28 to nearly 100	Flow rates should be 2-3 times minute ventilation: levels >60% may require additional oxygen bleed-in
Nonrebreather	90-95	Flow rates of 12-15 L/min; incorporates valve to reduce room air entrainment and rebreathing of expired air
Ventimask	24, 28, 31, 35, 40, or 50	Provides controlled FiO_2; useful in patients with chronic obstructive pulmonary disease to prevent depression of respiratory drive; poorly humidified gas at maximum FiO_2
Optiflow/Airvo	24-85	Flow rates of 2-60 L/min; delivers humidified air: more comfortable than mask ventilation
CPAP/BiPAP	Variable from 28 to nearly 100	CPAP, continuous positive pressure; BiPAP, higher positive pressure during inhalation; may be poorly tolerated, cause gastric distention/aspiration risk

FiO_2, fraction of inspired oxygen.

a. Volume-controlled modes—deliver a set tidal volume with airway pressures varying depending on lung compliance.

i. Intermittent mandatory ventilation

a) Delivers a preset tidal volume over a set time

b) Assists with any patient-initiated breaths up to a set rate, with any additional breaths unassisted

TABLE 4.3 Modes of Mechanical ventilation

Categories	Modes	Trigger	Control	Cycling	Inspiratory Flow
Volume-control modes	Assist-control ventilation (VC/AC)	Patient or time	Flow	Volume	Square, decelerating, or sinusoidal
	Intermittent mandatory ventilation (SIMV)	Patient or time	Pressure for patient breaths. Flow or pressure for ventilator breaths	Flow for patient breaths Volume or time for ventilator breaths	Square, decelerating, sinusoidal for patient breaths
Pressure-control modes	Pressure-control ventilation (PC/AC)	Patient or time	Pressure	Time	Decelerating
	Pressure-support ventilation (PSV)	Patient	None	Flow	Decelerating
Advanced ventilator settings	Airway pressure release ventilation (APRV)	Patient or time	Pressure and time (T_{high}, T_{low}, P_{high}, P_{low})	Time	Square

ii. Assist-control ventilation

a) Delivers a preset tidal volume over a set time at each patient-initiated breath and delivers additional ventilator-initiated breaths up to a set respiratory rate, if needed

b) This mode improves work of breathing by assisting all breaths but may be uncomfortable if the breaths are dyssynchronous.

b. Pressure-controlled modes—deliver a set airway pressure with tidal volume varying depending on compliance.

i. Pressure-support ventilation (PSV)

a) Delivers a preset inspiratory pressure without a set rate. This mode delivers constant inspiratory pressure until inspiratory flow drops below a predetermined value, allowing for exhalation

b) PSV is used for spontaneously breathing patients and is dependent on ongoing patient respiratory effort.

c) Low pressures (5-8 cm H_2O) are set routinely to overcome the resistance caused by the ET and the inspiratory demand valves.

d) This mode is often utilized to evaluate for extubation.

ii. Pressure-control ventilation (PCV)

a) Time-cycled mode of ventilation that delivers a preset inspiratory pressure at a set rate with each breath delivered over a set time

b) PCV allows maximum airway pressure to be set to minimize barotrauma.

c) This mode is used in patients with poor lung compliance, which requires a higher pressure.

iii. Airway pressure release ventilation

a) Allows spontaneous breathing throughout the ventilation cycle

b) It is time-cycled between two levels of positive airway pressure.

c) This mode increases the mean airway pressure without increasing the peak airway pressures.

d) More time spent in high-pressure portion of cycle recruits alveoli.

3. Ventilator management—adjustable variables include (**Figure 4.2**)

a. FiO_2—Fraction of inspired oxygen in delivered breath

i. Should be adjusted to ensure adequate oxygenation with the lowest possible levels to prevent pulmonary oxygen toxicity

b. Tidal volume (VT) —Volume of air that is delivered with each breath

c. Ventilatory rate (f) —Delivered breath cycles per minute

i. Once the tidal volume has been determined, the rate is chosen to provide adequate minute ventilation and adjusted to optimize arterial pH and $PaCO_2$.

d. Inspiratory–expiratory (I:E) ratio—Proportion of each breath cycle dedicated to inspiration vs. expiration

i. The normal I:E ratio is 1:2 to 1:3.

ii. Longer expiratory times allow patients with obstructive lung disease to exhale fully and prevent breath stacking.

iii. Longer inspiratory times are useful in patients with low pulmonary compliance.

iv. Inverse-ratio ventilation takes advantage of breath stacking, using I:E ratios from 1:1 to 4:1, by progressive alveolar recruitment with a higher mean airway pressure. It is used most commonly with PCV.

e. Positive end-expiratory pressure (PEEP)—Alveolar pressure above atmospheric pressure that exists at the end of expiration

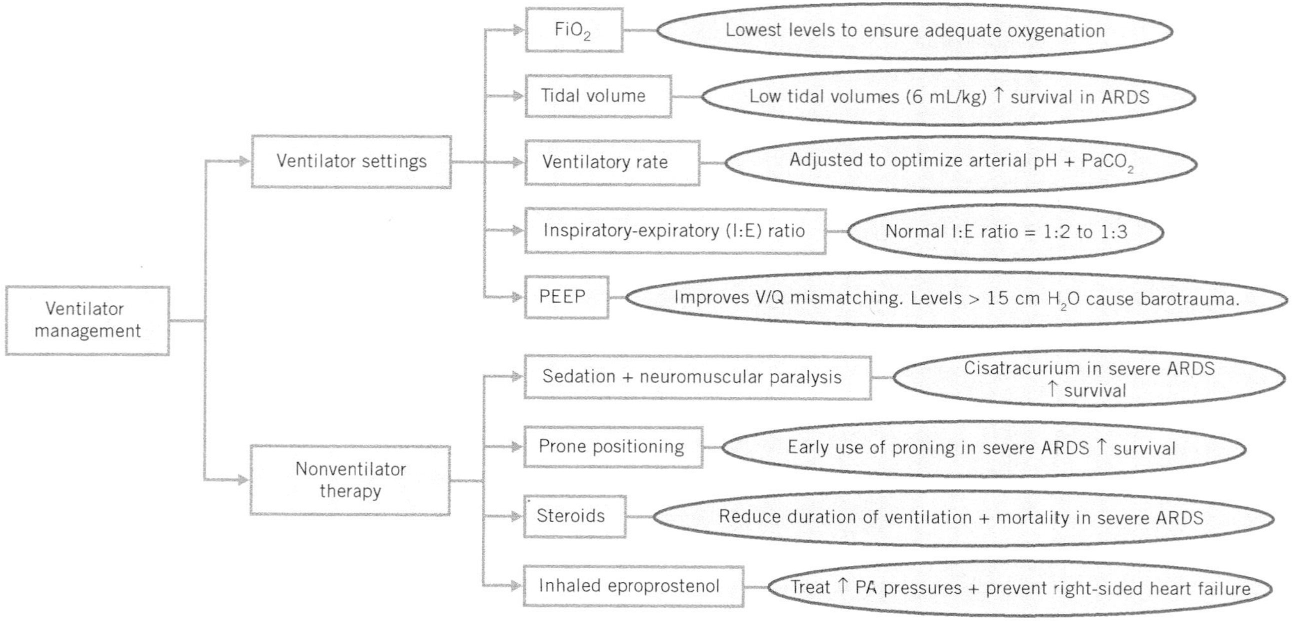

FIGURE 4.2 Management of ventilator in critically ill patients.

i. Increases functional residual capacity and improves V/Q matching by opening terminal airways and recruiting alveoli.
ii. PEEP of 5 cm H_2O is considered minimal; higher levels are used with hypoxemia.
iii. PEEP levels >15 cm H_2O increase risk of barotrauma and pneumothorax.

4. Sedation and neuromuscular paralysis
   a. Often necessary to control anxiety, synchronize breathing, and allow for rest.
   b. The minimum sedation necessary should be used—less sedation is associated with shorter ICU length of stay.[18]
5. Weaning from mechanical ventilation
   a. Prolonged ventilatory support may require a lengthened wean from the ventilator due to deconditioned respiratory muscles and time for lung recovery.
   b. Weaning should not be attempted during hemodynamic instability and high work of breathing.
   c. Reduction in the FiO_2 to 0.40 and PEEP to 5 cm H_2O should be attempted first.
   d. Daily PSV trials should be used to assess suitability for extubation.
   e. A common tool is the rapid shallow breathing index, calculated as respiratory rate/tidal volume, with a value >105 suggesting that discontinuation of assisted ventilation is unlikely to succeed.
6. Complications
   a. ET dislodgment and patient self-extubation can become an emergency. For this reason, restraint of the patient's upper extremities may be required.
   b. ET cuff leaks lead to a decreased airway pressure and return of expired volume. It may indicate that the ET needs to be advanced or exchanged.
   c. Barotrauma from high peak airway pressures can lead to subcutaneous emphysema, pneumomediastinum, and pneumothorax. A pneumothorax that develops on positive-pressure ventilation may result in tension physiology and should be treated with tube thoracostomy.
   d. Oxygen toxicity refers to high intra-alveolar oxygen concentration causing lung damage. The precise mechanism is unknown, but it likely involves oxidation of cell membranes due to oxygen radicals. FiO_2 should be weaned as soon as possible.

C. ARDS

1. Characterized by widespread inflammatory changes in the lungs and defined by poor lung compliance and poor oxygenation. Degree of severity classified based on Berlin criteria
   a. Mild—200 mm Hg < $PaO_2/FiO_2 \le 300$ mm Hg
   b. Moderate—100 mm Hg < $PaO_2/FiO_2 \le 200$ mm Hg
   c. Severe—$PaO_2/FiO_2 \le 100$ mm Hg
2. Etiology—can result from direct injury to the lung (i.e., trauma) or from severe systemic illness (i.e., sepsis).
3. Management

a. Ventilator management
   i. Randomized trial demonstrated improved survival in patients who were ventilated with low tidal volumes (6 mL/kg ideal body weight) compared with high tidal volumes (12 mL/kg).[19]
   ii. Tidal volumes should be set to maintain plateau pressures <30 cm H_2O to minimize barotrauma but >20 cm H_2O to minimize atelectasis.
b. Paralysis
   i. Paralysis may be necessary in patients with severe respiratory failure and decreased pulmonary compliance, as a study showed the use of cisatracurium in patients with severe ARDS improved survival.[20]
   ii. The extent of paralysis should be assessed with neuromuscular monitoring, and adequacy of anesthesia should be ensured with a processed EEG.
c. Prone positioning is a rescue strategy for patients with severe ARDS.
   i. Theoretical benefits include recruitment of dorsal lung units, improved mechanics, decreased V/Q mismatch, and increased secretion drainage.[21]
   ii. The PROSEVA study demonstrated a survival advantage with early use of prone positioning for patients with severe ARDS.[22]
d. Steroids have been shown to reduce duration of mechanical ventilation and overall mortality when given early in patients with moderate to severe ARDS.[23]
e. Inhaled epoprostenol (Veletri) may be used to treat patients with increased PA pressures in ARDS to improve oxygenation and decrease the risk of developing right-sided heart failure.

V. CARDIOVASCULAR

A. Cardiac arrhythmia: Associated with direct injury to the heart (i.e., myocardial ischemia) or various physiologic derangements from systemic illness (i.e., electrolyte abnormalities).
   1. Examples of arrhythmias
      a. Sinus tachycardia: Elevated heart rate originating from sinoatrial node
      b. Paroxysmal supraventricular tachycardia: Elevated heart rate arising from aberrations above the atrioventricular node.
         i. On ECG, unable to discern P waves
         ii. Conduction to ventricular system remains intact.
         iii. Heart rates are generally higher than in sinus tachycardia, and patients are more symptomatic.
      c. Atrial flutter and fibrillation: Originates from disordered conduction within atrial system. Not all atrial impulses will be conducted to ventricular system.
      d. Ventricular tachycardia and fibrillation: Disordered rhythm originating below the atrioventricular node.
      e. Bradyarrhythmias—often resulting from heart block (impaired conduction or nonconduction of atrial depolarizations to ventricles).

2. Management
   a. Supportive care: Electrolyte correction, circulatory support, treat underlying systemic illness
      i. Vagal maneuvers for supraventricular tachycardia (i.e., Valsalva maneuver, cardiac massage)
   b. Medical therapy
      i. Rate control: β-Blocker, calcium channel blocker
      ii. Supraventricular tachycardia: Adenosine
      iii. Ventricular tachycardia: Amiodarone
      iv. Bradycardia: Atropine
   c. Electrocardioversion is reserved for medically refractory tachyarrhythmia or if associated with hemodynamic instability
   d. Defibrillation: Pulseless ventricular tachycardia, ventricular fibrillation
   e. Transcutaneous pacing: For bradycardia or severe heart block
3. Cardiac arrest requires initiation of Basic Life Support and Advanced Cardiovascular Life Support protocols.

VI. CIRCULATORY FAILURE AND SHOCK

A. Defined by global tissue hypoxia that occurs when oxygen supply cannot meet metabolic demands.

B. Classification and recognition of shock—Early recognition and prompt intervention is critical. The patient's recent history, laboratory values, and physical examination are usually sufficient for determining the etiology (**Table 4.4**).

TABLE 4.4 Clinical Parameters in Shock

Shock Classification	Skin	Jugular Venous Distention	Cardiac Output	Pulmonary Capillary Wedge Pressure	Systemic Vascular Resistance	Mixed Venous Oxygen Content
Hypovolemic	Cool, pale	↓	↓	↓	↓	↓
Cardiogenic	Cool, pale	↑	↓	↑	↑	↓
Septic						
Early	Warm, pink	↑↓	↑	↓	↓	↑
Late	Cool, pale	↓	↓	↓	↑	↑↓
Neurogenic	Warm, pink	↓	↓	↓	↓	↓

1. Hypovolemic or hemorrhagic shock
   a. Results from loss of circulating blood volume caused by acute hemorrhage, fluid depletion, or dehydration
   b. Patients are peripherally vasoconstricted, tachycardic, and have low jugular venous pressure.
2. Distributive shock
   a. Hyperdynamic state consisting of tachycardia, vasodilation, decreased systemic vascular resistance (SVR), and increased CO
   b. Examples include sepsis, neurogenic shock, adrenal insufficiency, and anaphylaxis
   c. Septic shock described further in "Infection and Sepsis"
   d. Neurogenic shock results from interruption of the spinal cord at or above the thoracolumbar sympathetic nerve roots, which leads to vasodilation due to loss of sympathetic tone.
   e. Anaphylaxis is a type I hypersensitivity reaction to a specific antigen resulting in widespread vasodilation.
3. Obstructive shock
   a. Results from etiologies that prevent adequate CO but is not intrinsically cardiac in origin, such as PE, tension pneumothorax, or cardiac tamponade
   b. Jugular venous pressure is elevated in setting of peripheral vasoconstriction.
4. Cardiogenic shock
   a. Results from inadequate CO due to intrinsic cardiac failure
   b. Diagnosis may require echocardiography.
   c. These patients typically are peripherally vasoconstricted and tachycardic with an elevated jugular venous pressure.

C. Interventions common to all types of shock. The goal of therapy is to ensure adequate oxygen delivery. Because oxygen delivery is proportional to SaO_2, hemoglobin concentration, and cardiac output, each should be optimized.
1. SaO_2—Supplemental oxygen should be administered or an airway placed to achieve an SaO_2 >92%.
2. Hemoglobin concentration—maintain hemoglobin ≥7 g/dL. In ongoing myocardial infarction or severe ischemic cardiomyopathy, the threshold is 8 g/dL.[24]
3. Cardiac output—cardiac output depends on heart rate and stroke volume.
   a. Frequently assess with physical examination, continuous cardiac monitoring, and urine output.
   b. Correct tachy- and bradyarrhythmias.
   c. Support mean arterial pressure with volume resuscitation and correction of electrolyte and acid–base abnormalities.
   d. May require pharmacologic support (**Table 4.5**).
   e. Central venous catheters may be required for ongoing resuscitation and invasive cardiopulmonary monitoring.

TABLE 4.5 MvO_2, Mixed Venous Oxygen Saturation

Class and Drug	Blood Pressure	Systemic Vascular Resistance	Cardiac Output	Heart Rate	Inotrope Low Dose	Inotrope High Dose	Renal Blood Flow	Coronary Blood Flow	MvO_2
α Only									
Phenylephrine	↑↑	↑↑↑↑	↓	↓	±	±	↓↓↓↓	±↑↑	↑
α and β									
Norepinephrine	↑↑↑	↑↑↑↑	↑↑↑	↑±	↑	↑	↓↓↓↓	↑↑	↑↑
Epinephrine	↑↑↑	↑↑↑↑	↑↑↑↑	↑↑↑	↑↑	↑↑↑	↓±	↑↑	↑↑↑
Dopamine	↑↑	↑↑	↑↑↑	↑↑	±	↑↑	↑↑↑	↑↑	↑↑
β Only									
Dobutamine	±	↓↓↓	↑↑↑↑	↑↑	↑↑↑	↑↑↑	±	↑↑↑	↑↑↑
β-Blocker									
Metoprolol	↓	↓	↓↓	↓↓↓	↓↓	↓↓↓	±	↓↓	↓↓

(continued)

TABLE 4.5 $\dot{M}vO_2$, Mixed Venous Oxygen Saturation (*Continued*)

Class and Drug	Blood Pressure	Systemic Vascular Resistance	Cardiac Output	Heart Rate	Inotrope Low Dose	Inotrope High Dose	Renal Blood Flow	Coronary Blood Flow	MvO_2
Other									
Angiotensin II	↑↑	↑↑	↓	↑↑	±	±	↓↓	±	↓↓
Nitroglycerine	±↓	↓↓	↑↑	±	±	±	±↑	↓	↓↓
Hydralazine	↓↓	↓↓↓	↑↑	↑↑	±	±	±↑	↓	↓↓
Nitroprusside	↓↓↓	↓↓↓	↓↓↓	±↑	±	±	↑↑	±	↓↓
Vasopressin	↑↑	↑↑↑	↓↓	↓↓	±	±	↓↓	↓	±

Inotropes and vasoactive drugs and their specific actions.

f. Procedural approach: Central line placement in internal jugular vein

i. Use anatomical landmarks of the anterior cervical triangle to locate the internal jugular vein.

a) Inferior border: Clavicle

b) Lateral border: Clavicular head of sternocleidomastoid muscle

c) Medial border: Sternal head of sternocleidomastoid muscle)

ii. Use ultrasound to definitively identify the internal jugular vein and differentiate from the common carotid artery. Differences between internal jugular vein and common carotid artery are:

a) Internal jugular vein is lateral to the common carotid artery.

b) Internal jugular vein is wider than the common carotid artery.

c) Internal jugular vein is compressible and has nonpulsatile flow.

iii. Insert finder needle under ultrasound guidance into the internal jugular vein. Continuously aspirate as you advance the needle until venous blood is encountered.

iv. With the Seldinger technique, use a guidewire to exchange needle for a series of dilators to widen the tract, and place the catheter.

v. CXR is usually obtained to verify the tip of the catheter is at the junction of the right atrium and the superior vena cava.

D. Specific therapy

1. Hypovolemic or hemorrhagic shock

a. Therapy focuses on control of ongoing loss and restoration of intravascular volume.

b. Patients with blood losses of <20% can be resuscitated using crystalloid solutions.

c. Patients in whom diaphoresis, ashen facies, and hypotension develop have lost 30% or more of their blood volume and require transfusion.

d. To achieve rapid infusion rates, two large-bore peripheral intravenous access and/or central line are indicated.

e. Fluids and blood products should be warmed to prevent hypothermia, which can impair oxygen unloading and compromise coagulation.

2. Cardiogenic shock

a. Management is directed toward maintaining adequate myocardial perfusion and CO with volume expansion and vasoactive medications.

b. Initial treatment is often guided by CVP measurements or PA catheter data. CVP in this setting is useful for assessment of right ventricle function.[25]

c. Intra-aortic balloon counterpulsation or mechanical circulatory support may be necessary before and during recovery from definitive surgical treatment.

3. Distributive shock

a. Septic shock (see "Infection and Sepsis").

b. Anaphylactic shock: Supportive care. May need renal replacement therapy to remove offending agent.

c. Neurogenic shock: Volume and vasopressor support. Dopamine should be considered first line for patients with neurogenic shock with bradycardia.

i. Because patients with spinal shock tend to equilibrate body temperature with their environment, fluids and room temperature must be kept warm.

E. Obstructive shock

1. Tension pneumothorax is treated by needle decompression followed by tube thoracostomy.
2. Pericardial tamponade is treated by needle decompression, often with catheter placement for drainage.
3. The treatment of PE varies based on the degree of hemodynamic compromise. Options include systemic anticoagulation, thrombolysis, and surgical clot removal.

VII. FLUIDS, ELECTROLYTES, AND RENAL FUNCTION

A. Electrolyte abnormalities—occur with fluid shifts and renal dysfunction

1. Hyponatremia
   a. Symptoms: Lethargy, headaches, seizures, coma
   b. Occurs with syndrome of inappropriate antidiuretic hormone secretion
   c. Treatment: Controlled correction with infusion of isotonic or hypertonic fluids. Rapid correction can cause central pontine myelinolysis.
2. Hypernatremia
   a. Central diabetes insipidus—Can be seen in patients with traumatic brain injuries
      i. Results from decreased release of antidiuretic hormone from hypothalamus
      ii. Leads to increased serum sodium and decreased urine osmolality
   b. Treatment: Free water restriction, controlled infusion of hypotonic fluids. Rapid correction can lead to cerebral edema.
3. Hypokalemia
   a. Symptoms: Weakness, ileus, cardiac arrhythmia
   b. Etiology: High-volume gastrointestinal (GI) losses, alkalosis (drives potassium intracellularly)
4. Hyperkalemia
   a. Symptoms: Cardiac arrhythmias, cardiac arrest. Noted by peaked T waves on ECG.
   b. Treatment
      i. Calcium to stabilize myocardium
      ii. Treatment with insulin and glucose, β-agonists, and sodium bicarbonate drives potassium intracellulary
      iii. Diuretics and sodium polystyrene sulfonate promote excretion of potassium in urine and stool, respectively

5. Hypocalcemia
   a. Signs include
      i. Chvostek sign: Muscle spasm after tapping on the facial nerve
      ii. Trousseau sign: Muscle spasm of extremity after squeezing of blood pressure cuff
   b. Etiology: Tumor lysis syndrome, hypoparathyroidism (monitor for hypocalcemia following parathyroidectomy)
6. Hypercalcemia
   a. Symptoms—"bones, stones, moans, and groans"—bony pain, nephrolithiasis, abdominal pain, lethargy. In acute setting, usually associated with polyuria and dehydration.
   b. Etiology: Hyperparathyroidism, bony metastatic disease
   c. Treatment: Crystalloid resuscitation
7. Hyperphosphatemia
   a. Symptoms: Asymptomatic
   b. Etiology: Renal insufficiency, rhabdomyolysis, tumor lysis syndrome
   c. Treatment: Renal replacement therapy (if associated with renal failure)
8. Hypophosphatemia
   a. Symptoms: Muscle weakness, cardiac arrhythmias
   b. Etiology: Alkalosis, refeeding syndrome

B. Acid–base disorders
1. Metabolic acidosis
   a. Anion gap acidosis: Results from accumulation of acid, resulting in high anion gap. Example is lactic acidosis.
      i. Etiology: Decreased oxygen delivery as seen in shock, leading to increased reliance on anaerobic respiration.
      ii. Treatment: Resuscitation
   b. Nonanion gap metabolic acidosis: Results from acid–base imbalance with preservation of normal anion gap. Example is high-volume lower GI losses.
2. Metabolic alkalosis
   a. Associated with electrolyte abnormalities, such as hypokalemia
   b. Example is high-volume emesis
      i. Excretion of high concentration of hydrogen ions (H^+)
      ii. Stimulates aldosterone secretion, which promotes uptake of H^+ in exchange for potassium in distal tubule of nephrons.
      iii. Results in hypochloremic, hypokalemic metabolic alkalosis
3. Respiratory acidosis
   a. Etiology: Hypoventilation and accumulation of carbon dioxide
   b. Treatment: Increase ventilation (increase tidal volume, frequency)
4. Respiratory alkalosis
   a. Etiology: Hyperventilation and decreased concentration of carbon dioxide.

C. Acute kidney injury and renal failure
1. Acute kidney injury—reduction in renal function within 7 days, characterized by reduced urine output, increased serum creatinine, increased blood urea nitrogen

2. Etiology
   a. Prerenal: Decreased renal perfusion. Examples—hypovolemia, shock
   b. Intrinsic renal: Renal parenchymal injury. Examples—glomerular disease, acute tubular necrosis
   c. Postrenal: Obstruction of urinary tract. Examples—nephrolithiasis, ureteral stricture.
3. Diagnosis
   a. Serum and urine tests: Basic metabolic panel, urinalysis, urine electrolytes
   b. Fractional excretion of sodium (FE_{Na})—percent of filtered sodium that is excreted in urine. Help determine etiology of acute kidney injury.
      i. FE_{Na} < 1% consistent with prerenal disease
      ii. FE_{Na} distorted by diuretic use. For patients on diuretics, calculate fractional excretion of urea (FE_{Urea})
   c. Imaging to rule out obstructive pathology: Renal ultrasound, noncontrast CT imaging
   d. Renal biopsy to diagnose parenchymal disease
4. Treatment
   a. Maintain renal perfusion.
   b. Avoid nephrotoxic agents.
   c. Address obstructive pathology (i.e., ureteral stent for stricture).
5. Renal replacement therapy
   a. Indications—"AEIOU"—acidosis, electrolyte abnormalities, intoxicants, overload (fluid), uremia
   b. Modalities
      i. Hemodialysis: Blood filtered through dialysis machine to filter toxins and remove excess fluid
      ii. Peritoneal dialysis: Filtered by peritoneal lining, waste collected and removed in fluid instilled into peritoneal cavity
      iii. Hemodialysis more common modality if renal replacement therapy is urgently indicated.
   c. In setting of hemodynamic instability, hemodialysis can be performed continuously vs. intermittently for more gentle fluid removal.

$$\text{FENa} = \frac{Urine\ Na \times Plasma\ Cr}{Plasma\ Na \times Urine\ Cr}$$

VIII. ABDOMEN AND GASTROINTESTINAL TRACT

A. Nutritional support
1. Indications for nutritional support
   a. Unable to have adequate oral intake (i.e., intubated patient)
   b. Severe systemic illness, such as sepsis or extensive burns, that require nutritional supplementation
2. Enteral nutrition
   a. Preferred modality if adequate GI function

b. Access
   i. Temporary access can be achieved with nasogastric or nasojejunal tubes.
   ii. If nutritional support is required for extended period of time, consider placing gastrostomy or jejunostomy tubes.
c. **Procedural approach: Insertion of percutaneous endoscopic gastrostomy tube (PEG).**
   i. Assess anatomy of esophagus and stomach with upper endoscopy.
   ii. Ideal gastrostomy tube placement is in the upper abdomen approximately two fingerbreadths below the costal margin.
   iii. Transilluminate endoscopic light through the abdominal wall and insert finder needle into abdominal wall. Continuously aspirate through needle until air is encountered and needle is visualized endoscopically.
   iv. Using Seldinger technique, a guidewire is inserted into the stomach percutaneously and snared by the gastroscope.
   v. The gastrostomy tube can either be "pulled" (tube is pulled down esophagus into stomach and out of abdominal wall) or "pushed" (tube is pushed into abdominal wall and stomach along the guidewire).
d. Complications
   i. Wound complications from leaking around tube
   ii. Perforation: Transverse colon can come be damaged by percutaneous access.
   iii. Dislodgment: If tube is removed before tract has matured (within 7 days of placement), can lead to peritonitis from free leakage of gastric contents.

3. Parenteral nutrition
   a. Indications: Unable to use GI tract safely. Examples—bowel obstruction, high-output gastroenteric fistula
   b. Complications
      i. Central line-associated bloodstream infection
      ii. Liver injury from cholestasis and steatosis

B. Upper GI hemorrhage prophylaxis
   1. Risk factors for GI bleeding
      a. Head injury (Cushing ulcers)
      b. Burns (Curling ulcers)
      c. Prolonged mechanical ventilation
      d. History of peptic ulcer disease
      e. Use of NSAIDs or steroids
      f. Presence of shock, renal failure, portal hypertension, or coagulopathy
   2. An H_2-receptor antagonist should be used to maintain mucosal integrity in these patients. Proton-pump inhibitors are preferred by some, and they should be used in patients who bleed despite H_2-receptor antagonists.
   3. The use of stress ulcer prophylaxis for a patient without an above-listed risk factor should be avoided due to an increased risk of *Clostridium difficile*–associated diarrhea.[26]

C. Acute liver injury and liver failure
  1. Acute liver injury is defined as
    a. Onset of hepatic encephalopathy
    b. Impaired synthetic function (i.e., elevated international normalized ratio)
    c. Symptom onset within 26 weeks
  2. Causes—Examples include
    a. Acetaminophen toxicity
    b. Other drug or toxin-mediated liver injury
    c. Viral hepatitis
    d. Hypoperfusion leading to ischemia
  3. Treatment
    a. N-acetylcysteine for acetaminophen toxicity
    b. Serial neurologic examination, management of hyperammonemia for hepatic encephalopathy
    c. Correction of coagulopathy if active bleeding is present
    d. Coagulopathy is treated only if patient is bleeding.
    e. Evaluation for liver transplant

IX. INFECTION AND SEPSIS

A. Definition—
  1. Systemic inflammatory response syndrome (SIRS) can be seen with infectious or noninfectious etiologies. The clinical definition of SIRS requires two of the following:
    a. Temperature >38 °C or <36 °C,
    b. Heart rate >90 beats/min,
    c. Respiratory rate >20/min or $PaCO_2$ <32, and
    d. White blood cell count >12 or <4 or >10% bands.
  2. Sepsis is defined as life-threatening organ dysfunction due to dysregulated host response to infection.
  3. Severe sepsis is multiple-organ dysfunction or hypoperfusion resulting from infection.

B. Diagnosis
  1. Cultures should be obtained as part of the initial evaluation, at least one of which should be drawn percutaneously, prior to the initiation of antibiotics.
  2. Comprehensive laboratory analysis including complete blood count, serum lactate, comprehensive metabolic panel, coagulation studies, and arterial blood gas may be obtained during initial evaluation.

C. Treatment (per Surviving Sepsis Guidelines[27])
  1. Supportive care
    a. Stabilization of airway and correction of hypoxemia should be immediately performed, if necessary, in patients presenting in presumed septic shock.
    b. Volume resuscitation
      i. Tissue perfusion is achieved by aggressive fluid resuscitation (IV crystalloid solution, 30 mL/kg), started during the first hour and completed by hour 3 of presentation.

ii. Previous early goal-directed therapy consisted of volume resuscitation for a CVP of 8 to 12, mean arterial pressure (MAP) >65, urine output >0.5 mL/kg/h, and mixed SvO_2 >70%, although this protocol not found to improve survival over standard medical judgment.[28,29]

c. Vasoactive medications

i. Patients with sepsis who fail to achieve hemodynamic stability with fluids are started on a vasoactive medication, for initial MAP goal >65 mm Hg.

ii. Norepinephrine is commonly selected for its vasoconstrictive properties as well as its ability to increase CO.

iii. Dopamine is still used by some, but it is associated with higher rate of dysrhythmias.[30,31]

iv. The addition of low-dose vasopressin increases MAP, SVR, and urine output in patients with sepsis who are hyporesponsive to catecholamines.

2. Steroids should be administered when vasopressor therapy reaches >0.25 μg/kg/min after 4 hours of initiation. IV Hydrocortisone and PO Fludrocortisone can be administered for a 7-day course.[32]

a. Routine use of corticosteroids in septic shock may not offer a survival advantage.[33]

3. Antibiotic therapy

a. Broad-spectrum intravenous antibiotics should be initiated within the first hour.[34]

i. Sepsis from presumed pneumonia is commonly treated with vancomycin and cefepime.

ii. For suspected intra-abdominal infections, vancomycin and piperacillin/tazobactam may be used.

b. Infection with resistant organisms is more common with prior antibiotic treatments, prolonged hospitalizations, and presence of invasive devices.

c. The use of antifungal therapies and agents directed at highly resistant gram-negative rods, methicillin-resistant *Staphylococcus aureus*, vancomycin-resistant enterococcus, and resistant pneumococcus should be guided by the clinical situation and local susceptibility patterns.

4. Source control: Drainage, debridement, or removal of the infectious source (including lines) is imperative.

X. GLYCEMIC CONTROL AND ENDOCRINE DYSFUNCTION

A. Management of hyper- and hypoglycemia: Optimal range 110 to 180 mg/dL3[35]

1. Conventional glucose targets (180-200 mg/dL) linked to poorer perioperative outcomes (i.e., increased risk of infection, poor wound healing).

2. Intensive insulin therapy (goal 80-120 mg/dL) can lead to increased morbidity and mortality associated with hypoglycemia; can lead to further episodes of hypoglycemia, which can be life-threatening and result in poor outcomes.

B. Critical illness–related corticosteroid insufficiency can result from adrenal insufficiency or glucocorticoid resistance.
   1. The use of corticosteroids is not without risk and increases the risk of infection.[36]
   2. Adrenal insufficiency is best diagnosed by an increase in cortisol level of <9 μg/dL after a cosyntropin stimulation test or random total cortisol level <10 μg/dL.
   3. Patients with primary adrenal insufficiency or those in septic shock refractory to vasopressors should be treated with hydrocortisone prior to performing cosyntropin stimulation test.[37]

XI. HEMATOLOGY

A. Anemia
   1. The prospective Transfusion Requirements in Critical Care (TRICC) trial reported that transfusing all patients to a hemoglobin of 10 mg/dL either has no effect or may actually decrease survival in the critically ill.[24]
   2. A restrictive transfusion strategy (Hg < 7 mg/dL) is recommended in critically ill patients, except in those with acute coronary syndrome, severe hypoxemia, or active hemorrhage (Hg < 8 mg/dL).
   3. Recombinant erythropoietin has not been shown to reduce the rate of transfusion or mortality in critically ill patients, but increased the risk of thrombotic events.[38]

B. Venous thromboembolism (VTE) prophylaxis
   1. Critically ill patients are considered high risk for VTE, even after routine prophylactic anticoagulation.
   2. Use of low-molecular-weight heparin may be more effective than unfractionated heparin in preventing deep vein thrombosis in critically ill patients.[39]

C. Heparin-induced thrombocytopenia (HIT)
   1. HIT is caused by autoantibodies directed against heparin-PF4 (platelet factor 4), resulting in platelet activation.
   2. Thrombocytopenia is common in critically ill patients, but HIT is rare.
   3. 4 T score can be calculated to assess pretest probability of HIT. Points are assigned for[40]
      a. Degree of thrombocytopenia
      b. Timing of onset after heparin administration
      c. Presence of thrombosis
      d. No other cause of thrombocytopenia
   4. Diagnose with HIT antibody testing and serotonin release assay.

XII. MEDICATIONS

Medications commonly used in ICU are described in **Table 4.6**.

TABLE 4.6 Drugs Commonly Used in the Intensive Care Unit

Drug	Dilution (Concentration)	Loading Dose	Dose	Comments
Amiodarone	150 mg/100 mL D5W (1.5 mg/mL)	150 mg	0.5-1 mg/min	Contraindicated in cardiogenic shock or sinus node dysfunction AV block. Prolongs QT interval. Associated with pulmonary fibrosis
Angiotensin II	2.5 mg/mL 0.9% NaCl (5,000 ng/mL)		0.05-1.6 μg/kg/min	May cause thromboembolic events, thrombocytopenia, and tachycardia
Diltiazem	125 mg/125 mL 0.9% NaCl or D5W (1 mg/mL)	0.25 mg/kg (followed by 0.35 mg/kg if needed)	5-15 mg/h	May cause hypotension
Dobutamine	250 mg/100 mL 0.9% NaCl (2,500 μg/mL)		2-20 μg/kg/min	Selective inotropic (β) effect; may cause tachycardia and arrhythmias
Dopamine	400 mg/250 mL 0.9% NaCl or D5W (1,600 μg/mL)		Dopa 1-3 μg/kg/min; α, 3-10 μg/kg/min, β, 10-20 μg/kg/min	Clinical response is dose and patient dependent, may cause arrhythmias and tachycardia
Epinephrine	5 mg/500 mL 0.9% NaCl or D5W, or 4 mg/100 mL 0.9% NaCl or D5W		0.01-0.05 μg/kg/min	Mixed α and β effects; use central line; may cause tachycardia and hypotension
Esmolol	2.5 g/250 mL 0.9% NaCl or D5W (10 mg/mL)	500 μg/kg/min for 1 min (optional)	50-300 μg/kg/min	Selective β_1-blocker: $T_{1/2}$ 9 min; not eliminated by hepatic or renal routes, may cause hypotension

(continued)

TABLE 4.6 Drugs Commonly Used in the Intensive Care Unit (*Continued*)

Drug	Dilution (Concentration)	Loading Dose	Dose	Comments
Heparin	25,000 U 250 mL 0.45% NaCl (100 U/mL)	60 U/kg	14 units/kg/h	Obtain PTT every 4-6 h until PTT is 1.5-2 times control; may cause thrombocytopenia
Lidocaine	1 mg/kg (can repeat two times if needed)	1–4 mg min		Dose should be decreased in patients with hepatic failure, acute MI, CHF, or shock
Nitroglycerin	50 mg 250 mL D5W (200 ng/mL)		5-20 µg/min	Use cautiously in right-sided MI
Nitroprusside	50 mg 250 mL D5W (200 µg/mL)		0.25-10 mg/kg/min	Signs of toxicity include metabolic acidosis, tremors, seizures, and coma; thiocyanate may accumulate in renal failure
Norepinephrine	8 mg 500 mL D5W (16 µg/mL)	0.01-2 µg/kg/min		Potent α effects; mainly β_1 effects at lower doses, use central line
Phenylephrine	10 mg/250 mL 0.9% NaCl or D5W (40 µg/mL)	10-100 µg/min	0-4 µg/kg/min	Pure α effects; use central line; may cause reflex bradycardia and decreased cardiac output
Vasopressin	20 U/100 mL NS (0.2 units/mL)	0-0.06 U/min		Do not titrate; higher doses may cause myocardial ischemia

CHF, congestive heart failure; D5W, 5% dextrose in water; MI, myocardial infarction; PTT, partial thromboplastin time; $T_{1/2}$, terminal half-life.

Key References

Citation	Summary
Young D, Harrison DA, Cuthbertson BH, Rowan K; TracMan Collaborators. Effect of early vs. late tracheostomy placement on survival in patients receiving mechanical ventilation: the TracMan randomized trial. *J Am Med Assoc.* 2013;309(20):2121-2129.	• A total of 909 patients identified as likely requiring mechanical ventilation >7 d randomized to early tracheostomy (within 4 d) or late tracheostomy (after 10 d). • There was no significant difference in 30-d mortality between the two groups. Ability for physicians to accurately predict which patients required extensive mechanical ventilation was limited.
Acute Respiratory Distress Syndrome Network; Brower RG, Matthay MA, et al. Ventilation with lower tidal volumes as compared with traditional tidal volumes for acute lung injury and the acute respiratory distress syndrome. *N Engl J Med.* 2000;342(18):1301-1308.	• A total of 861 patients with ARDS randomized to traditional ventilatory support (tidal volume 12 mL/kg of predicted body weight) vs. lower tidal volume (6 mL/kg of predicted body weight). • Patients randomized to lower tidal volume group had lower mortality compared with traditional group (31.0% vs. 39.8%, $P = .007$).
Evans L, Rhodes A, Alhazzani W, et al. Executive summary: surviving sepsis campaign. International guidelines for the management of sepsis and septic shock 2021 [published correction appears in *Crit Care Med.* 2022;50(4):e413-e414]. *Crit Care Med.* 2021;49(11):1974-1982.	• Guidelines for management of sepsis and septic shock.
NICE-SUGAR Study Investigators; Finfer S, Chittock DR, et al. Intensive versus conventional glucose control in critically ill patients. *N Engl J Med.* 2009;360(13):1283-1297.	• A total of 6,104 ICU patients assigned to intensive glucose control (81-108 mg/dL) vs. conventional control (<180 mg/dL). • At 90 d, patients randomized to intensive control group had higher mortality than conventionally treated group (27.5% vs. 24.9%).

CHAPTER 4: CRITICAL CARE

Review Questions

1. The side effects of propofol, a common sedative used in critical care, include?
2. What are the different types of shock?
3. How do you confirm proper airway placement (endotracheal tube, tracheostomy)?
4. What are complications of PEG placement?
5. How do "SIRS" and "sepsis" differ?
6. Optimal glycemic control in critically ill patients is?
7. Prophylaxis of stress-induced GI bleeding is indicated for patients with

REFERENCES

1. Lee BH, Inui D, Suh GY, et al. Association of body temperature and antipyretic treatments with mortality of critically ill patients with and without sepsis: multi-centered prospective observational study. *Crit Care.* 2012;16(1):R33.
2. Scheer B, Perel A, Pfeiffer UJ. Clinical review: complications and risk factors of peripheral arterial catheters used for haemodynamic monitoring in anaesthesia and intensive care medicine. *Crit Care.* 2002;6(3):199-204.
3. Nuttall G, Burckhardt J, Hadley A, et al. Surgical and patient risk factors for severe arterial line complications in adults. *Anesthesiology.* 2016;124(3):590-597.
4. Binanay C, Califf RM, Hasselblad V, et al. Evaluation study of congestive heart failure and pulmonary artery catheterization effectiveness: the ESCAPE trial. *J Am Med Assoc.* 2005;294(13):1625-1633.
5. Keren H, Burkhoff D, Squara P. Evaluation of a noninvasive continuous cardiac output monitoring system based on thoracic bioreactance. *Am J Physiol Heart Circ Physiol.* July 2007;293(1):H583-H589.
6. Pandharipande PP, Sanders RD, Girard TD, et al. Effect of dexmedetomidine versus lorazepam on outcome in patients with sepsis: an a priori-designed analysis of the MENDS randomized controlled trial. *Crit Care.* 2010;14(2):R38.
7. Erdman MJ, Doepker BA, Gerlach AT, Phillips GS, Elijovich L, Jones GM. A comparison of severe hemodynamic disturbances between dexmedetomidine and propofol for sedation in neurocritical care patients. *Crit Care Med.* 2014;42(7):1696-1702.
8. Mirzakhani H, Nozari A, Ehrenfeld JM, et al. Case report: profound hypotension after anesthetic induction with propofol in patients treated with rifampin. *Anesth Analg.* 2013;117(1):61-64.
9. Schroeppel TJ, Fabian TC, Clement LP, et al. Propofol infusion syndrome: a lethal condition in critically injured patients eliminated by a simple screening protocol. *Injury.* 2014;45(1):245-249.
10. Brook AD, Ahrens TS, Schaiff R, et al. Effect of a nursing-implemented sedation protocol on the duration of mechanical ventilation. *Crit Care Med.* 1999;27(12):2609-2615.
11. Devlin JW, Skrobik Y, Gélinas C, et al. Clinical practice guidelines for the prevention and management of pain, agitation/sedation, delirium, immobility, and sleep disruption in adult patients in the ICU. *Crit Care Med.* S2018;46(9):e825-e873.

12. Salluh JI, Soares M, Teles JM, et al. Delirium epidemiology in critical care (DECCA): an international study. *Crit Care.* 2010;14(6):R210.

13. Devlin JW, Roberts RJ, Fong JJ, et al. Efficacy and safety of quetiapine in critically ill patients with delirium: a prospective, multicenter, randomized, double-blind, placebo-controlled pilot study. *Crit Care Med.* 2010;38(2):419-427.

14. Reade MC, Eastwood GM, Bellomo R, et al. Effect of dexmedetomidine added to standard care on ventilator-free time in patients with agitated delirium: a randomized clinical trial. *J Am Med Assoc.* 2016;315(14):1460-1468.

15. Wijdicks EF, Varelas PN, Gronseth GS, Greer DM; American Academy of Neurology. Evidence-based guideline update: determining brain death in adults. Report of the Quality Standards Subcommittee of the American Academy of Neurology. *Neurology.* 2010;74(23):1911-1918.

16. Freeman BD, Borecki IB, Coopersmith CM, Buchman TG. Relationship between tracheostomy timing and duration of mechanical ventilation in critically ill patients. *Crit Care Med.* 2005;33(11):2513-2520.

17. Young D, Harrison DA, Cuthbertson BH, Rowan K; TracMan Collaborators. Effect of early vs late tracheostomy placement on survival in patients receiving mechanical ventilation: the TracMan randomized trial. *J Am Med Assoc.* 2013;309(20):2121-2129.

18. Strøm T, Martinussen T, Toft P. A protocol of no sedation for critically ill patients receiving mechanical ventilation: a randomised trial. *Lancet.* 2010;375(9713):475-480.

19. Acute Respiratory Distress Syndrome Network; Brower RG, Matthay MA, Morris A, Schoenfeld D, Thompson BT, Wheeler A. Ventilation with lower tidal volumes as compared with traditional tidal volumes for acute lung injury and the acute respiratory distress syndrome. *N Engl J Med.* 2000;342(18):1301-1308.

20. Papazian L, Forel JM, Gacouin A, et al. Neuromuscular blockers in early acute respiratory distress syndrome. *N Engl J Med.* 2010;363(12):1107-1116.

21. Fan E, Needham DM, Stewart TE. Ventilatory management of acute lung injury and acute respiratory distress syndrome. *J Am Med Assoc.* 2005;294(22):2889-2896.

22. Guérin C, Reignier J, Richard JC, et al. Prone positioning in severe acute respiratory distress syndrome. *N Engl J Med.* 2013;368(23):2159-2168.

23. Villar J, Ferrando C, Martínez D, et al. Dexamethasone treatment for the acute respiratory distress syndrome: a multicentre, randomised controlled trial. *Lancet Respir Med.* 2020;8(3):267-276.

24. Hébert PC, Wells G, Blajchman MA, et al. A multicenter, randomized, controlled clinical trial of transfusion requirements in critical care. Transfusion requirements in Critical Care Investigators, Canadian Critical Care Trials Group. *N Engl J Med.* 1999;340(6):409-417.

25. Marik PE, Baram M, Vahid B. Does central venous pressure predict fluid responsiveness? A systematic review of the literature and the tale of seven mares. *Chest.* 2008;134(1):172-178.

26. Buendgens L, Bruensing J, Matthes M, et al. Administration of proton pump inhibitors in critically ill medical patients is associated with increased risk of developing *Clostridium difficile*-associated diarrhea. *J Crit Care.* 2014;29(4):696.e11-696.e15.

27. Evans L, Rhodes A, Alhazzani W, et al. Executive summary. Surviving sepsis campaign: international Guidelines for the management of sepsis and septic shock 2021. *Crit Care Med.* 2021;49(11):1974-1982.

28. Rivers E, Nguyen B, Havstad S, et al. Early goal-directed therapy in the treatment of severe sepsis and septic shock. *N Engl J Med.* 2001;345(19):1368-1377.

29. ProCESS Investigators; Yealy DM, Kellum JA, et al. A randomized trial of protocol-based care for early septic shock. *N Engl J Med.* 2014;370(18):1683-1693.

30. De Backer D, Biston P, Devriendt J, et al. Comparison of dopamine and norepinephrine in the treatment of shock. *N Engl J Med.* 2010;362(9):779-789.

31. Patel GP, Grahe JS, Sperry M, et al. Efficacy and safety of dopamine versus norepinephrine in the management of septic shock. *Shock.* 2010;33(4):375-380.

32. Annane D, Renault A, Brun-Buisson C, et al. Hydrocortisone plus Fludrocortisone for adults with septic shock. *N Engl J Med.* 2018;378(9):809-818.

33. Wang C, Sun J, Zheng J, et al. Low-dose hydrocortisone therapy attenuates septic shock in adult patients but does not reduce 28-day mortality: a meta-analysis of randomized controlled trials. *Anesth Analg.* 2014;118(2):346-357.

34. Ibrahim EH, Sherman G, Ward S, Fraser VJ, Kollef MH. The influence of inadequate antimicrobial treatment of bloodstream infections on patient outcomes in the ICU setting. *Chest.* 2000;118(1):146-155.

35. NICE-SUGAR Study Investigators; Finfer S, Chittock DR, et al. Intensive versus conventional glucose control in critically ill patients. *N Engl J Med.* 2009;360(13):1283-1297.

36. Sprung CL, Annane D, Keh D, et al. Hydrocortisone therapy for patients with septic shock. *N Engl J Med.* 2008;358(2):111-124.

37. Marik PE, Pastores SM, Annane D, et al. Recommendations for the diagnosis and management of corticosteroid insufficiency in critically ill adult patients: consensus statements from an international task force by the American College of Critical Care Medicine. *Crit Care Med.* 2008;36(6):1937-1949.

38. Corwin HL, Gettinger A, Fabian TC, et al. Efficacy and safety of epoetin alfa in critically ill patients. *N Engl J Med.* 2007;357(10):965-976.

39. Fernando SM, Tran A, Cheng W, et al. VTE prophylaxis in critically ill adults: a systematic review and network meta-analysis. *Chest.* 2022;161(2):418-428.

40. Lo GK, Juhl D, Warkentin TE, Sigouin CS, Eichler P, Greinacher A. Evaluation of pretest clinical score (4 T's) for the diagnosis of heparin-induced thrombocytopenia in two clinical settings. *J Thromb Haemost.* 2006;4(4):759-765.

5 Trauma Resuscitation and Adjuncts

Emily J. Onufer and Jessica Kramer McCool

I. INTRODUCTION

A. Epidemiology
1. Injury is a leading cause of death and disability around the world, especially among young patients.
2. Trauma deaths have a trimodal distribution.
   a. Immediate death
      i. At the time of traumatic event.
      ii. Common etiologies are profound blood loss or devastating neurologic injury.
      iii. Cannot be prevented by interventions from trauma providers
   b. Early death
      i. Within the first few hours of traumatic event
      ii. Can be prevented with prompt trauma assessment and intervention
   c. Late death
      i. Days to weeks after the initial injury due to secondary complications
      ii. Examples include sepsis, acute respiratory distress syndrome, multiple organ dysfunction and failure.
      iii. Can be prevented with prompt trauma resuscitation and comprehensive posttraumatic care

B. Guidelines established by **Advanced Trauma Life Support (ATLS)** provide a standardized comprehensive approach to minimize morbidity and mortality related to traumatic injuries.

II. PREHOSPITAL CARE

Prehospital care of the trauma patient is provided by a wide range of emergency medical service personnel with varying levels of training (first responders, emergency medical technicians, and paramedics). Main objectives are

A. Injury assessment and patient triage
1. Identify patients with survivable injuries.
2. Triage patients based on severity of injuries and clinical stability.
3. Distribute patients to appropriate trauma centers. Levels of trauma centers are determined by state and regional authorities but generally include the following.
   a. Level I
      i. Twenty-four-hour in-house general surgeons trained to treat traumatic injuries

ii. Subspecialty providers (orthopedic surgery, neurosurgery, maxillofacial surgery, etc.) are readily available.
iii. Established referral network from community hospitals
iv. Leaders in trauma research, education, and quality improvement

b. Level II
i. Twenty-four-hour coverage by general surgeons
ii. Access to specialty services (anesthesiology, radiology, critical care, etc.) that can provide comprehensive care to most patients
iii. Patients requiring subspecialty tertiary care needs will still require transfer to level I centers.

c. Level III
i. Twenty-four-hour availability of emergency medicine and/or general surgery personnel who can promptly assess and stabilize injured patients
ii. Have established relationships with level I and level II centers for prompt transfers of critically ill patients and patients with specialty needs

d. Level IV
i. Able to implement ATLS protocols to quickly assess and stabilize trauma patients prior to transfer to higher-level centers

B. Patient stabilization
1. Secure airway with tracheal intubation or laryngeal mask airway
2. Bag mask and provide supplemental oxygen.
3. Establish vascular access and begin resuscitation.
4. Immobilize spine on a backboard and place a properly fitted cervical collar in patients with suspected spinal injuries.

C. Transfer of care to trauma center
1. Communication
a. Description of trauma event. Helps providers determine the pattern and severity of expected injuries (**Table 5-1**).
b. Vital signs and quick neurologic assessment
c. Inventory of injuries noted by first responders. *Patients still require a thorough assessment at the trauma center to ensure all injuries are noted.*
d. List treatments given en route to the trauma center and summarize patient response to these treatments.

D. Trauma center preparation
1. Prepare trauma bay
a. Collect and check all necessary resources, such as airway equipment, warmed intravenous fluids, and other supplies, to address specific injury patterns.
b. Ensure trauma bay is at an appropriate temperature to minimize risk of hypothermia, which can worsen acidosis and coagulopathy.
2. Mobilization of all trauma team personnel and resources
a. Designate team leader to lead trauma resuscitation.
b. Assign roles to other providers.
i. Assess and establish airway.
ii. Obtain vascular access and collect blood for laboratory tests.

TABLE 5-1 Mechanism of Trauma With Possible Associated Injuries

Mechanism	Impact	Possible Associated Injuries
Front-end car collision	Direct impact between driver's knees and dashboard	• Patellar fracture • Posterior knee dislocation (with popliteal artery injury) • Femoral shaft fracture • Posterior acetabular rim fracture
Feet-first fall from significant height	Axial loading	• Calcaneal fracture • Lower extremity long bone fracture • Acetabular injury • Lumbar spine compression fracture
Pedestrian struck by motor vehicle	Impact on car bumper, windshield, hood, or pavement	• Injury to tibia and fibula (striking bumper) • Head injury (striking windshield/hood) • Injury to upper extremity (extended arm hitting pavement)

Child struck by motor vehicle	Impact on car bumper, windshield, hood, or pavement	• Waddell triad:
		  • Femur fracture (striking bumper)
		  • Abdominal solid organ injury (liver or spleen; striking fender)
		  • Opposite side head injury (landing on pavement)

iii. Perform procedures, such as tube thoracostomy, that will immediately address life-threatening injuries.

c. All team members should wear proper personal protection equipment.

d. Protocols to ensure prompt response by laboratory and radiology personnel should be activated.

e. Operating room staff and critical care providers should also be notified when patients have severe injury patterns or will need immediate operative intervention.

III. PRIMARY SURVEY

A. Overview

1. Systematic, rapid evaluation for immediate threats to life
2. Follows *ABCDE* mnemonic
   a. Airway with cervical spine control
   b. Breathing and ventilation
   c. Circulation and hemorrhage control

    d. Disability
    e. Exposure and environmental control
3. History is obtained (if possible) following the acronym *AMPLE*.
    a. Allergies
    b. Medications
    c. Past medical history
    d. Last oral intake
    e. Events surrounding the injury

B. Airway

1. Assessment
    a. A patient who is able to respond verbally in a clear voice has a patent airway.
    b. In nonverbal patients, rapidly assess for and remove obvious causes of obstruction.
    c. Even without signs of obvious obstruction, patients with Glasgow Coma Score (GCS) < 8 are unable to protect their airway. (For more information on GCS, please see Disability.)
2. Basic maneuvers
    a. Suctioning
    b. Jaw-thrust to displace tongue anteriorly away from the pharyngeal inlet
    c. Place oropharyngeal (or, in the absences of facial trauma, nasopharyngeal) airway to mechanically displace tongue anteriorly
3. Tracheal intubation
    a. Preferred method to establish a secure airway.
    b. Rapid sequence induction (**Figure 5-1**) can prepare a patient for intubation within a few minutes.
    c. It is important to closely monitor the patient's hemodynamic status as many induction agents can alter vital signs.
4. Cricothyrotomy
    a. Emergency surgical airway in adults after unsuccessful orotracheal attempts or with massive facial trauma.
    b. **Surgical technique: Cricothyrotomy**
        i. Make a longitudinal skin incision on the anterior neck between the cricoid and thyroid cartilages over the cricothyroid membrane.
        ii. Access the airway through the cricothyroid membrane. Bluntly expand defect using scalpel handle or tracheal spreader.
        iii. An endotracheal or tracheostomy tube is inserted into the trachea through the cricothyrotomy.
5. Percutaneous transtracheal ventilation
    a. Indicated in children younger than 12 years, who are at increased risk for airway stenosis from cricothyrotomy.
    b. Small cannula, such as a 14-gauge intravenous catheter, is placed through the cricothyroid membrane.
6. Patients with cricothyrotomy or percutaneous transtracheal ventilation systems should be revised to a definitive secure airway (orotracheal intubation vs. surgical tracheostomy) when it is safe to do so.

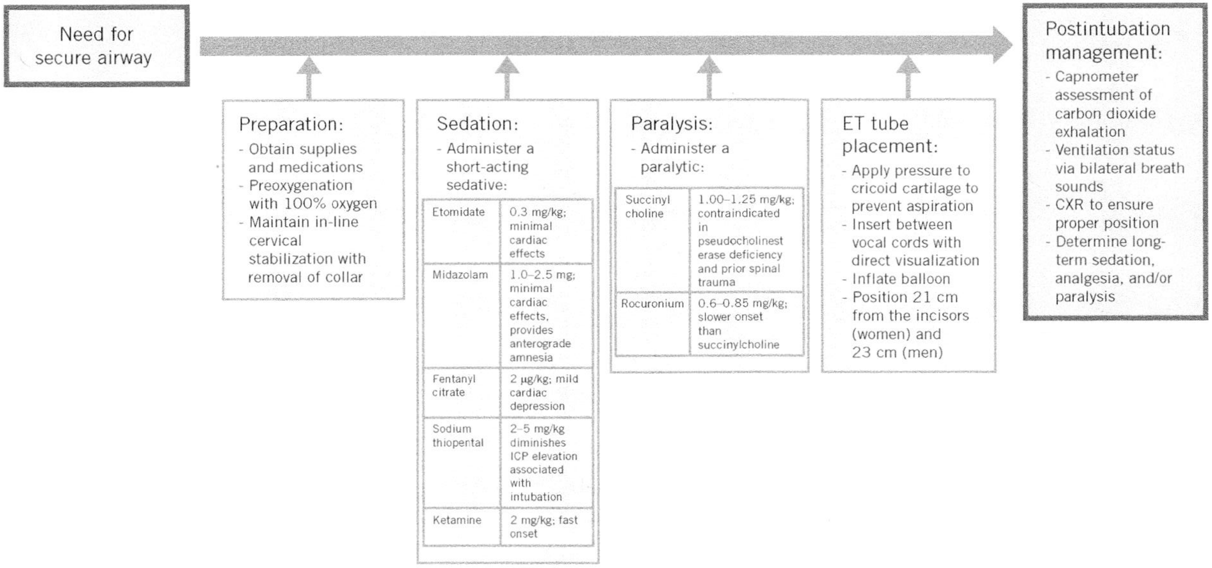

Need for secure airway
Preparation:
- Obtain supplies and medications
- Preoxygenation with 100% oxygen
- Maintain in-line cervical stabilization with removal of collar
Sedation:
- Administer a short-acting sedative:
Etomidate
0.3 mg/kg; minimal cardiac effects
Midazolam
1.0–2.5 mg; minimal cardiac effects, provides anterograde amnesia
Fentanyl citrate
2 μg/kg; mild cardiac depression
Sodium thiopental
2–5 mg/kg diminishes ICP elevation associated with intubation
Ketamine
2 mg/kg; fast onset
Paralysis:
- Administer a paralytic:
Succinyl choline
1.00–1.25 mg/kg; contraindicated in pseudocholinesterase deficiency and prior spinal trauma
Rocuronium
0.6–0.85 mg/kg; slower onset than succinylcholine
ET tube placement:
- Apply pressure to cricoid cartilage to prevent aspiration
- Insert between vocal cords with direct visualization
- Inflate balloon
- Position 21 cm from the incisors (women) and 23 cm (men)
Postintubation management:
- Capnometer assessment of carbon dioxide exhalation
- Ventilation status via bilateral breath sounds
- CXR to ensure proper position
- Determine long-term sedation, analgesia, and/or paralysis

FIGURE 5-1 Rapid sequence intubation to achieve endotracheal intubation.

C. Breathing

1. Assessment

a. Every trauma patient should have oxygen administered (via nasal cannula or bag valve facemask) and a pulse oximeter placed.

b. Signs of dysfunctional breathing include abnormal or unequal breath sounds, accessory muscle usage, or abnormal chest wall motion.

c. In the unstable patient, treatment should be immediate and not be delayed for imaging studies.

2. Pneumothorax or hemothorax

a. Definitions

i. Pneumothorax: Injuries in the lung parenchyma cause air to leak into the pleural space.

ii. Hemothorax: Injuries in lung parenchyma cause blood to leak into the pleural space.

iii. Tension pneumothorax: Entrapment of air within the pleural space, resulting in increased pressure that can compress other intrathoracic structures, severely reducing cardiac and respiratory function.

a) *Can cause hemodynamic instability and should be promptly recognized and treated.*

iv. Open pneumothorax, or sucking chest wound: Any chest wound communicating with the pleural space that preferentially draws air into the pleural cavity

b. Treatment

i. Needle decompression

a) Place a 14-gauge intravenous catheter in the second intercostal space in the midclavicular line or through the 4th intercostal space in the midaxillary line.

b) A tube thoracostomy should promptly follow decompression.

ii. **Surgical technique: Tube thoracostomy placement**

a) Position the patient in a semi-lateral decubitus position. The "safe triangle" for tube thoracostomy placement is marked by (i) the lateral border of the pectoralis major muscle, (ii) anterior border of the latissimus dorsi muscle, and (iii) level of the nipple of inframammary fold.

b) Make a transverse incision through the skin and subcutaneous tissue and bluntly enter the pleural cavity with a curved clamp. It is important to direct the instrument over the top of the rib to minimize the risk of injury to the intercostal neurovascular bundle.

c) Insert the thoracostomy tube through this tract and direct it superiorly and posteriorly.

d) When the tube is positioned and secured properly, it should be immediately connected to an underwater seal-suction device.

e) A CXR is obtained to assess for lung re-expansion and tube position.

iii. Sucking chest wounds must be covered with a partially occlusive bandage secured on *three* sides, forming a one-way valve and preventing development of a tension pneumothorax.

3. Flail chest
   a. Definition: Three or more ribs with two or more fractures per rib. Often associated with underlying pulmonary contusion
   b. Characterized by paradoxical chest wall motion with spontaneous respirations (chest moves in with inspiration and out with expiration)
   c. Treatment
      i. Adequate pain control (often with epidural analgesia)
      ii. Respiratory support. Many of these patients will require early mechanical ventilatory support.
      iii. Aggressive pulmonary toilet to prevent lung consolidation and pneumonia
4. Tracheobronchial disruption
   a. Definition: Injury of the airway structures (trachea and main bronchi)
   b. Characterized by severe subcutaneous emphysema with respiratory compromise and often associated with pneumothorax
   c. Treatment
      i. Intubate unaffected bronchus.
      ii. Tube thoracostomy on the affected side to evacuate escaped air.
      iii. Diagnostic bronchoscopy and operative repair provide definitive therapy.

D. Circulation

1. Assessment
   a. Vital signs
   b. Mental status
   c. On physical examination, assess capillary refill, temperature, and skin turgor
   d. With placement of Foley catheter, urine output can also be used to assess circulation and guide resuscitation.
   e. Ensure patient has adequate vascular access to promptly initiate resuscitation if needed.
2. **Hemorrhagic shock**
   a. Overview
      i. This is the most common type of shock and occurs as a result of decreased intravascular volume secondary to hemorrhage (**Table 5-2**).
      ii. Hemorrhagic shock is the presumed etiology of hemodynamic instability in all trauma patients until proven otherwise.
   b. External hemorrhage control
      i. Common areas of external hemorrhage that can be easily missed include the posterior scalp, axillae, perineum, and posterior trunk.
      ii. Techniques to control external hemorrhage include direct pressure, tourniquet, and reduction of large bony injuries.

TABLE 5-2 Estimated Blood Loss by Initial Hemodynamic Variables

	Class I	Class II	Class III	Class IV
Blood loss (mL)	Up to 750	750-1,500	1,500-2,000	>2,000
Blood loss (% blood volume)	Up to 15%	15%-30%	30%-40%	>40%
Pulse rate	<100	>100	>120	>140
Blood pressure (mm Hg)	Normal	Normal	Decreased	Decreased
Pulse pressure (mm Hg)	Normal or increased	Decreased	Decreased	Decreased
Urinary output (mL/h)	>30	20-30	5-15	Negligible

c. Vascular access
   i. Peripheral access: Two large-bore intravenous lines placed (14 or 16 gauge), preferably in the antecubital fossae.
   ii. Central venous access: 8.5 Fr. catheter (Cordis catheter) placed via Seldinger technique into a major blood vessel, such as femoral vein or subclavian vein.
   iii. Intraosseous access: Placement of special hollow bore needle through the cortex of a long bone (i.e., tibia, humerus, sternum) into the medullary space.

d. Resuscitation
   i. Permissive hypotension (systolic blood pressure goal 80-90 mm Hg) has been proven to increase survival in the trauma patient.[1]
   ii. Early resuscitation with blood products prevents dilutional coagulopathy and treats intrinsic acute traumatic coagulopathy.
   iii. Institutional protocols should be established to determine indications for massive transfusion.
   iv. If time has not allowed proper cross-matching (as is frequently the case), type O blood should be used. Premenopausal women should receive Rh− blood. Men and postmenopausal women can receive either Rh− or Rh+ blood.
   v. In addition to hemorrhage, trauma can also lead to transient hyperfibrinolysis.
      a) CRASH-2 trial: Tranexamic acid, an antifibrinolytic, was found to improve survival when administered early in patients with known or suspected massive hemorrhage.[2]

e. Internal hemorrhage control

i. Pelvic hemorrhage. If blood loss is suspected secondary to severe pelvic trauma, a pelvic binder or a sheet should be placed around the greater trochanters of the femur.

ii. Resuscitative thoracotomy ("Emergency Department Thoracotomy," EDT) allows for identification and control of both intrathoracic and subdiaphragmatic hemorrhage and is a procedure of last resort in a moribund patient.

iii. Surgical technique: Resuscitative thoracotomy

a) Position the patient supine with the left arm elevated and then perform a left anterolateral thoracotomy at the fifth intercostal space from the left sternocostal junction to the latissimus dorsi muscle.

b) Elevate the left lung medially to locate and dissect the descending aorta and place a vascular clamp across it.

c) If cardiac injury is suspected, open the pericardial sac and evacuate any blood clots and identify any cardiac lacerations.

d) If there is active bleeding in the pulmonary hilum, apply a vascular clamp across it.

e) Once injuries have been temporized, proceed immediately to the operating room for definitive management.

iv. Indications[3,4]–Table 5-3

a) Penetrating trauma

1) Witnessed arrest during resuscitation

2) Pulseless and have only received cardiopulmonary resuscitation for less than 15 minutes

b) Blunt trauma

1) Witnessed arrest during resuscitation

v. Contraindications

a) No signs of life at scene of trauma

b) Prolonged pulselessness (more than 15 minutes)

c) Has nonsurvivable injuries

d) Definitive injury management is not readily available.

TABLE 5-3 EAST Recommendations to Perform EDT

Strongly Recommended	Conditionally Recommended
• Patients who arrive pulseless *with signs of life* after *penetrating thoracic injury*	• Patients who arrive pulseless *without signs of life* after *penetrating thoracic injury* • Patient who arrive pulseless *with or without signs of life* after *penetrating extrathoracic injury* • Patients who arrive pulseless *with or without signs of life* after *blunt injury*

EAST, Eastern Association for the Surgery of Trauma.

vi. Resuscitative endovascular balloon occlusion of the aorta (REBOA) is a minimally invasive technique using a balloon catheter to occlude the aorta for control of noncompressible torso hemorrhage.
   a) Indicated for hemorrhagic control of life-threatening subdiaphragmatic injuries
   b) The use of REBOA is currently limited to certified institutions and trained physicians.
   c) Technique
      1) Using ultrasound guidance, place a 7 Fr or larger sheath into the common femoral artery. Can also be achieved via femoral artery cutdown. An appropriately placed femoral arterial line can be upsized to a REBOA. Avoid cannulation of the superficial femoral artery, which can lead to limb loss.
      2) The balloon should be inflated in the distal thoracic aorta (zone 1) to control intra-abdominal or retroperitoneal hemorrhage or those in arrest. For those with pelvic, junctional, or lower extremity hemorrhage, the balloon catheter should be inflated at the distal abdominal aorta (zone 3).
   d) Prolonged balloon inflation can cause end-organ ischemia or spinal cord injury from ischemia; therefore, definitive hemorrhage control must be performed immediately.

3. Cardiogenic shock

a. Definition: Occurs when cardiac output is inadequate to perfuse peripheral tissues, either by extrinsic compression (tension pneumothorax, cardiac tamponade) or myocardial injury

b. Diagnosis
   i. On physical examination, signs of cardiogenic shock include:
      a) Cool, pale skin
      b) Distended jugular veins
      c) Transient response to initial resuscitation
   ii. Bedside echocardiogram can evaluate for external compression from pericardial effusion and assess overall cardiac function.
   iii. Electrocardiogram and serum troponin levels can be obtained if blunt cardiac injury is suspected.
   iv. In the operating room, a subxiphoid pericardial window can be made to assess for hemopericardium. If blood is detected, myocardial injury is presumed and will usually require operative exploration via a median sternotomy.

c. Treatment
   i. Emergent decompression with tube thoracostomy or needle decompression is required if tension pneumothorax is suspected.
   ii. Resuscitative thoracotomy may be needed to identify and temporize the injury if the patient has a witnessed arrest and does not have an extended period of pulselessness.
   iii. Penetrating myocardial injuries require operative intervention.
   iv. Patients with blunt cardiac injury often require close monitoring for development of arrhythmias and cardiac dysfunction

4. **Neurogenic shock**
   a. Definition: Occurs as a result of loss of peripheral sympathetic tone after neurologic (i.e., spinal cord) injury. This leads to increase in venous capacitance and decreased venous return.
   b. Signs of neurogenic shock include:
      i. Warm skin
      ii. Absent rectal tone
      iii. Inappropriate bradycardia
   c. Treatment
      i. Fluid resuscitation
      ii. Pharmacologic support with vasopressors to help restore sympathetic tone

E. Disability
1. Assessment
   a. The Glasgow Coma Scale (GCS) is a clinical tool to quickly assess a patient's level of consciousness following a traumatic injury. See **Table 5-4** for an overview of the GCS.

TABLE 5-4 Glasgow Coma Scale Based on ATLS Guidelines, 10th Edition

Scale	Score
Eye Opening (E)	
Spontaneous	4
To sound	3
To pressure	2
None	1
Nontestable	NT
Verbal Response (V)	
Oriented	5
Confused	4
Words	3
Sounds	2
None	1
Nontestable	NT
Best Motor Response (M)	
Obeys commands	6
Localizing	5
Normal flexion	4
Abnormal flexion	3
Extension	2
None	1
Nontestable	NT

b. A thorough neurologic examination can be performed as part of the secondary survey and includes evaluation of pupillary response, ability to follow commands, and gross asymmetry of limb movement to painful stimuli.
c. Severe neurologic injuries require urgent evaluation and are either intracranial or spinal in origin.

2. **Intracranial injuries**
   a. Signs
      i. Asymmetric pupillary changes can indicate impending herniation.
      ii. Altered mental status
      iii. Can often be asymptomatic
   b. Diagnosis
      i. CT scan of the head is the most sensitive test to diagnose intracranial injuries.
   c. Treatment
      i. The objective is to prevent secondary injury by optimizing cerebral perfusion pressure (CPP).
      ii. CPP is defined as the difference between mean arterial pressure (MAP) and intracranial pressure (ICP): CPP = MAP − ICP.
      iii. Goal CPP (>60-70 mm Hg)
      iv. Supporting MAP
         a) Resuscitation to prevent hypovolemia
         b) Pharmacologic support may be needed to further increase MAP.
      v. Minimizing ICP
         a) ICP can be measured via subarachnoid pressure monitor ("bolt").
         b) Mannitol (1 g/kg) or hypertonic saline should be emergently administered in the trauma bay to prevent herniation if elevated ICP is suspected.
         c) General measures used to prevent an increase in the ICP include
            i. Elevating the head of the bed to 30° to 45°
            ii. Maintaining the patient's head in the midline position to prevent obstruction of jugular venous outflow
            iii. Permissive hypercarbia can promote cerebral vasodilation.
            iv. Intraventricular catheter placed in the nondominant lateral ventricle can also be used and has the advantage of draining cerebrospinal fluid, if needed.
3. **Spinal cord injuries**
   a. Signs of spinal cord injuries
      i. Neurogenic shock
      ii. Loss of sensory and/or motor function
   b. Management
      i. Optimize spinal cord perfusion with resuscitation and vasopressors
4. Neurosurgical consultation is required for all patients with severe neurologic injuries.

F. Exposure
1. Exposure: Complete visual inspection is crucial.
   a. Logroll the patient to examine posteriorly while maintaining spinal stability
   b. Splaying of the legs to examine the perineum, and elevation of the arms to inspect the axillae
   c. In penetrating trauma, ballistic injuries should be counted and positions noted. This provides information on projectile trajectory, which can indicate certain injury patterns.
2. Environmental control: Minimize heat loss in exposed trauma patients
   a. Keep resuscitation room warm.
   b. Promptly cover patient once survey has been completed.
   c. All resuscitation fluids should be warmed.

IV. ADJUNCTS TO THE PRIMARY SURVEY

A. Radiographs
1. Overview
   a. Quickly diagnose potentially fatal injuries.
   b. Evaluate radiographs for suspected pathology based on the patient's history and correlate with pertinent findings of primary survey.
   c. Radiographs should not delay treatment (i.e., needle decompression, pelvic binder placement) if warranted based on mechanism and presentation.
2. CXR: Should be read in a stepwise fashion.
   a. Trachea and bronchi
      i. Assess for position of an endotracheal tube, if placed.
      ii. Tracheal lacerations present with pneumomediastinum, pneumothorax, or subcutaneous emphysema along the neck.
      iii. Bronchial disruptions present with massive pneumothoraces with a persistent air leak on placement of a tube thoracostomy.
   b. Pleural spaces and lung parenchyma
      i. Assess the pleural spaces for abnormal collections of fluid (effusion or hemothorax) or air (pneumothorax).
      ii. Assess the lung parenchyma for infiltrates or areas of consolidation (pulmonary contusion, aspiration).
      iii. Be aware that overlying structures (backboards, ECG leads) can obscure lung apices and should be cleared away, if possible.
   c. Mediastinum
      i. Look for air or blood between tissue planes, indicating injury.
      ii. Air or blood in the pericardium leads to an enlarged cardiac silhouette.
      iii. If suspected based on mechanism and examination, a widened mediastinum is concerning for a great vessel injury and should lead to a CT angiography of the chest to assess the mediastinal vessels (if the patient is stable) or immediate operative intervention (if the patient is unstable).

d. Diaphragm
   i. To assess for rupture, the diaphragm should be assessed for elevation, obliteration, or irregularity.
   ii. Examine for air- or Orogastric/Nasogastric tube-containing stomach or mass-like density (bowel, omentum, spleen, etc.) above the diaphragm.

e. Bony thorax
   i. Assess the clavicle, scapula, sternum, and ribs for fractures.
   ii. Clavicular, scapular, and sternal fracture and 1st to 3rd rib fractures are associated with great vessel injuries.
   iii. The 4th to 12th ribs should be carefully examined for two or more contiguous rib fractures in two places, indicating flail chest.
   iv. Lower rib fractures (9th-12th) can be associated with intra-abdominal injuries, such as spleen, liver, or kidney.

f. Soft tissues
   i. Assess soft tissues for disruption of tissue planes and presence of subcutaneous air.

g. Tubes, lines, and foreign bodies
   i. Assess placement and position of *all* lines and tubes.
   ii. Assess location of foreign bodies and correlate this with physical examination; this is especially important to know if a projectile crosses the midline and could result in a great vessel injury.
   iii. Radiopaque markers placed adjacent to ballistic injuries on the skin surface can assist with determining trajectory.

3. Pelvic radiograph: Assess for large pelvic fractures that can lead to massive internal hemorrhage.
   a. Bony pelvis
      i. Assess all pelvic bones and bilateral femurs for fracture.
      ii. Open-book pelvic fracture in a patient with hypotension should be treated with immediate placement of a pelvic binder.

B. Focused Assessment Sonography in Trauma (FAST) examination
1. The FAST examination is a noninvasive way to identify hemorrhage using a bedside ultrasound and helps triage whether the patient should go to the operating room, the CT scanner, or the angiography suite.
2. The FAST examination is particularly important in the unstable blunt trauma patient—identification of free fluid on these patients should direct these patients to the operating room (**Figure 5-2**).
3. The following images are obtained:
   a. Pericardial sac using a subxiphoid or parasternal view
   b. Hepatorenal fossa using a midaxillary view at the 10th or 11th rib space
   c. Splenorenal fossa using a midaxillary view at the 8th or 9th rib space
   d. Pelvis or pouch of Douglas using a suprapubic view

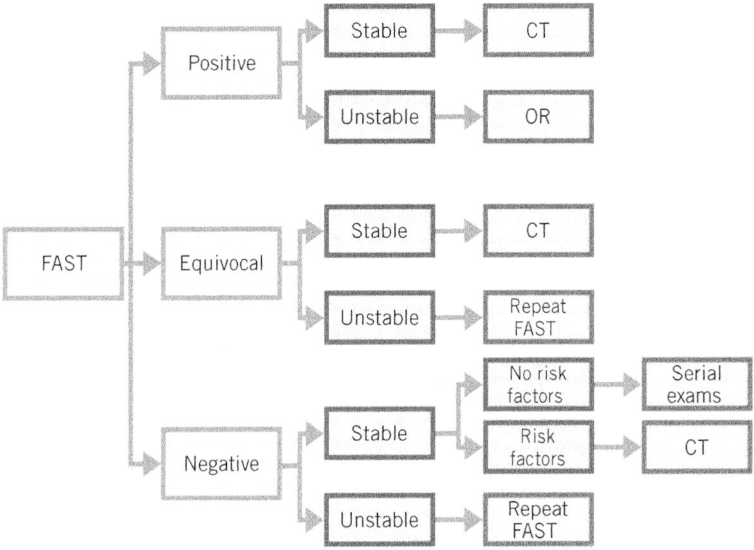

FIGURE 5-2 FAST algorithm for blunt abdominal trauma.

C. Invasive monitoring
1. Arterial blood gas, end-tidal CO_2 monitoring, and central venous pressure monitoring can be used to assess cardiovascular and respiratory function.
2. Foley catheterization
   a. Allows for assessment for hematuria, indicating possible renal and/or urologic trauma.
   b. Allows continuous monitoring of renal perfusion (adequate resuscitation volume replacement should produce a urinary output of at least 0.5 mL/kg/h in adults and 1 mL/kg/h in children), which is an indication of overall circulation and can guide resuscitation.
   c. Contraindications for Foley placement without radiographic confirmation of an intact urethra include blood at the urethral meatus or a high-riding, mobile, or nonpalpable prostate.

V. SECONDARY SURVEY

The secondary survey follows the primary survey. It is a complete head-to-toe examination of the patient designed to inventory all injuries sustained in the trauma. Thoroughness is the key to finding all injuries, and a systematic approach is required. Diagnostic evaluation is necessary for making decisions about subsequent interventions or evaluations.

Key References

Citation	Summary
Cotton BA, Au BK, Nunez TC, Gunter OL, Robertson AM, Young PP. Predefined massive transfusion protocols are associated with a reduction in organ failure and postinjury complications. *J Trauma.* 2009;66(1):41-49.	• Trauma patients requiring massive transfusion (>10 units of blood within 24 h of injury) have lower rates of multiorgan failure and infectious complications when blood products are delivered early and in a balanced ratio.
Holcomb JB, Tilley BC, Baraniuk S, et al. Transfusion of plasma, platelets, and red blood cells in a 1:1:1 vs a 1:1:2 ratio and mortality in patients with severe trauma: the PROPPR randomized clinical trial. *JAMA.* 2015;313(5):471-482.	• Although severely injured patients randomized to receive plasma, platelets, and red blood cells in a 1:1:1 ratio compared to those receiving products in a 1:1:2 ratio did not have a statistically significant improvement in 24-h or 30-d mortality, they were more likely to achieve hemostasis and experienced fewer deaths due to exsanguination.
CRASH-2 trial collaborators, Shakur H, Roberts I, et al. Effects of tranexamic acid on death, vascular occlusive events, and blood transfusion in trauma patients with significant haemorrhage (CRASH-2): a randomised, placebo-controlled trial. *Lancet.* 2010;376(9734):23-32.	• In this randomized placebo-controlled trial, adult trauma patients randomized to receive tranexamic acid vs placebo had significantly reduced all-cause mortality.
Gonzalez E, Moore EE, Moore HB, et al. Goal-directed hemostatic resuscitation of trauma-induced coagulopathy: a pragmatic randomized clinical trial comparing a viscoelastic assay to conventional coagulation assays. *Ann Surg.* 2016;263(6):1051-1059.	• In this randomized clinical trial, goal-directed massive transfusion utilizing TEG improved patient survival compared to massive transfusion directed by conventional coagulation assays.

CHAPTER 5: TRAUMA RESUSCITATION AND ADJUNCTS

Review Questions

1. What are the components of the primary survey?
2. What are the signs and symptoms of a tension pneumothorax?
3. Where on the chest should a tube thoracostomy be placed?
4. How do you diagnose cardiac tamponade? How do you treat it?

5. What are the components of your circulation assessment?
6. What is a contraindication to Foley placement in the trauma patient? What sign on physical examination will make you suspect this?
7. What are the components of the Glasgow Coma Scale?

REFERENCES

1. Schreiber MA, Meier EN, Tisherman SA, et al. A controlled resuscitation strategy is feasible and safe in hypotensive trauma patients: results of a prospective randomized pilot trial. *J Trauma Acute Care Surg.* 2015;78(4):687-695; discussion 695-697.
2. CRASH-2 trial collaborators; Shakur H, Roberts I, Bautista R, et al. Effects of tranexamic acid on death, vascular occlusive events, and blood transfusion in trauma patients with significant haemorrhage (CRASH-2): a randomised, placebo-controlled trial. *Lancet.* 2010;376(9734):23-32.
3. Seamon MJ, Haut ER, Van Arendonk K, et al. An evidence-based approach to patient selection for emergency department thoracotomy: a practice management guideline from the Eastern Association for the Surgery of Trauma. *J Trauma Acute Care Surg.* 2015;79(1):159-173.
4. Panossian VS, Nederpelt CJ, El Hechi MW, et al. Emergency resuscitative thoracotomy: a nationwide analysis of outcomes and predictors of futility. *J Surg Res.* 2020;255:486-494.
5. Cotton BA, Au BK, Nunez TC, Gunter OL, Robertson AM, Young PP. Predefined massive transfusion protocols are associated with a reduction in organ failure and postinjury complications. *J Trauma.* 2009;66(1):41-48; discussion 48-49.
6. Holcomb JB, Tilley BC, Baraniuk S, et al. Transfusion of plasma, platelets, and red blood cells in a 1:1:1 vs a 1:1:2 ratio and mortality in patients with severe trauma: the PROPPR randomized clinical trial. *JAMA.* 2015;313(5):471-482.
7. Gonzalez E, Moore EE, Moore HB, et al. Goal-directed hemostatic resuscitation of trauma-induced coagulopathy: a pragmatic randomized clinical trial comparing a viscoelastic assay to conventional coagulation assays. *Ann Surg.* 2016;263(6):1051-1059.

6 Head, Neck, and Spinal Trauma

Erin G. Andrade and Jessica K. Staszak

I. INITIAL TRAUMA EVALUATION

A. Primary Survey: Glasgow Coma Scale (GCS) is an important tool to quickly assess neurologic function, determine additional diagnostics, and predict neurologic recovery.

1. Eye opening response
4: Eyes open spontaneously
3: Eyes open to verbal command
2: Eyes open to pain
1: No eye opening

2. Verbal response
5: Answers questions appropriately
4: Disoriented but still able to converse
3: Inappropriate responses but still verbalizes words
2: Incomprehensible speech or sounds
1: No verbal response

3. Motor response
6: Obeys commands
5: Purposeful movement to pain
4: Withdraws from pain
3: Decorticate (flexion) positioning.
2: Decerebrate (extension) positioning
1: No motor response

B. Secondary survey

1. Complete neurologic examination

2. Head and face

a. Facial soft tissue and bone examination

i. Lacerations

ii. Bony deformities, instability, or step offs indicate fractures.

iii. Ecchymosis over the mastoid process (Battle's sign) can indicate skull fracture.

b. Eye examination

i. Evaluate globus and orbit structure. Signs of trauma include periorbital instability or conjunctival hemorrhage.

ii. Unilateral pupillary dilatation may herald the onset of early brain herniation.

iii. Periorbital hematoma (raccoon eyes) may signify basal skull fractures.

iv. Extraocular movement examination assesses for entrapment.

c. Nasal examination
   i. Signs of nasal bone fractures include septal deviation and epistaxis.
   ii. Cerebrospinal fluid (CSF) rhinorrhea is sign of a basal skull fracture.
d. Ear examination
   i. The ears should be assessed for ruptured tympanic membranes, hemotympanum, and otorrhea, which can be signs of basal skull fracture.
e. Oral cavity examination
   i. The oral cavity should be assessed for missing dentition, mucosal or glossal violations, and foreign bodies.

3. Spine examination
   a. Following blunt trauma, patients with potential cervical spine injuries require cervical spine immobilization. For proper examination, remove the cervical collar and maintain the neck in a neutral position.
   b. The entire spine should be assessed for posterior midline tenderness and palpated for deformities.

II. RADIOGRAPHIC EVALUATION OF HEAD AND FACIAL INJURIES

A. Noncontrasted CT of the head
   1. Penetrating trauma: Determine trajectory of injury
   2. Blunt head trauma
      a. Noncontrasted head CT indicated for patients with GCS < 13 or with a decline in neurologic examination during observation.
      b. For patients with GCS 13 to 15, the Canadian CT Head Rule is used to determine who warrants head CT.[1] See **Table 6.1** for an overview of these indications.
      c. The indications for imaging in patients on anticoagulation are the same; however, these patients should undergo a longer observation period prior to discharge to rule out delayed hemorrhage.

B. Noncontrasted CT of the face
   1. Patients with significant craniofacial soft-tissue injury or clinical signs of facial fractures, such as bony deformities, instability, or step offs, require radiographic evaluation to determine bony integrity.
   2. Facial CT has generally supplanted facial plain films for this purpose.

III. TYPES OF HEAD INJURIES

A. Epidural hematomas (EDHs)
   1. Classically present with a "lucid interval" after injury, followed by rapid deterioration.
      a. Nonspecific sign as this can also be seen with other forms of severe brain injury.
   2. EDHs typically result from laceration of the middle meningeal artery due to fracture of the squamosal portion of the temporal bone.
   3. CT imaging: Biconvex hyperdensities that typically respect the suture lines (**Figure 6.1A** and **B**).

TABLE 6.1 Canadian CT Head Rule (Initial GCS 13-15)[a]
Age ≥ 65 years
GCS < 15 after 2 h
Open/depressed skull fracture
Signs of basal skull fracture
>Two episodes of emesis
Amnesia ≥ 30 min
Significant mechanism (peds vs. auto, ejected passenger, fall ≥ 3 ft or five stairs)

[a]The Canadian CT rule applies to patients who present with a GCS of 13 to 15, loss of consciousness, amnesia, or confusion, and any of the manifestations in the table (*JAMA*. 2005;294(12):1511-1518).

B. Acute subdural hematomas

1. Result from high-speed acceleration or deceleration trauma and portend severe underlying intracranial injury, leading to shearing or tearing forces.
2. Affected blood vessels are small bridging (emissary) veins that drain the underlying neural tissue into the dural sinuses.
3. CT imaging: Hyperdense crescents representing blood interspersed between the brain surface and dura (**Figure 6.1C**).

C. Chronic SDHs

1. Manifest days to weeks after the initial head injury, especially in the elderly and alcoholic populations.
2. Symptoms include focal neurologic deficits, mental status changes, metabolic abnormalities, and/or seizures. May also be asymptomatic.
3. CT imaging: Crescentic collection tracking between the dura and the brain, hypodense (**Figure 6.1D**).

D. Cerebral contusions

1. Contusion patterns
   - **a.** "Coup" pattern: Injury to the cerebral cortex occurs in the region immediately underlying the site of impact.
   - **b.** "Contrecoup" pattern: Injury to cerebral cortex resulting when brain comes into contact with the opposite side of the skull following the initial impact.
2. CT imaging: Small, punctate hyperdensities that are commonly located in the basal frontal and temporal lobes (**Figure 6.1E**). Small contusions are better visualized on MRI.

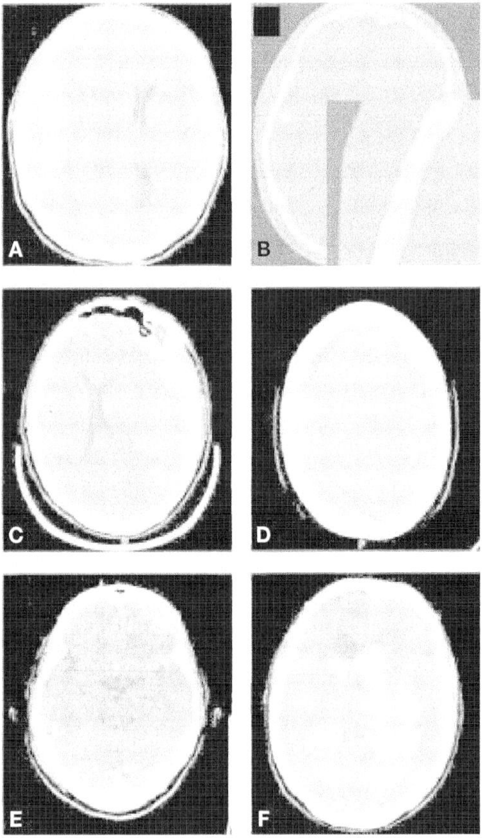

FIGURE 6.1 Noncontrasted head CTs. A, Large right-sided epidural hematoma with mass effect and midline shift; B, bone windows from "A" demonstrating associated linear temporal bone fracture (*asterisk*, see inset); C, left-sided acute subdural hematoma with significant midline shift; D, bilateral mixed-density subdural hematomas with both acute (hyperdense) and chronic (hypodense) components; E, bilateral frontal and right-sided temporal hemorrhagic contusions with surrounding edema (hypodense); and F, large left-sided basal ganglia intraparenchymal hemorrhage (nontraumatic, likely related to hypertension) with intraventricular extension resulting in acute hydrocephalus.

E. Intraparenchymal hemorrhages
   1. Result from lacerations of larger cerebral vessels
      a. May progress to brain herniation in severe cases.
      b. Extension of bleeding into the ventricular system may result in intraventricular hemorrhage, which can lead to hydrocephalus due to impaired CSF reabsorption.
   2. CT imaging: Focal areas of hyperdensity, typically with hypodensity surrounding areas of edema (**Figure 6.1F**)

F. Skull and facial fractures
1. Classification
a. Open vs. closed
i. Open: Associated with overlying laceration.
ii. Closed: Bony injury is not exposed by overlying soft tissue injury.
b. Depressed vs. nondepressed
i. Depressed: Skull is sunken into intracranial cavity. Higher risk of underlying cerebral contusion.
ii. Nondepressed: Intracranial cavity is not violated by fracture.
2. Management
a. Closed, nondepressed fractures are often managed nonoperatively.
b. Open, depressed fractures may require elevation and debridement of depressed bony fragments as well as devitalized tissue, followed by a course of antibiotics.

IV. MANAGEMENT OF HEAD INJURIES

This section focuses on the initial management of head injuries. For a more in-depth discussion of this topic, please refer to the guidelines for the management of severe traumatic brain injury (TBI).[2] Neurosurgical consultation should be sought immediately when these injuries are identified.

A. Preservation of cerebral perfusion

The goal is preservation of cerebral perfusion in order to prevent secondary injury. This is achieved by maintaining intracranial pressure (ICP) < 20 mm Hg and cerebral perfusion pressure (CPP) between 60 and 70 mm Hg (CPP = mean arterial pressure − ICP).

1. Monitoring and treatment of elevated ICP
a. ICP monitoring (i.e., bolt) is recommended if serial neurologic examinations cannot be used as a reliable indicator of progressive intracranial pathology.
b. Management of elevated ICP
i. Initial steps in the management of elevated ICP, as listed in **Table 6.2**, include sedation, pain control, osmotic diuretics, head of bed elevation, and hyperventilation.
ii. In a randomized clinical trial (RESCUEicp), decompressive craniectomy in patients with TBI and refractory intracranial hypertension resulted in lower mortality but were more likely to experience severe disability.[3]
2. Maintain adequate mean arterial pressure
a. Hemorrhage control, maintenance of normovolemia, and vasopressor use
b. Hypotension (systolic blood pressure < 90 mm Hg) is associated with poor outcomes in severely head-injured patients.

B. Coagulopathy
1. Occurs in one-third of patients and should be corrected expeditiously to minimize intracranial hematoma expansion[4]
2. Correction guidelines

TABLE 6.2 Therapies for Intracranial Hypertension

Therapeutic Modality	Usage
Mannitol	• Dose: 0.25-1 g/kg IV q2–6h in hemodynamically stable patients with adequate renal function • Monitor electrolytes • Keep serum osmolarity < 320 • Strict ins and outs
Hypertonic saline 3%	• Dose: 250-mL bolus IV q6h (30-60 mL IV q6h if 23.4% hypertonic saline is used) or continuous infusion 1 mL/kg/h • Place central line • Keep Na < 160 mmol/L
Hyperventilation ($PaCO_2$ 30-35 mm Hg)	• Limit use to acute and emergent situations, until other interventions take effect • This may worsen cerebral ischemia
Sedation	• To prevent agitation, pain, and patient–ventilator dyssynchrony
Metabolic suppression (barbiturate coma)	• Usually reserved for refractory elevation of ICP • Adequate hemodynamic monitoring is needed to prevent hypotension
Surgical decompression	Consider for patients with: • Mass lesions • Uncontrollable ICPs • Deteriorating neurologic examination
Temperature control	• Normothermia: avoid fevers (antipyretics, cooling blankets, etc.)
Other	• Elevate the head of the bed to 30° • CSF drainage by ventriculostomy

a. International normalized ratio ≤1.4
b. Partial thromboplastin time < 40 seconds
c. Platelets ≥ 100,000

3. Thromboelastography with platelet mapping can provide more specific metrics for resuscitation and has been associated with lower mortality.[5]
4. Anticoagulants and antiplatelet agents should be discontinued and reversed (if applicable).

C. Functional recovery

1. After moderate to severe TBI, approximately a quarter of patients who undergo inpatient rehabilitation will achieve disability-free recovery by 1 year.[6]

2. Medical therapy
   a. Catecholaminergic agents and stimulants have been trialed to assess for increased neurologic recovery following TBI.
   b. Amantadine has been shown to increase the rate of functional recovery of patients with TBI undergoing rehabilitation.[7]

V. INJURIES OF THE NECK AND CERVICAL SPINE

A. Penetrating neck injury (**Figure 6.2**)
   1. Associated with vascular and aerodigestive injuries
   2. Physical examination
      a. Hard signs—indications for immediate surgical exploration
         i. Shock
         ii. Pulsatile bleeding or expanding hematoma
         iii. Audible bruit of palpable thrill
         iv. Airway compromise
      b. Soft signs
         i. Minor hemoptysis and hematemesis
         ii. Nonexpanding hematoma
         iii. Dysphonia
         iv. Dysphagia
   3. Classification of penetrating neck injuries
      a. Classification based on anatomic landmarks:
         i. **Zone I**, the thoracic inlet, from the manubrium to the cricoid cartilage
         ii. **Zone II**, the mid neck, from the cricoid cartilage to the angle of the mandible
         iii. **Zone III**, the upper neck, from the angle of mandible to the base of the skull
   4. Diagnosis
      a. Patients with penetrating neck injuries who are hemodynamically stable should undergo CT angiography (CTA) to determine the trajectory of the injury and to plan the operative approach.
      b. If an esophageal injury is suspected and CTA is equivocal, esophagoscopy and esophagography may be performed.
      c. Bronchoscopy should be performed if tracheal injury is suspected.
   5. Management
      a. In the unstable patient, ATLS algorithms should be followed to secure an airway and tamponade of any active bleeding should be attempted. If patients are not able to lie flat, or are not sufficiently stable to undergo diagnostic imaging, they should undergo emergent neck exploration.
      b. Surgical techniques: Operative approach is generally based on location of injury (see **Table 6.3**).
         i. Median sternotomy: Indicated for surgical management of zone 1 injuries.
            a) Skin incision is made between sternal notch and the xiphoid process.

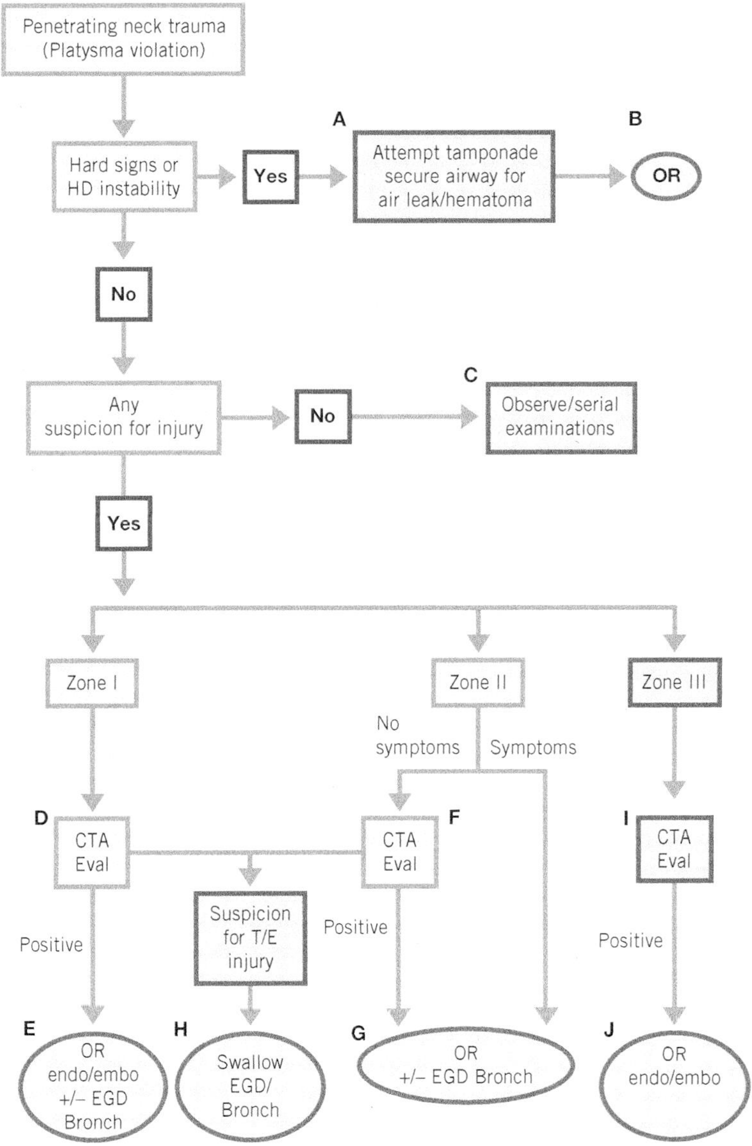

FIGURE 6.2 Western Trauma Association management algorithm for penetrating neck trauma. EGD, esophagogastroduodenoscopy; HD, hemodynamic; OR, Operating room; T/E, trachea/esophagus. *(Adapted from Sperry JL, Moore EE, Coimbra R, et al. Western Trauma Association critical decisions in trauma: penetrating neck trauma. J Trauma Acute Care Surg. 2013;75(6):936-940.)*

TABLE 6.3 Zones of Penetrating Neck Injury

Zone	Operative Approach
1	Median sternotomy with possible extension along sternocleidomastoid or supraclavicular incision
2	Transverse cervical collar incision or anterior sternocleidomastoid incision
3	Preferably endovascular, difficult to control operatively, need to dislocate mandible

b) The incision is extended through the subcutaneous tissue to expose the sternum.
c) The periosteum is lifted off the sternum.
d) Using a sternal saw or a Lebsche knife, the sternum is divided to expose mediastinal structures.

ii. Transverse cervical collar incision or anterior sternocleidomastoid incision: Indicated for surgical management of zone 2 injuries. Technique for exposure via anterior sternocleidomastoid incision:

a) Longitudinal skin incision is made along the anterior border of sternocleidomastoid muscle.
b) Incision is carried through the platysma.
c) Initial structures that are encountered are the internal jugular vein and the carotid sheath.
d) During the dissection, special attention should be paid to the preservation of cranial nerves (vagus, glossopharyngeal, hypoglossal, marginal mandibular branch of facial nerve).

iii. Endovascular approach

a) Useful approach for zone 3 injuries, as open exposure may require dislocation of mandible.

B. Cervical spine

1. Radiographic evaluation

a. Guidelines such as the Canadian C-Spine Rule and NEXUS are used to determine who can be clinically cleared and who should undergo imaging.

i. NEXUS criteria—cervical spine imaging is not indicated if[8]:

a) No posterior midline tenderness
b) No intoxication or altered mental status

c) No focal deficit
d) No painful distracting injuries

ii. For the Canadian C-Spine Rule, see **Figure 6.3**.[9]

b. Use of a standardized protocol significantly increases detection rates, although more data are emerging to determine which injuries need intervention.

2. Spine immobilization in the setting of penetrating trauma is associated with increased mortality, likely due to delayed recognition of injuries, and of no benefit for decreasing progression of neurologic injuries.[10]

VI. MANAGEMENT OF BLUNT CEREBROVASCULAR INJURY

A. Introduction

1. Blunt cerebrovascular injury (BCVI) to the carotid or vertebral arteries carries significant morbidity, including the possibility of cerebral hemorrhage or stroke (CVA).
2. See **Table 6.4** for classification of BCVI.[11,12]
3. Such injuries are commonly a result of hyperextension or hyperflexion with rotation of the neck or a direct blow to the cervical region.

B. Diagnosis

1. CTA should be obtained if patients meet Denver criteria for BCVI as listed in **Table 6.5**.[13]

C. Management of BCVI

1. Grades I-IV receive antithrombotic therapy or anticoagulation and an interval follow-up CTA.
   a. EAST 2020 guidelines recommend antithrombotic therapy over anticoagulation based on the CADISS trial, which showed no difference between the two groups.[14]
   b. A more recent randomized noninferiority trial (TREAT-CAD) was unable to show noninferiority of aspirin compared with coumadin.[15]
2. Endovascular stenting was previously used routinely for grade II and grade III injuries, but due to a high risk of complications including in-stent thrombosis, it is now only used in the setting of worsening injury.[16]
3. Grade V injuries require surgical or endovascular intervention for bleeding control.

VII. THORACOLUMBAR SPINAL INJURIES

A. Diagnostic imaging

1. Patients with back pain, thoracolumbar spine tenderness, neurologic deficits, or known or suspected high-energy mechanisms in which spinal trauma might be sustained should be screened with a CT scan of the axial spine to include the thoracic, lumbar, and sacral regions.

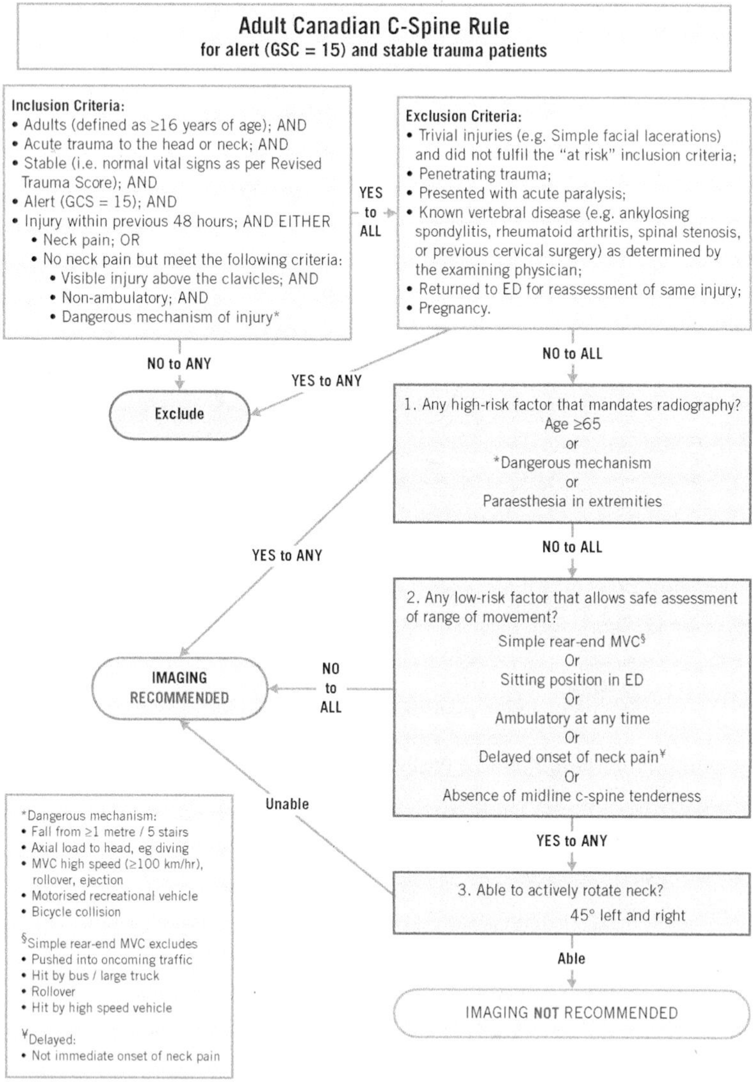

FIGURE 6.3 An example of a decision support flowchart illustrating the Canadian Adult C-Spine Rule (adult cervical spine trauma). ED, emergency department; MVC, motor vehicle collision. *(From Saragiotto BT, Maher CG, Lin CWC, Verhagen AP, Goergen S, Michaleff ZA. Canadian C-spine rule and the National Emergency X-Radiography Utilization Study (NEXUS) for detecting clinically important cervical spine injury following blunt trauma. Cochrane Database Syst Rev. 2018;2018(4):CD012989. Copyright 2018, The Cochrane Collaboration.)*

TABLE 6.4 Blunt Cerebral Vascular Injury Grading System

Grade	Imaging Description
1	Luminal irregularity or dissection with <25% luminal narrowing
2	Dissection or intramural hematoma with >25% luminal narrowing, intraluminal thrombus, or raised intimal flap
3	Pseudoaneurysm
4	Occlusion
5	Transection with free extravasation

Also referred to as Denver or Biffl scale.

2. A CT scan should be considered for patients with a known or suspected injury to the cervical spine, or any other region of the spine, due to the high incidence of concurrent spinal injuries.

B. Types of spinal injuries

The spinal column is divided into the anterior, middle, and posterior columns. The **anterior column** contains the anterior longitudinal ligament,

TABLE 6.5 Updated Denver Screening Criteria for BCVI

Signs and Symptoms

- Arterial hemorrhage from neck/nose/mouth
- Cervical bruit in patient <50 year old
- Expanding cervical hematoma
- Focal neurologic defect: transient ischemic attack, hemiparesis, vertebrobasilar symptoms, Horner syndrome
- Neurologic deficit inconsistent with head CT
- Ischemic stroke on CT or MRI

Risk Factors

- High-energy transfer mechanism with
- LeFort II or III fracture
- Cervical spine fracture with subluxation, fractures extending into the transverse foramen, or fractures of C1–C3
- Basilar skull fracture with carotid canal involvement
- Near hanging with anoxic brain injury
- Diffuse axonal injury with GCS ≤ 6

anterior half of the annulus fibrosus, and vertebral body. The **middle column** consists of the posterior ligament, posterior half of the annulus fibrosus, and vertebral body, and the **posterior column** consists of the ligamentum flavum, articulating facets, lamina, and spinous processes. As a generalized rule, an injury affecting one column is stable; however, an injury affecting two or more columns is unstable.

1. Compression fractures
   a. Mechanism of injury: Axial loading forces on the spinal column, resulting in height loss of the anterior portion of the vertebral body.
   b. These are usually stable injuries because only one column is usually affected. In some patients, there is a >50% loss in height of the anterior vertebral body, which places the posterior column under significant strain.
   c. Management: C-collar/thoracic brace vs. surgical fixation procedures on an individualized basis.
2. Burst fractures
   a. Mechanism of injury axial loading.
   b. These fractures involve both the anterior and middle columns. Burst fractures are potentially unstable and carry a high incidence of associated neurologic injuries.
   c. Management of these injuries is individualized.
3. Penetrating injuries to the neck and torso
   a. May result in fractures of the spine or penetration of the spinal canal.
   b. While these injuries are often stable, indications for surgery include deterioration of neurologic status, spinal compression, or cauda equina syndrome, as well as complications related to presence of a foreign body.

Key References

Citation	Summary
Hutchinson PJ, Kolias AG, Timofeev IS, et al. Trial of decompressive craniectomy for traumatic intracranial hypertension. *N Engl J Med*. 2016; 375(12):1119-1130.	• The RESCUEicp Trial demonstrated that decompressive craniectomy in patients with refractory intracranial hypertension resulted in not only lower rates of mortality but also an increase in the proportion of patients in the following categories at 6 mo: vegetative state, "lower severe disability" (defined as independent at home), and "upper severe disability" (defined as dependent on others for care).

Citation	Summary
Cannon JW, Dias JD, Kumar MA, et al. Use of thromboelastography in the evaluation and management of patients with traumatic brain injury: a systematic review and meta-analysis. *Crit Care Explor.* 2021;3(9):e0526.	• Abnormalities in thromboeslastography (TEG) and thromboelastopgraphy with platelet mapping (TEG-PM) are associated with poor outcomes in patients with TBI. • TEG and TEG-PM can provide more precise data to guide resuscitation.
Giacino JT, Whyte J, Bagiella E, et al. Placebo-controlled trial of amantadine for severe traumatic brain injury. *N Engl J Med.* 2012;366(9):819-826.	• A total of 184 patients with severe TBI were randomized to receive either amantadine or placebo. • After approximately 4 wk of follow-up, patients treated with amantadine achieved improved functional recovery based on the Disability Rating Scale compared with those receiving placebo.
Markus HS, Levi C, King A, Madigan J, Norris J; Cervical Artery Dissection in Stroke Study (CADISS) Investigators. Antiplatelet therapy vs anticoagulation therapy in cervical artery dissection: the Cervical Artery Dissection in Stroke Study (CADISS) randomized clinical trial final results. *JAMA Neurol.* 2019;76(6):657-664.	• A total of 250 patients with traumatic cervical dissection were randomized to receive either antiplatelet or anticoagulation (heparin followed by warfarin) for 3 mo. • After 1 y of follow-up, the risk of stroke for either group was approximately 2.5%. There was no significant difference between the two groups.
Engelter ST, Traenka C, Gensicke H, et al. Aspirin versus anticoagulation in cervical artery dissection (TREAT-CAD): an open-label, randomised, non-inferiority trial. *Lancet Neurol.* 2021;20(5):341-350.	• Noninferiority trial design: 194 patients with traumatic cervical dissections were randomized to receive aspirin vs. vitamin K antagonist. The primary endpoint was composite outcome of stroke, major hemorrhage, and death. • The primary endpoint occurred in 23% of the aspirin group vs. 15% of the vitamin K antagonist group, which did not meet predetermined noninferiority criteria.

CHAPTER 6: HEAD, NECK, AND SPINAL TRAUMA

Review Questions

1. What are the signs of a potential blunt cerebral vascular injury?
2. Does decompressive craniectomy among those with severe TBI and refractory intracranial hypertension result in more survivors in a vegetative state?
3. Is the use of a cervical collar indicated in penetrating neck trauma?
4. Which type of head injury typically presents with a lucid interval prior to a worsening neurologic examination?
5. How do epidural and subdural hematomas appear on noncontrasted head CT?
6. If a penetrating neck injury requires an operative intervention, what is the operative approach based on zone of injury?

REFERENCES

1. Stiell IG, Clement CM, Rowe BH, et al. Comparison of the Canadian CT head rule and the New Orleans criteria in patients with minor head injury. *JAMA*. 2005;294(12):1511-1518.
2. Carney N, Totten AM, O'Reilly C, et al. Guidelines for the management of severe traumatic brain injury, fourth edition. *Neurosurgery*. 2017;80(1):6-15.
3. Hutchinson PJ, Kolias AG, Timofeev IS, et al. Trial of decompressive craniectomy for traumatic intracranial hypertension. *N Engl J Med*. 2016;375(12):1119-1130.
4. Simmons JW, Pittet JF, Pierce B. Trauma-induced coagulopathy. *Curr Anesthesiol Rep*. 2014;4(3):189-199.
5. Cannon JW, Dias JD, Kumar MA, et al. Use of thromboelastography in the evaluation and management of patients with traumatic brain injury: a systematic review and meta-analysis. *Crit Care Explor*. 2021;3(9):e0526.
6. Schneider EB, Sur S, Raymont V, et al. Functional recovery after moderate/severe traumatic brain injury: a role for cognitive reserve? *Neurology*. 2014;82(18):1636-1642.
7. Giacino JT, Whyte J, Bagiella E, et al. Placebo-controlled trial of amantadine for severe traumatic brain injury. *N Engl J Med*. 2012;366(9):819-826.
8. Hoffman JR, Mower WR, Wolfson AB, Todd KH, Zucker MI. Validity of a set of clinical criteria to rule out injury to the cervical spine in patients with blunt trauma. National Emergency X-Radiography Utilization Study Group. *N Engl J Med*. 2000;343(2):94-99.
9. Stiell IG, Wells GA, Vandemheen KL, et al. The Canadian C-spine rule for radiography in alert and stable trauma patients. *JAMA*. 2001;286(15):1841-1848.
10. Velopulos CG, Shihab HM, Lottenberg L, et al. Prehospital spine immobilization/spinal motion restriction in penetrating trauma: a practice management guideline from the Eastern Association for the Surgery of Trauma (EAST). *J Trauma Acute Care Surg*. 2018;84(5):736-744.
11. Fabian TC, George SM Jr, Croce MA, Mangiante EC, Voeller GR, Kudsk KA. Carotid artery trauma: management based on mechanism of injury. *J Trauma*. 1990;30(8):953-961; discussion 961-3.
12. Foreman PM, Griessenauer CJ, Kicielinski KP, et al. Reliability assessment of the Biffl scale for blunt traumatic cerebrovascular injury as detected on computer tomography angiography. *J Neurosurg*. 2017;127(1):32-35.

13. Burlew CC, Biffl WL, Moore EE, Barnett CC, Johnson JL, Bensard DD. Blunt cerebrovascular injuries: redefining screening criteria in the era of noninvasive diagnosis. *J Trauma Acute Care Surg.* 2012;72(2):330-335; discussion 336-337, quiz 539.

14. Markus HS, Levi C, King A, Madigan J, Norris J; Cervical Artery Dissection in Stroke Study CADISS Investigators. Antiplatelet therapy vs anticoagulation therapy in cervical artery dissection: the Cervical Artery Dissection in Stroke Study (CADISS) randomized clinical trial final results. *JAMA Neurol.* 2019;76(6):657-664.

15. Engelter ST, Traenka C, Gensicke H, et al. Aspirin versus anticoagulation in cervical artery dissection (TREAT-CAD): an open-label, randomised, non-inferiority trial. *Lancet Neurol.* 2021;20(5):341-350.

16. Kim DY, Biffl W, Bokhari F, et al. Evaluation and management of blunt cerebrovascular injury: a practice management guideline from the Eastern Association for the Surgery of Trauma. *J Trauma Acute Care Surg.* 2020;88(6):875-887.

7 Chest Trauma

Hannah M. Phelps, Jordan M. Kirsch, and
Melissa K. Stewart

I. INTRODUCTION

Thoracic injuries occur in 20% to 25% of all traumas and may contribute to as many as 75% of trauma-related deaths. As such, prompt diagnosis and management of injuries to the heart, lungs, great vessels, and other mediastinal structures is essential.

A. Initial workup
  1. Advanced Trauma Life Support protocols should be followed.
  2. Specific to thoracic trauma, as part of the primary and secondary surveys, the physical examination should evaluate for absence of breath sounds, presence of chest wall contusion/crepitus, flail segments, penetrating injuries, and evidence of prior thoracic surgery (thoracotomy/sternotomy scar).
  3. In addition, as adjuncts to the primary survey, the patient should undergo CXR and focused assessment with sonography for trauma (FAST)/extended focused assessment with sonography for trauma to evaluate for life-threatening injuries in need of immediate intervention.

B. Anatomy
  1. Heart and pericardium
     a. The heart is a mediastinal structure positioned with the left and right ventricles facing anteriorly, causing these to be the most commonly injured chambers. The left atrium lies posteriorly and is least commonly injured.
     b. The pericardium is a thin membranous sac surrounding the heart composed of parietal and visceral layers with an intervening potential space (up to 30 mL of fluid in space is physiologically normal).
     c. Phrenic nerves run along the lateral aspect of the pericardium.
     d. The vagus nerve runs posterior to the pericardium and lung root.
  2. Lungs and pleura
     a. The parietal pleura lines the chest wall, and the visceral pleura covers the lungs. Between the pleural layers there is a potential space.
     b. The right lung has three lobes; the left lung has two lobes.
  3. Tracheobronchial tree
     a. The trachea enters the thoracic inlet down to the carina, located at T4, where it then splits into right and left mainstem bronchi.
  4. Esophagus
     a. Four segments
        i. Cervical esophagus: Cricoid to suprasternal notch, deviates left
           a) Blood supply: Esophageal branches of inferior thyroid artery
        ii. Upper thoracic esophagus: Suprasternal notch to carina, courses right of the aorta

a) Blood supply: Esophageal branches of bronchial arteries

iii. Midthoracic esophagus: Carina to gastroesophageal (GE) junction, weaves under left mainstem bronchus

a) Blood supply: Esophageal branches of bronchial arteries

iv. Lower/abdominal esophagus: GE junction at the diaphragmatic hiatus (T11)

a) Blood supply: Left gastric and phrenic arteries

5. Chest wall and diaphragm

a. Twelve ribs articulate posteriorly with transverse and costal facets of thoracic vertebrae. Ribs 1 to 6 (true ribs) articulate directly with the sternum anteriorly, ribs 6 to 10 (false ribs) fuse costal cartilages to articulate with the inferior sternum, ribs 11 to 12 (floating ribs) do not articulate with the sternum.

i. The neurovascular bundle runs inferior to ribs.

b. Three major diaphragmatic foramina allow for passage of key structures: IVC at T8, esophagus at T10, aorta at T12

i. The phrenic nerve arises from C3, C4, C5 and runs through posterolateral mediastinum to diaphragm.

C. Physiology

1. Cardiac tamponade physiology (occurs in three phases)

a. Phase 1: Increasing pericardial pressure decreases diastolic ventricular filling → reduction in subendocardial blood flow → tachycardia

b. Phase 2: Decreased diastolic filling, stroke volume, and coronary perfusion → anxiety, diaphoresis, pallor

c. Phase 3: Compensatory mechanisms fail → loss of cardiac perfusion → cardiac arrest

2. Tension pneumothorax physiology

a. Continuous accumulation of air in the pleural space → increased pleural/intrathoracic pressure → decreased return of blood to the heart (preload) → cardiopulmonary compromise and eventual arrest

II. CARDIAC INJURY

A. Epidemiology/Etiology/Classification

1. Blunt cardiac injury

a. Caused by direct energy transfer to the heart via compression of the heart between sternum and vertebral column or direct injury from sternal or rib fracture

b. May manifest as free septal rupture, free wall rupture, coronary artery thrombosis, cardiomyopathy, dysrhythmia, or rupture of chordae tendinae/papillary muscles

c. See **Figure 7.1** for algorithmic approach to blunt cardiac injury

2. Penetrating cardiac injury

a. Right ventricle most commonly injured due to anterior position

b. Causes obstructive or hemorrhagic shock depending on integrity of pericardial sac

i. Classic presentation of acute pericardial tamponade: **Beck's triad** = hypotension, diminished heart sounds, distended neck veins

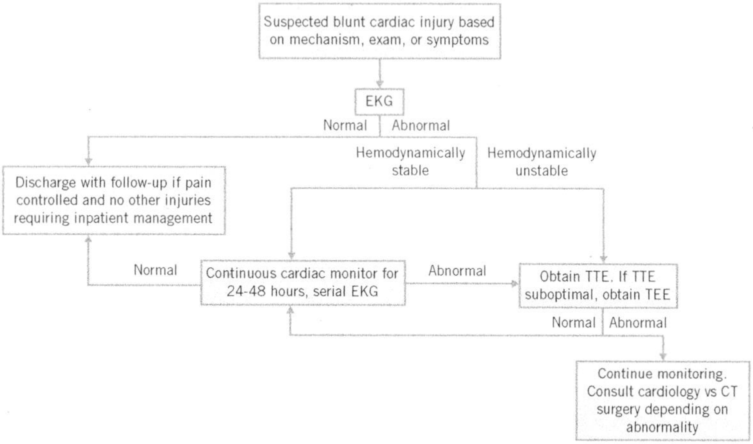

FIGURE 7.1 Workup and management of blunt cardiac injury. TEE, transesophageal echocardiogram; TTE, transthoracic echocardiogram.

c. See **Figure 7.2** for algorithmic approach to penetrating cardiac injury.
d. The subxiphoid window is a useful technique to evaluate for suspected cardiac injury during abdominal exploration.
e. **Surgical technique: Subxiphoid window**
   i. A subxiphoid window can be made during trauma exploratory laparotomy to evaluate for hemopericardium and possible cardiac injury. Extend the midline incision superiorly up to the tip of the xiphoid process.
   ii. Excise the xiphoid process, retract the sternum anteriorly, and bluntly dissect the anterior diaphragm until the cardiophrenic fat pad is exposed.
   iii. Make a small vertical incision in the pericardium. Be careful to identify and preserve the phrenic nerves.
   iv. If blood is encountered, further exploration to identify and manage a cardiac injury is warranted through a median sternotomy.

B. Diagnosis/Testing
1. Laboratory studies
   a. No laboratory test can diagnose cardiac injury in isolation.
   b. Elevation of cardiac enzymes (troponin) in conjunction with EKG changes can suggest blunt cardiac injury, although the role of cardiac enzymes in evaluating for blunt cardiac injury remains controversial.[1]
2. Imaging
   a. Ultrasound, traditionally via subxiphoid view of FAST examination, can be used to assess for pericardial effusion in trauma bay
      i. Note poor negative predictive value with concomitant hemothorax
   b. Formal echocardiography (transthoracic or transesophageal) used to assess structural injuries

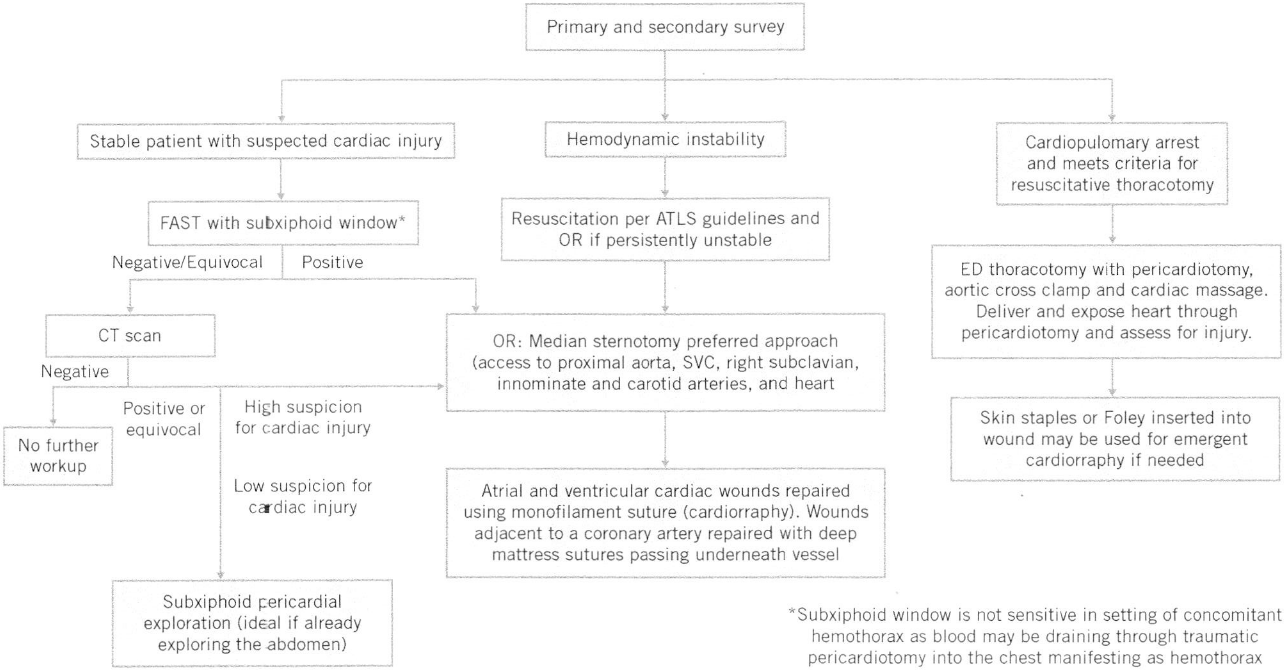

FIGURE 7.2 Workup and management of penetrating cardiac injury. OR, Operating room; SVC, Superior vena cava.

c. Chest CT should *not* be used for patients with suspected tamponade as emergent intervention is required.

3. Other

a. EKG findings of blunt cardiac trauma: Dysrhythmias (sinus tachycardia most common), bundle branch block, ST changes

i. If EKG is normal, no additional workup is indicated.

C. Treatment

1. Blunt cardiac injury

a. **Figure 7.1** outlines workup and management of blunt cardiac injury

b. Optimize cardiac function in cases of new heart failure or dysrhythmia

c. Structural injury generally requires operative intervention.

i. Cardiac rupture best repaired via median sternotomy

ii. Assess for pericardial tamponade (note that these windows are only diagnostic in the context of chest trauma; positive findings require operative exploration)

a) Subxiphoid window, or classic "pericardial window"

b) Transdiaphragmatic pericardial window if laparotomy is also indicated

2. Penetrating cardiac injury

a. **Figure 7.2** outlines workup and management of penetrating cardiac injury

b. As with blunt cardiac injury, decompression is required in setting of pericardial tamponade

c. Source of hemorrhage must be directly controlled.

d. Left anterolateral thoracotomy with possible bilateral extension (clamshell thoracotomy) preferred approach for trauma resuscitation

D. Outcomes/Complications

1. Pericarditis

a. Presents with fever, chest pain, pericardial rub

b. EKG: Diffuse ST elevation and PR depression in most leads (I, II, III, aVL, aVF)

c. Treat with NSAID

III. CHEST WALL, PLEURAL, AND DIAPHRAGM INJURIES

A. Epidemiology/Etiology/Classification

1. Pneumothorax and hemothorax

a. Pneumothorax: Air enters the thorax from hole in lung or chest wall causing air to accumulate between the parietal and visceral pleura. As the pleural pressure increases, the lung collapses.

i. Tension pneumothorax: Develops when air is trapped between parietal and visceral pleura causing increased intrathoracic pressure, displacement of mediastinal structures to contralateral hemithorax, and decreased venous return to the heart

a) Triad: Absent breath sounds on affected side, tachycardia, hypotension refractory to fluid resuscitation

ii. Open pneumothorax ("sucking chest wound"): Occurs when soft tissue defect >2/3 tracheal circumference is present and air is preferentially drawn into the pleural space via the chest defect when negative intrathoracic pressure is created for inspiration
b. Hemothorax: Accumulation of blood between parietal and visceral pleura
2. Boney injury of thoracic cage
a. Rib fractures
i. May cause acute respiratory failure, particularly in elderly
ii. Flail segment: Fracture of at least two adjacent ribs in at least two places causing paradoxical movement of "flail" segment of chest wall during inspiration
b. Fracture of sternum, clavicle, and/or scapula
3. Diaphragm injury
a. Can be difficult to diagnose but high risk of bowel herniation if not repaired

B. Diagnosis/Testing
1. Laboratory studies
a. None specific
b. Obtain basic trauma laboratory tests including complete blood count (CBC), comprehensive metabolic panel (CMP), clotting studies, type and screen (T&S), urinalysis (UA)
2. Imaging
a. CXR: Used to assess lung parenchyma (contusion) and pleura (hemothorax, pneumothorax), trachea and bronchi (deviation, subcutaneous emphysema), rib and bone fractures; may be able to identify diaphragm injury (viscera in the chest)
b. Chest CT: In stable patients, can help distinguish between pleural fluid collections and pulmonary contusion; also has increased sensitivity for detecting rib fractures and pneumothorax in stable patient
c. Pleural ultrasound: Used to detect pneumothorax/hemothorax and may be more readily available than CXR in certain situations

C. Treatment
1. Pneumothorax and hemothorax
a. **Figure 7.3** outlines the workup and management of hemo/pneumothorax.
b. Tension physiology requires immediate needle decompression or finger thoracostomy.
c. Immediate treatment for open pneumothorax involves supplemental oxygen, three-sided occlusive dressing, and chest tube remote from site of wound.
d. Traditional teaching called for 36 to 38 Fr chest tube for traumatic hemo/pneumothorax in adults; however, recent data show no difference in outcomes with smaller tubes (20-32 Fr) or pigtail catheters.[2]

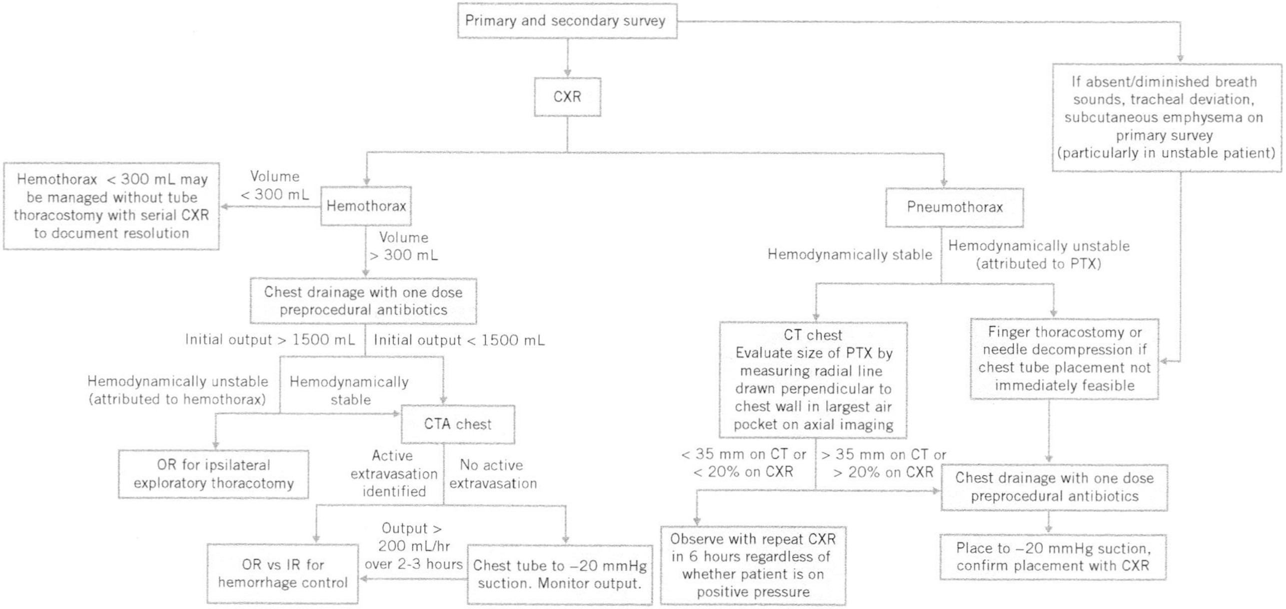

FIGURE 7.3 Workup and management of traumatic hemo/pneumothorax. PTX, pneumothorax.

e. Monitor chest tube output—if initial output >1.5 L or continued output of >200 mL/h for 4 hours → obtain CT angiography chest if patient is stable and consider emergent thoracotomy or angioembolization (for intercostal artery bleeding).

f. Pulmonary tractotomy is used to treat deep penetrating lung injury and involves opening the tract of the injury and ligating open blood vessels and bronchi.

2. Boney injuries of thoracic cage

a. Management of rib fractures

i. Aggressive pulmonary toilet, incentive spirometry, and multimodal pain management (both systemic and locoregional) are critical to preventing hypoventilation, atelectasis, and pneumonia.

ii. **Figure 7.4** outlines when to consider surgical stabilization of rib fractures (SSRF).

b. Management of sternal fractures

i. Operative fixation is recommended for unstable fracture or fractures associated with infection or chronic pain.

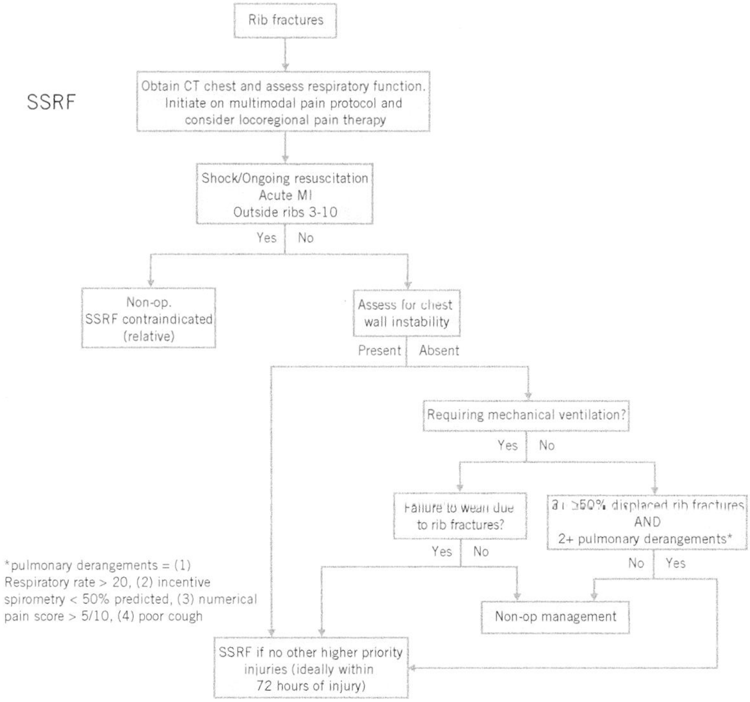

FIGURE 7.4 Indications for surgical stabilization of rib fractures (SSRF). *(Adapted from Chest Wall Injury Society Guideline for SSRF Indications, Contraindications, and Timing.)*

3. Diaphragm injury
   a. Acute diaphragmatic injury is best repaired via abdominal approach because one can evaluate for other intra-abdominal injuries. Chronic diaphragmatic injuries are best repaired via thoracic approach.

D. Outcomes/Complications
1. Pneumonia
   a. Occurs when patients hypoventilate with resultant atelectasis secondary to pain from rib fractures
2. Retained hemothorax
   a. Blood left within the thoracic cavity tends to form stable clot that is not amenable to tube drainage and can progress to pneumonia and empyema
   b. Video-assisted thoracoscopic surgery (VATS) can be performed with high success rates.
   c. Surgical technique: VATS
      i. VATS is indicated 3 to 7 days post injury for retained hemo- or pneumothorax, persistent air leak/bronchopleural fistula, posttraumatic empyema, intrapulmonary abscess, and foreign body removal.
      ii. One or more ports are placed through the lateral chest wall in the fourth or fifth intercostal space.
      iii. After thorough inspection, the pathology is addressed (evacuate effusion, identify and control active bleeding, decortication for persistent pneumothorax, repair or resection of pulmonary lacerations).
      iv. Upon completion, thoracostomy tube is placed under thoracoscopic guidance to optimize drainage of pleural fluid.
3. Empyema
   a. Infection of pleural space diagnosed by positive pleural cultures or frank purulence
   b. Treated with antibiotics (usually long term) and pleural washout and drainage via VATS or thoracotomy
      i. VATS is typically used in earlier stages and thoracotomy for later-stage or failed initial therapy.
4. Persistent air leak and bronchopleural fistula
   a. Persistent air leak is one that lasts beyond 5 to 7 days.
   b. Causes
      i. True bronchopleural fistula is a centrally located communication between the pleural space and a lobar or segmental bronchus, which can happen with injury to major bronchus or following pulmonary resection but is overall uncommon.
      ii. Most posttraumatic air leaks result from communication between lung parenchyma and pleural space.
   c. Can be managed with autologous blood pleurodesis, commercially available sealants, endobronchial one-way valves, or resection

IV. ESOPHAGEAL INJURY

A. Epidemiology/Etiology/Classification

1. Epidemiology
   a. <1% of esophageal injuries are due to blunt force.
      i. Perforation of cervical esophagus may occur with blunt blow to hyperextended neck.
      ii. Sudden force on distended stomach may cause distal esophageal injury.
   b. Most traumatic esophageal injuries occur at cervical esophagus due to close proximity to skin.

B. Diagnosis/Testing

1. Laboratory studies
   a. None are specific.
   b. Obtain basic trauma laboratory tests including CBC, CMP, clotting studies, T&S, UA.
2. Imaging
   a. CXR: May show pneumomediastinum, pleural effusion
   b. Contrast study: Start with water-soluble (diatrizoate meglumine and diatrizoate sodium [Gastrografin]); if negative, follow with dilute barium study.
   c. Esophagoscopy: Useful for diagnosing esophageal injury in operating room but can miss up to 40% of esophageal injuries, so should be performed in conjunction with contrast imaging.

C. Treatment

1. Small, contained cervical esophageal injuries can be managed conservatively.
2. See **Figure 7.5** for basic treatment algorithm when esophageal injury is suspected.
3. Rarely, esophageal injuries will require operative repair.
4. **Surgical technique: Operative repair of esophageal injuries**
   a. Key principles of esophageal injury management are infection control with adequate source control and antimicrobial treatment, clear identification and repair of injury, and establishment of nutritional support.
   b. Incision and exposure will depend on location of injury.
      i. Upper third: Left collar or left anteromedial sternocleidomastoid muscle incision
      ii. Middle third: Right posterolateral thoracotomy at fifth intercostal space
      iii. Lower third: Left thoracotomy at seventh intercostal space
   c. Irrigate the area thoroughly and place drains.
   d. Assess need for feeding tube placement—typically feeding jejunostomy with decompressive gastrostomy (if distal injury).

D. Outcomes/Complications

1. Requires nothing by mouth with operative drainage/decompression and consideration for distal feeding access. Successful repair is confirmed with repeat esophagram.

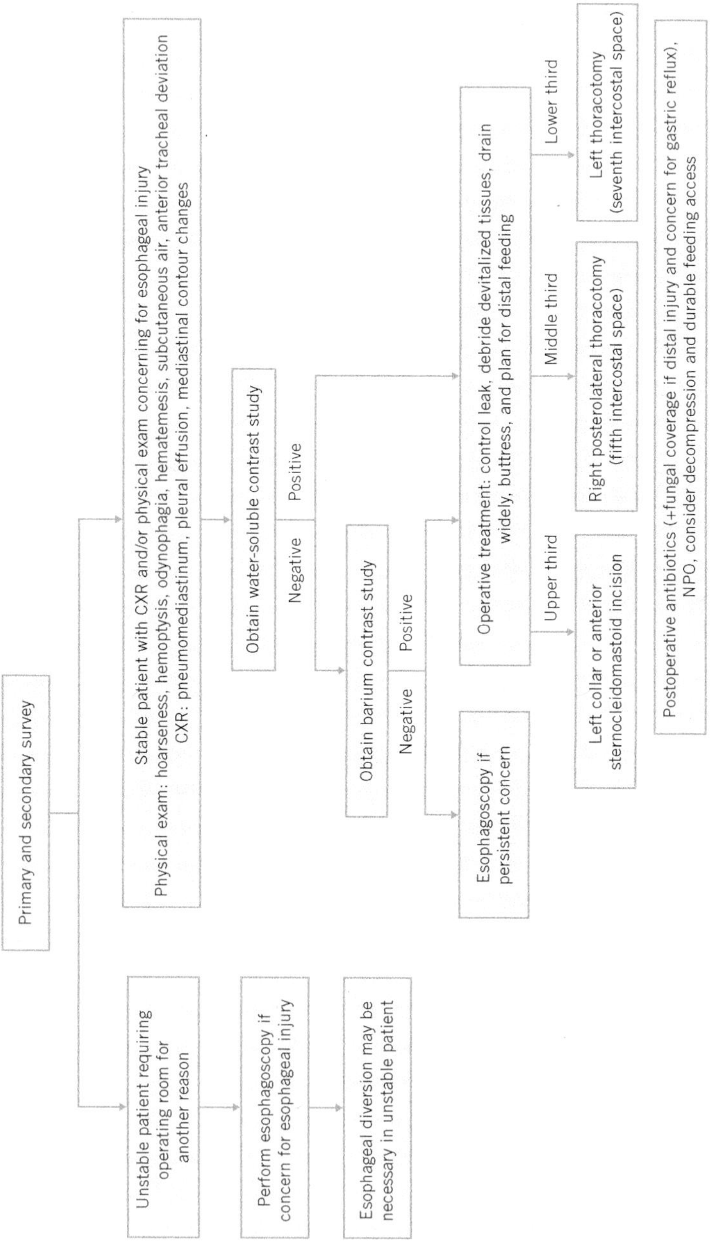

FIGURE 7.5 Workup and management of traumatic esophageal injury.

2. High complication rate following esophageal injury and repair including leak, infection (mediastinitis/empyema), or Tracheoesophageal fistula
3. Delayed diagnosis increases mortality.
   a. Untreated cervical esophageal injuries may progress to swelling, fever, erythema, increasing crepitus, airway distress, or frank abscess.
   b. Untreated thoracic esophageal injuries may progress to mediastinitis, empyema, and septic shock.

V. TRACHEOBRONCHIAL AND LUNG INJURY

A. Epidemiology/Etiology/Classification
   1. Pulmonary laceration
      a. Often caused by broken ribs
      b. May result in hemothorax and/or pneumothorax requiring placement of chest tube (see **Figure 7.3**)
   2. Pulmonary contusion
      a. When lung parenchyma absorbs a force, alveolar hemorrhage and tissue edema may occur, resulting in pulmonary contusion.
      b. Resultant impairment in oxygenation and ventilation peaks around 24 hours, but can progress for up to 3 days.
   3. Tracheobronchial injury may manifest as extensive subcutaneous emphysema, large/continuous air leak after chest tube placement, hemoptysis.

B. Diagnosis/Testing
   1. Laboratory studies
      a. None specific
      b. Obtain basic trauma laboratory tests including CBC, CMP, clotting studies, T&S, UA
   2. Imaging
      a. Pulmonary contusion may not be evident on initial imaging and may take days to "blossom."
      b. If tracheobronchial injury is suspected, bronchoscopy is gold standard for diagnosis.

C. Treatment
   1. See **Figure 7.6** for algorithmic approach to suspected tracheobronchial injuries.
   2. Tracheobronchial injuries <1/3 the circumference of the bronchus may be managed nonoperatively if air leak is controlled by chest tube.
   3. Pulmonary contusion is typically managed nonoperatively and may require mechanical ventilation in severe cases. Judicious fluid management is essential.

D. Outcomes/Complications
   1. Complications of lung injury may include pneumonia, empyema, intrapulmonary abscess, retained hemothorax, persistent air leak, and/or bronchopleural fistula.
      a. Management may be amenable to treatment with VATS (see operative procedures).

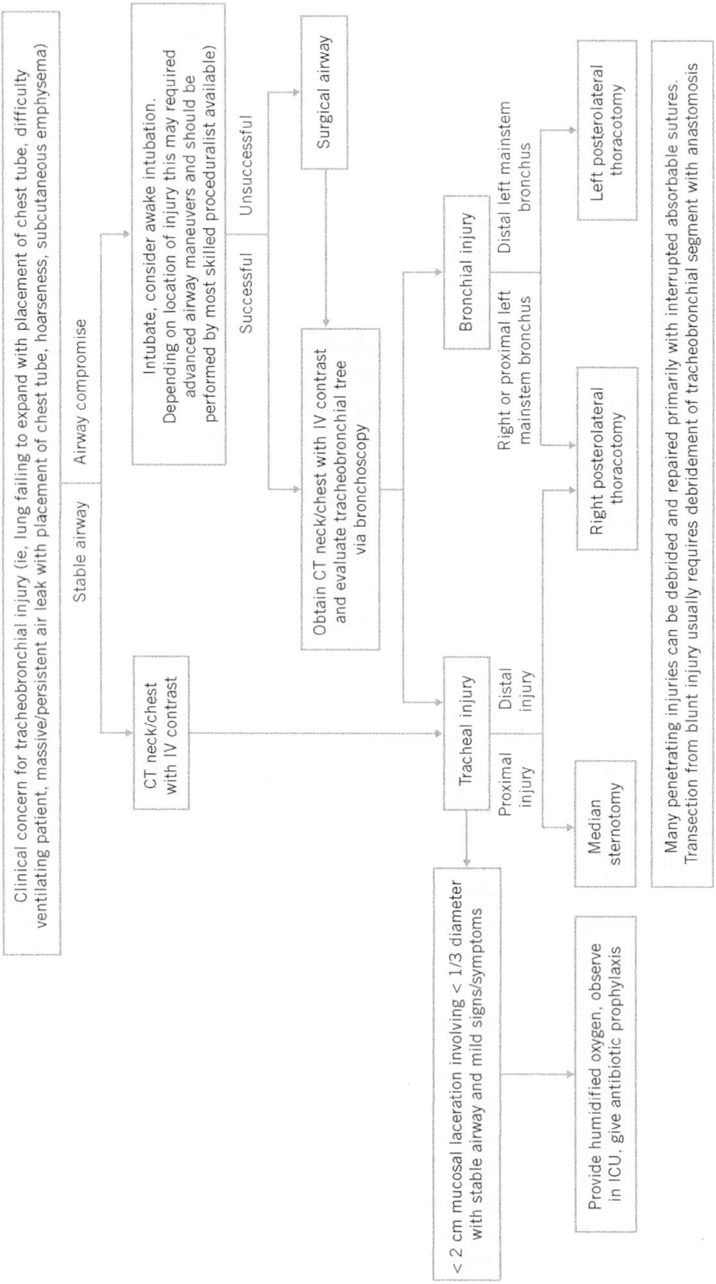

FIGURE 7.6 Workup and management of traumatic tracheobronchial injury.

Key References

Citation	Summary
Moore EE, Knudson MM, Burlew CC, et al. Defining the limits of resuscitative emergency department thoracotomy: a contemporary Western Trauma Association perspective. *J Trauma.* 2011; 70(2):334-339.	• Prospective multicenter study aimed to identify injury patterns and physiologic profiles compatible with survival after emergency department (ED) thoracotomy. • Authors conclude that ED thoracotomy can be considered futile in (1) patients suffering blunt trauma with >10 min prehospital cardiopulmonary resuscitation (CPR) without response, (2) patients suffering penetrating trauma with >15 min CPR without response, and (3) patients in asystole on arrival to ED without evidence of tamponade.
Bulger EM, Arneson MA, Mock CN, Jurkovich GJ. Rib fractures in the elderly. *J Trauma.* 2000;48(6):1040-1047.	• Retrospective cohort study aimed to assess morbidity and mortality of rib fractures in elderly patients. • Authors conclude that elderly patients (age 65 years and older) with rib fractures as a result of blunt trauma have twice the mortality and thoracic morbidity of their younger counterparts and that for each additional rib fracture mortality increases by 19% and risk of pneumonia by 27%.
Salim A, Velmahos GC, Jindal A, et al. Clinically significant blunt cardiac trauma: role of serum troponin levels combined with electrocardiographic findings. *J Trauma.* 2001;50(2):237-243.	• Prospective trial aimed to evaluate the utility of serum troponin I and electrocardiogram in identifying patients with blunt cardiac injury. • Authors conclude that combination of electrocardiogram and serum troponin I reliably predicts significant blunt cardiac injury; patients with abnormal EKG and troponin I should be closely monitored for at least 24 h, whereas patients with normal EKG and troponin I can be safely discharged in absence of other injuries.

CHAPTER 7: CHEST TRAUMA

Review Questions

1. What is the immediate treatment of a patient s/p gun shot wound to the right chest with HR 125, SBP 80, notable tracheal deviation to the left, and absent breath sounds on the right?
2. What parameters help guide decision to proceed to the operating room for emergent thoracotomy following chest tube placement for hemothorax?
3. What are indications for resuscitative (ED) thoracotomy?
4. What studies should be obtained to evaluate for blunt cardiac injury in a patient suffering a blow to the chest?
5. What is the first step in the workup of esophageal injury in a stable patient?
6. Tension pneumothorax and cardiac tamponade cause which type of shock?
7. What are the components of Beck's triad and what pathology do they suggest?

REFERENCES

1. Clancy K, Velopulos C, Bilaniuk JW, et al. Screening for blunt cardiac injury: an Eastern Association for the Surgery of Trauma practice management guideline. *J Trauma Acute Care Surg*. 2012;73(5 suppl 4):S301-S306.
2. Inaba K, Lustenberger T, Recinos G, et al. Does size matter? A prospective analysis of 28-32 versus 36-40 French chest tube size in trauma. *J Trauma Acute Care Surg*. 2012;72(2):422-427.
3. Moore EE, Knudson MM, Burlew CC, et al. Defining the limits of resuscitative emergency department thoracotomy: a contemporary Western Trauma Association perspective. *J Trauma*. 2011;70(2):334-339.
4. Bulger EM, Arneson MA, Mock CN, Jurkovich GJ. Rib fractures in the elderly. *J Trauma*. 2000;48(6):1040-1046; discussion 1046-7.
5. Salim A, Velmahos GC, Jindal A, et al. Clinically significant blunt cardiac trauma: role of serum troponin levels combined with electrocardiographic findings. *J Trauma*. 2001;50(2):237-243.

8 Abdominal Trauma

Kerry A. Swanson and Douglas J. Schuerer

I. INTRODUCTION

A. Anatomy: The abdominal cavity extends from the diaphragm to the pelvic floor, corresponding to the space between the nipples and the inguinal creases on the anterior aspect of the torso.

B. Trauma resuscitation management (for more information, see Chapter 5—Trauma Resuscitation)

1. All trauma patients should immediately have two large-bore IV lines (14 or 16 gauge).
2. Laboratory samples may be sent at the time of initial access with **type and screen** being the most important.
3. All patients should be assumed to be in hemorrhagic shock until proven otherwise (see Chapter 5, Table 5.4 for classes of shock).
   a. Resuscitation with blood products, preferably in a 1:1:1 ratio of packed red blood cells–fresh frozen plasma–platelets.
   b. A massive transfusion protocol (MTP) should be in place at each institution.
   c. Crystalloid, colloid, and hypertonic saline should be avoided.
   d. Permissive hypotension prior to definitive control of bleeding reduces overall transfusion requirements and coagulopathy.[1]
   e. Target blood pressure should be tailored to patients age and medical history as elderly patients may not tolerate the same degree of hypotension as younger patients.

C. Injury classification (**Table 8.1** and **Figure 8.1**)

D. Imaging modalities in abdominal trauma (**Table 8.2**)

E. Trauma laparotomy (**Table 8.3**)

1. Successful operative management of trauma in a hemodynamically unstable patient requires a team approach, with close communication between the attending surgeon, surgical assistants, anesthesiologist, circulating nurse, and surgical technologist.
   a. The surgeon should clearly communicate the plan to the rest of the team. Management of specific injuries will be discussed in the next section.
2. Damage control
   a. Close communication with the anesthesiologist about the hemodynamic status of the patient is important to determine if the operation should be temporarily interrupted either allowing continued

TABLE 8.1 Injury Classification

Stab Wounds	**A.** Only one-third of stab wounds to anterior abdomen penetrate peritoneal cavity and cause significant injury **B.** Options for evaluation **a.** Local exploration **b.** Laparoscopy **c.** Laparotomy **d.** Observation
Gunshot wounds	**A.** High probability of significant injury **B.** Often require laparotomy **a.** Stable hemodynamics without peritoneal signs on examination may be an exception with use of single-contrast CT with selective use of oral or rectal contrast and serial examination for at least 24 h (*Am J Roentgenol.* 2018;210:761-765).
Blunt trauma	**A.** Physical signs of significant organ injury often absent **B.** A number of algorithms have been proposed to exclude serious injury. See **Figure 8.1** for one suggested algorithm **a. Unstable patients without other injuries** should undergo immediate laparotomy **b. Unstable patients with multiple injuries**, FAST may be useful to determine if abdomen is the source of shock; if CT scan is readily available head and abdomen/pelvis scan may be obtained if patient is fairly stable **c. Awake, unimpaired patients without abdominal complaints** may be safely observed without abdominal imaging with admission and serial abdominal examinations as long as no plans to undergo anesthetic during admission **d. Stable patients with multiple injuries** should undergo CT evaluation to identify presence of occult intra-abdominal injury, which may determine need for laparotomy. Laparoscopy has also been proposed as an adjunct in this situation

resuscitation prior to continuing or controlling bleeding and enteric spillage with temporary abdominal closure with plans to continue resuscitation in an intensive care setting.

II. SOLID ORGAN INJURIES

A. Diaphragmatic injuries

1. Occur most commonly as a result of penetrating thoracic or abdominal trauma; however, blunt trauma can produce rupture secondary to rapid elevation of intra-abdominal pressure
2. Diagnosis: Most commonly made during laparotomy, but can be recognized on CXR or CT

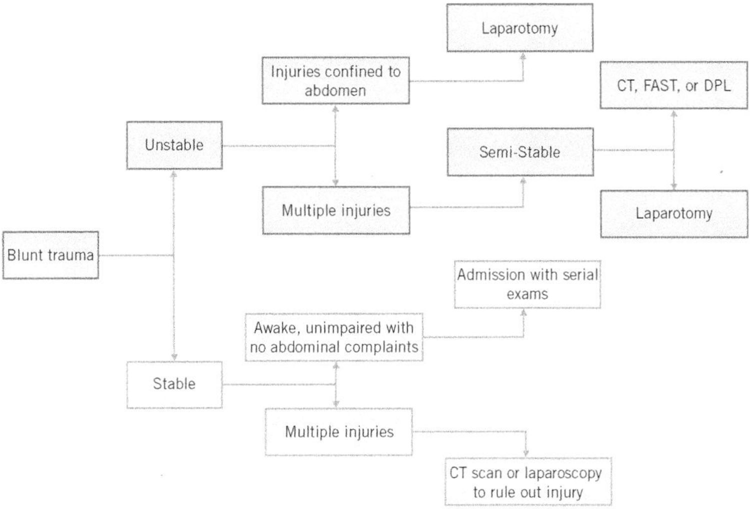

FIGURE 8.1 Suggested algorithm in treatment of patient with suspected blunt abdominal trauma. DPL, diagnostic peritoneal lavage.

TABLE 8.2	Imaging Modalities in Abdominal Trauma
Trauma ultrasonography—Focused Abdominal Sonography for Trauma (FAST)	**A.** FAST commonly initial radiographic screening evaluation in all traumas following the primary survey—**most useful in blunt abdominal trauma with hypotension** **B.** Purpose is to identify free intraperitoneal and/or pericardial fluid in six standard areas **a.** Right paracolic gutter **b.** Left paracolic gutter **c.** Morrison pouch (hepatorenal recess) **d.** Pericardium **e.** Perisplenic region **f.** Suprapubic region **C.** Limitations in children and penetrating trauma **D** Highly specific, but **does not exclude** major intra-abdominal injury or evaluate retroperitoneal bleeding
CT	**A.** Useful to evaluate anatomy and injuries in great detail **B.** Decreases the number of unnecessary laparotomies decreasing morbidity and cost **C.** Triple-contrast CT (oral, IV, rectal) is traditional, but oral and rectal contrast may be selectively utilized with high-resolution scanner (*Am J Roentgenol.* 2018;210: 761-765).

TABLE 8.3

Surgical Approach: Trauma Laparotomy

1. Position patient supine with both arms at 90°
2. Foley catheter and nasogastric tube should be placed
3. Patient should be prepped and draped widely from chin to both knees
4. Antibiotics: A single dose of a broad-spectrum antibiotic with aerobic and anaerobic coverage should be given, keeping in mind that the initial dosage may need to be increased and repeated after transfusion of 10 units of blood products[2]
5. Midline incision
6. Small bowel evisceration and packing of all four quadrants with laparotomy pads
7. Deliberate unpacking, identification, and repair of injuries

3. Management: Operative repair, urgency based on size and acuity
4. Operative repair: Primary repair using permanent sutures in an interrupted figure-of-eight fashion.

B. Hepatic injuries
1. Liver is the most common injured solid organ.
2. Use of CT has increased diagnosis of occult liver injury.
3. Diagnosis: Laparotomy or CT with IV contrast
4. Management: Laparotomy, angiography with embolization, or observation.
   a. Hemodynamically unstable patients *require* operative exploration.
   b. Penetrating trauma
      i. *Nonoperative management may be acceptable in the setting of trauma isolated to the liver in a hemodynamically normal patient.*[3]
   c. Blunt trauma
      i. *Stable patients without alternative indication for laparotomy should be admitted for close hemodynamic monitoring and serial laboratory tests.*
   d. Ongoing blood loss in the stable patient warrants angiographic evaluation and embolization.
   e. Damage control
      i. Interventional radiology consultation for evaluation and intervention upon arterial bleeding after packing or as a part of damage control should be considered.
5. Operative repair
   a. Hemorrhage from hepatic trauma can be massive.
   b. Rapid mobilization of injured lobe with perihepatic compression for initial hemostasis.
   c. Complex injuries may be best managed with damage control, packing, intensive care unit admission, and resuscitation.
   d. Temporary control maneuvers: Pringle maneuver, total vascular isolation, atriocaval shunt.

e. Definitive hemostasis can be obtained with a combination of cautery, chromic suture, topical hemostatic agents, finger fracture and ligation, and omental packing.
f. Formal anatomic resection should be avoided due to high associated morbidity and mortality.
g. Closed suction drains should be placed near injury to help identify and control bile leaks.

C. Gallbladder injuries
1. Frequently coexist with hepatic, portal triad, and pancreaticoduodenal injuries
2. Diagnosis: Laparotomy, CT scan with IV contrast
3. Operative treatment: Cholecystectomy
   a. This also provides effective access to biliary tree integrity via cholangiography.

D. Common bile duct injuries
1. Most frequently due to penetrating trauma and associated with other injuries in the right upper quadrant
2. Diagnosis: Laparotomy, intraoperative cholangiography if biliary involvement suspected
3. Management: Operative repair and drainage
4. Operative repair: Primary repair of injured duct over a T-tube

E. Splenic injuries
1. Spleen is the second most common injured solid organ.
2. Diagnosis: Laparotomy or CT scan with IV contrast
3. Management (**Figure 8.2**)
4. Unstable patients should undergo operative exploration
5. Nonoperative management
   a. Blunt trauma: Hemodynamically stable patients without alternative indication for laparotomy may undergo close observation of vital signs and serial hematocrit determinations.
   b. Patients with CT evidence of a contrast "blush" or evidence of continued blood loss who remain stable should undergo embolization.
   c. Patients with failure of nonoperative management (e.g., requiring continuing transfusion) should undergo operative exploration.
6. Postsplenectomy vaccination
   a. All patients following splenectomy or embolization should receive immunization against *Streptococcus pneumoniae, Haemophilus influenzae*, and *Neisseria meningitidis.*
   b. Recommended to be given 14 days following splenectomy; however, should be given prior to hospital discharge if concerns about patient follow-up.
7. Operative repair
   a. Minor injuries contained within splenic capsule require no intervention.
   b. Bleeding from small capsular lacerations can be controlled with direct pressure or topical hemostatic agents.
   c. Stable patients: Splenorrhaphy has been advocated in the past, but most requiring intervention should undergo splenectomy.

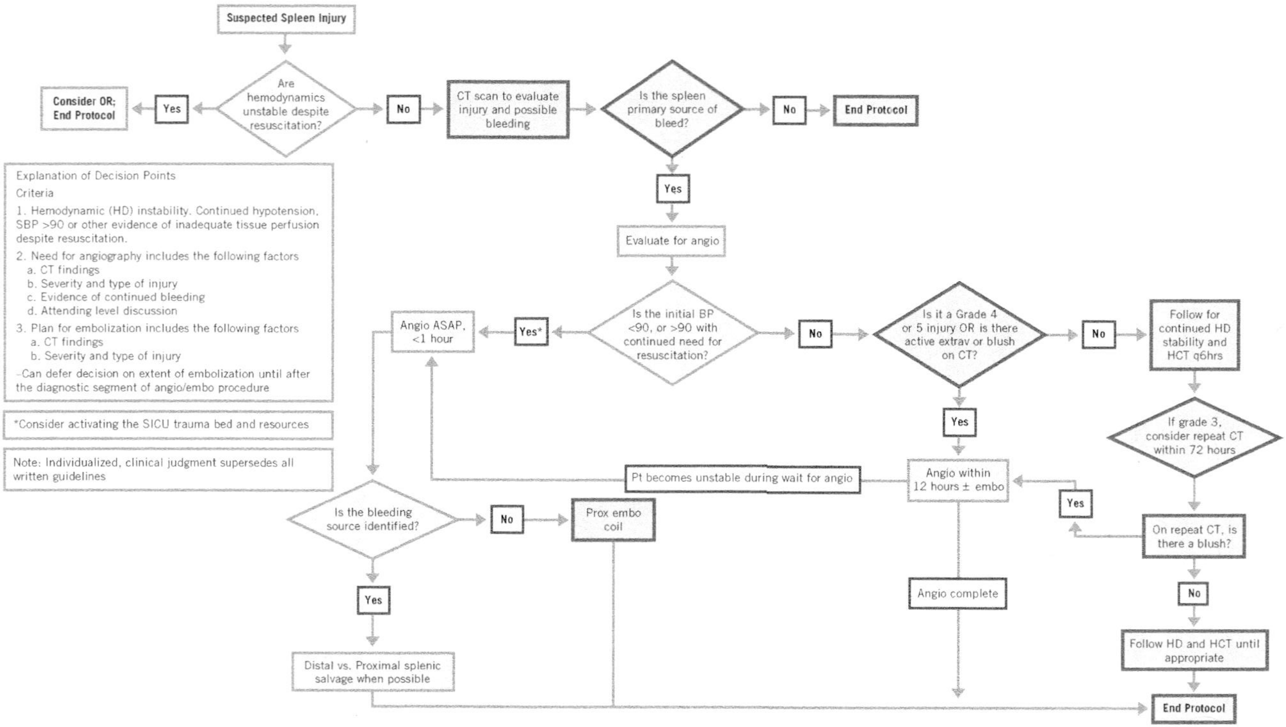

FIGURE 8.2 Splenic trauma algorithm.

   d. Unstable patients or those with failed splenic salvage should have rapid splenectomy.
      i. Control of splenic hilum with clamps followed by ligation of splenic arteries and veins as close to hilum as possible to avoid injury to pancreas

F. Pancreatic injuries
   1. Most often due to penetrating trauma.
   2. Isolated pancreatic trauma is rare; typically associated with injury to the stomach or liver.
   3. Diagnosis: CT is the best imaging modality. Magnetic resonance cholangiopancreatography or Endoscopic retrograde cholangiopancreatography can be used to identify ductal injuries in stable patients or following laparotomy.
      a. Pancreatic enzymes are not helpful in diagnosis.
   4. Management: Treatment focuses on determining the presence and location of major ductal involvement.
   5. Operative repair
      a. Exposure by performing Kocher maneuver and transecting the gastrohepatic and gastrocolic ligaments to inspect the body and tail of the pancreas
         i. Duct intact: Treat with closed suction drains.
         ii. Transected duct requires debridement and/or resection combined with closed suction drainage.
         iii. Pancreatic head injuries, especially in conjunction with duodenal and biliary trauma, may require pancreaticoduodenectomy but usually not during the initial operation where the goal is to control hemorrhage and drain widely.

G. Gastric injuries
   1. Most common in penetrating trauma
   2. Diagnosis: Laparotomy, bloody drainage from gastric tube should raise suspicion for gastric injury.
   3. Management: Definitive operative repair and gastric decompression
   4. Operative repair
      a. Simple lacerations can be repaired in two layers or stapled.
      b. Massive devitalization may require formal resection with restoration of continuity via gastroenterostomy.
      c. Vagotomy may be helpful to reduce risk of marginal ulcer.

H. Duodenal injuries
   1. Frequently coexist with devastating gastrointestinal (GI) and abdominal vascular trauma.
   2. Type and severity of duodenal injury determine management.
   3. Diagnosis: Modality of choice is CT with IV contrast; however, diagnosis may be challenging.
   4. Duodenal hematoma typically occurs after blunt trauma to upper abdomen.
      a. CT or upper GI fluoroscopy with Gastrografin can typically diagnose these injuries.
   5. Duodenal perforation can be difficult to diagnose.
      a. Patient may have vague back or flank pain and symptoms may evolve slowly.

b. Modality of choice is CT with oral contrast.
c. Upper GI fluoroscopy with water-soluble contrast may show evidence of a leak.

6. Management
   a. Duodenal hematoma can be managed nonoperatively the majority of time with long-term nasogastric decompression and nutritional support (parenteral or enteral distal to the level of injury).
      i. Operative evacuation may be necessary if obstruction persists for more than 14 days, and CT reimaging confirms persistent hematoma.
   b. Duodenal perforation requires definitive operative management with drainage and decompression.
7. Complex duodenal injuries
   a. Operative management depends on degree of injury; however, Kocher maneuver is essential for proper visualization and repair.
   b. Most defects (80%) can undergo primary transverse closure in two layers to avoid luminal narrowing with closed suction drainage to control any anastomotic leak followed by nasoduodenal decompression.
   c. Alternatively, antegrade or retrograde (preferred) tube duodenostomy can be performed in conjunction with tube gastrostomy and feeding jejunostomy, the so-called triple tube drainage.[4]
   d. Pancreaticoduodenectomy (Whipple procedure) should be reserved for the most complex injuries including duodenal devascularization or severe combined injuries involving pancreatic head or bile ducts.
      i. *Very high morbidity and mortality in trauma setting*

I. Intestinal injuries:
   1. Common in both penetrating and blunt trauma
   2. Diagnosis: Laparotomy
   3. Management: Definitive operative repair, diversion
      a. Small bowel repair: Primary repair or segmental resection with anastomosis
   4. Large-bowel injuries: Primary repair of colonic injury unless patient has prolonged intraoperative hypotension or massive colonic destruction.
   5. Rectal injury: Often associated with genitourinary or pelvic vascular trauma
      a. Operative repair: Primary repair of accessible injuries, diverting colostomy

J. Abdominal genitourinary injuries
   1. Renal injuries
      a. Most common in blunt trauma.
      b. Diagnosis: CT with IV contrast, CT pyelogram, laparotomy
      c. Management: Conservative management may be attempted in a hemodynamically stable patient without expanding or pulsatile hematoma within Gerota's fascia.
      d. Urologic complications of conservative management can often be treated by endourological or percutaneous interventions.
      e. In penetrating injuries nonoperative treatment in hemodynamically stable patients without other injuries when completely staged with

CT or IV pyelogram. There must be a high index of suspicion to avoid ureteral injuries.

f. Unstable patients: Exploration or angioembolization is indicated for vascular injury with extravasation with deep or complex renal lacerations.

g. Operative management:
   i. In blunt trauma, operative exploration should be considered for patients with major blunt injury with devascularized segments, hypotensive patients, or those with expanding or pulsatile hematomas.
   ii. In penetrating trauma, high-grade injuries have high risk of delayed bleeding. Exploration should be considered if laparotomy is indicated for other injuries.

2. Ureteral injuries
   a. Most common in penetrating trauma
   b. Diagnosis: CT with IV contrast with delayed images, laparotomy
   c. Operative repair
      i. Lacerations: Debridement of devitalized tissue and primary spatulated repair over ureteral stent in stable patients; in unstable patients may leave temporary urinary drainage followed by delayed repair
      ii. Contusions: Ureteral stenting or resection and primary repair

3. Bladder injuries
   a. Most common in blunt trauma, often associated with pelvic fractures
   b. Diagnosis: High suspicion in stable patient with gross hematuria and pelvic fracture; retrograde cystography, laparotomy
   c. Management: Surgical repair and/or catheter drainage
      i. Intraperitoneal bladder rupture should undergo operative repair
      ii. Extraperitoneal bladder rupture
         a) Uncomplicated can be managed with catheter drainage.
         b) Complicated extraperitoneal bladder injury should undergo surgical repair.
   d. Operative repair: Repair in one or two layers followed by catheter drainage

K. Vascular injuries

1. Abdominal vascular injury is often lethal with penetrating mechanisms with mortality ranging from 20% to 60%.
2. Early deaths result from hemorrhage, and late deaths are related to multisystem organ failure.[5]
3. Free rupture presents volume-unresponsive hemorrhagic shock, while a hematoma may present with hemodynamic stability or with transient responsiveness to resuscitation.
   a. Free intraperitoneal bleeding often presents with an unstable patient who without immediate surgical intervention will rapidly deteriorate.
4. Operative repair: Following trauma laparotomy and packing, hemorrhage may be temporarily managed with several techniques.

a. Aortic access via left anterior thoracotomy above the fifth rib space after dividing the inferior pulmonary ligament and retracting the lung anteriorly. Manual compression or T bar at the hiatus to control hemorrhage.
b. Intra-abdominal T bar at the level of the hiatus.
c. Supraceliac clamping of the aorta by dividing the gastrohepatic ligament and right crus of the diaphragm while retracting the stomach and esophagus.
d. Resuscitative balloon occlusion of the aorta (REBOA)
   i. The REBOA is inserted via a femoral puncture and positioned based on the location of suspected bleeding.
e. Retroperitoneal hematomas
   i. The retroperitoneum is divided into three zones. See **Figure 8.3** for suggested management.
      a) Central abdominal hematomas (zone I) contain the aorta, inferior vena cava (IVC), or major branches including the celiac and superior and inferior mesenteric arteries.
      b) Flank hematomas (zone II) are in the paracolic gutters containing the renal vessels and kidneys; management depends on mechanism and signs of ongoing bleeding.
      c) Pelvic hematomas (zone III) begin at sacral promontory and contain iliac arteries and veins. In blunt trauma, they are usually due to pelvic fractures.

L. Abdominal trauma in pregnancy
1. Responsible for approximately 50% of all deaths in pregnant women
   a. Interpersonal violence is the highest nonobstetric cause of death in pregnant women.
   b. A gravid uterus displaces the majority of the intra-abdominal organs and thus relatively protects the mother from penetrating abdominal injury.
2. In general, pregnant patients should be managed similarly to nonpregnant patients, following the dictum that the best way to take care of the fetus is to take care of the mother.
   a. Fetal well-being should not preclude any urgent operative or radiologic investigations.
   b. In pregnancies 20 weeks of gestation or greater, or unknown gestation, fetal heart monitoring and urgent obstetrical consultation should be obtained.
   c. If possible, mother should be positioned in *left lateral decubitus position* to off-load pressure on the IVC and should be given supplemental oxygen.
   d. Placental abruption is the most common cause of fetal demise and typically presents with vaginal bleeding.
   e. If the patient expires in the trauma bay or operating room and the fetus is at least 26 weeks of gestation, postmortem caesarean section should be performed expediently.

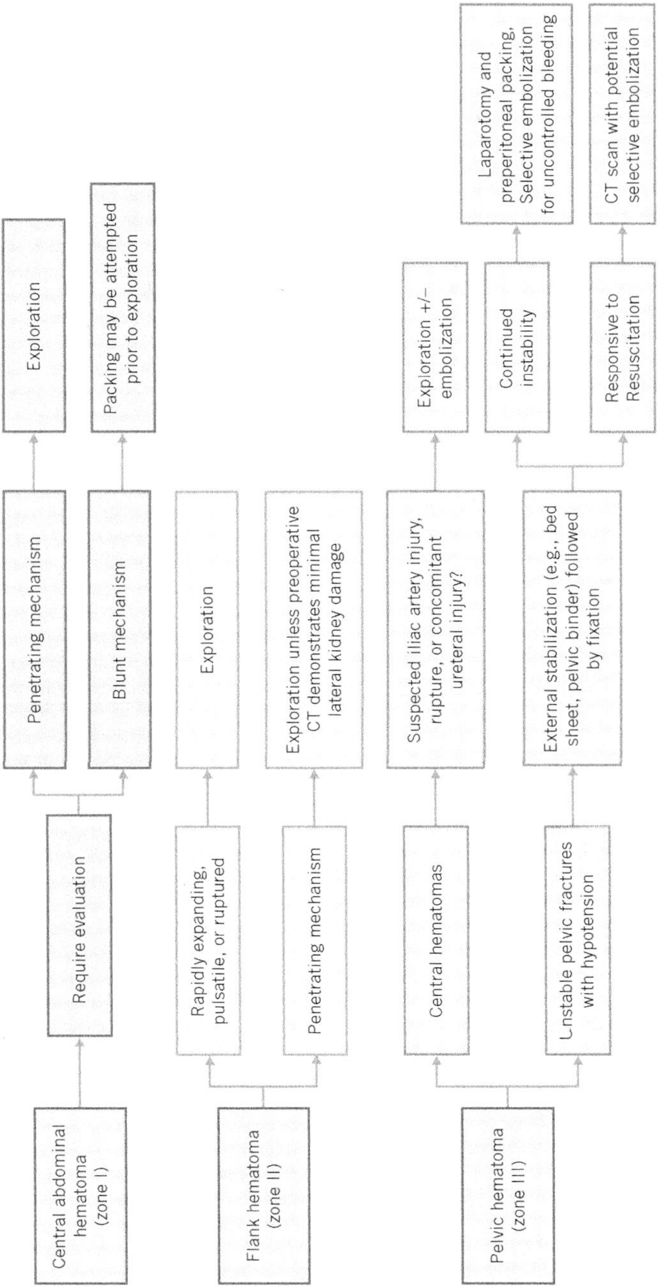

FIGURE 8.3 Management of retroperitoneal hematomas.

Key References

Citation	Summary
Rotondo MF, Schwab CW, McGonigal MD, et al. "Damage control": an approach for improved survival in exsanguinating penetrating abdominal injury. *J Trauma*. 1993;35(3):375-383.	• Retrospective review of patients comparing definitive laparotomy (DL) with "damage control" (DC) in the treatment of penetrating abdominal wounds with combined vascular and visceral injuries found that, in patients with major vascular injury and two or more visceral injuries (maximum injury subset), DC had increased survival compared with DL.
Rozycki GS, Ballard RB, Feliciano DV, Schmidt JA, Pennington SD. Surgeon-performed ultrasound for the assessment of truncal injuries: lessons learned from 1540 patients. *Ann Surg*. 1998;228(4):557-567.	• Prospective study evaluating accuracy in Focused Assessment for the Sonographic examination of the Trauma Patient (FAST) to identify clinical conditions in which FAST is most accurate. This study found that FAST was most accurate in patients with precordial or transthoracic injuries (sensitivity 100%, specificity 99.3%) and those with hypotensive blunt abdominal trauma (sensitivity 100%, specificity 100%) and should be the initial diagnostic modality in these patients as immediate surgical intervention is justified in these patients.
Holcomb JB, Tilley BC, Baraniuk S, et al. Transfusion of plasma, platelets, and red blood cells in a 1:1:1 vs a 1:1:2 ratio and mortality in patients with severe trauma: the PROPPR randomized clinical trial. *JAMA*. 2015;313(5):471-482.	• Randomized controlled trial of severely injured patients predicted to require MTP comparing blood product ratios of plasma, platelets, and red blood cells in a 1:1:1 vs. 1:1:2 ratio found that the use of a 1:1:1 ratio did not result in mortality differences at 24 h or 30 d; however, the 1:1:1 group achieved hemostasis and fewer deaths due to exsanguination by 24 h.

CHAPTER 8. ABDOMINAL TRAUMA

Review Questions

1. What patients may be safely observed following blunt trauma?
2. FAST is most useful in what subset of patients?
3. What antibiotics should be given and when should they be redosed?
4. What vaccinations should be given as postsplenectomy prophylaxis?
5. What is the focus for treating pancreatic injuries?
6. What is the typical management of a duodenal hematoma?

7. What imaging is indicated in a stable patient with a suspected renal or ureteral injury?
8. What retroperitoneal hematomas require operative exploration?
9. At what gestational age do pregnant trauma patients require fetal monitoring and obstetrics consultation?

REFERENCES

1. Morrison CA, Carrick MM, Norman MA, et al. Hypotensive resuscitation strategy reduces transfusion requirements and severe postoperative coagulopathy in trauma patients with hemorrhagic shock: preliminary results of a randomized controlled trial. *J Trauma*. 2011;70(3):652-663.
2. Goldberg SR, Anand RJ, Como JJ, et al. Prophylactic antibiotic use in penetrating abdominal trauma: an Eastern Association for the Surgery of Trauma practice management guideline. *J Trauma Acute Care Surg*. 2012;73(5 suppl 4):S321-S325.
3. Como JJ, Bokhari F, Chiu WC, et al. Practice management guidelines for selective nonoperative management of penetrating abdominal trauma. *J Trauma*. 2010;68(3):721-733.
4. Stone HH, Fabian TC. Management of duodenal wounds. *J Trauma*. 1979;19(5):334-339.
5. Kobayashi LM, Constantini TW, Coimbra R. *Clinical Review of Vascular Trauma*. 1st ed. Springer Berlin; 2014.
6. Rotondo MF, Schwab CW, McGonigal MD, et al. "Damage control": an approach for improved survival in exsanguinating penetrating abdominal injury. *J Trauma*. 1993;35(3):375-382; discussion 382-383.
7. Rozycki GS, Ballard RB, Feliciano DV, Schmidt JA, Pennington SD. Surgeon-performed ultrasound for the assessment of truncal injuries: lessons learned from 1540 patients. *Ann Surg*. 1998;228(4):557-567.
8. Holcomb JB, Tilley BC, Baraniuk S, et al. Transfusion of plasma, platelets, and red blood cells in a 1:1:1 vs a 1:1:2 ratio and mortality in patients with severe trauma: the PROPPR randomized clinical trial. *JAMA*. 2015;313(5):471-482.

9 Extremity Trauma

Andrea Tian and Christopher M. McAndrew

I. COMMON ORTHOPEDIC TERMS

A. *Fracture*—a broken bone (**Figure 9.1**)
 1. Simple: Single fracture line and well aligned for reduction, a "stable" fracture
 2. Comminuted: Multiple fracture lines
 3. Unstable: Complex fractures due to multiple fracture lines, displacement, malalignment, or soft tissue injury. Often require surgical intervention.
 4. Segmental: At least two fracture lines (i.e., three fracture fragments) with an intact ring of cortical bone in between
 5. Avulsion: Small piece of bone is torn from main bone, usually results from pulling from ligament or tendon.
 6. Articular: Involves a joint surface.

B. *Dislocation*—incongruity between normally apposed joint surfaces

C. *Reduction*—realign fracture or dislocation to restore length, alignment, and rotation of the bone or joint. Can be closed (incisionless) or open (operative intervention for direct visualization and manipulation of bone).

D. *Fixation*—implementation of hardware to stabilize extremity
 1. Internal: Surgical implantation of fixation devices into bone
 2. External: Application of external stabilization apparatus, attached to fracture fragments via percutaneous pins

E. *Splint vs. Cast*—Rigid dressing, usually composed of plaster or fiberglass, used to immobilize injured extremity.
 1. Casts are placed circumferentially around injured extremity, while splints have gaps that allow for swelling.
 2. *Braces* are applied across a joint space.

F. *Epiphysis vs. Metaphysis vs. Diaphysis*—components of a long bone
 1. Epiphysis: End of the bone, capped with articular cartilage that forms joints
 2. Diaphysis: Shaft of the bone
 3. Metaphysis: Neck of bone, contains growth plates

G. *Malunion vs. Nonunion*
 1. Malunion: Fracture that has healed in a suboptimal position
 2. Nonunion: Lack of fracture healing after 9 months

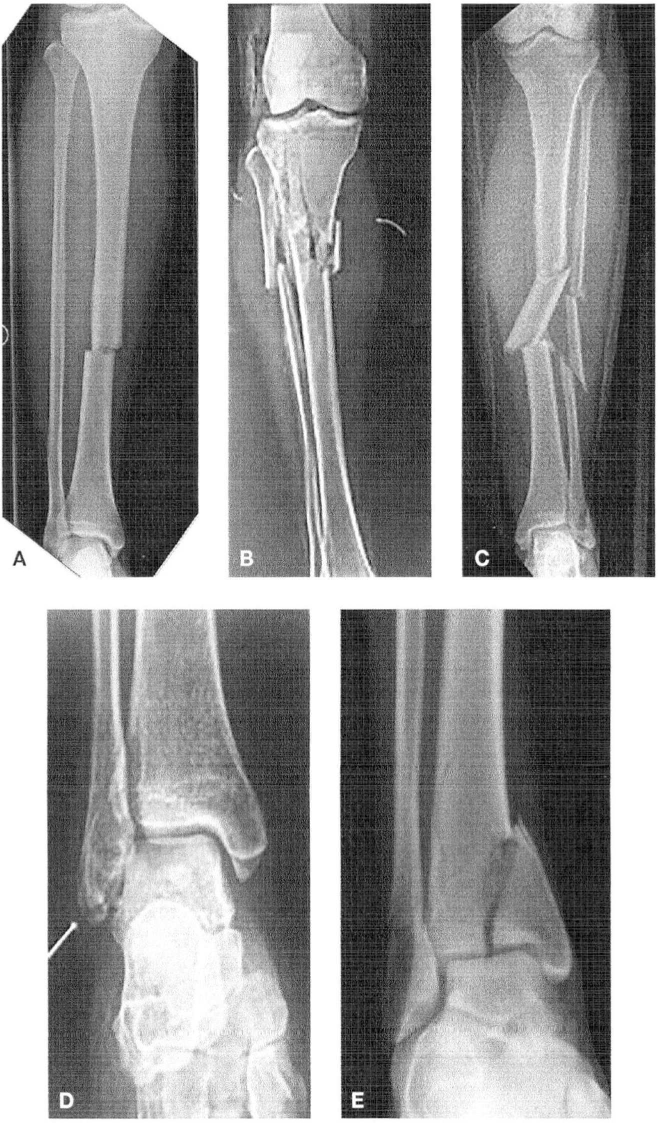

FIGURE 9.1 Fracture Patterns. A, Simple. B, Comminuted. C, Segmental. D, Avulsion. E, Articular.

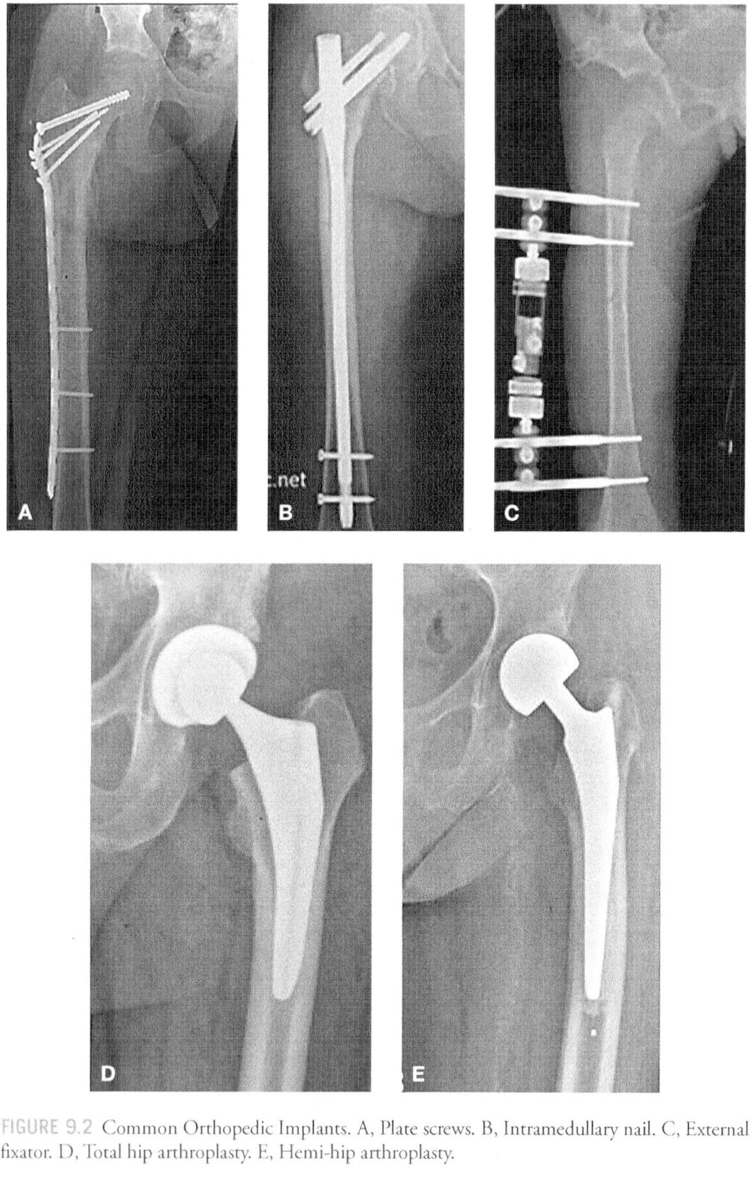

FIGURE 9.2 Common Orthopedic Implants. A, Plate screws. B, Intramedullary nail. C, External fixator. D, Total hip arthroplasty. E, Hemi-hip arthroplasty.

II. COMMON ORTHOPEDIC IMPLANTS (FIGURE 9.2)

A. *Screws*—simple machine that converts torque into compression. Often used in conjunction with plates for internal fixation.
B. *Nails*—cylindrical implants placed into the marrow space of long bones and fixed at both ends with interlocking screws. Component of internal fixation.
C. *External fixators*—combination of bars and rings that stabilize a fracture from outside of the body.
D. *Arthroplasty*—joint replacement
   1. Total joint arthroplasty: Replacement of both sides of the joint
   2. Hemiarthroplasty: Replacement of just one side of the joint

III. INITIAL ASSESSMENT AND MANAGEMENT OF EXTREMITY TRAUMA

A. History
   1. Mechanism of injury, especially the relative energy associated with the injury—low-energy fall vs. high-energy motor vehicle collision (MVC)
   2. Preinjury functional level, including occupation/hobbies, ambulatory status, and hand dominance in patients with upper-extremity injuries
   3. History of prior orthopedic interventions
B. Physical examination
   1. Systematic examination of extremity reduces risk of missed injury.[1]
      a. Inspect for bruising, swelling, lacerations, abrasions, and deformity
      b. Palpate for tenderness, crepitus, and deformity of the underlying bone
      c. Compare with contralateral (uninjured) extremity and evaluate for asymmetry
   2. Vascular examination
      a. Palpate for pulses or Doppler arterial signals.
      b. Inspect capillary refill, temperature, color.
      c. The ankle-brachial index (ABI) is the ratio of systolic pressure of lower extremity to systolic pressure of upper extremity. Trauma patients with ABI < 0.9 should be further evaluated with diagnostic imaging. Technique for calculating ABI
         i. Measure systolic blood pressure of upper extremities: Locate brachial artery with Doppler transducer and inflate blood pressure cuff over the upper arm. Slowly deflate the cuff and note the pressure at which Doppler signal of brachial artery returns.
         ii. Measure systolic blood pressure of affected lower extremity: Locate dorsalis pedis and posterior tibia arteries of the foot with Doppler transducer and inflate blood pressure cuff over calf. Slowly deflate the cuff and note the pressures at which Doppler signals of pedal arteries return.
         iii. Calculate ABI by dividing the *highest pressure in foot* by the *higher pressure of the two arms.*
         iv. Elderly patients may have chronically low ABI due to peripheral vascular disease.
   3. Sensorimotor evaluation (**Table 9.1**)

TABLE 9.1 Peripheral Nerve Examination

Nerve	Sensory	Motor	Muscle
Deep peroneal (DP)	Web space between great and second toe	Ankle and great toe dorsiflexion	Tibialis anterior (TA), extensor hallucis longus (EHL)
Superficial peroneal	Lateral dorsum of foot	Eversion of hindfoot	Peroneus brevis and longus
Tibial (T)	Plantar surface of foot	Ankle and great toe plantar flexion	Gastrocnemius and soleus (GS), flexor hallucis longus (FHL)
Axillary (A)	Lateral deltoid	Shoulder abduction	Deltoid
Radial (R)	Dorsal web space between thumb and index	Extension of thumb IP joint	Extensor pollicis longus (EPL)
Median (M)	Two-point discrimination of thumb, index, long	Abduct thumb perpendicular to palm, flex index DIP joint	Abductor pollicis brevis (APB), flexor digitorum profundus to index (FDP2)
Ulnar (U)	Two-point discrimination of ring, small	Spread fingers apart, flex small finger DIP joint	Interossei (IO), flexor digitorum profundus to small (FDP5)

DIP, distal interphalangeal; IP, interphalangeal.

C. Imaging
   1. See **Table 9.2** for recommendations for injury-specific radiographic assessment.
   2. Include imaging of the joints above and below the injury
   3. Certain injuries (pelvic injuries and injuries involving joint spaces) often require further advanced imaging with CT.

D. Management: Certain conditions require immediate intervention and should be recognized by all trauma providers.
   1. Pelvic fractures and zone III retroperitoneal hematoma
      a. See Chapter 8 Abdominal Trauma for more information on retroperitoneal hematoma.
      b. Can present with hemorrhagic shock.
      c. Initial management with resuscitation and pelvic immobilization with binder or sheet.

TABLE 9.2 Imaging Examinations for Orthopedic Injuries

Conditions	X-Ray	Advanced Imaging
Clavicle fracture	Two views of the clavicle with both clavicles on the same exposure to evaluate length of the contralateral side	
Proximal humerus fracture	Shoulder series: AP/Grashey (true AP)/scapular Y/axillary view of the shoulder	
Scapula fracture	Shoulder series	CT
Shoulder dislocation	Shoulder series	
AC dislocation	Shoulder and clavicle series	
Sternoclavicular dislocation	Clavicle series	CT to evaluate displacement and visualize adjacent neurovascular structures
Humeral shaft fracture	Two orthogonal views of the humerus, full shoulder, and elbow series	
Distal humerus fracture	Elbow series: AP/lateral/oblique views of the elbow	
Radial head fracture	Elbow series	
Olecranon fracture	Elbow series	
Elbow dislocation	Elbow series	
Radius and ulna fracture	AP/lateral radiographs for the forearm, elbow, and wrist	
Distal radius fracture	Wrist series: PA/lateral/oblique	CT to evaluate comminuted intra-articular fractures
Scaphoid fracture	PA/lateral/ulnar deviation view/bilateral clenched fists on same exposure	

TABLE 9.2 Imaging Examinations for Orthopedic Injuries (*Continued*)

Conditions	X-Ray	Advanced Imaging
Hand finger fractures	PA/lateral of the hand	
Pelvic fracture	AP pelvis, inlet and outlet views	CT to evaluate pelvic, sacral, and lumbar fractures
Pubic rami fracture	AP pelvis, inlet and outlet views	CT
Acetabular fracture	AP pelvis. Judet views	CT
Femoral neck fracture	AP pelvis, cross-table lateral	MRI or CT if history suggests fracture, but none seen on radiograph
Intertrochanteric fracture	AP pelvis, cross-table lateral, traction view	MRI or CT if history suggests fracture, but none seen on radiograph
Femoral shaft fracture	AP/lateral of the femur, including AP/pelvis and AP lateral knee films	
Hip dislocation	AP pelvis, cross-table lateral. May require Judet views if acetabular fracture is present	CT scan for native hip dislocations post reduction
Distal femur fracture	AP/lateral knee, AP/lateral femur	
Patella fracture	AP/lateral knee	
Tibial plateau fracture	AP/lateral knee, AP/lateral tibia	CT scan prior to definitive fixation
Tibial shad fracture	AP/lateral tibia, AP/lateral knee, foil ankle series	
Knee dislocation	AP/lateral knee	CT angio to evaluate for vascular injury. MRI to evaluate for ligamentous injury (nonurgent)

(*continued*)

TABLE 9.2 Imaging Examinations for Orthopedic Injuries (*Continued*)

Conditions	X-Ray	Advanced Imaging
Pilon fracture	Ankle series: AP/lateral/ mortise views, consider full foot series	
Ankle fracture/ dislocation	Ankle series, may require stress view	
Calcaneus fracture	Lateral foot view, axial view of calcaneus. Consider lumbar spine films if patient has back pain	
Talus fracture/ dislocation	Ankle series, foot series	CT scan
Metatarsal fracture	Foot series: AP/lateral/ oblique	MRI or bone scan if concern for stress fracture
Lisfranc fracture	Foot series performed while weightbearing	CT or MRI if high suspicion and radio-graph negative

AC, acromioclavicular; AP, anterior–posterior; PA, posterior–anterior.

   d. Control of bleeding with angiogram/embolization or surgical packing of preperitoneal space is indicated if there is transient or no response to resuscitation.[2]

2. Open fractures—fractures associated with overlying soft tissue injury and break in skin.
   a. Require urgent administration of IV antibiotics (ideally within *1 hour*) and surgical debridement to prevent infection.[3]
3. Compartment syndrome—increased compartmental pressures resulting from hemorrhage into compartments or reperfusion injury. Can lead to irreversible damage of neurovascular structures and muscle necrosis.
   a. Pain is the most sensitive symptom/sign. Sensorimotor dysfunction is a late finding.
   b. Although there are tools that can objectively measure compartmental pressure, compartment syndrome is a clinical diagnosis and treatment should not be delayed for additional diagnostics.
   c. Treatment is fasciotomy to surgically release compartments. Prophylactic fasciotomy is indicated for limbs with reperfusion following prolonged ischemia from neurovascular injury.
   d. Technique of lower leg[4]

i. Adequate release of the four compartments of the lower leg (anterior, lateral, superficial posterior, deep posterior) can be achieved with two incisions.

ii. Medial incision is made about one fingerbreadth medial to tibia, extending from tibial tuberosity to medial malleolus. To access the deep posterior compartment, the soleus muscle is separated from the tibia.

iii. Lateral incision is made about one fingerbreadth anterior to the fibula, extending from fibular head to lateral malleolus. Adequate decompression can be achieved with an "H"-shaped incision into the anterior and lateral compartments and across the intermuscular septum.

iv. Following fasciotomy, the muscles should be assessed regularly for viability. Necrotic muscle should be promptly debrided.

v. Closure of fasciotomy incisions varies and includes primary closure and split-thickness skin grafts.

4. Mangled extremity—extremity with significant injury to the vascular, bony, soft tissue and/or nervous structures.

a. Salvageability of mangled extremity depends on several clinical factors, such as patient's clinical status, the ability to revascularize the limb within a timely fashion, and the overall presumed functional status of the limb if it is able to be salvaged. Management is complex and requires a multidisciplinary approach. Algorithm presented in **Figure 9.3** provides a simple overview of limb salvage.

b. Mangled extremity severity score (MESS) can help predict when limb salvage is feasible (**Table 9.3**).[5,6]

IV. INJURIES BY LOCATION

A. *Shoulder*

1. **Clavicle fractures**

a. Mechanism: Fall or direct blow to the shoulder

b. Treatment: Nonoperative with sling

2. **Proximal humerus fractures**

a. Mechanism: Low-energy fall, usually seen in the elderly

b. Treatment: Nonoperative with sling

i. Internal fixation should be considered if there is evidence of neurovascular compromise or humeral head avascular necrosis.

ii. Shoulder arthroplasty may be considered if stable internal fixation cannot be achieved.

3. **Scapula fractures**

a. Mechanism: High-energy chest trauma. Suspect thoracic injuries if scapula fracture is present.

b. Treatment is typically conservative management with sling. Surgery is required if intra-articular glenoid displacement is present.

4. **Shoulder (glenohumeral) dislocations**

a. Classification

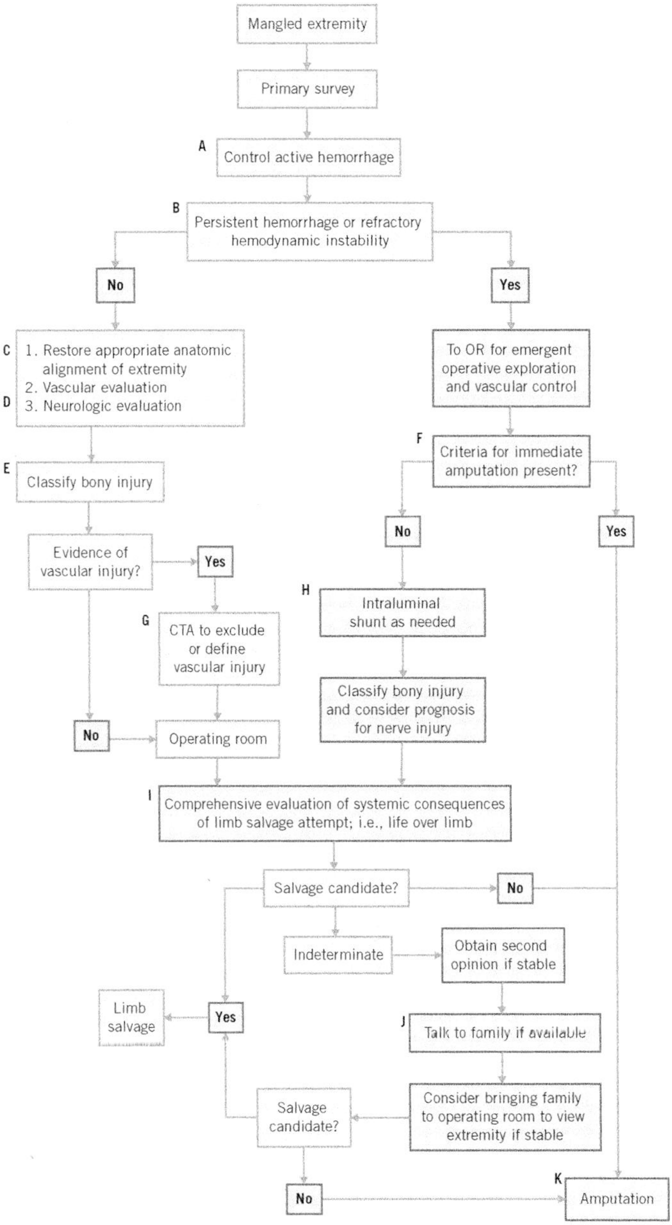

FIGURE 9.3 Algorithm for management of patients with mangled extremities. *(Reprinted with permission from Scalea TM, DuBose J, Moore EE, et al. Western Trauma Association critical decisions in trauma: management of the mangled extremity. J Trauma Acute Care Surg. 2012;72(1):86-93.)*

TABLE 9.3 Mangled Extremity Severity Score (MESS)

Mechanism of Injury	
Low energy (stab, simple fracture)	1
Medium energy (dislocation, comminuted fracture)	2
High energy (MVC, shotgun)	3
Very high energy (gross contamination)	4
Limb Ischemia (double if >6 h)	
No ischemia (palpable pulse)	0
Mild ischemia (reduced or absent pulse with normal perfusion)	1
Moderate ischemia (reduced capillary refill)	2
Severe ischemia (cold, paresthesia, no capillary refill)	3
Shock Present	
No hypotension	0
Transient hypotension	1
Persistent hypotension	2
Age (years)	
<30	0
30-50	1
≥50	2

MVC, motor vehicle collision.

MESS was originally designed to predict which injured extremities will ultimately require amputation. Traditionally, limbs with MESS ≥ 7 are considered unsalvageable. Although the more recent literature now advocate a multidisciplinary approach to limb salvage assessment and management, MESS still remains an important prognostic tool.

i. Anterior shoulder dislocations occur with forced shoulder abduction and/or external rotation.

b. Associated with injuries to axillary nerve and artery

i. Posterior shoulder dislocations are associated with seizure and electrical shock.

c. Treatment involves early reduction with axial traction and full abduction above the head.

5. **Acromioclavicular dislocations**
   a. Mechanism: A fall or direct blow to the shoulder
   b. Presentation: Pain with cross-body adduction
   c. Treatment: Nonoperative with sling
6. **Sternoclavicular (SC) dislocations**
   a. Mechanism: High-energy direct loads through the shoulder or upper chest
   b. Presentation
      i. Localized pain, swelling, and tenderness
      ii. Hoarseness, dyspnea, dysphagia, or engorged neck veins are red flags for posterior sternoclavicular joint dislocations with neurovascular compromise.
   c. Treatment
      i. Anterior SC dislocations: Conservative management
      ii. Posterior dislocations: Require reduction because of potential injury to mediastinal structures

B. *Upper arm and elbow*

1. **Humeral shaft fractures**
   a. Mechanism: Fall, direct blow to the arm, or rotational injury
   b. Associated with injury to radial nerve[7]
   c. Treatment
      i. Nonoperative management for closed fractures
      ii. Indications for surgical fixation include open fractures, concurrent injury below the elbow ("floating elbow"), or a body habitus that is not amenable to nonoperative management.
2. **Distal humerus fractures**
   a. Mechanism: Fall onto an outstretched hand or directly onto the elbow.
   b. Associated with injuries to median, radial, and ulnar nerves
   c. Treatment
      i. Operative intervention to prevent elbow joint stiffness
      ii. Comminuted articular fractures in the elderly population may benefit from total elbow arthroplasty if stable internal fixation cannot be achieved.
3. **Radial head fractures**
   a. Presentation: Limited elbow range of motion, pain with forearm rotation
   b. Treatment
      i. Nonoperative management if minimal involvement of the articular surface
      ii. Comminution or displacement may require operative intervention with internal fixation, radial head arthroplasty, or radial head excision.
4. **Elbow dislocations (ulnohumeral)**
   a. Mechanism: Posterolateral dislocations are most common, resulting from fall onto outstretched hand.

b. Treatment: Reduction and assessment of stability through gentle passive range of motion

C. *Forearm, wrist, and hand*

1. **Radial and ulnar shaft fractures**
   - **a.** Radial and ulnar fractures often occur together. These require operative intervention.
   - **b.** Isolated ulnar shaft fracture can occur following a direct blow to ulna.
   - **c.** Monteggia injury: Ulnar fracture with dislocation of radial head
   - **d.** Galeazzi injury: Radial fracture with distal radioulnar joint dislocation
2. **Distal radius fractures**
   - **a.** Mechanism: Fall onto an outstretched hand
   - **b.** Associated with acute carpal tunnel syndrome due to swelling or hematoma compressing median nerve, resulting in pain and/or paresthesia in the median nerve distribution
   - **c.** Treatment
     - **i.** Conservative management with splinting and cast immobilization for 4 to 6 weeks
     - **ii.** Displacement and limb shortening are indications for surgical treatment.
     - **iii.** Acute carpal tunnel must be released urgently.
3. **Scaphoid fractures**
   - **a.** Mechanism: Fall onto an outstretched hand.
   - **b.** Presentation: Tenderness in the "anatomic snuffbox" (triangular depression of dorsal surface of hand below base of thumb)
   - **c.** Treatment
     - **i.** Nondisplaced fractures can be treated with splint.
     - **ii.** Displaced fractures and proximal pole fractures are at risk of nonunion and avascular necrosis. Surgery is indicated.
4. **Metacarpal and phalangeal fractures**
   - **a.** The most common fracture is of the distal fifth metacarpal, or "boxer's fracture."
   - **b.** Presentation: Swelling and bruising over knuckles
   - **c.** Treatment
     - **i.** Reduction and splinting, followed by reexamination in 1 to 2 weeks for rotational deformity.
     - **ii.** Operative intervention indicated for open fractures, malalignment, and joint space widening.

D. *Pelvic fractures*

1. Young–Burgess classification
   - **a.** Anterior–posterior compression: Force applied along the anterior–posterior axis, resulting in disruption of pelvic ring (widening of pubic symphysis and/or sacroiliac joint space)
   - **b.** Lateral compression: Force applied laterally to medially, resulting in fractures of pubic rami, sacral ala, and/or posterior ilium. Usually not associated with intrapelvic hemorrhage.
2. **Pelvic ring disruption** injuries typically result from high-energy mechanisms, such as motor vehicle collisions or a fall from height.

a. Can be associated with life-threatening hemorrhage from zone III retroperitoneal hematomas (see Chapter 8 Abdominal Trauma for more information on retroperitoneal hematomas).
b. Presentation
    i. Crepitus, pelvic instability, or pain with iliac wing compression
    ii. Associated soft-tissue (i.e., degloving or Morel–Lavallée lesion), rectal, gynecologic, and lower urogenital injuries
c. Treatment
    i. See "Initial Assessment and Management of Extremity Trauma" for management of hemorrhage.
    ii. External fixation of pelvis until patient is stable for definitive surgical management.

3. **Pubic rami fractures**
    a. Mechanism: Isolated fractures occur in elderly patients after falls.
    b. Presentation: Groin pain and pain with weightbearing
    c. Treatment: Early mobilization
4. **Sacral fractures**
    a. Mechanisms: High-energy injury (young), low-energy fall (elderly)
    b. Complete sacral fractures, in which the fracture line passes through the entirety of the sacrum, require operative intervention
5. **Acetabular fractures**: Fracture of the articular surface of hip
    a. Associated with hip dislocations
    b. Treatment: Fractures of weightbearing portion of acetabulum require operative intervention

E. *Hip and femur*

1. **Hip fractures (femoral neck and intertrochanteric fractures)**
    a. Mechanism: Fall onto hip
    b. Classic presentation: Shortened, externally rotated lower extremity. However, they can present with nonspecific groin or medial thigh pain (site of referred pain from the hip joint).
    c. Treatment
        i. Surgery is indicated to promote early mobilization and reduce risk of avascular necrosis of the femoral head.[8,9]
        ii. Stable femoral neck fractures are treated with internal fixation.
        iii. Unstable femoral neck fractures may require hip arthroplasty.
2. **Hip dislocations**
    a. Mechanism: Posterior dislocations are most common and result from MVC (i.e., impact of dashboard on knee).
    b. Presentation: Shortened, adducted, and internally rotated limb
    c. Associated with sciatic or peroneal nerve injury
    d. Treatment: Immediate closed reduction with gentle traction and internal rotation of affected limb
3. **Femoral shaft fractures**
    a. High-energy mechanisms, associated with polytrauma
    b. Treatment
        i. Immediate application of skeletal traction to stabilize fracture until surgical intervention
        ii. Preferred surgical intervention is reduction and internal fixation with intramedullary nail.

iii. In the clinically unstable patient, external fixation may be the initial treatment.[10]

F. *Knee and tibia*

1. **Distal femur fractures**
   a. Early reduction and immobilization prevent malalignment of distal femur, which greatly affects gait and force transfer through the lower extremity.
   b. Most will require surgical intervention.
2. **Patellar fractures**
   a. Mechanism: Direct fall onto the knee
   b. Presentation: Palpable defect, unable to perform a straight-leg raise
   c. Treatment
      i. Fractures with displacement, joint incongruity, or loss of active knee extension require surgical treatment.
      ii. Nondisplaced or vertical fractures can be treated with a knee immobilizer and weightbearing as tolerated.
3. **Knee dislocations**
   a. High-energy mechanisms
   b. Presentation: Deformity, ligamentous instability, and neurovascular compromise
   c. The incidence of concomitant vascular injury, usually of popliteal neurovascular bundle, is approximately 30%.
      i. Pedal pulse examination has a low sensitivity (79%) for detecting significant vascular injury.[11]
      ii. ABI testing and CT angiogram can be used for further evaluation.
   d. Treatment
      i. Emergent reduction to reduce risk of permanent neurovascular injury
      ii. If vascular repair is necessary, a spanning external fixator can be placed to stabilize the knee. After any vascular repair, prophylactic fasciotomy of the lower leg should be considered.
      iii. Delayed ligamentous reconstruction may be necessary to restore knee stability.[12]
4. **Tibial plateau fractures:** Fractures of tibia that involve the articular surface.
   a. Presentation: Knee effusions, swelling in the lower leg, ecchymosis, and deformity
   b. Treatment
      i. Nondisplaced fractures may be treated with brace and nonweightbearing.
      ii. Surgical intervention is required for articular incongruity, displacement, comminution, or instability.
      iii. If severe soft tissue swelling is present, external fixation is used until surgical fixation is feasible.[10]
5. **Tibial shaft fractures**
   a. High risk of open fractures
   b. Treatment
      i. Early debridement and administration of intravenous antibiotics for open fractures

ii. Most fractures require internal fixation with intramedullary nailing to promote early mobility.
iii. Since tibial shaft fractures are associated with neurovascular injuries, consider prophylactic fasciotomy.

G. **Distal tibia and ankle**

1. **Pilon fractures:** Intra-articular distal tibia fractures, often comminuted
   a. Mechanism: Axial loading mechanism such as a fall from height
   b. Associated with significant soft tissue injury, such as swelling and fracture blisters
   c. Treatment[13]
      i. Usually require operative intervention
      ii. Given soft tissue swelling, may require initial treatment with external fixation until operative intervention is feasible
   d. May result in significant posttraumatic ankle arthritis
2. **Ankle fractures**: Involve the lateral, medial, and/or posterior malleoli but lack the impaction and comminution seen in pilon fractures
   a. Twisting mechanism
   b. Treatment
      i. All fractures should be reduced in the emergency room with postreduction radiographs demonstrating adequate joint and fracture reduction.
      ii. Stable, nondisplaced fractures of the ankle can be treated with immobilization and protected weightbearing.
      iii. Unstable fractures (one with both medial and lateral injuries) and fractures with joint subluxation benefit from operative treatment.
3. **Achilles tendon ruptures**
   a. Mechanism: Running, jumping, or vigorous physical activity
   b. Presentation: Sudden posterior ankle pain and difficulty walking. Examination reveals palpable defect, weak plantar flexion.
      i. Thompson sign: No passive ankle plantar flexion on squeezing the patient's calf. Seen with complete rupture.
   c. Similar outcomes achieved with operative and nonoperative interventions.[14]

H. Foot

1. **Calcaneus fractures**
   a. Presentation: Axial load such as fall from height
   b. Associated with spine fractures
   c. Treatment is usually nonoperative with splint.
2. **Talus fractures**
   a. Mechanism: Forced dorsiflexion of foot (i.e., impact to foot from MVC)
   b. Associated with ankle dislocations
   c. Talar dislocations are treated with emergent reduction to decrease the risk of avascular necrosis, neurovascular injury, and skin compromise.
3. **Lisfranc injuries:** Disruptions of the Lisfranc ligament, which runs from the base of the second metatarsal to the medial cuneiform

a. Mechanism: Bending or twisting force through the midfoot
b. Presentation: Significant swelling and midfoot tenderness. Pathognomonic examination finding is plantar ecchymosis at the midfoot.
c. Lisfranc injuries are placed in a bulky splint and elevated in preparation for eventual operative treatment.

4. **Metatarsal fractures**
   a. Mechanism: Stress fractures (i.e., distance runners)
   b. Treatment
      i. Single metatarsal fractures can be treated nonoperatively.
         a) Jones fracture, or fracture of fifth metatarsal, occurs in vascular watershed area. Requires more aggressive treatment, including surgery.
      ii. Multiple metatarsal fractures: Closed reduction and percutaneous pinning
5. **Toe fractures** are best treated by "buddy taping" to the adjacent digit and giving the patient a hard-soled shoe for more comfortable ambulation.

Key References

Citation	Summary
Johansen K, Daines M, Howey T, Helfet D, Hansen ST Jr. Objective criteria accurately predict amputation following lower extremity trauma. *J Trauma.* 1990;30(5):568-573.	• Retrospective analysis of 25 patients with severe lower extremity injuries—9 limbs required amputation (mean MESS $< 9.11 \pm 0.51$); 17 limbs were salvaged (mean, 4.88 ± 0.27). • Prospective analysis demonstrated significant difference between 14 salvaged (mean, 4.00 ± 0.28) and 12 doomed (mean, 8.83 ± 0.53). • In both analysis, MESS ≥ 7 predicted amputation with 100% accuracy.
Gustilo RB, Anderson JT. Prevention of infection in the treatment of one thousand and twenty-five open fractures of long bones: retrospective and prospective analyses. *J Bone Joint Surg Am.* 1976;58(4):453-458.	• Meta-analysis evaluating effectiveness of antibiotics in the initial treatment of open fractures • Analysis of data from 913 patients has demonstrated use of antibiotics had a protective effect (reduced risk of early wound infection, chronic drainage, osteomyelitis, delayed union or nonunion, amputation, death) compared with no antibiotics.
Simunovic N, Devereaux PJ, Sprague S, et al. Effect of early surgery after hip fracture on mortality and complications: systematic review and meta-analysis. *CMAJ.* 2010;182(15):1609-1616.	• Meta-analysis of 13,478 elderly patients from 16 observational studies demonstrated early or surgical treatment (within 72 h) for hip fracture associated with significant reduction in mortality (relative risk 0.81, 95% confidence interval 0.68-0.98).

CHAPTER 9: EXTREMITY TRAUMA

Review Questions

1. Open fractures require administration of _______ within 1 hour of diagnosis to prevent infection.
2. What are the four compartments of the lower leg? How are these compartments decompressed with a two-incision fasciotomy?
3. Name three orthopedic injuries that often require surgical intervention.

REFERENCES

1. Pfeifer R, Pape HC. Missed injuries in trauma patients: a literature review. *Patient Saf Surg*. 2008;2:20.
2. Velmahos GC, Toutouzas KG, Vassiliu P, et al. A prospective study on the safety and efficacy of angiographic embolization for pelvic and visceral injuries. *J Trauma*. 2002;53(2):303-308; discussion 308.
3. Gustilo RB, Anderson JT. Prevention of infection in the treatment of one thousand and twenty-five open fractures of long bones: retrospective and prospective analyses. *J Bone Joint Surg Am*. 1976;58(4):453-458.
4. Bowyer MW. Lower extremity fasciotomy: indications and technique. *Current Trauma Reports*. 2015;1:35-44.
5. Johansen K, Daines M, Howey T, Helfet D, Hansen ST Jr. Objective criteria accurately predict amputation following lower extremity trauma. *J Trauma*. 1990;30(5):568-572; discussion 572-573.
6. Togawa S, Yamami N, Nakayama H, Mano Y, Ikegami K, Ozeki S. The validity of the mangled extremity severity score in the assessment of upper limb injuries. *J Bone Joint Surg Br*. 2005;87(11):1516-1519.
7. Shao YC, Harwood P, Grotz MR, Limb D, Giannoudis PV. Radial nerve palsy associated with fractures of the shaft of the humerus: a systematic review. *J Bone Joint Surg Br*. 2005;87(12):1647-1652.
8. Simunovic N, Devereaux PJ, Sprague S, et al. Effect of early surgery after hip fracture on mortality and complications: systematic review and meta-analysis. *CMAJ (Can Med Assoc J)*. 2010;182(15):1609-1616.
9. Zuckerman JD, Skovron ML, Koval KJ, Aharonoff G, Frankel VH. Postoperative complications and mortality associated with operative delay in older patients who have a fracture of the hip. *J Bone Joint Surg Am*. 1995;77(10):1551-1556.
10. Tuttle MS, Smith WR, Williams AE, et al. Safety and efficacy of damage control external fixation versus early definitive stabilization for femoral shaft fractures in the multiple-injured patient. *J Trauma*. 2009;67(3):602-605.
11. Mills WJ, Barei DP, McNair P. The value of the ankle-brachial index for diagnosing arterial injury after knee dislocation: a prospective study. *J Trauma*. 2004;56(6):1261-1265.
12. Mook WR, Miller MD, Diduch DR, Hertel J, Boachie-Adjei Y, Hart JM. Multiple-ligament knee injuries: a systematic review of the timing of operative intervention and postoperative rehabilitation. *J Bone Joint Surg Am*. 2009;91(12):2946-2957.
13. Watson JT, Moed BR, Karges DE, Cramer KE. Pilon fractures. Treatment protocol based on severity of soft tissue injury. *Clin Orthop Relat Res*. 2000;2000(375):78-90.
14. Uquillas CA, Guss MS, Ryan DJ, Jazrawi LM, Strauss EJ. Everything achilles: knowledge update and current concepts in management—AAOS exhibit selection. *J Bone Joint Surg Am*. 2015;97(14):1187-1195.

10 Burns

Oluseye Oduyale, Bracken A. Armstrong,
Jessica Kramer McCool, and John Kirby

I. INTRODUCTION

A. Burn injuries result from acute exposure—thermal, chemical, or electrical.

B. Burns compromise the skin's function as a barrier to injury and infection and as a regulator of body temperature and fluid loss.

C. Like trauma, mortality from burns occur in a multimodal pattern: Immediately after the injury or weeks later from sepsis and multiorgan failure.

II. ASSESSMENT OF BURN PATIENTS

A. Burns are often associated with traumatic injuries.

B. Initial assessment focuses on the primary and secondary survey (see Chapter 5 Trauma Resuscitation for more information).

C. Specific guidelines for the management of burns may also be found in the American Burn Association consensus statement[1] and the International Society of Burn Injury practice guidelines for burn care.[2,3] See **Figure 10.1** for an overview of assessment and management of burn injuries.

1. **Primary survey**
   a. **Airway**
      i. Suspect airway compromise in all patients, especially with injuries sustained in confined spaces or explosions.
      ii. Signs of airway compromise include hoarseness, stridor, facial burns, singed hair, carbonaceous sputum.
      iii. When appropriate, consider nasolaryngoscopy or bronchoscopy to assess for airway edema, erythema, and carbonaceous deposits.

   b. **Breathing**
      i. Severely burned patients develop early pulmonary insufficiency due to direct tracheobronchial injury or inflammatory responses leading to acute respiratory distress syndrome.
      ii. Signs of breathing compromise include increased work of breathing, wheezing, and desaturations. If on mechanical ventilation, monitor for higher FiO_2 to PaO_2 ratios, and higher peak or plateau pressures.

   c. **Circulation**
      i. Severely burned patients often suffer from a combination of hypovolemic and distributive shock as a result of insensible fluid losses, severe inflammation, and capillary leakage.

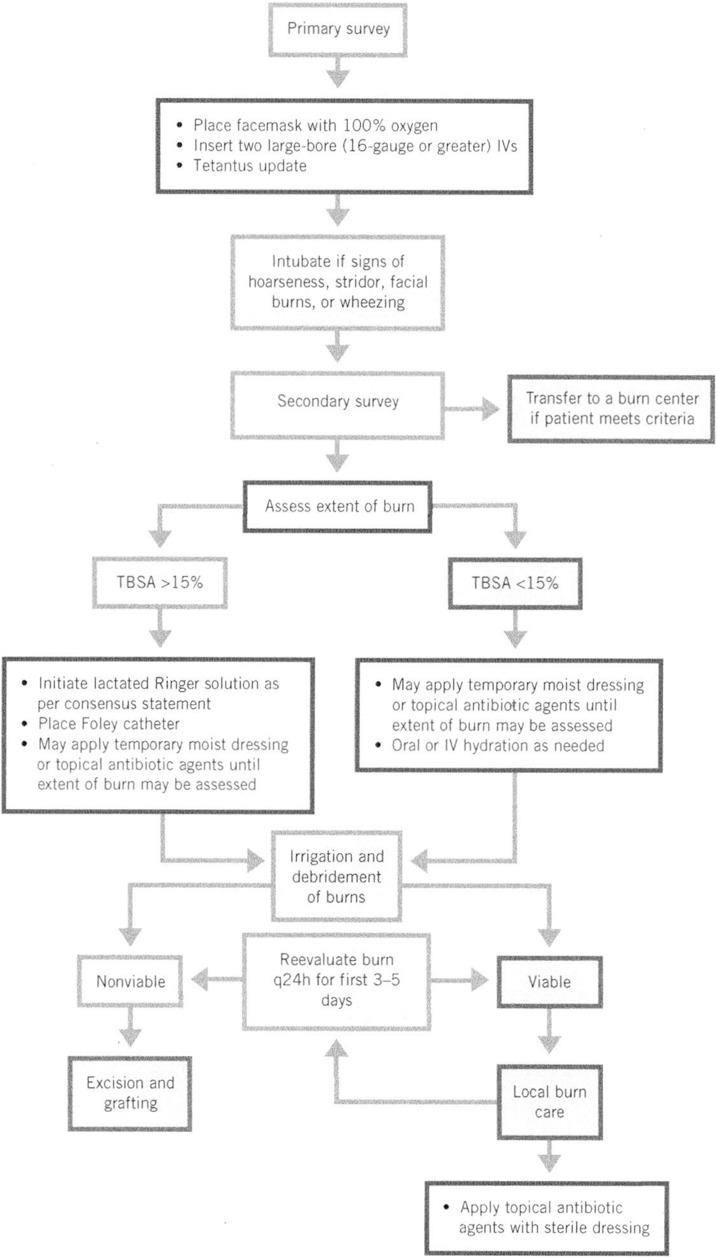

FIGURE 10.1 Algorithm for the evaluation and management of burns.

ii. Monitor signs of hemodynamic instability.
iii. Suspect compartment syndrome in circumferential burns of the trunk or extremities.

d. **Disability**
i. Calculate Glasgow Coma Scale and perform neurologic examination, including peripheral extremity neurological and functional examinations.

e. **Exposure**
i. Remove all clothing, including jewelry, to prevent any continued injury.
ii. Assess for signs of other traumatic injuries.

2. **Secondary survey**
a. **Depth:** See **Table 10.1** for overview of burn depths.
i. Classified based on the deepest layer of soft tissue involved
ii. Ranges from superficial, affecting only the epidermis, to full thickness and deeper, affecting muscle and bone

TABLE 10-1 Classification of burns according to injury depth, exam features, and clinical outcome.

Injury Class and Depth	Exam Features	Clinical Outcome
Superficial *Epidermis*	Dry with blanching erythema. Painful to touch.	Heals in <1 week without scarring.
Superficial partial-thickness *Papillary dermis*	Moist with blisters. Blanching erythema. Severe pain to touch.	Heals in <1 month without hypertrophic scarring. Expect return of full function.
Deep partial-thickness *Reticular dermis*	Easily unroofed blisters with blanching erythema or pale color. Pain to pressure only.	Heals in <2 months with scarring. Earlier and improved outcome expected with surgery.
Full-thickness and deeper *Subcutaneous fat, muscle, or bone*	Dry, waxy white, leathery gray or charred black with no capillary refill. Pain to deep pressure only.	Expect functional impairment and scarring without surgery.

b. Percent total body surface area (TBSA) estimation

i. Small areas: The area of patient's hand, including palm and fingers, is approximately 1% TBSA.[5]

ii. Large areas: Rule of 9's where each region represents a multiple of 9% TBSA.[6] See **Figure 10.2** to see how the rule of 9's is applied to adult and pediatric patients.

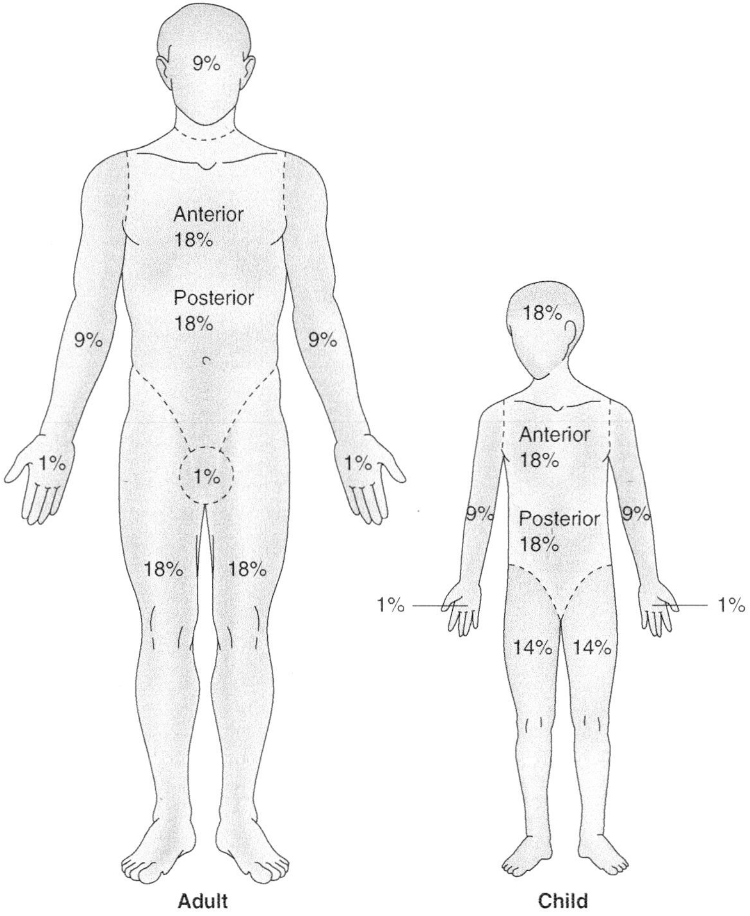

FIGURE 10.2 Estimation of percent area burned in adults and children using the rule of nines.

3. **Burn center referrals**

Per guidelines of the American Burn Association, patients with any of the following should be referred to a burn center with consideration given for possible transfer.[7]

a. Partial-thickness burns >10% TBSA.
b. Any full-thickness burn.
c. Burns that involve the face, hands, feet, genitalia, perineum, or major joints.
d. Inhalation, chemical, or electrical injury (including lightning).
e. Patients with preexisting conditions that could complicate management, prolong recovery, or affect mortality.
f. Significant associated mechanical trauma. Note, if the traumatic injury poses a greater threat to life, the patient should be stabilized at a trauma center before transfer to a burn unit.
g. Children in hospitals without qualified personnel or equipment for the care of children.
h. Patients requiring specialized rehabilitation, psychological support, or social services (including suspected neglect or child abuse).

III. MANAGEMENT OF BURN PATIENTS

A. Resuscitation

1. **Oxygen**
   a. All patients should receive at 100% O_2 via facemask until CO toxicity is ruled out or resolved if found.
   b. Major inhalation injuries require early intubation optimally with large-bore endotracheal tubes to assist with aggressive pulmonary toileting.
2. **IV fluids**
   a. At least two large-bore peripheral IV lines are required for administration of crystalloid in patients with burns >15% TBSA.
   b. IV lines placed near or through burnt tissue may need to be sutured in place to maintain their position with subsequent tissue swelling.
   c. Oral rehydration can be adequate for patients with minor injuries.
   d. American Burn Association consensus formula for initial resuscitation in burn patients:
      i. Give half of total volume in first 8 hours, then half over next 16 hours.
   e. Although estimated infusion needs are helpful, overresuscitation may be harmful and efforts should be continuously adjusted based on patient's clinical response.

$$2 \text{ to } 4 mLs * Weight \text{ in } kg * \%TBSA = Volume \text{ required in first } 24 \text{ hours}$$

B. Further management

1. **Pain control and sedation**
   a. Narcotics are often needed for acute pain control.
   b. Ketamine may have less hemodynamic effects for procedural pain control and sedation.

c. Dexmedetomidine is preferred for long-term sedation and reduces opioid requirement.
d. NSAIDs and other nonopioid analgesics are important adjuncts.

2. **Foley catheter**
   a. Monitor urine output for >1 mL/kg/h in children and 0.5 mL/kg/h in adults and adjust ongoing resuscitation accordingly.
3. **Naso- and orogastric tubes**
   a. Insert in the intubated patients and those who develop nausea and vomiting. This may also be necessary for enteral access for nutrition and medication.
4. **Continuous pulse oximetry**
   a. Falsely elevated levels can be seen in carbon monoxide poisoning.
5. **Diagnostic testing**
   a. Complete blood count, type and cross, basic metabolic panel, β-hCG (in women), arterial blood gas, lactate, arterial carboxyhemoglobin, and urinalysis.
   b. ECG is useful particularly in elderly patients or those with electrical burns or significant electrolyte derangements.
6. **Tetanus prophylaxis**
   a. Tetanus toxoid vaccine: Indicated if last booster ≥5 years
   b. Human tetanus immunoglobulin (Hyper-Tet): If unvaccinated or vaccination status unknown
7. **Treatment of associated injuries**
   a. In explosions, patients may suffer a wide range of thermal, blast, blunt, and penetrating injuries. It is necessary to address life-threatening injuries in conjunction with Advanced Trauma Life Support (ATLS) guidelines.

C. Local wound care

A surgical consultation should be obtained for all patients with significant injury.

1. **Irrigation and debridement**
   a. Blisters and bullae should be unroofed.
   b. Can be completed under bedside procedural sedation
   c. Remove superficial debris and necrotic tissue to assess true depth of injury. Removal of nonviable tissue also reduces bacterial colonization and subsequent infection and promotes wound healing
   d. Normal saline, sterile instruments, scrub brushes, towels may be used.
2. **Dressings and ointments**
   a. See **Table 10.2** for a brief description of topical antimicrobial agents.
   b. Clean burn wounds are covered with a nonadherent dressing, which serves as thermal insulation and as a barrier from particulates and micro-organisms.
   c. Dressings should be changed 1 to 2 times daily for the first 3 to 5 days.
   d. Choice of topical antimicrobial agent and dressing should be communicated with the burn center prior to transfer.

TABLE 10.2 Topical Antimicrobial Agents for Burns

Agent	Advantages	Disadvantages
Silver sulfadiazine (Silvadene)	Broad spectrum (gram-positive and negative, some fungal) Nonirritating Cream limits water and heat loss	*Pseudomonas* resistance Limits wound visibility Difficult to remove Reduces epithelialization rate Occasional transient leukopenia Contraindicated in sulfa allergy
Mafenide acetate (Sulfamylon)	Broad spectrum (including *Pseudomonas* and *Enterococcus* species) Good eschar penetration	Expensive in solution form Painful Allergic rash Metabolic acidosis via carbonic anhydrase inhibition Contraindicated in sulfa allergy
Polymyxin B sulfate, neomycin, bacitracin, mupirocin	Painless Clear ointment allows wound observation Tolerated well on facial burns Mupirocin-improved activity MRSA and gram-negative	Poor gram-negative coverage Poor eschar penetration
Silver nitrate	Good antimicrobial coverage Safe in sulfa allergy	Painful Stains tissue gray to black Hypotonic (can cause hypoNa) Nitrate toxicity can cause methemoglobinemia
Silver-impregnated dressings (Acticoat, Aquacel Ag, Mepilex Ag)	Easy application Good antimicrobial coverage Lasts up to 7 d	Expensive

MRSA, methicillin-resistant *Staphylococcus aureus.*

e. Early transfers may need solely clean dressings to allow for better assessment on burn center arrival without needing to remove topical creams or ointments.

D. Operative management

1. **Escharotomy**
   - a. Noncompliance of full-thickness circumferential burns and subsequent tissue edema can lead to compartment syndrome.
   - b. Longitudinal, full-thickness incisions in the eschar should be performed.
   - c. **Surgical technique: General principles of escharotomy**
     - i. Escharotomies are indicated in patients with circumferential deep dermal or full-thickness burns of torso or limbs that can compromise circulatory or respiratory function.
     - ii. Plan and mark incisions.
     - iii. Sharply incise the tissue into the subcutaneous fat. Bluntly open up the incision to ensure the wound edges are adequately separated.
     - iv. Incisions should be dressed with antimicrobial nonadherent dressings.
     - v. Patient should be closely monitored for restoration of circulatory and respiratory function.
2. **Burn excision**
   - a. Tangential excision is preferred as soon as tolerable given patient hemodynamics and other critical injuries.
   - b. For deep-partial and full-thickness burns, it is essential to remove nonviable tissue and provide well-perfused wound bed for healing or grafting.
   - c. Early excision and grafting have been shown to reduce hypermetabolism, infection rates, length of stay, and mortality.[8]
   - d. For each trip to the operating room, consider limiting burn excision to <20% TBSA or 2 hours of operating time.
   - e. **Surgical technique: Burn excision and skin grafting**
     - i. Deep burn injuries require excision of eschar and ischemic/necrotic tissue to expose healthy, well-perfused wound bed for closure vs. coverage. This usually occurs 24 to 72 hours after burn injury, as the primary objective immediately after injury is resuscitation and management of other traumatic injuries that may be life-threatening.
     - ii. The most common form of excision is tangential burn excision, which involves serial removal of layers of tissue until bleeding is encountered.
     - iii. Control blood loss from the wound bed with electrocautery (although this should be minimized to promote wound healing) or topical hemostatic agents such as fibrin sealants.
     - iv. Smaller wounds can be closed primarily.
     - v. For larger wounds, autologous skin grafting is a common technique to provide coverage.

a) Full-thickness skin grafting: Donor tissue is applied as is to wound bed. This is used around joints (minimize risk of contracture) and cosmetically sensitive areas such as the face and neck.

b) Split-thickness skin grafting: Donor tissue is meshed to increase surface area.

3. **Wound coverage**.

a. Direct wound closure is a good option for smaller wounds that can close with little tension.

b. For larger wounds, wound coverage restores native function of skin and can help with cosmesis.

c. Wound coverage should be applied to clean, well-perfused wounds.

d. Several options exist for temporary or permanent wound coverage, ranging from autologous skin grafts to synthetic substitutes. See **Table 10.3** for an overview of wound coverage options.

e. Temporary coverage materials are advantageous when donor sites are limited or physiology inadequate for permanent operative coverage.

TABLE 10.3 Overview of Wound Coverage Options for Burn Patients

	Notes	Disadvantages
Autograft	Harvested from patient, thus avoids immunologic rejection Split-thickness skin graft (STSG) • Harvested between 0.008 and 0.012 in and can be meshed up to 4:1. • Allows for reharvesting within 2-3 wk Full-thickness skin graft • Allows for better cosmesis and function in certain anatomic areas (e.g., face, hands, neck)	Limited availability in severely burned patients STSG likely to form contractures Creation of additional wounds Take rates variable
Allograft	Cadaveric skin grafts may help shrink wound size, facilitating autografting	Poorer take rates than autograft Expensive
Xenograft	Obtained from unrelated species Readily available and inexpensive	Poorer take rates than allograft
Synthetic/biosynthetic	E.g., Biobrane, Integra, Alloderm Combination of collagen, growth factors, and synthetic compounds formed into matrix or membrane to facilitate growth Helps prime wound bed for autografting	Higher rates of infection

f. **Skin grafting** should be applied to clean, noninfected, and granulating bed to facilitate adequate take and subsequent healing.
g. **Flap reconstruction** may be needed for complex wounds with deeper structures (muscle, bone, nerves, or vessels) exposed. For larger wounds, flap reconstruction can minimize contractures that can limit function.

E. Nutrition

Severe burns can induce a hypermetabolic state up to 200% the normal metabolic rate and lasting up to a year post injury. This may manifest long-term as persistent tachycardia, failure to thrive, and/or poor wound-healing capacity.[9,10]

1. Curreri formula for burn patients: Estimated metabolic requirements = (25 kcal × weight in kg) + (40 kcal × % TBSA)
2. **Early enteral feeds**
   a. Shown to decrease the hypermetabolic response, hospital stay, and infection rates[11]
   b. Nasogastric or nasojejunal tubes may be required for supplemental tube feeds in severely burned patients.
   c. Patients requiring frequent debridement may benefit from surgical postpyloric feeding access to maximize nutritional intake.
   d. Parenteral nutrition is recommended for patients who do not tolerate full caloric needs via enteral routes.
3. **Micronutrient supplementation**
   a. Although no formal guidelines on supplementation exist, trace elements (Cu, Zn, Se) and vitamins (A, C, E) decrease healing time and rates of infection.[12]
4. **Adjunctive therapies**
   a. Improved outcomes have been shown with use of β-blockade (propranolol) and anabolic steroids (oxandrolone, recombinant growth hormone) to offset catabolic state.[10]

F. Infection

Burn patients are at high risk for burn wound and non-burn-related infections (catheter-associated infections, pneumonia, etc.). Infections are the leading cause of death in burn patients.[13]

1. **Burn wound infection**
   a. Defined as $\geq 10^5$ organisms per gram of tissue.
   b. Gram-positive organisms are the most common pathogens in early burn wound infections. Burn wound infections with gram-negative organisms (i.e., *Pseudomonas*) and yeast can be seen later on during the hospitalization.
   c. The most common causal organism is *Staphylococcus aureus*.
   d. Atypical and fungal isolates increase mortality risks.
   e. See **Table 10.4** for classification and management of burn wound infections.
2. **Burn sepsis**
   a. Difficult to diagnose in burn patients as physiologic derangements from burns themselves can be similar to those from sepsis.
   b. Suspicion is based on rapid clinical changes and physical appearance of wounds (i.e., purulence, bullae, discoloration, malodor, fat liquefication).

TABLE 10.4 Management of Burn Wound Infection

	Characteristics	Management
Colonization	$<10^5$ organisms No wound changes	Local wound care and routine dressing changes Prophylactic antibiotics not indicated
Noninvasive infection	$>10^5$ organisms No organisms in unburned tissue Absence of systemic changes	Wound excision, topical antimicrobial therapy, local wound care Antibiotics are reserved for spreading erythema (gram-positive coverage, with MRSA or *Pseudomonas* coverage based on clinical suspicion)
Invasive infection	$>10^5$ organisms with Organisms in unburned tissue OR Systemic signs of sepsis	Resuscitation as indicated, broad-spectrum antibiotics, serial wide excision every 24-28 h until wound is clean and appears viable

Antibiotics may be started empirically but should ultimately be tailored to culture or histopathologic data as available.

MRSA, methicillin-resistant *Staphylococcus aureus*.

c. American Burn Association criteria for burn sepsis in adults:
   i. One of the following
      a) Culture-confirmed infection (blood, wound, urine, etc.)
      b) Pathologic tissue source ($>10^5$ organisms)
      c) Response to antimicrobial administration
   ii. **AND** three of the following:
      a) Temperature >39 or <36.5 °C
      b) Progressive tachycardia, heart rate > 110
      c) Progressive tachypnea, >25 breaths per min
      d) Leukocytosis or leukopenia
      e) Thrombocytopenia 3 days after initial resuscitation
      f) Hyperglycemia (in nondiabetics) or worsening insulin resistance
      g) Intolerance of enteral feeds >24 h

IV. SPECIAL CONSIDERATIONS

A. Inhalation injuries

This should be suspected in all burn patients, especially patients presenting with loss of consciousness, found in enclosed spaces, or exposed to flames or chemicals.

1. **Airway injuries**
   a. May present as hoarseness, stridor, facial burns, singed hair, carbonaceous sputum

b. Heat generally affects upper airway, while chemicals and steam travel further, damaging lower airway and lung parenchyma.
c. Treatment: Supportive care, early intubation
   i. Nebulized heparin has been shown to reduce the number of mechanical ventilation days for burn patients.[14]

2. **Carbon monoxide poisoning**
   a. Should be suspected in patients with inhalational injuries
   b. Falsely elevates pulse-oximetry readings
   c. Symptoms include headache, lethargy, nausea, and vomiting. Associated with "cherry-red lips."
   d. Normal CO-Hb values: <5% nonsmokers, <10% in smokers
   e. Treatment: Oxygen administration (via facemask or hyperbaric chamber) reduces half-life of CO-Hb.
3. **Hydrogen cyanide poisoning**
   a. Should be suspected in closed space interior fires in association with any CO poisoning
   b. Suspect in patients with persistent acidosis without other sources.
   c. Treatment: Empiric hydroxocobalamin (Cyanokit), sodium thiosulfate

B. Electrical injuries
1. Injury is proportional to voltage, current, duration of contact, and electrical resistance of tissues affected.
2. Severity is often underestimated as only entrance and exit wounds are visible.
3. Associated injuries include burns, rhabdomyolysis, cardiac injury, and fractures.
4. High suspicion for **compartment syndrome** in these patients

C. Chemical injuries
1. **Dry compounds**—brush off prior to copious irrigation
2. **Acidic compounds**—causes coagulative necrosis. Hydrofluoric (HF) acid is absorbed rapidly and may be cardiotoxic as it causes hypomagnesemia and hypocalcemia.
3. **Basic compounds**—penetrates deeply and causes liquefactive necrosis
4. **Management**—remove soiled clothing and debris, irrigate for 15 to 30 mins, consult to toxicology center for systemic toxicities. Neutralizing agents generally not to be recommended. Apply Ca gel for HF acid burns and IV Ca for HF acid toxicity.

D. Cold injuries
1. **Hypothermia:** See **Table 10.5** for classification of hypothermia.
   a. Body temperature < 35 °C. See **Table 10.5** for the stages of hypothermia.[16]
   b. **Passive rewarming:** Blankets or other forms of insulation
   c. **Active external warming:** Heating blankets, heated forced-air or water systems
   d. **Active internal rewarming** needed for severe hypothermia and includes the use of warmed intravenous fluids. Invasive rewarming methods can include warmed peritoneal/pleural lavage, extracorporeal membrane oxygenation, or heated hemodialysis.
2. **Frostbite**
   a. Results from intracellular ice crystals and microvascular occlusion

TABLE 10.5 Stages of Accidental Hypothermia and Clinical Findings

	Temperature (°C)	Clinical Findings
Cold stress	37-35	Shivering without significant physiologic changes
Stage I (mild)	35-32	Altered mentation, tachycardia, tachypnea, cold diuresis, shivering, coagulopathy
Stage II (moderate)	32-28	Lethargy, bradycardia, arrhythmias, hypoventilation, blunted shivering
Stage III (severe)	<28	Coma, v-fib, cardiac arrest, apnea, areflexia, oliguria

Stage IV hypothermia is defined as hypothermia with absent vitals. The risk of cardiac arrest increases <32 °C but is unlikely to be due solely to hypothermia until <28 °C.

b. Classification
   i. **First degree:** Hyperemia and edema, without skin necrosis
   ii. **Second degree:** Superficial vesicle formation containing clear or milky fluid surrounded by hyperemia, edema, and partial-thickness necrosis
   iii. **Third degree:** Hemorrhagic bullae and full-thickness necrosis
   iv. **Fourth degree:** Gangrene with full-thickness involvement of skin, muscle, and bone

c. Treatment: Warm water bath (40-42 °C) or moist heat, elevation, weightbearing precautions, escharotomy as indicated. Consider tissue plasminogen activator with or without heparin to improve perfusion.[15]

d. Frostbite wounds can evolve weeks after injury; thus, debridement or amputation should be delayed to allow wound to demarcate. More urgent surgical intervention is needed if dry gangrene develops into wet gangrene.

E. Long-term care

1. Burn survivors often suffer long-term issues related to pain, cosmesis, skin fragility, and/or itching, mental health illness, or permanent disability.
2. Long-term care of burn patients include
   a. Intensive physical rehabilitation
   b. Nutrition optimization
   c. Prompt management of wound complications like contractures and graft loss
   d. Psychosocial support

Key References

Citation	Summary
Ong YS, Samuel M, Song C. Meta-analysis of early excision of burns. *Burns*. 2006;32(2):145-50.	• Meta-analysis of randomized control trials comparing early excision (within 0-5 d) of burns to conservative treatment. • Early excision was shown to reduce mortality, and length of stay, although patients experienced increased transfusion requirements.
Mosier MJ, Pham TN, Klein MB, et al. Early enteral nutrition in burns: compliance with guidelines and associated outcomes in a multicenter study. *J Burn Care Res*. 2011;32(1):104-109.	• Retrospective review of 154 mechanically ventilated burn patients comparing outcomes of enteral nutrition started before or after 24 h. • No differences in abdominal compartment syndrome, hyperglycemia, or gastrointestinal bleeds; however, early nutrition decreased wound infection rates and intensive care unit length of stay.
Cox CL, McIntire AM, Bolton KJ, et al. A multicenter evaluation of outcomes following the use of nebulized heparin for inhalation injury (HIHI2 Study). *J Burn Care Res*. 2020;41(5):1004-1008.	• Multicenter, retrospective, case–control study comparing administration of nebulized heparin vs. control in patients with inhalation injury. • Patients who received nebulized heparin had 8-11 fewer days on the ventilator.
Herndon DN, Hart DW, Wolf SE, Chinkes DL, Wolfe RR. Reversal of catabolism by beta-blockade after severe burns. *N Engl J Med*. 2001;345(17):1223-1229.	• Randomized trial of 25 children comparing resting energy expenditure in patients who received propranolol vs. placebo. • Net muscle-protein balance increased by 82% over baseline in propranolol group while decreasing 27% in the placebo. Fat-free mass remained steady in the propranolol group, while decreasing 9% in the control group.

CHAPTER 10: BURNS

Review Questions

1. What is the most common causal organism in burn sepsis?
2. What is the most common cause of death in burn patients after initial resuscitation?
3. A patient presents to the ED after suffering severe burns to the face, neck, and arms. The next step in management should be__.

4. When should antibiotics be started for burn patients?

5. A patient presents with deep burns to 30% TBSA. After intubation and adequate resuscitation, he remains persistently acidotic. What should one be suspicious of, and what is the appropriate treatment?

6. A 42-year-old patient presents with second-degree burns to the anterior surface of both lower extremities and anterior torso. What is his approximate total percentage body surface area burn?

7. A patient receives a scald burn to his arm after spilling hot tea. The burn is red and blistered and is painful to touch. What is the depth of this burn?

REFERENCES

1. Gibran NS, Wiechman S, Meyer W, et al. Summary of the 2012 ABA burn quality consensus conference. *J Burn Care Res*. 2013;34(4):361-385.
2. ISBI Practice Guidelines Committee, Steering Subcommittee, Advisory Subcommittee. ISBI practice guidelines for burn care. *Burns*. 2016;42(5):953-1021.
3. ISBI Practice Guidelines Committee, Advisory Subcommittee, Steering Subcommittee. ISBI practice guidelines for burn care, Part 2. *Burns*. 2018;44(7):1617-1706.
4. Monafo WW. Initial management of burns. *N Engl J Med*. 1996;335(21):1581-1586.
5. Berry MG, Evison D, Roberts AH. The influence of body mass index on burn surface area estimated from the area of the hand. *Burns*. 2001;27(6):591-594.
6. Wachtel TL, Berry CC, Wachtel EE, Frank HA. The inter-rater reliability of estimating the size of burns from various burn area chart drawings. *Burns*. 2000;26(2):156-170.
7. Guerriero C, Cairns J, Jayaraman S, Roberts I, Perel P, Shakur H. Giving tranexamic acid to reduce surgical bleeding in sub-Saharan Africa: an economic evaluation. *Cost Eff Resour Alloc*. 2010;8(1):1.
8. Ong YS, Samuel M, Song C. Meta-analysis of early excision of burns. *Burns*. 2006;32(2):145-150.
9. Herndon DN, Hart DW, Wolf SE, Chinkes DL, Wolfe RR. Reversal of catabolism by beta-blockade after severe burns. *N Engl J Med*. 2001;345(17):1223-1229.
10. Williams FN, Jeschke MG, Chinkes DL, Suman OE, Branski LK, Herndon DN. Modulation of the hypermetabolic response to trauma: temperature, nutrition, and drugs. *J Am Coll Surg*. 2009;208(4):489-502.
11. Mosier MJ, Pham TN, Klein MB, et al. Early enteral nutrition in burns: compliance with guidelines and associated outcomes in a multicenter study. *J Burn Care Res*. 2011;32(1):104-109.
12. Adjepong M, Agbenorku P, Brown P, Oduro I. The role of antioxidant micronutrients in the rate of recovery of burn patients: a systematic review. *Burns Trauma*. 2016;4:18.
13. Greenhalgh DG, Saffle JR, Holmes JH, et al. American Burn Association consensus conference to define sepsis and infection in burns. *J Burn Care Res*. 2007;28(6):776-790.
14. Cox CL, McIntire AM, Bolton KJ, et al. A multicenter evaluation of outcomes following the use of nebulized heparin for inhalation injury (HIHI2 study). *J Burn Care Res*. 2020;41(5):1004-1008.
15. McIntosh SE, Hamonko M, Freer L, et al. Wilderness Medical Society practice guidelines for the prevention and treatment of frostbite. *Wilderness Environ Med*. 2011;22(2):156-166.
16. Paal P, Gordon L, Strapazzon G, et al. Accidental hypothermia-an update: the content of this review is endorsed by the International Commission for Mountain Emergency Medicine (ICAR MEDCOM). *Scand J Trauma Resusc Emerg Med*. 2016;24(1):111.

11 Wound Care

Tiffany K. Brocke and Bracken A. Armstrong

I. INTRODUCTION

As creators of wounds, surgeons require expertise in wound care. Acute wounds heal by an orderly physiologic process and often require little intervention. For chronic wounds, this process is deranged for a variety of reasons and may require extensive specialized time-intensive care. In modern high-resourced settings, a certified Wound, Ostomy, and Continence Nurse is an indispensable part of the multidisciplinary wound care team to assist surgeons with these endeavors. The spectrum of wound care options can be daunting. In this chapter, we outline effective strategies to combat and expedite wound healing across commonly encountered surgical diseases.

II. ACUTE WOUND HEALING

A. Physiology of the acute wound: See **Figure 11.1** for details.

1. **Early wound healing**
   a. **Hemostasis**
      i. The coagulation cascade produces fibrin matrix, activating platelets and serving as internal scaffold.
      ii. In later phases of wound healing, the fibrin matrix facilitates cell attachment and serves as a reservoir for cytokines.
   b. **Inflammatory phase** (days 1-4).
      i. Injury immediately activates three plasma-based systems:
         a) Coagulation cascade: Limit blood loss and achieve hemostasis
         b) Complement cascade: Recruit immune cells and enhance their activity
         c) Kinin cascade: Local hormonal system that plays a role in modulating immunity in microenvironment and, later on, scar formation[1]
      ii. **Polymorphonuclear leukocytes (PMNs)** are the dominant inflammatory cells in the wound for the first 24 to 48 hours.
         a) Phagocytize bacteria and damaged tissue
         b) Release cytokines such as TNF-α and interleukin-1 that further stimulate the inflammatory response and local vasodilation.
      iii. **Monocytes** migrate into the extravascular space through capillaries and differentiate into **macrophages**.
         a) Phagocytize bacteria and damaged tissue

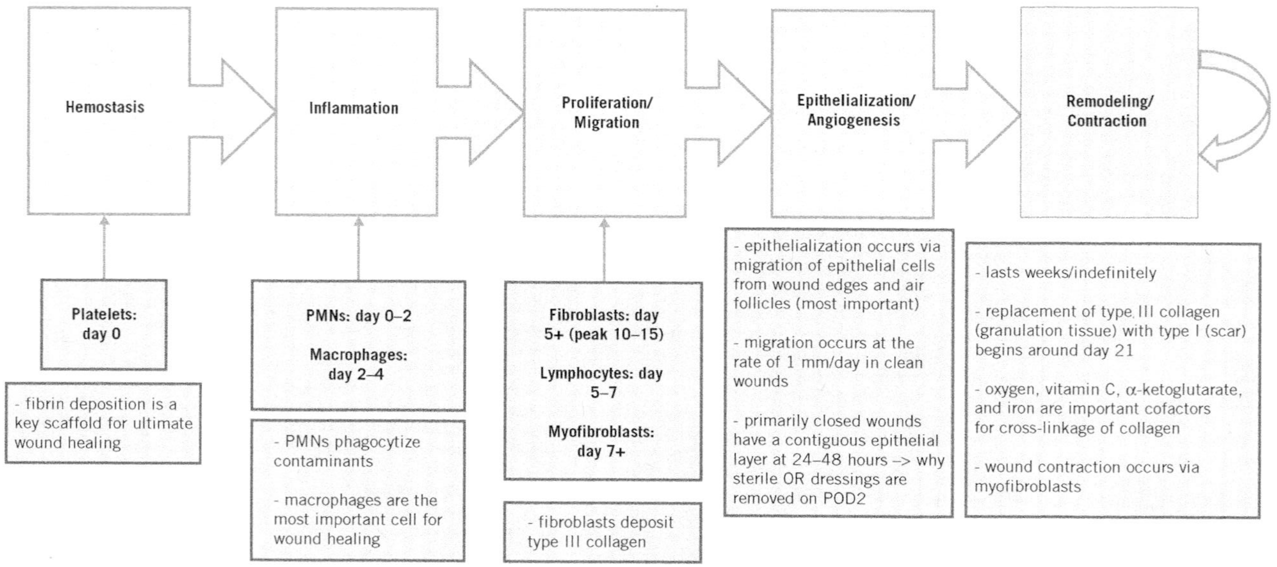

FIGURE 11.1 Timeline of physiologic wound healing. When tissue is disrupted, a well-organized cellular cascade is activated, designed to restore structural integrity to the injured tissue. OR, operating room; POD, postoperative day.

b) Secrete enzymes for the degradation of tissue
c) Release cytokines for inflammatory cell recruitment and fibroblast proliferation

iv. The inflammatory phase lasts a well-defined period of time in primarily closed wounds (~4 days), but it continues indefinitely to the end point of complete epithelialization in wounds that close by secondary or tertiary intention.

2. **Intermediate wound healing** involves mesenchymal cell migration and proliferation, angiogenesis, and epithelialization.
   a. **Fibroblasts** are recruited by chemotactic cytokines and migrate into the wound in 2 to 4 days after the injury.
   b. **Angiogenesis** takes place to restore the vasculature that has been disrupted by the wound.
   c. **Epithelialization** restores the barrier between the wound and the external environment.
      i. Occurs from edges of wound and from remaining epidermal appendages.
      ii. Migration of epithelial cells occurs at the rate of 1 mm/d in clean, open wounds.
      iii. Primarily closed wounds have a contiguous epithelial layer at 24 to 48 hours.
3. **Late wound healing** involves the deposition of collagen and other matrix proteins and wound contraction. The primary function of the fibroblast at this stage becomes protein synthesis.
   a. **Collagen** is the main protein secreted by fibroblasts.
      i. Provides strength and structure to wound.
      ii. **Type III** is the initial predominant collagen. Replaced by **type I collagen** at around 21 days.
      iii. Oxygen, vitamin C, α-ketoglutarate, and iron are important cofactors for the cross-linkage of collagen fibers.
   b. **Wound contraction** is a decrease in the size of the wound without an increase in the number of tissue elements that are present.
      i. Mediated by contraction of myofibroblasts
      ii. Wound contraction begins 4 to 5 days after wounding and continues for 12 to 15 days or longer if the wound remains open.
   c. The final wound-healing event is scar formation and remodeling.
      i. Type III collagen broken down and replaced by denser and more organized type I collagen
      ii. Wound reaches 60% of original tensile strength in 6 weeks.
      iii. Wound reaches 80% of original tensile strength in 3 to 6 months. *This is the maximum tensile strength wounds are able to recover.*

B. Effects of medications (i.e., chemotherapy agents and immunomodulators)[2]
   1. Examples of medications that have not been shown to have clinically significant impact on wound healing. Can be continued throughout the perioperative period.
      a. Methotrexate
      b. Mercaptopurine

c. Cyclosporine
d. Hydroxychloroquine

2. Examples of medications that can impede wound healing. Should be held in perioperative period.
   a. Sirolimus
   b. Doxorubicin
   c. Azathioprine
   d. Cisplatin
   e. Bevacizumab
3. Impact of steroids on wound healing depends on how long steroids have been administered.[3]
   a. Acute (<10 days): Little to no clinically significant impact on wound healing
   b. Chronic (>30 days): Can increase rate of wound complications

C. Scars

1. Physiologic scars—Patients often desire to minimize the appearance of physiologic incisional scars.
   a. Commonly recommended treatments include scar massage and use of silicone gel sheets to increase local moisture.
   b. Topical vitamin E ointment is often anecdotally recommended, but there are little data to support its use.[4]
2. Dysregulated scar formation
   a. Hypertrophic scar: Excessive scar tissue contained without site of injury
   b. Keloid: Excessive scar tissue that expands beyond site of injury
      i. Keloids are characterized by disorganized type I and III collagen.
      ii. Risk factors include hypertension, obesity, and black race or Hispanic ethnicity.
      iii. The most commonly accepted treatment is intralesional injection of triamcinolone, but other topical/local chemotherapeutic, immunomodulatory, and laser therapies have been attempted with variable success.[5]

III. SPECIAL CATEGORIES OF ACUTE WOUNDS

A. Hidradenitis suppurativa

1. Introduction
   a. Hidradenitis suppurativa (HS) is a chronic inflammatory disease of the hair follicles and apocrine sweat glands resulting in nodules, abscesses, scarring, and tunneling sinus tracts.
   b. Affects intertriginous areas including the axillae, inguinal creases, inframammary and infragluteal folds, perineum, and perianal regions.
2. Epidemiology
   a. Lifetime prevalence is 0.1% to 2%.
   b. Risk factors include African descent, obesity, smoking, type 2 diabetes, polycystic ovarian syndrome, and history of other autoimmune diseases.
3. Disease severity is described with the Hurley classification (**Table 11.1**).

TABLE 11.1 Hurley Classification of Hidradenitis Suppurativa Severity

Hurley Stage	Clinical Features
Hurley 1	Recurrent nodules/abscesses with minimal scar
Hurley 2	Limited sinuses/scarring in a single body region
Hurley 3	Multiple/extensive sinuses and scarring in multiple regions

4. Management
   a. Nonoperative management is reviewed in **Table 11.2**.[6,7]
   b. Operative management during disease flares should be limited to patients with evidence of superimposed infection, including cellulitis and fever.
      i. Abscesses may be treated with simple incision and drainage for patient comfort, with high risk of recurrence.
         a) **Surgical approach: Incision and drainage of abscess**
            1) Palpate abscess and identify area of fluctuance (i.e., thinnest epithelial coverage).
            2) Administer local anesthetic at the site and/or as a circumferential block.
            3) Make incision in area of fluctuance. May take a sample of abscess fluid for wound culture to help guide antibiotic therapy.
            4) Bluntly break up any loculations to allow for adequate drainage. Wash with copious sterile saline until effluent is clear.
            5) Wound cavity is left open and packed with dressing. For larger wounds, wound can be loosely closed over a Penrose drain to keep wound tract open for adequate drainage.
      ii. Hurley 2 or 3 disease has shown benefit from CO_2 laser excision of hair follicles.
      iii. Severely scarred disease may be treated with deroofing of lesions or true wide local excision, with comparable rates of recurrence, around 25%; excision is favored for tunneling disease.[7]
         a) The resultant wound may be managed with primary closure, negative pressure wound therapy, split-thickness skin grafting, or local flaps.
         b) The Limberg flap, locally transposed from the posterior axillary margin, has shown good recovery of functional outcomes after excision of axillary HS.[8]

B. Necrotizing Soft Tissue Infection
   1. **Introduction**
      a. Necrotizing soft tissue infections (NSTIs), formerly known as necrotizing fasciitis, comprise the set of skin and soft tissue infections characterized by rapid and extensive tissue destruction, involving skin, subcutaneous fat, and superficial fascia, up to and including muscular fascia.

TABLE 11.2 Medical Management of Hidradenitis Suppurativa

Therapy	Uses
Lifestyle Modifications	
Weight loss and smoking cessation	Including bariatric surgery if indicated
Avoiding tight clothing, shaving, and topical agents like antiperspirant over affected areas	Anecdotal recommendations, limited evidence base
Topical Antiseptics	
Chlorhexidine or zinc pyrithione washes	Daily or bid, expert opinion
Topical Therapy	
Clindamycin ointment	First line, risk for development of resistance
Intralesional triamcinolone	Injected for inflamed lesions
Systemic antibiotics	
Oral tetracycline	First line, either for flares or maintenance
Oral clindamycin/rifampin	Second line, 8- to 12-wk courses for flares
Parenteral ertapenem	Rescue therapy during surgical planning; systemic antibiotics are less effective in more severe disease
Hormonal Therapy	
Anti-androgen therapy (ethinyl estradiol, spironolactone)	Beneficial in women, especially with comorbid PCOS or menstrual flares
Immunotherapy	
Adalimumab (first line), infliximab (second line)	Growing evidence for benefit in moderate to severe disease

- i. Necrotizing fasciitis is specifically diagnosed intraoperatively by observed involvement of fascia with infection.
- b. The burden of disease is high with over 30% mortality worldwide for the syndrome.

2. **Pathophysiology**
   - a. Pathogens
     - i. Most commonly **polymicrobial**
     - ii. Most common single organism NSTI: Group A streptococcus (*Streptococcus pyogenes*, *Streptococcus aureus*)
       - a) Can be associated with toxic shock syndrome, characterized by erythematous macular rash.
     - iii. Gas-forming infection is classically caused by ***Clostridioides*** species; deep penetrating trauma, including injection drug use, and retained products of conception are particular risk factors for *Clostridioides* infection.[9]
     - iv. *Vibrio* species are a rarer etiology that should be considered with aggressive infection in the setting of exposure to untreated water.
   - b. More rarely, NSTI can develop following blunt trauma without violation of the skin, known as cryptogenic infection, thought to originate from transient bacteremia.
3. **Diagnosis**
   - a. Mainly a clinical diagnosis—A high index of clinical suspicion for NSTI should be maintained in any patient describing rapidly progressive severe pain or skin changes.
   - b. Examination may reveal bullae, erythema, petechiae, skin necrosis, crepitus, and hyperesthesia/allodynia, as well as tachycardia, fever, hypotension, and altered mental status.
   - c. A Laboratory Risk Indicator for Necrotizing Soft Tissue Infection (LRINEC) score may be calculated using values from routine laboratory tests to assist in risk assessment.[10] LRINEC score is calculated using:
     - i. C-reactive protein (CRP): NSTI is associated with elevated CRP.
     - ii. White blood cell count: NSTI is associated with leukocytosis.
     - iii. Hemoglobin: NSTI is associated with anemia.
     - iv. Sodium: NSTI is associated with hyponatremia.
     - v. Creatinine (Cr): NSTI is associated with elevated Cr.
     - vi. Glucose: NSTI is associated with hyperglycemia.
   - d. Radiographs or CT imaging may reveal gas in soft tissues but are not required for diagnosis.
     - i. Absent fascial enhancement on CT is specific for necrotizing fasciitis.[11]
   - e. **Treatment**
     - i. Early aggressive debridement of all necrotic tissue is critical for survival (**Figure 11.2**).
       - a) Tissue cultures should be sent intraoperatively to guide antibiotics.
       - b) If necrotizing infection is identified, return to the operating room should occur within the first 24 hours postoperatively to reassess for progression of infection and adequacy of debridement.

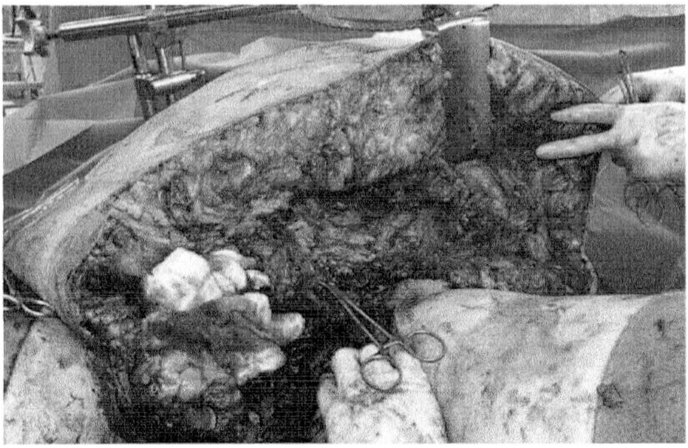

FIGURE 11.2 Necrotizing soft tissue infection. Initial debridement of necrotizing fasciitis in a patient who initially presented with fever and severe perineal pain. Examination revealed crepitus over the mons and inferior abdominal wall. Image taken from near the pannus, partially debrided in the foreground and held with a retractor, looking cephalad. Note the burden of necrotic tissue marked by the clamp inferiorly and the body wall retractor at image right. This patient survived and has been discharged from rehabilitation to home.

ii. Parenteral antibiotics are initiated as soon as NSTI is suspected.

a) Initial regimens should be broad for coverage of gram-positive and gram-negative aerobic and anaerobic organisms and methicillin-resistant *Staphylococcus aureus* (MRSA).

1) Examples include vancomycin or linezolid for MRSA, with piperacillin/tazobactam, a carbapenem, or ceftriaxone + metronidazole.

b) For rapidly progressive or severe infection, clindamycin or linezolid should be added to inhibit toxin production.[11]

iii. Supportive care. Patients with NSTI can present with septic shock. See Chapter 4 Critical Care for more details on management of septic shock.

iv. Wound management

a) Initial management with topical antimicrobial gauze (such as Dakin's solution) to allow for frequent reassessment

b) Once infection is controlled, surgeons may transition to use of negative pressure wound therapy, possibly with delayed primary closure, to reduce the burden of wound care (discussed below).

IV. CHRONIC WOUND HEALING

A. Physiology of the chronic wound: A chronic wound is a wound that fails to heal in a reasonable amount of time, usually 4 to 6 weeks, resulting from a disruption of the normal healing process. See **Table 11.3** for factors that contribute to derangements in wound healing.

1. Slowed or arrested in the inflammatory or proliferative phases of healing.

TABLE 11.3 Factors Leading to Derangement of the Healing Process, and Development and Persistence of Chronic wounds

Wound-Intrinsic or Local Factors	Systemic Factors
Infection: Prolongs inflammatory phase	Diabetes mellitus: Affects all stages of wound healing
Hypoxia: Decreases nutrient delivery, reduces collagen deposition	Smoking: Systemically decreased oxygen carrying capacity and vasoconstriction
Edema: Capillary distention and damage triggers inflammatory response	Steroid/antineoplastic/anti-inflammatory medications: Affect cellular migration and function
Lack of moisture: Decreases cellular migration	Congenital disease states: E.g., osteogenesis imperfecta (type I collagen defect), Marfan syndrome (fibrillin-1 defect)
Foreign bodies: Prolong inflammatory response	Nutrition: Both protein–calorie malnutrition and micronutrient deficiencies
Necrotic tissue: Increases local bioburden and prevents growth of new tissue	Chronic liver/kidney disease: Affect immune cell function
Radiation: Chronically depletes microvasculature and produces local proinflammatory changes	Aging: The physiologic aging process leads to altered skin/connective tissue cellular composition and slows cellular migration
Repetitive trauma: Inflammatory process resets with each new injury (e.g., weight bearing on foot wounds)	Denervation: Affects all stages of wound healing (Barker AR et al. *Ann Plast Surg*. 2006;57(3):339-342)
Malignancy: Malignant conversion of chronic inflammation permits evasion of the physiologic homeostatic process	Local anatomy: May contribute to repetitive trauma to wound (e.g., Charcot deformity)
Biofilms: Chronic low-virulence bacterial infections, often adherent to medical implants or chronic wounds via an extracellular matrix. Typically resistant to antibiotics	

2. Have increased levels of matrix metalloproteinases, which degrade cytokines and growth factors that contribute to wound healing.
3. Accumulation of excessive reactive oxygen species, which impair fibroblast function and contribute to a local proinflammatory cytokine milieu.

B. Principles of care for chronic wounds include
1. Multidisciplinary team care including surgeon, wound nurse, and recruitment of patient social resources, e.g., family
2. Biopsy to rule out malignant conversion of chronic inflammation (also known as a Marjolin's ulcer, classically observed in burns)
3. Optimization of underlying susceptibility
4. Judicious surgical intervention to convert a chronic wound into an acute wound, to treat infection, or to reduce burden of necrotic tissue
5. Choice of dressing to maintain a moist but not wet wound base

V. SPECIAL CATEGORIES OF CHRONIC WOUNDS

A. Diabetic foot ulcers
1. Pathogenesis: Diabetes impairs all stages of wound healing.
   a. Patients with diabetic neuropathy may not notice trauma that can lead to formation of wounds.
   b. Microvascular and macrovascular disease
      i. Leads to tissue hypoxia
      ii. Decreases phagocytosis, chemotaxis, mobilization of PMNs
      iii. Decreases secretion of growth factors
      iv. Impairs migration of skin fibroblasts
      v. Weakens collagen formation
2. Evaluation
   a. Thorough physical examination is crucial for early diagnosis of infection. **Figure 11.3** shows an example of an infected diabetic foot ulcer.
      i. Semmes–Weinstein monofilament measures tactile sensitivity and can be used to evaluate for neuropathy.
   b. Workup of diabetic foot ulcers should include plain radiographs of the foot to evaluate for osteomyelitis.
   c. Ankle-brachial index measurements are made to evaluate for vascular insufficiency.
3. Osteomyelitis is an important complication of diabetic foot wounds.
   a. Factors that increase the likelihood of osteomyelitis are ulcer size >2 cm^2, positive probe to bone test, and elevated erythrocyte sedimentation rate.[12]
   b. MRI is the most sensitive imaging modality to detect osteomyelitis.
   c. Bone biopsy with culture should be obtained to guide antibiotic therapy, and all infected bone removed if possible.
4. Treatment
   a. Supportive care
      i. Glycemic control to improve wound healing abilities.
      ii. Offload the ulcer with an appropriate diabetic shoe or other orthotic device.
      iii. Regular inspection and careful hygiene and foot care by the patient are key to preventing injuries and identifying wounds early.

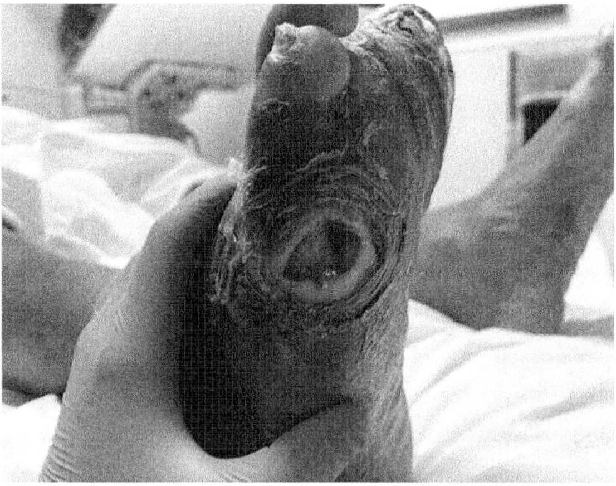

FIGURE 11.3 Diabetic foot ulcer. Signs of worsening odor, swelling of the foot, and sloughing of the surrounding skin are consistent with infected wound.

b. Surgical debridement and wound care
   i. Clean wounds
      a) Usually require only minimal debridement.
      b) Dress with damp gauze or hydrogel dressing.[13]
      c) Exudative wounds may benefit from alginate, hydrocolloid, or negative-pressure wound therapy (NPWT).
      d) In wounds that appear clean but are failing to progress with adequate treatment, consider quantitative bacterial wound culture. Bacterial levels $>10^6$ colony-forming unit (CFU)/g of tissue impede wound healing.[14]
   ii. Infected wounds
      a) Require prompt thorough surgical exploration, drainage of abscess cavities, and debridement of necrotic or devitalized tissue.

c. Antibiotic therapy
   i. For infected wounds, initial antibiotic therapy should include broad-spectrum coverage of MRSA and aerobic and anaerobic gram-negative rods.
   ii. Cellulitis surrounding diabetic foot ulcers is most commonly caused by gram-positive bacteria.
   iii. Superficial cultures are inaccurate. Deep wound cultures should be obtained during surgical debridement to guide antibiotic therapy.
   iv. Duration of therapy may be limited to 2 to 4 weeks in the case of osteomyelitis with resection of all involved bone, or 6 weeks or longer if infected bone persists.
   v. Consider consultation with an infectious disease specialist.

B. Chronic leg ulcers
   1. Arterial insufficiency ulcers
      a. Tend to occur distally on digits

b. Wounds often manifest as dry gangrene. Dry gangrene is managed with daily Betadine painting and dressings that prevent maceration of vulnerable tissue.
c. If the patient is found to have a component of critical limb ischemia contributing to tissue loss, optimization of inflow should precede resection of devitalized tissue, unless active infection is present. See Chapter 35 for further discussion of management.

2. Venous stasis ulcers
   a. Are more common than chronic leg ulcers from arterial disease.
   b. Typically occur in the supramedial malleolar location.
   c. Surgical debridement is avoided unless active infection is present. See Chapter 46 for a complete description of venous stasis ulcers and their treatment.

C. Pressure injuries
1. Epidemiology
   a. The prevalence of pressure ulcers is approximately 30% in the long-term acute care setting.[15]
   b. Pressure ulcers increase in-hospital mortality rates more than two-fold as well as increase the risk of hospital readmissions.[16]
2. Pathophysiology
   a. Prolonged pressure applied to soft tissue over bony prominences, usually caused by paralysis or immobility associated with severe illness, leads to ischemic ulceration and tissue breakdown, also known as decubitus ulcers.
   b. Ulcers frequently develop over the sacrum, ischium, greater trochanter, and heels. Pressure ulcers are described by stages (**Table 11.4**).

TABLE 11.4 National Pressure Ulcer Advisory Panel Classification Scheme

Stage	Description
I	Nonblanchable erythema of intact skin; wounds generally reversible at this stage with intervention
II	Partial-thickness skin loss involving epidermis or dermis; may present as an abrasion, blister, or shallow crater
III	Full-thickness skin loss involving damage or necrosis of subcutaneous tissue but not extending through underlying structures or fascia
IV	Full-thickness skin loss with damage to underlying support structures (i.e., fascia, tendon, or joint capsule)
Unstageable	Full-thickness tissue loss with actual depth of ulcer unknown due to slough and/or eschar in wound bed
Suspected deep tissue injury	Localized area of discolored skin or blood-filled blister due to damage of underlying tissue

   c. See **Figure 11.4** for an example of an unstageable sacral decubitus ulcer before and after debridement. The examiner must also look for underlying bony breakdown and osteomyelitis.
3. Prevention
   a. *Skin care:* Skin should be kept well moisturized but protected from excessive contact with extraneous fluids such as stool with use of barrier products as needed.
   b. *Frequent repositioning:* High-risk patients should be repositioned at a minimum every 2 hours, either while seated or in bed. The importance of patient and family buy-in and participation in this process cannot be overstated.
   c. *Appropriate support surfaces:* Adequate support surfaces redistribute pressure from the bony prominences that cause pressure ulcers. Static foam, air, gel, and water-overlay support surfaces are

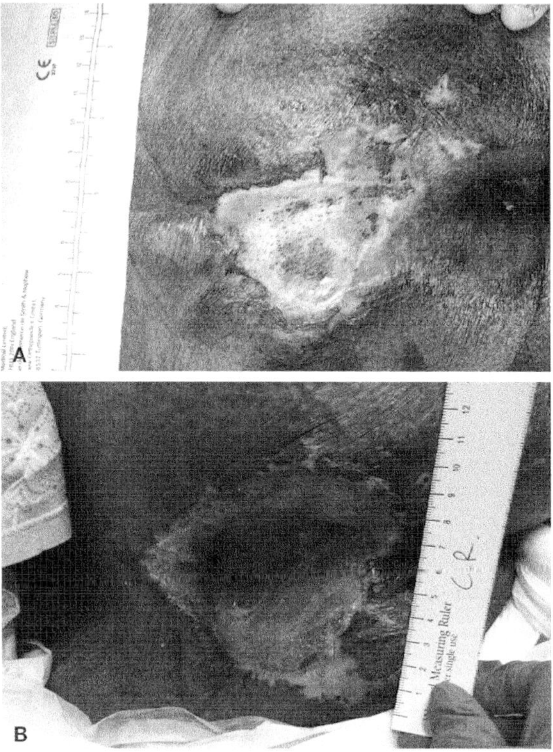

FIGURE 11.4 A, Sacral decubitus ulcer in a patient immobilized by chronic illness, covered with eschar and unstageable. B, The same ulcer following debridement and 1 month of NPWT; note the depth of the wound concealed by the original eschar.

appropriate for low-risk patients. Dynamic support surfaces are powered and actively redistribute pressure. These include alternating and low air-loss mattresses. These surfaces are appropriate for high-risk patients.

d. *Nutrition:* High-risk patients should also undergo nutritional screening to ensure that caloric and protein goals are met.

4. Treatment

a. Wound care

i. The base of uninfected ulcers should be cleaned with saline irrigation or a commercially available wound cleanser at each dressing change.

ii. For actively infected wounds, a short course (3-5 days) of damp-to-dry dressing changes with antiseptic solutions, such as Dakin's solution, may facilitate local bacterial control. *This does not take the place of appropriate debridement and systemic antibiotic therapy.*

iii. Dressing can be transitioned to NPWT once the wound is clean.

b. Control of infection and bacterial colonization

i. Evidence of active infection (purulence, surrounding cellulitis, or foul odor) should prompt re-exploration of the wound with debridement of any necrotic or infected tissue.

ii. Quantitative tissue cultures should be obtained from wounds that fail to heal.

iii. The underlying bone should be evaluated for osteomyelitis with appropriate imaging.

iv. Patients whose injuries are felt to be exacerbated by medically uncontrolled stool contamination may benefit from fecal diversion with a colostomy.

c. Nutrition

i. Successful treatment of pressure ulcers requires adequate nutrition. Patients should be provided with 30 to 35 kcal/kg body weight and 1.25 to 1.5 g protein/kg body weight.[17]

d. Debridement

i. Eschar and necrotic tissue should be debrided unless contraindicated.

ii. Sharp debridement of small wounds can be done at the bedside if pain is tolerable. Larger wounds require operative debridement for control of bleeding.

iii. Once the bulk of eschar and devitalized tissue is removed, debridement can be continued with wet-to-damp gauze dressings or with enzymatic debridement with topical agents such as collagenase.

e. Wound closure

i. Most pressure ulcers can heal spontaneously; some may need surgical closure.

ii. Surgical management may include simple closure, split-thickness skin grafting, or creation of a musculocutaneous flap.

iii. Recent studies have shown promising results in cohort case series with coverage of these relatively avascular structures with either acellular matrices or bioactive human skin allografts combined with NPWT.[18]

VI. WOUND CLOSURE AND CARE

A. Types of wound closure

1. Primary intention
   a. Wound is closed by direct approximation of the wound margins.
   b. This treatment is appropriate when the wound is clean and closure can be performed without tension in a timely fashion after injury, generally under 6 hours.
2. Secondary intention
   a. Occurs when a wound is left open and is allowed to close by epithelialization and contraction.
   b. This method is commonly used in the management of wounds with delayed presentation to care or tissue defects not amenable to reapproximation, or for heavily contaminated wounds at high risk for postclosure infection.
   c. Healing by secondary intention is characterized by prolonged inflammatory and proliferative phases of healing that continue until the wound has completely epithelialized.
3. Tertiary intention, or delayed primary closure
   a. Option for managing wounds that are too heavily contaminated for primary closure but appear clean and well vascularized after 4 to 5 days of open observation.
   b. Patient satisfaction, pain control, and return to normal function can be improved if patients can be provided with delayed primary closure rather than prolonged wound care for healing by secondary intention.

B. Open wound care options

Please find in **Table 11.5** a brief overview of dressing product categories for consideration in individualizing wound care regimens. We highlight some important options, but the entire array of topical treatments is beyond the scope of this chapter.

VII. NEGATIVE PRESSURE WOUND THERAPY

A. Introduction

1. Utilizes constant or intermittent vacuum applied over a wound to stimulate capillary ingrowth and the formation of granulation tissue, while maintaining a relatively clean wound environment.

TABLE 11.5 Common and Advanced Options for Wound Care Including Uses and Considerations for Particular Patient Populations

Dressing	Description	Example Brands	Uses	Notes
Topical ointments	Petroleum-based, antibiotic impregnated	Bacitracin, Polysporin, Neosporin	Accelerate epithelialization of approximated wounds by maintaining moisture and decreasing inflammation	
Iodine paint	Liquid 10% povidone iodine	Betadine	Prevent infection of dry gangrenous tissue	
Antiseptic solutions	Dakin's: 0.5%, 0.25%, or 0.125% sodium hypochlorite solution Vashe: Hypochlorous acid		Dakin's: Used to soak packing material or instilled in NPWT Vashe: Wound base cleanser between dressing changes	Dakin's is cytotoxic and inhibits healing; use for 3- to 5-d courses only in acutely infectec wounds
Enzymatic debriders	Topical collagenase or medical honey (oxidase)	Santyl, Medihoney	Facilitate removal of necrotic eschar or fibrinous exudate to restore healthy wound base	
Silver sulfadiazine	Topical silver-impregnated antibacterial ointment	Silvadene	Apply dime-thick layer to bum eschar. Wash off and reapply daily. Has antiseptic properties, but inhibits epithelialization	Increases risk of kernicterus → not safe in pregnant women near term or infants <2 mo. Other adverse effects: Neutrcpenia, hepatic renal failure

Mafenide acetate	Available as a liquid for soaking dry gauze dressing, or cream; antibacterial ointment	Sulfamylon	Prevent infection of burns after meshed graft placement; particularly useful over burned cartilage, e.g. pinna	Adverse effects: Metabolic alkalosis
Impregnated gauze	Petroleum-impregnated gauze	Xeroform	Maintain moisture	Contraindicated if infection is suspected
Gauze packing	Typically wet-to-damp gauze packed into open wound, often damped with sterile 0.9% saline		Prevents premature wound closure, facilitates drainage, provides gentle debridement. Greatest debridement from dry gauze packing, but painful and rarely indicated	Common for venous stasis ulcers
Hydrogels	Gel applied to wound base	IntraSite	Absorb exudate, facilitate debridement of necrotic tissue; cover with nonadherent nonabsorbent dressing	
Hydrocolloids	Occlusive wafers	Multiple manufacturers: McKesson, DuoDerm	Maintain moisture in shallow wounds with light exudate	Common for venous stasis ulcers
Hydrofibers	Strands packed into wounds, transform into gel in wound	Aquacel, Drawtex	Extremely absorptive for heavily draining wounds	

(continued)

TABLE 11.5 Common and Advanced Options for Wound Care Including Uses and Considerations for Particular Patient Populations (*Continued*)

Dressing	Description	Example Brands	Uses	Notes
Alginates	Seaweed-derived glucuronic acid dressings, transform into gel in wound	Kaltostat	Absorptive for heavily draining wounds; absorbable, useful for very deep wounds	
Adhesive films	Self-adherent plastic membranes	Tegaderm	Waterproof, but oxygen permeable; useful for clean partial-thickness wounds	E.g. Split-thickness skin graft donor sites
Growth factors	Topical human-recombinant platelet-derived growth factor		Promotes granulation tissue formation and epithelialization; best evidence in diabetic foot ulcers, used in difficult-to-heal wounds	Often cost-prohibitive
Skin substitutes	Xenograft: E.g., Permacol, Matriderm—animal-derived collagen matrix Allogeneic: E.g., AlloDerm, Strattice, Integra—cadaveric or acellular animal matrix Bioengineered living tissue: From neonatal (e.g., Dermagraft, Apligraf) or autologous skin (Epicel, Hyalograft)—living cultured keratinocytes on a structural mesh		Used to bridge skin soft tissue, fascial defects (e.g., large hernias in contaminated fields), facilitate healing of chronic wounds	Typically quite expensive; may be absorbable over time; use guided by individual properties

Medical larvae	5-10 larvae/cm^2 of wound within containment dressing, 48-72 h duration	Provide debridement, disinfection, stimulate granulation tissue, and eradicate biofilms. High rates of limb salvage in diabetic foot infections	Generally good patient acceptance (Sherman RA. *J Diabetes Sci Technol.* 2009;3(2):336-344)
Hyperbaric oxygen	90 min/d at 2 atm pressure of oxygen; typical course 5 d/wk ×30 treatments	Treats local hypoxia in wounds; commonly used in burns and diabetic foot wounds with improved limb salvage (PMR 2009:1:471)	Adverse effects: Middle ear trauma, barotrauma, fire risk, claustrophobia

2. There are many NPWT devices and setups. See **Figure 11.5** for an example of an institutionally created NPWT system.
3. NPWT may be applied to nearly any open wound provided that the wound bed is free of necrotic and nonviable tissue, is well perfused, and is free of active progressive infection.
4. NPWT dressings are changed approximately every 3 days and therefore should not be used in wounds requiring more frequent physical examination.
5. When used for chronic wounds, the chronic wound should be converted to an acute wound through enzymatic or surgical debridement prior to application of NPWT.

B. Uses of NPWT

1. NPWT is effective in the management of wounds as diverse as diabetic foot wounds, pressure and venous stasis ulcers, the open abdomen, closed incisions, and wounds including donor and recipient sites of split-thickness skin grafts, prosthetic mesh, or exposed bone or tendon.[19-22]
2. A meta-analysis of randomized controlled trials evaluating NPWT showed a reduction in dehiscence, seroma formations, and skin necrosis compared with standard care.[23]

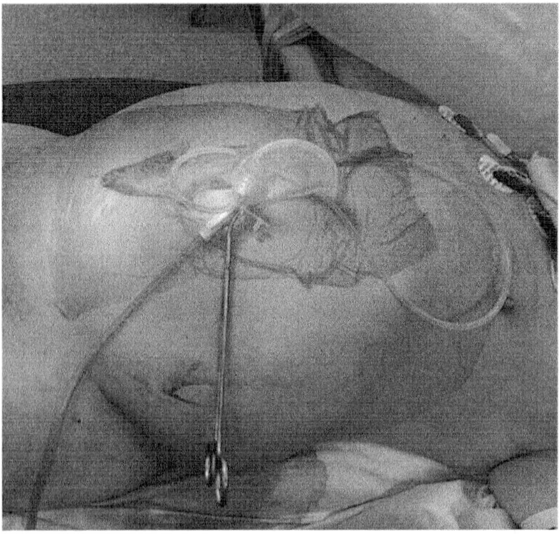

FIGURE 11.5 Institutionally created negative pressure wound therapy device for open abdomen. A clear plastic drape is used to cover the abdominal viscera; dry Kerlix gauze is layered over the plastic; a Jackson–Pratt drain is invested in the gauze; the wound is covered with adhesive plastic; the Jackson–Pratt bulb is connected to wall suction.

3. NPWT can be used to manage enteroatmospheric fistulae and increase fistula closure rates.[24] In the case of fistulae, surrounding wound burden can also be reduced when using NPWT in combination with fistula isolation devices.
4. NPWT is contraindicated for wounds with exposed major blood vessels, untreated osteomyelitis, or cancer.

C. **Technique to NPWT application**
1. Chronic or infected wounds should be debrided until healthy well-vascularized wound bed with granulation tissue is exposed.
2. Apply foam sponge to the wound bed.
    a. Typically, a black foam sponge is utilized to promote growth of granulation tissue.
    b. White foam sponges are denser and are used over tenuous abdominal fascial closures to reduce the risk of vacuum erosion into bowel and iatrogenic enterocutaneous fistula creation.
    c. For coverage of split-thickness skin graft sites, our preference is to apply a layer of Promogran Prisma between black sponge and tissue; this dressing is silver-impregnated cellulose and is valued for its antimicrobial activity, cost-effectiveness, and progranulation properties.
3. Adherent plastic film is applied over foam to create airtight seal for vacuum.
4. Vacuum device is connected to provide constant suction.
5. If suction is unexpectedly discontinued prior to next dressing change, NPWT should be discontinued and wound care transitioned to wet-to-dry gauze until new NPWT system can be applied.

D. NPWT with instillation (e.g., VeraFlow)
1. Has the additional component of intermittent irrigation of the wound via the vacuum system while off suction, typically with sterile normal saline or quarter-strength (0.125%) Dakin's solution.
2. Benefit is felt to arise from solubilizing devitalized tissue and assisting with removal of viscous exudate and bioburden.
3. Expert consensus recommends NPWT with instillation use in complex wounds with invasive infection or extensive biofilm.[25]
4. NPWT with instillation compared with classic NPWT has been shown to have superior effect on bacterial colonization in chronic wounds and decreased hospital length of stay and need for surgical intervention in infected wounds.[26]
5. It is contraindicated in untreated osteomyelitis, malignancy within the wound, and possible connection to thoracic or abdominal cavity and is not recommended over split-thickness skin graft recipient sites.[27]

Key References

Citation	Summary
Duane TM, Huston JM, Collom M, et al. Surgical Infection Society 2020 Updated Guidelines on the management of complicated skin and soft tissue infections. *Surg Infect (Larchmt).* 2021;22(4):383-399.	• Recommendations established by Surgical Infection Society, providing overview of treatment for complicated skin and soft tissue infections, including surgical debridement, antibiotic management, and wound care.
Edwards J, Stapley S. Debridement of diabetic foot ulcers. *Cochrane Database Syst Rev.* 2010;2010(1):CD003556. Published 2010.	• Meta-analysis compiling data from randomized controlled trials evaluating various surgical debridement and wound care interventions for diabetic foot ulcers. Findings suggest hydrogel dressings increased healing rate compared with gauze dressings.
Kim PJ, Attinger CE, Steinberg JS, et al. Negative-pressure wound therapy with instillation: international consensus guidelines. *Plast Reconstr Surg.* 2013;132(6):1569-1579.	• Guidelines established by multidisciplinary panel of podiatrists, general and plastic surgeons, burn specialists, and infectious disease experts on the use of NPTWi. Indications for NPTWi include "patients with multiple comorbidities, patients with an American Society of Anesthesiology Classification ≥2, severe traumatic wounds, diabetic foot infections, and wounds complicated by invasive infection or extensive biofilm."

CHAPTER 11: WOUND CARE

Review Questions

1. When does a well-healed wound reach the original strength of uninjured issue?
2. List five options for nonoperative management of hidradenitis suppurativa.
3. Quantitative bacterial wound culture results of ≥ _______ CFU/g tissue suggest that wound healing may be impeded by bacterial bioburden.
4. Describe the difference between healing by primary and secondary intention.
5. List four benefits of negative pressure wound therapy (NPWT).
6. Which cell type is most important for wound healing?
7. Describe the staging of pressure ulcers.

REFERENCES

1. Chao J, Shen B, Gao L, Xia CF, Bledsoe G, Chao L. Tissue kallikrein in cardiovascular, cerebrovascular and renal diseases and skin wound healing. *Biol Chem*. 2010;391(4):345-355.
2. Boyce M, Massicotte A. Practical guidance in perioperative management of immunosuppressive therapy for rheumatology patients undergoing elective surgery. *Can J Hosp Pharm*. 2020;73(3):218-224.
3. Wang AS, Armstrong EJ, Armstrong AW. Corticosteroids and wound healing: clinical considerations in the perioperative period. *Am J Surg*. 2013;206(3):410-417.
4. Liu A, Moy RL, Ozog DM. Current methods employed in the prevention and minimization of surgical scars. *Dermatol Surg*. 2011;37(12):1740-1746.
5. Ekstein SF, Wyles SP, Moran SL, Meves A. Keloids: a review of therapeutic management. *Int J Dermatol*. 2021;60(6):661-671.
6. Alikhan A, Sayed C, Alavi A, et al. North American clinical management guidelines for hidradenitis suppurativa: a publication from the United States and Canadian Hidradenitis Suppurativa Foundations—Part I—diagnosis, evaluation, and the use of complementary and procedural management. *J Am Acad Dermatol*. 2019;81(1):76-90.
7. Alikhan A, Sayed C, Alavi A, et al. North American clinical management guidelines for hidradenitis suppurativa: a publication from the United States and Canadian Hidradenitis Suppurativa Foundations—Part II—topical, intralesional, and systemic medical management. *J Am Acad Dermatol*. 2019;81(1):91-101.
8. Varkarakis G, Daniels J, Coker K, Oswald T, Akdemir O, Lineaweaver WC. Treatment of axillary hidradenitis with transposition flaps: a 6-year experience. *Ann Plast Surg*. 2010;64(5):592-594.
9. Duane TM, Huston JM, Collom M, et al. Surgical infection society 2020 updated guidelines on the management of complicated skin and soft tissue infections. *Surg Infect*. 2021;22(4):383-399.
10. Wong CH, Khin LW, Heng KS, Tan KC, Low CO. The LRINEC (Laboratory Risk Indicator for Necrotizing Fasciitis) score: a tool for distinguishing necrotizing fasciitis from other soft tissue infections. *Crit Care Med*. 2004;32(7):1535-1541.
11. Stevens DL, Bryant AE. Necrotizing soft-tissue infections. *N Engl J Med*. 2017;377(23):2253-2265.
12. Lam K, van Asten SA, Nguyen T, La Fontaine J, Lavery LA. Diagnostic accuracy of probe to bone to detect osteomyelitis in the diabetic foot: a systematic review. *Clin Infect Dis*. 2016;63(7):944-948.
13. Edwards J, Stapley S. Debridement of diabetic foot ulcers. *Cochrane Database Syst Rev*. 2010;2010(1):CD003556.
14. Lavery LA, Davis KE, Berriman SJ, et al. WHS guidelines update: diabetic foot ulcer treatment guidelines. *Wound Repair Regen*. 2016;24(1):112-126.
15. Wound, Ostomy and Continence Nurses Society-Wound Guidelines Task Force. WOCN 2016 guideline for prevention and management of pressure injuries (ulcers): an executive summary. *J Wound Ostomy Continence Nurs*. 2017;44(3):241-246.
16. Wald HL. Prevention of hospital-acquired geriatric syndromes: applying lessons learned from infection control. *J Am Geriatr Soc*. 2012;60(2):364-366.

17. Munoz N, Posthauer ME, Cereda E, Schols J, Haesler E. The role of nutrition for pressure injury prevention and healing: the 2019 international clinical practice guideline recommendations. *Adv Skin Wound Care.* 2020;33(3):123-136.

18. Flood MS, Weeks B, Anaeme KO, et al. Treatment of deep full-thickness wounds containing exposed muscle, tendon, and/or bone using a bioactive human skin allograft: a large cohort case series. *Wounds.* 2020;32(6):164-173.

19. Blume PA, Walters J, Payne W, Ayala J, Lantis J. Comparison of negative pressure wound therapy using vacuum-assisted closure with advanced moist wound therapy in the treatment of diabetic foot ulcers: a multicenter randomized controlled trial. *Diabetes Care.* 2008;31(4):631-636.

20. Attinger CE, Janis JE, Steinberg J, Schwartz J, Al-Attar A, Couch K. Clinical approach to wounds: débridement and wound bed preparation including the use of dressings and wound-healing adjuvants. *Plast Reconstr Surg.* 2006;117(7 suppl):72s-109s.

21. Roberts DJ, Zygun DA, Grendar J, et al. Negative-pressure wound therapy for critically ill adults with open abdominal wounds: a systematic review. *J Trauma Acute Care Surg.* 2012;73(3):629-639.

22. Virani SR, Dahapute AA, Bava SS, Muni SR. Impact of negative pressure wound therapy on open diaphyseal tibial fractures: a prospective randomized trial. *J Clin Orthop Trauma.* 2016;7(4):256-259.

23. Ge D. The safety of negative-pressure wound therapy on surgical wounds: an updated meta-analysis of 17 randomized controlled trials. *Adv Skin Wound Care.* 2018;31(9):421-428.

24. Wirth U, Renz BW, Andrade D, et al. Successful treatment of enteroatmospheric fistulas in combination with negative pressure wound therapy: experience on 3 cases and literature review. *Int Wound J.* 2018;15(5):722-730.

25. Kim PJ, Attinger CE, Crist BD, et al. Negative pressure wound therapy with instillation: review of evidence and recommendations. *Wounds.* 2015;27(12):S2-S19.

26. Faust E, Opoku-Agyeman JL, Behnam AB. Use of negative-pressure wound therapy with instillation and dwell time: an overview. *Plast Reconstr Surg.* 2021;147(1S-1):16S-26S.

27. Kim PJ, Attinger CE, Constantine T, et al. Negative pressure wound therapy with instillation: international consensus guidelines update. *Int Wound J.* 2020;17(1):174-186.

28. Kim PJ, Attinger CE, Steinberg JS, et al. Negative-pressure wound therapy with instillation: international consensus guidelines. *Plast Reconstr Surg.* 2013;132(6):1569-1579.

12 Acute Abdomen

Sophia H. Roberts and Obeid N. Ilahi

I. INTRODUCTION

A. Defined as the recent or sudden onset of severe abdominal pain
B. The most common emergent issue in general surgery and often presents with a vast differential diagnosis including both intra- and extraperitoneal processes.
C. A thorough history and physical examination combined with selective testing is critical for evaluating patients with acute abdominal pain.
D. While this chapter focuses on intra-abdominal etiologies of abdominal pain, it is important to be aware of other potential sources involving the abdominal wall (e.g., rectus sheath hematoma) or extra-abdominal organs (e.g., testicular torsion).

II. PATHOPHYSIOLOGY

A. Visceral pain is deep, dull, poorly localized pain that is triggered by inflammation, ischemia, and geometric changes such as distention, traction, and pressure.
   1. The general location of pain often correlates with the anatomic location of disease (**Figure 12.1**).
B. By contrast, **parietal pain** is sharp, severe pain that is well localized to a distinct abdominal quadrant due to (a) peritoneal irritation by localized inflammation of an organ in contact with the parietal peritoneum, (b) chemical peritonitis from a perforated viscus, or (c) mechanical stimulation as from a surgical incision or trauma (**Figure 12.2**).
   1. Parietal pain can correlate with local or diffuse peritonitis and usually signifies the need for surgical treatment.
C. Referred pain arises from a deep structure but is superficial at the painful site.
   1. Examples include biliary tract pain, which refers to the right inferior scapular area, renal colic referring down to the ipsilateral groin, or a ruptured aortic aneurysm or pancreatitis radiating to the back.
D. Epigastric pain corresponds with foregut-derived structures (stomach to second portion of duodenum, liver, biliary tract, pancreas, spleen).
E. Periumbilical pain corresponds with midgut-derived structures (second portion of duodenum to proximal two-thirds of transverse colon).
F. Suprapubic pain corresponds with hindgut-derived structures (distal transverse colon to anal verge).

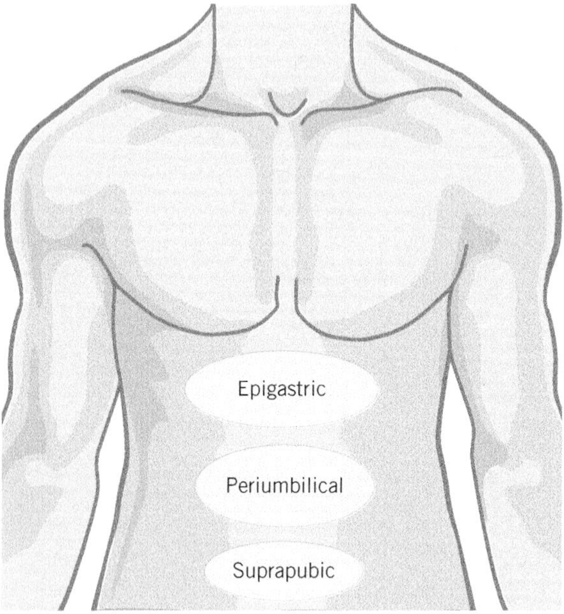

FIGURE 12.1 Visceral pain distribution correlates with location of intra-abdominal disease.

III. EVALUATION

A thorough history and physical examination with ancillary imaging and laboratory tests can guide the diagnostic and treatment process (**Figure 12.3**).

A. History of present illness provides a chronological description of the patient's signs and symptoms (**Table 12.1**).
   1. Past medical history
      a. Medical conditions precipitating intra-abdominal pathology
         i. Peripheral vascular disease or coronary artery disease may predispose patients to abdominal vascular disease, such as abdominal aortic aneurysm or mesenteric ischemia.
         ii. Cancer history should raise suspicion for bowel obstruction or perforation from progression or recurrence.
   2. Surgical history
      a. Following abdominal surgeries patients may develop adhesions predisposing them to bowel obstructions.
      b. If a patient has had prior abdominal surgery, it is important to be aware of anatomic variations (e.g., bowel resections, organ transplantation, bariatric surgery).

B. Medications
   1. Nonsteroidal anti-inflammatory medications, such as aspirin or ibuprofen, increase the risk of complicated peptic ulcer disease, namely, bleeding, obstruction, and perforation.

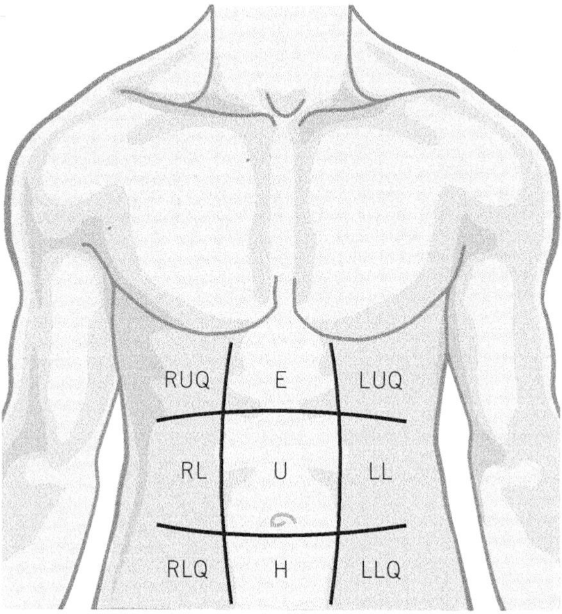

FIGURE 12.2 Parietal pain distribution, when localized, may correlate with inflammatory processes involving the underlying intra-abdominal structures. E, epigastric (gastric, pancreatic, biliary, hernia); H, hypogastric (bladder, appendiceal, colonic, pelvic); LL, left lumbar (renal, colonic); LLQ, left lower quadrant (colonic, pelvic, hernia); LUQ, left upper quadrant (splenic, gastric, duodenal, biliary, pancreatic); RL, right lumbar (renal, colonic, hernia); RLQ, right lower quadrant (appendiceal, colonic, pelvic, hernia); RUQ, right upper quadrant (biliary, gastric, pancreatic); U, umbilical (pancreatic, appendiceal, gastric, small bowel, hernia).

2. Corticosteroids often mask classic signs of inflammation such as fever and peritoneal signs.
3. Antibiotics may either attenuate abdominal symptoms due to treatment of the underlying disease process or cause diarrhea/abdominal pain from antibiotic-induced pseudomembranous colitis.

C. Physical examination
1. Overall appearance
   a. Patients with diffuse peritonitis appear acutely ill and tend to minimize stimulation to the abdomen by lying quietly and still.
   b. Colic causes intermittent pain, causing patients to be restless or writhing in pain, unable to find a comfortable position.
2. Vital signs
   a. Fever suggests inflammatory or infectious process; marked fever >39 °C suggests the presence of abscess, cholangitis, or pneumonia.
   b. Hypotension and/or tachycardia signal hypovolemia or sepsis.

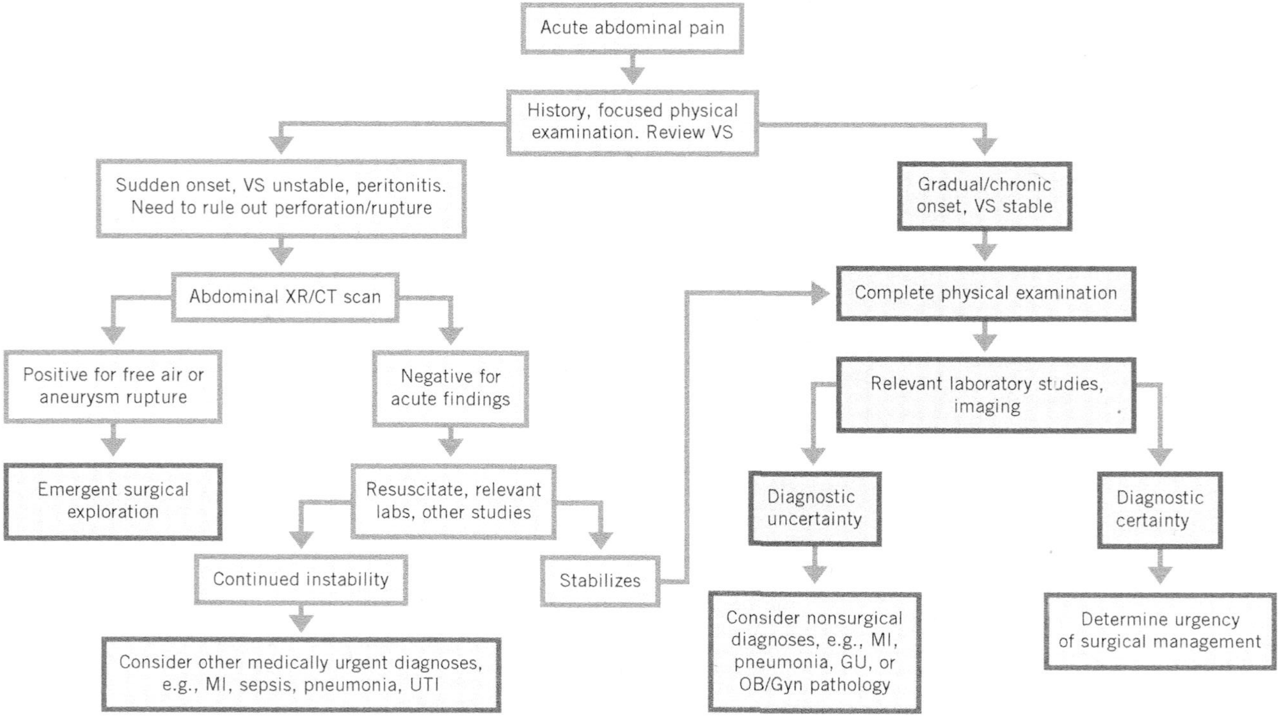

FIGURE 12.3 Diagnostic algorithm for the evaluation of acute abdominal pain. GU, genitourinary; MI, myocardial infarction; UTI, urinary tract infection; VS, vital signs.

TABLE 12.1 Findings to Elicit During History Taking and Differential Diagnoses to Consider

Findings on History	Differential Diagnosis
Onset/Duration	
• Sudden (within seconds)	• Perforated viscus, ruptured aneurysm, myocardial infarction, acute mesenteric occlusion
• Rapid acceleration (within minutes)	• Colic syndromes: Biliary, ureteral, bowel obstruction • Inflammatory: Appendicitis, pancreatitis, diverticulitis • Ischemic: Mesenteric ischemia, bowel strangulation, volvulus
• Gradual (over hours)	• Inflammatory: Appendicitis, cholecystitis • Obstructive: Nonstrangulated bowel obstruction, urinary retention • Other mechanical: Ectopic pregnancy, tumors
Character	
• Colicky, waxing, and waning	Hyperperistalsis of smooth muscle against mechanical obstruction (SBO, renal stone) Exception is biliary colic—constant, intense, lasting 30 min to 1 h
• Severe, persistent, steadily increasing	Infectious or inflammatory process
Location	Specific organs localizing to their respective quadrants, refer to Figure 12.2
Alleviating/aggravating factors	Diffuse peritonitis—worse with movement Colic—unable to find a comfortable position Obstruction—transient relief from vomiting Peptic ulcer—transient relief from food intake
Associated Symptoms	
• Nausea/vomiting	Vomiting after pain—appendicitis Vomiting before pain—gastroenteritis/food poisoning Bilious—distal to duodenum Hematemesis—peptic ulcer, gastritis
• Fevers/chills	Inflammation/infection
• Anorexia	Common symptom in acute abdominal pain

3. Abdominal examination should be done systematically. Analgesia administered prior to examination may alter findings but does not decrease diagnostic accuracy.
   a. Inspect abdomen for distention, scars, masses, or skin changes.
   b. Auscultation may reveal high-pitched bowel sounds of obstruction or the absence of sounds from ileus or diffuse peritonitis.
   c. Percussion may reveal tympanitic sounds from bowel distention or fluid wave of ascites; it is also useful for localizing tenderness and peritoneal irritation when clearly present so as not to expose the patient to deep palpation.
   d. Palpation should be performed with the patient supine.
      i. Begin at a site remote from the reported site of pain.
      ii. Note areas of tenderness and guarding.
      iii. Peritonitis can be evoked by rocking the patient's pelvis or shaking the bed and assessing for pain.
      iv. Pain out of proportion to examination is classic for mesenteric ischemia.
      v. Search for hernias and palpable masses.
      vi. Consider referred pain patterns.
   e. Rectal examination should be done routinely in all patients with suspected gastrointestinal (GI) bleeding, obstruction, or lower abdominal/pelvic pathology.
      i. Rectal mass may be an obstructing cancer; important to note the fraction of circumference involved, mobility, and distance from anal verge.
      ii. Occult blood in stool specimen indicates GI bleeding.
   f. Pelvic examination must be performed in all women of child-bearing age with lower abdominal pain.
      i. Important to note the appearance of the cervix and any discharge.
      ii. Bimanual examination should be performed for cervical motion tenderness, adnexal tenderness, or masses.
   g. Testicular/scrotal examination must be performed in all males with abdominal pain.
      i. Testicular torsion produces painful, swollen, and tender testicles that retract upward in the scrotum.
      ii. Epididymitis may coexist with urinary tract infection (UTI).

D. Laboratory evaluation
1. Complete blood count (CBC) with differential
   a. Leukocytosis indicates the likelihood of an infectious source.
   b. Left shift on the white count differential points to an inflammatory process in the setting of a normal white blood cell count.
   c. Hemoglobin and hematocrit can be elevated from volume contraction due to dehydration; conversely, they may be low from occult blood loss.
2. Electrolyte profile
   a. Hypokalemic, hypochloremic metabolic alkalosis classically appears in patients with prolonged vomiting and volume depletion.

   b. Metabolic acidosis with a low serum bicarbonate level suggests general tissue hypoperfusion and may suggest an underlying ischemic process.
   c. Elevated blood urea nitrogen or creatinine suggests volume depletion.
3. Liver function panel
   a. Mild transaminitis (<2× normal), elevation of alkaline phosphatase and total bilirubin are seen in acute cholecystitis.
   b. Moderate transaminitis (>3× normal) in the setting of acute right upper quadrant pain is most likely an obstructing stone in the common bile duct. Transaminitis precedes elevation of total bilirubin or alkaline phosphatase in the acute setting.
   c. Marked transaminitis (>1,000 IU/L) is likely due to acute hepatitis or ischemia.
4. Pancreatic enzymes, amylase, and lipase are measured when pancreatitis is suspected. The degree of elevation does not correlate with the severity of pancreatitis.
   a. Mild hyperamylasemia can be nonspecific, also being elevated in sialadenitis, perforated ulcer, cholecystitis, or bowel obstruction.
   b. Elevation of lipase is more specific for pancreatic parenchymal disease.
5. Lactic acid level is measured when intestinal ischemia is suspected.
   a. Serum lactate is a general indicator of tissue hypoxia due to impaired perfusion.
   b. Mild lactic acidosis is seen in patients with arterial hypotension.
   c. Ongoing elevation despite resuscitation is concerning for progressive tissue ischemia.
6. Urinalysis assesses urologic causes of abdominal pain.
   a. Bacteriuria, pyuria, and presence of leukocyte esterase or nitrites on urinalysis suggest the presence of UTI. Recurrent UTI in males is unusual and warrants further evaluation.
   b. Hematuria is seen with nephrolithiasis and renal or urothelial cancer.
7. Urine human chorionic gonadotropin must be obtained in all women of child-bearing age. A positive urine test should be followed by quantitated serum levels.
   a. Low level (<4,000 mIU) usually accompanies ectopic pregnancy.
   b. Higher levels (>4,000 mIU) indicate intrauterine pregnancy, usually detectable on ultrasound.

E. Radiographic evaluation, while an important component of a diagnostic workup, should be used selectively to minimize cost, radiation, and contrast exposure to the patient.
   1. Abdominal radiographs
      a. Presence of free air under the diaphragm suggests viscus perforation.
      b. Bowel distension with air fluid levels suggests obstruction.
   2. Abdominal ultrasound
      a. Visualization of the appendix
         i. Findings of appendicitis include a thick-walled or noncompressible appendix that is ≥6 mm in diameter, appendicolith, and periappendiceal fluid.

b. Visualization of the gallbladder
   i. Findings of acute cholecystitis include gallbladder wall thickening >3 mm, wall edema, gallbladder distension >40 mm, pericholecystic fluid, and positive sonographic Murphy sign.
c. Visualization of the common bile duct
   i. Upper limit of normal is 6 to 8 mm in diameter
   ii. Normal bile duct diameter varies with age
   iii. Bile duct dilation can be seen normally in patients post cholecystectomy.

3. CT
   a. IV contrast often improves the visualization of abdominal structures.
   b. PO contrast should be administered if the patient has a history of bariatric surgery to visualize possible anastomotic stenosis or leak.
   c. Look for the following abnormalities
      i. Free fluid—blood, succus, urine
      ii. Free air—perforation, fistula
      iii. Bowel or stomach dilation—obstruction
      iv. Bowel inflammation or ischemia
      v. Volvulus—cecal, sigmoid, or gastric
      vi. Masses
   d. Examine in the context of patient's prior surgical history—examine staple lines, anastomoses, foreign material
4. MRI
   a. Good for visualizing small bowel inflammation in the setting of active Crohn's

F. Differential diagnosis

Common etiologies of acute abdominal pain are described in **Table 12.2** and explored more in depth below. In general, patients with peritonitis on physical examination should be taken urgently for surgical intervention. For specific management, see respective chapters.

IV. COMMON ETIOLOGIES

A. Rectus sheath hematoma
1. Epidemiology/Etiology
   a. Caused by abdominal trauma or forceful contraction of the rectus, resulting in rupture of an epigastric artery or tear in rectus muscle
   b. Risk factors: Abdominal trauma, anticoagulation, abdominal surgery, coughing, chronic obstructive pulmonary disease, pregnancy
2. Presentation
   a. Acute abdominal pain with palpable abdominal wall mass
3. Diagnosis
   a. Imaging and invasive studies
      i. CT abdomen/pelvis with IV contrast (may see active extravasation)
   b. Laboratory testing
      i. Hemoglobin should be measured every 4 to 6 hours.
      ii. Prothrombin time (PT)/international normalized ratio and partial thromboplastin time should be obtained.

TABLE 12.2 Acute Abdomen Common Differential Diagnoses

Diagnosis	Presentation	Laboratory Findings	Radiologic Findings
Appendicitis	• Progressive, persistent RLQ pain • Anorexia • Mild fever and tachycardia	Leukocytosis, pyuria, albuminuria, hematuria	• Ultrasound—diameter > 6 mm, lack of luminal compressibility, presence of appendicolith • CT scan—distended, thick-walled appendix with streaking of periappendiceal fat
Acute cholecystitis	• Postprandial epigastric or RUQ pain • Nausea/vomiting • Positive Murphy sign	Possible leukocytosis, elevation in liver enzymes, elevated bilirubin (may suggest obstructed common bile duct)	• Ultrasound—gallbladder wall thickening, pericholecystic fluid, sonographic Murphy sign, increased bile duct size • HIDA scan—nonfilling of the gallbladder
Acute pancreatitis	• Severe epigastric pain radiating to the back • Tachycardia, fever, and hypotension, depending on the severity of the episode	Elevation of amylase, lipase, and serum transaminases	• Plain radiograph—may reveal a sentinel loop or pancreatic calcifications • CT scan with IV contrast to identify pancreatic necrosis or fluid collection
Perforated peptic ulcer	• Risk factors include smoking, alcohol consumption, and chronic use of NSAIDs or steroids • Sudden-onset, severe epigastric pain that progresses to peritonitis	Leukocytosis	Plain radiograph—free intraperitoneal air

(*continued*)

TABLE 12.2 Acute Abdomen Common Differential Diagnoses (*Continued*)

Diagnosis	Presentation	Laboratory Findings	Radiologic Findings
Gastric volvulus	• Sharp epigastric pain with severe nausea and retching, inability to vomit	Leukocytosis and lactic acidosis	Plain radiographs—distended stomach, intrathoracic gastric bubble, double air–fluid level CT scan—abnormally positioned stomach, gastric wall pneumatosis
Intestinal obstruction	• Sharp, crampy periumbilical pain with intervening pain-free periods • Nausea, vomiting, and obstipation • Abdominal distention, high-pitched or tinkling bowel sounds, and a variable degree of abdominal tenderness	Leukocytosis and lactic acidosis	Plain radiograph—dilated loops of small bowel, air–fluid levels, and paucity of gas distally in the colon and rectum
Mesenteric ischemia	• Sudden onset of severe, constant abdominal pain • Vomiting and diarrhea • Pain out of proportion to examination	Leukocytosis and lactic acidosis	Angiography may confirm the diagnosis; however, radiologic studies are not indicated if peritonitis is present on physical examination
Ruptured abdominal aortic aneurysm	• Sudden onset of abdominal pain with varying manifestations of radiation to the flank or back • May present with shock • Tender, pulsatile abdominal mass on examination	Leukocytosis	• Plain radiographs—calcification in the aortic wall • CT scan—gold standard for diagnosis (should only be performed in hemodynamically stable patients)

HIDA, hepatobiliary iminodiacetic acid; RLQ, right lower quadrant; RUQ, right upper quadrant.

4. Nonoperative treatment[1]
   a. Obtain type and screen and serial CBCs
   b. Resuscitation with fluids and blood products
   c. If applicable, anticoagulation should be reversed
   d. Patients may be observed with serial blood counts and serial abdominal examinations if they remain hemodynamically stable
5. Operative treatment
   a. Angiographic embolization should be attempted first, especially if active extravasation is seen on imaging.
   b. If embolization fails, surgical treatment involves evacuation of the hematoma and ligation of bleeding vessels.
6. Outcomes/Complications
   a. Mortality rate is <2%
   b. 80% of patients can be managed without invasive intervention
   c. The hematoma will usually reabsorb within 2 to 3 months

B. Mesenteric ischemic
1. Epidemiology/Etiology
   a. Arterial embolism accounts for 50% of cases.
      i. Risk factors: Atrial fibrillation, myocardial infarction, valvular heart disease
   b. Arterial thrombosis accounts for 20% of cases.
   c. Nonocclusive mesenteric ischemia (NOMI) accounts for 20%.
      i. Caused by hypoperfusion
   d. Mesenteric venous thrombosis accounts for 10% of cases.
2. Presentation
   a. Acute abdominal pain out of proportion that is poorly localized
3. Diagnosis
   a. Imaging and invasive studies
      i. CT angiography abdomen/pelvis including arterial and venous phase may show filling defect in the superior mesenteric artery (SMA), venous engorgement, pneumatosis, mesenteric edema, or portal venous gas.
      ii. Abdominal plain film may show small bowel distension and ileus. Late findings may include portal venous gas, pneumatosis, and thumbprinting.
   b. Laboratory testing
      i. Leukocytosis with left shift
      ii. Anion gap metabolic acidosis with increased lactic acid
4. Nonoperative treatment
   a. The treatment of NOMI is supportive and correction of the underlying reason for hypoperfusion.
   b. The treatment of mesenteric venous thrombosis is anticoagulation, unless there is necrotic bowel, which requires resection.
5. Operative treatment
   a. Arterial embolism and thrombosis require urgent surgical exploration for revascularization with resection of necrotic bowel.
      i. Embolism: SMA exploration, embolectomy
      ii. Thrombosis: SMA exploration, endarterectomy with possible bypass

b. Abdominal closure should be delayed allowing for a second look of the bowel within 24 to 48 hours.

6. Outcomes/Complications
   a. Overall mortality rate 60% to 80%
   b. Reperfusion injury can occur due to oxidative stress and generation of free radicals that promote necrosis.

C. Small bowel obstruction (SBO)

1. Epidemiology/Etiology
   a. The most common cause in Western societies is postoperative adhesions.
   b. The second most common cause is incarcerated hernia.
   c. Absence of hernia or prior surgery should prompt a workup for malignancy or Crohn's.
2. Presentation
   a. Nausea, vomiting
   b. Obstipation, abdominal distension
   c. Intermittent, cramping abdominal pain
3. Diagnosis
   a. Imaging and invasive studies
      i. Leukocytosis can be seen with partial SBO or closed-loop obstruction.
      ii. Vomiting may cause hypokalemic, hypochloremic metabolic alkalosis.
      iii. Elevated lactate may indicate bowel ischemia.
   b. Laboratory testing
      i. Abdominal radiograph may reveal distension of the bowel and stomach with air fluid levels.
      ii. CT abdomen/pelvis with IV contrast[2]
         a) Single transition point—complete or partial SBO
         b) Two transition points—closed-loop obstruction
      iii. Small bowel follow-through with water-soluble PO contrast
         a) Should be considered in all patients with partial SBO >48 hours
         b) Serial abdominal radiographs following PO contrast administration
         c) Both diagnostic and therapeutic, as PO contrast can hasten return of bowel function
4. Nonoperative treatment
   a. Nasogastric decompression, nothing by mouth, and IV fluids
   b. Small bowel follow-through with water-soluble PO contrast if symptoms do not resolve within 48 hours
   c. Not appropriate for closed-loop obstruction or strangulated bowel
5. Operative treatment[3]
   a. Should be considered if partial SBO has not resolved in 3 to 5 days.
   b. Laparoscopic abdominal exploration is a safe and acceptable alternative to open surgery, depending on the patient's status and the surgeon's experience.
   c. Changes in patient's status or abdominal examination may indicate worsening bowel ischemia and warrants surgical exploration.

d. Closed-loop obstructions require urgent exploration with resection of compromised bowel.

6. Outcomes/Complications
   a. Laparoscopic surgery is associated with earlier recovery of bowel function and shorter hospital length of stay.
   b. Single-band adhesive obstruction is associated with a higher rate of success in laparoscopic cases.
   c. Complications of delayed treatment include bowel perforation.
   d. Mortality rate for nonstrangulated obstruction is 2%.
   e. Mortality rate for strangulated obstruction is 8% to 25%.

D. Colitis—infectious and ischemic

1. Epidemiology/Etiology
   a. Ischemic colitis
      i. Caused by vascular occlusion by thrombus or emboli, vasospasm, or a low-flow state with decreased perfusion
      ii. Incidence of 4.5 to 44 cases per 100,000 person-years
      iii. Most commonly manifests as mesenteric ischemia
      iv. Slight female predominance
      v. More predominant in the elderly
      vi. The splenic flexure (Griffith point) and the rectosigmoid junction (Sudeck point) are the most susceptible to ischemia. These areas are known as watershed areas.
   b. Infectious colitis
      i. Caused by bacterial, viral, or parasitic pathogens
         a) *Salmonella, Shigella, Campylobacter,* enterohemorrhagic *Escherichia coli, Entamoeba histolytica, Clostridium difficile,* cytomegalovirus
      ii. *C. difficile*
         a) Colonizes the intestinal tract of 1% to 3% healthy adults and 20% of patients on antibiotics. However, only a fraction of these patients develop *C. difficile* colitis.
         b) Transmission is by ingestion of spores that are resistant to heat and antibiotics.
            1) Spores enter the colon the fecal–oral route and produce toxins A and B.
         c) Localized mucosal injury and necrosis result in formation of pseudomembranes.
         d) Increased fluid secretion from colonic enterocytes results in watery diarrhea
         e) Antibiotics disturb normal colonic flora and allow *C. difficile* to multiply.
            1) The most common antibiotics associated with *C. difficile* are clindamycin, fluoroquinolones, penicillins, and cephalosporins.

2. Presentation
   a. Abdominal pain ranging from vague to severe with peritonitis
      i. Embolic colon ischemia presents with acute-onset abdominal pain.

   - ii. Patients with chronic vascular insufficiency may have postprandial abdominal pain or weight loss.
- b. Diarrhea
   - i. Ischemic—bloody
   - ii. Infectious—watery with or without blood
- c. Patients may have a history of recent travel or immunosuppression.

3. Diagnosis
   - a. Imaging and invasive studies
      - i. CT abdomen/pelvis with IV contrast
         - a) Ischemic—bowel wall thickening, absent bowel wall enhancement, possible source of vascular occlusion
         - b) Infectious—hyperemia, mucosal edema, bowel wall thickening, pericolic fat stranding
            - 1) Colonic dilation >6 cm or cecal dilation >12 cm suggests toxic megacolon
      - ii. Unprepped colonoscopy or sigmoidoscopy
         - a) Contraindicated if the patient has peritonitis or free air is evident on CT
         - b) Ischemic—pale mucosa, sloughing, mucosal edema, ulcerations, hemorrhage, black mucosa if ischemia is full thickness
         - c) Not indicated for diagnosis of infectious colitis unless needed to rule out alternative diagnosis
            - 1) Presence of pseudomembranes in *C. difficile* colitis is pathognomonic.
   - b. Laboratory testing
      - i. CBC may show leukocytosis.
      - ii. Basic metabolic panel/comprehensive metabolic panel may show metabolic acidosis.
      - iii. Lactate may be elevated.
      - iv. Fulminant colitis—marked leukocytosis, lactic acidosis, hypoalbuminemia
      - v. Stool test for ova and parasites
      - vi. *C. difficile*
         - a) Stool sample assay for toxins A and B
         - b) Nucleic acid amplification testing by polymerase chain reaction for toxin B gene (may be positive in asymptomatic carriers)
4. Nonoperative treatment
   - a. Infectious—appropriate antibiotic therapy
      - i. *C. difficile*
         - a) PO vancomycin or PO fidaxomicin for 10 days
         - b) PO vancomycin and IV metronizadole for fulminant disease
5. Operative treatment
   - a. Ischemic—in the presence of peritonitis, clinical deterioration, perforation, or full-thickness ischemia on colonoscopy
      - i. Laparotomy with resection of nonviable bowel with or without stoma creation
   - b. Infectious—in the presence of peritonitis, clinical deterioration, perforation, or toxic megacolon
      - i. Laparotomy, total abdominal colectomy with end ileostomy

6. Outcomes/Complications
   a. Colonoscopy should be performed after resolution of ischemic or infectious colitis.
   b. Following ischemic colitis, some patients may develop a stricture.
   c. Mortality rate after surgery for *C. difficile* colitis is >50%.

V. OPERATIVE SUMMARY

A. Operative steps: Appendectomy

1. Three trocars are placed: 12 mm at the umbilicus, 5 mm left lower quadrant, and 5 mm suprapubic.
2. Adhesions to the appendix are divided and the appendix is elevated.
3. The mesoappendix is divided using LigaSure, staples, or cautery.
4. The appendix is stapled at the base and removed (via largest trocar site or additional incision, often through containment bag).
5. Irrigation is performed (if needed), drain can be considered in cases of significant perforation or purulence, pneumoperitoneum is reduced, and port sites are closed.

B. Operative steps: Exploratory laparotomy for SBO

1. Enter the abdomen with a midline laparotomy.
2. Inspect the affected bowel for the cause of the obstruction. Divide any adhesions obstructing the bowel. If there is an obstructing mass or signs of perforation or ischemia, resect the affected bowel.
3. To begin your small bowel resection, score the mesentery with electrocautery and make a window in the mesentery with a Kelly clamp.
4. Pass a GIA stapler on either side of the segment of bowel to be divided. Use a blue load (3.8 mm) to divide the bowel.
5. Divide the mesentery with electrocautery.
6. Position the two segments of bowel in the antimesenteric position. Cut off the adjacent corners of the staple lines. Insert a GIA-60 mm or GIA-80 mm cutting stapler with one end in the proximal small bowel segment and the other in the distal small bowel segment. Fire the stapler to create a side-to-side anastomosis.
7. Inspect the anastomosis and invert the staple line with a layer 3-0 silk interrupted Lembert sutures.
8. Run the bowel and ensure the mesentery is not twisted. Close the abdomen.

C. Operative steps: Incarcerated ventral hernia

1. Enter the abdomen with a midline laparotomy. Be cautious to not enter the hernia sac and injure the bowel.
2. Reduce the contents of the hernia.
3. Inspect the incarcerated bowel. If there are signs of perforation or ischemia, resect the affected segment of bowel. Run the bowel to look for any further injury.
4. Close the fascial defect primarily, if possible. Avoid using mesh if there is any suspicion for abdominal contamination.
5. Close the abdomen primarily.

Key References

Citation	Summary
Gallagher EJ, Esses D, Lee C, Lahn M, Bijur PE. Randomized clinical trial of morphine in acute abdominal pain. *Ann Emerg Med.* 2006;48(2):150-160, 160 e1-e4.	• This randomized, double-blinded, placebo-controlled clinical trial compared intravenous morphine with placebo in adult patients presenting to the emergency department to determine if morphine decreases the diagnostic accuracy. This study showed that appropriately dosed morphine reduces discomfort without reducing diagnostic accuracy.
Girard E, Abba J, Boussat B, et al. Damage control surgery for non-traumatic abdominal emergencies. *World J Surg.* 2018;42(4):965-973.	• This prospective series of 164 consecutive patients who underwent damage control surgery for non-traumatic abdominal emergencies demonstrated that patients with peritonitis and acute pancreatitis are those who benefited the most from damage control surgery.
Kao AM, Cetrulo LN, Baimas-George MR, et al. Outcomes of open abdomen versus primary closure following emergent laparotomy for suspected secondary peritonitis: a propensity-matched analysis. *J Trauma Acute Care Surg.* 2019;87(3):623-629.	• This retrospective, single-center study used a propensity-matched analysis to compare outcomes of primary closure vs. delayed abdominal closure in 534 nontrauma patients who underwent emergent laparotomy for peritonitis. This study demonstrated that patients with an open abdomen had increased postoperative complications, mortality, and longer median hospital length of stay.
Behman R, Nathens AB, Mason S, et al. Association of surgical intervention for adhesive small-bowel obstruction with the risk of recurrence. *JAMA Surg.* 2019;154(5):413-420.	• This longitudinal, propensity-matched, retrospective study compared the incidence of recurrent adhesive SBO in 27,904 patients undergoing operative management vs. conservative management at their initial hospital admission. This study demonstrated that operative management was associated with a significant reduction in risk of SBO recurrence. In patients initially treated with conservative management, the 5-y probability of recurrence increased with each episode until surgical intervention, which resulted in a 50% decrease in risk of subsequent recurrence.

CHAPTER 12: ACUTE ABDOMEN

Review Questions

1. Describe the onset and characterize the pain associated with perforated viscus.
2. How does perforated viscus present on abdominal radiograph?
3. Describe the onset and characterize the pain associated with small bowel obstruction.
4. What are the risk factors for peptic ulcer disease?
5. Where does biliary pain refer to?
6. What electrolyte and metabolic disturbances are observed with prolonged vomiting?

REFERENCES

1. Liao ED, Puckett Y. A proposed algorithm on the modern management of rectus sheath hematoma: a literature review. *Cureus*. 2021;13(11):e20008.
2. Sheedy SP, Earnest F, Fletcher JG, Fidler JL, Hoskin TL. CT of small-bowel ischemia associated with obstruction in emergency department patients: diagnostic performance evaluation. *Radiology*. 2006;241(3):729-736.
3. Paulson EK, Thompson WM. Review of small-bowel obstruction: the diagnosis and when to worry. *Radiology*. 2015;275(2):332-342.
4. Gallagher EJ, Esses D, Lee C, Lahn M, Bijur PE. Randomized clinical trial of morphine in acute abdominal pain. *Ann Emerg Med*. 2006;48(2):150-160.e1-e4.
5. Girard E, Abba J, Boussat B, et al. Damage control surgery for non-traumatic abdominal emergencies. *World J Surg*. 2018;42(4):965-973.
6. Kao AM, Cetrulo LN, Baimas-George MR, et al. Outcomes of open abdomen versus primary closure following emergent laparotomy for suspected secondary peritonitis: a propensity-matched analysis. *J Trauma Acute Care Surg*. 2019;87(3):623-629.
7. Behman R, Nathens AB, Mason S, et al. Association of surgical intervention for adhesive small-bowel obstruction with the risk of recurrence. *JAMA Surg*. 2019;154(5):413-420.

13 Esophagus

William D. Gerull and Bryan F. Meyers

I. STRUCTURAL AND FUNCTIONAL DISORDERS OF THE ESOPHAGUS

A. Hiatal hernia

1. **Epidemiology**
   - **a.** Hiatal hernias are common (up to 60% of individuals 50 years old).
   - **b.** While most are asymptomatic, patients with a hiatal hernia are more likely to have symptoms related to persistent gastroesophageal reflux disease (GERD).[1] Some patients will complain of pain.
2. The **type of hiatal hernia** is defined by the location of the gastroesophageal (GE) junction and the relationship of the stomach to the distal esophagus.
   - **a. Type I (sliding)** is the most common type of hiatal hernia, although usually asymptomatic. The distal esophagus and gastric cardia herniate up through the hiatus.
   - **b. Type II (paraesophageal)** is rare; the peritoneum and greater curvature of the stomach herniate along the distal esophagus, and the GE junction remains anchored within the abdomen.
   - **c. Type III (combination of types I and II)** is more common than pure type II and involves the herniation of both the greater curvature of the stomach and the GE junction into the chest.
   - **d. Type IV** hiatal hernias occur when abdominal organs (e.g., colon or spleen) other than or in addition to the stomach herniate through the hiatus into the chest.
3. **Symptoms**
   - **a.** Type I hiatal hernias are usually asymptomatic but may present with reflux.
   - **b.** Type II, III, and IV hiatal hernias frequently produce postprandial pain or bloating, early satiety, breathlessness with meals, and mild dysphagia.
     - **i.** The herniated stomach is susceptible to volvulus and can develop ischemic longitudinal ulcers.
4. **Diagnosis and evaluation**
   - **a.** A **CXR** with a retrocardiac soft-tissue mass, with or without an air–fluid level above the diaphragm, suggests a hiatal hernia.
     - **i.** Differential diagnosis includes mediastinal cyst, epiphrenic diverticulum, abscess, or a dilated obstructed esophagus.
     - **ii.** However, **retrocardiac air–fluid level** on two-view plain radiograph is pathopneumonic for a hiatal hernia.

b. A **barium swallow** confirms the diagnosis, delineates the type of hiatal hernia, and defines the anatomy (length and coexisting abnormalities such as strictures or ulcers).
   i. Patients with hiatal hernia are at increased risk for aspiration. For this reason, barium is the preferred agent for contrasted studies due to the risk of pneumonitis with aspirated water-soluble agents.
c. **Esophagogastroduodenoscopy (EGD)** is indicated in patients with symptoms of reflux or dysphagia to assess for the presence of esophagitis, stricture, or Barrett's esophagus. EGD also establishes the location of the GE junction in relation to the hiatus.
   i. A sliding hiatal hernia is defined as existing when greater than 2 cm of gastric mucosa is present between the diaphragmatic hiatus and the mucosal squamocolumnar junction.
d. **Esophageal manometry** evaluates esophageal motility in patients who are being considered for operative repair to assist in operative planning for a potential fundoplication.
e. **CT scan** is most valuable in the emergent setting to evaluate tissue viability and anatomy. In the nonemergent setting, CT may be useful for preoperative planning in patients with *large* type III or IV hernias or recurrent hernias.

5. **Management options**
   a. Asymptomatic type I hernias: No treatment.
   b. Symptomatic type I hernias (GERD) should undergo a trial of medical therapy. Patients who should be evaluated for an antireflux procedure (see Section II) and hiatal hernia repair include patients who have failed medical therapy, patients who have ongoing regurgitation or respiratory symptoms, patients who have Barrett esophagus, and young patients who would require lifelong proton-pump inhibitors (PPIs). Patients with *atypical* symptoms (chest pain, hoarseness, frequent pneumonias, or dysphagia) require further testing and continued medical therapy.
   c. Patients with a type II, III, or IV hiatal hernia should be considered for surgical repair via an abdominal or occasionally thoracic approach.
6. **Operative principles**
   a. Paraoesophageal hernia repair is most commonly performed through a laparoscopic, transabdominal approach.
   b. Robotic-assisted laparoscopy has become a promising safe and feasible approach.
      i. The robotic approach allows for greater access to the superior mediastinum, which can decrease the need for esophageal lengthening procedures such as a Collis gastroplasty via wedge fundectomy (see below) while achieving low, long-term recurrence rates.[2]
   c. Main surgical principles include the reduction of the hernia, resection of the sac, and closure of the hiatal defect.
   d. The hiatal defect is primarily repaired with suture, and the additional use of on-lay mesh reinforcement for this closure remains at

surgeon discretion, given limited current evidence to support significant symptom improvement.[3]

e. Collis gastroplasty is a technique used to lengthen a shortened esophagus (i.e., <3 cm of intra-abdominal esophagus after mobilization) to minimize tension on the antireflux repair.
   i. A gastric tube is formed from the upper lesser curvature of the stomach in continuity with the distal esophagus.
   ii. A gastroplasty can be considered in patients with minimal intra-abdominal esophagus despite adequate esophageal mobilization.[4]

B. Gastroesophageal reflux (GERD)

1. **Prevalence**
   a. Symptoms of heartburn and excessive regurgitation are relatively common in the US, occurring daily in 18% to 28% of the population.[5]
2. **Pathophysiology**
   a. Relates to the abnormal exposure of the distal esophagus to refluxed stomach contents. In 60% of patients, it is due to a mechanically defective lower esophageal sphincter (LES).[6]
   b. The classic symptom of GERD is postural aggravated epigastric burning pain that is readily relieved by antacids. Other symptoms include regurgitation and dysphagia. *Atypical symptoms* may mimic laryngeal, respiratory, cardiac, biliary, pancreatic, or gastric disease.
3. **Diagnosis and evaluation**
   a. EGD is the most direct method to evaluate symptomatic patients for objective evidence of GERD such as esophagitis and Barrett changes. Esophagitis is a clinical and pathologic diagnosis.
   b. Esophageal manometry guides the selection of the best antireflux procedure by defining the location and function of the LES.
      i. It helps exclude achalasia, scleroderma, and diffuse esophageal spasm.
      ii. Characteristics of a monometrically abnormal LES are (1) a resting pressure <6 mm Hg, (2) an overall length <2 cm, and (3) an abdominal length <1 cm.
   c. Esophageal pH testing over a 24-hour period is the gold standard in the diagnosis of GERD. **A DeMeester score less than 14.7 is normal.**
   d. Upper gastrointestinal (GI) radiography is useful for identifying anatomical abnormalities that may cause symptoms. However, only 33% of patients with GERD demonstrate spontaneous reflux on upper GI radiography, making this study insufficient as a standalone diagnostic study.
   e. A gastric emptying study can be useful in evaluating patients with previous esophageal surgery (rule out vagus nerve injury) or those with symptoms of gastroparesis.
      i. Patients with gastroparesis may benefit additionally from a pyloric drainage procedure (i.e., pyloroplasty or pyloromyotomy), and such a finding may influence the type of fundoplication performed.

4. **Complications**
   a. Approximately 20% of patients with GERD have complications, including esophagitis, stricture, or Barrett esophagus.
   b. Esophageal cancer can form in the setting of long-standing reflux disease.
5. **Treatment**
   a. *Medical treatment* aims to reduce the duration and amount of esophageal exposure to gastric acid.
   b. *Behavioral recommendations* include remaining upright after meals for at least 1 hour, sleeping with an elevated head of the bed, and avoiding bending or straining.
   c. *Dietary alterations* are aimed at maximizing LES pressure and decreasing stomach acidity. Patients are instructed to lose weight; eat small, frequent meals; and stop smoking. Fatty foods, alcohol, caffeine, chocolate, peppermint, and certain medications may exacerbate reflux.
   d. *Pharmacologic therapy* is indicated in patients who do not improve with postural or dietary measures and include antacids, H2-receptor antagonists, and PPIs.
6. **Surgical treatment**
   a. **Surgical approach: Laparoscopic paraoesophageal hernia repair and Nissen fundoplication**
      i. Position the patient supine, split leg, with body secured to allow for reverse Trendelenburg position. Place liver retractor.
      ii. Dissect the gastrohepatic ligament (pars flaccida). If present, a replaced left hepatic artery and/or accessory hepatic artery may be visible.
      iii. Identify the right crus and open the phrenoesophageal ligament.
      iv. Perform a blunt dissection of the crus off the esophagus anteriorly and circumferentially to the left crus (identify and preserve anterior vagus).
      v. Divide the short gastric vessels to improve caudal dissection.
      vi. Create a posterior window behind the esophagus (identify and protect posterior vagus).
      vii. Complete a sutured posterior crural closure with interrupted nonabsorbable suture.
      viii. Complete a sutured posterior crural closure with interrupted nonabsorbable suture.
      ix. Perform fundoplication.
         a) Bring the stomach fundus behind the esophagus.
         b) Perform the "shoeshine" maneuver.
         c) Place a 56 F or 60 F bougie.
         d) Perform a 360° wrap over the distal esophagus using three nonabsorbable sutures, incorporating the esophageal wall.
         e) Use a length of 2 to 3 cm, avoiding the anterior vagus nerve.
      x. Use esophagogastroduodenoscopy after completion to assess the adequacy of the wrap.

b. Should be considered in patients who have symptomatic reflux despite optimal medical management and manometric evidence of a defective LES.
c. It should also be considered in patients who have achieved relief with medical therapy but want to avoid a lifetime of medication.
d. Surgery consists of either a transabdominal or a transthoracic antireflux operation to replicate a competent LES and to keep the GE junction in the abdomen.
e. *A laparoscopic, transabdominal approach is most commonly utilized.* A transthoracic approach is a reasonable alternative in patients with esophageal shortening or stricture, coexistent pulmonary lesion, or prior antireflux repair.
f. Surgical wraps
   i. **Nissen fundoplication** (360° fundic wrap) is effective at preventing reflux but is associated with an inability to vomit, gas bloating, and dysphagia. During surgery, care must be taken to ensure that the wrap is not too tight and placed appropriately around the distal esophagus. Esophageal dysmotility on manometry is a contraindication for a Nissen.
   ii. **Toupet fundoplication** is a partial 270° posterior wrap, with the wrapped segment sutured to the crural margins and to the anterolateral esophageal wall. It is the preferred fundoplication for GERD patients with esophageal dysmotility, and recent data suggest that it should be strongly considered for most patients due to a lower incidence of postoperative dysphagia and equivalent or better relief of GERD symptoms when compared with Nissen fundoplication.[7]
   iii. **Dor fundoplication** is an anterior 180° fundal wrap with the gastric fundus folded over the anterior esophagus and secured to the right crura. A Dor is particularly useful following an anterior myotomy (i.e., Heller) to help cushion the exposed mucosa.
   iv. **Belsey Mark IV repair** consists of a 240° fundic wrap around 4 cm of distal esophagus performed through the *transthoracic approach.* In cases of esophageal neuromotor dysfunction, it produces less dysphagia than with a 360° wrap.

7. **Postoperative complications**
   a. Postoperative dysphagia can result from a fundoplication that is too tight, a misplaced or postoperatively slipped fundoplication, or an inappropriate complete fundoplication in the setting of poor esophageal contractile function.
   b. Recurrent reflux after surgery is increasingly common as time progresses, due to natural loosening of the wrap, and may require medical therapy.
      i. However, reflux occurring immediately or too soon after surgical repair may suggest an inadequate or disrupted repair.

c. Gas bloating can occur if the fundoplication is too tight or if there is unrecognized gastric outlet obstruction. Vagus nerve injury can lead to gastroparesis and bloating, often difficult to distinguish from the bloating of an excessively tight wrap.

II. FUNCTIONAL ESOPHAGEAL DISORDERS

A. Motor disorders of esophageal smooth muscle and LES

1. **Achalasia**
   - **a.** Although rare, it is the most common primary esophageal motility disorder.
   - **b.** Characterized by failure of the LES to relax with swallowing, and loss of effective esophageal body peristalsis, resulting in esophageal dilation.
   - **c.** Characteristically, pathology reveals alteration in the ganglia of Auerbach plexus.
   - **d.** Symptoms
     - **i.** Progressive dysphagia (~100%)
     - **ii.** Regurgitation immediately after meals (>70%)
     - **iii.** Odynophagia (30%)
     - **iv.** Aspiration with resultant bronchitis and pneumonia (10%)
     - **v.** Some patients experience chest pain due to esophageal spasms.
   - **e.** Diagnostic studies
     - **i.** Diagnostic CXR often shows a fluid-filled, dilated esophagus and absence of a gastric air bubble.
     - **ii.** A barium esophagogram demonstrates tapering ("bird's beak") of the distal esophagus and a dilated proximal esophagus (**Figure 13.1**).
     - **iii.** Esophageal manometry is the definitive diagnostic test for achalasia.
       - **a)** Characteristic manometric findings include the absence of peristalsis and limited or absent relaxation of the LES with swallowing.
     - **iv.** Endoscopy rules out benign strictures or malignancy.
       - **a)** When these symptoms are caused by secondary malignant or nonmalignant causes the syndrome is referred to as pseudoachalasia.
         - **1)** Possible nonmalignant etiologies of pseudoachalasia include pancreatic pseudocysts, aortic aneurysm, pancreatic pseudocyst, and post-surgical in the setting of vagotomy, bariatrics, or a Nissen fundoplication that was excessively tight.
   - **f.** Medical treatment
     - **i.** Aimed at decreasing the LES tone
       - **a)** Nitrates and calcium-channel blockers
       - **b)** Have limited effect overall and rarely used for long-term therapy

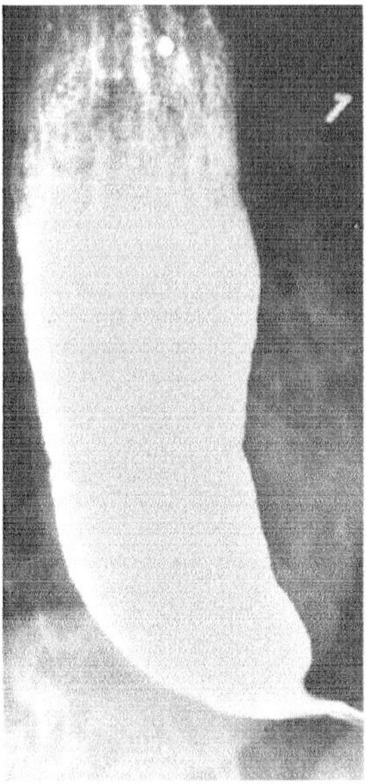

FIGURE 13.1 Upper GI study showing characteristic contrast layering seen ("bird's beak) in patients with achalasia.

g. Endoscopic treatment
  i. Endoscopic balloon dilation or bougie dilation may offer transient relief.
  ii. Botox injection can be effective, but the effects are short-lived.

h. Surgical treatment
  i. Heller esophagomyotomy
    a) Shown to produce excellent results in >90% of patients[8]
    b) A concomitant antireflux procedure (270° or 180° fundoplication) with the esophagomyotomy helps to avoid late stricture due to GERD caused by the incompetent LES.[9]
  ii. Peroral endoscopic myotomy (POEM)
    a) A newer endoscopic treatment option
    b) Steps include the creation of a submucosal tunnel; division of the circular muscle layer of distal esophagus, LES, and proximal stomach; and closing the submucosal tunnel with endoscopic clips.
    c) Dysphagia outcomes, postoperative pain, and symptomatic GERD are similar to laparoscopic Heller/fundoplication.[10]
    d) While POEM is highly effective in relieving symptoms of achalasia, patients more often experience significant GERD postoperatively as compared with a Heller myotomy.

2. **Diffuse esophageal spasm**
   a. Loss of the normal peristaltic coordination of the esophageal smooth muscle
   b. Primary symptoms: Severe spastic pain, dysphagia, regurgitation, and weight loss
   c. Diagnosis is confirmed with esophageal manometry—spontaneous activity, repetitive waves, and prolonged, high-amplitude contractions.
   d. Main treatment with calcium-channel blockers and nitrates
   e. Surgical treatment is very rare and may consist of a long esophagomyotomy and often a concomitant antireflux procedure.
3. **Nutcracker/jackhammer esophagus**
   a. Characterized manometrically by prolonged, high-amplitude peristaltic waves associated with chest pain that may mimic cardiac symptoms.
   b. Treatment with calcium-channel blockers and long-acting nitrates has been helpful.[11]
4. **Secondary dysmotility**
   a. Esophageal response to inflammatory injury or systemic disorders.
      i. Inflammation can produce fibrosis, which can lead to loss of peristalsis and esophageal contractility.
   b. The most common cause of secondary dysfunction is GERD, resulting in erosive esophagitis and stricture formation.
      i. Intensive medical treatment of reflux is essential before operation.
      ii. Toupet fundoplication with or without a Collis gastroplasty is preferred for these patients because of the presence of esophageal fibrosis, esophageal shortening, and impaired peristalsis.
5. **Progressive systemic sclerosis**
   a. Associated with esophageal manifestations in 60% to 80% of patients
   b. Esophagus is the earliest site of GI involvement.
   c. Smooth muscle atrophy and fibrosis results in absent contractions in the mid-distal esophagus.
   d. Contractility is preserved within the striated muscle of the proximal esophagus.

B. Esophageal strictures
1. **Esophageal strictures** can be either benign or malignant.
   a. Benign strictures are either congenital or acquired.
2. **Congenital**
   a. Congenital webs represent a failure of appropriate canalization of the esophagus during development and can occur at any level.
3. **Acquired strictures**
   a. Esophageal rings or webs occur at all levels.
      i. An example is Schatzki ring, which occurs in the lower esophagus at the junction of the squamous and columnar epitheliums due to GERD.
         a) A hiatal hernia is almost always present, although esophagitis is rarely present.

b) Treatment generally consists of medical management of reflux with periodic dilation for symptoms of dysphagia.

b. Strictures of the esophagus can result from any esophageal injury, including chronic reflux, previous perforation, infection, or inflammation.

4. **Symptoms**
   - **a.** Become increasingly common when the lumen narrows beyond 12 mm
   - **b.** Typically, progressive dysphagia to solid food. Regurgitation and weight loss may follow.
5. **Evaluation and treatment**
   - **a.** Must always exclude malignancy.
   - **b.** The diagnosis of stricture often is based on a barium swallow.
   - **c.** Esophagoscopy is essential to assess the location, length, size, and distensibility of the stricture and to obtain appropriate biopsies.
   - **d.** Most benign strictures are amenable to dilation to relieve symptoms, then focus is directed to correcting the underlying etiology.
   - **e.** Resection (esophagectomy) can be required for recurrent or persistent strictures or if malignancy cannot be ruled out.

C. Esophageal diverticula

1. Esophageal diverticula are acquired conditions of the esophagus found primarily in adults.
2. A pharyngoesophageal (or Zenker) diverticulum is a pulsion diverticulum.
   - **a.** It is the most common type of symptomatic diverticulum.
   - **b.** Caused by a hypertensive, poorly relaxing, upper esophageal sphincter (UES) or uncoordinated pharyngeal contraction and opening of the UES to result in increased pharyngeal intraluminal pressure.
   - **c.** Herniation of *only the mucosa and submucosa results in this false diverticulum*
   - **d.** Symptoms
     - **i.** Progressive cervical dysphagia, halitosis, cough on assuming a recumbent position, and spontaneous regurgitation of undigested food
   - **e.** Diagnosis
     - **i.** Usually diagnosed via barium swallow
   - **f.** Treatment
     - **i.** Cricopharyngeal myotomy and diverticulectomy or diverticulopexy
3. A traction (midesophageal or parabronchial) diverticulum
   - **a.** Typically occurs in the middle third of the esophagus and is an example of a true (full-thickness) diverticulum.
   - **b.** It occurs secondary to mediastinal inflammatory diseases (histoplasmosis or tuberculosis).
   - **c.** Symptoms are rare, but when present, may prompt operative excision of the diverticulum and the adjacent inflammatory mass.
4. Epiphrenic diverticulum
   - **a.** Is almost always associated with an underlying esophageal motility disorder.
   - **b.** While it can be located at almost every level of the esophagus, typical location occurs in the distal 10 cm of the thoracic esophagus.

c. Many patients are asymptomatic, and the diagnosis is made with a contrast esophagogram, although endoscopy and esophageal function studies are needed to define the underlying pathophysiology.

d. Operative treatment
   i. Indicated for patients with progressive or incapacitating symptoms
   ii. Standard treatment consists of diverticulectomy or diverticulopexy, along with an extramucosal esophagomyotomy to relieve distal obstruction

III. TRAUMATIC INJURY TO THE ESOPHAGUS

A. Esophageal perforation

1. **Background**
   a. Associated with a high mortality rate, upward of 20%
2. Causes
   a. Intraluminal causes
      i. Most common cause of esophageal injury
      ii. Instrumentation injuries (i.e., EGD, dilation) represent 75% of esophageal perforations and most commonly occur at anatomical narrowings of the esophagus.
      iii. Other less frequent intraluminal causes
         a) Foreign bodies can cause acute perforation, or more commonly follow an indolent course with late abscess formation in the mediastinum or development of empyema.
         b) Ingested caustic substances, such as alkali chemicals, can produce coagulation necrosis of the esophagus.
         c) Cancer of the esophagus may lead to perforation.
         d) Barotrauma induced by external compression, forceful vomiting (Boerhaave syndrome), seizures, childbirth, or lifting can produce esophageal perforation. Almost all of these injuries occur in the distal esophagus on the left side.
   b. Extraluminal causes
      i. Penetrating injuries to the esophagus can occur from stab wounds or, more commonly, gunshot wounds.
      ii. Blunt trauma may produce an esophageal perforation related to a rapid increase in intraluminal pressure or compression of the esophagus between the sternum and the spine.
      iii. Operative injury to the esophagus during an unrelated procedure occurs infrequently and may occur during spine surgery, aortic surgery, or mediastinoscopy.
   c. Signs and symptoms
      i. Dysphagia, pain, and fever, and quickly progress to sepsis if left undiagnosed or untreated.
      ii. Cervical perforations may present with neck stiffness and mediastinal or subcutaneous emphysema.
         a) Intrathoracic perforation presents with chest pain, subcutaneous or mediastinal emphysema, dyspnea, and a pleural effusion (right sided in proximal perforations, left in distal perforations).

b) Intra-abdominal perforations present with peritonitis.

d. Diagnosis

i. Pneumomediastinum, pleural effusion, pneumothorax, atelectasis, and soft-tissue emphysema on CXR or mediastinal air and fluid on CT scan.

a) Rapid evaluation with water-soluble contrast (Gastrografin) or dilute barium contrast esophagography (10% false-negative rate) is mandatory.

b) Intramural perforation after endoscopic procedures appears to have a thin collection of contrast material parallel to the esophageal lumen without spillage into the mediastinum.

c) Esophagoscopy is used primarily as an adjunctive study and can miss sizable perforations.

e. Initial management

i. (1) adequate drainage of the leak, (2) intravenous antibiotics, (3) aggressive fluid resuscitation, (4) adequate nutrition, (5) relief of any distal obstruction, (6) diversion of enteric contents past the leak, and (7) restoration of GI integrity.

ii. Patients are kept nil per os (NPO), a nasogastric tube is carefully placed, and they receive intravenous hydration and broad-spectrum antibiotics.

f. Definitive management

i. Generally requires operative repair, although a carefully selected group of nontoxic patients with a locally contained perforation may be observed.

ii. Esophageal stent placement and appropriate drainage has been effective for some spontaneous perforations and anastomotic leaks.[12]

g. Location-specific treatment

i. Cervical and upper thoracic perforations usually are treated by cervical drainage alone or in combination with esophageal repair.

ii. Thoracic perforations should be closed primarily and buttressed with healthy tissue, and the mediastinum should be drained widely. If primary closure is not possible, options include wide drainage alone or in conjunction with resection, or with exclusion and diversion in cases of severe traumatic injury to the esophagus.

iii. Abdominal esophageal perforations typically require an upper abdominal midline incision.

iv. Perforations associated with intrinsic esophageal disease (e.g., carcinoma, hiatal hernia, or achalasia) require addressing the perforation and surgically correcting the associated esophageal disease.

B. Caustic ingestion

1. **Background**

a. Liquid alkali solutions (e.g., drain cleaners, lye) are responsible for most of the serious caustic esophageal and gastric injuries, producing coagulation necrosis in both organs.

b. Acid ingestion is more likely to cause isolated gastric injury.

2. **Initial Management**
    a. The first step is to evaluate the airway and ensure hemodynamic stability.
    b. Airway compromise or significant burns may require tracheostomy.
    c. Fluid resuscitation and broad-spectrum antibiotics.
    d. *Do not induce* vomiting, place on NPO, and give patients an oral suction device.
3. **Evaluation**
    a. Water-soluble contrast esophagography and gentle esophagoscopy should be done early to assess the severity and extent of injury and to rule out esophageal perforation or gastric necrosis.
4. **Management**
    a. Without perforation, management is supportive, with acute symptoms generally resolving over several days.
    b. Perforation, unrelenting pain, or persistent acidosis mandate surgical intervention.
        i. A transabdominal approach is recommended to allow evaluation of the patient's stomach and distal esophagus.
5. Late complications include the development of strictures and an increased risk (×1,000) of esophageal carcinoma.

IV. ESOPHAGEAL TUMORS

A. Barrett esophagus

1. **Introduction**
    a. Barrett esophagus occurs when columnar epithelium (intestinal type metaplasia) replaces the normal squamous epithelium.
    b. Typically, a complication of chronic GERD; histologically demonstrates intestinal-type metaplasia.
2. **Prevalence**
    a. Barrett esophagus is diagnosed in approximately 2% of all patients undergoing esophagoscopy and in 10% to 15% of patients with esophagitis.
    b. Middle-aged white men is the most common demographic.
3. **Symptoms**
    a. Arise from chronic GERD and includes heartburn (50%), dysphagia (75%), and bleeding (25%)[13]
4. **Diagnosis**
    a. Requires correlation between endoscopic and histologic appearances
5. **Complications**
    a. Esophageal ulceration and stricture are more likely to occur in patients with Barrett esophagus than in those with GERD alone.
    b. Barrett ulcers, like gastric ulcers, penetrate the metaplastic columnar epithelium and can occur in up to 50% of patients with Barrett esophagus.
    c. Benign strictures occur in 30% to 50% of patients with Barrett esophagus.
        i. The stricture is located at the squamocolumnar junction, which may be found proximal to the GE junction.

d. The metaplastic columnar epithelium of Barrett esophagus is prone to development of dysplasia.
   i. Low-grade dysplasia is present in 5% to 10% of patients with Barrett esophagus.
   ii. Malignant degeneration from benign to dysplastic to malignant epithelium occurs in Barrett esophagus.
e. Adenocarcinomas above the normal GE junction are characteristic of malignant degeneration of Barrett esophagus.
   i. The risk of development of adenocarcinoma in Barrett esophagus is *50 to 100 times that of the general population*; yet adenocarcinoma is still a rare event in a Barrett patient.
   ii. Approximately 0.12% to 0.43% per year will progress from Barrett to adenocarcinoma.[14]

6. **Treatment (Figure 13.2)**
   a. Uncomplicated Barrett esophagus in asymptomatic patients requires endoscopic surveillance and biopsy annually or even less frequently *in the absence of dysplasia.*
   b. Uncomplicated Barrett esophagus in symptomatic patients should be managed as in patients with GERD, and they should have periodic endoscopic surveillance with four-quadrant biopsies.
   c. Elimination of reflux with an antireflux procedure may halt progression of the disease, heal ulceration, and prevent stricture formation but will not reverse the columnar metaplasia of Barrett.
      i. Patients who undergo antireflux disease still require surveillance.
   d. Barrett ulcers
      i. Frequently, 8 weeks of treatment with a PPI are necessary to achieve complete healing.
      ii. Ulcers that fail to heal or recur despite 4 months of medical therapy are an indication for rebiopsy and antireflux surgery.
   e. Barrett-associated strictures
      i. Managed with periodic esophageal dilation combined with medical management.
      ii. Recurrent or persistent strictures warrant an antireflux operation combined.
      iii. Rarely, strictures unable to be dilated require resection.

7. **Dysplasia**
   a. Low-grade dysplasia requires frequent (every 3-6 months) surveillance esophagoscopy and biopsy.
      i. Medical therapy for GERD is recommended in these patients, even when asymptomatic.
   b. High-grade dysplasia is pathologically indistinguishable from carcinoma in situ and until recently was an indication for esophagectomy.
      i. Esophageal-sparing options are increasingly utilized such as endoscopic mucosal resection and radiofrequency ablation.
      ii. Resection via esophagectomy is reserved for failure of these less-invasive approaches.
   c. Adenocarcinoma in patients with Barrett esophagus is an indication for esophagogastrectomy.

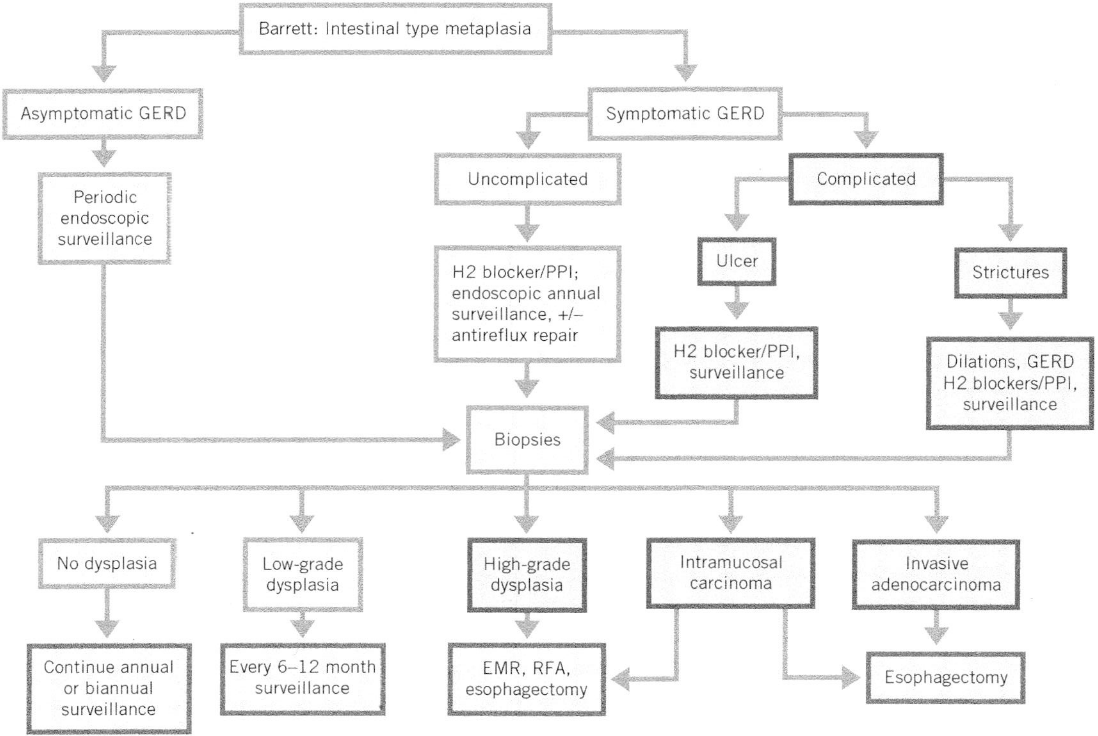

FIGURE 13.2 Algorithm for surveillance and management of Barrett esophagus. EMR, endoscopic mucosal resection; RFA, radiofrequency ablation.

i. Early detection offers the best opportunity to improve survival after resection, which is 20% at 5 years for all patients with cancer but far higher in those detected by surveillance and screening.

B. Benign esophageal neoplasms

1. Benign esophageal neoplasms are rare: The most common lesions are mesenchymal tumors (leiomyomas and some GI stromal tumors) and polyps.
2. Clinical features depend primarily on the location of the tumor within the esophagus.
   a. Intraluminal tumors, like polyps, cause esophageal obstruction, and patients present with dysphagia, vomiting, and aspiration.
   b. Intramural tumors, like leiomyomas, are typically asymptomatic but can produce dysphagia or chest pain if large.
3. Diagnosis usually involves a combination of barium swallow, esophagoscopy, and perhaps CT scanning or magnetic resonance scan studies.
4. Treatment of all symptomatic or enlarging tumors is surgical removal.
   a. Intraluminal tumors can usually be removed endoscopically.
   b. Intramural tumors usually can be enucleated from the esophageal muscular wall without entering the mucosa.

C. Esophageal carcinoma

1. **Epidemiology**
   a. Adenocarcinoma and squamous cell carcinoma of the esophagus represent 1% of all cancers in the US.
   b. It is more common in men (4:1) and most frequently diagnosed between **ages 65 and 74 years.**
2. **Risk factors**
   a. Squamous cell carcinoma: African American race; alcohol and cigarette use; achalasia; caustic esophageal injury; and geographic locations of China, South Africa, France, and Japan
   b. Adenocarcinoma: White race, GERD, Barrett esophagus, obesity, and cigarette smoking
3. **Pathology**
   a. Squamous cell carcinoma is multicentric and most frequently involves the middle third of the esophagus.
   b. Adenocarcinoma constitutes the majority of malignant esophageal tumors in the US.
      i. It typically exhibits extensive proximal and distal submucosal invasion, is not often multicentric, and commonly involves the distal esophagus.
   c. Less common malignant esophageal tumors include small-cell carcinoma, melanoma, leiomyosarcoma, lymphoma, and esophageal involvement by metastatic cancer.
4. **Symptoms**
   a. Most patients with early-stage disease are asymptomatic or may have symptoms of reflux, dysphagia, odynophagia, and weight loss.
   b. Hoarseness, abdominal pain, persistent bone pain, hiccups, and respiratory symptoms may indicate a more advanced stage.

c. Approximately 50% of presenting patients have unresectable primary tumors or distant metastasis at the time of diagnosis.

5. **Diagnosis**
   a. Barium swallow or CT with IV and PO contrast demonstrating esophageal mass or stricture and confirmed with esophagoscopy and biopsy.
6. **Staging**
   a. Esophageal adenocarcinoma and squamous cell carcinoma are staged differently; squamous cell carcinoma has the additional variable of anatomical location.
   b. Evaluation for lymph node and distant-organ metastatic disease is performed by positron emission tomography (PET)-CT.
   c. Endoscopic ultrasonography is most accurate for determining the depth of wall invasion and the involvement of peritumoral lymph nodes in patients without evidence of M1 disease on PET-CT.
   d. Lesions above the carina in M0 disease require bronchoscopy to evaluate the airway for involvement.
7. **Treatment**
   a. Surgical resection remains a mainstay of curative treatment of patients with localized disease.
   b. Total esophagectomy with a cervical esophagogastric anastomosis and subtotal resection with a high intrathoracic anastomosis have become the most common resections and produce the best long-term functional results as well as the best chance for cure. Options for esophageal replacement include the stomach, colon, and jejunum.
8. **Complications of esophagectomy**
   a. Aspiration pneumonia, anastomotic leak, and atrial fibrillation.
   b. Respiratory complications, including pneumonia, can be reduced by using retrograde drainage of the conduit (retrograde tube gastrostomy), instead of a nasogastric tube.[15]
   c. Management of an anastomotic leak is based on the size of the leak, the location of the anastomosis, and the clinical status of the patient.
      i. Cervical anastomotic leaks can usually be managed by opening the incision to allow drainage. Occasionally, the leak tracks below the thoracic inlet into the mediastinum, necessitating evaluation of ischemic injury to the stomach and wider debridement and drainage.
      ii. Intrathoracic anastomotic leaks are associated with a high mortality rate, and large or poorly drained leaks require operative exploration.
9. **Adjuvant therapy**
   a. Preoperative chemotherapy or chemoradiotherapy may enhance local control and resectability.
      i. For localized squamous carcinoma of the thoracic esophagus, preoperative chemoradiation followed by resection is the preferred approach.[16]
      ii. Optimal treatment of squamous cell esophageal cancers remains controversial with the current literature suggesting that chemoradiotherapy may be a definitive therapy option rather than only an adjuvant for surgically fit patients.[17]

iii. For patients with adenocarcinoma who undergo neoadjuvant chemoradiation and esophageal resection or for patients with GE junction cancers, nivolumab is recommended as adjuvant chemotherapy.[18]

b. Patients with dysphagia and or severe malnutrition may require feeding tube placement to optimize nutrition during neoadjuvant therapy.

c. Radiotherapy is used worldwide for attempted cure and palliation of patients with squamous cell esophageal cancer deemed unsuitable for resection. The 5-year survival rate is 5% to 10%.
   i. Palliative treatment is used to relieve obstruction and mitigate dysphagia.
   ii. Radiotherapy and chemotherapy work best in patients with squamous cell carcinoma above the carina. Adenocarcinoma is less responsive to radiation.

d. Intraluminal prostheses intubate the esophagus and stent the obstruction.
   i. Potential complications include perforation, erosion, or migration of the stent and obstruction of the tube.

e. Endoscopic laser techniques (photodynamic therapy) can restore an esophageal lumen successfully 90% of the time, with only a 4% to 5% perforation rate.

Key References

Citation	Summary
van Hagen P, Hulshof MC, van Lanschot JJ, et al. Preoperative chemoradiotherapy for esophageal or junctional cancer. *N Engl J Med.* 2012;366(22):2074-2084.	• Randomized control trial comparing outcomes for patients with resectable esophageal cancer receiving surgery alone or neoadjuvant chemoradiotherapy followed by surgery. Preoperative chemoradiotherapy improved survival among patients with potentially curable esophageal or esophagogastric junction cancer.
Kelly RJ, Ajani JA, Kuzdzal J, et al. Adjuvant nivolumab in resected esophageal or gastroesophageal junction cancer [published correction appears in *N Engl J Med.* 2023;388(7):672]. *N Engl J Med.* 2021;384(13):1191-1203.	• Randomized control trial survival for resected esophageal or GE junction cancer who had received neoadjuvant chemoradiotherapy and had residual pathological disease to receive adjuvant nivolumab or placebo. For patients with adenocarcinoma who underwent neoadjuvant chemoradiation and resection of esophageal or GE junction cancers, nivolumab is recommended as adjuvant chemotherapy for 1 y as disease-free survival was significantly longer for those who received adjuvant nivolumab.

CHAPTER 13: ESOPHAGUS

Review Questions

1. Which type of hiatal hernia does not need to be repaired?
2. During a hiatal hernia repair after extensive mediastinal dissection, how can more esophageal length be created if needed?
3. Which procedure reduces the incidence of postoperative dysphagia in patients with GERD who also have abnormal esophageal motility?
4. Which is the most common symptom of achalasia?
5. Which esophageal motility disorder has manometry with prolonged high-amplitude peristaltic waves and chest pain?
6. How is esophageal leiomyoma in the esophageal muscular wall surgically removed?
7. How do you rule out malignancy on preoperative workup for dysphagia?

REFERENCES

1. Petersen H, Johannessen T, Sandvik AK, et al. Relationship between endoscopic hiatus hernia and gastroesophageal reflux symptoms. *Scand J Gastroenterol.* 1991;26(9):921-926.
2. Gerull WD, Cho D, Kuo I, Arefanian S, Kushner BS, Awad MM. Robotic approach to paraesophageal hernia repair results in low long-term recurrence rate and beneficial patient-centered outcomes. *J Am Coll Surg.* 2020;231(5):520-526.
3. Tam V, Winger DG, Nason KS. A systematic review and meta-analysis of mesh vs suture cruroplasty in laparoscopic large hiatal hernia repair. *Am J Surg.* 2016;211(1):226-238.
4. Hoang CD, Koh PS, Maddaus MA. Short esophagus and esophageal stricture. *Surg Clin North Am.* 2005;85(3):433-451.
5. El-Serag HB, Sweet S, Winchester CC, Dent J. Update on the epidemiology of gastro-oesophageal reflux disease: a systematic review. *Gut.* 2014;63(6):871-880.
6. Zaninotto G, DeMeester TR, Schwizer W, Johansson KE, Cheng SC. The lower esophageal sphincter in health and disease. *Am J Surg.* 1988;155(1):104-111.
7. Amer MA, Smith MD, Khoo CH, Herbison GP, McCall JL. Network meta-analysis of surgical management of gastro-oesophageal reflux disease in adults. *Br J Surg.* 2018;105(11):1398-1407.
8. Mattioli S, Ruffato A, Lugaresi M, Pilotti V, Aramini B, D'Ovidio F. Long-term results of the Heller-Dor operation with intraoperative manometry for the treatment of esophageal achalasia. *J Thorac Cardiovasc Surg.* 2010;140(5):962-969.
9. Elakkary E, Duffy A, Roberts K, Bell R. Recent advances in the surgical treatment of achalasia and gastroesophageal reflux disease. *J Clin Gastroenterol.* 2008;42(5):603-609.
10. Dirks RC, Kohn GP, Slater B, et al. Is peroral endoscopic myotomy (POEM) more effective than pneumatic dilation and Heller myotomy? A systematic review and meta-analysis. *Surg Endosc.* 2021;35(5):1949-1962.
11. Roman S, Kahrilas PJ. Management of spastic disorders of the esophagus. *Gastroenterol Clin North Am.* 2013;42(1):27-43.
12. Dasari BV, Neely D, Kennedy A, et al. The role of esophageal stents in the management of esophageal anastomotic leaks and benign esophageal perforations. *Ann Surg.* 2014;259(5):852-860.
13. Skinner DB, Walther BC, Riddell RH, Schmidt H, Iascone C, DeMeester TR. Barrett's esophagus. Comparison of benign and malignant cases. *Ann Surg.* 1983;198(4):554-565.

14. Falk GW. Barrett's oesophagus: frequency and prediction of dysplasia and cancer. *Best Pract Res Clin Gastroenterol.* 2015;29(1):125-138.

15. Puri V, Hu Y, Guthrie T, et al. Retrograde jejunogastric decompression after esophagectomy is superior to nasogastric drainage. *Ann Thorac Surg.* 2011;92(2):499-503.

16. Ajani JA, D'Amico TA, Almhanna K, et al. Esophageal and esophagogastric junction cancers, version 1.2015. *J Natl Compr Canc Netw.* 2015;13(2):194-227.

17. Chen CY, Li CC, Chien CR. Neoadjuvant vs definitive concurrent chemoradiotherapy in locally advanced esophageal squamous cell carcinoma patients. *World J Surg Oncol.* 2018;16(1):141.

18. Tanzawa S, Makiguchi T, Tasaka S, et al. Prospective analysis of factors precluding the initiation of durvalumab from an interim analysis of a phase II trial of S-1 and cisplatin with concurrent thoracic radiotherapy followed by durvalumab for unresectable, locally advanced non-small cell lung cancer in Japan (SAMURAI study). *Ther Adv Med Oncol.* 2022;14:17588359221116603.

19. van Hagen P, Hulshof MC, van Lanschot JJ, et al. Preoperative chemoradiotherapy for esophageal or junctional cancer. *N Engl J Med.* 2012;366(22):2074-2084.

20. Adjuvant nivolumab in resected esophageal or gastroesophageal junction cancer. *N Engl J Med.* 2023;388(7):672.

14 Stomach

Alston James and William Hawkins

I. INTRODUCTION

A. Anatomy

1. Derived from embryonic foregut
2. Divisions of the stomach (**Figure 14.1**)[1]
   a. Most proximal region—cardia, immediately distal to lower esophageal sphincter
   b. Fundus is the superior aspect and is floppy and distensible.
   c. Angle of His (formed by the fundus and the left margin of the abdominal esophagus) plays an important role as an anatomical sphincter to prevent reflux.
   d. The right border of the stomach body is the lesser curvature, left border is greater curvature.
   e. Sharp right angle of lesser curvature marks the angularis incisura, at which point the body ends and the antrum (distal stomach) begins.
   f. Pylorus connects the distal stomach (antrum) to the duodenum.
3. Blood supply
   a. Majority derived from celiac artery—(**Figure 14.2**)[2]
      i. Left and right gastric arteries
      ii. Left and right gastroepiploic arteries
      iii. About 15% to 20% of patients have aberrant left hepatic artery arising from left gastric artery—proximal ligation of left gastric artery can result in acute left-sided hepatic ischemia.
   b. Extensive anastomotic connections exist between these major vessels.
      i. Typically stomach perfusion is not compromised if at least one is intact, assuming arcades are intact.
   c. Venous anatomy mirrors arterial—the right and left gastric veins drain into the portal vein while the right gastroepiploic vein drains into the superior mesenteric vein and the left gastroepiploic vein drains into the splenic vein.

B. Physiology

1. Primary function is to prepare ingested food for digestion and absorption.
2. While fasting → peristalsis occurs via the migrating myoelectric complex (MMC); one cycle is 90 to 120 minutes, ensuring frequent clearance of gastric contents during fasting.
3. During meals → stomach stores food through receptive relaxation of proximal stomach.
4. Liquids: Pass easily from stomach to duodenum along the lesser curve

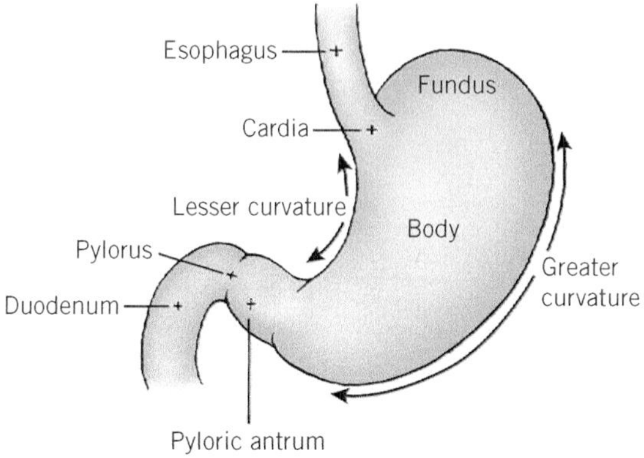

FIGURE 14.1 Gastric anatomy.

5. Solids: Actively propelled through pylorus by the antrum; pumps against closed pylorus to create thoroughly mixed meal prior to passage through pylorus
6. Acid production
   a. Chief responsibility of parietal cell via the H^+/K^+ adenosine triphosphatase (ATPase) acid-secreting pump
   b. Acid production is **positively influenced** by three stimuli:
      i. **Acetylcholine** (neurotransmitter used by vagus nerve and parasympathetic ganglion)—stimulates parietal cells directly as well as indirectly by stimulating G-cells (gastrin) and Enterochromaffin-like (ECL) cells (histamine)
      ii. **Gastrin**—produced by G-cells in the gastric antrum; has direct effects on parietal cell and indirect effects via ECL cells (histamine)
      iii. **Histamine**—released by ECL cells
   c. **Histamine** stimulates acid production in parietal cell by increasing **intracellular cAMP** and directly activating the ATPase; whereas **Gastrin** and **Acetylcholine** stimulate **phospholipase C**, increasing intracellular calcium and indirectly activating the ATPase.
   d. Acid production is negatively influenced by **somatostatin**, made by D-cells.
   e. Three phases of acid secretory response—**cephalic** (anticipation of food), **gastric** (food enters the stomach—accounts for majority of acid production), and **intestinal** (food enters the proximal small bowel)
   f. Critical line of immunologic defense, preventing colonization of the upper gastrointestinal (GI) tract with bacteria
7. Plays small role initiating enzymatic digestion, the majority of which continues in small bowel

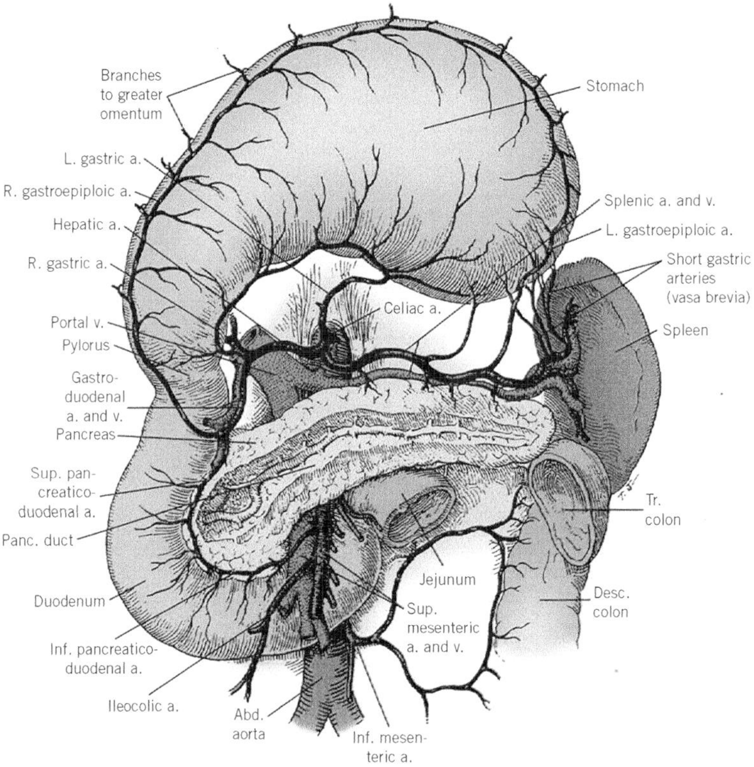

FIGURE 14.2 Gastric blood supply.

a. Starches are broken down by salivary **amylase**.
b. **Pepsin** initiates protein digestion (converted from pepsinogen to pepsin by gastric acid).

8. Regulation
   a. Neural (sympathetic and parasympathetic)
      i. Parasympathetic (vagus nerves)
         a) Branches of the vagus coalesce into the right and left vagus nerve just above esophageal hiatus.
         b) At the gastroesophageal junction, the left vagus is anterior and the right vagus is posterior.
         c) Left vagus—gives branches to the liver and continues along lesser curvature as the nerve of Latarjet
         d) Right vagus—gives branches to stomach, first branch is "criminal nerve of Grassi," which if left undivided can be responsible for recurrent peptic ulcer disease (PUD)

e) Ninety percent of vagal nerve fibers are afferent.
f) Ten percent are efferent—influencing gastric motor function and gastric secretion.
g) Receptive relaxation mediated by vagus nerve

ii. Sympathetic (celiac plexus) and intrinsic nervous system (Auerbach and Meissner autonomic plexuses)
a) Incompletely understood
b) Myogenic control—excitatory membranes of gastric smooth muscle cells

b. Hormonal
i. Ghrelin
a) Produced by endocrine cells in the stomach, increases gastric emptying and motility, and increases gastric acid secretion

C. Histology

1. Outer to inner: Serosa → muscularis propria → **submucosa** → mucosa
2. Submucosa → collagen-rich layer of connective tissue—**strongest layer of the gastric wall**
3. Gastric mucosa → simple columnar epithelia interrupted by gastric pits containing one or more gastric glands (cellular composition of the glands varies by location)
4. Cells that control digestion
   a. Parietal cells—predominantly in the body of stomach, responsible for acid production
   b. Chief cells—secrete pepsinogen
   c. Mucus-secreting cells
5. Cells that control function
   a. G-cells (gastrin)—predominantly in the antrum
   b. D-cells (somatostatin)—generally slows digestion

II. FUNCTIONAL DISORDERS OF THE STOMACH

A. Gastroparesis

1. **Epidemiology/etiology/classification**
   a. Gastroparesis—delayed gastric emptying in the absence of mechanical gastric outlet obstruction
   b. Owing to loss of antral pump function, gastroparesis predominantly affects solid food transit in stomach

i. **The most common etiology is idiopathic** (50%)

ii. *Medical* causes: Diabetes mellitus, viral infection (cytomegalovirus or Epstein–Barr virus [EBV]), neurologic disease (multiple sclerosis, cerebrovascular accident, Parkinson's), medications such as tricyclic antidepressants, calcium channel blockers, and cyclosporine

iii. *Surgical* causes: Related to intentional or accidental vagotomy—resulting in the loss of the receptive relaxation and gastric accommodation in response to meal ingestion (accelerated emptying of liquids, delayed emptying of solids)

iv. In addition, delayed gastric emptying is common following some surgeries like a Whipple (pancreaticoduodenectomy), 10% to 40% incidence.

2. **Presentation/symptoms**
   a. Symptoms of abnormal gastric motility are nausea, emesis, postprandial fullness, early satiety, abdominal pain, bloating.
3. **Diagnosis/testing**
   a. **Imaging**—the principal goal is to rule out mechanical obstruction
      i. Esophagogastroduodenoscopy (EGD)
      ii. Upper GI
      iii. Gastric-emptying study (once mechanical obstruction is ruled out)
         a) Radionucleotide scan—using meal of radiolabeled food
            1) Scans are performed immediately after food is ingested and at 1, 2, and 4 hours after the meal, and percentage of meal retained in the stomach at 4 hours is calculated.
            2) Retention of >10% of food at 4 hours is considered abnormal.
4. **Nonoperative treatment**
   a. First line—regardless of cause → dietary modification
      i. Small, frequent meals
      ii. More liquid than solid
      iii. Low fat, low fiber
      iv. Stop meds that slow gastric emptying (opioids, CCBs, TCAs, and dopamine agonists)
      v. Optimize glycemic control in diabetic patients
   b. Pharmacologic therapy
      i. Metoclopramide (Reglan)
         a) Dopamine 2 receptor antagonist that stimulates antral contractions and decreases postprandial relaxation of the fundus
      ii. Macrolide antibiotics (erythromycin and azithromycin)
         a) Stimulate fundal contraction via MMC
5. **Operative treatment**
   a. Rarely required, only indicated in refractory symptoms despite maximal medical therapy
   b. Palliative options: Surgical venting gastrostomy, jejunostomy for nutrition
   c. Therapeutic options
      i. Pyloromyotomy/pyloroplasty—lower outflow resistance
      ii. Surgical implantation of gastric electrostimulators for refractory idiopathic and diabetic gastroparesis
         a) Leads placed in antrum laparoscopically and connected to subcutaneously placed stimulator
      iii. Gastric peroral endoscopic myotomy
      iv. Surgical approach: Gastrostomy
         a) The patient is positioned supine on the table with arms extended.
         b) An upper midline incision exposes the stomach.
         c) The optimal location of the gastrostomy on the anterior surface of the mid-stomach is identified.
         d) Using 3-0 PDS, sew two purse-string sutures in concentric circles with inner diameter of approximately 1 and 2 cm, respectively.

e) Identify the location on the abdominal wall for tube exit site through the middle of the rectus muscle in the left upper quadrant and at least 2 fingerbreadths below the left costal margin. A tract is created here and the tube is passed into the abdominal cavity.

f) If fixation is desired, place four separate stitches through the seromuscular layer of stomach and the peritoneum of the abdominal wall, surrounding the point where the tube exits the abdominal wall.

g) Create a small gastrotomy in the center of the concentric circles and pass the tube into the stomach.

h) Tie the two purse-string sutures (inner one first) around the catheter.

i) Close abdomen in standard fashion, suture the tube to the skin in two places with a nylon suture to prevent dislodgement.

III. GASTRIC ADENOCARCINOMA

A. Epidemiology/etiology

1. More common worldwide than in the US (5th vs. 14th)
2. In the US, only 25% of patients present with localized disease.
3. Overall 5-year survival rate in the US is poor (28%)[3]
4. Risk factors
   - **a.** *H. pylori* infection (especially **cytotoxin-associated gene A–positive** strains)
   - **b.** More common and higher mortality in African Americans, Asian Americans, and Hispanics compared with white patients
   - **c.** Male gender
   - **d.** Family history
   - **e.** Low socioeconomic status
   - **f.** Diets high in nitrates, salted/pickled foods
   - **g.** Hereditary diffuse gastric cancer (*CDH1* mutation)
   - **h.** Smoking
5. Ninety-five percent of cancers are adenocarcinomas, arising from mucus-producing cells in gastric mucosa.

B. Classification

1. The **Lauren Classification** system is the most widely used and divides gastric cancers into two subtypes:
   - **a. Intestinal-type cancers** are glandular and arise from the gastric mucosa.
     - **i.** More common in elderly men and in the distal stomach
     - **ii.** Are associated with *H. pylori* and other environmental exposures that lead to chronic gastritis, intestinal metaplasia, and dysplasia
     - **iii.** Hematogenous metastatic spread to distant organs is seen.
   - **b. Diffuse-types of cancers** arise from the lamina propria and are associated with an invasive growth pattern with rapid submucosal spread of signet ring cells.

i. They occur more commonly in association with inherited syndromes, as well as in younger patients, females, and the proximal stomach.
ii. Transmural and lymphatic spread is common, with early metastases.
iii. Prognosis is poorer.

2. As part of The Cancer Genome Atlas project an updated classification schema was created.[4]
   a. **Microsatellite unstable** (**MSI-H**, 20%) characterized by mismatch repair gene MLH1 silencing, leading to a high mutation rate
   b. **EBV–positive** (10%) tumors seen more often in male patients, often in the stomach fundus or body. Tumors often overexpress PD-L1.
   c. **Chromosomally unstable** (50%) tumors characterized by intestinal histology, with high somatic copy number variation, and p53 and RAS mutations
   d. **Genomically stable** (20%) tumors have low somatic copy number variation. Often have CDH1 mutations and diffuse histology.
3. **Presentation**
   a. Vague, nonspecific, epigastric abdominal pain
   b. Weight loss
   c. Nausea/vomiting
   d. Anorexia/fatigue
   e. Dysphagia → Proximal tumors
   f. Gastric outlet obstruction → Distal tumors
4. **Diagnosis/testing**
   a. **Imaging/invasive testing**
      i. Diagnosis most commonly made via EGD
      ii. Screening not common in the US
   b. **Staging**
      i. **CT scan of chest/abdomen/pelvis** with oral and IV contrast is the best initial test for detecting locoregional and metastatic disease.
      ii. **Positron emission tomography (PET)/CT** can detect nodal and distant metastatic disease not apparent on CT alone (only 50% of gastric adenocarcinomas are PET avid).
      iii. **Endoscopic ultrasound (EUS)** is indicated for further staging in patients with locoregional disease and delineates depth of tumor invasion in the gastric wall and adjacent structures.
         a) EUS is a good predictor of advanced (T3/4 or >N0) disease, with a positive predictive value for advanced disease of 76% and a negative predictive value for low-risk disease (T1-2, N0) of 91%.[5]
      iv. **Laparoscopic staging** can detect occult distant metastases in 31% of patients.[6]
         a) Peritoneal washings with cytology should be performed for clinical stage $T3^{+}$ or N^{+} patients.
5. **Treatment**
   a. **Curative intent**
      i. Often relies on combination of surgery and chemotherapy for local/locoregional disease

ii. **Surgical therapy** necessitates complete resection with negative microscopic margins (>4 cm).
   a) **Proximal tumors** (nearly half of all cancers) require total gastrectomy or proximal subtotal gastrectomy. Total gastrectomy with Roux-en-Y esophagojejunostomy is preferred to avoid reflux esophagitis and impaired gastric emptying.
   b) **Surgical approach: Gastrectomy—partial**
      1) The patient is positioned supine with arms extended. Abdomen is entered through an upper midline incision.
      2) If performing for cancer, liver and peritoneum are inspected for the presence of metastatic disease before proceeding.
      3) Mobilize the greater curvature of the stomach, separate greater omentum from transverse colon, and divide the short gastrics to the level of planned gastric resection.
      4) Mobilize the hepatic flexure of the colon and complete the separation of the greater omentum from transverse mesocolon. Identify the gastrocolic trunk and divide the right gastroepiploic vein.
      5) Divide the lesser omentum as close to the liver as possible, taking care to avoid injury of a replaced or accessory left hepatic artery. Circumferentially dissect 2 to 3 cm distal to pylorus and divide with a stapler.
      6) Transect the stomach with the stapler approximately 4 to 6 cm proximal to the level of the lesion.
      7) If performing for cancer, divide the gastric arteries at their origin and take associated nodal packets including the right gastric artery, the right gastroepiploic artery, and left gastric arteries.
      8) Reconstruction with a retrocolic Roux-en-Y gastrojejunostomy is performed, using a Roux limb of at least 40 cm.
   c) **Midbody tumors** (comprise 15%-30%) generally require total gastrectomy.
   d) **Distal tumors** are approached by subtotal gastrectomy, which has a similar outcome but decreased complications vs. total gastrectomy.[7]
   e) **Early gastric cancers** confined to the mucosa (T1a) that are <2 cm and have clear margins with no lymph node involvement and are well to moderately differentiated on pathology have limited propensity and may be treated by **endoscopic mucosal resection.**[8]
   f) **Laparoscopic gastric resections** have advantages of reduced pain, shorter hospitalization, and improved quality of life.[9]

iii. **Lymphadenectomy** entails removal of ≥15 nodes, with a *D2 lymphadenectomy* being preferred in the Western hemisphere and conferring improved survival over *D1 dissection.*[10,11]

a) A D2 lymphadenectomy includes a D1 dissection (perigastric nodes) + celiac, left gastric, common hepatic, and splenic artery lymph nodes.

iv. **Systemic therapy**

a) Critical as the majority of patients with locoregional disease are at high risk for local or systemic recurrence following curative surgery.

b) **Perioperative systemic chemotherapy** improves overall and disease-free survival rates in patients with resected gastric cancer treated with epirubicin/cisplatin/5-fluorouracil (ECF) chemotherapy.

1) In the MAGIC trial, perioperative ECF therapy, consisting of three cycles of **neoadjuvant** and three cycles of **adjuvant** chemotherapy, led to 36% vs. 23% 5-year survival in resected gastric cancer.[12]

2) Potential benefits of delivering chemotherapy in the **neoadjuvant** setting include increased tumor downstaging and R0 resection rate, as well as the ability to guide therapeutic response and prognosis.[13]

3) Alternatively, **adjuvant chemoradiotherapy** can be given alone with good results.[14]

c) New avenues of treatment for patients who present with **advanced/metastatic disease**

1) For patients with tumors overexpressing HER2 (20%), trastuzumab can be given with chemotherapy and improve survival for advanced disease by nearly 3 months.[15]

2) In a recent phase II trial of anti-PD-1 therapy for metastatic gastric cancer, in a small number of patients with EBV^+ and MSI-H tumors, 100% and 86% of EBV^+ and MSI-H patients, respectively, responded to therapy, two of which achieved complete response.[16]

v. **Palliation**

a) Important role due to overall low historic cure rates from systemic therapy. Patients with peritoneal disease, hepatic or nodal metastases, or other poor prognostic factors benefit most from endoscopic palliation.

IV. UPPER GI BLEEDING

A. Epidemiology/etiology/classification

1. More common in men than in women and increases with age
2. Differential is broad—peptic ulcer disease, esophagitis, gastritis/duodenitis, portal hypertension (varices and portal hypertensive gastropathy).
3. Less common causes include vascular lesions (angiodysplasia), traumatic lesions (Mallory–Weiss, Cameron lesions, iatrogenic), upper GI tumors, and hemobilia.

4. Historically, >50% of upper GI bleeding were secondary to peptic ulcer disease; however, in recent decades this is likely an overestimation (now closer to 20%-25%).[17-19]

B. Presentation/symptoms
1. Commonly presents with hematemesis and/or melena, hematochezia only in severe cases
2. Epigastric pain or anorexia, especially if bleeding related to an ulcer

C. Diagnosis/testing
1. **Laboratory studies**
   a. Complete blood count, basic metabolic panel, liver function tests, blood type and crossmatch coagulation studies
   b. Note that, with extreme hemorrhage, the initial hemoglobin may not reflect the true nature of blood loss; over time, hemoglobin levels will drop as blood becomes increasingly diluted.
   c. Elevated blood urea nitrogen to creatinine ratio or urea to creatinine ratio is also indicative of acute upper GI bleed.
      i. Values of >30:1 or >100:1, respectively, suggest upper GI bleed as the cause.
2. **Imaging**—upper endoscopy is the diagnostic modality of choice for acute upper GI bleeding.
   a. High sensitivity and specificity for locating and identifying bleeding in the upper GI tract
   b. *Modified Forrest Classification* stratifies risk of rebleeding based on observed ulcer characteristics on endoscopy:
      i. Class Ia—spurting hemorrhage
      ii. Class Ib—oozing hemorrhage
      iii. Class IIa—nonbleeding visible vessel
      iv. Class IIb—adherent clot
      v. Class IIc—flat pigmented spot
      vi. Class III—clean ulcer base

D. Nonoperative treatment
1. Initial approach standard for hypovolemic blood loss:
   a. Large-bore IV access ×2
   b. Resuscitation with fluid and blood products
   c. Close monitoring of vital signs
2. Early initiation of IV proton-pump inhibitor (PPI)
3. Early upper flexible endoscopy, ideally within 24 hours
4. If high risk on endoscopy (class I or IIa,b), treatment is required—thermal coagulation, hemoclips, or sclerosant injection.
   a. Epinephrine injection can be used as an adjunct but no longer recommended as monotherapy.
5. Routine repeat endoscopy is not recommended if no continued signs of bleeding.
6. Second episode of rebleeding after initially successful endoscopy is treated with repeat endoscopy.
7. If GI bleed is felt to be secondary to portal hypertension, portal decompression with transjugular intrahepatic portosystemic shunt can be considered.

E. Operative treatment
1. Rarely indicated, but can be effective for 5% to 10% of patients with endoscopically refractory bleeding or for patients who are hemodynamically unstable
   a. The most common etiology is bleeding from gastroduodenal artery (GDA) from ulcer in the posterior wall of duodenum.
   b. Can be approached laparoscopically or open
      i. Kocherize duodenum, open the duodenal bulb, and oversew GDA with three-point U stitch technique—ligating the main vessel and preventing back bleeding from side branches.

V. GASTROINTESTINAL STROMAL TUMORS—BASICS

A. Epidemiology/etiology/classification
1. The most common sarcomatous tumor of the GI tract
   a. The most common GI tract location is the stomach (60%).
2. Vast majority arise from **intestinal pacemaker cells—so-called interstitial cells of Cajal.**
3. Most patients are >50 year old with a slight male predominance.
4. Frequently display prominent extraluminal growth and can get very large before becoming symptomatic

B. Presentation/symptoms
1. Often asymptomatic and found incidentally
2. Can present with vague abdominal pain secondary to mass effect and hemorrhage
3. If large enough, can cause symptoms of gastric outlet obstruction

C. Diagnosis/testing
1. **Imaging/invasive testing**
   a. EGD/EUS demonstrates a round, smooth **submucosal** tumor.
   b. Biopsy (if performed) shows spindle cell or epithelioid appearance and stains positive for CD117, CD34, and PDGFRA.
2. **Staging**
   a. According to tumor size and histologic frequency of mitoses (low grade <5 mitoses/5 mm^2)
   b. Staging accomplished by CT abdomen/pelvis, with chest imaging reserved for larger (>2 cm)/high-grade lesions

D. Nonoperative treatment
1. For tumors **<2 cm with no high-risk EUS features,** regular surveillance can be considered.

E. Operative treatment
1. Open or laparoscopic surgical resection with **2-cm margins** of grossly normal gastric wall
2. En bloc resection of structures involved by local invasion should be attempted, **but lymphadenectomy is not indicated.**

F. Adjuvant therapy
1. Most gastrointestinal stromal tumors (GISTs) express the **c-kit** receptor (CD117), a tyrosine kinase that acts as a growth factor receptor.

a. **Imatinib** (**Gleevec**) is a small-molecule inhibitor of the c-kit receptor that is first-line therapy for metastatic or recurrent GIST and can also be used to downsize bulky disease prior to resection.

2. Imatinib should be given in the adjuvant setting for intermediate or high-risk disease: >5 cm tumor and/or >10 mitoses.[20,21]
3. Prior to imatinib therapy, tumors should be sent for *KIT* (CD117) and *PDGFRA* gene testing, whereby *KIT* exon 11 mutation predicts a 90% response rate to imatinib, *KIT* exon 9 mutation predicts a 50% response rate, PDGFRA mutation leads to variable response depending on exact mutation, and wild-type *KIT* and *PDGFRA* genes predict <50% response rate.[22]

G. Outcomes/complications

1. Local recurrence and metastasis via hematogenous spread are common and are frequently treated with imatinib or second-line tyrosine kinase inhibitor.

VI. PEPTIC ULCER DISEASE

A. Epidemiology

1. Lifetime worldwide prevalence 5% to 10%
2. Related to lifestyle and infectious causes
   a. *H. pylori*: Associated with 95% of duodenal and 75% of gastric ulcers
   b. NSAID use
   c. Cigarette smoking
   d. Acid hypersecretion (including due to gastrin-secreting tumors)
   e. Physiologic stress (hospitalized patient for life-threatening, nonbleeding illness), e.g., Cushing (central nervous system injury) and Curling (severe burn) ulcers
3. Incidence is declining in developed countries in recent decades likely due to increased detection and eradication of *H. pylori*, decreased NSAID use, and environmental factors.

B. Classification

1. Type 1: Located along the lesser curvature, normal/decreased acid secretion, along with *H. pylori* injection in majority (60%-70%)
2. Type 2: Body of stomach/incisura and duodenal, high acid secretion (15%)
3. Type 3: Prepyloric, associated with high acid secretion (20%)
4. Type 4: Proximal stomach/cardia, low mucosal protection, as well as normal or decreased acid secretion
5. Type 5: Anywhere in stomach, medication induced (often associated with NSAIDs and/or steroids)

C. Presentation

1. Most patients are asymptomatic.
2. Burning or gnawing epigastric pain
3. Duodenal ulcers—pain decreases with food intake.
4. Gastric ulcers—pain increases with food intake.
5. Complications include bleeding, gastric outlet obstruction, fistulization and perforation.

D. Diagnosis/testing
1. **Laboratory studies**
   a. Fasting serum gastrin levels should be obtained if concern for gastric hypersecretion.
   b. *H. pylori* infection testing can be performed by urea breath test, stool antigen testing, or serologic antibody testing.
2. **Imaging/invasive studies**
   a. EGD is the most sensitive and specific test and allows for concomitant biopsy.
   b. Endoscopic biopsy can be obtained to rule out malignancy as well as test for *H. pylori.*

E. Nonoperative treatment
1. *H. pylori* eradication
   a. Triple therapy: PPI + two antibiotics (often clarithromycin + amoxicillin or metronidazole) for 10 to 14 days
2. Antisecretory medicines
   a. PPIs, which prevent acid secretion by irreversibly binding and inhibiting the H^+/K^+ ATPase on the parietal cell
   b. H2 receptor antagonists prevent acid secretion by inhibiting the Histamine-2 (H2) receptor on parietal cells.
3. Smoking cessation promotes healing
4. Follow-up endoscopy for gastric ulcers given risk of malignancy

F. Operative treatment
1. Operative treatment is reserved for patients who fail medical management or present with complicated disease (bleeding, perforation, strictures).
2. Increasingly rare with improved recognition of *H. pylori* and antisecretory therapy
3. For ulcers associated with increased acid output, options include truncal vagotomy with drainage procedure, selective vagotomy with drainage, highly selective vagotomy.
4. Increasing selectivity of vagotomy is associated with increasing rates of recurrence but with lower associated rates of delayed gastric emptying.
5. **Surgical approach: Repair of Gastroduodenal perforation**
   a. The patient is positioned supine on the table with arms extended. The abdomen is entered in the upper midline and the liver is retracted.
   b. Cultures of the peritoneal fluid are sent for microbiology.
   c. Identify the location of the perforated ulcer:
      i. If duodenal, close the ulcer loosely with silk sutures, using the tails to fasten a tongue of omentum as a buttress (modified Graham patch).
      ii. If gastric, excise the ulcer completely, if possible, and send for pathology to exclude malignancy and test for *H. pylori.* An omental buttress may also be used to reinforce the staple line.
   d. Leak test may be performed either by endoscopic insufflation or instillation of methylene blue into the orogastric or nasogastric tube.

Key References

Citation	Summary
Joensuu H, Eriksson M, Sundby Hall K, et al. One vs three years of adjuvant imatinib for operable gastrointestinal stromal tumor: a randomized trial. *JAMA*. 2012;307(12):1265-1272.	• Randomized control trial studying the role of imatinib administration duration as adjuvant therapy for high-risk GIST. Trial results suggest that 36 mo of treatment compared with 12 improves recurrence-free survival.
Dematteo RP, Ballman KV, Antonescu CR, et al. Adjuvant imatinib mesylate after resection of localised, primary gastrointestinal stromal tumour: a randomised, double-blind, placebo-controlled trial [published correction appears in *Lancet*. 2009;374(9688):450]. *Lancet*. 2009;373(9669):1097-1104.	• Randomized control trial comparing 1 y of adjuvant imatinib to placebo following resection of GIST of at least 3 cm in size found that adjuvant imatinib therapy significantly improved recurrence-free survival.
Abdelfatah MM, Barakat M, Lee H, et al. The incidence of lymph node metastasis in early gastric cancer according to the expanded criteria in comparison with the absolute criteria of the Japanese Gastric Cancer Association: a systematic review of the literature and meta-analysis. *Gastrointest Endosc*. 2018;87(2):338-347.	• Review of patients who underwent gastrectomy and lymph node dissection for early gastric cancer found that, while lymph node metastasis for standard criteria patients was 0.2%, the rate for expanded criteria (undifferentiated mucosal lesions < 2 cm or differentiated lesions < 3 cm with slight submucosal invasion—T1b) patients was significantly higher.

CHAPTER 14: STOMACH

Review Questions

1. What are the four main sources of blood supply to the stomach?
2. Which ulcer location is more commonly associated with *H. pylori*, gastric or duodenal?
3. What is strongest layer of the gastric wall?
4. What is the most common etiology of gastroparesis?
5. Which ulcer location is more commonly associated with malignancy, gastric or duodenal?
6. How many lymph nodes are recommended when performing surgery to remove a GIST?
7. What are the indications for adjuvant imatinib therapy following GIST resection?

REFERENCES

1. Yeo C. Shackelford's surgery of the alimentary tract. In: Wilson R, Stevenson C, eds. *Figure 563—Regions of the Stomach*. 8th ed. Elsevier; 2019:634-646.
2. Yeo C. Shackelford's surgery of the alimentary tract. In: Wilson R, Stevenson C, eds. *Figure 565—Vascular Supply of the Foregut*. 8th ed. Elsevier; 2019:634-648.
3. National Cancer Institute. *Surveillance, Epidemiology, and End Results Program*. https://seer.cancer.gov/statistics/
4. Cancer Genome Atlas Research Network. Comprehensive molecular characterization of gastric adenocarcinoma. *Nature*. 2014;513(7517):202-209.
5. Bentrem D, Gerdes H, Tang L, Brennan M, Coit D. Clinical correlation of endoscopic ultrasonography with pathologic stage and outcome in patients undergoing curative resection for gastric cancer. *Ann Surg Oncol*. 2007;14(6):1853-1859.
6. Sarela AI, Lefkowitz R, Brennan MF, Karpeh MS. Selection of patients with gastric adenocarcinoma for laparoscopic staging. *Am J Surg*. 2006;191(1):134-138.
7. Bozzetti F, Marubini E, Bonfanti G, Miceli R, Piano C, Gennari L. Subtotal versus total gastrectomy for gastric cancer: five-year survival rates in a multicenter randomized Italian trial. Italian Gastrointestinal Tumor Study Group. *Ann Surg*. 1999;230(2):170-178.
8. Han S, Hsu A, Wassef WY. An update in the endoscopic management of gastric cancer. *Curr Opin Gastroenterol*. 2016;32(6):492-500.
9. Kim HH, Han SU, Kim MC, et al. Long-term results of laparoscopic gastrectomy for gastric cancer: a large-scale case-control and case-matched Korean multicenter study. *J Clin Oncol*. 2014;32(7):627-633.
10. Bilimoria KY, Talamonti MS, Wayne JD, et al. Effect of hospital type and volume on lymph node evaluation for gastric and pancreatic cancer. *Arch Surg*. 2008;143(7):671-678; discussion 678.
11. Songun I, Putter H, Kranenbarg EM, Sasako M, van de Velde CJ. Surgical treatment of gastric cancer: 15-year follow-up results of the randomised nationwide Dutch D1D2 trial. *Lancet Oncol*. 2010;11(5):439-449.
12. Cunningham D, Allum WH, Stenning SP, et al. Perioperative chemotherapy versus surgery alone for resectable gastroesophageal cancer. *N Engl J Med*. 2006;355(1):11-20.
13. Newton AD, Datta J, Loaiza-Bonilla A, Karakousis GC, Roses RE. Neoadjuvant therapy for gastric cancer: current evidence and future directions. *J Gastrointest Oncol*. 2015;6(5):534-543.
14. Smalley SR, Benedetti JK, Haller DG, et al. Updated analysis of SWOG-directed intergroup study 0116: a phase III trial of adjuvant radiochemotherapy versus observation after curative gastric cancer resection. *J Clin Oncol*. 2012;30(19):2327-2333.
15. Bang YJ, Van Cutsem E, Feyereislova A, et al. Trastuzumab in combination with chemo therapy versus chemotherapy alone for treatment of HER2-positive advanced gastric or gastro-oesophageal junction cancer (ToGA): a phase 3, open-label, randomised controlled trial. *Lancet*. 2010;376(9742):687-697.
16. Wong GS, Zhou J, Liu JB, et al. Targeting wild-type KRAS-amplified gastroesophageal cancer through combined MEK and SHP2 inhibition. *Nat Med*. 2018;24(7):968-977.
17. Boonpongmanee S, Fleischer DE, Pezzullo JC, et al. The frequency of peptic ulcer as a cause of upper-GI bleeding is exaggerated. *Gastrointest Endosc*. 2004;59(7):788-794.

18. Enestvedt BK, Gralnek IM, Mattek N, Lieberman DA, Eisen G. An evaluation of endoscopic indications and findings related to nonvariceal upper-GI hemorrhage in a large multicenter consortium. *Gastrointest Endosc.* 2008;67(3):422-429.

19. Loperfido S, Baldo V, Piovesana E, et al. Changing trends in acute upper-GI bleeding: a population-based study. *Gastrointest Endosc.* 2009;70(2):212-224.

20. Dematteo RP, Ballman KV, Antonescu CR, et al. Adjuvant imatinib mesylate after resection of localised, primary gastrointestinal stromal tumour: a randomised, double-blind, placebo-controlled trial. *Lancet.* 2009;373(9669):1097-1104.

21. Joensuu H, Eriksson M, Sundby Hall K, et al. One vs three years of adjuvant imatinib for operable gastrointestinal stromal tumor: a randomized trial. *JAMA.* 2012;307(12):1265-1272.

22. (NCCN) NCCN. *NCCN Guidelines Version 2.2022 Gastrointestinal Stromal Tumors (GISTs).* 2022.

23. Abdelfatah MM, Barakat M, Lee H, et al. The incidence of lymph node metastasis in early gastric cancer according to the expanded criteria in comparison with the absolute criteria of the Japanese Gastric Cancer Association: a systematic review of the literature and meta-analysis. *Gastrointest Endosc.* 2018;87(2):338-347.

15 The Surgical Management of Obesity

Ina Chen and Francesca Dimou

I. OBESITY, MORBID OBESITY, AND METABOLIC SYNDROME

A. Definition
   1. Obesity is defined as a body mass index [BMI = weight (kg)/height (m^2)] ≥30 kg/m^2.
   2. See **Table 15.1** for obesity classification.
   3. Obesity is associated with several comorbidities. Patients in higher classes of obesity are at higher risk of obesity-related morbidity and mortality. See **Table 15.2** for examples of obesity-related comorbidities.

B. Epidemiology
   1. The etiology of morbid obesity is poorly understood with debate as to the role of genetic, psychosocial, and environmental factors.
   2. Obesity is a disease process that has drastically increased in prevalence over the past few decades. From 1999 to 2020, obesity prevalence in the US increased from 30.5% to 41.9%, reaching epidemic proportions. The prevalence of severe obesity increased from 4.7% to 9.2%.[1]
   3. Obesity impacts all health groups. Nearly one of five children and adolescents are obese.[2]

C. Treatment for obesity includes lifestyle modifications, pharmacotherapy, and endoscopic management. See **Table 15.3** for an overview of nonsurgical management of obesity.

D. For patients with severe obesity, surgery is the most effective treatment. See **Table 15.4** for the indications and contraindications of bariatric surgery.

E. Several clinical trials have described the health benefits of bariatric surgery for patients with severe obesity.
   1. The Swedish Obese Subjects (SOS) study is a long-term prospective interventional study comparing weight-loss surgery vs nonoperative management.[3-5]

TABLE 15.1 Obesity Classification

Body Mass Index	Classification
30 to <35	Class 1 obesity
35 to <40	Class 2 obesity
≥40	Class 3 obesity, or "severe" obesity

TABLE 15.2 Obesity-Related Comorbidities

Cardiac	Pulmonary
Hypertension Sudden cardiac death (myocardial infarction) Coronary artery disease Deep venous thrombosis Heart failure Venous stasis	Obesity hypoventilation syndrome Asthma Obstructive sleep apnea
Metabolic	**Musculoskeletal**
Type II diabetes Hyperlipidemia Hypercholesterolemia Nonalcoholic steatohepatitis	Degenerative joint disease Lumbar disc disease Osteoarthritis Ventral hernias
Gastrointestinal	**Genitourinary/Gynecologic**
Cholelithiasis Gastroesophageal reflux disease	Stress incontinence Polycystic ovarian syndrome Menstrual irregularities
Infectious	**Neurologic**
Fungal infections Necrotizing soft tissue infections	Pseudotumor cerebri Stroke

TABLE 15.3 Nonsurgical Management of Morbid Obesity

Lifestyle Modifications and/or Medical Therapy	Endoscopic Therapy
Self-guided or structured diet and exercise	Gastric balloon
GLP-1 agonists (liraglutide, semaglutide)	Endoscopic sleeve gastroplasty
Antidepressants (bupropion, topiramate)	
Phentermine	
Orlistat	

TABLE 15.4 Indications and Contraindications of Weight Loss Surgery

Indications	Contraindications
Failed medical weight loss	Untreated/uncontrolled severe psychiatric illness
BMI > 40	Active alcohol or drug abuse
BMI > 35 with obesity-related comorbidities	Prohibitive operative risks secondary to severe medical disease
	Inability to comprehend nature of surgical intervention or comply with required postoperative nutritional and lifestyle changes
	For women of child-bearing age—patients actively pregnant or intending to get pregnant within 12-18 mo postop

   a. Patient recruitment began in 1994, and of the recruited patients, 2,010 elected to have operation who were then compared with a matched group of 2,037 control patients (baseline BMI of each group was 41.8 and 40.9 kg/m^2, respectively).
   b. Surgical interventions for the 2,010 patients were gastric bypass (13%), gastric banding (19%), and vertical banded gastroplasty (68%).
   c. Data after 10 and 20 years of follow-up showed that patients treated with bariatric surgery benefited from greater weight loss vs controls.
      i. Surgical patients also had higher rates of diabetes mellitus (DM) remission.
      ii. Most importantly, surgery was demonstrated to be associated with reduction in overall mortality compared with nonoperative management.
   d. Criticisms of the SOS study include weaknesses in study design, outdated surgical techniques, and homogeneous sample population.
2. The STAMPEDE Trial is a randomized-controlled trial comparing bariatric surgery vs intensive medical therapy for the treatment of DM.
   a. A total of 150 obese patients with uncontrolled type 2 DM were randomized to intensive medical therapy vs bariatric surgery (gastric bypass vs sleeve gastrectomy). The primary endpoint was proportion of patients with hemoglobin A1C (HbA1C) < 6%.
   b. After 1 year, 12% medical therapy vs 42% gastric bypass/37% sleeve achieved a HbA1C < 6. In addition, surgery patients had more weight loss and decreased use of medications for hyperglycemia/dyslipidemia/hypertension.[6]

c. Three-year outcomes: 5% medical group vs 38% bypass/24% sleeve achieved HbA1C < 6.[7]
d. Five-year outcomes: 5% medical vs 29% bypass/23% sleeve achieved HbA1C < 6.[8]

II. PREOPERATIVE EVALUATION AND OPTIMIZATION

Statements released by the American Society for Metabolic and Bariatric Surgery and the National Institutes of Health (NIH) provide guidelines for preoperative evaluation and optimization prior to bariatric surgery. However, this process is highly variable between institutions. Below are some recommendations that are widely considered to be important for patient selection and optimization.[9,10]

A. Patient selection
  1. Based on the 1991 NIH guidelines, BMI is the primary component to qualify for bariatric surgery. Specifically, those with a BMI of 40 or those with a BMI of 35 to 39 with an associated comorbid condition are considered for surgery.
  2. Only patients who can tolerate a major operation should be offered weight loss surgery. Standard perioperative risk assessment applies. These include the following:
    a. Tests such as CXR and electrocardiography can be used to assess overall cardiopulmonary health.
    b. Clinical scores assessing the risk of perioperative thromboembolic events can be used to identify high-risk patients who may benefit from extended prophylactic anticoagulation.
    c. Verify patient is up to date on cancer screening.
    d. Women of child-bearing age should not be pregnant at the time of their surgery and are advised to remain on contraception for at least 1 year postoperatively. Weight loss surgery is associated with elevated risk of fetal anomalies and demise during this time.
  3. Baseline nutritional evaluation includes
    a. A thorough dietary and weight history
    b. Nutritional laboratory work
      i. Basic electrolytes
      ii. Liver function tests
      iii. Albumin and prealbumin
      iv. Iron panel
      v. Vitamin levels: B12, folic acid, vitamin D
      vi. Lipid profile
  4. The above components are considered the framework for selecting those eligible for bariatric surgery. Additional workup depends on the patient's insurance plan and their past medical and surgical history.

B. Assess for obesity-related comorbidities
  1. Obstructive sleep apnea
    a. Screen with clinical questionnaire, such as STOP-BANG, and verify with sleep study if indicated.
  2. DM
  3. Hypertension
  4. Dyslipidemia

C. Tests for operative planning
   1. Upper endoscopy, pH monitoring
      a. Recommended for patients undergoing sleeve gastrectomy, considering this operation may exacerbate gastroesophageal reflux disease.
      b. Evaluate for objective signs of reflux, such as esophagitis and Barrett's esophagus.
   2. *Helicobacter pylori*
      a. Diagnose and treat prior to surgery to minimize the risk of ulcer formation.
      b. It is especially important in patients undergoing gastric bypass as the excluded stomach will be difficult to access postoperatively.
D. Preoperative optimization
   1. Smoking cessation: Smoking increases the risk of perioperative and postoperative complications, such as marginal ulcers, wound healing, and anastomotic leak. Some centers do not offer bariatric surgery in active smokers.
   2. Preoperative weight loss: The surgeon may recommend weight loss prior to bariatric surgery depending on the patient's preoperative weight, the operation, and their overall surgical risk. Weight loss prior to surgery is not indicative of greater weight loss after surgery but more important for minimizing perioperative surgical risk.
   3. Nutritional optimization and education: Most centers require patients to meet with a certified dietitian preoperatively to review macro- and micronutrient requirements following surgery.
   4. Psychosocial assessment and optimization
      a. Patients are counseled on the lifestyle changes associated with surgery.
      b. Eating behaviors and patterns are identified preoperatively to better help patients adapt to eating behaviors after surgery as this can result in a drastic change.
      c. Untreated or suboptimally treated mental illness is identified and/or addressed prior to surgery.

III. BARIATRIC SURGERY TECHNIQUES

The more common types of bariatric surgery are given in **Table 15.5**:

A. Gastric band surgery
   1. A fluid-filled silicone band is placed around the stomach. The degree of restriction can be modified by adjusting the amount of fluid via a subcutaneous port.
   2. Gastric band surgery has fallen out of favor as many patients experience suboptimal weight loss.
B. Sleeve gastrectomy (**Figure 15.1**)
   1. The sleeve gastrectomy is the most common bariatric operation done in the US. Approximately 70% to 80% of the stomach is resected resulting in a smaller residual stomach.
   2. This is accomplished by mobilizing the greater curve of the stomach from the gastrocolic ligament. The branches of the gastroepiploic and short gastric vessels are divided up to the angle of His.

TABLE 15.5 Overview of Bariatric Surgical Procedures

	Sleeve Gastrectomy (SG)	Roux-en-Y Gastric Bypass (RYGB)	Biliopancreatic Diversion and Duodenal Switch (BPD-DS)
Mechanism of weight loss	Restrictive	Restrictive and malabsorptive	Malabsorptive[a]
Expected weight loss after 1 y (% loss of excess body weight)[b]	50%-60%	60%-70%	>70%
Prevalence[c]	60%	20%	<2%

[a]While BPD-DS does have some weight loss due to restriction from sleeve gastrectomy, most of the weight loss is attributed to malabsorptive mechanisms as most of the small bowel length is bypassed in the biliopancreatic limb.

[b]Excess body weight is defined as the amount of weight that exceeds calculated ideal body weight based on height, gender, and age.

[c]Other weight loss procedures include gastric banding, endoscopic procedures, and surgical revisions.

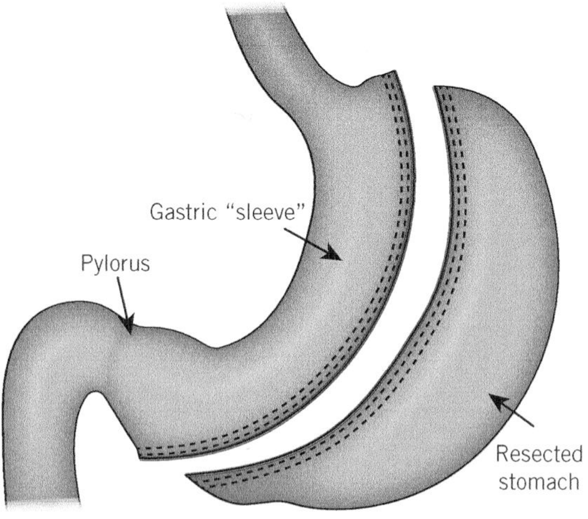

FIGURE 15.1 Sleeve gastrectomy. *(Reprinted from https://commons.wikimedia.org/wiki/File:GVL.png; https://creativecommons.org/licenses/by-sa/4.0/.)*

3. The distal extent of sleeve gastrectomy is measured 4 to 6 cm proximal to the pylorus. An anatomic landmark that can be used is the second branch of the right gastroepiploic artery.
4. The sleeve gastrectomy is created with serial firings of a surgical stapler over a bougie from distal landmark toward angle of His. Staple line reinforcements, such as bovine pericardium, can be used to decrease risk of staple line bleed.[11]
5. A leak test is then recommended, which can be done in several ways including endoscopic insufflation, air, and/or methylene blue.
6. The resected stomach is removed from the abdomen and the abdomen is closed.

C. Roux-en-Y gastric bypass (RYGB) (**Figure 15.2**)

1. The RYGB is an efficient weight loss operation given it is restrictive and malabsorptive.
2. The technical approach for an RYGB varies among surgeons, but there are important technical goals to achieve regardless of approach:
   a. The proximal stomach is constructed to hold approximately 30 mL, resulting in caloric restriction.
   b. The small intestine that is brought to the proximal stomach can be done so in either an antecolic or retrocolic orientation.
   c. The small intestine brought to the proximal stomach creates the gastrojejunostomy. This is the Roux limb and typically measured to be 100 to 150 cm long.
   d. The biliopancreatic limb (BP) is measured from the ligament of Treitz and should be at least 50 cm in length.
   e. The measured Roux limb is then anastomosed to the BP limb to create the jejunojejunostomy. Distal to this anastomosis is known as the common channel.

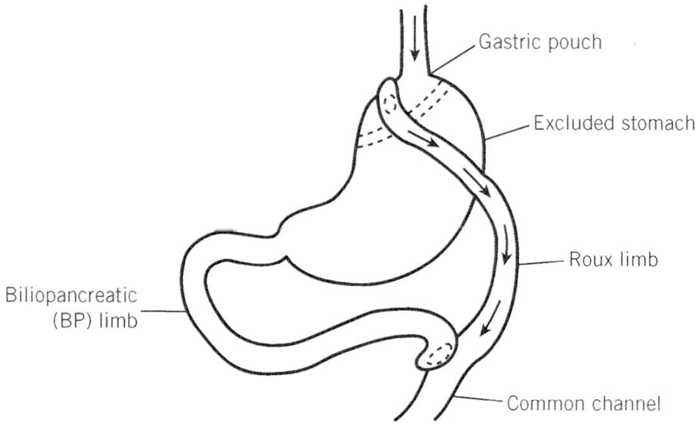

FIGURE 15.2 Gastric bypass.

3. It is important to close the mesenteric defects given the long-term possibility of internal hernia that may result in bowel obstruction and bowel ischemia. These defects should be closed with nonabsorbable suture.

D. Biliopancreatic diversion with duodenal switch (BPD-DS) (**Figure 15.3**)

1. The BPD-DS accounts for 2% of bariatric operations in the US. It is the most efficient weight loss operation and also more technically challenging with a greater risk of perioperative complications.
2. The bowel is measured 50 cm from the ileocecal valve to mark the distal anastomosis (ileoileostomy) and then 200 cm to the proximal anastomosis (duodenoileostomy). These measurements and limb lengths are not necessarily consistent, however, given the changes in weight loss and alterations in technique over the years.
3. A sleeve gastrectomy is then completed.
4. Dissection is then taken along the inferior portion of the distal stomach at the level of the pylorus. A retroduodenal dissection is completed with care not to injure the pancreas or duodenum. It is important to identify the gastroduodenal artery as a landmark and remain proximal to this. The dissection is taken 2 to 3 cm distal to the pylorus where it is then transected. It is also important to ensure the common bile duct is not injured or transected during this step.

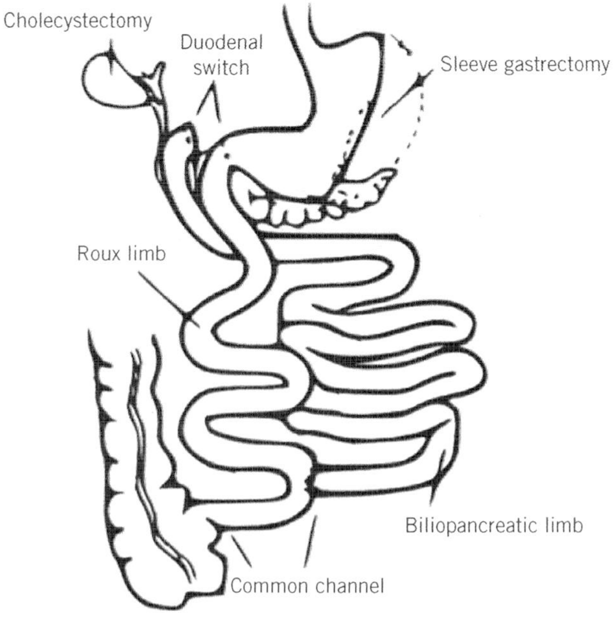

FIGURE 15.3 BPD-DS.

5. The small bowel that was marked as the duodenoileostomy is then anastomosed to the transected duodenum. The small bowel is then transected distal to this anastomosis to create the Roux limb.
6. The distal end of the biliopancreatic limb is then anastomosed to the Roux limb creating the ileoileostomy.
7. A cholecystectomy should be performed at the time of the duodenal switch given the risk of postoperative gallstone disease. Specifically, common bile duct stones. Given the altered anatomy of the duodenal switch, access to the biliary tree can be risky and complicated in these patients.
8. An alternative to the BPD-DS is the single anastomosis duodenal ileostomy, which is gaining popularity given it is only a single anastomosis resulting in shorter operative time. However, the long-term implications of this operation need to be further investigated.

IV. POSTOPERATIVE MANAGEMENT

As weight loss surgery becomes more common, many institutions have adopted enhanced recovery after surgery (ERAS) pathways to standardize care and provide an evidence-based approach to perioperative management.[12] Major components of ERAS pathways for the management of patients undergoing bariatric surgery include:

A. Pain control
   1. Multimodal approach, including regional analgesia
   2. Avoid NSAIDs, which can increase risk of ulcer formation.

B. Early ambulation
   1. Decrease risk of venous thromboembolic (VTE) events.
   2. Decrease risk of perioperative pulmonary complications.

C. Postoperative oxygenation
   1. Patients on noninvasive positive-pressure ventilation (NPPV) prior to their operation should continue using their devices in the perioperative period.
   2. NPPV should also be used liberally in patients with obesity hypoventilation syndrome.

D. Early nutrition and diet progression
   1. Most patients can initiate a clear liquid diet on postoperative day 0 and gradually advance over the next few weeks.
   2. Micronutrient supplementation, including multivitamin, vitamins B1 and B12, and calcium, should be initiated by postoperative day 1.
   3. Patients should receive nutritional counseling to discuss adequate hydration, macronutrient, and micronutrient requirements.

E. VTE prevention
   1. Morbidly obese patients are at increased risk for perioperative VTE and should be started on weight-adjusted chemical prophylaxis in the perioperative period if there is no contraindication due to active bleeding.

F. Prophylactic antacid therapy
   1. Given risk of marginal ulcer formation with an RYGB, it is recommended patients receive at least 90 days of proton pump inhibitor therapy as prevention.

V. POSTOPERATIVE ISSUES AND COMPLICATIONS

Bariatric surgery has become increasingly safe with improved understanding of the physiology of obesity and improved surgical procedures. However, surgeons must be mindful of postoperative complications as signs are often subtle and nonspecific. Any severe or persistent gastrointestinal complaints warrant further examination, typically employing radiographic imaging studies and possible surgical intervention (**Figure 15.4**). Tachycardia in the postoperative setting can often be the first sign of a serious postoperative complication and should warrant investigation (**Figure 15.5**).

A. Anastomotic leaks
   1. Associated with high morbidity and mortality rates
   2. Clinical findings include tachycardia, leukocytosis, and fever. Typical findings of peritonitis and sepsis may be absent until late in the patient's clinical course.
   3. Management of leaks is time dependent and can include surgical closure of the defect, drainage, or placement of an intraluminal stent.

B. Small bowel obstruction
   1. Patients present with abdominal pain, nausea and vomiting, and minimal bowel function.
   2. Etiologies include anastomotic edema and/or hematoma, adhesions, abdominal wall hernias, and intussusception.
   3. Internal hernia is an etiology of bowel obstruction unique to operations involving intestinal bypass.
      a. Locations for internal hernias following an RYGB include:
         i. Transverse mesocolon (if a retrocolic Roux limb)
         ii. The small bowel mesenteric defect at the jejunojejunostomy site
         iii. Petersen's space: A defect between the small bowel limbs, the transverse mesocolon and the retroperitoneum
      b. Treatment of obstruction is prompt surgical exploration to prevent bowel ischemia and necrosis.

C. Gallstone formation
   1. Rapid weight loss increases the risk of gallstone formation.
   2. Use of ursodeoxycholic acid during the rapid weight loss period is recommended.[13]
   3. Concomitant cholecystectomy has fallen out of favor for most patients undergoing weight loss surgery as rate of patients requiring subsequent cholecystectomy for gallstone pathology following weight loss surgery is <10%.[14]

D. Dumping syndrome
   1. Results from patients' inability to regulate gastric emptying of simple carbohydrates or other osmotic loads.
   2. Types of dumping syndrome
      a. Early
         i. Occurs within 30 minutes of eating.
         ii. Results from dumping of large osmotic load into the intestine.
         iii. Symptoms include crampy pain from intestinal distention and osmotic diarrhea.
      b. Late
         i. Occurs a few hours after eating.
         ii. Results from increased insulin release in response to carbohydrate load

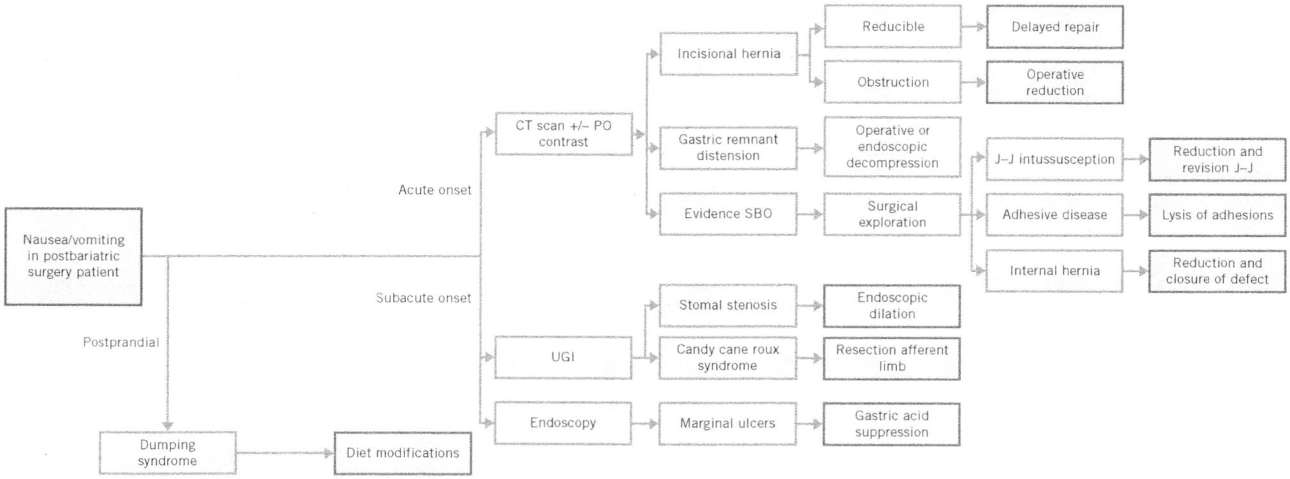

FIGURE 15.4 Algorithm for general workup of gastrointestinal symptoms in patients who have undergone bariatric surgery. J-J, Jejuno-jejunal anastomosis; SBO, small bowel obstruction; UGI, upper gastrointestinal series.

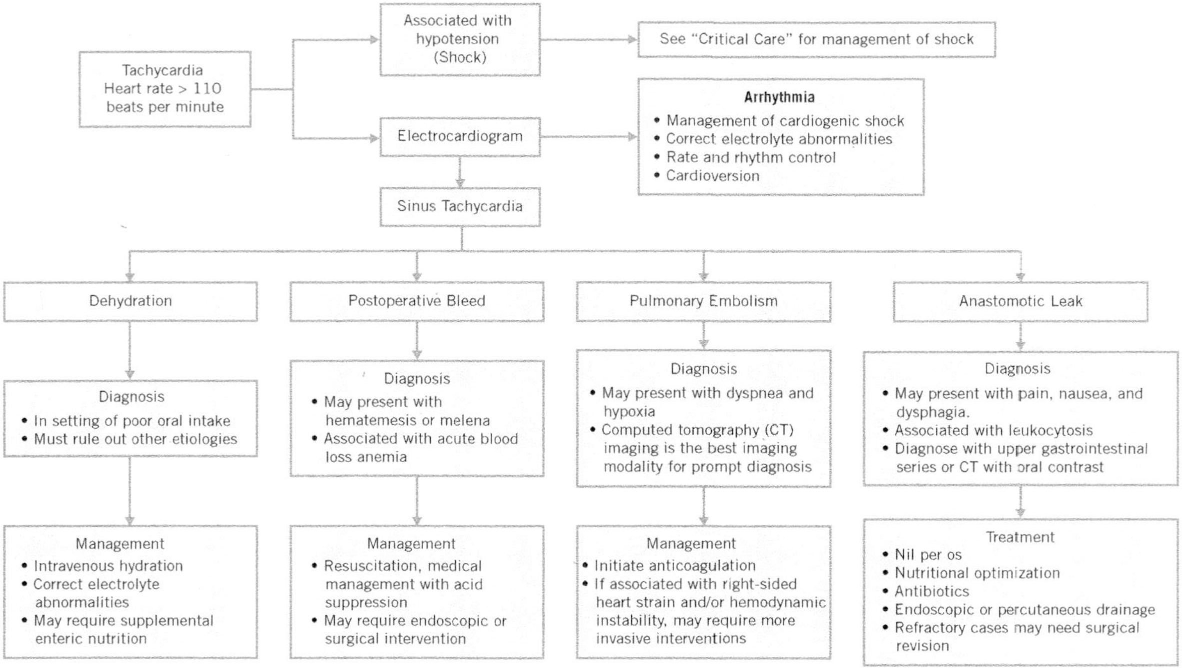

FIGURE 15.5 Algorithm for evaluation and management of postoperative tachycardia.

iii. This leads to symptoms of hypoglycemia, such as tachycardia and diaphoresis.

3. Treatment may involve dietary measures including high-protein diets, acarbose and somatostatin analogues, or surgical reintervention for refractory cases.[15]

E. Nutritional deficiencies

1. A risk after any procedure with a malabsorptive component, and the risk increases with the amount of small intestine bypassed.
2. The most common postoperative deficiencies seen are iron, calcium, and vitamin B12. Vitamin B1 (thiamine) deficiency can present as Wernicke–Korsakoff syndrome, which can lead to permanent neurologic deficits.
3. BPD-DS and its variant procedures carry the additional risk of fat-soluble vitamin deficiencies (vitamins A, D, E, K).

VI. LONG-TERM SURVEILLANCE AFTER BARIATRIC SURGERY

Patients undergoing bariatric surgery must participate in long-term surveillance to optimize weight-loss outcomes and to monitor for complications associated with malnutrition.

A. Monitor weight loss progress.

1. The most common etiology of suboptimal weight loss is nonadherence to lifestyle modifications. Routine surveillance visits are essential in reinforcing these habits.
2. However, anatomical etiologies, such as gastrogastric fistula, will need to be addressed with surgery.[16]

B. Monitor for improvements or resolution of obesity-related comorbidities.

1. Medical therapy for obesity-related comorbidities (i.e., hypertension, DM, and hyperlipidemia) should be titrated under medical supervision as weight loss progresses.

C. Monitor for macro- and micronutrient deficiencies.

1. Routine laboratory work monitoring macro- and micronutrient levels can identify deficiencies early before the development of symptoms. For an overview of the most common postoperative deficiencies, please refer guidelines published by the American Society for Metabolic and Bariatric Surgery.[17]

D. Monitor for other long-term complications of bariatric surgery.

1. Marginal ulcers
   a. Ulcer formation at gastrojejunostomy in RYGB.
   b. Symptoms include postprandial pain, dysphagia, nausea, and vomiting.
   c. Major risk factors include smoking, NSAIDs, and steroids.
   d. Diagnosed with an upper endoscopy.
   e. The mainstay of treatment is medical therapy (i.e., acid reduction with proton pump inhibitors). Rarely, medically refractory ulcers will need surgical revision.
2. Gastrogastric (GG) fistula
   a. Fistula between gastric pouch and excluded stomach.
   b. Can increase the risk of marginal ulcer formation. However, in many cases it may be asymptomatic. Providers should have a high index of suspicion for GG fistula in postoperative patients with suboptimal weight loss.
   c. Treatment is surgical revision.

Key References

Citation	Summary
Sjöström L, Lindroos AK, Peltonen M, et al. Lifestyle, diabetes, and cardiovascular risk factors 10 years after bariatric surgery. *N Engl J Med.* 2004;351(26):2683-2693.	• Ten-year results of Swedish Obese Subjects (SOS) prospective study, in which morbidly obese patients undergoing bariatric surgery were compared with conventionally treated patients. • After 10 y, patients undergoing bariatric surgery were more likely to recover from obesity-related comorbidities such as diabetes, dyslipidemia, hypertension.
Schauer PR, Kashyap SR, Wolski K, et al. Bariatric surgery versus intensive medical therapy in obese patients with diabetes. *N Engl J Med.* 2012;366(17):1567-1576.	• Prospective observational study comparing bariatric surgery vs medical therapy alone in improvement of type 2 diabetes. • In obese patients with poorly controlled type 2 diabetes, bariatric surgery resulted in improved glycemic control compared with medical therapy alone.
Aiolfi A, Gagner M, Zappa MA, et al. Staple Line Reinforcement During Laparoscopic Sleeve Gastrectomy: Systematic Review and Network Meta-analysis of Randomized Controlled Trials. Obes Surg. 2022;32(5):1466-1478.	• Sleeve gastrectomy remains the most prevalent weight loss surgery. • Meta-analysis of randomized controlled trials evaluating staple line reinforcements showed decreased risk of bleeding and staple line leak. • There was no significant difference in surgical site infection, sleeve stenosis, and mortality.
Salminen P, Helmiö M, Ovaska J, et al. Effect of laparoscopic sleeve gastrectomy vs laparoscopic Roux-en-Y gastric bypass on weight loss at 5 years among patients with morbid obesity: The SLEEVEPASS randomized clinical trial. *JAMA.* 2018;319(3):241-254.	• A total of 240 patients randomized to sleeve gastrectomy vs gastric bypass. Primary endpoint was percentage excess weight loss. • After 5 y, gastric bypass was associated with greater percentage excess weight loss, although the difference did not meet prespecified equivalence margins. • Follow-up data after 7 and 10 y showed similar results, in which patients who underwent gastric bypass experienced greater percentage excess weight loss compared with patients with sleeve gastrectomy. Both surgeries did result in sustained clinically significant weight loss and remain viable options for patients.

Citation	Summary
Peterli R, Wölnerhanssen BK, Vetter D, et al. Laparoscopic sleeve gastrectomy versus Roux-Y-gastric bypass for morbid obesity-3-Year outcomes of the prospective randomized Swiss Multicenter Bypass Or Sleeve Study (SM-BOSS). *Ann Surg.* 2017;265(3):466-473.	• After 3 y, patients who underwent sleeve gastrectomy vs gastric bypass experienced similar weight loss, improvements in quality of life, and complication rates. • Patients who underwent gastric bypass experienced improvements in reflux disease and dyslipidemia compared with those who underwent sleeve gastrectomy.

CHAPTER 15: THE SURGICAL MANAGEMENT OF OBESITY

Review Questions

1. What are the indications of bariatric surgery?
2. Name three obesity-related comorbidities.
3. According to the American Society of Metabolic and Bariatric Surgery, what is the most common bariatric surgery performed in the US?
4. In Roux-en-Y gastric bypass (RYGB), what are the three mesenteric defects that should be closed to prevent internal hernias?
5. Sinus tachycardia in the postoperative period may be the only sign of serious postoperative complications, such as:
6. In patients who have undergone RYGB, what are the major risk factors of marginal ulcer formation?

REFERENCES

1. Rauova L, Zhai L, Kowalska MA, Arepally GM, Cines DB, Poncz M. Role of platelet surface PF4 antigenic complexes in heparin-induced thrombocytopenia pathogenesis: diagnostic and therapeutic implications. *Blood.* 2006;107(6):2346-2353.
2. Stein PD, Fowler SE, Goodman LR, et al. Multidetector computed tomography for acute pulmonary embolism. *N Engl J Med.* 2006;354(22):2317-2327.
3. Sjöström L, Lindroos AK, Peltonen M, et al. Lifestyle, diabetes, and cardiovascular risk factors 10 years after bariatric surgery. *N Engl J Med.* 2004;351(26):2683-2693.
4. Carlsson LM, Peltonen M, Ahlin S, et al. Bariatric surgery and prevention of type 2 diabetes in Swedish obese subjects. *N Engl J Med.* 2012;367(8):695-704.
5. Sjöström L. Review of the key results from the Swedish Obese Subjects (SOS) trial: a prospective controlled intervention study of bariatric surgery. *J Intern Med.* 2013;273(3):219-234.
6. Schauer PR, Kashyap SR, Wolski K, et al. Bariatric surgery versus intensive medical therapy in obese patients with diabetes. *N Engl J Med.* 2012;366(17):1567-1576.
7. Schauer PR, Bhatt DL, Kirwan JP, et al. Bariatric surgery versus intensive medical therapy for diabetes—3-year outcomes. *N Engl J Med.* 2014;370(21):2002-2013.
8. Schauer PR, Bhatt DL, Kirwan JP, et al. Bariatric surgery versus intensive medical therapy for diabetes—5-year outcomes. *N Engl J Med.* 2017;376(7):641-651.
9. NIH. Gastrointestinal surgery for severe obesity consensus development conference statement. 2022. https://consensus.nih.gov/1991/1991gisurgeryobesity084html.htm

10. Mechanick JI, Youdim A, Jones DB, et al. Clinical practice guidelines for the perioperative nutritional, metabolic, and nonsurgical support of the bariatric surgery patient—2013 update: cosponsored by American Association of Clinical Endocrinologists, the Obesity Society, and American Society for Metabolic & Bariatric Surgery. *Obesity.* 2013;21(suppl 1):S1-S27.

11. Aiolfi A, Gagner M, Zappa MA, et al. Staple line reinforcement during laparoscopic sleeve gastrectomy: systematic review and network meta-analysis of randomized controlled trials. *Obes Surg.* 2022;32(5):1466-1478.

12. Stenberg E, Dos Reis Falcão LF, O'Kane M, et al. Guidelines for perioperative care in bariatric surgery: Enhanced Recovery After Surgery (ERAS) Society recommendations—A 2021 update. *World J Surg.* 2022;46(4):729-751.

13. Adams LB, Chang C, Pope J, Kim Y, Liu P, Yates A. Randomized, prospective comparison of ursodeoxycholic acid for the prevention of gallstones after sleeve gastrectomy. *Obes Surg.* 2016;26(5):990-994.

14. Warschkow R, Tarantino I, Ukegjini K, et al. Concomitant cholecystectomy during laparoscopic Roux-en-Y gastric bypass in obese patients is not justified: a meta-analysis. *Obes Surg.* 2013;23(3):397-407.

15. Tack J, Deloose E. Complications of bariatric surgery: dumping syndrome, reflux and vitamin deficiencies. *Best Pract Res Clin Gastroenterol.* 2014;28(4):741-749.

16. Herron DM, Birkett DH, Thompson CC, Bessler M, Swanström LL. Gastric bypass pouch and stoma reduction using a transoral endoscopic anchor placement system: a feasibility study. *Surg Endosc.* 2008;22(4):1093-1099.

17. Parrott J, Frank L, Rabena R, Craggs-Dino L, Isom KA, Greiman L. American Society for metabolic and bariatric surgery integrated health nutritional guidelines for the surgical weight loss patient 2016 update: micronutrients. *Surg Obes Relat Dis.* 2017;13(5):727-741.

16 Small Intestine

Cameron Casson and Radhika Smith

I. SMALL BOWEL OBSTRUCTION

A. Definition

1. Obstruction is the mechanical occlusion of the intestinal lumen.
   a. **Partial obstruction:** Some distal passage of fluid or gas
   b. **Complete obstruction:** Lumen is fully occluded
      i. Can lead to **strangulation**, where the involved small intestine has vascular compromise leading to **infarction** and eventual perforation of the intestinal wall
2. **Ileus** occurs when there is a failure of peristalsis, thus resulting in a "functional obstruction" rather than a mechanical obstruction.
   a. Common causes: Recent abdominal operations, electrolyte disturbances, trauma, peritonitis, intra-abdominal abscess, systemic infections, bowel ischemia, and medications

B. Etiology: There are many causes of small bowel obstruction (SBO), see **Table 16.1**.

1. Most common etiology in the US: Adhesions following an abdominal operation, accounting for up to 70% of cases
2. Most common etiology worldwide: Incarcerated hernias (second leading cause in the US)

C. Presentation

1. Signs and symptoms
   a. Nausea and emesis (proximal obstructions tend to present with bilious emesis and distal obstructions with feculent emesis)
   b. Abdominal distention
   c. Colicky, poorly localized abdominal pain
   d. **Obstipation** (inability to pass stool or gas)
   e. With a persistent obstruction, hypovolemia progresses due to impaired intestinal absorption, increased secretion, and fluid losses from emesis. Electrolyte abnormalities associated with dehydration can also be seen.
2. Physical examination
   a. Abnormal vital signs are generally indicative of hypovolemia (e.g., tachycardia and hypotension)
   b. Abdominal distension
   c. Tympani to percussion
   d. Prior surgical scars, masses, or hernias
   e. Peritonitis mandates prompt surgical treatment due to the concern for bowel strangulation and/or perforation.

TABLE 16.1 Etiology of Small Bowel Obstruction

Etiology	Description
Adhesions	Due to prior abdominal operations (or rarely isolated congenital adhesions/bands)
Incarcerated hernias	Bowel can become incarcerated within a variety of hernias (ventral, inguinal, femoral, internal, etc.)
Intussusception	One portion of bowel (the intussusceptum) telescopes into another (the intussuscipiens); the lead point can be due to tumors, polyps, enlarged lymph nodes, or a Meckel diverticulum. This results in luminal occlusion and proximal obstruction and can be seen incidentally on CT in asymptomatic patients as well. Adults: Requires further workup to evaluate for malignancy or other source Children: Often unknown etiology and treated nonoperatively (see Chapter 39)
Volvulus	Rotation of a segment of bowel around its vascular pedicle; often caused by adhesions or congenital anomalies
Strictures	Due to ischemia, inflammation (such as in Crohn's disease), radiation, or prior operations
Gallstone ileus	Complication of cholecystitis with fistulization between the biliary tree and small bowel allows one or more gallstones to travel distally and obstruct the lumen, typically at the ileocecal valve
Bowel compression	Can be internal or external compression due to tumors, abscesses, hematomas, or other intra-abdominal masses
Foreign bodies	Typically pass without incident or can be endoscopically retrieved, but if not, may require operative intervention

D. Diagnosis

1. **Laboratory evaluation**
   - **a.** In the early stages of SBO, laboratory values may be normal. As the process progresses, laboratory values commonly reflect dehydration (hypochloremic, hypokalemic contraction alkalosis).
   - **b.** Elevated white blood cell count and/or serum lactate levels are concerning for possible strangulation/ischemia.

2. **Radiologic evaluation**
   a. **Abdominal plain films** may demonstrate dilated loops of small intestine, air–fluid levels, and paucity of colorectal gas. These findings may be absent in early, proximal, and/or closed-loop obstructions.
      i. **Pneumatosis intestinalis** and/or portal venous gas suggests a strangulated obstruction and bowel necrosis.
      ii. Free intra-abdominal air indicates hollow viscus perforation.
      iii. Air in the biliary tree and a radiopaque gallstone in the right lower quadrant are pathognomonic of **gallstone ileus.**
      iv. **Paralytic ileus** appears as gaseous distention uniformly distributed throughout the stomach, small intestine, and colon.
   b. **CT** can localize and characterize the obstruction and provides information regarding etiology of SBO and presence of other intra-abdominal pathologies.
      i. Small bowel feces sign ("fecalization") is the presence of gas and liquid/solid mixed within dilated small bowel related to stasis and is seen with high-grade obstructions.

E. Management of SBO has been outlined in guidelines provided by the Eastern Association for the Surgery of Trauma as well as the Bologna Guidelines.[1,2] A sample treatment algorithm is given in **Figure 16.1**.
   1. If the patient is clinically stable with no concerns for strangulated obstruction or peritonitis, then nonoperative management can be attempted.
   2. Early evaluation of patients with a water-soluble oral contrast agent may be useful in differentiating patients who will spontaneously resolve their obstruction from patients who will require operative intervention, resulting in a shorter length of stay.[3]
   3. Signs of shock, intestinal strangulation or perforation, or failure to improve with nonoperative management are indications for operative intervention. Diagnostic laparoscopy or exploratory laparotomy are both acceptable approaches.
   4. The goal of surgery is to identify and treat the origin of obstruction, which may require extensive adhesiolysis and/or resection. Enteroenteric or enterocolic bypass or palliative decompressive gastrostomy tube may be needed for unresectable obstructing lesions.

II. MECKEL'S DIVERTICULUM

A. The most common congenital anomaly of the gastrointestinal (GI) tract.

B. "True" diverticulum in that it contains all layers of the bowel wall.

C. "Rule of Twos": 2% incidence, a 2:1 male:female ratio, 2 inch in length, located 2 ft from the ileocecal valve (antimesenteric border of the ileum), typically presenting before 2 years of age, and often containing one of two types of heterotopic mucosa (gastric or pancreatic)

D. Presentation
   1. The vast majority of cases are asymptomatic.
   2. The most common presenting symptom: Painless, episodic bleeding from a peptic ulcer of adjacent normal ileum on the mesenteric border

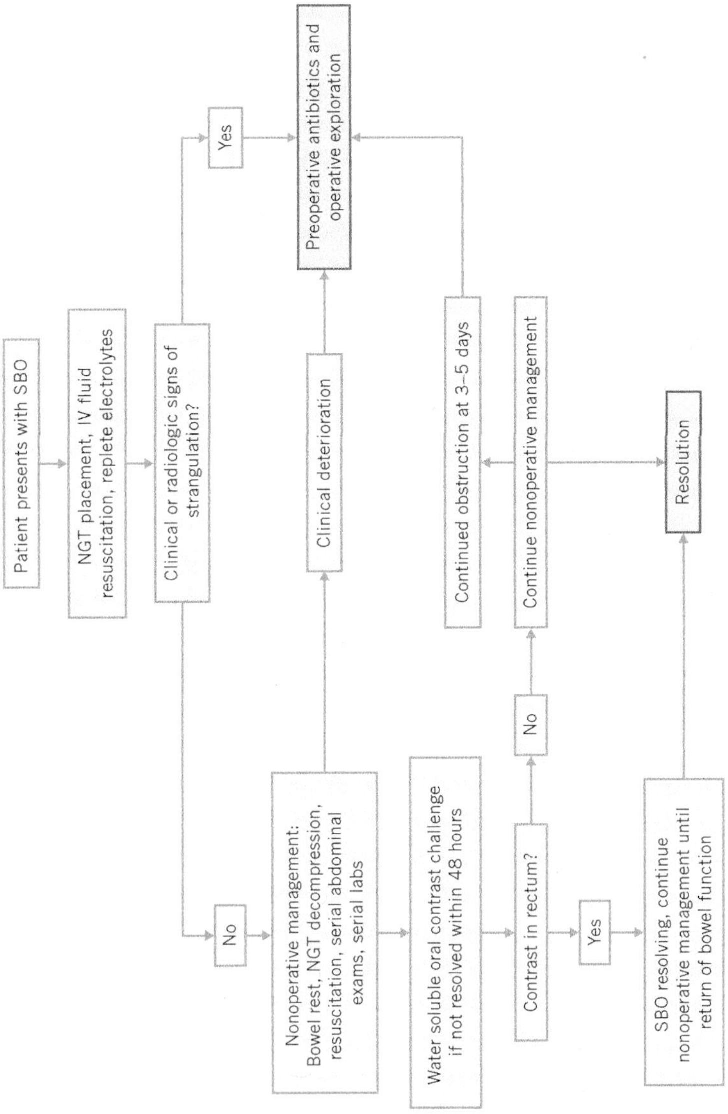

FIGURE 16.1 Algorithm of management of small bowel obstruction.

of the bowel caused by acid secretion from gastric mucosa within the diverticulum.

3. The second most common presentation: Intestinal obstruction due to intussusception or incarcerated hernia (**Littré hernia**)
   a. Obstruction can also occur due to volvulus of small bowel around a fibrous band connecting the diverticulum to the anterior abdominal wall.
4. **Meckel's diverticulitis** occurs in 20% of symptomatic patients and is often mistaken for acute appendicitis.

E. Diagnosis
1. In adults, clinical diagnosis of a Meckel's diverticulum is extremely difficult except in the presence of bleeding.
2. **Meckel scan:** Radionucleotide study based on the uptake of Tc-99m pertechnetate by ectopic gastric mucosa.
   a. In children, this test is the most accurate (90%) for diagnosing a Meckel's diverticulum but is less accurate (46%) in adults because of reduced prevalence of ectopic gastric mucosa within the diverticulum.
3. **Tagged red blood cell scan:** Can be useful in the presence of bleeding.
4. **Contrast studies**, such as small bowel follow through (SBFT), are diagnostic in up to 75% patients.
5. **CT** and **sonography** are typically of little value because distinguishing between a diverticulum and intestinal loops can be very difficult unless diverticulitis is present.

F. Treatment: Resection is indicated in symptomatic patients. Incidental diverticulectomy during surgery for other abdominal pathology *is not indicated* as lifelong morbidity associated with the presence of a Meckel's diverticulum is extremely low.
1. **Simple diverticulectomy:** For patients with an obstruction
2. **Segmental small-bowel resection:** For patients with acute diverticulitis, a wide-based diverticulum, volvulus with necrotic bowel, or bleeding from a mesenteric ulcer

III. FISTULAS

A. Introduction: A fistula is defined as an abnormal communication between two epithelialized surfaces. Fistulas are categorized according to anatomy, output, and etiology.

B. Anatomic considerations
1. Fistulas can be characterized by what organ systems are involved and the location of this abnormal connection: External vs. internal and proximal vs. distal (**Table 16.2**).
2. Fistulas can also be characterized by their outputs (**Table 16.3**). High-output fistulas are more likely to lead to complications such as fluid and electrolyte losses, malnutrition, and the inability to close without operative intervention.

C. Etiology: Fistulas can also be categorized by their etiologies. The most common cause is iatrogenic following an abdominal operation. Other common etiologies can be seen in **Table 16.4**.

TABLE 16.2 Anatomic Classification of Small Bowel Fistulas

Anatomic Location	Classification
External	Connection between internal organ to skin (enterocutaneous fistula) or internal organ to open wound (enteroatmospheric fistula)
Internal	Connection between two hollow viscera (e.g., enteroenteric fistula)
Proximal	Stomach, duodenum, or jejunum Associated with high outputs
Distal	Ileum or colon Associated with lower outputs

D. Pathophysiology

1. Loss of GI contents leads to hypovolemia as well as acid/base and electrolyte abnormalities. High-output fistulas release large volumes of fluid leading to dehydration and intravascular volume depletion.
2. Malnutrition is often due to both insufficient caloric intake and functional exclusion of portions of the GI tract limiting absorptive capacity.

E. Diagnosis

1. **Imaging**
   a. CT with oral and IV contrast to help characterize the location of the fistula and to evaluate for associated intra-abdominal abscesses or undrained fluid collections.
   b. **Fistulography** ("fistulogram") where contrast is injected into the fistula to provide visualization of all tracts and sites of enteral communication.
      i. Oral contrast studies, such as an upper GI with SBFT, can demonstrate contrast extravasation through the fistula but are less sensitive.

TABLE 16.3 Classification of Small Bowel Fistulas by Output

Output	Amount (mL/d)	Associated Anatomic Locations
Low	<200	Distal (ileum or colon)
Moderate	200-500	Distal or proximal
High	>500	Proximal (stomach, duodenum, or jejunum)

TABLE 16.4 Etiology of Small Bowel Fistulas

Etiology	Characteristics
Prior abdominal operations	Leading cause of fistula formation Increased risk in the setting of complex operations including extensive intestinal adhesions or in the setting of malnutrition and/or immunosuppression
Crohn's disease	Common cause of enterocutaneous fistulas, ileosigmoid fistulas, and enteroenteric fistulas
Diverticular disease	Form when localized abscess drains into adjacent organs
Malignancy	Form when tumors perforate or invade adjacent structures Will not heal if cancer is present
Radiation enteritis	Predisposes to fistula formation after an operation, regardless of the temporal proximity of radiation exposure
Trauma	Penetrating injuries, missed enteric injuries during an operation, or injuries repaired in a contaminated field are prone to leak and subsequent fistula formation
Foreign body	Mesh or suture may cause erosion into adjacent organs and fistula formation
Infectious diseases	Amebiasis, tuberculosis, or *Actinomyces*

c. Contrast enema may be helpful in the evaluation of rectal or colonic fistulas.

2. **Endoscopy:** Endoscopy is useful to assess the bowel for underlying pathology, such as peptic ulceration, inflammatory bowel disease (IBD), or cancer, but is unlikely to specifically identify a fistula.

F. Nonoperative treatment

1. Spontaneous closure

a. Depending on the etiology and underlying pathology, approximately 40% of enterocutaneous fistulas will close spontaneously in 4 to 6 weeks with adequate nutritional support and control of sepsis.

i. Increased rates of spontaneous closure in fistulas with low output, long tracts (>2 cm), small orifices (<1 cm^2), absence of malnutrition, abscess, sepsis, or active IBD.

b. Common conditions under which fistulas fail to spontaneously close can be remembered using the mnemonic "**FRIENDS**": <u>F</u>oreign body, **R**adiation, **I**nflammation or **I**nfection, **E**pithelialization, **N**eoplasm or lack of **N**utrition, **D**istal obstruction, and/or **S**teroids (immunosuppression).

2. Fluid resuscitation and electrolyte correction: IV fluid administration is typically necessary because adequate enteral replacement of fistula output is difficult.
3. **Sepsis control:** Sepsis remains the primary determinant of fistula mortality. Sepsis accompanying fistulas is caused by undrained enteric leaks or abscesses. Percutaneous abscess drainage should be performed if present.
   a. IV antibiotics directed against bowel flora are indicated.
   b. Operation for source control may be required to manage continuous bacterial seeding from the GI tract.
   c. Infected wounds are opened and packed to allow complete drainage, debridement, and healing by secondary intention.
4. Nutritional support: Nutritional support is essential to facilitate spontaneous closure and to optimize the patient for operative repair if the fistula does not heal on its own.
   a. **Complete bowel rest** with initial nil per os status reduces fistula drainage and simplifies the evaluation and stabilization of the patient.
   b. **Enteral feeding** is preferred as long as fistula output does not increase significantly.
      i. Low-output colonic or distal small intestine fistulas are often safely fed with standard enteral formulas/diets.
      ii. Proximal fistulas may be fed distal to the fistula (e.g., feeding jejunostomy tube for a gastric fistula).
   c. **Total parenteral nutrition (TPN)** provides nourishment when enteral feeding is not possible.
      i. Indications: Intolerance to enteral nutrition, high-output fistulas, and proximal fistulas where distal enteral access is not possible
      ii. Complications: Biliary stasis, hepatic dysfunction, trace element (zinc, copper, chromium) and essential fatty acid deficiencies, as well as central venous catheter-related complications, such as infections
5. Decrease of fistula output: H_2-receptor antagonists or proton-pump inhibitors are used to reduce gastric secretions, and thus gastric and duodenal fistula output, and provide stress ulceration prophylaxis.
   a. Somatostatin and its analogs have mixed results in decreasing fistula output and fistula closure.[4]
6. Skin protection: Fistula effluent is corrosive to the skin and must be controlled.
   a. Dressings may be used to simply absorb effluent from low-output fistulas but may impede healing and cause skin breakdown if prolonged contact occurs.
   b. Barrier/ostomy devices are useful as they isolate the effluent away from the skin and allow for quantification of output.

c. Vacuum-assisted wound closure devices may help control skin irritation and speed fistula closure.[5]

d. Early involvement of an enterostomal therapist is critical in the management of patients with fistula.

G. Operative management

1. Indications: Failure to heal with nonoperative management or inadequate sepsis control
2. Delaying reoperation allows adhesions to attenuate and the patient to recover nutritional status and general health, ideally at least 4 to 6 months from the time of last laparotomy.
3. Operative goals are to eradicate the fistula tract and to restore the epithelial continuity of the associated organ systems.
4. Enteral feeding tubes placed at the time of definitive repair may facilitate postoperative management and maintenance of nutrition.
5. Operative approach varies by fistula location, as seen in **Table 16.5**.

IV. SHORT BOWEL SYNDROME

A. Short-bowel syndrome (SBS) is a malabsorptive state and symptom complex following massive resection of the small intestine (either at one time or through sequential resections over time).

1. In adults, the normal length of the small intestine varies from 300 to 600 cm and correlates directly with body surface area. Functional bowel <200 cm or **<30%** of the initial small intestine length are at high risk of developing SBS. With an end stoma, resection resulting in <100 cm of intact small intestine generally leads to SBS. However, in patients

TABLE 16.5 Operative Approaches to Fistula Management

Fistula Location	Surgical Approach	Considerations
Gastric fistulas	Primary repair with serosal and/or omental patch placement	Low-output fistulas will often close spontaneously (e.g., after gastrostomy tube removal)
Duodenal fistulas	Small: Primary closure Moderate to large: Serosal patch or a Roux-en-Y duodenoenterostomy	Primary closure of large defects can lead to duodenal stricture
Small bowel fistulas	Bowel resection with primary anastomosis	
Large bowel fistulas	Bowel resection with primary anastomosis	High spontaneous closure rates

with an intact ileocecal valve and one-third of the colon, SBS may not develop until <75 cm of small intestine remains.

2. Children tend to develop SBS when <30% of normal small intestine length for age remains. Infants may survive resection of up to 85% of their bowel because of enhanced adaptation and growth.
3. SBS may be seen with greater lengths of remaining bowel if an underlying disease, such as CD or radiation enteritis, is present.
4. Because the ileum has specialized absorptive function, complete resection is not well tolerated, whereas the entire jejunum may be resected with lower risk of serious adverse nutritional sequela.

B. Etiology: The leading causes of massive intestinal resection resulting in SBS are as follows:

1. In children: Necrotizing enterocolitis, congenital intestinal atresia, midgut volvulus, and gastroschisis (see Chapter 39)
2. In adults: Mesenteric ischemia, trauma, IBD, strangulated hernia, neoplasm, volvulus, and portal vein thrombosis

C. Pathophysiology

1. The small intestine undergoes **adaptation** in response to massive resection in an attempt to counteract the development of SBS. Slower transit and increased nutrient absorption occurs through functional adaptations.
   a. The distal small intestine has the greatest adaptive potential and can assume nearly all of the absorptive properties of the proximal gut.
   b. Colonic adaptation manifests as increased absorption and colonocyte degradation of carbohydrates into short-chain fatty acids, which increases caloric uptake up to 50%. In addition, the colon can absorb a significant amount of the increased fluid and electrolytes it encounters in the setting of adaptation to SBS.
2. Despite these adaptive changes, there are still several complications with malabsorption and malnutrition in SBS, as seen in **Figure 16.2**.

D. Acute phase management: Management in the initial 4 weeks after small intestinal resection includes stabilization as metabolic, respiratory, and cardiovascular derangements frequently accompany massive small bowel resection.

1. Close monitoring of fluid balance and serum electrolytes is critical.
2. **Prolonged ileus** is common and TPN should be provided until GI function resumes.
3. Early initiation of nutritional support promotes a positive nitrogen balance, wound healing, and adaptation of remnant bowel.
   a. **Enteral nutrition** has positive trophic effects on bowel mucosa and should be initiated, if possible. Feeding tubes placed at the time of the intestinal resection are often necessary.
   b. Initial feeds should be gradual, continuous, low volume, low fat, and isosmotic.

E. Maintenance phase management: Maintenance therapy in SBS focuses on long-term nutritional goals, support of adaptation that takes place over the first 1 to 2 years, and addressing various clinical issues that may arise.

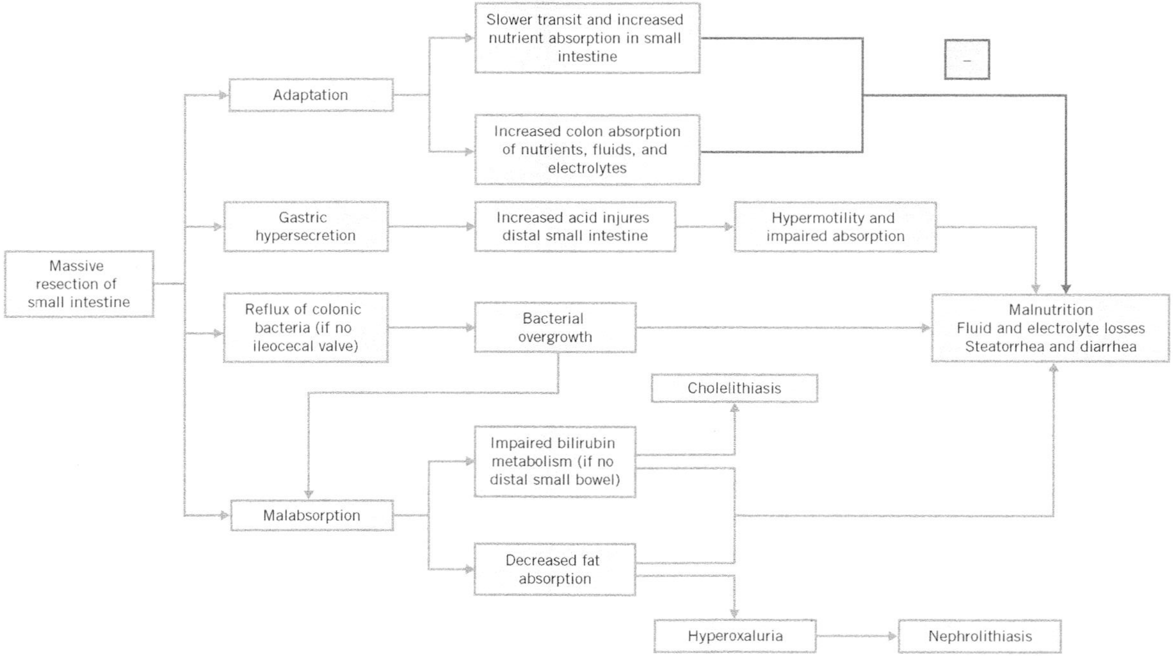

FIGURE 16.2 Pathophysiology in short-bowel syndrome (SBS). Diagram demonstrates pathophysiologic changes in the small bowel and colon following massive resection with subsequent clinical effects (each arrow represents "leads to" and the "-" represents "prevents").

1. **Nutritional support** with supplemental electrolytes (potassium, magnesium), vitamins (A, D, E, K, B_{12}), trace elements and minerals (zinc, selenium, and iron), and essential fatty acids (linoleic acid) should be given parenterally until adequate enteral absorption is achieved.
   a. A glucagon-like peptide (GLP-2) analogue, teduglutide, has been shown to increase adaptation and decrease TPN dependence.[6] The use of growth hormone and glutamine remains controversial.
2. **Diarrhea** is often multifactorial, and dietary modifications can improve symptoms. Medications such as H_2-receptor blockers, bile-chelating resins (cholestyramine), antisecretory medications (loperamide, somatostatin analogs), and low-dose narcotics (diphenoxylate hydrochloride and atropine [Lomotil], codeine, or tincture of opium) are useful for decreasing output.
3. **Late complications** are common and include nephrolithiasis, cholelithiasis, nutritional deficiencies (anemia, bone disease, and coagulopathy), liver dysfunction, as well as TPN and central access–related complications. Anastomotic leaks, fistulas, strictures, and late bowel obstructions can also occur beyond the postoperative period, depending on the underlying pathology.

F. Operative management: Various surgical procedures have been described for the management of SBS but have not been widely adopted.
1. Intestinal lengthening procedures may decrease TPN dependence, increase oral caloric intake, and reverse liver disease.
2. The most common procedures are the **serial transverse enteroplasty procedure** and the **Bianchi** (longitudinal intestinal lengthening and tailoring) **procedure**, both with similar efficacy.
3. **Isolated small-bowel transplants** or **multivisceral transplantations** are rare but may be additional options for SBS. These options have been limited by the high immunogenicity of the small intestine requiring prohibitively high doses of immunosuppression to prevent rejection.

V. NEOPLASMS

A. Benign tumors
1. Small-bowel neoplasms are relatively uncommon, and benign tumors are more common than malignant tumors.
2. Benign neoplasms are often discovered incidentally.
3. See **Table 16.6** for the types of benign small intestine tumors.
4. Other rare benign tumors include **neurofibromas and fibromas** that can cause intussusception. **Endometriosis**, implants that appear as puckered, bluish-red, serosal-based nodules, can cause intestinal bleeding or obstruction.

B. Malignant tumors
1. Malignant tumors account for <2% of all intestinal cancers.
2. Most malignant tumors eventually become symptomatic with weight loss, abdominal pain, obstruction, perforation, and/or hemorrhage. Small-bowel neoplasms can also be a lead point for intussusception.
3. **Table 16.7** outlines the characteristic factors, diagnosis, and treatment of the most commonly seen malignant neoplasms of the small intestine.

TABLE 16.6 Benign Tumors of the Small Intestine

Tumor	Pathogenesis/Risk Factors	Presentation	Treatment	Additional Comments
Leiomyoma	Mesenchymal cells; grow in the submucosal plane	Smooth, eccentric filling defects on imaging	Segmental bowel resection; need pathology to differentiate from malignant stromal tumors	**Most common benign tumor**
Adenoma	Subtypes: Simple tubular, Brunner gland, **villous adenoma** (only subtype with high malignant potential)	Can cause intermittent pain secondary to obstruction, intussusception, or bleeding	Endoscopic removal if possible, otherwise small bowel resection	Sporadic or familial (**familial adenomatous polyposis** syndrome)
Hamartoma	Associated with **Peutz–Jeghers syndrome**, an autosomal-dominant syndrome characterized by mucocutaneous hyperpigmentation and multiple GI polyps	Can cause intermittent pain secondary to obstruction, intussusception, or bleeding	Resect if >1 cm or symptomatic Local excision or endoscopic treatment preferred over segmental resection	Increased risk for de novo small intestine/colonic adenocarcinomas and require frequent endoscopic screening; most frequently in **jejunum**
Lipoma	Benign growth of fatty tissue	Can cause intermittent pain secondary to obstruction, intussusception, or bleeding	Bowel resection only if symptomatic (no malignant potential)	Most frequently in **ileum**
Hemangioma	Associated with **Osler–Weber–Rendu** disease (or hereditary hemorrhagic telangiectasia)	Can cause GI bleeding	Bowel resection only if symptomatic	Rare in small bowel

TABLE 16.7 Malignant Tumors of the Small Intestine

Tumor	Pathogenesis/Risk Factors	Presenting Symptoms	Diagnosis	Treatment	Additional Comments
Adenocarcinoma	Risk factors include villous adenomas, polyposis syndromes, Crohn's disease (CD), and hereditary nonpolyposis colorectal cancer (HNPCC) or **Lynch syndrome**	Periampullary tumors: Painless jaundice, duodenal obstruction, or bleeding Distal tumors: Abdominal pain and weight loss from progressive obstruction	CT scan, endoscopy with or without ERCP	Surgical resection *En bloc* resection with associated mesenteric nodal basin • Terminal ileum tumors: Also undergo right colon resection • Duodenum cancer: Pancreaticoduodenectomy Adjuvant 5-FU chemotherapy often used	**Most common malignant tumor** Most frequently in the **duodenum**
Gastrointestinal stromal tumor (GIST)	Mutations in **c-kit** (CD117, a tyrosine kinase)	Intermittent pain secondary to obstruction, intussusception, or bleeding	CT scan, endoscopy/EUS	Segmental bowel resection with negative margins (no lymphadenectomy as tumors rarely metastasize to lymph nodes). Chemoradiation not effective, but Adjuvant **imatinib mesylate (Gleevec)**, a tyrosine kinase inhibitor, can cause radiographic and histologic regression of metastatic lesions and improve recurrence-free survival in high-risk patients (tumor rupture, tumor >5 cm, >10 mitosis per HPF, tumor 2.1-5 cm with >5 mitosis per HPF, or metastatic disease)	Equal bowel distribution Histologic grade and tumor size predict survival Risk factors for recurrence include tumor size, a high mitotic rate, and tumor rupture

Primary small-bowel lymphomas	Majority are non-Hodgkin, B-cell lymphomas (NHL); arise de novo or in association with a preexisting systemic condition (celiac disease, CD, or immune suppression)	Highly variable, nonspecific	CT scan, endoscopy, PET scan Operation is frequently required for histologic confirmation	Based on subtype, similar to lymphoma arising in the periphery Surgery may be indicated for bowel obstruction, bleeding, or perforation	Most frequently in the **ileum**
Neuroendocrine tumor (NET)	Arise from enterochromaffin cells of intestinal crypts	Asymptomatic until advanced disease causes local symptoms (obstruction, pain, bleeding) or metastasis results in **carcinoid syndrome**	Gold standard: 24-h urinary 5-hydroxy-indoleacetic acid **(5-HIAA)**. Serum chromogranin A (high sensitivity); multiphasic CT; 68-Ga DOTATATE PET/CT or 111-In pentetreotide (OctreoScan) to evaluate for metastasis	Operative resection with examination of the entire bowel as 30% of cases have **synchronous lesions** • Jejunum/ileum tumors: Surgical segmental bowel resection • Duodenal/periampullary tumors: Pancreaticoduodenectomy • Locally advanced disease requires aggressive resection • Metastasis: Solitary liver lesions should be resected Chemoradiation minimally effective **Octreotide**, a somatostatin analogue, used palliatively for carcinoid syndrome	Most occur within 2 ft of the **ileocecal valve** More likely to metastasize than other GI NETs

ERCP, endoscopic retrograde cholangiopancreatography; EUS, endoscopic ultrasound; 5-FU, 5-fluorouracil; HPF, high power field; PET, positron emission tomography.

4. **Carcinoid syndrome** occurs when there has been metastatic spread of a neuroendocrine tumor to the liver in sufficient volume to lead to hormone release and systemic symptoms.
   a. Hormones released by carcinoid tumors are normally metabolized by the liver and produce no symptoms; however, hormones released by hepatic metastases drain into the systemic circulation causing diarrhea and flushing of the face, neck, and upper chest when there is tumor in sufficient volume. Tachycardia, hypotension, bronchospasm, and coma may be observed. In long-standing carcinoid syndrome, patients develop right-sided heart endocardial and valvular fibrosis.

C. Metastatic disease
1. Metastases from different cancers can spread to the small bowel, and palliative resection, diversion, or bypass may be appropriate for symptomatic relief.
   a. Several primary cancers are known to metastasize to the small intestine including melanoma, colorectal, gynecologic, breast, stomach, lung, prostate, and renal cancers.
2. Median survival is poor, and cases should be considered individually.
3. Palliative gastrostomy with or without TPN may be appropriate in advanced cases.

VI. CROHN'S DISEASE

A. Crohn's disease (CD) is an idiopathic, chronic, granulomatous IBD that can affect any part of the GI tract from mouth to anus.
1. CD is incurable, slowly progressive, and may be characterized by episodes of exacerbation and remission.
2. Incidence of CD varies by geography with lower rates in Asia and the Middle East and higher rates in Europe and North America.

B. Etiology/bowel involvement
1. The cause of CD is unknown but is believed to involve both genetic and environmental factors.
   a. CD is 25 times more common among patients with a family history and has a concordance rate of 60% in monozygotic twins.
   b. Environmental aspects, such as smoking, also increase the risk of developing CD.
2. Pathogenesis likely relates to a defective mucosal barrier and/or dysregulated intestinal immunity leading to chronic inflammation within the intestinal wall. Intestinal dysbiosis has been recognized in CD, but it is unknown if it is a cause or effect of the disease.
3. The **terminal ileum** is the most common site of disease. Disease affecting both the small and large intestines (primarily ileum) occurs in 55% of patients. Small bowel–only disease occurs in 30% of patients, whereas colonic-only disease occurs in 15% to 20%. **Perianal** involvement commonly coexists with more proximal forms, and isolated anorectal disease is rare.

C. Clinical presentation
1. CD has a highly variable presentation.
2. Physical examination: No physical signs are pathognomonic for CD, although the appearance of the perineum, if multiple fistulas and skin tags are present, may be highly suggestive.

3. **Diarrhea** occurs in almost all patients. Patients with ileal disease may present with SBO symptoms or have **steatorrhea** secondary to bile salt deficiency.
4. **Abdominal pain** typically is colicky, worse after meals, relieved by defecation, and poorly localized.
5. **Weight loss** occurs as a result of decreased oral intake, malabsorption, protein-losing enteropathy, and/or steatorrhea when small bowel is involved (less likely with isolated colonic disease). Children with CD may develop vitamin and mineral deficiencies and stunted growth and development.
6. Constitutional symptoms such as malaise and fever are common.
7. Anorectal disease may precede intestinal symptoms.
8. **Extraintestinal manifestations** can be numerous, including conjunctivitis, iritis, uveitis, pyoderma gangrenosum, erythema nodosum multiforme, arthritis, and ankylosing spondylitis.

D. Diagnosis

1. **Endoscopy:** Lower, and sometimes upper, endoscopy is crucial for determination of location and severity of disease as well as diagnostic biopsies. Those with long-standing colitis (>7-10 years) are at increased risk for **adenocarcinoma**, and surveillance colonoscopy for cancer is imperative (see Chapter 23).
   a. The Simple Endoscopic Score for Crohn's Disease (SES-CD) is an **endoscopic scoring system** used in the diagnosis of CD.[7] The ileum, right colon, transverse colon, left colon, and rectum are each scored on a scale of 0 to 3 for the following endoscopic parameters: Ulcer size, ulcerated and affected surfaces, and stenosis. A higher score indicates more severe disease.
   b. Other indices exist, such as Crohn's Disease Endoscopic Index of Severity and the Rutgeerts' score for postoperative CD.[8]
2. **Pathology/histology:** CD is characterized by **transmural inflammation**.
   a. Grossly, the bowel is thickened with creeping fat, corkscrew vessels, and a shortened fibrotic mesentery with lymphadenopathy.
   b. Mucosal changes include pinpoint hemorrhages, aphthous ulcers, deep linear fissures, crypt abscesses, and/or **cobblestoning.**
   c. These findings commonly occur segmentally, causing **skip lesions** along the intestine, but can be continuous.
   d. **Granulomas (noncaseating)** are found in the bowel wall in 40% to 60% of patients.
3. **Imaging**
   a. **CT enterography** (CTE) and **magnetic resonance enterography** (MRE) are imaging modalities of choice to evaluate the small bowel in CD.
      i. MRE is typically favored as it avoids radiation exposure in patients who will likely require multiple evaluations over the course of their lifetime.
      ii. Enterography, or the use of a contrast agent to distend the bowel, is useful in evaluating bowel inflammation, disease distribution, and complications such as strictures.

b. SBFT is another frequently utilized imaging modality. Although less sensitive than MRE or CTE, SBFT allows for visualization of CD features such as narrowing of the bowel lumen, cobblestoning, and fistula formation.

E. Treatment

1. **Medical management** is the first-line treatment for CD to palliate symptoms and reduce inflammation.
   a. Treatment is dictated by the disease location, severity, presence of complications, and treatment goal (to induce or maintain disease remission).
   b. We recommend the following published guidelines regarding management of these patients: American Gastroenterological Association (AGA) and European Crohn's and Colitis Organisation (ECCO).[9,10]
      i. Glucocorticoids, with or without addition of a thiopurine, are often used to **induce remission**. In patients with severe or fulminant colitis, patients are hospitalized for treatment, which includes bowel rest, TPN, and IV glucocorticoids. Patients who are steroid dependent or steroid resistant may require treatment **with immunomodulator or biologic therapies** (or resection).
      ii. A summary of these medications can be found in **Table 16.8**.
2. **Surgical management** is indicated when medical therapy has failed or to address complications such as high-output fistulas, perforation, intra-abdominal abscess, severe colitis, bleeding, obstruction from fibrotic strictures, or dysplasia/malignancy.
   a. **Small bowel resection/ileocolic resection:** At the time of operation, the most important principle is to correct the complication while *preserving bowel length* to prevent SBS.
      i. Resection to histologically negative margins does not reduce the likelihood of disease recurrence; therefore, grossly normal margins are acceptable.[11]
      ii. **Surgical approach: Small intestinal resection/ileocolic resection**
         a) Resection can be performed via open or minimally invasive (laparoscopic or robotic) techniques.
         b) After initial access/exploration, mobilize the cecum/ascending colon if ileocolic resection, transect the small intestine/colon on either side of the affected bowel segment, typically using a stapling device, with grossly negative margins (more extensive for malignancy).
         c) The associated mesentery is then divided, using either clamps and ties or an energy device. For cancerous lesions, the mesentery is resected down to the base while preserving mesentery to the remaining bowel.
         d) The anastomosis is then created. Commonly, a side-to-side enteroenterostomy is created using a stapling device, although a hand-sewn anastomosis is also acceptable.
         e) Abdomen is closed.
      iii. In the absence of free perforation, large abscesses, massively dilated bowel, severe malnutrition, or high-dose immunosuppression, primary anastomosis is safe.

TABLE 16-8 Drugs Used in the Medical Management of Crohn's Disease

Drug Class	Mechanism of Action	Route	Use
Glucocorticoids Budesonide Prednisone Prednisolone Methylprednisolone	Represses expression of proinflammatory cytokines and adhesion molecules by immune cells	Oral or IV (severe disease)	Inducing remission, bridge to immunomodulator or biologic therapy
Aminosalicylates (5-ASA) Sulfasalazine Mesalamine	Immunomodulator: Interferes with the metabolism of arachidonic acid to prostaglandins and leukotrienes	Oral	Second-line induction/maintenance in mild to moderate colonic or ileocolonic disease
Thiopurines Azathioprine 6-mercaptopurine	Immunomodulator: Incorporated into DNA to halt cellular replication	Oral	Maintaining remission; reduce immunogenicity against biologic therapy
Methotrexate (MTX)	Immunomodulator: Binds to dihydrofolate reductase to inhibit folate synthesis and subsequently inhibits DNA synthesis, repair, and cellular replication	IM/SC, then transition to oral	Maintaining remission; reduce immunogenicity against biologic therapy
Antitumor necrosis factor-alpha (anti-TNF) antagonists Infliximab (Remicade) Adalimumab (Humira) Certolizumab (Cimzia)	Monoclonal antibody: Binds to TNF-alpha to prevent induction of proinflammatory cells and cytokines	IV, SC	Induction and maintenance in patients who have an inadequate response to above
Anti-integrin antibodies Natalizumab (Tysabri) Vedolizumab (Entyvio)	Monoclonal antibody: Binds to integrin and prevents migration of lymphocytes from the vasculature into inflamed tissue	IV	Induction and maintenance in patients who have an inadequate response to above
Anti-interleukin antibodies Ustekinumab (Stelara)	Monoclonal antibody: Binds to interleukin 12 and 23 to prevent natural killer cell activation and T-cell differentiation and activation	IV, SC	Induction and maintenance in patients who have an inadequate response to above

iv. If primary anastomosis is not able to be completed at the time of resection, an ileostomy may be needed (or a loop ileostomy to divert proximal to threatened/tenuous anastomosis), and then closure of the stoma can be completed later when conditions for wound healing are improved.

b. **Surgical approach: Brooke ileostomy creation**

i. If possible, prior to the operation, the patient should be marked for stoma location in the lying, sitting, and standing positions. The stoma should be located on a flat surface, in a position where the patient can see the stoma, and free from any areas of crease or the beltline, ideally through the rectus abdominis.

ii. Excise a circular skin opening at the stoma site, approximately 2 to 3 cm in diameter.

iii. Vertically incise the subcutaneous fat (excise some, if needed) and the anterior rectus sheath (cruciate incision acceptable).

iv. Split the rectus muscle vertically and incise the posterior rectus sheath and/or peritoneum depending on the location on the abdominal wall.

v. Via open or laparoscopic approach, bring the ileum up through the opening until there is adequate projection of ileum above the skin. Ensure that the mesentery is in proper orientation and is not twisted when the bowel is brought up to the abdominal wall (**Figure 16.3**).

vi. Open the distal end of the ileum and place absorbable sutures in four quadrants with a full-thickness bite of the distal open end of the bowel, a seromuscular bite of the bowel at the skin level, followed by a bite of the dermis using a single stitch (**Figure 16.4**). When these sutures are tied, the distal mucosa is everted. Place interrupted sutures from the open end of the bowel to the dermis in between the four quadrant stitches (**Figure 16.5**). The final everted stoma can be seen in **Figure 16.6**.

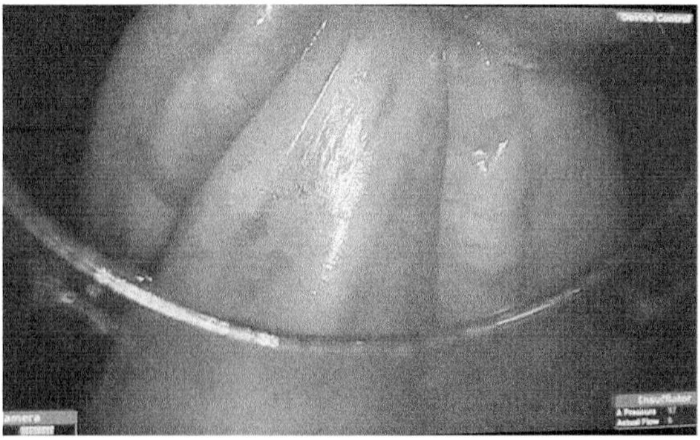

FIGURE 16.3 Confirming loop ileostomy bowel orientation laparoscopically.

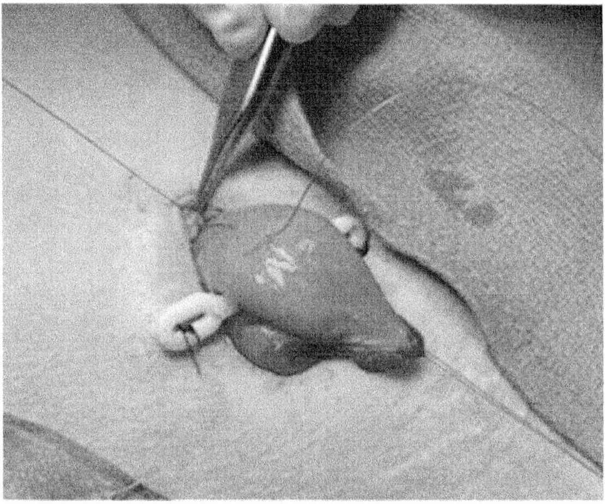

FIGURE 16.4 Placement of three-point everting sutures.

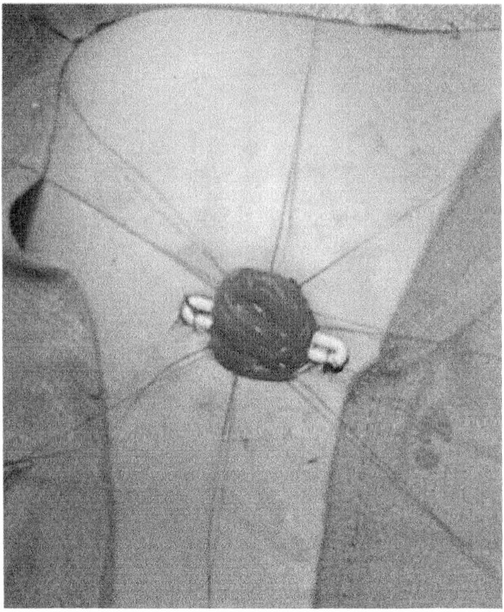

FIGURE 16.5 Ileostomy eversion with stay sutures in place.

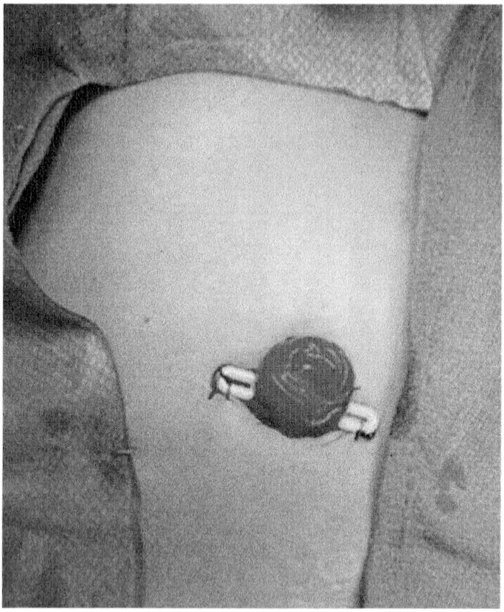

FIGURE 16.6 Completed loop ileostomy.

c. **Surgical approach: Local loop ileostomy closure**
   i. A loop ileostomy closure can be completed in a stapled or a hand-sewn fashion.
   ii. The bowel is dissected away from the skin and cleared from the subcutaneous tissues and fascia, any abdominal adhesions at the site are freed, and the bowel is elevated to the abdominal wall (**Figure 16.7**). The ileostomy itself can be excised and sent to pathology depending on the state of that bowel and its usefulness for the anastomosis.
   iii. A side-to-side anastomosis is created in routine fashion (**Figures 16.8** and **16.9**). If performing a hand-sewn closure, the defect in the bowel wall that was made to create the ostomy is closed.
   iv. Once anastomosis is returned to the abdomen and fascia closed, the skin can be partially closed (wicks or drains optional) to allow for continued drainage from the wound during healing (**Figure 16.10**).

d. **Surgical approach: End ileostomy closure**
   i. Can be completed via open or minimally invasive techniques, depending on the circumstances.
   ii. The patient can be in supine positioning for planned anastomosis to the left or transverse colon, whereas the patient should

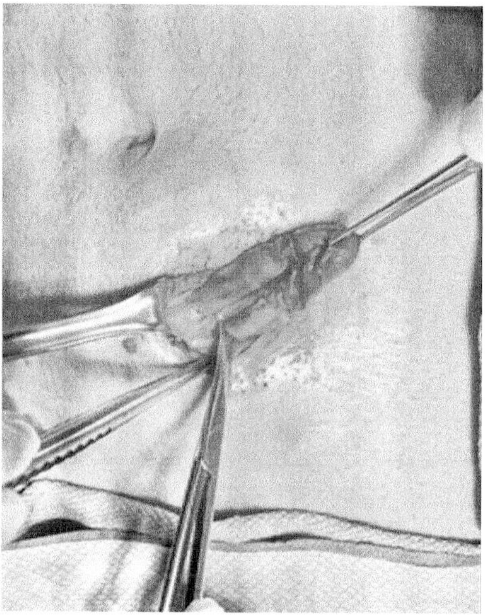

FIGURE 16.7 Ileostomy closure: freeing subcutaneous tissues.

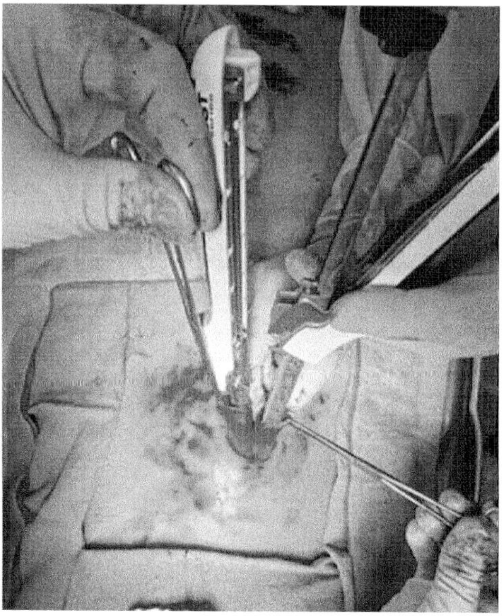

FIGURE 16.8 Ileostomy closure: initial stapling to create side-to-side anastomosis.

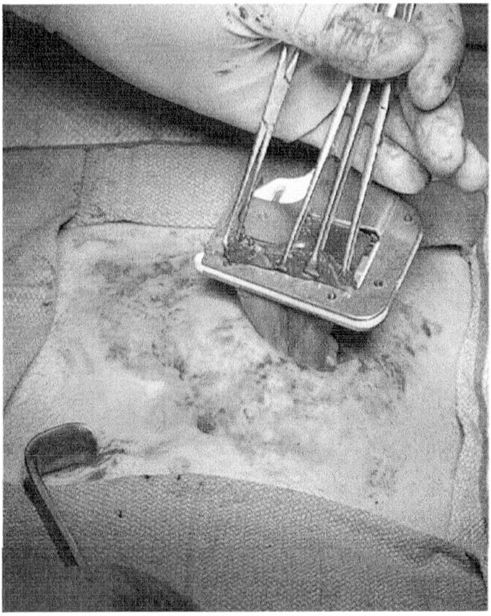

FIGURE 16.9 Ileostomy closure: completing the stapled anastomosis.

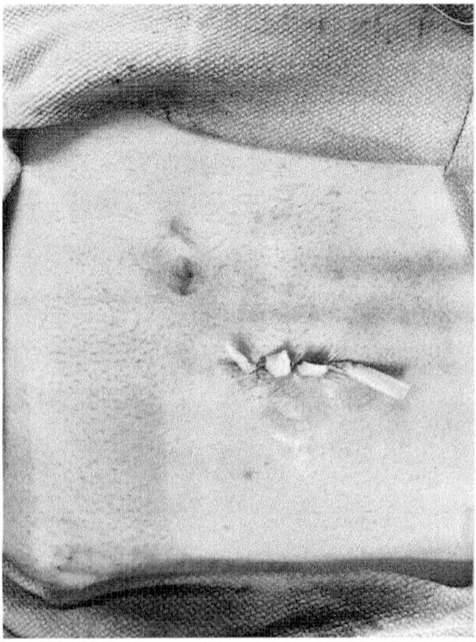

FIGURE 16.10 Ileostomy closure: final wound with drain wicks in place.

be in lithotomy position if an ileorectal or ileoanal anastomosis with J-pouch is to be completed.

iii. The distal bowel ("target") is identified in the abdomen before the ostomy is taken down.

iv. The ileostomy is then taken down, returned to the abdomen, and anastomosed to the distal bowel in either a stapled or hand-sewn fashion.

v. The abdomen is closed, and the stoma site is managed as with loop ileostomy closure of the skin above.

e. Laparoscopic resections are safe alternatives to open procedures.

f. Strictures of appropriate length and type can be treated with **stricturoplasty** to preserve bowel length (**Figure 16.11**).

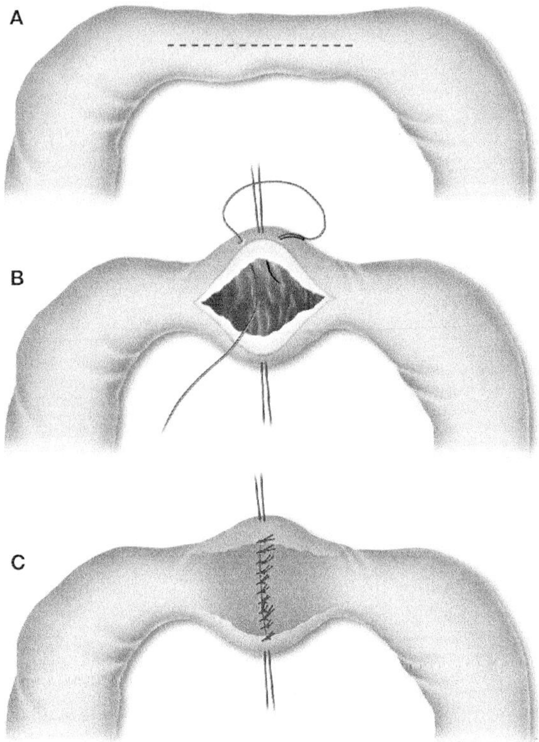

FIGURE 16.11 Stricturoplasty A, Full-thickness, longitudinal incision is made on the antimesenteric border of the strictured segment of bowel. B and C, The incision is closed transversely in one (B) or two (C) layers to relieve any obstruction while preserving bowel length. *(Reprinted with permission from Yeo H, Michelassi F. Heineke-Mikulicz, finney, and michelassi strictureplasty. In: Wexner SD, Fleshman JW, eds. Colon and Rectal Surgery: Abdominal Operations. 2nd ed. Wolters Kluwer; 2019:653-660. Figure 70-1.)*

g. Unfortunately, there are high rates of recurrent stricture at the anastomosis following resection for CD. The **Kono-S anastomosis (Figure 16.12)**, which is a functional end-to-end anastomosis, is gaining popularity as a reconstruction option after small bowel resection in patients with CD in attempts to reduce recurrence.[12]
   i. Early studies have demonstrated this configuration to be effective in reducing the risk of surgical recurrence in CD.[13]
h. Patients undergoing operation for presumed acute appendicitis but are found to have Crohn's ileitis should undergo appendectomy if the cecum is not inflamed. The terminal ileum should not be removed at that time unless absolutely necessary.

F. Prognosis: CD is a chronic, pan-intestinal disease that currently has no cure and requires chronic, lifelong treatment, with operation reserved for severe complications.

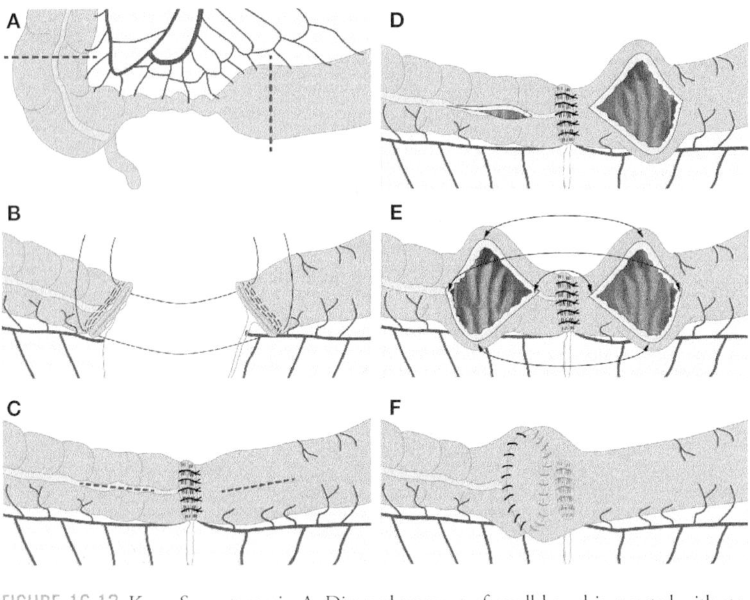

FIGURE 16.12 Kono-S anastomosis. A, Diseased segment of small bowel is resected with staplers placed perpendicular to the mesentery. B, The bowel stumps are then sutured together with absorbable suture to form a supporting column. C, Starting approximately 0.5 mm-1 cm from the support column on either side (D) the bowel is opened longitudinally at the antimesenteric border. E, The longitudinal incisions are closed transversely in a hand-sewn fashion. F, Completed anastomosis with support column to help reduce recurrent postoperative strictures. *(Reprinted from Horisberger K, Birrer DL, Rickenbacher A, et al. Experiences with the Kono-S anastomosis in Crohn's disease of the terminal ileum-a cohort study. Langenbecks Arch Surg. 2021;406(4):1173-1180. http://creativecommons.org/licenses/by/4.0/.)*

Key References

Citation	Summary
Maung AA, Johnson DC, Piper GL, et al. Evaluation and management of small-bowel obstruction: An Eastern Association for the Surgery of Trauma practice management guideline. *J Trauma Acute Care Surg*. 2012;73(5 suppl 4):S362-S369.	• The Eastern Association for the Surgery of Trauma (EAST) evidence-based guidelines for the management of SBO. Unless patients have signs of peritonitis, clinical deterioration, or evidence of bowel ischemia on imaging, patients can safely undergo initial nonoperative management for partial or complete SBO. Water-soluble contrast study should be done in 48-72 h if obstruction is not resolved for diagnostic and therapeutic purposes.
Zielinski MD, Haddad NN, Cullinane DC, et al. Multi-institutional, prospective, observational study comparing the Gastrografin challenge versus standard treatment in adhesive small bowel obstruction. *J Trauma Acute Care Surg*. 2017;83(1):47-54.	• Patients receiving Gastrografin for adhesive small bowel obstruction had lower rates of exploration and shorter hospital length of stay compared with patients who did not.
Daperno M, D'Haens G, Van Assche G, et al. Development and validation of a new, simplified endoscopic activity score for Crohn's disease: the SES-CD. *Gastrointest Endosc*. 2004;60(4):505-512.	• The Simple Endoscopic Score for Crohn's Disease is a reproducible and easy-to-use endoscopic scoring system for Crohn's disease, which is used to monitor disease progression and treatment efficacy.
Feuerstein JD, Ho EY, Shmidt E, et al. AGA clinical practice guidelines on the medical management of moderate to severe luminal and perianal fistulizing Crohn's disease. *Gastroenterology*. 2021;160(7):2496-2508.	• The American Gastroenterological Association (AGA) evidence-based guidelines for the medical management of Crohn's disease.
Torres J, Bonovas S, Doherty G, et al. ECCO guidelines on therapeutics in Crohn's disease: medical treatment. *J Crohns Colitis*. 2020;14(1):4-22.	• The European Crohn's and Colitis Organisation (ECCO) evidence-based guidelines for the medical management of Crohn's disease.
Kono T, Fichera A, Maeda K, et al. Kono-S anastomosis for surgical prophylaxis of anastomotic recurrence in crohn's disease: an international multicenter study. *J Gastrointest Surg*. 2016;20(4):783-790.	• The Kono-S anastomosis, or antimesenteric functional end-to-end handsewn anastomosis, is a safe and effective technique in reducing the risk of surgical recurrence of Crohn's disease.

CHAPTER 16: SMALL INTESTINE

Review Questions

1. What is the first-line treatment for a partial small bowel obstruction (pSBO) in a stable patient without peritonitis?
2. Stable patients with SBO who do not have return of bowel function within 48 hours after adequate decompression should undergo what diagnostic and possibly therapeutic intervention?
3. Patients who have high-output fistulas (more than 500 mL daily) should use what mode of nutrition?
4. What are factors that might prevent spontaneous fistula closure?
5. What is the mechanism of action of imatinib mesylate (Gleevec) used in the treatment of GIST tumors?
6. What is the preferred imaging modality to best assess the extent and other abdominal pathologies associated with ileal Crohn's disease?
7. What is the preferred surgical approach for a short-segment small bowel stricture in a patient who has had multiple resections and is at risk for short bowel syndrome?

REFERENCES

1. Maung AA, Johnson DC, Piper GL, et al. Evaluation and management of small-bowel obstruction: an Eastern Association for the Surgery of Trauma practice management guideline. *J Trauma Acute Care Surg*. 2012;73(5 suppl 4):S362-S369.
2. Ten Broek RPG, Krielen P, Di Saverio S, et al. Bologna guidelines for diagnosis and management of adhesive small bowel obstruction (ASBO): 2017 update of the evidence-based guidelines from the world society of emergency surgery ASBO working group. *World J Emerg Surg*. 2018;13:24.
3. Zielinski MD, Haddad NN, Cullinane DC, et al. Multi-institutional, prospective, observational study comparing the Gastrografin challenge versus standard treatment in adhesive small bowel obstruction. *J Trauma Acute Care Surg*. 2017;83(1):47-54.
4. Stevens P, Burden S, Delicata R, Carlson G, Lal S. Somatostatin analogues for treatment of enterocutaneous fistula. *Cochrane Database Syst Rev*. 2019;2019(6):CD010489.
5. Gribovskaja-Rupp I, Melton GB. Enterocutaneous fistula: proven strategies and updates. *Clin Colon Rectal Surg*. 2016;29(2):130-137.
6. Kochar B, Long MD, Shelton E, et al. Safety and efficacy of teduglutide (Gattex) in patients with Crohn's disease and need for parenteral support due to short bowel syndrome-associated intestinal failure. *J Clin Gastroenterol*. 2017;51(6):508-511.
7. Daperno M, D'Haens G, Van Assche G, et al. Development and validation of a new, simplified endoscopic activity score for Crohn's disease: the SES-CD. *Gastrointest Endosc*. 2004;60(4):505-512.
8. Hart L, Bessissow T. Endoscopic scoring systems for the evaluation and monitoring of disease activity in Crohn's disease. *Best Pract Res Clin Gastroenterol*. 2019;38-39:101616.
9. Feuerstein JD, Ho EY, Shmidt E, et al. AGA clinical practice guidelines on the medical management of moderate to severe luminal and perianal fistulizing Crohn's disease. *Gastroenterology*. 2021;160(7):2496-2508.
10. Torres J, Bonovas S, Doherty G, et al. ECCO guidelines on therapeutics in Crohn's disease: medical treatment. *J Crohns Colitis*. 2020;14(1):4-22.

11. Fazio VW, Marchetti F, Church M, et al. Effect of resection margins on the recurrence of Crohn's disease in the small bowel. A randomized controlled trial. *Ann Surg.* 1996;224(4):563-571; discussion 571-573.

12. Horisberger K, Birrer DL, Rickenbacher A, Turina M. Experiences with the Kono-S anastomosis in Crohn's disease of the terminal ileum-a cohort study. *Langenbeck's Arch Surg.* 2021;406(4):1173-1180.

13. Kono T, Fichera A, Maeda K, et al. Kono-S anastomosis for surgical prophylaxis of anastomotic recurrence in Crohn's disease: an International multicenter study. *J Gastrointest Surg.* 2016;20(4):783-790.

17 Surgical Diseases of the Liver

Sandra Garcia Aroz and William C. Chapman

I. INTRODUCTION

Liver lesions whether benign or malignant may cause symptoms prompting workup or remain asymptomatic until incidentally detected by imaging. Although some lesions are appropriate for surveillance and conservative management, surgery often plays an important role.

A. Segmental and surgical anatomy
   1. **Cantlie line**, extending from the gallbladder fossa to the inferior vena cava (IVC), is the functional plane between the left and right liver.
   2. French surgeon Claude **Couinaud** delineated the functional anatomy of the liver into eight segments with distinct arterial, venous, and biliary inflow and outflow (**Figure 17.1**).
   3. The **Brisbane Terminology** has further standardized segmental and surgical anatomy (**Table 17.1**).

B. Anatomic features
   1. Inflow
      a. **Venous**
         i. The **portal vein** (PV) supplies 75% of vascular inflow
      b. **Arterial**
         i. The **hepatic artery** (HA) supplies 25% of vascular inflow
            a) Celiac axis → **common HA** → **proper HA**, which runs anteriorly and medially within the porta hepatis.
            b) A **replaced** (or accessory) **right HA** arises from the superior mesenteric artery in about 20% of cases and courses posterior to the bile duct and lateral to the PV.
            c) A **replaced** (or accessory) **left HA** arises from the left gastric artery in around 15% of cases and runs in the gastrohepatic ligament.
   2. Outflow
      a. **Venous**
         i. Three **hepatic veins** drain into the IVC.
         ii. In most cases, the **left** and **middle hepatic veins** join just prior to insertion into the IVC.
      b. **Biliary**
         i. The **common bile duct** lies anterior and lateral in the porta. Similar to the PV, the **left hepatic duct** takes a longer extrahepatic course than the **right hepatic duct**.

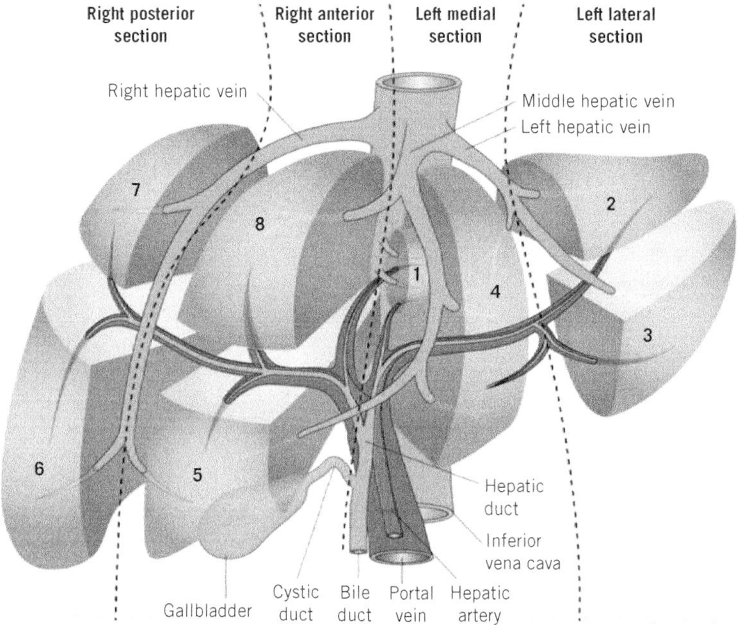

FIGURE 17.1 Schematic of liver anatomy separating the parenchyma into eight anatomic segments. Each segment has its own blood supply and biliary drainage. *(Reprinted from López-Terrada D, Alaggio R, de Dávila MT, et al. Towards an international pediatric liver tumor consensus classification: proceedings of the Los Angeles COG liver tumors symposium. Mod Pathol. 2014;27(3):472-491. Copyright 2014, United States & Canadian Academy of Pathology. With permission.)*

C. Physiology

1. **Bilirubin**
   a. Product of heme catabolism.
   b. Heme is conjugated to glucuronic acid by glucuronyl transferase, generating water-soluble **conjugated (direct) bilirubin,** which is excreted in bile.
2. **Bile**
   a. Liver produces approximately 1 L of bile a day.
   b. >90% of excreted bile salts are absorbed in the terminal ileum and transported back to the liver (**enterohepatic circulation**).
   c. The liver controls several metabolic processes including gluconeogenesis, glycogenolysis, and protein metabolism.
3. **Laboratory testing (Figure 17.2)**
4. **Liver failure and cirrhosis**
   a. Grading
      i. **Child–Pugh score** was originally used to predict surgical mortality and is now widely used to classify liver failure severity and predict survival (**Table 17.2**).

TABLE 17.1 Brisbane Terminology of Liver Anatomy and Resections

Segment	Second-Order Division	First-Order Division
I (Caudate)		
II	Left lateral section	Left liver or left hemiliver
III		
IV	Left medial section	
V	Right anterior section, along with Section VIII	Right liver or right hemiliver
VI	Right posterior section	
VII		
VIII	Right anterior section, along with Section V	

ii. **Model for End-Stage Liver Disease (MELD)** is employed by the United Network for Organ Sharing (UNOS) for prioritization on the liver transplant waitlist. The equation incorporates serum **bilirubin, international normalized ratio (INR), and creatinine.**

a) Patients with scores ≥10 should be referred to a hepatologist for management and consideration of organ transplantation.

b. Portal hypertension

i. The gold standard measurement is **hepatic venous pressure gradient** (difference between free and wedged hepatic venous pressures).

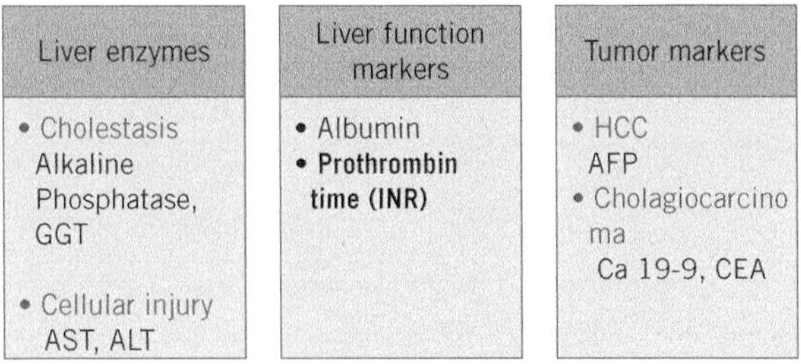
Liver enzymes
• Cholestasis
Alkaline Phosphatase, GGT
• Cellular injury
AST, ALT
Liver function markers
• Albumin
• Prothrombin time (INR)
Tumor markers
• HCC
AFP
• Cholagiocarcinoma
Ca 19-9, CEA

FIGURE 17.2 Laboratory testing. AFP, alpha fetoprotein; ALT, alanine aminotransferase; AST, aspartate aminotransferase; Ca 19-9, carbohydrate antigen 19-9; CEA, carcinoembryonic antigen; GGT, gamma-glutamyl transferase; HCC, hepatocellular carcinoma; INR, international normalized ratio.

TABLE 17.2 Child–Pugh Classification of Severity of Cirrhosis

	Points Assigned		
Parameter	1	2	3
Ascites	Absent	Slight	Moderate
Bilirubin	<2 mg/dL (<34.2 μmol/L)	2-3 mg/dL (34.2-51.3 μmol/L)	>3 mg/dL (>51.3 μmol/L)
Albumin	>3.5 g/dL (35 g/L)	2.8-3.5 g/dL (28-35 g/L)	<2.8 g/dL (<28 g/L)
Prothrombin time	<4	4-6	>6
INR	<1.7	1.7-2.3	>2.3
Encephalopathy	None	Grade 1-2	Grade 3-4

Class A (5-6, least severe), B (7-9, moderately severe), or C (10-15, most severe).

a) **≥8 mm Hg** suggests intrinsic liver disease.
b) Varices develop ≥10 mm Hg.
c) Treatment goal is reduction to <12 mm Hg.

II. BENIGN LIVER TUMORS

A. Hemangioma

1. **Presentation**
   a. The most common benign liver tumor
   b. Flat, red-blue, well circumscribed, soft, and compressible
   c. Uncommon, but occurs in up to 5% of the population.
   d. Malignant degeneration does not occur.
   e. Rupture is extremely rare.
2. **Diagnosis**
   a. Multiphase contrast-enhanced CT and MRI are almost always diagnostic, eliminating the need for biopsy.
      i. Peripheral **centripetal enhancement** progressing to confluence over time (**Figure 17.3**).
      ii. Marked T2 hyperintensity (bright signal) on MRI
3. **Management**
   a. Asymptomatic lesions can be observed.
   b. Intervention is reserved for hemorrhage or in cases of diagnostic uncertainty.
   c. Can be enucleated under careful vascular control.
   d. Acute hemorrhage is typically treated with embolization.

B. Focal nodular hyperplasia (FNH)

1. **Presentation**
   a. The second most common benign hepatic tumor

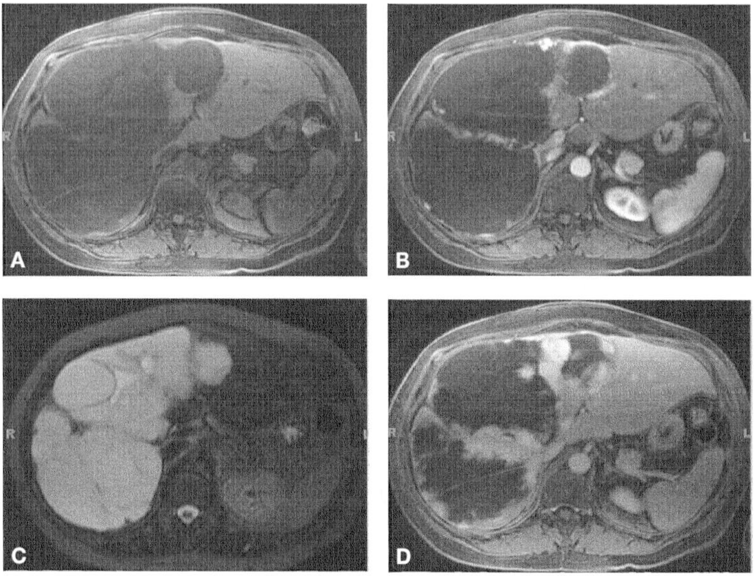

FIGURE 17.3 Large cavernous hemangioma. Characteristic peripheral interrupted puddling that progresses during dynamic imaging (A, B, and D) along with the characteristically bright signal intensity on T2-weighted imaging (C) provides a definitive diagnosis of hemangioma on MRI.

b. Predominantly in women of child-bearing age (association between FNH and hormonal exposure is not as strong as for hepatic adenomas).
c. Solitary lesions, well circumscribed, lobulated, and unencapsulated.
d. Rarely symptomatic, with pain, palpable mass, or rupture.

2. **Diagnosis**
   a. MRI with gadoxetate disodium (Eovist, Bayer) or gadobenate dimeglumine (MultiHance, Bracco) is the test of choice with near 100% specificity
   b. **Homogeneous enhancement on the arterial phase**
   c. **Central "stellate" fibrous scar** with delayed enhancement on MRI with hepatobiliary phase imaging (**Figure 17.4**)
3. **Management**
   a. No role for resection except if symptomatic (e.g., pain) or with diagnostic uncertainty despite adequate imaging

C. Hepatic adenoma

1. **Presentation**
   a. Benign proliferations of hepatocytes
   b. Frequently found in young women due to **association with synthetic estrogen and progesterone use**, most commonly oral contraceptive pills
   c. Solitary, round, well-circumscribed, unencapsulated lesions

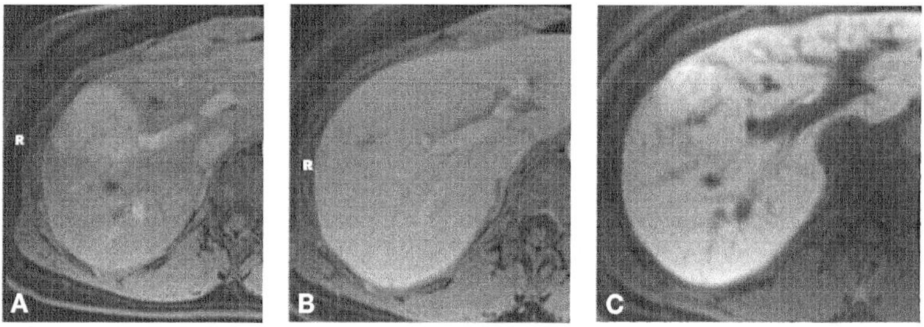

FIGURE 17.4 Focal nodular hyperplasia (FNH). Arterial phase hyperenhancement (A) and equilibration during portal venous (B) or later postcontrast phases, along with retention of contrast similar to or brighter than the background liver during the hepatobiliary phase (C), are classic features of FNH. MRI performed with hepatobiliary contrast agents can provide definitive diagnosis of FNH.

d. Pathologic examination reveals sheets of normal hepatocytes separated by dilated sinusoids without **bile ductules, distinguishing adenomas from FNH**.
e. Asymptomatic or vague abdominal pain/discomfort and fullness
f. Can present with severe pain in cases of **rupture and hemorrhage**
g. Bleeding can occur at high rates (>50%) depending on the size and location of the lesions.[1]

2. **Diagnosis**
   a. Multiphasic MRI or CT
      i. Heterogeneity due to hemorrhage, necrosis, and fat content
      ii. Hyperenhancing on arterial phase with variable enhancement patterns including washout or delayed central enhancement during portal venous and delayed phase imaging
3. **Management**
   a. Consideration of resection for lesions >5 cm and/or with rupture

III. ABSCESSES AND CYSTIC DISEASE

A. Pyogenic abscesses

1. **Presentation**
   a. From direct spread of bacteria via the biliary tree (cholangitis, biliary empyema) or from gastrointestinal source (diverticulitis)
   b. Immunocompromised patients are at risk for fungal abscesses.
   c. Fever and abdominal pain
2. **Diagnosis**
   a. Laboratory studies can reveal leukocytosis and elevated alkaline phosphatase, although this is nonspecific.
   b. Ultrasonography and CT can be used to characterize the size and location of disease as well as biliary duct stones or strictures that may require intervention.

3. **Management**
   a. Systemic antibiotics and resuscitation
   b. **Percutaneous drainage** with aspirated fluid cultures to guide antibiotic selection
   c. Operative drainage may be required if percutaneous access is unsafe or not feasible.

B. Amebic abscesses
1. **Presentation**
   a. Caused by hematogenous spread via the portal system of gastrointestinal infection by the protozoan *Entamoeba histolytica*
   b. Persistent fever and right upper quadrant (RUQ) pain
   c. Intestinal manifestations of amebiasis such as diarrhea may also be present.
2. **Diagnosis**
   a. Serologic antibody testing
   b. Needle aspiration can be performed when the diagnosis is unclear, yielding "anchovy paste" fluid, a combination of proteinaceous debris and necrotic hepatic tissue.
   c. Imaging reveals a cystic hypoechoic or hypoenhancing mass with peripheral enhancement.
      i. Chronic or treated lesions may be calcified.
3. **Management**
   a. Metronidazole orally or intravenously for 7 to 10 days.
   b. Drainage is rarely required.

C. Echinococcal cysts (hydatid cysts)
1. **Presentation**
   a. The most common parasitic hepatic cystic lesion
   b. RUQ pain and hepatomegaly
2. **Diagnosis**
   a. Imaging is the preferred diagnostic test.
   b. Aspiration should not be performed as the initial diagnostic test, as spillage of cyst contents can result in spread of the organisms throughout the peritoneal cavity.
3. **Management**
   a. Cyst aspiration, including cyst injection with sclerosing agents (hypertonic saline, alcohol)
   b. Careful resection to prevent spillage should be performed, if necessary, after preoperative treatment with albendazole.

D. Intrahepatic biliary cysts (simple cysts)
1. **Presentation**
   a. Found in >10% of the population
   b. More common with increasing age
   c. Often present incidentally
   d. Larger cysts can result in increased abdominal girth, abdominal discomfort, and early satiety.
2. **Diagnosis**
   a. Ultrasonography, CT, or MRI shows homogeneous hypodense lesions with smooth rounded borders.

3. **Management**
   a. Although cysts can be drained percutaneously, they frequently recur.
   b. Operative management includes fenestration, in which the cyst is unroofed, or complete enucleation.
      i. Enucleation or resection should be performed if there is concern for neoplastic cystic lesions (biliary cystadenoma, cystadenocarcinoma).
      ii. Irregular or abnormally thickened walls and mural nodules should increase suspicion for malignancy.
   c. Liver transplantation may be necessary for cases of marked hepatomegaly in the setting of polycystic liver disease not amenable to fenestration or resection.

IV. METASTATIC DISEASE

Metastatic disease is the most common malignancy affecting the liver in the US. Many gastrointestinal cancers metastasize to the liver via the portal drainage.

A. Colorectal cancer (CRC)

1. **Presentation**
   a. The most common primary malignancy responsible for metastases to the liver is CRC.
   b. Fifty percent of patients with CRC present with or develop hepatic metastases during the course of their disease.
2. **Diagnosis**
   a. Contrasted CT/MRI
      i. Homogeneous **hypoattenuating** lesions on portal venous phase imaging
3. **Management**
   a. In carefully selected cases, surgical resection is associated with 5-year survival of up to 50%, much greater than the 5-year survival for patients not undergoing resection (<20%).[2]
   b. Resection should aim for microscopically negative margins (R0 resection).
   c. For synchronous primary colorectal and metastatic hepatic disease:
      i. Two disease sites can be resected simultaneously or sequentially, with no inferior strategy in terms of morbidity or mortality.[3]
         a) Generally sequential resection is preferred when major hepatectomy would be required concurrently with a major colorectal procedure.
      ii. For high tumor burden or for tumors in close proximity to vital structures, bridging the patient to surgery can be attempted with systemic therapy or procedural treatments such as radiofrequency ablation (RFA) (see section VII: Additional Treatments).
      iii. Postoperatively, repeat physical examinations, imaging, and carcinoembryonic antigen levels should be obtained every 3 to 4 months for 2 years, then every 6 months for 3 additional years.

B. Neuroendocrine tumors

1. **Presentation**
   a. Up to 75% of patients with neuroendocrine tumors develop liver metastasis.
   b. Poorer prognosis (<50% 5-year overall survival vs. >75% for patients without metastases).[4]
   c. Once hepatic metastases occur, they can become symptomatic due to systemic release of hormonal factors resulting in flushing, diarrhea, and/or nausea.
2. **Diagnosis**
   a. MRI: **Hypervascular, hyperenhancing** lesions
3. **Management**
   a. Indications for resection
      i. Symptomatic palliation
      ii. Treatment due to limited effective chemotherapeutic options and improved long-term survival
   b. R0 (negative margins) resection has not been associated with improved survival.
   c. Regional therapy also considered for unresectable hepatic metastases.

V. MALIGNANT LIVER TUMORS

A. Hepatocellular carcinoma (HCC)

1. **Presentation**
   a. The most common primary liver tumor
   b. Annual incidence in the US of approximately 6 cases per 100,000 individuals[5]
   c. Rising incidence, attributable to increased rates of cirrhosis from several primary diagnoses
   d. Hepatitis B viral infection is a major risk factor, even in the absence of cirrhosis.
   e. Presenting symptoms for HCC are vague and may include weight loss, weakness, and dull, persistent epigastric or RUQ pain.
2. **Diagnosis**
   a. For high-risk patients (particularly those with chronic hepatitis B or cirrhosis), screening by ultrasonography with or without alpha fetoprotein (AFP) is recommended[6]; AFP elevations are nonspecific but should prompt additional studies.
   b. **Pathologic diagnosis is not necessary**
      i. Diagnosis and treatment decisions can often be made based on imaging alone.
   c. Multiphasic CT or MRI: Hyperenhancement relative to the background liver on the arterial phase **with contrast washout** (hypoenhancement) relative to the background liver in **portal venous or delayed phases (Figure 17.5)**.
   d. The **Liver Reporting and Data System (LI-RADS)** provides the criteria for HCC diagnosis.[7]

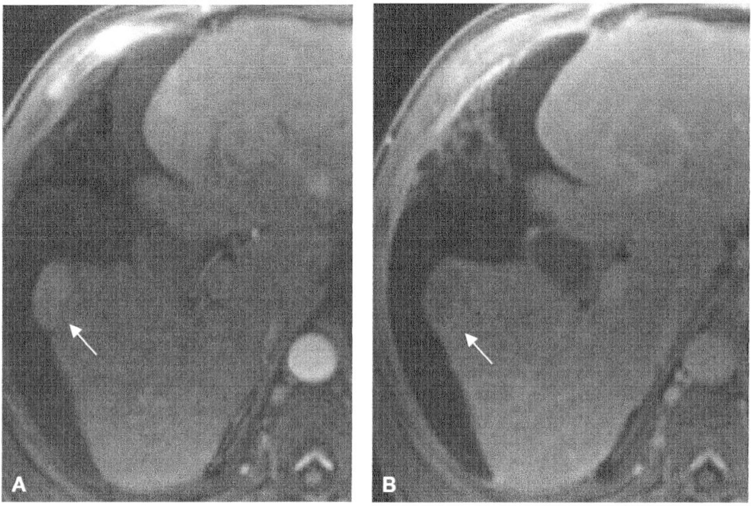

FIGURE 17.5 Hepatocellular carcinoma (HCC)—multiphase liver MRI shows mass hyperenhancement on arterial phase image (A, arrow) and washout appearance on portal venous phase image (B, arrow) relative to background liver. Dynamic multiphase imaging is essential for demonstrating features of HCC. These features in combination allow for noninvasive definitive diagnosis of HCC.

i. Categories range from "definitely benign" (LR-1) to "definitely HCC" (LR-5) based on size/growth, arterial phase hyperenhancement, "washout," and delayed enhancing capsule appearance.

3. **Management**
   a. Without treatment, HCC has a poor prognosis.
   b. Treatment depends on resectability and the patient's overall condition including suitability for transplantation.
   c. **Surgical resection**
      i. Preoperative careful assessment of future liver remnant (FLR)
      ii. Surgeons should aim for complete anatomic resections with negative 1-cm margins.
      iii. Five-year overall survival rates after resection are >50%, although recurrence rates are high.[8]
   d. **Orthotopic liver transplantation**
      i. **Milan criteria**
         a) UNOS primary metric for transplant eligibility
         b) **Single tumor <5 cm or three or fewer tumors with the largest measuring <3 cm,** without vascular invasion or metastases.
      ii. Regional therapies can be used as a bridge to transplantation (see section Additional Treatments) or for downstaging purposes.
   e. **Sorafenib**, a tyrosine kinase inhibitor, has shown modest benefit in patients with advanced HCC, with median survival prolongation of 2.8 months.
   f. **Immunotherapy is being evaluated for nontransplant candidates**.

B. Cholangiocarcinoma

1. **Presentation**
   a. The second most common primary hepatic malignancy
   b. Intrahepatic cholangiocarcinoma (ICC) accounts for 10% of all cholangiocarcinoma.
      i. Presents as dull RUQ pain, weight loss, and laboratory abnormalities including elevated alkaline phosphatase
   c. More commonly, cholangiocarcinoma involves the extrahepatic ducts (extrahepatic cholangiocarcinoma): 65% are located distally in the bile duct and are treated like periampullary tumors. These usually present with jaundice.
   d. Twenty-five percent are hilar and when resectable require combined liver and biliary tract resection.
   e. Patients with primary sclerosing cholangitis are at increased risk for cholangiocarcinoma and usually unresectable at presentation due to associated biliary strictures.
2. **Diagnosis**
   a. Unlike HCC, imaging is not considered definitive.
   b. Tissue biopsy is performed for diagnostic confirmation.
   c. Multiphase contrast-enhanced MRI/Magnetic resonance cholangiopancreatography (MRCP) or CT
      i. Peripheral arterial phase hyperenhancement, delayed central enhancement, peripheral washout, and targetoid appearance on hepatobiliary phase imaging and diffusion[7]
      ii. Other features that favor ICC include peripheral capsular retraction, ductal dilation, severe ischemia/necrosis, and marked diffusion restriction.
   d. MRI/MRCP and CT can be helpful in defining the extent of bile duct involvement (Bismuth–Corlette) and vascular involvement for surgical planning.
3. **Management**
   a. Resection is the only potential curative therapy.
   b. Radiation and chemotherapy with gemcitabine plus cisplatin are commonly employed, although overall prognosis remains poor.[9,10]

VI. SPECIFIC RESECTIONS

The type of resection is chosen based on lesion location and the ability to achieve a tumor-negative margin while leaving adequate FLR. They are divided into anatomical and nonanatomical resections (**Figure 17.6**).

A. Wedge resections

1. Nonanatomical resections
2. Used for benign or small malignant lesions located in the periphery
3. If lesions are located at the edge of the liver surface, the shape of a "V" is marked with electrocautery. This mark is used as the limit around which the parenchyma is transected.
4. When the lesion is located at the dome or in a more central location, a circle is used to mark the limit of the resection.

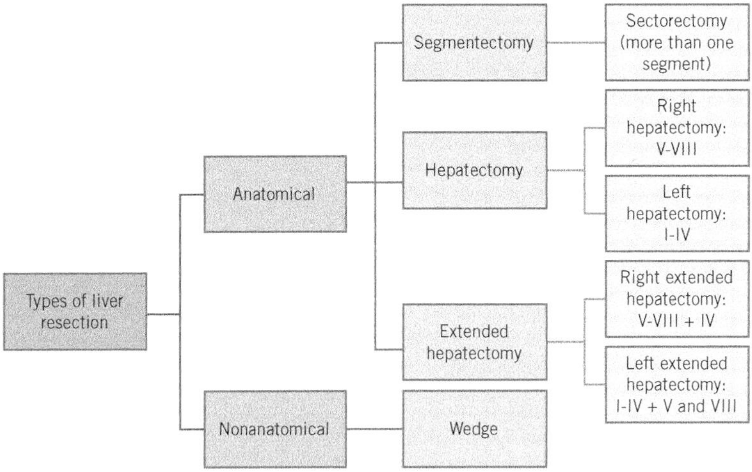

FIGURE 17.6 Types of hepatic resections.

B. Segmental resections
1. Anatomic resections refer to the resection of one or more liver segments to obtain tumor-free margins.
2. Surgical approach
   a. Intraoperative ultrasonography to confirm lesion location and margins
   b. Cholecystectomy if the resection plane extends into the gallbladder fossa, or in the setting of gallstones
   c. Dissection of the porta hepatis structures
   d. Transection plane marking is performed with the assistance of ultrasonography to identify important structures and anatomic relationships
   e. Parenchymal transection (see hepatic transection below) until the segmental blood supply is reached
   f. Confirmation of adequate blood flow to the remaining liver (temporarily clamp segmental vessels, ultrasonography)
   g. Segmental artery, portal vein, and bile duct division
   h. Segmental hepatic vein identification and division

C. Hepatectomy
1. Removal of the right (right hepatectomy) or left hemiliver (left hepatectomy)
   a. **Surgical approach**
      i. Steps a-c are performed as above.
      ii. Right/left portal vein and hepatic artery ligation as required for major hepatectomy.
      iii. Mark the transection plane using liver discoloration as transection line.
      iv. Ligate and divide the right/left hepatic duct, usually intrahepatically, once identified.

v. Identify right/left hepatic vein. Once isolated suture-ligation or vascular stapler can be considered for extrahepatic control.
vi. Finalize the parenchymal transection and check for hemostasis and bile leaks.

D. Hepatic transection

1. Many possible techniques
   a. Clamp–crush
   b. Electrocautery
   c. Water-jet dissector
   d. Devices employing ultrasonography technology (e.g., cavitron ultrasonic surgical aspirator), radiofrequency, or other electrosurgical sealing techniques
2. Vessels or bile duct branches are divided using these devices or ties, clips, or staples.
3. The **Pringle maneuver** (isolation of the portal triad and **cross-clamping** of hepatic inflow) can aid in control of bleeding.
   a. Extended periods of inflow occlusion can lead to hepatic injury, ischemia, and systemic reperfusion injury.
   b. Ideally, no more than 15 to 20 minutes of Pringle clamping at a time, with at least 5 minutes between clamping and cumulative clamp time of <120 minutes.
4. **Minimally invasive** hepatectomy
   a. Laparoscopy has become increasingly common, with excellent results, including lower morbidity and length of stay compared with open procedures.[11]
   b. Patient selection and surgeon experience play an important role in optimizing outcomes and selecting the safest surgical approach.

E. Complications

1. **Posthepatectomy bile leak**
   a. Bilirubin concentration in drain fluid at least three times serum bilirubin on or after postoperative day 3, or the need for radiologic or operative intervention due to biliary collections or bile peritonitis[12]
   b. Occurs in approximately 10% of patients and is a major cause of postoperative morbidity and extended length of stay
2. Posthepatectomy liver failure
   a. Major cause of perioperative mortality and represents impaired ability of the remnant liver to perform synthetic, excretory, and detoxifying functions
   b. Defined as an elevated INR and hyperbilirubinemia on or after postoperative day 5; if these values are elevated preoperatively, increasing INR and bilirubin on or after postoperative day 5 is used.[13]

VII. ADDITIONAL TREATMENTS

A. Portal vein embolization

1. FLR can be increased by about 10% at 1 month post embolization of the hemiliver planned for resection, with additional growth, thereafter, depending on underlying liver function.[14]

B. Two-stage hepatectomy
   1. Resectable lesions on both sides of the liver
   2. One side is resected and, following an interval of systemic therapy as necessary, the second side may be amenable to resection with sufficient FLR.

C. Associating liver partition and portal vein ligation for staged hepatectomy (ALPPS)
   1. Newer approach to improve the FLR in a short duration
   2. First, portal vein ligation is performed with hepatic artery inflow preservation to the planned future site for resection, along with hepatic transection (phase I).
   3. Following adequate hepatic hypertrophy, usually within 1 to 2 weeks, a second surgery is performed to resect the diseased liver (phase II).

D. A number of other procedures can be performed as definitive treatments in patients who are not surgical candidates or as a bridge to surgery or transplant.
   1. Trans arterial chemoembolisation, RFA, Y-90 radioembolization, and stereotactic body radiation.

Key References

Citation	Summary
Dueland S, Syversveen T, Solheim JM, et al. Survival following liver transplantation for patients with nonresectable liver-only colorectal metastases. *Ann Surg.* 2020;271(2):212-218.	• Prospective randomized controlled trial including patients with unresectable CRC liver-only metastasis. The study investigates whether more strict selection criteria can be used to obtain overall survival after liver transplantation that is comparable with that observed for conventional indication for liver transplant.
Mazzaferro V, Regalia E, Doci R, et al. Liver transplantation for the treatment of small hepatocellular carcinomas in patients with cirrhosis. *N Engl J Med.* 1996;334(11):693-699.	• Prospective study that includes patients with HCC who underwent liver transplantation (LT). The study selects patients who will achieve good outcomes after LT and defines the Milan criteria for LT. Single tumor <5 cm or three or fewer tumors with the largest measuring <3 cm, without vascular invasion or metastases.

Citation	Summary
Mazzaferro V, Citterio D, Bhoori S, et al. Liver transplantation in hepatocellular carcinoma after tumour downstaging (XXL): a randomised, controlled, phase 2b/3 trial [published correction appears in *Lancet Oncol*. 2020;21(8):e373]. *Lancet Oncol*. 2020;21(7):947-956.	• Randomized control trial comparing survival after liver transplantation vs. other therapies, in patients with HCC outside Milan criteria.
Llovet JM, Ricci S, Mazzaferro V, et al. Sorafenib in advanced hepatocellular carcinoma. *N Engl J Med*. 2008;359(4):378-390.	• Prospective, multicenter, phase 3, double-blind, randomized, placebo-controlled trial that includes patients with advanced hepatocellular carcinoma. The study compares overall survival and progression of disease after administration of sorafenib vs. placebo.

CHAPTER 17: SURGICAL DISEASES OF THE LIVER

Review Questions

1. Which CT feature is characteristic of hepatocellular carcinoma?
2. What is the best management for a simple hepatic abscess?
3. A liver mass exhibits peripheral nodular enhancement on arterial phase followed by progressive centripetal fill-in on portal venous phase. What does the lesion most likely represent?

REFERENCES

1. Bieze M, Phoa SS, Verheij J, van Lienden KP, van Gulik TM. Risk factors for bleeding in hepatocellular adenoma. *Br J Surg*. 2014;101(7):847-855.
2. Kopetz S, Chang GJ, Overman MJ, et al. Improved survival in metastatic colorectal cancer is associated with adoption of hepatic resection and improved chemotherapy. *J Clin Oncol*. 2009;27(22):3677-3683.
3. Lykoudis PM, O'Reilly D, Nastos K, Fusai G. Systematic review of surgical management of synchronous colorectal liver metastases. *Br J Surg*. 2014;101(6):605-612.
4. Lesurtel M, Nagorney DM, Mazzaferro V, Jensen RT, Poston GJ. When should a liver resection be performed in patients with liver metastases from neuroendocrine tumours? A systematic review with practice recommendations. *HPB (Oxford)*. 2015;17(1):17-22.
5. El-Serag HB, Kanwal F. Epidemiology of hepatocellular carcinoma in the United States: where are we? Where do we go? *Hepatology*. 2014;60(5):1767-1775.
6. Heimbach JK, Kulik LM, Finn RS, et al. AASLD guidelines for the treatment of hepatocellular carcinoma. *Hepatology*. 2018;67(1):358-380.
7. Fowler KJ, Potretzke TA, Hope TA, Costa EA, Wilson SR. LI-RADS M (LR-M): definite or probable malignancy, not specific for hepatocellular carcinoma. *Abdom Radiol (NY)*. 2018;43(1):149-157.

8. Lim KC, Chow PK, Allen JC, Siddiqui FJ, Chan ES, Tan SB. Systematic review of outcomes of liver resection for early hepatocellular carcinoma within the Milan criteria. *Br J Surg*. 2012;99(12):1622-1629.
9. Valle JW, Wasan H, Johnson P, et al. Gemcitabine alone or in combination with cisplatin in patients with advanced or metastatic cholangiocarcinomas or other biliary tract tumours: a multicentre randomised phase II study—the UK ABC-01 Study. *Br J Cancer*. 2009;101(4):621-627.
10. Ben-Josef E, Guthrie KA, El-Khoueiry AB, et al. SWOG S0809: a phase II intergroup trial of adjuvant capecitabine and gemcitabine followed by radiotherapy and concurrent capecitabine in extrahepatic cholangiocarcinoma and gallbladder carcinoma. *J Clin Oncol*. 2015;33(24):2617-2622.
11. Bagante F, Spolverato G, Strasberg SM, et al. Minimally invasive vs. open hepatectomy: a comparative analysis of the national surgical quality improvement program database. *J Gastrointest Surg*. 2016;20(9):1608-1617.
12. Koch M, Garden OJ, Padbury R, et al. Bile leakage after hepatobiliary and pancreatic surgery: a definition and grading of severity by the International Study Group of Liver Surgery. *Surgery*. 2011;149(5):680-688.
13. Rahbari NN, Garden OJ, Padbury R, et al. Posthepatectomy liver failure: a definition and grading by the International Study Group of Liver Surgery (ISGLS). *Surgery*. 2011;149(5):713-724.
14. Leung U, Simpson AL, Araujo RL, et al. Remnant growth rate after portal vein embolization is a good early predictor of post-hepatectomy liver failure. *J Am Coll Surg*. 2014;219(4):620-630.
15. Dueland S, Syversveen T, Solheim JM, et al. Survival following liver transplantation for patients with nonresectable liver-only colorectal metastases. *Ann Surg*. 2020;271(2):212-218.
16. Mazzaferro V, Regalia E, Doci R, et al. Liver transplantation for the treatment of small hepatocellular carcinomas in patients with cirrhosis. *N Engl J Med*. 1996;334(11):693-699.
17. Mazzaferro V, Citterio D, Bhoori S, et al. Liver transplantation in hepatocellular carcinoma after tumour downstaging (XXL): a randomised, controlled, phase 2b/3 trial. *Lancet Oncol*. 2020;21(7):947-956.
18. Llovet JM, Ricci S, Mazzaferro V, et al. Sorafenib in advanced hepatocellular carcinoma. *N Engl J Med*. 2008;359(4):378-390.

18 Surgical Diseases of the Biliary Tree

Heidy Cos and Adeel S. Khan

I. BENIGN BILIARY OBSTRUCTION

A. Asymptomatic cholelithiasis
   1. Epidemiology/etiology
      a. Prevalence 10% to 15%
      b. Made of cholesterol, bile salts, or bilirubin
   2. Presentation
      a. Found incidentally on imaging (CT, ultrasonography)
   3. Diagnosis
      a. Abdominal ultrasonography, CT, MRI
   4. Management
      a. Nonoperative, observation

B. Symptomatic cholelithiasis (biliary colic)
   1. Epidemiology/etiology
      a. About 1% to 3% of patients with gallstones are symptomatic
      b. Risk factors: Obesity, female gender, age
      c. Intermittent obstruction of the cystic duct
   2. Presentation
      a. Epigastric and right upper quadrant (RUQ) pain
      b. Related to fatty meals or while sleeping
   3. Diagnosis
      a. See **Figure 18.1** for diagnostic workup of RUQ pain.
      b. RUQ ultrasonography: Gallstones, normal gallbladder wall
      c. Normal liver function tests
   4. Management
      a. Elective cholecystectomy: Laparoscopic vs. robot-assisted
      b. Critical view of safety: Pioneered at Washington University in St. Louis. Comprises three criteria that should be met prior to division of the cystic duct and artery[1]:
         i. Hepatocystic triangle clear of fat and fibrous tissue
         ii. Lower third of the gallbladder dissected off the cystic plate
         iii. Two and only two structures entering the gallbladder (cystic duct and artery).

C. Acute calculous cholecystitis
   1. Epidemiology/etiology
      a. Risk factors: Obesity, female gender, age
      b. Continuous obstruction of the cystic duct secondary to impacted gallstone
   2. Presentation

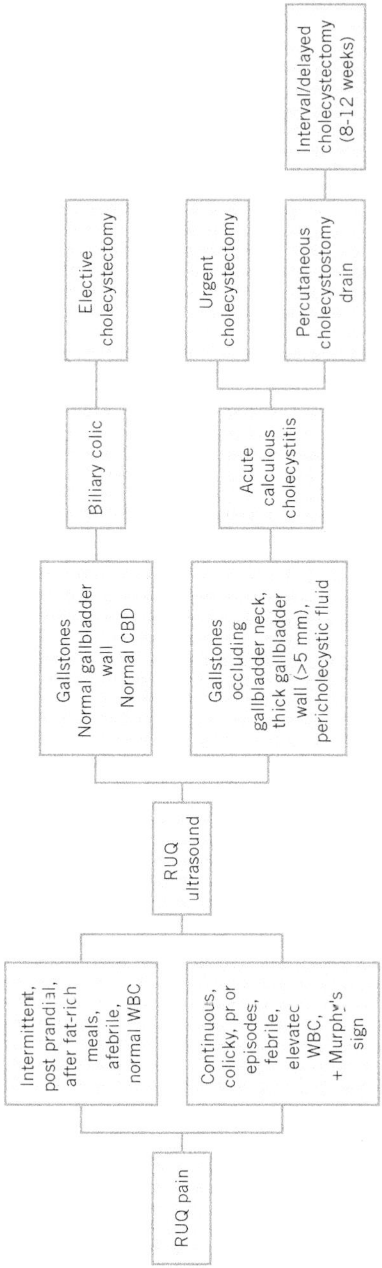

FIGURE 18.1 Algorithm for management of RUQ pain.

a. Acute-onset (<72 h) nonremitting epigastric and RUQ pain
b. Often precipitated by a large fatty meal
c. History of cholelithiasis and/or biliary colic
d. Fever
e. Murphy's sign: Inspiratory arrest during deep palpation of the RUQ

3. Diagnosis
   a. RUQ ultrasonography
      i. Gallbladder wall thickening (>5 mm)
      ii. Pericholecystic fluid
      iii. With sonographic Murphy's sign (tenderness with compression of the gallbladder by the ultrasonography probe)
      iv. Gallstones or sludge in the gallbladder
   b. Tokyo Guidelines[2]
      i. See **Table 18.1**
   c. CT of the abdomen and pelvis: Less sensitive. Can show gallbladder wall thickening, gallstones, pericholecystic fluid
   d. Hepatobiliary iminodiacetic acid (HIDA) scan or radionuclide cholescintigraphy: Radioactive tracer is injected intravenously. Failure of the gallbladder to fill with the tracer 4 hours after injection is diagnostic of acute cholecystitis.
   e. Severity grading
      i. Grade I: Acute cholecystitis that does not meet other criteria
      ii. Grade II: ≥1 of the following
         a) White blood cells >18K
         b) Palpable tender mass in the RUQ
         c) Duration of pain >72 hours
         d) Marked local inflammation (gangrene, abscess, biliary peritonitis, emphysematous cholecystitis)
      iii. Grade III: Cholecystitis with evidence of ≥1 organ system dysfunction

TABLE 18.1 Tokyo Guidelines for Acute Cholecystitis

Criteria	
Part A—Local signs of inflammation	RUQ mass, pain, or tenderness Murphy's sign
Part B—Systemic signs of inflammation	Fever, elevated CRP, elevated WBC
Part C—Imaging	Imaging findings characteristic of acute cholecystitis

Diagnosis is suspected when ≥1 condition from A and ≥1 from B or C and definite if ≥1 in A, B, and C.

CRP, C-reactive protein; WBC, white blood cell.

4. Management
   a. IV antibiotics, fluid resuscitation
   b. Urgent laparoscopic cholecystectomy
      i. See Section V
   c. For patients who are high risk/poor surgical candidates/in need for optimization general management is with percutaneous cholecystostomy drain followed by elective interval cholecystectomy 8 to 12 weeks after additional optimization.
   d. A meta-analysis of outcomes in over 1,600 patients showed that laparoscopic cholecystectomy within 7 days of symptom onset resulted in a lower incidence of wound infection and a shorter hospital stay than delayed surgery, with no difference in mortality, morbidity, biliary injury, or conversion to open operation.[3]

D. Acalculous cholecystitis
1. Epidemiology/etiology
   a. Severely ill/hospitalized patients (intubated, pressor support)
   b. Sepsis
   c. Patients on total parenteral nutrition/prolonged nil per os time
2. Presentation
   a. Fever and leukocytosis
   b. Can present with RUQ pain if patient is awake
3. Diagnosis
   a. RUQ ultrasonography: Pericholecystic fluid, thickened gallbladder wall, NO gallstones
   b. HIDA scan: Failure of the gallbladder to fill with tracer
4. Management
   a. Intravenous antibiotics
   b. Management of comorbidities
   c. Percutaneous cholecystostomy drain
      i. Interval cholecystectomy can be performed after resolution of critical illness.

E. Choledocholithiasis
1. Epidemiology/etiology
   a. Gallstones that originate in the gallbladder pass through the cystic duct, and become lodged in the common bile duct (**Figure 18.2**).
2. Presentation
   a. RUQ pain
   b. Jaundice
   c. History of biliary colic
3. Diagnosis
   a. Laboratory tests
      i. Elevated direct bilirubin and alkaline phosphatase
   b. Imaging
      i. RUQ ultrasonography: Dilated common bile duct (CBD) (>5 mm), CBD stone
      ii. Cross-sectional imaging: Magnetic resonance cholangiopancreatography (MRCP) more sensitive than CT

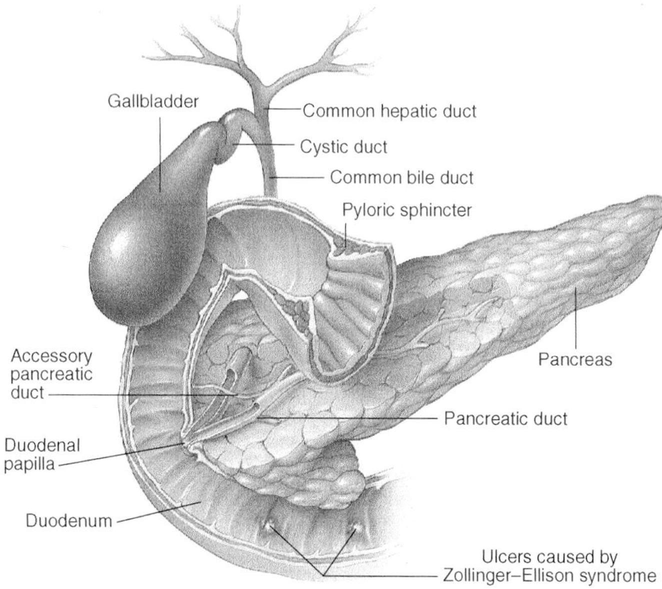

FIGURE 18.2 Biliary anatomy. *(Reprinted with permission from Escott-Stump S. Nutrition and Diagnosis-Related Care. 7th ed. Wolters Kluwer Health/Lippincott Williams & Wilkins; 2011.)*

   iii. Endoscopic retrograde cholangiopancreatography (ERCP): Nonfilling of the biliary tree proximal to the CBD obstruction

4. Management
 a. Stone extraction by ERCP with/without sphincterotomy followed by cholecystectomy
 b. If ERCP not readily available: Cholecystectomy with intraoperative cholangiogram and adjuncts such as irrigation/flushing of the stone, intravenous glucagon, or choledochoscopy can be used.
  i. See Biliary Operations section for bile duct exploration.
 c. Patients with ultrasonography evidence of a CBD stone, bilirubin >4 mg/dL, clinical ascending cholangitis, or dilated CBD with a bilirubin >1.8 mg/dL are considered high risk for choledocholithiasis and should undergo ERCP prior to cholecystectomy.[4]

F. Acute cholangitis

1. Epidemiology/etiology
 a. Bacterial infection of the biliary tree, associated with obstruction of the ductal system
 b. Causes: Choledocholithiasis, benign and malignant strictures, biliary-enteric anastomosis, occlusion of indwelling stents or tubes

2. Presentation
 a. Charcot's triad: Fever, jaundice, RUQ pain. Present in 50% to 70% of patients

b. Reynold's pentad: Charcot's triad with hypotension and altered mental status. Present in <10% of patients
c. Sepsis
3. Diagnosis
a. Laboratory: Leukocytosis, increased bilirubin (direct > indirect)
b. Imaging
i. RUQ ultrasonography: Gallstones, bile duct dilation
ii. ERCP or percutaneous transhepatic cholangiography (PTC): Diagnostic and therapeutic
4. Treatment
a. IV fluid resuscitation
b. IV antibiotics: Coverage of gram-negative and anaerobic organisms
c. Biliary decompression: ERCP, PTC
i. Ability to stent strictures if encountered

II. BILIARY STRICTURES AND CYSTS

A. Biliary strictures
1. Etiology
a. Pancreatitis
b. Choledocholithiasis
c. Primary sclerosing cholangitis (PSC)
d. Prior hepatic transplantation
e. Trauma or iatrogenic injury after instrumentation or operation
f. Biliary malignancy
2. Treatment
a. Dependent upon etiology—see below
B. Primary sclerosing cholangitis
1. Epidemiology/etiology
a. Autoimmune disorder characterized by progressive fibrous structuring of the biliary tree and cholestasis
b. Present in 1% to 5% of patients with inflammatory bowel disease
c. About 10% to 20% of patients with PSC will develop cholangiocarcinoma
d. Median time from diagnosis to liver failure: 10 to 12 years
2. Presentation
a. Jaundice, pale/acholic stools, dark urine
b. Progressive liver failure
c. RUQ pain, pruritus, fatigue, weight loss, bouts of cholangitis
3. Diagnosis
a. Laboratory
i. Elevation in alkaline phosphatase, aspartate transaminase, alanine transaminase
ii. Perinuclear anti-neutrophil cytoplasmic antibodies positive in 80% of patients. Highly suggestive, but not specific
b. Imaging
i. Gold standard: Cholangiography via ERCP or PTC
a) Diffuse and irregular narrowing of the entire biliary tree with short, annular strictures resulting in beaded appearance
ii. CT or MRCP

4. Management
   a. Medical
      i. Immunosuppression: Steroids, azathioprine, cyclosporine, methotrexate
   b. Surgical
      i. Liver transplant if progression to liver failure occurs

C. Choledochal cyst
1. Etiology
   a. Congenital dilations of the biliary tree that may occur in any bile duct but characteristically involve the common hepatic duct and CBD.
   b. Associated with anomalous pancreaticobiliary junction in 30% to 70% of cases and thought to be due to exposure of the biliary epithelium to digestive and pancreatic enzymes
2. Presentation
   a. Clinical course ranges from biliary obstruction in neonates to jaundice and abdominal pain in older children.
   b. Choledocholithiasis, cholangitis, portal hypertension
   c. Cholangiocarcinoma may develop in up to 30% of cysts.
   d. Cysts may be entirely asymptomatic.
3. Diagnosis
   a. Initial diagnosis is often made with ultrasonography and/or CT, but additional evaluation of the cyst should be performed with specific biliary imaging such as ERCP or MRCP.
   b. An anatomic classification scheme has identified five distinct types (**Table 18.2**).

TABLE 18.2 Choledochal Cyst Classification

Cyst Type	Frequency	Anatomy	Treatment
I	50%-85%	Fusiform dilation of the CBD	Excision with Roux-en-Y hepaticojejunostomy
II	2%	Saccular cysts of the extrahepatic bile ducts	Simple excision
III	1%-5%	Cysts of the intraduodenal portion of the CBD	Endoscopic unroofing or excision with sphincterotomy
IV	15%-35%	Multiple intra- and extrahepatic cysts	Excision with Roux-en-Y hepaticojejunostomy
V (Caroli disease)	20%	Multiple intrahepatic cysts	Resection (if isolated to a portion of the liver) or transplantation

CBD, common bile duct.

4. Treatment
   a. Primarily surgical and depends on the cyst type (see table above)

III. BILE DUCT INJURY

A. Epidemiology/etiology
   1. Can be related to pancreatitis, choledocholithiasis, primary sclerosing cholangitis, liver transplant, trauma, ERCP/instrumentation of the biliary tree, as complication of laparoscopic cholecystectomy
   2. Classification of bile duct injuries (see **Figure 18.3**)

B. Presentation
   1. Intraoperatively: Only 25% identified intraoperatively generally by unexpected bile leakage or abnormal intra-operative cholangiogram
   2. Postoperatively: Within 1 week of cholecystectomy. RUQ pain, fever, with or without jaundice

C. Diagnosis
   1. Laboratory: With or without leukocytosis, with or without increased direct bilirubin
   2. Imaging
      a. CT or MRI: Biloma from small bile duct leak
      b. MRCP with angiography should be performed if CBD injury is suspected, delineates biliary tree anatomy and identifies presence of concurrent vascular injury.
      c. HIDA scan: Will detect presence vs. absence of bile leak
      d. Cholangiogram (via endoscopy/ERCP or percutaneous/PTC): Can be diagnostic and therapeutic due to ability to place stents across injury

D. Management
   1. See **Table 18.3**
   2. Roux-en-Y hepaticojejunostomy: Identification and debridement of the bile duct to viable tissue followed by tension-free mucosa to mucosa anastomosis with fine absorbable suture

IV. BILIARY NEOPLASMS

A. Gallbladder cancer
   1. Epidemiology
      a. Gallbladder cancer is the most common malignancy of the biliary tract.
      b. Poor prognosis with median survival of 5 to 8 months
      c. Strong correlation with gallstones (95%)
      d. Nearly all gallbladder cancers are adenocarcinomas.
      e. Concomitant cholecystitis is frequently present.
      f. Tumors spread primarily by direct extension into liver segments IV and V and also via lymphatics along the cystic duct to the CBD.
   2. Presentation
      a. Generally advanced stage at presentation.

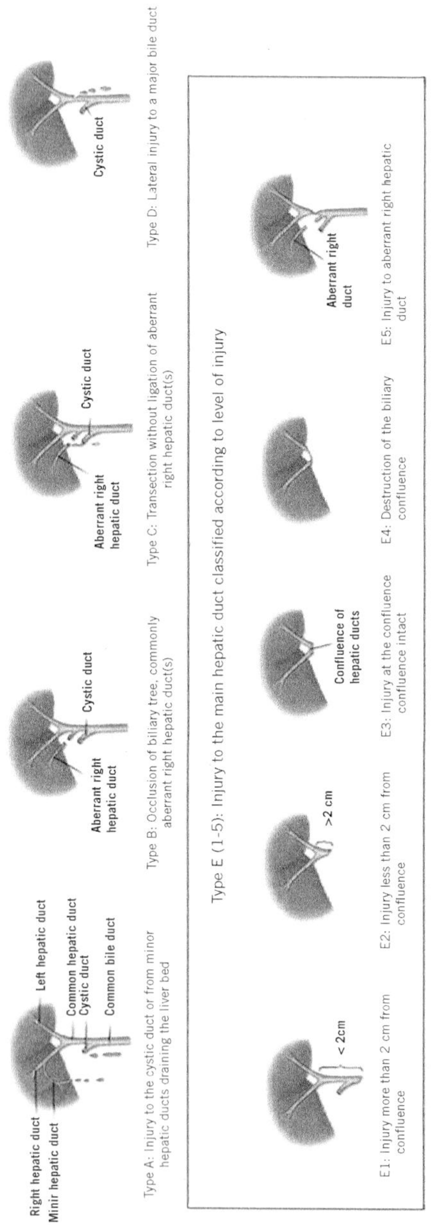

FIGURE 18.3 Strasberg classification of bile duct injuries.

TABLE 18.3 Typical Management of Biliary Injuries by Classification

Biliary Injury Classification	Definition	Typical Management
A	Leak from cystic duct stump or duct of Luschka	ERCP with sphincterotomy and stenting
B	Occlusion of aberrant right hepatic duct	Hepaticojejunostomy reconstruction
C	Transection without ligation of aberrant right hepatic duct	Hepaticojejunostomy reconstruction
D	Lateral injury to major bile duct	<50%, nonelectrocautery—primary repair with T-tube placement >50% or electrocautery—hepaticojejunostomy reconstruction
E1	Common hepatic duct division >2 cm from bifurcation	Hepaticojejunostomy reconstruction
E2	Common hepatic duct division <2 cm from bifurcation	Hepaticojejunostomy reconstruction—may require reconstruction to R and L duct separately
E3	Common hepatic duct division at the bifurcation with confluence preserved	Hepaticojejunostomy reconstruction—may require reconstruction to R and L duct separately
E4	Hilar stricture, involvement of the confluence, and loss of communication between right and left hepatic ducts	Hepaticojejunostomy reconstruction to R and L duct separately
E5	Involvement of aberrant right hepatic duct with or without CBD stricture	Hepaticojejunostomy reconstruction to involved segment

CBD, common bile duct; ERCP, endoscopic retrograde cholangiopancreatography; L, left; R, right.

   b. Polyps ≥1.5 cm have a 46% to 70% prevalence of cancer, whereas in those <1 cm, the risk of malignancy is <5%.[5]
   c. Malignant polyps tend to be sessile and echogenic on ultrasonography.
3. Diagnosis
   a. Usually diagnosed incidentally after cholecystectomy

b. Symptoms of stage I and II gallbladder cancer are often due to the presence of gallstones, whereas stage III and IV cancers present with weight loss and symptoms of CBD obstruction.
c. Suggestive ultrasonography findings include thickening or irregularity of the gallbladder, a polypoid mass, or diffuse wall calcification indicative of porcelain gallbladder.
d. Tumor markers (carbohydrate antigen 19-9 [CA 19-9]) may be elevated in patients with gallbladder cancer.

4. Treatment
   a. Prophylactic cholecystectomy should be considered for polyps >1 cm in size or those meeting morphologic criteria.
   b. Mucosal disease confined to the gallbladder wall (Tis and T1a tumors) is often identified after routine laparoscopic cholecystectomy. Because the overall 5-year survival rate is as high as 80%, cholecystectomy with negative margins is adequate therapy.
   c. Patients with a preoperative suspicion of gallbladder cancer should undergo open cholecystectomy because port site recurrences and late peritoneal metastases (associated with bile spillage) have been reported.
   d. For patients with incidentally discovered T2 gallbladder cancer after laparoscopic cholecystectomy, re-resection including segments IVb and V of the liver as well as portal lymphadenectomy should be performed.
      i. Routine port-site or bile duct resection is not indicated.
   e. Preoperatively diagnosed T2 tumors are treated by radical cholecystectomy including the gallbladder, gallbladder bed of the liver (segments IVb and V), hepatoduodenal ligament, and nodal tissue including paraduodenal, peripancreatic, hepatic artery, and celiac lymph nodes.
   f. Lymph node metastases or extension of disease beyond the gallbladder wall requires more radical resection.
   g. Depending on the extent of local invasion, extirpation may range from wedge resection of the liver adjacent to the gallbladder bed to trisectionectomy. Improvement in survival has been demonstrated after radical resection.[6]
   h. Because of the aggressive nature of this malignancy, adjuvant chemoradiation is often recommended; however, efficacy is limited.
      i. Adjuvant regimens include gemcitabine and cisplatin (ABC-02), capecitabine (BILCAP), and oxaliplatin (PRODIGE-12).
   i. Extensive liver involvement or discontiguous metastases preclude surgical resection.
   j. Jaundice may be palliated by percutaneous or endoscopically placed biliary stents.
   k. Duodenal obstruction can be surgically bypassed if present.

B. Cholangiocarcinoma
   1. Epidemiology
      a. Cholangiocarcinomas arise from the bile duct epithelium and can occur anywhere along the course of the biliary tree.

b. Classified according to anatomic location
  i. Intrahepatic (20%)
  ii. Extrahepatic upper duct (hilar or Klatskin tumor, 40%)
    a) Bismuth–Corlette classification scheme (**Table 18.4**)
  iii. Extrahepatic lower duct (40%)
c. Tumors are locally invasive, spreading along bile ducts, and often metastasize to regional lymph nodes, the liver, and the peritoneum.
d. Predisposing conditions include male gender, PSC, choledochal cysts, intrahepatic stones, and parasitic infestations such as *Clonorchis* species.

2. Presentation
  a. Jaundice, weight loss, and pain
3. Diagnosis
  a. CA 19-9 is the most used marker in the diagnosis of cholangiocarcinoma, although inflammation and cholestasis may also elevate the levels.
  b. Abdominal MRI or MRCP: Can demonstrate the tumor in relation to the portal structures and is sensitive for intrahepatic metastases.
  c. Ultrasonography or CT: May be used if magnetic resonance is contraindicated or not tolerated.
  d. ERCP: Valuable for diagnosing extrahepatic tumors via biliary brushings or biopsy and can also be used for preoperative biliary decompression, which has the advantage of improving liver function prior to resection but carries the risk of cholangitis and increased postoperative infection.
4. Treatment
  a. Resection remains the primary treatment, although only 15% to 20% are resectable at presentation.
  b. Intrahepatic tumors are best treated with hepatectomy.
    i. Resectability is assessed with a goal of 1-cm tumor-free margins and maintenance of an adequate future liver remnant (FLR) (see Chapter 17).
    ii. If there is risk of insufficient FLR, volume optimizing strategies such as preoperative portal vein embolization can be used to promote hyperplasia of the FLR.
  c. For hilar tumors, surgical resection typically involves removal of the bile duct bifurcation, ipsilateral hemiliver, and often the caudate lobe, especially with left-sided tumors.

TABLE 18.4 Bismuth–Corlette Classification of Hilar Cholangiocarcinoma

Type I	Tumor remains below the confluence of the right and left hepatic ducts
Type II	Tumor involves the confluence of the right and left hepatic ducts
Type III	Tumor involves either the right or the left hepatic duct and extends to secondary radicals
Type IV	Tumor involves secondary radicals of both the right and left hepatic ducts

i. The goal of resection is to obtain an R0 resection (complete, margin-negative resection).
ii. Biliary reconstruction is then performed as a Roux-en-Y hepaticojejunostomy.
iii. Whipple operation may be necessary in some cases to obtain a negative distal CBD margin.

d. Vascular involvement is not an absolute contraindication to resection as portal vein and hepatic artery resection may be feasible in select cases at high-volume centers.
e. Contraindications to resection include bilateral intrahepatic ductal spread, extensive arterial or portal vein involvement, vascular involvement with evidence of contralateral ductal spread, and significant lymph node involvement or distant spread.
f. Liver transplant with neoadjuvant chemoradiation is currently considered for carefully selected patients in selected US centers for early-stage, unresectable perihilar cholangiocarcinomas with excellent results in this highly selected population.[7]
g. Tumors in the middle of the extrahepatic bile duct may be approached with segmental bile duct excision, cholecystectomy, and portal lymphadenectomy. However, a Whipple operation or liver resection may be required to achieve R0 resection.
h. Distal bile duct cholangiocarcinomas are treated the same as pancreatic head malignancies with a Whipple operation in the absence of locally advanced or metastatic disease (see Chapter 19).

5. Palliation for patients with unresectable disease involves surgical, radiologic, or endoscopic biliary decompression.

V. BILIARY OPERATIONS

A. Cholecystectomy

1. Minimally invasive (laparoscopic or robot-assisted)

a. **Operative approach to laparoscopic cholecystectomy**

i. After port placement and establishment of pneumoperitoneum, the abdomen is explored to rule out the presence of other disease.
ii. The gallbladder fundus is retracted cephalad and the infundibulum laterally.
iii. Using a combination of cautery and blunt dissection, the lower third of the gallbladder is dissected off the liver bed and the triangle of Calot is dissected free of fat, fibrous, and areolar tissue.
iv. The critical view of safety is obtained demonstrating two and only two structures entering the gallbladder, the bottom one-third of the liver is dissected off the liver bed, and the hepatocystic triangle is cleared of fat and fibrous tissue.
v. Cystic artery and cystic duct are clipped and transected.
vi. The gallbladder is removed from the cystic plate.
vii. Gallbladder is extracted using an endocatch bag, and port sites are closed.

b. Bailout procedures
   i. Consider conversion to open (see below) or a laparoscopic bail-out procedure if unable to obtain the critical view of safety
      a) Fenestrating subtotal cholecystectomy—distal gallbladder is transected and left open with a closed cystic duct.
      b) Reconstituting subtotal cholecystectomy—distal gallbladder is transected and then closed.
c. Complications
   i. Bile duct injury (see Section III)
   ii. Hepatic artery injury

2. Open
   a. Indications for conversion to open
      i. Failure to progress
      ii. Inability to achieve a critical view of safety
      iii. Biliary injury
      iv. Inability to control bleeding
   b. Technique
      i. Right subcostal incision
      ii. Gallbladder is cauterized off the liver bed in "top-down" fashion, starting at the fundus.
      iii. Two ties are placed at the level of the cystic duct and artery, and these structures are cut to complete the cholecystectomy.

B. Common bile duct exploration (CBDE)

1. Transcystic CBDE
   a. Less effective than transcholedochal but less risk for strictures[8]
   b. **Operative approach to transcystic CBDE**
      i. Perform a cholangiogram
      ii. Using the ductotomy from the cholangiogram, pass a stone extraction implement or choledochoscope
      iii. Saline flushing of the cystic duct or glucagon can be used to flush stones or debris into the duodenum.
      iv. A Fogarty balloon can be used to extract impacted stones.
2. Transcholedochal CBDE
   a. Laparascopic or open
   b. **Operative approach to transcholedochal CBDE**
      i. Dissect cystic duct to the junction with the CBD
      ii. Dissect the peritoneal layer overlying the anterior surface of the supraduodenal CBD for approximately 2 cm
      iii. Make a longitudinal choledochotomy to avoid injury to the blood supply to the CBD (located at the 3- and 9-o'clock positions along the duct)
      iv. Once the CBD is entered, stones may spontaneously spill out. Use suction–irrigation or external pressure to remove additional stones, then consider evaluation of the duct with choledochoscopy or fluoroscopy for residual stones.
      v. Unlike the transcystic approach, a choledochotomy allows the choledochoscope to be inserted proximally into the common, left, and right hepatic ducts or distally into the common duct.

vi. A stone retrieval wire basket can be used via the choledochoscope's working channel to retrieve any remaining stones.
vii. Primarily close the ductotomy using 4-0 or 5-0 absorbable sutures in a running or interrupted fashion.

Key References

Citation	Summary
Primrose JN, Fox RP, Palmer DH, et al. Capecitabine compared with observation in resected biliary tract cancer (BILCAP): a randomised, controlled, multicentre, phase 3 study [published correction appears in Lancet Oncol. 2019 April 2;:]. *Lancet Oncol.* 2019;20(5):663-673.	• A randomized, controlled, multicenter, phase 3 study was done across 44 specialist hepatopancreatobiliary centers in the UK. Aimed to determine whether adjuvant capecitabine improved overall survival compared with observation following surgery for biliary tract cancer in patients with histologically confirmed cholangiocarcinoma or muscle-invasive gallbladder cancer who had undergone a macroscopically complete resection. Although this study did not meet its primary endpoint of improving overall survival in the intention-to-treat population, the prespecified sensitivity and per-protocol analyses suggest that capecitabine can improve overall survival in patients with resected biliary tract cancer when used as adjuvant chemotherapy following surgery and could be considered as standard of care. Furthermore, the safety profile is manageable, supporting the use of capecitabine in this setting.
Strasberg SM, Hertl M, Soper NJ. An analysis of the problem of biliary injury during laparoscopic cholecystectomy. *J Am Coll Surg.* 1995;180(1):101-125.	• Original paper describing the development of the critical view of safety to prevent biliary injury during laparoscopic cholecystectomy.
Michael Brunt L, Deziel DJ, Telem DA, et al. Safe cholecystectomy multi-society practice guideline and state-of-the-art consensus conference on prevention of bile duct injury during cholecystectomy. *Surg Endosc.* 2020;34(7):2827-2855.	• Society guidelines for strategies to minimize the risk of bile duct injury during laparoscopic cholecystectomy.

CHAPTER 18: SURGICAL DISEASES OF THE BILIARY TREE

Review Questions

1. What is Murphy's sign?
2. Describe the typical ultrasonography findings in acute cholecystitis.
3. Describe Charcot's triad for cholangitis.
4. Describe Reynold's pentad for cholangitis.
5. What are the three elements of the critical view of safety?
6. What are the two approaches in which common bile duct exploration can be performed?

REFERENCES

1. Berci G, Morgenstern L. An analysis of the problem of biliary injury during laparoscopic cholecystectomy. *J Am Coll Surg.* 1995;180(5):638-639.
2. Yokoe M, Hata J, Takada T, et al. Tokyo Guidelines 2018: diagnostic criteria and severity grading of acute cholecystitis (with videos). *J Hepatobiliary Pancreat Sci.* 2018;25(1):41-54.
3. Wu XD, Tian X, Liu MM, Wu L, Zhao S, Zhao L. Meta-analysis comparing early versus delayed laparoscopic cholecystectomy for acute cholecystitis. *Br J Surg.* 2015;102(11):1302-1313.
4. Barkun AN, Barkun JS, Fried GM, et al. Useful predictors of bile duct stones in patients undergoing laparoscopic cholecystectomy. McGill Gallstone Treatment Group. *Ann Surg.* 1994;220(1):32-39.
5. Koga A, Watanabe K, Fukuyama T, Takiguchi S, Nakayama F. Diagnosis and operative indications for polypoid lesions of the gallbladder. *Arch Surg.* 1988;123(1):26-29.
6. Hong EK, Kim KK, Lee JN, et al. Surgical outcome and prognostic factors in patients with gallbladder carcinoma. *Korean J Hepatobiliary Pancreat Surg.* 2014;18(4):129-137.
7. Sapisochin G, Fernandez de Sevilla E, Echeverri J, Charco R. Liver transplantation for cholangiocarcinoma: current status and new insights. *World J Hepatol.* 2015;7(22):2396-2403.
8. Zerey M, Haggerty S, Richardson W, et al. Laparoscopic common bile duct exploration. *Surg Endosc.* 2018;32(6):2603-2612.
9. Primrose JN, Fox RP, Palmer DH, et al. Capecitabine compared with observation in resected biliary tract cancer (BILCAP): a randomised, controlled, multicentre, phase 3 study. *Lancet Oncol.* 2019;20(5):663-673.
10. Strasberg SM, Hertl M, Soper NJ. An analysis of the problem of biliary injury during laparoscopic cholecystectomy. *J Am Coll Surg.* 1995;180(1):101-125.
11. Brunt LM, Deziel DJ, Telem DA, et al. Safe cholecystectomy multi-society practice guideline and state-of-the-art consensus conference on prevention of bile duct injury during cholecystectomy. *Surg Endosc.* 2020;34(7):2827-2855.

19 Pancreas

Katharine E. Caldwell and Chet Hammill

I. ANATOMY

The pancreas has four sections: Head/uncinate, neck, body, and tail. It is a retroperitoneal organ located in the lesser sac. The head is cradled by the C-loop of the duodenum, while the tail sits near the splenic hilum, anterior to the left adrenal gland (**Figure 19.1**).

A. The pancreatic neck lies anterior to mesenteric vessels and the portal vein.

B. The body begins left of the superior mesenteric vein (SMV) and lies anterior to the splenic vein.

II. BLOOD SUPPLY

A. Arterial (**Figure 19.1**)

1. Pancreatic head: Superior pancreaticoduodenal arteries (from celiac artery via gastroduodenal artery) and the inferior pancreaticoduodenal arteries (from the superior mesenteric artery)
2. Distal pancreas: Branches of splenic artery—superior (dorsal) pancreatic, greater pancreatic, and transverse pancreatic arteries

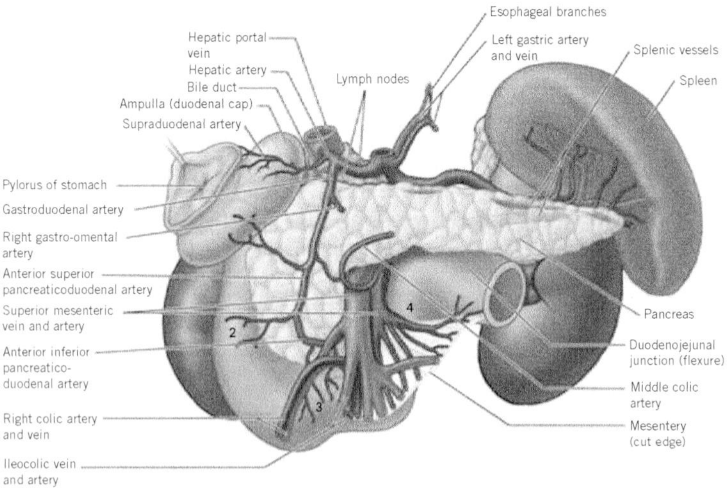

FIGURE 19.1 Anatomic relationships of the pancreas to surrounding organs and vasculature.

B. Venous drainage (**Figure 19.1**)
   1. Pancreaticoduodenal and splenic veins drain into the portal venous system
C. Lymphatic drainage
   1. Anterior pancreatic head and neck: Pancreaticoduodenal and pyloric lymph nodes to the celiac and hepatic lymph node basis
   2. Posterior pancreatic head, neck, and uncinate: Retropancreatic nodes to celiac and hepatic or superior mesenteric lymph nodes
   3. Body and tail: Celiac nodal plexus
   4. Pancreatic surface directly in contact with the retroperitoneum: Posterior abdominal wall or perineural lymphatic channels

III. EMBRYOLOGY

The pancreas forms from ventral and dorsal outpouchings of the duodenum, each with an individual drainage duct. In the most common final configuration, the ventral duct joins with the dorsal duct at the neck of the pancreas and the dorsal duct regresses.

A. Other anatomic configurations
   1. **Pancreas divisum**—failure of fusion of the ventral and dorsal pancreatic buds leading to a dominant dorsal duct draining through a second duodenal ampulla and ventral duct draining through the typical ampulla of Vater (**Figure 19.2**).
      a. The most common congenital abnormality of the pancreas (4%-14% of population)

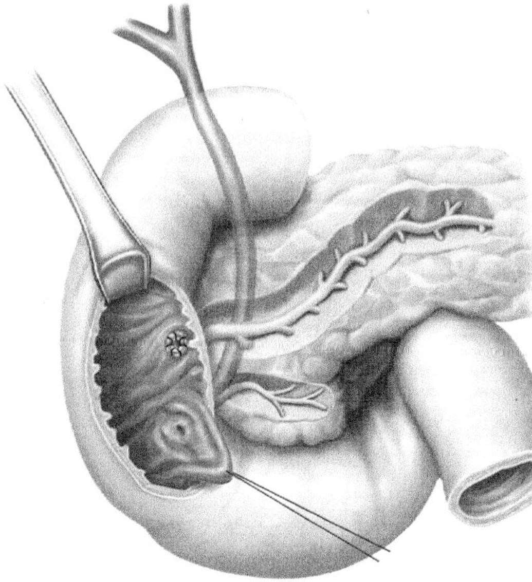

FIGURE 19.2 Pancreas divisum.

b. Thought to be associated with increased risk of pancreatitis due to relationship to certain genetic mutations (CFTR) suggesting a cumulative effect[1]
c. Minor papilla sphincterotomy may be required for patients with recurrent episodes of pancreatitis

2. **Annular pancreas**—malrotation of the ventral portion of the pancreas leads to a band of pancreatic tissue surrounding the duodenum
a. Can lead to duodenal obstruction, generally early in life that requires duodenoduodenostomy or duodenojejunostomy to bypass the obstruction.
b. Resection of pancreatic band is generally not recommended due to the risk of postoperative pancreatic fistula.

IV. PANCREATIC DUCTAL ADENOCARCINOMA

A. Etiology and epidemiology
1. The third leading cause of cancer-related mortality in the US.[2]
2. Over 50% of patients have metastatic disease at the time of diagnosis.
3. Five-year survival rate has steadily improved over time, although it is still very poor with only about 10% of patients surviving to 5 years.[2]
4. Five-year survival is significantly better (43.9%) for patients who present with surgically resectable localized disease.
5. Median age of diagnosis is 65 years.
6. Pancreatic ductal adenocarcinoma represents over 90% of pancreatic malignancies.
7. Risk factors
a. Ninety percent of pancreatic ductal adenocarcinoma (PDAC) is sporadic
b. Smoking[3]
c. Family history
d. Intraductal papillary mucinous neoplasms and pancreatic intraepithelial neoplasms[4] (see Section VII)
e. Germline cancer gene mutations (ATM, BRCA2, MSH2, MSH6, TP53)[5]
f. Chronic pancreatitis

B. Diagnosis
1. Signs and symptoms
a. Generally nonspecific and gradual in onset
b. Epigastric or back pain
c. Weight loss
d. Steatorrhea—if pancreatic duct obstruction due to cancer exists
e. Diabetes—New-onset diabetes within a year prior to diagnosis is present in 15% of patients with PDAC[6]
f. Trousseau sign—migratory thrombophlebitis
g. Cancer of the head (70% of all PDAC) may lead to bile duct obstruction → painless jaundice, pruritus, dark urine, pale stools
h. Cancer of the body (20%) or tail (10%) of the pancreas generally presents with predominant pain or weight loss

2. Laboratory tests
   a. Markers of biliary obstruction may be elevated for masses causing bile duct obstruction: Serum bilirubin, alkaline phosphatase, aspartate transaminase/alanine transaminase
   b. Tumor markers: carbohydrate antigen (CA) 19-9 and carcinoembryonic antigen (CEA)
      i. Fifteen percent of patients with PDAC will demonstrate normal CA19-9 levels.
      ii. CA19-9 is not specific for disease and may be elevated in other benign conditions associated with biliary obstruction,[7] but it is often used for assessing disease response and correlates with resectability[8] and CA19-9 normalization after therapy correlates with prognosis.[9]
      iii. CEA levels are elevated (>5 ng/mL) in 40% to 50% of patients with PDAC.
3. Imaging
   a. CT
      i. Fine cut (≤3-mm slices) "pancreatic protocol" CT with both arterial and venous phases is necessary to evaluate the relationship of a mass to vascular structures to determine resectability.
      ii. PDAC often appears as a hypoattenuating mass that distorts normal glandular architecture.
      iii. Dilated pancreatic and biliary ducts ("double duct sign") can be present.
   b. MRI/magnetic resonance cholangiopancreatography (MRCP)
      i. Provide similar information to conventional CT and may help delineate relationship to vascular or surrounding structures
   c. Endoscopic ultrasound (EUS)/ endoscopic retrograde cholangiopancreatography (ERCP)
      i. May assist in diagnosis of a mass poorly seen on CT or when tissue diagnosis is necessary (e.g., diagnostic uncertainty, prior to initiation of neoadjuvant therapy)
      ii. ERCP can also assist in biliary drainage for patients with biliary obstruction at the time of diagnosis.
         a) As preoperative cholangitis is associated with increased mortality,[10] preoperative biliary stenting is indicated for patients with complications associated with obstruction.
   d. Staging laparoscopy
      i. Routine staging laparoscopy remains an area of debate.
      ii. May be used routinely at certain centers and may reduce the nontherapeutic laparotomy rate and assist in selection for neoadjuvant in patients with borderline resectable or locally advanced PDAC.[11]
4. Categorization
   a. National guidelines are utilized to categorize PDAC as resectable, borderline resectable, or locally advanced, on the basis of imaging findings.

C. Treatment

1. Neoadjuvant chemotherapy

   a. Neoadjuvant therapy with FOLFIRINOX or gemcitabine/nanoparticle albumin-bound paclitaxel (nab-paclitaxel) has become increasingly utilized due to demonstrated benefits in survival, R0 resection rates, and downstaging leading to improved rates of resection.[12]

   b. Neoadjuvant FOLFIRINOX in borderline resectable PDAC demonstrates prolonged overall survival and improved R0 resection.[13]

   c. Gemcitabine/nab-paclitaxel has been demonstrated to have potential to convert unresectable, locally advanced disease to surgically resectable disease.[14]

   d. No difference has been demonstrated in overall survival between FOLFIRINOX and gemcitabine/nab-paclitaxel, and FOLFIRINOX may offer increased toxicity.[15]

2. Resection

   a. Pancreatoduodenectomy (Whipple procedure)

      i. En bloc resection of the head of the pancreas, distal common bile duct (CBD), duodenum, proximal jejunum, and gastric antrum with reconstruction via gastrojejunostomy, hepaticojejunostomy, and pancreaticojejunostomy (**Figure 19.3**).

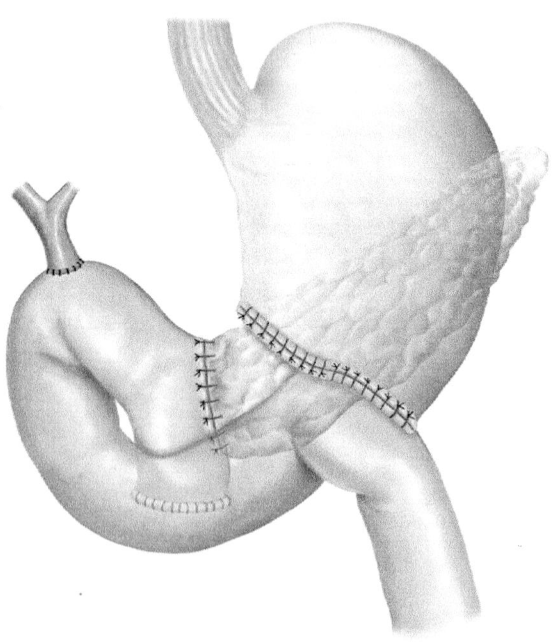

FIGURE 19.3 Whipple anatomy.

ii. Pylorus-sparing Whipple procedures are also possible, although without proven benefit in morbidity or survival.
iii. Morbidity and mortality has declined rapidly in the last several years with specialized centers now demonstrating mortality rates <3%.[16]

b. Distal pancreatectomy
   i. Used for malignant lesions of the body and tail
   ii. Resection of the pancreas at the SMV laterally to include the spleen
   iii. Modifications of this procedure, including the radical antegrade modular pancreatosplenectomy procedure to perform a more extensive lymph node dissection and resection of the ipsilateral adrenal gland may demonstrate improved R0 resection rates[17]
   iv. **Procedural approach: Distal Pancreatectomy**
      a) Safe laparoscopic entry with placement of multiple trochars to allow for camera placement as well as several working ports including a port for a laparoscopic stapler.
      b) Entry into the lesser sac through the gastrocolic ligament
      c) Laparoscopic ultrasound or palpation can be used to identify the location of the tumor
      d) Divide the short gastric vessels
      e) Mobilize the splenic flexure to expose the tail of the pancreas
      f) Incise the peritoneum from the inferior edge of the pancreas to the inferior pole of the spleen to mobilize the pancreas and retract medially
      g) Isolate and divide the splenic artery and vein
      h) Divide the pancreas with a stapler
      i) Mobilize the suspending splenic ligaments
      j) Remove the specimen

c. Minimally invasive pancreatectomy
   i. Laparoscopic distal pancreatectomy is now standard of care for candidates with amenable lesions.
   ii. Rates of laparoscopic and robotic Whipple procedures are increasing.
   iii. Minimally invasive resection for pancreatic cancer is feasible with similar R0 resection rates and survival rates,[18] although it is largely performed at high-volume centers with appropriate surgical expertise.

3. Adjuvant therapy
   a. Efficacy of adjuvant therapy was established in the CONKO-001 trial demonstrating improved survival after resection for patients treated with gemcitabine vs. observation alone[19]
   b. Gemcitabine/nab-paclitaxel improved median overall survival from 6.7 months in the gemcitabine only group to 8.5 months in the combination gemcitabine/nab-paclitaxel group. Demonstrates prolonged survival benefit over gemcitabine for patients with resected pancreas cancer[20]

4. Radiation therapy
    a. Historically used only in the adjuvant setting or as treatment for nonresectable disease, now more frequently in use in the neoadjuvant setting in select patients due to improved R0 resection rate and ability to improve resectability of patients with borderline resectable pancreatic ductal adenocarcinoma (PDAC)[21]

D. Complications
1. Postoperative considerations
    a. Delayed gastric emptying (20%) generally managed conservatively with appropriate decompression and watchful waiting
    b. Pancreatic fistula (20%)
        i. Fistula risk score
            a) Several validated risk scores to predict the development of post-op pancreatic fistula have been developed[22-24]
            b) These scores frequently include pancreas texture, duct diameter, blood loss, and other factors
    c. Surgical site infection (10%-15%)
    d. Hemorrhage (<10%) while relatively rare, contributes significantly to postoperative death
        i. Most commonly due to gastroduodenal artery stump bleeding or pseudoaneurysm formation
        ii. Generally managed with angiography and embolization
    e. Mortality
        i. Thirty-day mortality is approximately 3%.
        ii. Ninety-day mortality is double 30-day mortality.
        iii. Mortality rates are approximately 4 times higher at low-volume (<5 procedures/year) centers.[25]

V. PANCREATIC NEUROENDOCRINE TUMORS

A. Etiology
1. Pancreatic neuroendocrine tumors (pNETs) are a heterogeneous group of tumors that arise from the endocrine tissue of the pancreas.
2. They are rare, with increasing detection over time due to improved imaging techniques
3. Ten percent are associated with familial endocrine tumor syndromes
    a. Multiple endocrine neoplasia type 1
    b. Von Hippel–Lindau disease
    c. Neurofibromatosis type 1
    d. Tuberous sclerosis
4. Defined by the hormone they secrete (**Table 19.1**)

B. Diagnosis
1. Laboratory levels
    a. Hormone levels (pancreatic polypeptide, insulin, glucagon, and vasoactive intestinal peptide)
    b. Chromogranin A level—generally used to monitor recurrence after resection
2. CT
    a. Has lower sensitivity than DOTATATE positron emission tomography (PET) or EUS

TABLE 19.1 Neuroendocrine Tumors

Tumor	Typical Location	Secreted Hormone	Malignant	Clinical Presentation	Treatment
Insulinoma	Anywhere in the pancreas	Insulin	10%	Hypoglycemic symptoms	Enucleation or resection depending on location
Gastrinoma	Gastrinoma triangle[a]: Duodenum (70%) Pancreas (25%)	Gastrin	60%-90%	Zollinger–Ellison syndrome (refractory GERD, duodenal ulcers)	Resection
Glucagonoma	Pancreatic tail	Glucagon	50%-80%	Rash, diabetes, necrolytic migratory erythema	Resection
Somatostatinoma	Pancreas (55%) Duodenum/jejunum (45%)	Somatostatin	>70%	Diabetes, cholelithiasis, diarrhea	Resection
VIPoma	Pancreatic tail	Vasoactive intestinal peptide	40%-70%	Watery diarrhea, hypokalemia, achlorhydria	Resection
Nonfunctional	Anywhere in the pancreas	None	Varies by size	None	Resection vs. observation depending on size and growth rate

GERD, gastroesophageal reflux disease.

[a]Gastrinoma triangle: Triangle formed by junction of cystic duct and CBD, junction of 2nd/3rd portion of duodenum, junction of body and neck of pancreas.

b. Generally discovered incidentally during workup for other gastrointestinal complaints
c. Appearance: Generally well circumscribed, homogenously enhancing, and hypervascular
3. EUS/fine needle aspiration (FNA)
a. Generally indicated to establish tissue diagnosis or if tumor was not well visualized by CT
4. DOTATATE PET
a. Uses radioisotopes which bind to the somatostatin receptor
b. Highly sensitive for the detection of pNETs

C. Treatment
1. Resection remains the mainstay of treatment for functional or larger tumors
a. <1 cm, nonfunctional with imaging characteristics consistent with pNET → observation
b. 1 to 2 cm, nonfunctional pNET → observe or resect based on patient factors
c. >2 cm or functional → resection[26]
2. Surgical resection of isolated liver metastasis should be considered due to improved survival.[27]
3. Chemotherapy may be used for patients with intermediate- or high-grade pNETs.
4. Somatostatin analogues may help control symptoms for patients with functional pNETs and prevent growth.[28]

VI. RARE NEOPLASMS AND PSEDUOTUMORS OF THE PANCREAS

A. Acinar cell carcinoma
1. Treated with surgical resection and often only differentiated by PDAC on surgical pathology
2. Improved prognosis vs. PDAC

B. Solid pseudopapillary tumor
1. Most commonly seen in young women
2. Generally large at presentation
3. Treated by resection with favorable prognosis

C. Metastatic tumors
1. Most common: Renal cell carcinoma (RCC)
a. When isolated to the pancreas, RCC metastatic resection has 60% 5-year survival rates[29]
2. Less common: Ovarian, colon, melanoma

D. Lymphoma
1. Primary or metastatic to the pancreas
2. Treated with multimodal chemotherapy and radiation therapy without surgical resection

E. Lymphoplasmacytic sclerosing pancreatitis
1. Often misdiagnosed as pancreatic cancer
2. Young patients 30 to 50 years old with associated autoimmune disorders (Sjögren's, ulcerative colitis, sclerosing cholangitis)
3. Biopsy reveals plasma cells.
4. Patients may have increased levels of IgG4.[30]

VII. CYSTIC DISEASE OF THE PANCREAS

Cysts of the pancreas can present a diagnostic challenge as they can be either benign or premalignant and may require several imaging or testing modalities to appropriately diagnose. With the advent of advanced imaging techniques, more patients are having incidental pancreatic cysts discovered. Several society guidelines exist for the management and observation of these cysts[31-33] (**Figure 19.4**).

A. Pancreatic pseudocyst
  1. Etiology
    a. Disruption of the pancreatic duct generally after an episode of acute pancreatitis or direct trauma
    b. Cyst wall is made up of inflammatory tissue not a true epithelial-lined sac.
  2. Diagnosis
    a. Signs and symptoms
      i. Recurrent or persistent upper abdominal pain
      ii. Nausea/vomiting or early satiety due to gastric compression
    b. Imaging
      i. CT scan
        a) Radiographic study of choice
        b) Findings on CT can predict cysts unlikely to spontaneously resolve.
          1) Size > 4 cm
          2) Wall calcifications
          3) Thick walls
      ii. MRI/MRCP
        a) May be useful to delineate ductal anatomy
      iii. ERCP
        a) Determination of pancreatic duct anatomy
        b) Simultaneous ability for therapeutic intervention (stenting of proximal stricture, etc.)
  3. Treatment
    a. Cysts <6 cm and present for <6 weeks should be observed
      i. High rate of resolution
      ii. Intervention before 6 weeks increases complication risk
    b. Indications for intervention
    c. Symptomatic—obstructive symptoms (satiety, weight loss), pain
      i. Infection
  4. Drainage options
    a. Percutaneous drainage
      i. Indicated for patients whose cyst does not communicate with the duct and has no appropriate window for endoscopic drainage
      ii. Can also be used for nonmature (<6 weeks old) cysts that are infected
    b. Endoscopic internal drainage (cystoenteric drainage)
      i. Cyst-gastrostomy or cyst-duodenostomy
      ii. The first treatment of choice for mature cysts with appropriate window for endoscopic drainage

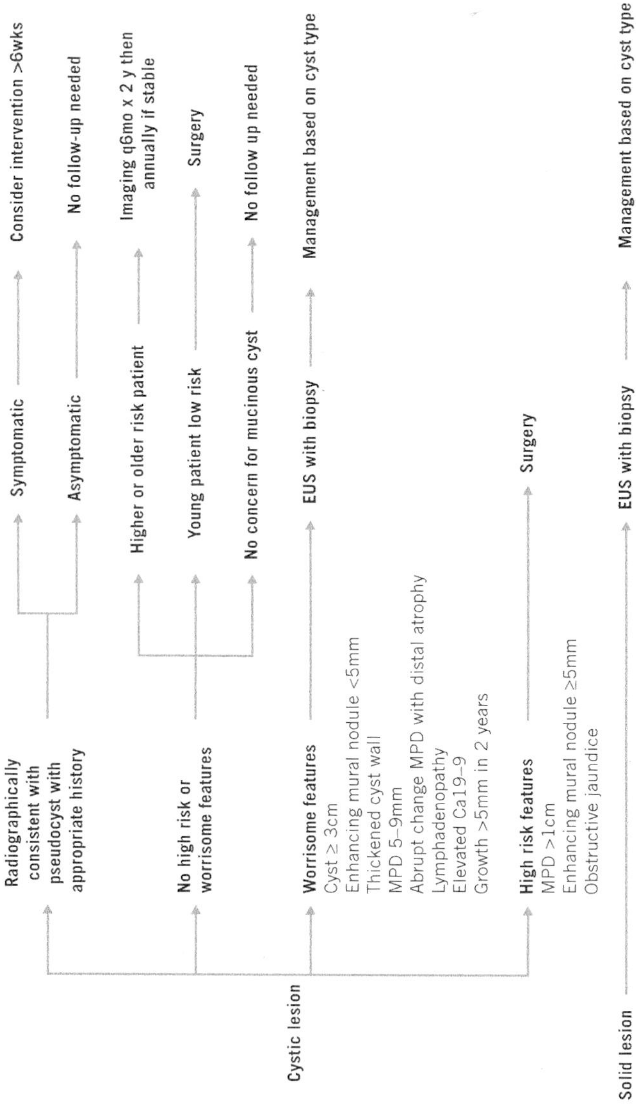

FIGURE 19.4 Management of cystic diseases of the pancreas.

c. Surgical internal drainage
   i. Roux-en-Y cyst-jejunostomy, loop cyst-jejunostomy, cyst-gastrostomy
   ii. Rarely indicated—reserved for patients who cannot have endoscopic drainage or fail endoscopic drainage
   iii. Obtain a biopsy of the cyst wall at time of drainage to rule out malignancy

5. Complications
   a. Infection
      i. Present in 5% to 20% of pseudocysts
      ii. Managed with drainage
   b. Hemorrhage
      i. Due to erosion into surrounding vessels
      ii. Most commonly involved vessels: Splenic artery (45%) > gastroduodenal artery (18%)/pancreaticoduodenal arteries (18%)
      iii. Treatment: Immediate angiographic embolization
   c. Obstruction
      i. Compression of stomach, small bowel, or colon
   d. Rupture
      i. Generally, can be treated nonoperatively with TPN and symptomatic paracentesis
   e. Enteric fistula
      i. Can result in spontaneous cyst resolution

B. Intraductal papillary mucinous neoplasm (IPMN)

1. Etiology
   a. Cyst communicating with the pancreatic ductal system and classified according to the type of ductal involvement[34]
      i. Main duct IPMN
      ii. Branched duct IPMN
      iii. Mixed-type IPMN
   b. >50% of all resected cystic neoplasms
2. Diagnosis
   a. Imaging
      i. Pancreatic protocol CT/MRCP
         a) Classic appearance on imaging with involvement of main or branch pancreatic ducts
      ii. EUS/FNA
         a) Indicated to further assess lesions in patients with any "worrisome features" on imaging
   b. Cyst fluid analysis (**Table 19.2**)
      i. Viscous fluid with elevated CEA and amylase
      ii. Elevated CA19-9 in the cyst may indicate malignancy
3. Treatment
   a. Due to the potential for occult malignancy, when surgery is indicated, standard oncologic resection (pancreaticoduodenectomy or distal pancreatectomy) with lymph node dissection should be performed (**Figure 19.5**)

TABLE 19.2 Pancreatic Cyst Fluid Analysis

	Amylase	CEA
Pseudocyst	High	Low
SCA	Low	Low
MCN	Low	High
IPMN	High	High

C. Mucinous cystic neoplasm (MCN)
1. Etiology
   a. Premalignant lesions making up 25% of all resected cystic neoplasms
   b. Generally located in the pancreatic body or tail
   c. About 90% to 95% found in women
2. Diagnosis
   a. Imaging
      i. Unilocular, macrocystic
      ii. No involvement of the pancreatic duct
   b. Cyst fluid analysis (**Table 19.2**)
      i. Viscous fluid, elevated CEA, low amylase
3. Treatment
   a. Traditionally, resection has been recommended at the time of identification due to the risk of invasive cancer with 10% to 40% malignancy risk[35]; however, new data indicate the potential for observation of cysts with low-risk features (size <5 cm, absence of mural nodules or enhancing walls)[36]
   b. Greater malignancy risk is associated with
      i. Size >4 cm
      ii. Age <55 years

D. Serous cystadenoma (SCA)
1. Etiology
   a. Benign lesion making up 16% of all resected cystic neoplasms
   b. Generally located in the pancreatic head
2. Diagnosis
   a. Imaging
      i. Generally diagnosed based on appearance on CT with an epithelial lining with "honeycomb" microcystic appearance and central calcified scar
   b. Cyst fluid analysis
      i. Nonviscous fluid, CEA low, amylase low
3. Treatment
   a. No intervention required
   b. Do not require additional surveillance imaging

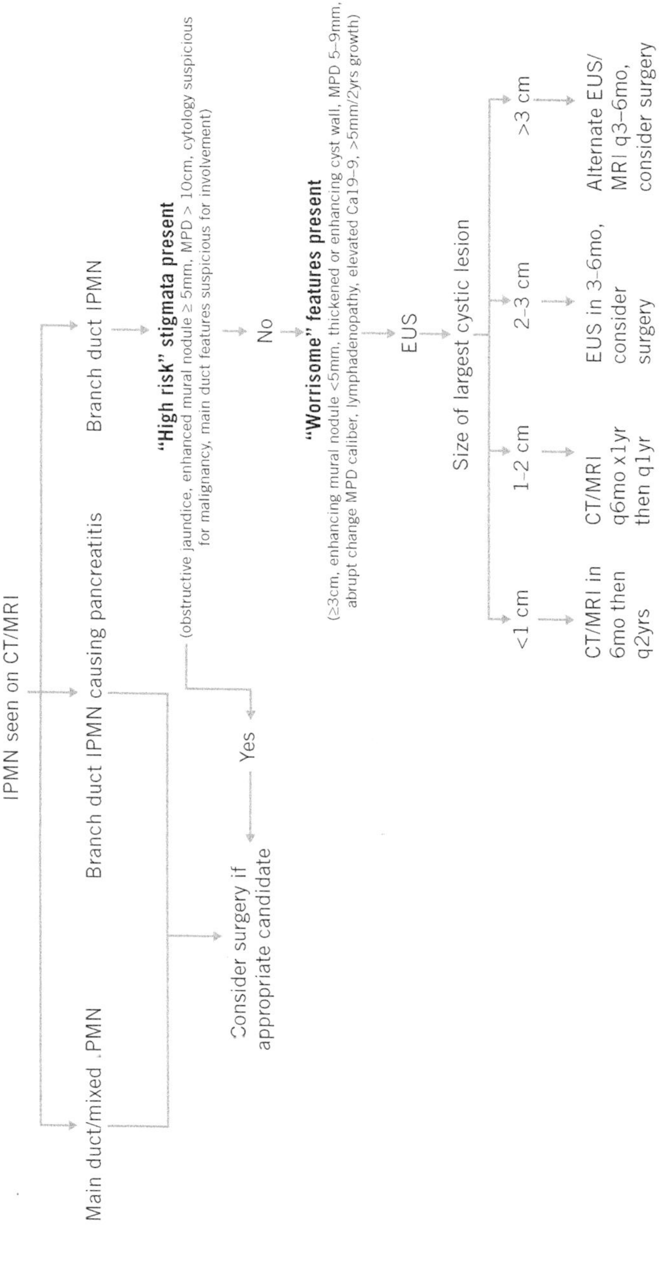
IPMN seen on CT/MRI
Branch duct IPMN
Branch duct IPMN causing pancreatitis
Main duct/mixed IPMN
"High risk" stigmata present
(obstructive jaundice, enhanced mural nodule ≥ 5mm, MPD > 10cm, cytology suspicious for malignancy, main duct features suspicious for involvement)
Yes
Consider surgery if appropriate candidate
No
"Worrisome" features present
(≥3cm, enhancing mural nodule <5mm, thickened or enhancing cyst wall, MPD 5–9mm, abrupt change MPD caliber, lymphadenopathy, elevated Ca19-9, >5mm/2yrs growth)
EUS
Size of largest cystic lesion
<1 cm
1–2 cm
2–3 cm
>3 cm
CT/MRI in 6mo then q2yrs
CT/MRI q6mo x1yr then q1yr
EUS in 3–6mo, consider surgery
Alternate EUS/MRI q3–6mo, consider surgery

FIGURE 19.5 Management of IPMN.

c. Indications for resection
   i. Symptoms (generally no symptoms unless >4 cm)
   ii. Inability to rule out malignancy

VIII. ACUTE PANCREATITIS

Acute pancreatitis is an inflammatory condition of variable severity. Approximately 80% of patients develop mild or moderately severe disease without associated organ failure, while the remaining patients develop severe disease, which carries an approximately 20% mortality rate.[37]

A. Etiology
   1. Gallstones (40%-45%)
   2. Alcohol and smoking (30%-35%)[38]
   3. ERCP associated (2%-5%)
   4. Metabolic abnormalities (e.g., hypertriglyceridemia, hypercalcemia)
   5. Drugs (e.g., azathioprine, sulfamethoxazole–trimethoprim, furosemide, valproic acid
   6. Toxins (e.g., scorpion stings, organophosphates)
   7. Infections (e.g., mumps, Coxsackie virus B, Epstein–Barr virus, cytomegalovirus)
   8. Neoplasms (benign or malignant)
   9. Trauma
   10. Autoimmunity (e.g., IgG4-associated lymphoplasmacytic pancreatitis, Sjögren's syndrome, lupus, primary biliary cirrhosis)
   11. Idiopathic

B. Diagnosis
   1. Atlanta criteria[39]
      a. Diagnosis can be made if two of the following three criteria are met
         i. Upper abdominal pain
         ii. Threefold increase in amylase or lipase
         iii. Radiographic evidence of acute pancreatitis
   2. Classification and severity scoring
      a. The Atlanta classification is the standard system for the classification of mild, moderately severe, and severe pancreatitis (**Table 19.3**).

TABLE 19.3 Atlanta Classification for Pancreatitis

Revised Atlanta Classification	Definition
Mild	No organ failure or systemic complications
Moderately severe	Transient organ failure (<48 h) or local systemic complications without persistent organ failure
Severe	Persistent organ failure (>48 h)

b. Multiple scoring systems exist (Ranson's criteria, APACHEII, BISAP) for evaluating the severity and associated risk of pancreatitis.

3. Signs and symptoms
   a. Epigastric pain radiating to the back
   b. Nausea, vomiting
   c. Evidence of systemic effects may be present in severe cases (e.g., acute renal failure, hypotension)
   d. Evidence of retroperitoneal hemorrhage
      i. Flank ecchymosis (Gray Turner sign)
      ii. Periumbilical ecchymosis (Cullen sign)
      iii. Inguinal ecchymosis (Fox's sign)
4. Laboratory findings
   a. Lipase—highly sensitive (95%)
   b. Amylase—Less sensitive than amylase and not frequently used in the modern context
   c. Acute phase proteins (C-reactive protein, tumor necrosis factor alpha, and interleukin 6)
   d. Hypocalcemia—due to complexing with fatty acids produced by activated lipase
   e. Elevated markers of biliary obstruction (hyperbilirubinemia, elevated aspartate aminotransferase/alanine aminotransferase, alkaline phosphatase)
5. Imaging
   a. CT
      i. Parenchymal enlargement and edema, necrosis, blurring of fat planes, peripancreatic fluid collections, bowel distension, mesenteric edema
      ii. Sensitivity and specificity of 90% and 100%.
      iii. Gold standard test for diagnosis
      iv. Not necessary to establish a diagnosis; however, can be important for identifying extent of pancreatic necrosis or signs of infected pancreatic necrosis
      v. Can also identify associated complications: Pleural effusions, pancreatic pseudocysts, splenic vein thrombosis
6. Ultrasound
   a. Indicated to evaluate for biliary etiology of acute pancreatitis (e.g., gallstones)
7. MRI
   a. May be used to evaluate for other complex causes of biliary pathology leading to pancreatitis (e.g., choledocholithiasis, CBD anomalies, pancreatic malignancies)
8. ERCP
   a. Indications for ERCP
      i. Patients with jaundice, biliary pancreatitis, and cholangitis not improving 24 hours after admission for stone extraction and endoscopic sphincterotomy
      ii. Patients with no identifiable cause on other imaging modalities to rule out strictures, neoplasms, or other occult causes

iii. Suspected pancreatic ductal disruption with need for stenting
iv. The multicenter APEC trial demonstrated that routine use of ERCP with biliary sphincterotomy for patients with gallstone pancreatitis without concomitant cholangitis did not reduce mortality or complications in patients with severe biliary pancreatitis[40]

C. Treatment
1. Supportive care
a. Volume resuscitation
i. Use isotonic fluid and target urine output of ≥0.5 mL/kg/h
b. Nutrition
i. Enteral nutrition significantly reduces the risk of multiorgan failure and mortality as compared with parenteral nutrition when started within 48 hours of admission.[41]
ii. The multicenter PYTHON trial found that tube feeding was not superior to on-demand feeding to reduce the rate of mortality.[42]
c. Analgesics
i. No specific analgesic regimen is superior in terms of efficacy or safety.[43]
d. Respiratory monitoring
i. Pulmonary complications may occur in up to 50% of patients.
e. Antibiotics are generally not indicated.
i. Routine use of antibiotics is not indicated and should be given only for confirmed or clinically suspected secondary infection.[44]
2. Interventional and surgical treatment
a. Indications
i. Clinical deterioration
ii. Gastric outlet or intestinal obstruction with failure to thrive beyond 6 to 8 weeks
iii. Infected pancreatic necrosis
b. Step-up approach[45]
i. Whenever possible, surgical debridement of pancreatic necrosis should be delayed ~3 to 4 weeks after onset of symptoms to allow for sequestration of necrosis.
ii. The step up approach advocates for the most minimally invasive possible treatment option with escalation to more maximally invasive options only after failure of prior attempted therapies.
a) Percutaneous drainage of necrotic or large fluid collection
b) Endoscopic drainage via transgastric stenting
c) Video-assisted retroperitoneal debridement
d) Open surgical debridement
iii. The step-up approach was associated with a 30% to 40% decrease in morbidity vs. primary open necrosectomy.
3. Treatment of gallstone pancreatitis
a. Cholecystectomy during the same hospitalization is advised to prevent disease recurrence due to reduced rates of gallstone complications and mortality.[46]

D. Complications of acute pancreatitis
1. Necrotizing pancreatitis
   a. Occurs in 10% to 20% of acute pancreatitis
2. Infected necrotizing pancreatitis
   a. CT finding of gas associated with an area of pancreatic necrosis is indicative.
   b. Historically FNA sampling has been used to assess; however, it has a high false-negative rate of up to 25%.[47] Can still be used for patients with no clear evidence of infection on CT and prolonged course of pancreatitis.
3. Pseudocyst
   a. See Section VII
4. Pseudoaneurysm
   a. Associated with necrotizing pancreatitis
   b. Pancreatic enzymes autodigest the walls of pancreatic and visceral arteries leading to wall defects.
   c. Most commonly involves splenic, gastroduodenal, and pancreaticoduodenal arteries
   d. Rupture may lead to life-threatening bleeding.
   e. Generally treated with angiography and embolization
5. Abdominal compartment syndrome
   a. Defined as the presence of intra-abdominal hypertension (intra-abdominal pressure >12 mm Hg) with acute organ dysfunction (respiratory failure, renal failure)
   b. Multifactorial development in pancreatitis: Due to visceral edema from large volume resuscitation, ascites, and space-occupying retroperitoneal and peripancreatic fluid collections
   c. Treatment: Volume removal (diuretics or dialysis), nasogastric tube placement, sedation, and neuromuscular blockade
      i. If more conservative strategies fail, decompressive laparotomy may be required
6. Portal system thrombosis
   a. Often asymptomatic and discovered incidentally on imaging
   b. Can result in chronic portal hypertension and varices
   c. Complete superior mesenteric or portal vein thromboses can lead to acute massive ascites, bowel infarction, or encephalopathy
   d. Splenic vein thrombosis may result in gastric varices
   e. Treatment: Anticoagulation with bridge to oral anticoagulation for 3 to 6 months
7. Ductal disruption
   a. Necrosis of a portion of the mid-pancreas can result in a portion of pancreatic tail that is no longer connected.
   b. This can result in recurrent pseudocyst formation, pancreatic fistula formation.
   c. Treatment: Endoscopic pancreatic duct stenting, surgical resection of the disconnected segment or drainage into a roux limb of jejunum

IX. CHRONIC PANCREATITIS

Chronic pancreatitis is a progressive inflammatory disorder characterized by destruction of pancreatic parenchyma with subsequent fibrosis. Commonly, this results in chronic abdominal pain and endocrine or exocrine pancreatic insufficiency.

A. Etiology
   1. Can be discussed according to TIGAR-O risk factors[48]
      a. Toxic-metabolic (e.g., Alcohol, tobacco)
         i. Tobacco now is the most commonly identified risk factor (59%) more common than alcohol (53%)
      b. Idiopathic
      c. Genetic (e.g., PRSS1, SPINK1, CFTR genes)
      d. Autoimmune
      e. Recurrent pancreatitis (multiple episodes of prior acute pancreatitis)
      f. Obstructive (e.g., pancreas divisum, tumor associated)

B. Diagnosis
   1. Signs and symptoms
      a. Upper mid-epigastric abdominal pain radiating to the back, generally postprandial and progressive over time
      b. Changes in bowel habits and bloating
      c. Steatorrhea
      d. Diabetes
      e. Weight loss and food avoidance
      f. Jaundice if associated with CBD stricturing
   2. Laboratory testing
      a. Lipase and amylase are generally normal
      b. Blood glucose levels[49]
         i. More than 30% of patients with chronic pancreatitis will develop diabetes with increased risk of development associated with older age, obesity, concurrent exocrine insufficiency, presence of calcifications, and history of pancreas surgery.
      c. Secretin stimulation tests
         i. Assesses pancreatic exocrine function by evaluation of duodenal bicarbonate levels after intravenous administration of secretin
      d. Seventy-two-hour evaluation of fecal fat
         i. Nonspecific, generally not used
      e. Fecal elastase 1[50]
         i. Reliable, noninvasive method for screening for exocrine insufficiency
   3. Imaging
      a. CT
         i. Sensitivity 75%; specificity 91%
         ii. Demonstrates pancreatic atrophy, pancreatic calcifications, pancreatic duct irregularity or dilation
         iii. Also useful for identification of associated causes (e.g., malignancy) and complications (e.g., pseudocysts, fistulas)

b. MRI
   i. Sensitivity 78%; specificity 96%
   ii. Generally not utilized for initial diagnosis but may be useful for delineation of the biliary system
c. ERCP/EUS
   i. Highest sensitivity and specificity for diagnosis of chronic pancreatitis (ERCP 92% and 94%, EUS 81% and 90%)
   ii. Generally, only utilized when CT/MRI is nondiagnostic or when needed for therapeutic intervention
   iii. Endoscopic ultrasound
      a) Rosemont criteria[51] define chronic pancreatitis as one major A and three minor, or one major A and major B, or two major A criteria
         1) Major A criteria
            - Hyperechoic features with shadowing
            - Main pancreatic duct calcification
         2) Major B criteria
            - Lobularity with honeycombing
         3) Minor criteria
            - Lobularity without honeycombing
            - Hyperechoic features without shadowing
            - Pseudocyst
            - Stranding
            - Irregular main pancreatic duct
            - Hyperechoic main pancreatic duct wall

C. Treatment
1. Medical management
   a. Malabsorption or steatorrhea—generally managed with pancreatic enzyme supplementation.
   b. Nutritional support—malnutrition is common due to postprandial pain and food avoidance as well as malabsorption.
   c. Diabetes—may be initially responsive to good nutrition and dietary control; however, oral hypoglycemic agents may be required.
   d. Pain control—Multimodal approach is generally recommended.
      i. In select patients, tricyclic antidepressants or gabapentin may be effective in reducing the need for narcotic pain medications.[52]
      ii. Adequate enzyme supplementation and nutritional therapy do not contribute directly to pain relief.
   e. Alcohol and tobacco cessation—can improve pain control and progression of disease and should be encouraged.
   f. Management of associated pleural effusions or ascites—tube thoracostomy or paracentesis may be required for pancreatitis-associated pleural effusion or pancreatic ascites.
2. Endoscopic therapy
   a. Endoscopic sphincterotomy, stenting, stone retrieval, or lithotripsy may be used for patients with ductal complications with pancreatitis.
   b. Endoscopic celiac plexus block may be considered for improving symptoms for patients with severe pain.

3. Surgical management
   a. Indications for surgery[53]
      i. Unremitting pain
      ii. Failure to thrive
      iii. Inability to rule to neoplasm
      iv. Management of associated complications (pseudocyst, aneurysm, stricture, fistula, gastric or intestinal obstruction)
   b. Resection procedures
      i. Whipple
         a) Resection of the pancreatic head, duodenum, and distal bile duct (as discussed in Section IV)
         b) Used for patients with an enlarged pancreatic head and no downstream biliary ductal dilation, patients with biliary or duodenal obstruction, or those in whom malignancy is suspected
      ii. Distal pancreatectomy
         a) Resection of the body and tail of the pancreas
         b) Used for patients with isolated distal disease
      iii. Total pancreatectomy and islet autotransplantation (TPIAT)
         a) Has historically been reserved for patients who have failed other treatment options or those who have small duct disease, although with expanding data now indicating that early surgery may be indicated in some conditions and may improve outcomes as compared with late surgery[54]
         b) Patients with hereditary and genetic pancreatitis treated with upfront TPIAT may have improved quality of life over other procedures.
   c. Drainage procedures (**Figure 19.6**)
      i. Lateral pancreatojejunostomy (Puestow)
         a) Pancreatic duct is opened longitudinally along the anterior aspect of the pancreas, and a side-to-side pancreatojejunostomy is created to a Roux-en-Y limb of jejunum
         b) Pancreatic duct size must exceed 5 mm with no associated pancreatic head enlargement
   d. Drainage/resection procedures
      i. Frey procedure
         a) Pancreatic ductal dilation with associated pancreatic head enlargement
         b) Combines lateral pancreatojejunostomy and local pancreatic head resection
         c) May have lower morbidity than Whipple or Beger procedure in meta analysis[55]
      ii. Beger procedure
         a) Pancreatic neck is divided and subtotal resection of the pancreatic head is performed.
         b) A Roux limb is anastomosed in a side-to-side fashion with the pancreatic head and an end-to-side fashion with the pancreatic body/tail.

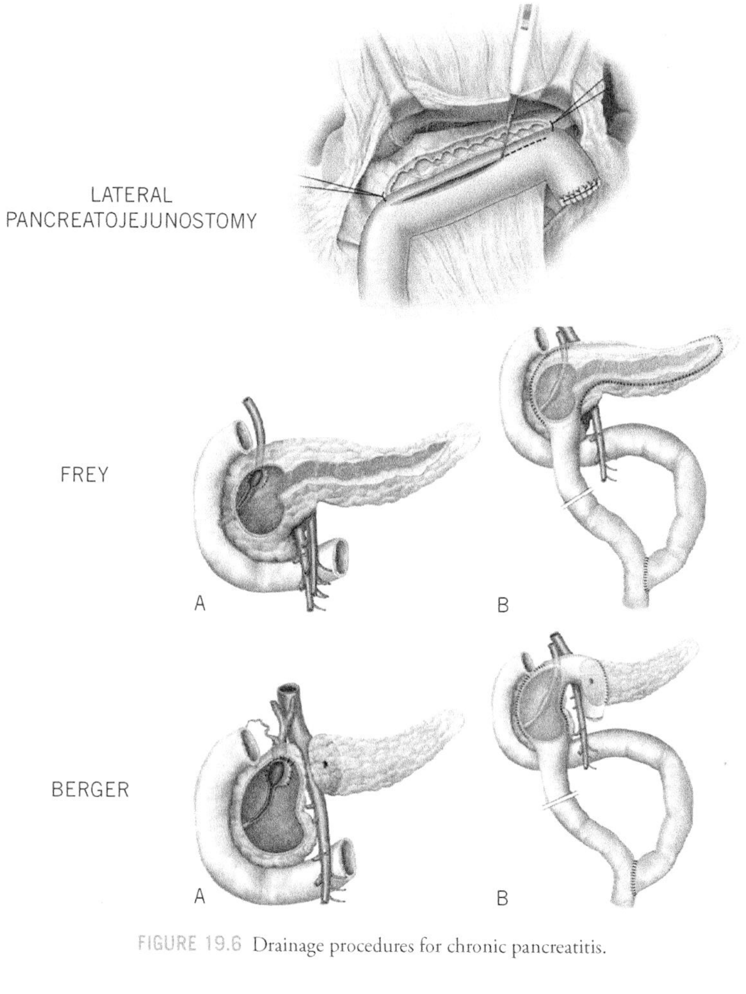

FIGURE 19.6 Drainage procedures for chronic pancreatitis.

- **e.** Celiac plexus block
  - **i.** Can be performed in isolation or as part of another surgical procedure
  - **ii.** Ganglionectomy or injection of sclerosing agents is possible.
  - **iii.** Less commonly performed due to rise of endoscopic techniques

D. Complications

- **1.** CBD obstruction
  - **a.** Associated strictures are common and when present must be distinguished from malignancy.

2. Pancreaticoenteric fistula
    a. Due to drainage of pancreatic abscess or pseudocyst into stomach, duodenum, transverse colon, or biliary tract
    b. May become infected or result in hemorrhage
3. Pancreaticopleural fistula
    a. Due to communication between the duct and pleural space
4. Pseudocyst (see Section VII)
5. Splenic vein thrombosis (see above)
6. Pancreatic cancer
    a. Chronic pancreatitis carries a relative risk between 6 and 11 for the development of pancreatic cancer[56]

Key References

Citation	Summary
van Santvoort HC, Bakker OJ, Bollen TL, et al. A conservative and minimally invasive approach to necrotizing pancreatitis improves outcome. *Gastroenterology*. 2011;141(4):1254-1263.	• This prospective multicenter study evaluated data from patients with necrotizing pancreatitis who underwent treatment with surgical drainage or drainage catheter placement and demonstrated that delayed intervention and catheter drainage as first treatments improve outcomes and surgery should be reserved for patients who have failed more conservative approaches.
Tanaka M, Fernández-Del Castillo C, Kamisawa T, et al. Revisions of international consensus Fukuoka guidelines for the management of IPMN of the pancreas. *Pancreatology*. 2017;17(5):738-753.	• This international consensus guideline outlines the strategies for management of IPMN including indications for surgical resection and recommendations for surveillance screening intervals.
Oettle H, Neuhaus P, Hochhaus A, et al. Adjuvant chemotherapy with gemcitabine and long-term outcomes among patients with resected pancreatic cancer: the CONKO-001 randomized trial. *J Am Med Assoc*. 2013;310(14):1473-1481.	• This phase 3 randomized control trial was the first to demonstrate the efficacy of adjuvant gemcitabine to prolong overall survival in patients with pancreatic cancer who had previously undergone complete resection.
Howe JR, Merchant NB, Conrad C, et al. The North American neuroendocrine tumor society consensus paper on the surgical management of pancreatic neuroendocrine tumors. *Pancreas*. 2020;49(1):1-33.	• This consensus guideline outlines the management of pancreatic neuroendocrine tumors including the recommendation for observation for tumors <1 cm, resection for tumors >2 cm, and decision making for when to consider resection for tumors between 1 and 2 cm.

CHAPTER 19: PANCREAS

Review Questions

1. What syndrome is a common manifestation of a gastrinoma?
2. What drainage procedure would be indicated for a patient with chronic pancreatitis and a dilated duct and no head enlargement?
3. What is the first-line treatment for acute pancreatitis?
4. What treatment should be recommended for a patient with a main duct IPMN?
5. What three anastomoses are made during a Whipple procedure?
6. For a patient with gallstone pancreatitis, when should cholecystectomy be performed?

REFERENCES

1. Bertin C, Pelletier AL, Vullierme MP, et al. Pancreas divisum is not a cause of pancreatitis by itself but acts as a partner of genetic mutations. *Am J Gastroenterol.* 2012;107(2):311-317.
2. Siegel RL, Miller KD, Fuchs HE, Jemal A. Cancer statistics, 2021. *CA Cancer J Clin.* 2021;71(1):7-33.
3. Bosetti C, Lucenteforte E, Silverman DT, et al. Cigarette smoking and pancreatic cancer: an analysis from the international pancreatic cancer case-control consortium (Panc4). *Ann Oncol.* 2012;23(7):1880-1888.
4. Oyama H, Tada M, Takagi K, et al. Long-term risk of malignancy in branch-duct intraductal papillary mucinous neoplasms. *Gastroenterology.* 2020;158(1):226.e5-237.e5.
5. Hu C, LaDuca H, Shimelis H, et al. Multigene hereditary cancer panels reveal high-risk pancreatic cancer susceptibility genes. *JCO Precis Oncol.* 2018;2:PO.17.00291.
6. Aslanian HR, Lee JH, Canto MI. AGA clinical practice update on pancreas cancer screening in high-risk individuals: expert review. *Gastroenterology.* 2020;159(1):358-362.
7. Marrelli D, Caruso S, Pedrazzani C, et al. CA19-9 serum levels in obstructive jaundice: clinical value in benign and malignant conditions. *Am J Surg.* 2009;198(3):333-339.
8. Hartwig W, Strobel O, Hinz U, et al. CA19-9 in potentially resectable pancreatic cancer: perspective to adjust surgical and perioperative therapy. *Ann Surg Oncol.* 2013;20(7):2188-2196.
9. Truty MJ, Kendrick ML, Nagorney DM, et al. Factors predicting response, perioperative outcomes, and survival following total neoadjuvant therapy for borderline/locally advanced pancreatic cancer. *Ann Surg.* 2021;273(2):341-349.
10. Darnell EP, Wang TJ, Lumish MA, et al. Preoperative cholangitis is an independent risk factor for mortality in patients after pancreatoduodenectomy for pancreatic cancer. *Am J Surg.* 2021;221(1):134-140.
11. Ta R, O'Connor DB, Sulistijo A, Chung B, Conlon KC. The role of staging laparoscopy in resectable and borderline resectable pancreatic cancer: a systematic review and meta-analysis. *Dig Surg.* 2019;36(3):251-260.
12. Chawla A, Molina G, Pak LM, et al. Neoadjuvant therapy is associated with improved survival in borderline-resectable pancreatic cancer. *Ann Surg Oncol.* 2020;27(4):1191-1200.
13. Murphy JE, Wo JY, Ryan DP, et al. Total neoadjuvant therapy with FOLFIRINOX followed by individualized chemoradiotherapy for borderline resectable pancreatic adenocarcinoma: a phase 2 clinical trial. *JAMA Oncol.* 2018;4(7):963-969.

14. Philip PA, Lacy J, Portales F, et al. Nab-paclitaxel plus gemcitabine in patients with locally advanced pancreatic cancer (LAPACT): a multicentre, open-label phase 2 study. *Lancet Gastroenterol Hepatol.* 2020;5(3):285-294.
15. Sohal DPS, Duong M, Ahmad SA, et al. Efficacy of perioperative chemotherapy for resectable pancreatic adenocarcinoma: a phase 2 randomized clinical trial. *JAMA Oncol.* 2021;7(3):421-427.
16. Panni RZ, Panni UY, Liu J, et al. Re-defining a high volume center for pancreaticoduodenectomy. *HPB (Oxford).* 2021;23(5):733-738.
17. Chun YS. Role of radical antegrade modular pancreatosplenectomy (RAMPS) and pancreatic cancer. *Ann Surg Oncol.* 2018;25(1):46-50.
18. de Rooij T, Lu MZ, Steen MW, et al. Minimally invasive versus open pancreatoduodenectomy: systematic review and meta-analysis of comparative cohort and registry studies. *Ann Surg.* 2016;264(2):257-267.
19. Oettle H, Neuhaus P, Hochhaus A, et al. Adjuvant chemotherapy with gemcitabine and long-term outcomes among patients with resected pancreatic cancer: the CONKO-001 randomized trial. *JAMA.* 2013;310(14):1473-1481.
20. Conroy T, Hammel P, Hebbar M, et al. FOLFIRINOX or gemcitabine as adjuvant therapy for pancreatic cancer. *N Engl J Med.* 2018;379(25):2395-2406.
21. Van Buren G II, Ramanathan RK, Krasinskas AM, et al. Phase II study of induction fixed-dose rate gemcitabine and bevacizumab followed by 30 Gy radiotherapy as preoperative treatment for potentially resectable pancreatic adenocarcinoma. *Ann Surg Oncol.* 2013;20(12):3787-3793.
22. Mungroop TH, van Rijssen LB, van Klaveren D, et al. Alternative fistula risk score for pancreatoduodenectomy (a-FRS): design and international external validation. *Ann Surg.* 2019;269(5):937-943.
23. Callery MP, Pratt WB, Kent TS, Chaikof EL, Vollmer CM Jr. A prospectively validated clinical risk score accurately predicts pancreatic fistula after pancreatoduodenectomy. *J Am Coll Surg.* 2013;216(1):1-14.
24. Kantor O, Talamonti MS, Pitt HA, et al. Using the NSQIP pancreatic demonstration project to derive a modified fistula risk score for preoperative risk stratification in patients undergoing pancreaticoduodenectomy. *J Am Coll Surg.* 2017;224(5):816-825.
25. Swanson RS, Pezzi CM, Mallin K, Loomis AM, Winchester DP. The 90-day mortality after pancreatectomy for cancer is double the 30-day mortality: more than 20,000 resections from the national cancer data base. *Ann Surg Oncol.* 2014;21(13):4059-4067.
26. Howe JR, Merchant NB, Conrad C, et al. The North American neuroendocrine tumor society consensus paper on the surgical management of pancreatic neuroendocrine tumors. *Pancreas.* 2020;49(1):1-33.
27. Saxena A, Chua TC, Perera M, Chu F, Morris DL. Surgical resection of hepatic metastases from neuroendocrine neoplasms: a systematic review. *Surg Oncol.* 2012;21(3):e131-e141.
28. Caplin ME, Pavel M, Ćwikła JB, et al. Lanreotide in metastatic enteropancreatic neuroendocrine tumors. *N Engl J Med.* 2014;371(3):224-233.
29. Konstantinidis IT, Dursun A, Zheng H, et al. Metastatic tumors in the pancreas in the modern era. *J Am Coll Surg.* 2010;211(6):749-753.
30. Hochwald SN, Hemming AW, Draganov P, Vogel SB, Dixon LR, Grobmyer SR. Elevation of serum IgG4 in Western patients with autoimmune sclerosing pancreatocholangitis: a word of caution. *Ann Surg Oncol.* 2008;15(4):1147-1154.
31. European Study Group on Cystic Tumours of the Pancreas. European evidence-based guidelines on pancreatic cystic neoplasms. *Gut.* 2018;67(5):789-804.

32. Elta GH, Enestvedt BK, Sauer BG, Lennon AM. ACG clinical guideline: diagnosis and management of pancreatic cysts. *Am J Gastroenterol.* 2018;113(4):464-479.

33. Vege SS, Ziring B, Jain R, Moayyedi P; Clinical Guidelines Committee; American Gastroenterology Association. American gastroenterological association institute guideline on the diagnosis and management of asymptomatic neoplastic pancreatic cysts. *Gastroenterology.* 2015;148(4):819-822; quize12-13.

34. Tanaka M, Fernandez-Del Castillo C, Kamisawa T, et al. Revisions of international consensus Fukuoka guidelines for the management of IPMN of the pancreas. *Pancreatology.* 2017;17(5):738-753.

35. van Huijgevoort NCM, Del Chiaro M, Wolfgang CL, van Hooft JE, Besselink MG. Diagnosis and management of pancreatic cystic neoplasms: current evidence and guidelines. *Nat Rev Gastroenterol Hepatol.* 2019;16(11):676-689.

36. Marchegiani G, Andrianello S, Crippa S, et al. Actual malignancy risk of either operated or non-operated presumed mucinous cystic neoplasms of the pancreas under surveillance. *Br J Surg.* 2021;108(9):1097-1104.

37. Forsmark CE, Vege SS, Wilcox CM. Acute pancreatitis. *N Engl J Med.* 2016;375(20):1972-1981.

38. Yuhara H, Ogawa M, Kawaguchi Y, Igarashi M, Mine T. Smoking and risk for acute pancreatitis: a systematic review and meta-analysis. *Pancreas.* 2014;43(8):1201-1207.

39. Banks PA, Bollen TL, Dervenis C, et al. Classification of acute pancreatitis–2012: revision of the Atlanta classification and definitions by international consensus. *Gut.* 2013;62(1):102-111.

40. Schepers NJ, Hallensleben NDL, Besselink MG, et al. Urgent endoscopic retrograde cholangiopancreatography with sphincterotomy versus conservative treatment in predicted severe acute gallstone pancreatitis (APEC): a multicentre randomised controlled trial. *Lancet.* 2020;396(10245):167-176.

41. Petrov MS, Pylypchuk RD, Uchugina AF. A systematic review on the timing of artificial nutrition in acute pancreatitis. *Br J Nutr.* 2009;101(6):787-793.

42. Bakker OJ, van Brunschot S, van Santvoort HC, et al. Early versus on-demand nasoenteric tube feeding in acute pancreatitis. *N Engl J Med.* 2014;371(21):1983-1993.

43. Meng W, Yuan J, Zhang C, et al. Parenteral analgesics for pain relief in acute pancreatitis: a systematic review. *Pancreatology.* 2013;13(3):201-206.

44. Baron TH, DiMaio CJ, Wang AY, Morgan KA. American gastroenterological association clinical practice update: management of pancreatic necrosis. *Gastroenterology.* 2020;158(1):67-75 e1.

45. van Santvoort HC, Bakker OJ, Bollen TL, et al. A conservative and minimally invasive approach to necrotizing pancreatitis improves outcome. *Gastroenterology.* 2011;141(4):1254-1263.

46. da Costa DW, Bouwense SA, Schepers NJ, et al. Same-admission versus interval cholecystectomy for mild gallstone pancreatitis (PONCHO): a multicentre randomised controlled trial. *Lancet.* 2015;386(10000):1261-1268.

47. Working Group IAP/APA Acute Pancreatitis Guidelines. IAP/APA evidence-based guidelines for the management of acute pancreatitis. *Pancreatology.* 2013;13(4 suppl 2):e1-e15.

48. Whitcomb DC; North American Pancreatitis Study Group. Pancreatitis: TIGAR-O version 2 risk/etiology checklist with topic reviews, updates, and use primers. *Clin Transl Gastroenterol.* 2019;10(6):e00027.

49. Bellin MD, Whitcomb DC, Abberbock J, et al. Patient and disease characteristics associated with the presence of diabetes mellitus in adults with chronic pancreatitis in the United States. *Am J Gastroenterol.* 2017;112(9):1457-1465.

50. Dominguez-Munoz JE, D Hardt P, Lerch MM, Lohr MJ. Potential for screening for pancreatic exocrine insufficiency using the fecal elastase-1 test. *Dig Dis Sci.* 2017;62(5):1119-1130.

51. Catalano MF, Sahai A, Levy M, et al. EUS-based criteria for the diagnosis of chronic pancreatitis: the Rosemont classification. *Gastrointest Endosc.* 2009;69(7):1251-1261.

52. Drewes AM, Bouwense SAW, Campbell CM, et al. Guidelines for the understanding and management of pain in chronic pancreatitis. *Pancreatology.* 2017;17(5):720-731.

53. Kempeneers MA, Issa Y, Ali UA, et al. International consensus guidelines for surgery and the timing of intervention in chronic pancreatitis. *Pancreatology.* 2020;20(2):149-157.

54. Abu-El-Haija M, Anazawa T, Beilman GJ, et al. The role of total pancreatectomy with islet autotransplantation in the treatment of chronic pancreatitis: a report from the International Consensus Guidelines in chronic pancreatitis. *Pancreatology.* 2020;20(4):762-771.

55. Zhou Y, Shi B, Wu L, Wu X, Li Y. Frey procedure for chronic pancreatitis: evidence-based assessment of short- and long-term results in comparison to pancreatoduodenectomy and Beger procedure. A meta-analysis. *Pancreatology.* 2015;15(4):372-379.

56. Beyer G, Habtezion A, Werner J, Lerch MM, Mayerle J. Chronic pancreatitis. *Lancet.* 2020;396(10249):499-512.

20 Spleen

Keenan J. Robbins and Maria Bernadette Doyle

I. INTRODUCTION

A. Splenic Anatomy

1. Oblong organ with a purple hue that resides in the left upper quadrant of the abdomen, deep to ribs 9 to 12.
2. Measures 7 to 13 cm on its long axis and weighs between 100 and 200 g.
3. The posterosuperior aspect of the spleen is convex and abuts the diaphragm, while the inferomedial surface is concave and is intimately associated with the pancreatic tail and splenic flexure of the colon.
4. Multiple ligaments maintain the spleen's position in the abdomen and are of particular relevance when mobilizing the spleen intraoperatively (**Figure 20.1**).
   a. The gastrosplenic ligament links the stomach and spleen and contains the short gastric and gastroepiploic vessels.
   b. The splenorenal ligament connects the spleen and left kidney, housing the splenic vessels and pancreatic tail.
   c. The splenocolic ligament and phrenicosplenic ligament connect the spleen to the transverse colon and diaphragm, respectively, and are avascular.
   d. The phrenicocolic ligament (sustentaculum lienis) is a band of peritoneum that bridges the diaphragm and transverse colon, contributing additional support to the spleen.
5. In the setting of **portal hypertension**, collaterals may develop within these otherwise avascular ligaments.

B. Abnormal development/anatomy

1. Abnormal development of the suspensory ligaments of the spleen can result in a wandering spleen, which may undergo torsion leading to infarction requiring splenectomy.
2. **Accessory spleen**: Splenic tissue exists apart from the main corpus of the spleen.
   a. Found in 10% to 20% of the population and does not require intervention unless the splenic tissue is contributing to a pathologic process (discussed later).
   b. Accessory spleens are typically found in the splenic hilum or along the pedicle of the splenic vessels.

C. Vascular supply

1. The primary vascular supply to the spleen comes from the splenic artery, usually a branch of the celiac axis.

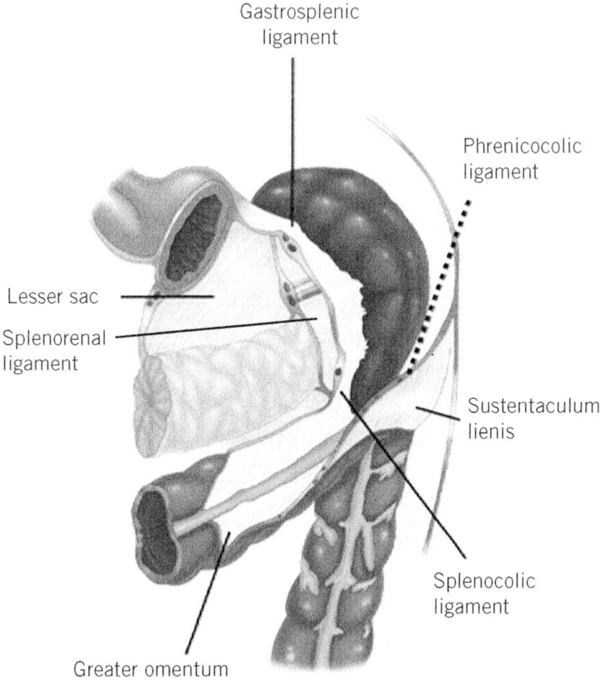

FIGURE 20.1 Suspensory ligaments of the spleen. *(Modified with permission from Poulin EC, Thibault C. The anatomical basis for laparoscopic splenectomy. Can J Surg. 1993:36(5):484-488. Copyright 1993, Canadian Medical Association.)*

2. As the splenic artery enters the splenic hilum it terminally branches in one of two fashions:
   a. A distributed-type splenic artery branches early with several long branches.
   b. A magistral-type splenic artery branches later into a few larger trunks that may complicate hilar dissection.

D. Splenic physiology

1. The spleen has hematologic and immunologic roles.
   a. During gestation and the first few months of life, the spleen plays a role in physiologic hematopoiesis.
      i. In adults, the spleen can contribute to extramedullary hematopoiesis in disease states that cause chronic anemia.
      ii. The venous sinuses and red pulp also serve as reservoirs for red blood cells (RBCs), which can be released during periods of distress and raise the hematocrit several points.
      iii. As part of the reticuloendothelial system (RES), the red pulp of the spleen filters hemoglobin and other components from lysed RBC.

b. The phagocytic nature of the RES also plays a role in the spleen's immunologic function, removing pathogens from the blood.
   i. Overly robust splenic phagocytosis, leading to pancytopenia, is called **hypersplenism** and is often an indication for splenectomy.
   ii. The white pulp of the spleen houses a significant portion of the body's white blood cells, which are released during an immune response.

II. HEMATOLOGIC DISEASES OF THE SPLEEN

A. Congenital disorders
  1. Hemoglobinopathies
    a. Sickle cell disease (SCD)
      i. Etiology
        a) Autosomal recessive defect in β-globin gene.
        b) In low-oxygen environments, hemoglobin polymerizes and assumes sickled shape, leading to hemolysis, microvascular obstruction, and tissue ischemia.
        c) Repeated episodes lead to infarction, autosplenectomy, and functional asplenia.
      ii. Presentation
        a) Hemolytic anemia
        b) Vaso-occlusive crisis (tissue ischemia causing pain, organ failure)
        c) Sequestration crisis (RBCs rapidly engorge spleen, causing hypovolemia and shock)
      iii. Diagnosis
        a) Complete blood count (CBC)—anemia, reticulocytosis
        b) Peripheral blood smear—sickled RBCs, reticulocytes
        c) Comprehensive metabolic panel—hyperbilirubinemia
      iv. Nonoperative management
        a) Avoid precipitants of vaso-occlusive crisis (e.g., dehydration)
        b) Hydroxyurea
        c) Blood transfusion
        d) Hematopoietic stem cell transplant (HSCT)
      v. Operative management
        a) Splenectomy rarely required; indicated for abscess, sequestration crisis, hypersplenism
        b) Debridement may be required for leg ulcers
      vi. Outcomes
        a) Children with SCD who undergo splenectomy are not at increased risk of death or infectious complications.[1]
    b. Thalassemia
      i. Encompasses multiple autosomal dominant (AD) mutations that result in decreased synthesis of hemoglobin chains.
      ii. RBC production is impaired, and hemolysis, anemia, and tissue hypoxia may follow.

iii. The thalassemias are the most common genetic disorder in humans.

iv. β-Thalassemia

a) **Etiology**

1) Decreased or absent β-globin synthesis

b) **Presentation**

1) β-Thalassemia minor—asymptomatic, mild microcytic anemia

2) β-Thalassemia major—symptomatic in the first year of life; transfusion-dependent anemia, impaired growth, hepatosplenomegaly secondary to extramedullary hematopoiesis

c) Diagnosis

1) Family history

2) CBC, fractionated bilirubin, haptoglobin

3) Genetic testing

d) Nonoperative management

1) Serial blood transfusions with chelators

2) HSCT

e) Operative management

1) Splenectomy indicated if excessive transfusion requirements, thalassemia-related growth impairment, hypersplenism, or symptomatic splenomegaly.

2) Ideally delayed until after 5 years of age to decrease risk of postsplenectomy infection.

f) Outcomes

1) Splenectomy decreases transfusion requirement and, ideally, prevents the development of extramedullary hematopoiesis.[2]

v. α-Thalassemia

a) Secondary to the underproduction of α-globin chains.

b) Symptoms parallel the severity of the anemia, ranging from death in utero to mild asymptomatic anemia.

c) Diagnosis and management are similar to β-thalassemia.

2. **Hemolytic anemias**

a. **Hereditary spherocytosis** (most common congenital anemia)

i. **Etiology**

a) AD defect in membrane proteins (spectrin, ankyrin, band 3 protein) causes RBCs to assume spherical shape, making them more vulnerable to splenic hemolysis.

ii. **Presentation**

a) Symptoms range from asymptomatic to severe anemia with jaundice, cholelithiasis with pigmented stones, and symptomatic splenomegaly.

iii. **Diagnosis**

a) CBC (elevated mean corpuscular hemoglobin concentration)

b) Peripheral blood smear (spherocytes)

c) Osmotic fragility test

iv. **Nonoperative management**
   a) Phototherapy (infants)
   b) Folate supplementation
   c) Blood transfusion
v. **Operative management**
   a) Splenectomy indications: Growth impairment, anemia-induced organ dysfunction, and extramedullary hematopoiesis.
   b) If preoperative right upper quadrant (RUQ) ultrasound imaging (US) demonstrates cholelithiasis, concomitant cholecystectomy indicated.
vi. **Outcomes**
   a) Splenectomy curative for most patients.[3] Refractory disease should prompt investigation for accessory splenic tissue.

b. **Hereditary elliptocytosis**
   i. Mutations in RBC surface proteins that render cells prone to splenic hemolysis.
   ii. The structural defects are less pronounced than in hereditary spherocytosis, and the disease course is milder.
   iii. Splenectomy is indicated for symptomatic anemia and is often curative.

c. **Enzymatic deficiencies**
   i. **Pyruvate kinase deficiency**
      a) **Etiology**
         1) Impaired glycolytic pathways result in ATP deficiency, rendering RBCs less deformable and more prone to hemolysis in the spleen.
      b) **Presentation**
         1) Often present with hemolytic anemia and jaundice in infancy
         2) Physiologic stress (e.g., infection, pregnancy) may unmask or exacerbate condition.
         3) Pigmented gallstones, hemochromatosis (delayed presentation)
      c) **Diagnosis**
         1) CBC with pronounced reticulocytosis
         2) Peripheral blood smear (spiculated RBC, possibly)
         3) Biochemical testing (pyruvate kinase activity), genetic testing (*PKLR* mutation)
      d) **Nonoperative management**
         1) Phototherapy (infants)
         2) Transfusion with chelators
      e) **Operative management**
         1) Symptomatic splenomegaly and ongoing transfusion requirement are indications for splenectomy, which is ideally delayed until 5 years of age.
      f) **Outcomes**
         1) Splenectomy decreases transfusion requirement.[4]

ii. **Glucose-6-phosphate dehydrogenase (G6PD) deficiency**
a) **Etiology**
1) X-linked recessive mutation imparts increased susceptibility to oxidative stress and hemolysis.
b) **Presentation**
1) Increased oxidative stress (e.g., infection, sulfa-based drugs, fava bean ingestion) leads to intermittent episodes of hemolysis and anemia.
c) **Diagnosis**
1) Biochemical testing (G6PD activity)
2) Peripheral blood smear—deformed RBCs (bite cells), inclusions of denatured hemoglobin (Heinz bodies)
d) **Nonoperative management**
1) Avoidance of oxidative stress.
2) Transfusion for severe anemia.
3) Chronic disease may require serial transfusions.
e) **Operative management**
1) Ongoing transfusion requirement, symptomatic splenomegaly, and hypersplenism are indications for splenectomy.
f) **Outcomes**
1) Splenectomy may reduce, if not resolve, transfusion requirement.[5]

B. Acquired disorders

1. **Immune-mediated hemolytic anemias** are caused by antibody-mediated RBC destruction. While this family of disorders is often called "autoimmune hemolytic anemia," not all are of autoimmune etiology and may be secondary to drug exposure, infection, or malignancy.
a. **Warm antibody hemolytic anemia** (75%-85% of immune-mediated hemolytic anemias)
i. **Etiology**
a) IgG-mediated hemolysis in the spleen
ii. **Presentation**
a) Typically, between 40 and 70 years old with anemia, jaundice, splenomegaly
b) In children, may present after viral illness and run a 2- to 3-week course before spontaneous resolution
iii. **Diagnosis**
a) Direct antiglobulin test (DAT) (direct Coombs test) identifies IgG bound to RBCs.
iv. **Nonoperative management**
a) Transfusion for severe or symptomatic anemia
b) Corticosteroids (e.g., prednisone). Monoclonal antibody vs. CD20 (rituximab) may be added. About 75% to 90% will respond to this regimen.
v. **Operative management**
a) Splenectomy indicated for disease refractory to medical therapy.

vi. **Outcomes**

a) Seventy-five percent of patients will have a complete response to splenectomy.[6]

b. **Cold antibody hemolytic anemia** (15%-25% of the immune-mediated hemolytic anemias)

i. Hemolysis occurs due to IgM binding RBCs at temperatures below body temperature (e.g., extremities, ears, nose).

ii. DAT is negative for IgG but positive for complement C3d.

iii. The initial intervention is to avoid cold temperatures, with plasmapheresis and transfusion indicated in severe disease.

iv. Steroids are not typically used and, as the liver is the site of hemolysis, splenectomy does not play a role in treatment.

2. **Myeloproliferative/myelodysplastic disorders** are the result of aberrant production of myeloid cells by the bone marrow. Either a pathologic excess of mature blood cell types exists (MPD), or the maturation process of myeloid precursors is dysfunctional (MDD).

a. **Acute myeloid leukemia**

i. **Etiology**

a) Overproduction of immature myeloblasts, crowding out normal marrow, resulting in ineffectual hematopoiesis and pancytopenia

ii. **Presentation**

a) Fatigue, infection, bleeding diathesis

iii. **Diagnosis**

a) CBC (anemia, neutropenia, thrombocytopenia)

b) Bone marrow biopsy augmented by flow cytometry and mutational analysis

iv. **Nonoperative management**

a) Cytotoxic chemotherapy

b) HSCT

v. **Operative management**

a) Splenectomy rarely indicated but may be utilized in the case of splenic rupture if less invasive measures not feasible[7]

vi. **Outcomes**

a) Splenectomy may be lifesaving in acute splenic rupture.

b. **Chronic myeloid leukemia (CML)**

i. **Etiology**

a) Myeloproliferative disorder that results in overproduction of granulocytes (basophils, eosinophils, neutrophils)

b) In most patients, translocation between chromosomes 9 and 22, t(9;22), results in *BCR-ABL* fusion oncogene on chromosome 22 (the Philadelphia chromosome) and constitutively active tyrosine kinase.

ii. **Presentation**

a) Chronic phase—asymptomatic laboratory test abnormalities, splenomegaly

b) Accelerated phase—tyrosine kinase inhibitors (TKIs)-refractory disease

c) Blast crisis—rapid proliferation of myeloblasts, clinical decline, abbreviated survival

iii. **Diagnosis**
   a) Fluorescence in situ hybridization
   b) Reverse transcriptase-polymerase chain reaction

iv. **Nonoperative management**
   a) BCR-ABL TKIs (e.g., imatinib)
   b) HSCT

v. **Operative management**
   a) Splenectomy indicated for symptomatic splenomegaly or treatment-limiting hypersplenism.

vi. **Outcomes**
   a) Splenectomy decreases hypersplenism-related transfusion requirement and improves mechanical symptoms.[8]

c. **Polycythemia vera (PCV)**

i. **Etiology**
   a) JAK2 mutation drives erythropoietin (EPO)-independent development of RBC precursors

ii. **Presentation**
   a) Hypertension, headache, blurry vision, pruritus
   b) Cyanosis, plethora, symptoms of hyperuricemia
   c) Thrombotic events
   d) Spent phase—marrow fibrosis and massive splenomegaly due to extramedullary hematopoiesis

iii. **Diagnosis**
   a) CBC (elevated hemoglobin and hematocrit)
   b) Bone marrow biopsy (hypercellularity)
   c) Diminished serum EPO levels (vs. secondary polycythemia)

iv. **Nonoperative management**
   a) Phlebotomy
   b) Aspirin
   c) Myelosuppression (e.g., hydroxyurea)

v. **Operative management**
   a) Splenectomy indicated for symptomatic splenomegaly

vi. **Outcomes**
   a) Splenectomy can increase thrombotic risk, and postoperative antiplatelet and anticoagulation therapy is indicated.

d. **Myelofibrosis**

i. **Etiology**
   a) Bone marrow replaced by fibrotic tissue
   b) Associated with JAK2 mutation

ii. **Presentation**
   a) Fatigue, fever, bone pain, night sweats
   b) Hepatomegaly, marked splenomegaly (extramedullary hematopoiesis); may lead to portal hypertension

iii. **Diagnosis**
   a) Peripheral blood smear (anisocytes, dacrocytes, poikilocytosis)
   b) Circulating $CD34^+$ cells[9]
   c) Bone marrow biopsy

iv. **Nonoperative management**
a) Supportive—transfusion, TKIs (e.g., ruxolitinib), hydroxyurea
b) Curative—HSCT

v. **Operative management**
a) Symptomatic splenomegaly, hypersplenism with transfusion requirement, splenic infarction, and portal hypertension are among the indications for splenectomy.

vi. **Outcomes**
a) Splenectomy for myelofibrosis less effective in resolving symptoms compared with other diseases, and there is considerable risk of perioperative morbidity and mortality.[10]

3. **Lymphoproliferative disorders** encompass multiple disease states characterized by the abnormal expansion of lymphocyte populations.

a. **Non-Hodgkin lymphoma (NHL)** is a collection of multiple subtypes that, taken together, represents the most common lymphoma.

i. **Etiology**
a) Acquired genetic changes result in abnormal proliferation of lymphocytes (B cells, T cells, or NK cells).

ii. **Presentation**
a) Indolent lymphadenopathy with splenomegaly, hepatomegaly, and laboratory test abnormalities (e.g., follicular lymphoma)
b) Aggressive disease with B symptoms (fever, night sweats, weight loss), rapidly enlarging nodal or extranodal mass, splenomegaly, hepatomegaly (e.g., diffuse large B-cell lymphoma [DLBCL])

iii. **Diagnosis**
a) Lymph node biopsy (excisional biopsy often required to ensure adequate tissue)
b) Immunophenotyping, flow cytometry

iv. **Nonoperative management**
a) Cytotoxic chemotherapy with or without anti-CD20 monoclonal antibody (i.e., rituximab)
b) Radiation

v. **Operative management**
a) Splenectomy indicated for symptomatic splenomegaly, hypersplenism-mediated cytopenias, or diagnostic uncertainty.

vi. **Outcomes**
a) Cytopenias resolved in the majority of patients who underwent splenectomy.[11]

b. **Hodgkin lymphoma**

i. Proliferation of characteristic malignant lymphocytes (Reed–Sternberg cells)

ii. It is often related to Epstein–Barr virus and presents with painless lymphadenopathy in the fourth decade of life.

iii. Historically, splenectomy was utilized for diagnostic purposes, but now indications for splenectomy mirror those of NHL.

c. **Chronic lymphocytic leukemia (CLL)** (most common adult leukemia)
   i. **Etiology**
      a) Increased production of mature B lymphocytes
   ii. **Presentation**
      a) Most often, asymptomatic lymphocytosis
      b) Painless lymphadenopathy
      c) Splenomegaly, hepatomegaly
      d) B symptoms (5%-10%)
   iii. **Diagnosis**
      a) CBC (lymphocytosis)
      b) Flow cytometry (B-cell antigens)
   iv. **Nonoperative management**
      a) Observation
      b) TKIs (e.g., ibrutinib), anti-CD20 monoclonal antibodies (i.e., rituximab)
      c) HSCT
   v. **Operative management**
      a) Symptomatic splenomegaly and hypersplenism are indications for splenectomy.
      b) Transformation to aggressive DLBCL (Richter syndrome) may also require operative intervention in the case of splenic rupture.
   vi. **Outcomes**
      a) Cytopenias resolve in 70% of patients after splenectomy.[12]

d. **Hairy cell leukemia**
   i. **Etiology**
      a) Rare subtype of CLL in which memory B cells acquire a BRAF V600E mutation and proliferate, accumulating in bone marrow and the spleen.
      b) Malignant cells develop distinctive cytoplasmic projections that give the disease its name.
   ii. **Presentation**
      a) Signs of pancytopenia (anemia, infection, bleeding diathesis)
      b) Symptoms related to massive splenomegaly (25%)
      c) Spleen is palpable in 80% to 90% of patients.
   iii. **Diagnosis**
      a) Bone marrow biopsy
      b) Peripheral blood smear (hairy cells)
      c) Flow cytometry, immunophenotyping
   iv. **Nonoperative management**
      a) Observation if asymptomatic
      b) Purine analogues (e.g., cladribine, pentostatin)
      c) Monoclonal antibodies (e.g., rituximab)
   v. **Operative management**
      a) Splenectomy, once first-line therapy, now reserved for refractory disease or symptomatic splenomegaly

vi. **Outcomes**
   a) Nearly all patients will have improvement of blood counts after splenectomy, but about one-third will recur.[13]

4. **Platelet disorders**
   a. **Chronic idiopathic thrombocytopenic purpura (ITP)**
      i. **Etiology**
         a) Autoantibodies bind platelet glycoproteins, and platelets are destroyed in the spleen.
         b) May be secondary to autoimmune disorder (e.g., lupus, antiphospholipid syndrome), infection (e.g., hepatitis C, HIV), or malignancy (e.g., CLL)
      ii. **Presentation**
         a) Asymptomatic thrombocytopenia
         b) Bruising, petechiae, mucosal bleeding if platelet count <20,000.
      iii. **Diagnosis**
         a) Physical examination (signs of bruising, bleeding)
         b) Peripheral blood smear (exclude other disorders)
         c) Hepatitis C and HIV testing
         d) Ultimately, ITP is a diagnosis of exclusion.
      iv. **Nonoperative management**
         a) Treat for symptoms, not for platelet counts
         b) Corticosteroids (e.g., prednisone)
         c) Intravenous immunoglobulin therapy
      v. **Operative management**
         a) For patients with refractory disease, splenectomy indicated
      vi. **Outcomes**
         a) The bulk of patients have prolonged response to splenectomy, but around one-fourth will have recurrent disease.[14]
   b. **Acute ITP**
      i. Typically, a disease of childhood in which symptoms appear after a viral illness, only to resolve within 6 months.
      ii. Vital to wait up to a year before performing splenectomy in the setting of ITP
   c. **Thrombotic thrombocytopenic purpura**
      i. **Etiology**
         a) Impairment of ADAMTS13 protease leads to decreased cleavage of von Willebrand factor (vWF), resulting in platelet aggregation and microvascular thrombosis.
         b) Usually autoimmune but may be secondary to drugs, infection, malignancy, or pregnancy. Rarely, an inherited condition.
      ii. **Presentation**
         a) Fatigue, bruising, petechiae
         b) Central nervous system symptoms (e.g., dizziness, focal deficits), gastrointestinal symptoms (e.g., nausea, vomiting)
         c) Microangiopathic hemolytic anemia, severe thrombocytopenia, fever, neurological symptoms, and renal failure is a

textbook constellation of symptoms but actually appears in <10% of patients.[15]

iii. **Diagnosis**
   a) CBC (anemia, severe thrombocytopenia, reticulocytosis)
   b) Fractionated bilirubin (elevated indirect bilirubin), haptoglobin (low), lactate dehydrogenase (elevated), DAT (negative)
   c) Peripheral blood smear (schistocytes)
   d) ADAMTS13 activity

iv. **Nonoperative management**
   a) Plasma exchange
   b) Corticosteroids (e.g., prednisone, methylprednisolone for severe disease)
   c) Monoclonal antibodies (e.g., anti-CD20, rituximab; anti-vWF, caplacizumab)
   d) Platelet transfusion not contraindicated[16]

v. **Operative management**
   a) Splenectomy plays a role in relapsed or refractory disease.

vi. **Outcomes**
   a) Splenectomy has low morbidity and mortality if performed during periods of clinical stability and provides extended relapse-free survival.[17]

III. SPLENIC ABSCESS, CYSTS, AND NEOPLASM

A. Splenic abscess

1. **Etiology**
   a. Usually due to hematogenous seeding from distant site of infection (e.g., endocarditis) but occasionally local spread (e.g., peripancreatic collection, perforated diverticulitis, pyelonephritis)
   b. *Staphylococcus*, *Streptococcus*, *Enterococcus*, *Escherichia coli*, fungal (immunocompromised)
2. **Presentation**
   a. Fever, left upper quadrant pain
3. **Diagnosis**
   a. US (hypoechoic)
   b. CT (hypoattenuating, potentially with ring enhancement)
4. **Nonoperative management**
   a. Broad-spectrum antibiotics, narrow when cultures return
   b. Percutaneous drainage (unilocular)
5. **Operative management**
   a. Splenectomy (multilocular)
6. **Outcomes**
   a. Trend toward fewer complications and lower mortality in percutaneous drainage compared with splenectomy.[18]

B. Cystic disease

1. **Parasitic**
   a. **Etiology**
      i. *Echinococcus granulosus* (hydatid cyst)
      ii. Rare in high-income countries

b. **Presentation**
   i. Asymptomatic
   ii. Mass effect
   iii. Rupture
c. **Diagnosis**
   i. US (calcification in cyst wall, daughter cysts)
   ii. Serologic testing
d. **Nonoperative management**
   i. Antiparasitic agents (e.g., albendazole)
   ii. Percutaneous aspiration, injection, reaspiration
e. **Operative management**
   i. Cysts >5 cm, multiloculated, or otherwise complicated cysts require cystectomy or splenectomy. May inject hypertonic saline or alcohol preoperatively to reduce chances of rupture and spillage.
f. **Outcomes**
   i. More aggressive surgical approaches are associated with higher rates of complications but result in fewer recurrences.[19]

2. **Nonparasitic**
   a. **Etiology**
      i. Primary (true) cysts (10% of nonparasitic cysts) have epithelial lining
         a) Congenital
         b) Epithelioid
         c) Mesenchymal
         d) Dermoid
      ii. Secondary cysts (pseudocyst)
         a) E.g., splenic peliosis (sinusoidal dilatation results in blood-filled cyst-like cavities)
         b) E.g., posttraumatic, abscess, infarct
   b. **Presentation**
      i. Incidental finding on imaging
      ii. Left upper quadrant pain
   c. **Diagnosis**
      i. US, CT
      ii. Percutaneous biopsy
   d. **Nonoperative management**
      i. Observation if asymptomatic and stable
      ii. Percutaneous aspiration/drainage
   e. **Operative management**
      i. Operative intervention (e.g., unroofing, splenectomy) indicated for symptoms of diagnostic uncertainty.
   f. **Outcomes**
      i. Higher recurrence rate after unroofing, compared with resection. Splenic preservation should be pursued when possible.[20]

C. Neoplasm
1. **Etiology**
   a. Primary
      i. Vascular (red pulp)

a) Hemangioma (most common benign tumor)
   1) Risk for rupture and bleeding when >2 cm
b) Hamartoma
c) Angiosarcoma (most common nonhematopoietic malignancy of the spleen)
   1) Poor prognosis

ii. Lymphoid (white pulp)
a) Lymphangioma (children, mostly)
b) Lymphoma (most common malignant tumor of spleen)
   1) Usually, NHL
   2) Secondary involvement more common than primary involvement

b. Secondary
i. Metastases (rare)
a) Melanoma, lung, breast, ovarian, pancreas, colon, gastric

2. **Presentation**
   a. Splenomegaly
   b. Rupture, bleeding
3. **Diagnosis**
   a. Imaging (CT, positron emission tomography [PET], MRI, US)
   b. Biopsy
   c. Splenectomy may be indicated if biopsy inconclusive and diagnostic uncertainty exists
4. **Nonoperative management**
   a. Observation
5. **Operative management**
   a. Splenectomy can be considered in symptomatic or oligometastatic disease.
6. **Outcomes**
   a. Strong data are lacking, but resection is a reasonable approach for symptomatic or low-volume metastatic disease with acceptable outcomes.[21]

IV. OTHER SPLENIC DISORDERS REQUIRING SURGICAL MANAGEMENT

A. Trauma
1. Increasing trend toward nonoperative management.[22]
2. Discussed in more detail in abdominal trauma chapter.

B. Splenic artery aneurysm
1. **Etiology**
   a. Most common visceral arterial aneurysm
   b. More common in women
   c. Associated with vascular disease, connective tissue disease, portal hypertension, and pregnancy
2. **Presentation**
   a. Incidental finding on imaging
   b. Abdominal pain, nausea, splenomegaly
   c. In extremis after rupture

3. **Diagnosis**
   a. Duplex US
   b. CT/magnetic resonance angiography
4. **Nonoperative management**
   a. Observation (<2 cm)
5. **Operative management**
   a. Symptoms, enlarging aneurysms, and **aneurysms in women of child-bearing age are indications for intervention.**
   b. Endovascular approach more common in the elective setting with open repair or splenectomy more common in the emergent setting.
6. **Outcomes**
   a. Elective endovascular therapy delivers high rates of success (>95%) with rare complications (<10%).[23]

C. Felty syndrome
   1. Is a complication of rheumatoid arthritis manifesting as neutropenia and splenomegaly.
   2. These patients are plagued by recurrent infections.
   3. Splenectomy indicated for refractory wounds and recurrent infections.
   4. Neutropenia resolves in nearly 90% of patients after splenectomy.

V. PREOPERATIVE CONSIDERATIONS

A. Imaging
   1. CT with IV contrast
      a. Preferred study
      b. Helps to clarify relationship of spleen and pancreatic tail, vascular anatomy, and presence of accessory spleens
   2. US
      a. RUQ US to identify presence of gallstones in patients with hemolytic disorders
   3. PET or tagged white cell scan
      a. May be useful if concern for metastasis or infectious disorder.

B. Vaccination
   1. For patients undergoing elective splenectomy, vaccination against encapsulated organisms (e.g., *Streptococcus pneumoniae*, *Haemophilus influenzae* type B, *Neisseria meningitidis*) at least 2 weeks prior to operation, although some data suggest this is not a hard cutoff.
   2. Given their preeminent role in the key perioperative period, surgeons should assume responsibility for the delivery of vaccinations.[24]

C. Transfusion
   1. Patients with chronic transfusion requirements should be typed and screened well in advance of elective splenectomy.
   2. Ideally, platelet count should be >20,000 prior to splenectomy.[25]
   3. Patients with severe thrombocytopenia should have platelets available in the operating room.
   4. If required, **platelets should be administered after the splenic artery is ligated to avoid consumption by the spleen.**

D. Deep vein thrombosis prophylaxis
1. Splenectomy carries an **increased risk for venous thromboembolism events** compared with other abdominal operations.[26]
2. Mechanical (i.e., sequential compression devices) and chemical (e.g., low-dose unfractionated heparin, low-molecular-weight heparin) prophylaxis should be employed in patients who are not at risk of major bleeding events.[27]

E. Other considerations
1. Preoperative stress-dose steroids should be considered for patients on chronic corticosteroids.
2. For patients with massive splenomegaly, preoperative splenic artery embolization may improve intra- and postoperative outcomes.[28]

VI. SPLENECTOMY

(Table 20.1)

A. Surgical approach: Open splenectomy
1. Indications include trauma and massive splenomegaly.
   a. Patient is positioned in reverse Trendelenburg and right side tilted down.
   b. Abdomen is entered via midline or left subcostal incision.
   c. Splenic mobilization begins by taking down the splenocolic ligament; lesser sac is entered via the gastrocolic ligament.
   d. Splenophrenic ligament divided, and a plane is developed posterior to the spleen and pancreatic tail.
   e. Gastrosplenic ligament divided and short gastrics taken down.
   f. Splenorenal ligament dissected, avoiding pancreatic tail, and the splenic vessels are identified and individually ligated and divided. Alternatively, vascular control and ligation may be pursued early to aid management of a very large spleen.
   g. Spleen is removed, and the abdomen surveyed for accessory splenic tissue before closing.

B. Surgical approach: Minimally invasive splenectomy
1. A minimally invasive approach has been associated with shorter length of stay and fewer postoperative complications.[29]
   a. Absolute contraindications to minimally invasive splenectomy include trauma, massive splenomegaly, and portal hypertension.
   b. Relative contraindications include moderate splenomegaly, severe cytopenias, splenic vein thrombosis, and bulky hilar adenopathy.
2. Procedure
   a. The patient is positioned in right lateral decubitus, with the space between their iliac crest and costal margin over the break in the bed.
   b. Camera port is placed at the umbilicus, and working ports are placed in the epigastrium and left anterior axillary line at the costal margin. Additional larger port is placed along the costal margin in the left axillary line to accommodate laparoscopic stapler.
   c. Laparoscopic resection involves similar steps as open splenectomy.
   d. The spleen is morcellated within a bag and removed in a piecemeal fashion.

TABLE 20.1 Summary of Indications and Outcomes for Splenectomy

Condition	Indication	Outcomes
Sickle cell disease	Abscess, sequestration crisis, hypersplenism	No increased risk of infectious complications or death for children w/SCD who undergo splenectomy
Thalassemia	Ongoing transfusion requirement, growth impairment, hypersplenism, symptomatic splenomegaly	Decreased transfusion requirement, preventing extramedullary hematopoiesis
Hereditary spherocytosis	Growth impairment, organ dysfunction, extramedullary hematopoiesis	Curative
Hereditary elliptocytosis	Symptomatic anemia	Curative
Pyruvate kinase deficiency	Ongoing transfusion requirement, symptomatic splenomegaly	Decreased transfusion requirement
G6PD deficiency	Ongoing transfusion requirement, hypersplenism, symptomatic splenomegaly	Decreased transfusion requirement
Warm antibody hemolytic anemia	Refractory disease	Complete response (75%)
Acute myeloid leukemia	Splenic rupture	Lifesaving
Chronic myeloid leukemia	Hypersplenism, symptomatic splenomegaly	Decreased transfusion requirement, improved symptoms
Polycythemia vera	Symptomatic splenomegaly	Increased risk of postoperative thrombotic events
Myelofibrosis	Symptomatic splenomegaly, hypersplenism-related transfusion requirement, splenic infarction, portal hypertension	Less effective than for other disease processes. High risk of morbidity and mortality

(continued)

TABLE 20.1 Summary of Indications and Outcomes for Splenectomy (*Continued*)

Condition	Indication	Outcomes
Non-Hodgkin lymphoma	Symptomatic splenomegaly, hypersplenism, diagnostic uncertainty	Resolution of cytopenias
Hodgkin lymphoma	Symptomatic splenomegaly, hypersplenism, diagnostic uncertainty	Resolution of cytopenias
Chronic lymphocytic leukemia	Symptomatic splenomegaly, hypersplenism, splenic rupture (transformation to DLBCL)	Resolution of cytopenias (70%)
Hairy cell leukemia	Refractory disease, symptomatic splenomegaly	Improved blood counts in most; significant recurrence rate (33%)
Chronic idiopathic thrombocytopenic purpura	Refractory disease	Prolonged response in most; significant recurrence rate (25%)
Thrombotic thrombocytopenic purpura	Relapse, refractory disease	Extended relapse-free survival
Splenic abscess	Multilocular cyst	Fewer complications with percutaneous drainage, if feasible
Parasitic cyst disease	>5 cm, multilocular, or otherwise complicated cysts	Less recurrence, but more morbidity, with aggressive surgical approaches
Nonparasitic cyst disease	Symptomatic disease, diagnostic uncertainty	Lower recurrence rate with splenectomy (vs. unroofing)
Splenic neoplasm	Diagnostic uncertainty, symptomatic disease, oligometastatic disease	Acceptable outcomes for resection of symptomatic or low-volume metastatic disease

TABLE 20.1 Summary of Indications and Outcomes for Splenectomy (*Continued*)

Condition	Indication	Outcomes
Splenic artery aneurysm	Symptomatic disease, enlarging aneurysm, women of child-bearing age	Elective endovascular approach has high rate of success and low rate of complications
Felty syndrome	Refractory wounds, recurrent infection	Resolution of neutropenia (90%)

3. Robotic splenectomy has been associated with some improved intra- and postoperative metrics, but this also significantly increased costs.

C. Intraoperative complications
1. Bleeding—the most commonly encountered intraoperative complication, may necessitate conversion to open splenectomy.
2. Pancreatic injury—if pancreatic tail injury is suspected, leave drain and check drain amylase before removal.
3. Colonic injury—may be primarily repaired.
4. Gastric injury—thermal injury can lead to delayed presentation of gastric perforation. Areas of concern can be oversewn.
5. Diaphragmatic injury—can be primarily repaired.

VII. POSTOPERATIVE CONSIDERATIONS

A. Early complications
1. Pulmonary complications (e.g., atelectasis, pneumonia, pleural effusion) are the most common complications, but significantly less common following a laparoscopic splenectomy.
2. Subphrenic abscess—treatment includes IV antibiotics and potentially percutaneous drainage.
3. Ileus
4. Wound complications (e.g., hematoma, seroma, surgical site infection)
5. Thrombotic complications—reactive thrombocytosis common
   a. Portal vein/mesenteric venous thrombosis is more common in laparoscopic splenectomy; splenomegaly and thrombocytosis are risk factors.[30]

B. Late complications
1. Overwhelming postsplenectomy infection
   a. May occur at any time in patients with impaired splenic function.
   b. Patients are at risk for fulminant infections from encapsulated bacteria.
   c. While the risk is highest in patients under 5 years, and within the first two postoperative years, the risk remains elevated throughout the life of the patient.

d. Presentation
   i. Nonspecific symptoms requiring a high index of suspicion
   ii. Aggressive supportive care including empiric antibiotics is required to prevent rapid progression and death.
e. Vaccination against encapsulated bacteria and seasonal influenza is recommended for patients with impaired or absent splenic function (**Table 20.2**).
f. Routine prophylaxis with daily antibiotics is recommended for certain high-risk patients.

TABLE 20.2 Vaccination for Patients Undergoing Splenectomy

Vaccine Target	Delivered Before Splenectomy (e.g., Elective Splenectomy)	Delivered Post Splenectomy (e.g., Trauma Splenectomy)
Streptococcus pneumoniae	PCV13 (10 wk preop, if unvaccinated) + PPSV23 (2 wk preop) + PPSV23 (5 y postop)	PCV13 (2 wk postop, if unvaccinated) + PPSV23 (10 wk postop) + PPSV23 (5 y postop) If vaccinated, PPSV23 (2 wk postop) + PPSV23 (5 y postop)
Haemophilus influenzae type B	If unvaccinated, Hib conjugate x1	If unvaccinated, Hib conjugate x1
Neisseria meningitidis	If < 2 y old, conjugated bivalent or conjugated quadrivalent meningococcal series If > 2 y old or if unvaccinated, quadrivalent meningococcal vaccine x1 For all, booster dose every 5 y	If < 2 y old, conjugated bivalent or conjugated quadrivalent meningococcal series If > 2 y and unvaccinated, two-dose quadrivalent meningococcal series 8-12 wk apart For all, booster dose every 5 y
Seasonal influenza	Annually Patients with sickle cell disease—inactivated vaccine All others—live attenuated vaccine	Annually Patients with sickle cell disease—inactivated vaccine All others—live attenuated vaccine

Data from Rubin LG, Schaffner W. Clinical practice. Care of the asplenic patient. *N Engl J Med.* 2014;371(4):349-356.

i. All asplenic patients should have a supply of emergency antibiotics (penicillin or fluoroquinolone) for febrile episodes and should receive prophylaxis when undergoing invasive procedures of the upper or lower respiratory tract.

2. Splenosis results from the intraperitoneal dissemination of splenic tissue after splenic rupture. When this occurs, it is commonly during morcellation and removal of the spleen, so great care should be taken during this component of laparoscopic splenectomy.

Key References

Citation	Summary
Skandalakis PN, Colborn GL, Skandalakis LJ, Richardson DD, Mitchell WE Jr, Skandalakis JE. The surgical anatomy of the spleen. *Surg Clin North Am.* 1993;73(4):747-768.	• Overview of surgically relevant splenic anatomy
Rodríguez-Luna MR, Balagué C, Fernández-Ananín S, Vilallonga R, Targarona Soler EM. Outcomes of laparoscopic splenectomy for treatment of splenomegaly: a systematic review and meta-analysis. *World J Surg.* 2021;45(2):465-479.	• Minimally invasive splenectomy safe and beneficial in the setting of splenomegaly
Iolascon A, Andolfo I, Barcellini W, et al. Recommendations regarding splenectomy in hereditary hemolytic anemias. *Haematologica.* 2017;102(8):1304-1313.	• Summary of recommendations for the use of splenectomy in hereditary hemolytic anemias

CHAPTER 20: SPLEEN

Review Questions

1. What causes hepatosplenomegaly in the thalassemias?
2. Patients with hemolytic disorders should undergo what additional diagnostic procedure in the preoperative period?
3. Where are RBCs destroyed in cold antibody hemolytic anemia?
4. What are indications for splenectomy in CML?
5. What may result from bag rupture during morcellation at the conclusion of laparoscopic splenectomy?
6. What is the preferred study for suspected splenic disorders?
7. Patients undergoing splenectomy should be vaccinated against which bacteria?

REFERENCES

1. Wright JG, Hambleton IR, Thomas PW, Duncan ND, Venugopal S, Serjeant GR. Postsplenectomy course in homozygous sickle cell disease. *J Pediatr.* 1999;134(3):304-309.
2. Rachmilewitz EA, Giardina PJ. How I treat thalassemia. *Blood.* 2011;118(13):3479-3488.
3. Englum BR, Rothman J, Leonard S, et al. Hematologic outcomes after total splenectomy and partial splenectomy for congenital hemolytic anemia. *J Pediatr Surg.* 2016;51(1):122-127.
4. Chonat S, Eber SW, Holzhauer S, et al. Pyruvate kinase deficiency in children. *Pediatr Blood Cancer.* 2021;68(9):e29148.
5. Hamilton JW, Jones FG, McMullin MF. Glucose-6-phosphate dehydrogenase Guadalajara —A case of chronic non-spherocytic haemolytic anaemia responding to splenectomy and the role of splenectomy in this disorder. *Hematology*. Aug 2004;9(4):307-309.
6. Barcellini W, Fattizzo B, Zaninoni A, et al. Clinical heterogeneity and predictors of outcome in primary autoimmune hemolytic anemia: a GIMEMA study of 308 patients. *Blood.* 2014;124(19):2930-2936.
7. Gnanapandithan K. Atraumatic splenic rupture in acute myeloid leukemia. *Cleve Clin J Med.* 2019;86(11):715-716.
8. Mesa RA, Elliott MA, Tefferi A. Splenectomy in chronic myeloid leukemia and myelofibrosis with myeloid metaplasia. *Blood Rev.* 2000;14(3):121-129.
9. Barosi G, Viarengo G, Pecci A, et al. Diagnostic and clinical relevance of the number of circulating CD34(+) cells in myelofibrosis with myeloid metaplasia. *Blood.* 2001;98(12):3249-3255.
10. Tefferi A, Mesa RA, Nagorney DM, Schroeder G, Silverstein MN. Splenectomy in myelofibrosis with myeloid metaplasia: a single-institution experience with 223 patients. *Blood.* 2000;95(7):2226-2233.
11. Brodsky J, Abcar A, Styler M. Splenectomy for non-Hodgkin's lymphoma. *Am J Clin Oncol.* 1996;19(6):558-561.
12. Dearden C. Disease-specific complications of chronic lymphocytic leukemia. *Hematology Am Soc Hematol Educ Program.* 2008;2008:450-456.
13. Magee MJ, McKenzie S, Filippa DA, Arlin ZA, Gee TS, Clarkson BD. Hairy cell leukemia. Durability of response to splenectomy in 26 patients and treatment of relapse with androgens in six patients. *Cancer.* 1985;56(11):2557-2562.
14. Chaturvedi S, Arnold DM, McCrae KR. Splenectomy for immune thrombocytopenia: down but not out. *Blood.* 2018;131(11):1172-1182.
15. Joly BS, Coppo P, Veyradier A. Thrombotic thrombocytopenic purpura. *Blood.* 2017;129(21):2836-2846.
16. Swisher KK, Terrell DR, Vesely SK, Kremer Hovinga JA, Lammle B, George JN. Clinical outcomes after platelet transfusions in patients with thrombotic thrombocytopenic purpura. *Transfusion.* 2009;49(5):873-887.
17. Kappers-Klunne MC, Wijermans P, Fijnheer R, et al. Splenectomy for the treatment of thrombotic thrombocytopenic purpura. *Br J Haematol.* 2005;130(5):768-776.

18. Gutama B, Wothe JK, Xiao M, Hackman D, Chu H, Rickard J. Splenectomy versus imaging-guided percutaneous drainage for splenic abscess: a systematic review and meta-analysis. *Surg Infect.* 2022;23(5):417-429.

19. Brunetti E, Kern P, Vuitton DA; Writing Panel for the WHO-IWGE. Expert consensus for the diagnosis and treatment of cystic and alveolar echinococcosis in humans. *Acta Trop.* 2010;114(1):1-16.

20. Mertens J, Penninckx F, DeWever I, Topal B. Long-term outcome after surgical treatment of nonparasitic splenic cysts. *Surg Endosc.* 2007;21(2):206-208.

21. de Wilt JH, McCarthy WH, Thompson JF. Surgical treatment of splenic metastases in patients with melanoma. *J Am Coll Surg.* 2003;197(1):38-43.

22. Coccolini F, Montori G, Catena F, et al. Splenic trauma: WSES classification and guidelines for adult and pediatric patients. *World J Emerg Surg.* 2017;12:40.

23. Lakin RO, Bena JF, Sarac TP, et al. The contemporary management of splenic artery aneurysms. *J Vasc Surg.* 2011;53(4):958-964; discussion 965.

24. Casciani F, Trudeau MT, Vollmer CM Jr. Perioperative immunization for splenectomy and the surgeon's responsibility: a review. *JAMA Surg.* 2020;155(11):1068-1077.

25. Keidar A, Feldman M, Szold A. Analysis of outcome of laparoscopic splenectomy for idiopathic thrombocytopenic purpura by platelet count. *Am J Hematol.* 2005;80(2):95-100.

26. Mukherjee D, Lidor AO, Chu KM, Gearhart SL, Haut ER, Chang DC. Postoperative venous thromboembolism rates vary significantly after different types of major abdominal operations. *J Gastrointest Surg.* 2008;12(11):2015-2022.

27. Gould MK, Garcia DA, Wren SM, et al. Prevention of VTE in nonorthopedic surgical patients. Antithrombotic therapy and prevention of thrombosis, 9th ed: American College of Chest Physicians Evidence-Based Clinical Practice Guidelines. *Chest.* 2012;141(2 suppl):e227S-e277S.

28. Wu Z, Zhou J, Pankaj P, Peng B. Comparative treatment and literature review for laparoscopic splenectomy alone versus preoperative splenic artery embolization splenectomy. *Surg Endosc.* 2012;26(10):2758-2766.

29. Winslow ER, Brunt LM. Perioperative outcomes of laparoscopic versus open splenectomy: a meta-analysis with an emphasis on complications. *Surgery.* 2003;134(4):647-653; discussion 654-655.

30. Pietrabissa A, Moretto C, Antonelli G, Morelli L, Marciano E, Mosca F. Thrombosis in the portal venous system after elective laparoscopic splenectomy. *Surg Endosc.* 2004;18(7):1140-1143.

21 Abdominal Transplantation

Jessica Lindemann and Jason R. Wellen

I. INTRODUCTION TO PHYSIOLOGIC IMMUNITY

A. Innate immune system
   1. Direct, nonspecific responses
   2. Lacks memory
   3. **Mediators**
      a. **Complement:** A cascade of proteins that form the **membrane attack complex** resulting in cell lysis. Byproducts of the complement cascade opsonize pathogens, promoting phagocytosis by **antigen-presenting cells** (APCs).
      b. **Natural killer cells:** Recognize cells that lack a self–**major histocompatibility complex** (MHC) and are part of the body's immunosurveillance for cancer.

B. Adaptive immune system
   1. Recognizes specific, pathogenic antigens in the context of the MHC
      a. MHC helps the immune system distinguish "self" from "nonself."
      b. In humans, these complexes are referred to as **human leukocyte antigens (HLAs)** and are located on chromosome 6.
   2. **Classes of HLA**
      a. **Class I (A, B, C):** Present on all nucleated cells, targets for cytotoxic T cells (CD8).
      b. **Class II (DR, DP, and DQ):** Present on APCs (B cells, dendrites, and macrophages), targets for helper T cells (CD4), trigger an antibody-mediated (humoral) immune response.
   3. **Adaptive immune responses**
      a. **Cell mediated:** Antigens in the peripheral tissues are presented to T cells located in lymph nodes and the spleen.
         i. **T-cell receptors** recognize a specific antigen in the context of the MHC.
         ii. T cells are selected based on their ability to bind self-MHC without activating a response.
         iii. MHC encountered in the tissues not recognized as self, activates an immune response. ***This is the basis of alloreactivity.***
            a) **CD4:** Recognize exogenous antigens presented in the context of MHC class II. Activation releases interleukin (IL)-2 and IL-4 causing B-cell and T-cell maturation, respectively.
            b) **CD8:** Recognize endogenous pathogens (e.g., TB, viruses) presented in the context of MHC class I.

b. **Antibody mediated (humoral)**
   i. B cells (bone) activate antibody-mediated (humoral) immunity.
   ii. IL-4 from helper T cells transforms B cells into **plasma cells**, which secrete antibodies specific to the offending pathogen.

II. TRANSPLANT IMMUNOLOGY

A. Isografts: Tissue transfer from genetically identical individuals (e.g., identical twins)
B. Xenografts: Tissue transfer between species
C. Allografts: Tissue transfer among members of the same species
   1. **Alloreactivity/histocompatibility**
      a. **ABO** blood compatibility is necessary for all transplants, except liver.
      b. **HLA-A, HLA-B, and HLA-DR** are the most important for compatibility.
         i. HLA-DR is the most important overall.
   2. **Cross-matching** detects preformed antibodies against donor HLA.
      a. It involves mixing recipient serum with donor lymphocytes.
      b. **Panel reactive antibodies** (PRAs) help to predict the likelihood of a positive cross-match by testing the potential recipient's serum against a panel of cells of various HLA specificities.
      c. The percentage of specificities in the panel with which the patient's sera react is the PRA.
      d. Patients who have been exposed to other HLAs via blood transfusion, pregnancy, or prior transplantation will have higher PRAs.

III. TRANSPLANT REJECTION

A. Types of rejection
   1. **Hyperacute rejection**
      a. Due to preformed anti-HLA antibodies that bind the allograft endothelium, causes vascular thrombosis and ischemic necrosis
      b. Treatment: Immediate removal of endograft
      c. Extraordinarily uncommon in the modern era of cross-matching
   2. **Accelerated rejection**
      a. Caused by sensitized T cells that produce a secondary immune response
      b. Generally occurs within 1 week of transplantation
      c. Treatment: Pulse steroids
   3. **Acute cellular rejection** (ACR)
      a. Cell mediated, involves T lymphocytes
      b. Typically occurs 1 week to 1 month after transplantation
      c. Treatment: High-dose methylprednisolone and an antilymphocyte preparation
   4. **Chronic rejection**
      a. Poorly understood phenomenon; emerging evidence suggests that the humoral immune response is an important contributor
      b. Can occur weeks to years after transplantation
      c. Treatment: Plasmapheresis, IV immunoglobulin, and rituximab

IV. IMMUNOSUPPRESSION

A. Definition: Medications that are used for induction, maintenance, and treatment of rejection
B. In general, steroids and antithymocyte agents are used for induction, with the aim of lymphocyte depletion and immune system downregulation.
C. An ideal maintenance therapy regimen includes a calcineurin inhibitor (CNI), an antiproliferative agent, and steroids.
D. In the treatment of rejection, it is important to choose medications that target the underlying mechanism.
E. Doses given in **Table 21.1** are typical for kidney transplant recipients; however, specific combinations of medications and dosages are tailored for the patient and organ transplanted.
F. Classes of immunosuppressive drugs (**Figure 21.1**, **Table 21.1**)

TABLE 21.1 Dosing and Indications for Immunosuppressive Medications

Drug	Indication	Dose
Corticosteroids		
Methylprednisolone (Solu-Medrol)	Induction	Up to 1 g IV initial dose, followed by taper
	Rejection	7 mg/kg IV qday for 3 d, then resume previous steroid dose
Prednisone	Maintenance	1 mg/kg PO qday for days 1-3, 20 mg qday for days 4-14, reduce by 5 mg weekly until 5 mg qday
	Rejection	3 mg/kg PO qday divided into 2-4 doses for 3-5 d, then resume previous steroid dose
Antiproliferative Agents/Antimetabolites		
Azathioprine (Imuran)	Maintenance	1-2 mg/kg PO qday or 2-3 mg/kg PO qday if used alone, max dose 200 mg/d
Mycophenolate Mofetil (CellCept)	Maintenance	1-3 g PO qday, divided over two doses
Mycophenolic acid (Myfortic)	Maintenance	360-1080 mg PO bid. Use 360 mg bid with tacrolimus, leukopenia diarrhea or in the first week posttransplant

(continued)

TABLE 21.1 Dosing and Indications for Immunosuppressive Medications (*Continued*)

Drug	Indication	Dose
Calcineurin Inhibitors (CNIs)		
Cyclosporine (CsA, Sandimmune, Neoral, Gengraff)	Maintenance	2-3 mg/kg PO bid as starting dose, titrate to trough of 300 ng/mL initially, target trough of 150 ng/mL from 6 wk posttransplant
Tacrolimus (FK506, Prograf)	Maintenance	0.1 mg/kg PO bid, titrate dose for target trough level of 5-7 ng/mL. Trough >15 ng/mL is considered toxic
mTOR Inhibitors		
Sirolimus (Rapamune)	Maintenance	6 mg PO loading dose on posttransplant day 1, 2 mg PO qday after, titrate to trough of 8 to 12 ng/mL for the first year
Everolimus (Zortress)	Maintenance	1 mg PO bid, titrate to trough level between 3 and 8 ng/mL
Costimulation Blockade		
Belatacept (Nulojix)	Maintenance	10 mg/kg IV loading dose posttransplant day 1, second dose on days 4 and 5, then once monthly 5 mg/kg IV
Antithymocyte Antibodies		
Thymoglobulin	Premedication needed	Diphenhydramine 50 mg PO, acetaminophen 650 mg PO, hydrocortisone 200 mg IV, given 1 h before infusion
	Induction	4.5 mg/kg IV over 4-6 h given on days 0, 1, and 2 posttransplant
	Rejection	2-3 mg/kg IV over 4-6 h for 3-4 d
Basiliximab (Simulect)	Induction	20 mg IV qday on posttransplant days 1 and 4

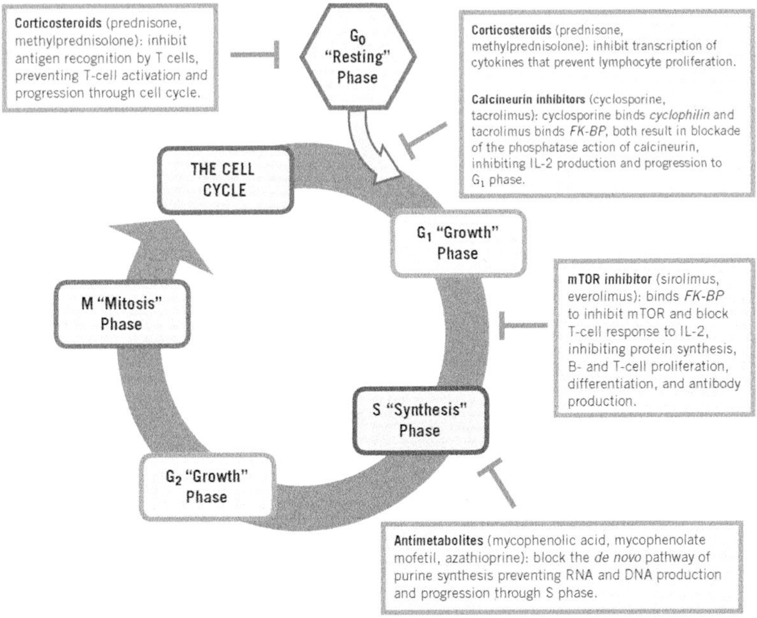

FIGURE 21.1 Classes of immunosuppressant medications and sites of action within the cell cycle.

G. Corticosteroids
   1. Play the broadest role in immunomodulation
   2. Prevent lymphocytes proliferation and neutrophils migration, as well as dampen the inflammatory response
   3. Used for induction, maintenance, and treatment of rejection
   4. Toxicities include poor wound healing, hyperglycemia, infections, cataracts, hypertension, weight gain, and osteoporosis

H. Antiproliferative agents/antimetabolites
   1. **Azathioprine**
      a. Purine analog that alters DNA and RNA synthesis inhibiting T- and B-lymphocyte proliferation
      b. Used for maintenance therapy only
      c. Toxicity: Myelosuppression (leukopenia and thrombocytopenia)
   2. **Mycophenolic acid**
      a. Inhibitor of purine synthesis, depleting guanosine triphosphate stores and preventing DNA synthesis in activated B and T lymphocytes
      b. Used for maintenance therapy only
      c. Toxicities: Gastrointestinal (GI) disturbance and leukopenia

I. Calcineurin inhibitors
   1. **Cyclosporine**
      a. Inhibits IL-2 production, preventing the initiation of T-cell proliferation
      b. Used for maintenance therapy only

c. Toxicities: Nephrotoxicity, hypertension, tremors, seizures, hyperkalemia, hyperuricemia, hypercholesterolemia, gingival hyperplasia, and hirsutism

2. **Tacrolimus**
    a. Acts similarly to CsA but is 10 to 100 times more potent
    b. Used for maintenance therapy only
    c. Toxicities: Similar to CsA, more GI and neurologic changes

J. mTOR inhibitors
1. **Sirolimus**
    a. Inhibits the mTOR molecule, blocking T-cell signal transduction
    b. Used as maintenance therapy and dosing adjustments are made based on concomitant use of a CNI
    c. Toxicity includes thrombocytopenia, hyperlipidemia, oral ulcers, anemia, proteinuria, and impairment of wound healing.
2. **Everolimus**
    a. Mechanism of action similar to sirolimus, but with greater bioavailability and a shorter half-life
    b. Used for maintenance therapy in combination with low-dose tacrolimus to minimize CNI toxicity
    c. Toxicity: Similar to sirolimus

K. Costimulation blockade (**Figure 21.2**)
1. **Belatacept**
    a. Prevents costimulation required for T-cell activation, resulting in T-cell antigen-specific tolerance (anergy)
    b. FDA-approved in 2011 for maintenance therapy in renal transplant; however, due to a 2014 clinical trial demonstrating increased risk of graft loss,[1] only off-label in liver transplantation
    c. Associated with posttransplant lymphoproliferative disorder (PTLD) and should be avoided in patients who are Epstein–Barr virus (EBV) seronegative

L. Antithymocyte antibodies (**Figure 21.2**)
1. **Thymoglobulin**
    a. Causes rapid T-cell depletion
    b. The most commonly used antithymocyte antibody in the US
    c. Derived from rabbit serum after exposure to human thymocytes or T cells
    d. Used as induction or rescue therapy following ACR, with premedication to avoid cytokine release syndrome
    e. Side effects: Allergic reaction, leukopenia, increased cytomegalovirus infection, and lymphomas
2. **Basiliximab** (Simulect)
    a. Binds to T-cell IL-2 receptor (CD25) only
    b. Used for induction therapy, but less often than thymoglobulin
        i. Usually reserved for patients with low risk of rejection and preoperative leukopenia, thrombocytopenia, and/or hypotension
    c. Side effects are minimal due to binding specificity.

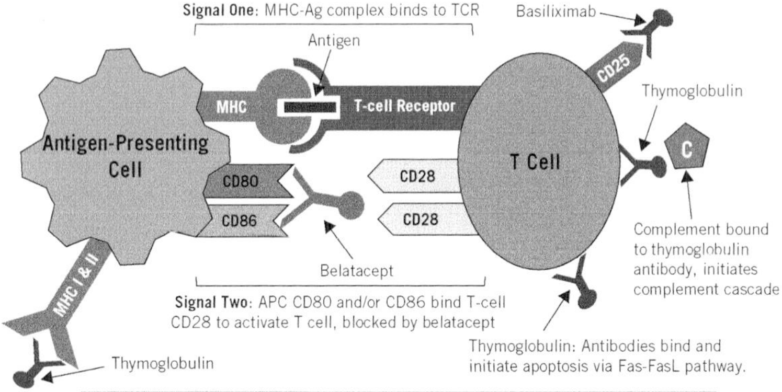

Costimulation Blockade (belatacept): blocks the binding of APC CD80 and/or CD86 to T-cell CD28, preventing Signal Two and inhibiting T-cell activation. Belatacept is a fusion protein composed of the Fc component of human IgG1 and CTLA-4 (CD27 analog) that competitively binds with CD80 and CD86.

Antithymocyte Antibodies (thymoglobulin, basiliximab): Thymoglobulin is a polyclonal antibody that causes rapid lymphocyte depletion via complement-dependent lysis and apoptosis. It also modulates T-cell activation and homing functions, interferes with APC function, and induces regulatory T cells and natural killer cells. Basiliximab is a non-T-cell depleting monoclonal antibody that competitively binds CD25, the IL-2 receptor on T cells, preventing T-cell proliferation and activation of B cells by T cells.

MHC – major histocompatibility complex, Ag – antigen, TCR – T-cell receptor, C – complement, APC – antigen-presenting cell

FIGURE 21.2 Mechanism of action for costimulation blockade and antithymocyte antibodies.

V. COMPLICATIONS OF IMMUNOSUPPRESSION

A. Bacterial infections
   1. Pneumonia and urinary tract infections (UTIs) are common after transplantation.
   2. Infectious complications from opportunistic organisms are now uncommon because of appropriate prophylactic strategies.

B. Viral infections
   1. **Cytomegalovirus (CMV)**
      a. Most common 1 to 4 months posttransplant in the absence of prophylaxis but may occur any time
      b. Can infect the recipient's liver, lungs, or GI tract
      c. Signs and symptoms: Fever, chills, malaise, anorexia, nausea, vomiting, cough, abdominal pain, hypoxia, leukopenia, and elevation in transaminases
      d. Diagnosis: CMV peripheral blood polymerase chain reaction or serologic assays
      e. Prophylaxis is useful in any patient who receives a CMV-positive allograft.
      f. Treatment: Decreasing immunosuppression and administering ganciclovir

2. **EBV**
   a. Can occur at any time after transplantation and may be associated with the development of PTLD (a monoclonal B-cell-originated lymphoma)
   b. Infects B cells
   c. Infiltration of the hematopoietic system, central nervous system (CNS), lungs, or other solid organs may occur
   d. Signs and symptoms: Fever, chills, sweats, enlarged lymph nodes, and elevated uric acid
   e. Diagnosis: Physical examination, EBV serology, CT scan of the head/chest/abdomen, and biopsy of potential sites or lesions
   f. Treatment: Reducing or withdrawing immunosuppression
3. **Herpes simplex virus**
   a. Signs and symptoms: Characteristic ulcers on the oral mucosa, in the genital region, and in the esophagus
   b. Renal transplant patients, if not on ganciclovir, are given prophylactic acyclovir
   c. Treatment: Decreasing the patient's immunosuppression and instituting acyclovir therapy
4. **BK virus**
   a. A member of the polyoma virus family
   b. Approximately 90% of individuals are seropositive.
   c. BK viruria develops in 30% of kidney transplant recipients and progresses to viremia in 15% of recipients within the first year. Persistent viremia leads to BK nephropathy, which occurs in up to 10% of kidney transplant recipients during the first year.
   d. Treatment: Reduction of immunosuppression, which may help clear the infection.

C. Fungal infections
1. Range from asymptomatic colonization to lethal invasive infections
2. Oral **candidiasis** can be prevented and treated with oral nystatin or fluconazole.
3. Esophageal candidiasis can be treated with a short course of IV amphotericin B or fluconazole.
4. Serious fungal infections are treated with amphotericin B, although use of less nephrotoxic agents such as caspofungin and anidulafungin is increasing.

D. Malignancies: Cancers that occur at a higher frequency in transplant recipients include squamous cell carcinoma, basal cell carcinoma, Kaposi sarcoma, lymphomas, hepatobiliary carcinoma, and cervical carcinoma.

VI. ORGAN ALLOCATION

A. Over 100,000 individuals in the US are currently waiting for organ donation. The gap between supply and demand grows daily, so a system exists that allocates solid organs to individuals based on two overarching themes:
1. **Justice:** Each candidate is given fair consideration based on individual circumstances and medical need.

2. **Utility:** The system tries to maximize the number of transplants performed and the survival of both patients and allografts.

B. The **United Network for Organ Sharing (UNOS)** is the organization contracted by the federal government to oversee organ allocation in the United States. Fifty-seven local Organ Procurement Organizations serve 11 UNOS regions.

C. **Kidney allocation**

1. Allocation factors include waiting time, pediatric status, being a prior living donor, how far the recipient lives from the donor hospital, and survival benefit (https://optn.transplant.hrsa.gov/governance/policies/).
2. Priority is given to candidates with less common blood types and a high calculated PRA score.
3. Survival benefit is in part predicted by the kidney donor profile index (KDPI).
    a. KDPI is calculated for deceased donor kidneys only and provides a measure of donor quality.
    b. Includes 10 donor factors and results in a score reported as a percent.
    c. Lower KDPI is associated with longer predicted graft survival.
    d. Recipient consent is required to receive a kidney with a KDPI > 85%.
    e. KDPI should not be used in isolation when determining whether to use a kidney for transplantation. Recipient factors and donor characteristics not included in the calculation should be considered.
    f. Additionally, KDPI was developed using kidney transplant outcomes in an adult population and should be used with caution in the pediatric recipient.[2]
4. In March 2021, the Organ Procurement and Transplantation Network initiated a new policy for kidney allocation to increase equity in access.
    a. Under this policy, kidneys are offered first to candidates listed at transplant centers within 250 nautical miles of the donor hospital.
    b. Offers not accepted by those candidates are then extended to potential recipients outside of the 250 nautical mile radius.
    c. Candidates also receive proximity points based on the distance between their transplant program and donor hospital, with the aim of improving efficiency in organ placement by prioritizing candidates closer to the donor hospital.

D. **Liver allocation**

1. Livers are allocated based on the Model for End-Stage Liver Disease (**MELD**) scoring system, which predicts 3-month mortality in patients with liver disease.
2. The MELD score is derived from a logarithmic formula that incorporates bilirubin, serum creatinine, and international normalized ratio (INR) and ranges from 6 to 40 (www.unos.org/resources/allocation-calculators/).
3. For patients with an initial MELD score > 11, the MELD score is recalculated with an adjustment formula for serum sodium (Na), as hyponatremia was found to be an independent predictor of mortality in liver transplant candidates.[3] Incorporating Na into the MELD score increases its predictive accuracy, particularly in patients with ascites.[4]

4. Special exception points may be granted, such as in cases of hepatocellular carcinoma (HCC), hilar cholangiocarcinoma, hepatopulmonary syndrome, or hepatorenal syndrome.
5. Children receive a Pediatric End-Stage Liver Disease score, which additionally considers the size of a child and serum albumin.[5]

VII. ORGAN DONATION

A. Types of organ donation
1. **Living donation**
   a. Given the significant number of candidates on the waiting list, living donation is important to increasing the donor pool.
   b. Advantages: Improved short- and long-term graft survival (1-year survival >95%), improved immediate allograft function, planned operative timing to allow for medical optimization, and, often, avoidance of dialysis.
   c. The evaluation of potential living donors includes assessment of their overall health, comorbid conditions, and psychosocial influences.
   d. Compatibility with their intended recipient is determined though ABO blood typing and HLA histocompatibility.
   e. Donors who are not compatible with their intended recipient may still donate through paired exchange and ABO-incompatible protocols.
   f. Living kidney donors undergo removal of one kidney. Living kidney grafts have an anticipated median survival of 19.2 years as compared to 11.2 years for deceased donor grafts.[6]
   g. Living donation for liver involves removal of either the right or the left hemiliver, and care must be taken that sufficient liver volume is available for both the recipient and the donor.
2. **Deceased donation**
   a. **Donation after brain death (DBD)**
      i. Strict criteria for establishing brain death include irreversible coma and the absence of brain stem reflexes (i.e., pupillary, corneal, vestibulo-ocular, and gag reflexes).
      ii. Other useful diagnostic tests include blood flow scan, arteriography, and an apnea test.
   b. **Donation after cardiac death (DCD)**
      i. Potential organ donors who do not meet strict brain death criteria but are considered to have nonrecoverable devastating neurologic insults.
      ii. Life support is discontinued in the operating room, and organ procurement is initiated after a specified interval following cardiac asystole.
      iii. While effectively increasing the donor pool, 16% to 28% of DCD livers have biliary complications, including ischemic cholangiopathy.[7]
      iv. However, there is a growing body of evidence to suggest that in high-volume centers and selected recipients, comparable outcomes can be achieved.[8]

v. Recent work had demonstrated no long-term differences in graft survival for recipients of DCD and DBD donors.[9]

B. Suitability for transplantation

1. Contraindications

a. **Active infection**

i. TB is an absolute contraindication to organ donation, and individuals with active tuberculosis are not candidates for organ transplantation.

ii. HIV was formally a contraindication; however, after the HOPE (HIV Organ Policy Equity) Act was implemented in 2015, it became possible for HIV+ donors to donate to HIV+ recipients.

iii. Localized infections (UTIs, pneumonia), in the absence of dissemination, are routinely given consideration.

iv. Even in the presence of bacteremia, appropriate initiation of antibiotic therapy ensures a small risk of transmission.

b. **Cancer**

i. With the exception of primary CNS tumors, active cancer, whether treated or not, is an absolute contraindication to organ donation.

a) The blood–brain barrier protects CNS tumor cells from widespread dissemination in the heavily immunosuppressed patient.

ii. Depending on the type of cancer, recipients may be listed after a cancer-free wait time ranging from 2 to 5 years.

C. General considerations

1. **Age**

a. As experience with marginal donors has grown, it has become apparent that arbitrary upper limits on donor age for DCD and DCB donation are unnecessary.

i. Individuals under the age of 18 years are prohibited from being living donors.

b. Good allograft function has been achieved with kidney and liver donors with advanced age.

2. **Overall health**

a. As the donor pool ages, systemic diseases that can affect specific organ function must be considered.

b. Hypertension and atherosclerosis can hinder the suitability of kidney allografts, while obesity with hepatic steatosis limits the suitability of liver allografts.

3. **Social behaviors**

a. All donors are tested for HIV, hepatitis, and other viral infections.

b. Donors who engage in high-risk behaviors may still transmit an infection if donation were to occur within the period prior to seroconversion.

c. Potential recipients are counseled regarding socially high-risk donors and given the option to consider organs allocated from this group.

VIII. ORGAN PROCUREMENT AND PRESERVATION

A. **Surgical procedure: Deceased donor procurement operation**

1. A midline laparotomy is made from xiphoid to pubis and a midline sternotomy is made.
2. Initial dissection aims to control the abdominal aorta and inferior mesenteric vein for the placement of cannulas.
3. Identification of hepatic hilar structures aids later dissection in the cold.
4. After cross-clamping the supraceliac aorta, the abdominal viscera are flushed and cooled with University of Wisconsin preservation solution or histidine–tryptophan–ketoglutarate.
5. The organs are packed with ice in the donor while the solution infuses.
6. Evacuation of blood into the chest via the inferior vena cava (IVC).
7. The donor liver is removed with its diaphragmatic attachments, a cuff of aorta surrounding the celiac axis and the superior mesenteric artery (SMA), and a portion of the supra- and infrahepatic IVC.
8. The donor kidneys are removed separately or *en bloc*.
9. The ureters are dissected widely to minimize devascularization and are divided near the bladder.
10. The pancreas may also be removed for transplantation, with the pancreas, duodenum, and spleen removed *en bloc*.
    a. The blood supply for the pancreas allograft comes from the donor splenic artery and SMA, and outflow is via the portal vein.

B. Organ preservation

1. With the advent of modern preservation solutions, donor livers can be preserved for up to 12 hours before reperfusion (kidneys up to 40 hours), with a low incidence of allograft dysfunction.
2. Ideally, cold ischemia time is minimized to <6 hours for livers and <24 hours for kidneys.
3. Recently, the use of machine perfusion for donor organs has increased.
    a. Hypothermic machine perfusion (HMP) involves placement of the graft on a pump that circulates cold preservation solution through the organ while awaiting transplantation (**Figure 21.3**).
    b. For kidney allografts, HMP was found to be superior to static cold storage resulting in decreased rates of delayed graft function.[10]
    c. Machine perfusion preservation in liver transplantation is being investigated with promising results.[11]

C. Organ transplantation

1. Kidney transplantation
    a. **Indications:** End-stage renal disease is the consequence of multiple disease processes; however, diabetes, hypertension, and polycystic kidney disease account for majority of cases (**Table 21.2**).
    b. **Surgical procedure: Kidney recipient operation (Figure 21.4)**
        1. Foley catheter is inserted and the bladder is irrigated with antibiotic-containing solution.
        2. A curvilinear paramedian (Gibson, "hockey-stick") incision is made in the right lower quadrant, the retroperitoneal space is entered, and the recipient external iliac artery and vein are identified and isolated.

3. An end-to-side donor renal vein to recipient external iliac vein anastomosis is performed.
4. The arterial anastomosis is created in a similar fashion, most often using a Carrel patch.
5. Mannitol and furosemide are administered IV prior to reperfusion. Care is taken to maintain the patient's systolic blood pressure above 120 mm Hg to ensure optimal perfusion of the transplanted kidney.
6. The ureteroneocystostomy is performed with imbrication of the bladder muscularis over the anastomosis to create an antireflux valve. Alternatively, the donor ureter can be anastomosed to the recipient ipsilateral ureter. Both are fashioned over a double-J ureteral stent.

c. **Postoperative considerations**

i. **IV fluid replacement**

a) Patients should be kept euvolemic or mildly hypervolemic in the early posttransplantation period with a goal of 120 mm Hg systolic blood pressure to ensure adequate perfusion to the new allograft.

b) Hourly urine output is replaced with one-half normal saline on a milliliter-for-milliliter basis as sodium concentration of the urine from a newly transplanted kidney is 60 to 80 mEq/L (normal is 20 mEq/L).

ii. **Renal allograft function or nonfunction**

a) If the patient's urine output is low in the early postoperative period (<50 mL/h), perfusion to the new allograft must be assessed.

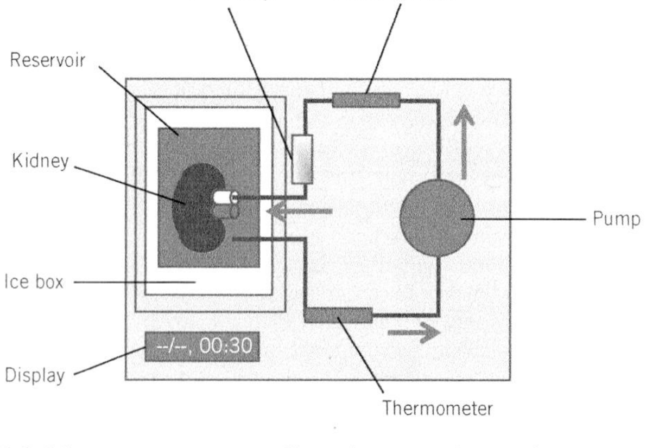

FIGURE 21.3 Schematic representation of hyperthermic machine perfusion in kidney transplantation. *(Figure 1 from O'Callaghan JM, Morgan RD, Knight SR, et al. Systematic review and meta-analysis of hypothermic machine perfusion versus static cold storage of kidney allografts on transplant outcomes. Br J Surg. 2013;100(8):991-1001. Reproduced by permission of British Journal of Surgery Society Ltd.)*

TABLE 21.2 Most Common Causes of Renal Failure Requiring Transplantation

Type	Characteristics
Congenital	Aplasia, obstructive uropathy
Hereditary	Alport syndrome (hereditary nephritis), polycystic kidney disease, tuberous sclerosis
Neoplastic	Postresection for renal cell carcinoma, Wilms tumor, other renal malignancies
Progressive	Diabetic nephropathy, chronic pyelonephritis, Goodpasture syndrome (antiglomerular basement membrane disease), hypertension, chronic glomerulonephritis, lupus nephritis, nephrotic syndrome, obstructive uropathy, scleroderma, amyloidosis
Traumatic	Vascular occlusion, parenchymal destruction

b) After volume resuscitation, low-dose (≤5 mg/h) dopamine infusion may be added to augment vasomotor tone and perfusion pressure.

c) Early poor function of a transplanted kidney is most commonly due to reversible **acute tubular necrosis (ATN)** secondary to reperfusion injury.

   1) Before the diagnosis of ATN can be made, noninvasive studies (renal Doppler ultrasonography or technetium-99m renal scan) demonstrating vascular patency/

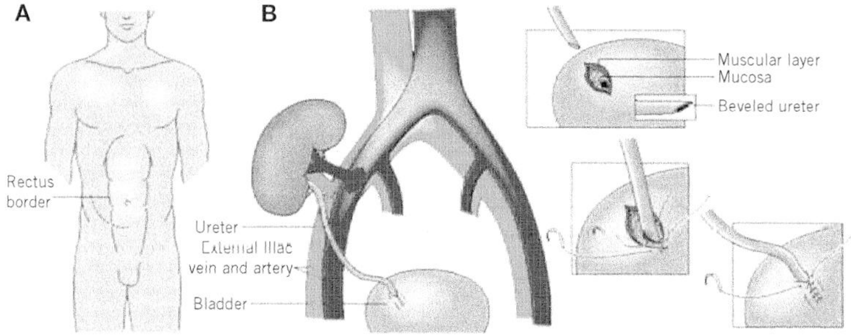

FIGURE 21.4 Anatomy of a renal transplant. A, Curvilinear iliac fossa incision used for the kidney transplant recipient procedure. B, Vascular anastomoses completed between the recipient external iliac artery and vein and donor renal artery and vein. Insets: Ureteral anastomosis performed using the external ureteroneocystostomy technique. *(Reprinted with permission from Freise CE, Stock PG. Renal transplantation. In: Mulholland MW, Lillemoe KD, Doherty GM, et al., eds. Greenfield's Surgery: Scientific Principles and Practice. 6th ed. Wolters Kluwer; 2017:541-551. Figure 36-3.)*

good renal blood flow in the absence of hydronephrosis or urinary leak must be obtained.
2) If adequate renal blood flow is confirmed, dialysis can be continued until allograft function recovers.

d. Complications

i. Lymphoceles

a) Collections due to lymphatic leaks in the retroperitoneum
b) Present one to several weeks after transplantation
c) Signs and symptoms: Generally asymptomatic and identified incidentally
d) Diagnosis: Ultrasound
e) Treatment:
 1) Indicated for symptomatic lymphoceles
 2) Drainage into the peritoneum, via laparoscopic or open methods

ii. Renal artery and vein thrombosis

a) Arterial and venous thromboses most often occur in the first 1 to 3 days after transplantation.
b) Signs and symptoms: Sudden cessation of urine output, rapid rise in serum creatinine, graft swelling, local pain
c) Diagnosis: Technetium-99m renal scan or Doppler ultrasound
d) Treatment: Immediate operative exploration and repair to prevent graft loss

iii. Urine leak

a) Generally due to anastomotic leak or ureteral sloughing secondary to ureteral blood supply disruption
b) Signs and symptoms: Pain, rising creatinine, and possibly urine draining from the wound
c) Diagnosis: Renal scan demonstrates radioisotope outside the urinary tract.
d) Treatment: Placement of a bladder catheter to reduce intravesical pressure and subsequent surgical exploration

iv. Rejection

a) Infrequent and inversely correlated with degree of HLA matching
b) Diagnosis: Renal biopsy
c) Treatment: Pulse steroids, and antithymocyte preparations can be used for steroid-resistant rejection and plasmapheresis should be considered for antibody-mediated rejection.

v. Graft surveillance

a) After the initial 3-month period, when ACR becomes less of a risk, tacrolimus and steroid doses are tapered.
b) Chronic long-term immunosuppression can be maintained at lower levels than those required for induction.
c) Very rarely, immunosuppression can be discontinued completely ("tolerance").

2. **Liver transplant**
   a. **Indication:** Complications attributable to end-stage liver disease (ESLD).
      i. While hepatitis C has been the leading contributor to ESLD, nonalcoholic steatohepatitis (NASH) has become increasingly prevalent.
         a) Newer antiviral treatments for hepatitis C have demonstrated sustained virologic response in 95% of treated individuals, decreasing the risk of advanced liver disease/need for transplant.
         b) In the largest single institution experience, liver transplantation for NASH increased fivefold from 2002 to 2011.[12]
         c) Although outcomes were comparable with other indications for orthotopic liver transplantation (OLT), there are significantly more health care resources consumed by this group of recipients.
   b. **Transplantation for hepatic malignancy**
      i. Cirrhosis is a risk factor for HCC.
      ii. The **Milan criteria** are guidelines for considering OLT in patients who present with early (stage I or II) HCC and underlying cirrhosis (**Table 21.3**).
      iii. Given the concern for HCC progression while awaiting transplantation, candidates receive MELD exception points, but only after 6 months of being listed.
      iv. At 6 months, candidates with an approved extension receive a MELD of 28, which increases with each extension to a maximum MELD score of 34.

TABLE 21.3 Most Common Indications for Orthotopic Liver Transplantation

Adults	
Chronic hepatitis C	Primary biliary cirrhosis
Alcoholic liver disease	Primary sclerosing cholangitis
Chronic hepatitis B	Autoimmune hepatitis
Children	
Extrahepatic biliary atresia	Primary hepatic tumors
α_1-Antitrypsin deficiency	Metabolic liver disease
Cystic fibrosis	

c. **Surgical procedure: Liver recipient operation** (**Figure 21.5**). There are many variations on the standard surgical technique for deceased donor transplant, which may involve the use of veno-venous bypass or creation of a portocaval shunt. A summary of the critical steps includes the following:

1. An upper abdominal transverse incision ("chevron," "Mercedes") followed by dissection and removal of the recipient's diseased liver with preservation of the retrohepatic IVC in the "piggy-back" technique.
2. Anastomosis of the donor suprahepatic IVC to the cuff of the hepatic veins off the recipient IVC in the "piggy-back" technique or donor suprahepatic followed by infrahepatic IVC anastomoses in the bicaval approach.
3. An end-to-end portal vein anastomosis followed by reperfusion of the liver allograft.
4. Creation of the hepatic artery anastomosis, typically end-to-end; additional reconstruction for aberrant arterial anatomy may be required.
5. Biliary reconstruction, preferably in an end-to-end donor-to-recipient fashion unless significant size mismatch or a diseased recipient bile duct (e.g., primary sclerosing cholangitis, biliary atresia, or secondary biliary cirrhosis). In those scenarios, a Roux-en-Y choledochojejunostomy is performed.

d. **Postoperative considerations**

i. **Hepatic allograft function**

a) Monitoring of hepatic allograft function begins intraoperatively after reperfusion.

1) Signs of satisfactory graft function: Hemodynamic stability normalization of acid–base status, normothermia, improving coagulopathy, euglycemia, and bile production

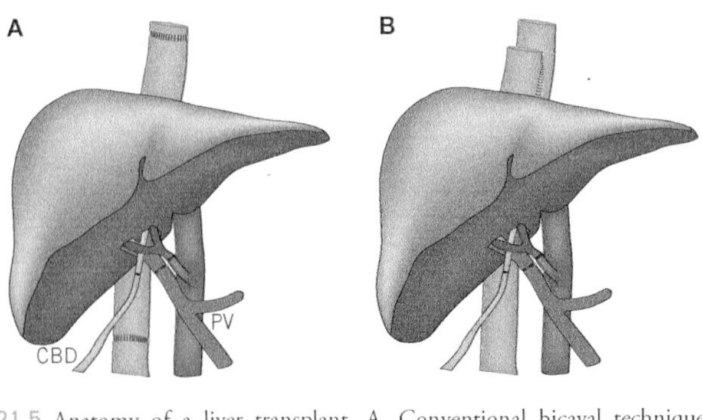

FIGURE 21.5 Anatomy of a liver transplant. A, Conventional bicaval technique for liver transplantation. B, Piggy-back technique for liver transplantation. CBD, common bile duct; PV, portal vein. *(Figure 1 adapted by permission from Nature: Zarrinpar A, Busuttil RW. Liver transplantation: past, present and future. Nat Rev Gastroenterol Hepatol. 2013;10(7):434-440. Copyright 2013, Springer Nature.)*

b) Postoperatively, satisfactory graft function is indicated by improving coagulation profile, decreasing transaminase levels, euglycemia, hemodynamic stability, adequate urine output, bile production, and clearance of anesthesia.
    1) Early elevations of bilirubin and transaminase levels may be indicators of preservation injury.

c) Peak levels of aspartate transaminase (AST) and alanine transaminase (ALT) are usually <2000 U/L and should decrease rapidly over the first 24 to 48 hours postoperatively.

d) Persistent transaminitis should prompt a liver Doppler ultrasound to assess vessel patency and flow.

e. Complications

i. Primary nonfunction

a) Hemodynamic instability, poor quantity and quality of bile, renal dysfunction, failure to regain consciousness, increasing coagulopathy, persistent hypothermia, and lactic acidosis despite patent vascular anastomoses (as demonstrated by Doppler ultrasound).

b) The incidence is approximately 1% and is fatal without retransplantation.

c) Risk factors include older donor age, longer cold ischemic time, fatty changes on donor liver biopsy, and smaller donor liver size.

ii. Hepatic artery thrombosis

a) Early posttransplantation period

b) Risk factors include vessel size mismatch between donor and recipient arteries, small vessels, prolonged ischemic time, and errors in surgical technique.

c) Presentation: Fever, hemodynamic instability, and rapid deterioration, with marked transaminase elevation
    1) Associated bile leak may be due to loss of the main vascular supply of the bile duct.

d) Treatment: Acute thrombosis may be treated by thrombectomy; however, this is usually unsuccessful and retransplantation is needed.

iii. Portal vein stenosis or thrombosis

a) Rare

b) Risk factors include hypercoagulability, history of portosystemic shunt, and errors in surgical technique.

c) Presentation: Hepatic dysfunction, ascites, renal failure, and hemodynamic instability

d) Treatment: Although surgical thrombectomy may be successful, urgent retransplantation is often necessary.

iv. Biliary stricture

a) Presentation: Hyperbilirubinemia

b) Risk factors: Bile duct ischemia, bile duct size mismatch between donor and recipient, and error in surgical technique

c) Diagnosis: Cholangiography via percutaneous transhepatic cholangiography, magnetic resonance cholangiopancreatography, or endoscopic retrograde cholangiopancreatography

d) Treatment:
   1) Single short bile duct stricture: Percutaneous or retrograde balloon dilation
   2) Long stricture: Revision of the biliary anastomosis

f. **Rejection**
   i. ACR can occur in 15% to 25% of patients
   ii. Diagnosis: Liver biopsy
   iii. Treatment: Pulse steroids, then antithymocyte preparations, tacrolimus, or anti-CD3 monoclonal antibodies can be used for patients with steroid-resistant rejection

3. **Pancreas transplant**

a. **Indications**
   i. Most patients who are evaluated for a pancreas transplant in conjunction with kidney transplantation are with type 1 diabetes and concomitant nephropathy.
   ii. Whole-organ pancreas transplantation represents the only therapeutic option for long-term insulin independence. Pancreatic allo islet cell transplantation is currently only allowed in the setting of a clinical trial.
   iii. Ninety-five percent of all pancreas transplants are performed in conjunction with renal transplant.
   iv. **Simultaneous kidney–pancreas transplantation** (**SKP**) is considered in patients with insulin-dependent diabetes who are dialysis dependent (or imminent) and have a creatinine clearance <30 mL/min.
   v. **Pancreas after kidney transplantation (PAK):** Patients with living kidney donors can be listed separately for deceased pancreas transplantation.
   vi. **Pancreas alone transplantation** (**PAT**) is reserved for patients with severe diabetes with life-threatening hypoglycemic episodes due to lower rates of graft survival when compared to simultaneous kidney–pancreas transplant.

b. **Surgical procedure: Pancreas recipient operation** (**Figure 21.6**). The most widely accepted technique uses whole-organ pancreas with venous drainage into the systemic circulation and enteric exocrine drainage, although there is wide variation across transplant centers. The pancreas transplant is typically placed in the right paracolic gutter, and if simultaneous kidney transplantation is performed, it is done on the left side.
   1. A midline laparotomy incision is made, and the right external iliac artery and vein are identified and isolated.
   2. The donor portal vein is anastomosed to the recipient external iliac vein in an end-to-side fashion.
   3. The donor splenic artery and SMA are reconstructed with a donor iliac artery Y-bifurcation autograft and anastomosed in an end-to-side fashion to the external iliac artery.
   4. The second portion of the duodenum is used to create a duodenojejunostomy. Alternatively, the duodenal segment can be anastomosed to the bladder.

c. **Postoperative considerations**

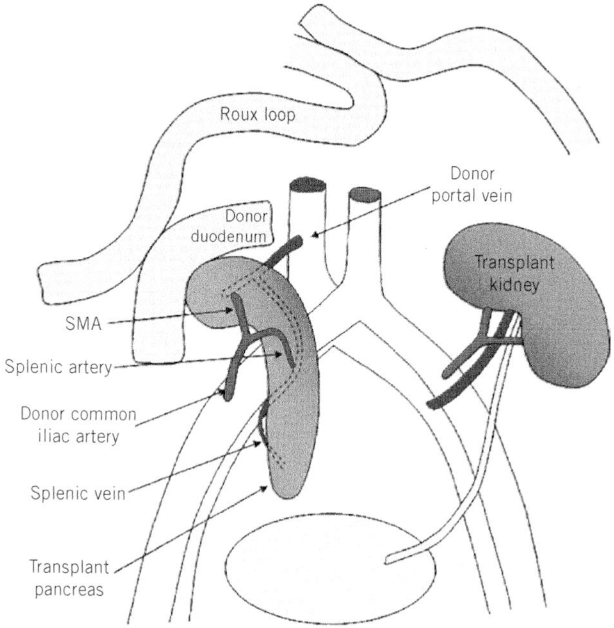

FIGURE 21.6 Anatomy of a simultaneous kidney–pancreas transplant. SMA, superior mesenteric artery. *(Reprinted from Hampson FA, Freeman SJ, Ertner J, et al. Pancreatic transplantation: surgical technique, normal radiological appearances and complications. Insights Imaging. 2010;1(5-6):339-347. https://creativecommons.org/licenses/by/2.0.)*

i. **Serum glucose**
   a) Followed during and after transplantation
   b) IV insulin infusions can generally be stopped intraoperatively or within the first few hours after pancreas transplantation.
   c) Posttransplant elevations may indicate graft failure.

ii. **Rejection**
   a) Suggested by a rise in serum amylase or a fall in urinary amylase.
   b) Rejection of pancreas and kidney transplants usually occurs in parallel.
   c) When indicated, biopsy of the pancreas transplant is performed percutaneously.

iii. **Graft-related complications**
   a) Metabolic acidosis and dehydration due to loss of sodium and bicarbonate into the urine from the transplanted duodenum.
   b) Other common complications include pancreatitis, UTIs, urethritis, and anastomotic leak from the duodenocystostomy.

c) 5-year graft survival for SKP is 91.3%, PAK 100%, and only 74% for PAT.

4. **Small intestine transplant**
   a. Replacement of small intestine for chronic intestinal failure most commonly due to short bowel syndrome and inability to be maintained on total parenteral nutrition.
   b. Very rare and only performed at highly specialized centers.
   c. Can be performed in combination with transplant of other organs, most commonly liver.
   d. Small intestine transplants carry many challenges including the need for high rates of immunosuppression due to the naturally occurring innate immune system within the gut, higher rates of PTLD, and higher infection risk within recipients when compared to other transplant recipients.
5. **Lung and heart transplant**
   a. Please see Chapters 31 and 32 for discussion of lung and heart transplant.

Key References

Citation	Summary
A comprehensive risk quantification score for deceased donor kidneys: the kidney donor risk index Rao PS, Schaubel DE, Guidinger MK, et al. A comprehensive risk quantification score for deceased donor kidneys: the kidney donor risk index. *Transplantation.* 2009;88(2):231-236.	• In this retrospective trial, data from over 69,000 kidney transplants were reviewed to develop a risk index for graft failure and independent associations were found between donor age, race, history of hypertension, history of diabetes, serum creatinine, cold ischemia time, and other factors with risk of graft failure.
Characteristics associated with liver graft failure: the concept of a donor risk index Feng S, Goodrich NP, Bragg-Gresham JL, et al. Characteristics associated with liver graft failure: the concept of a donor risk index. *Am J Transplant.* 2006;6(4):783-790.	• In this retrospective trial, data from over 20,000 liver transplants was reviewed to develop a donor risk index, which found that several factors independently predicted graft failure, including donor age over 40 years, donation after cardiac death, and split or partial grafts.
Liver transplantation for nonalcoholic steatohepatitis: the new epidemic Agopian VG, Kaldas FM, Hong JC, et al. Liver transplantation for nonalcoholic steatohepatitis: the new epidemic. *Ann Surg.* 2012;256(4):624-633.	• In this retrospective review, the authors evaluated the results of 144 patients with NASH and found that the incidence of liver transplant for NASH was increasing and that while outcomes were comparable, health care resource utilization was significantly higher.

CHAPTER 21: ABDOMINAL TRANSPLANTATION

Review Questions

1. What are the classes of HLA most important in determining a match for organ transplantation?
2. What are the four types of organ transplant rejection?
3. What are the categories of immunosuppressive drugs used in transplantation and what is one example of each?
4. List the categories of potential complications related to immunosuppression and give one example for each.
5. What factors are considered in UNOS kidney allocation?
6. What scoring system is used to allocate liver grafts and what recipient factors are included in the calculation of the score?
7. List the different types of organ donors.
8. List the potential complications after kidney transplantation and name one investigation to diagnose each.
9. List the potential complications after liver transplantation and the appropriate treatment for each.
10. List the different types of pancreas transplantation.

REFERENCES

1. Klintmalm GB, Feng S, Lake JR, et al. Belatacept-based immunosuppression in de novo liver transplant recipients: 1-year experience from a phase II randomized study. *Am J Transplant.* 2014;14(8):1817-1827.
2. Rao PS, Schaubel DE, Guidinger MK, et al. A comprehensive risk quantification score for deceased donor kidneys: the kidney donor risk index. *Transplantation.* 2009;88(2):231-236.
3. Kim WR, Biggins SW, Kremers WK, et al. Hyponatremia and mortality among patients on the liver-transplant waiting list. *N Engl J Med.* 2008;359(10):1018-1026.
4. Biggins SW, Kim WR, Terrault NA, et al. Evidence-based incorporation of serum sodium concentration into MELD. *Gastroenterology.* 2006;130(6):1652-1660.
5. McDiarmid Sv., Anand R, Lindblad AS; Principal Investigators and Institutions of the Studies of Pediatric Liver Transplantation SPLIT Research Group. Development of a pediatric end-stage liver disease score to predict poor outcome in children awaiting liver transplantation. *Transplantation.* 2002;74(2):173-181.
6. Poggio ED, Augustine JJ, Arrigain S, Brennan DC, Schold JD. Long-term kidney transplant graft survival-Making progress when most needed. *Am J Transplant.* 2021;21(8):2824-2832.
7. Mourad MM, Algarni A, Liossis C, Bramhall SR. Aetiology and risk factors of ischaemic cholangiopathy after liver transplantation. *World J Gastroenterol.* 2014;20(20):6159-6169.
8. Retraction. *Liver Transpl.* 2018;24(6):279-789. Accessed March 5, 2023. https://pubmed.ncbi.nlm.nih.gov/?term=Liver+Transpl.+2018%3B24%286%29%3A279%E2%80%93789
9. Müller AK, Breuer E, Hübel K, et al. Long-term outcomes of transplant kidneys donated after circulatory death. *Nephrol Dial Transplant.* 2022;37(6):1181-1187.

10. Tingle SJ, Figueiredo RS, Moir JAG, Goodfellow M, Talbot D, Wilson CH. Machine perfusion preservation versus static cold storage for deceased donor kidney transplantation. *Cochrane Database Syst Rev.* 2019;3(3):CD011671.

11. van Rijn R, Schurink IJ, de Vries Y, et al. Hypothermic machine perfusion in liver transplantation: a randomized trial. *N Engl J Med.* 2021;384(15):1391-1401.

12. Agopian VG, Kaldas FM, Hong JC, et al. Liver transplantation for nonalcoholic steatohepatitis: the new epidemic. *Ann Surg.* 2012;256(4):624-633.

13. Feng S, Goodrich NP, Bragg-Gresham JL, et al. Characteristics associated with liver graft failure: the concept of a donor risk index. *Am J Transplant.* 2006;6(4):783-790.

22 Appendix

Paul Kepper and Sean C. Glasgow

I. ANATOMY

A. The appendix is located on the inferior border of the cecum at the convergence of the three teniae coli of the ascending colon.
B. The **appendicular artery**, a branch of the ileocolic artery, supplies the appendix and is located in the **mesoappendix**.
C. The appendix is a "true diverticulum" (i.e., with all bowel layers) and is histologically differentiated from the colon by lymphoid aggregates in the submucosa.

II. APPENDICITIS

A. Epidemiology/etiology
   1. Approximately 300,000 cases annually in the US with highest incidence in patients aged 10 to 19 years (23.3 per 10,000 population).
   2. Lifetime risk is 9% in the US.[1,2]
   3. Caused by luminal obstruction (e.g., lymphoid hyperplasia, fecalith, tumor) followed by increased intraluminal and intramural pressure impairing venous drainage, resulting in wall ischemia, inflammation, and superimposed infection.
   4. If left untreated, the appendix may become necrotic and perforate, forming a periappendiceal phlegmon or abscess.

B. Presentation
   1. Periumbilical pain that evolves to the right lower quadrant (RLQ) with associated tenderness on examination
   2. Anorexia, nausea/vomiting, and low-grade fever are common. Pain usually precedes these symptoms.
   3. Variant locations of the appendiceal tip (retrocecal, pelvic, and retroperitoneal) may lead to unique presentations of acute appendicitis.

C. Diagnosis
   1. **Physical examination**
      a. Tenderness at **McBurney point**, located one-third of the distance from the anterior iliac spine to the umbilicus on the right, may suggest focal peritoneal signs.
      b. **Obturator sign** is pain with internal rotation of right leg flexed at the knee, suggestive of irritation of the obturator internus due to inflammation over the pelvic brim/pelvis on the right.
      c. **Psoas sign** is pain with extension of right leg at the hip suggestive of inflammation on the right psoas, perhaps due to a retrocecal appendicitis.

d. **Rovsing sign** is RLQ pain with palpation of the left lower quadrant with pain due to localized peritonitis on the right being stimulated by the peritoneal motion from the left.

2. **Laboratory evaluation**
   a. Complete blood cell count—white blood cell count >10,000 cells/μL
   b. Urinalysis—abnormalities may indicate bladder irritation but rule out urinary tract infection.
   c. Serum electrolytes, blood urea nitrogen, creatinine—abnormalities may indicate dehydration.
   d. Serum or urine pregnancy test in ovulating females

3. **Imaging**
   a. **CT** is the most commonly ordered imaging test to diagnose acute appendicitis.
      i. Positive CT findings—distension with inflammatory streaking of periappendiceal fat, appendicoliths/fecaliths
      ii. Patients with perforated appendicitis may have a phlegmon or abscess (**Figure 22.1**).
   b. **Ultrasound imaging** is preferred in children but often nondiagnostic in pregnant women, especially in the third trimester.
      i. Positive ultrasound imaging findings for appendicitis include appendiceal diameter > 6 mm, lack of luminal compressibility, appendicolith/fecalith.
   c. **MRI** can be done if ultrasound imaging is equivocal.
      i. MRI may be limited by availability (especially after hours), time to complete the examination, and patient factors (e.g., claustrophobia, inability to lie flat for extended periods of time, patient size too large).[3]

D. Treatment

1. An appendicitis treatment algorithm is available in **Figure 22.2**.
2. Initial treatment involves IV fluid resuscitation and antibiotics to provide coverage for *Escherichia coli*, *Klebsiella*, *Streptococcus* spp., and *Enterococcus* spp.

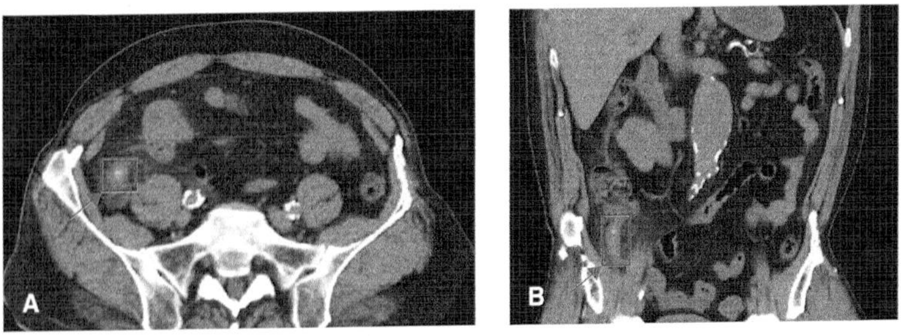

FIGURE 22.1 Axial (A) and coronal (B) CT images of patient with unperforated appendicitis (denoted by arrows/boxes). Acute appendicitis can be diagnosed on CT imaging by the presence of thickened appendiceal wall, fecalith, and/or periappendiceal fat stranding.

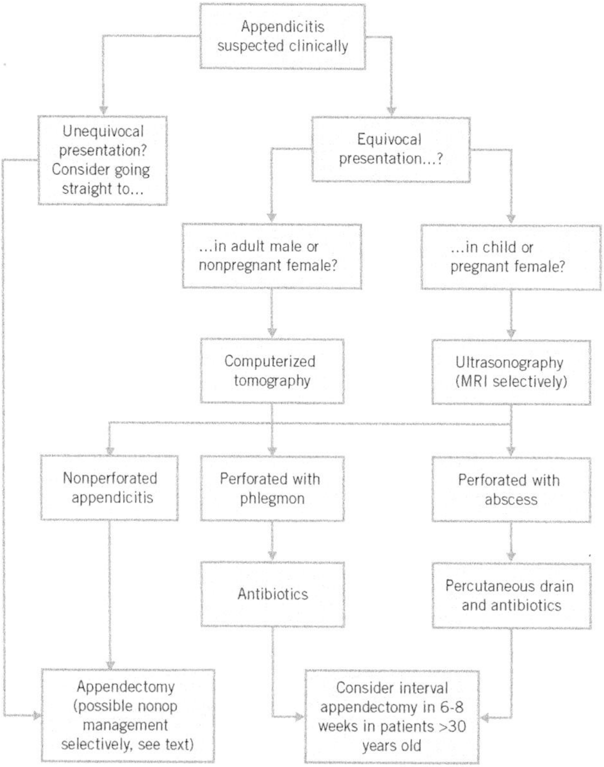

FIGURE 22.2 Appendicitis algorithm.

3. **Nonoperative management of uncomplicated appendicitis**
   a. Antibiotics alone are inferior to surgery for the treatment of uncomplicated appendicitis; 39.1% of patients treated with antibiotics alone have appendicitis recurrence within 5 years (APPAC trial, see landmark trials below).
   b. Nonoperative management is currently offered as an alternative to a minority of patients with either a prior history of surgical complications or mild, uncomplicated presentation of acute appendicitis with the absence of a fecalith.[2]
4. **Appendectomy** remains the standard of care for uncomplicated acute appendicitis.

a. **Surgical approach: Laparoscopic appendectomy**
   i. Three ports are placed: 10 mm at the umbilicus, 5 mm in the left lower quadrant, and 5 mm at the suprapubic midline.
   ii. Adhesions to the appendix are divided and the appendix is lifted.
   iii. The mesoappendix is divided using an energy device, stapler, or cautery.
   iv. The appendix is stapled at its base and removed through the largest incision (often through a containment bag).
   v. Irrigation is performed (if needed), drain can be considered in cases of significant perforation or purulence, pneumoperitoneum is reduced, and port sites are closed.

b. **Surgical approach: Open appendectomy**
   i. A transverse incision over McBurney point is made. The external and internal oblique and transversus abdominis muscle layers are split in the direction of their fibers.
   ii. The cecum is identified and teniae coli are traced to the appendix (or the ileum is identified by the antimesenteric fat or "ligament (or fold) of Treves" and traced back to the cecum).
   iii. The mesoappendix is divided, the appendiceal base ligated, and the appendix excised and delivered through the wound.
   iv. Irrigation is performed (if needed), drain can be considered in cases of significant perforation or purulence, and abdomen is closed (skin left open to close by secondary intention, if needed).

5. **Perforated appendicitis**
   a. Immediate appendectomy is rarely indicated.
   b. Start IV antibiotics covering gram-negative rods, gram-positive cocci, and anaerobes.
   c. Periappendiceal abscesses >2 cm diameter are percutaneously drained, if technically feasible, to achieve source control.
   d. Duration of antibiotic therapy depends on source control.
      i. After adequate source control (via drain or, rarely, surgery), 4 days of antibiotics is sufficient.[4]
      ii. With lack of source control, antibiotic therapy should not exceed 5 to 7 days; patients who do not clinically improve are reevaluated for source control intervention (laparoscopic appendectomy vs. drain) or for another diagnosis.[5]
   e. Interval appendectomy is recommended in patients aged 30 years and older due to increasing risk of malignancy with increased age in patients with complicated appendicitis.[6]

6. **Appendicitis in special populations**
   a. **Appendicitis in pregnancy**
      i. Appendicitis is the most common nongynecologic surgical emergency during pregnancy with an incidence of approximately 1 per 1,500.[7]
      ii. Ultrasound imaging is preferred as the initial diagnostic test, although its ability to accurately diagnose appendicitis decreases

in the third trimester; MRI should be considered if ultrasound imaging findings are equivocal.

iii. Appendectomy is safe during pregnancy and the preferred treatment of acute appendicitis in pregnant women, regardless of the trimester of pregnancy (see Chapter 40 for more details including approach, positioning, and monitoring recommendations).

7. **Appendicitis in children**
   a. The most common indication for emergency abdominal operation in childhood.
   b. The most common cause in children is lymphoid hyperplasia.
   c. Presentation varies with age.
      i. Children <5 years of age often present with nonspecific symptoms (diffuse abdominal pain, irritability, and/or diarrhea) leading to delay in diagnosis and a higher prevalence of perforation.
      ii. Adolescents have a presentation similar to that of adults.
   d. Clinical evaluation and ultrasound imaging are preferred to CT, with equal diagnostic accuracy as CT while reducing exposure to ionizing radiation.[8,9]
8. **Appendiceal neoplasms (Table 22.1)**
   a. **Neuroendocrine tumor (NET)**
      i. NET (previously "carcinoid tumors") are the most common appendiceal neoplasms, accounting for up to two-thirds of appendiceal tumors.
      ii. Most are asymptomatic but can cause obstruction and appendicitis.
      iii. Lymph node metastases present in 15% of tumors <1 cm, 47% of tumors between 1 and 2 cm, and 84% of tumors >2 cm.[10]
      iv. Tumors that metastasize to the liver release serotonin, causing **carcinoid syndrome:** Flushing, diarrhea, bronchoconstriction, and valvular heart disease.
      v. **Treatment**
         a) Surgical management determined by size
            1) <1 cm, appendectomy is curative
            2) >2 cm require formal right hemicolectomy to evaluate for and treat lymph node metastases.
            3) 1 to 2 cm are tailored based on patient and tumor characteristics.
         b) Factors that suggest poor prognosis that may warrant a right hemicolectomy for tumors <2 cm include mesoappendiceal invasion >3 mm, advanced grade consisting of elevated mitotic index (>2 mitoses per high-power field) or Ki-67 index (>3%) and lymphatic or vascular invasion.[11]
      vi. **Surveillance**
         a) NETs can be monitored for recurrence every 6 to 12 months for a total of 10 years using both biochemical and imaging studies.

TABLE 22.1 Appendiceal Tumors

Tumor	Features	Characteristics	Treatment
Neuroendocrine tumor	Most common appendiceal tumor	Release serotonin; carcinoid syndrome if metastasized beyond first pass effects of liver	<1 cm appendectomy is curative; >2 cm require hemicolectomy; Intermediate (1-2 cm) tumors are treated based on patient and histopathologic characteristics
Appendiceal mucinous neoplasms	Low-grade (LAMN) vs. high-grade (HAMN), mucinous adenocarcinoma	Appendiceal rupture leads to pseudomyxoma peritonei	Unruptured LAMN and HAMN require appendectomy alone, adenocarcinoma requires hemicolectomy Rupture associated with appendiceal mucinous neoplasia often requires cytoreductive surgery with hyperthermic intraperitoneal chemotherapy (HIPEC)
Adenocarcinoma	Mucinous, intestinal, signet ring, goblet cell	Rare	Right hemicolectomy with or without adjuvant chemotherapy

b) Serum chromogranin A or 24-hour 5-hydroxyindoleacetic acid levels along with CT or MRI is used to monitor recurrence.[11]

b. Appendiceal mucinous neoplasms

i. Produce mucin and are categorized based on histology: Low-grade appendiceal mucinous neoplasms (LAMN) and high-grade (HAMN).

ii. Malignant lesions are called **mucinous adenocarcinoma**.[12]

iii. **Clinical presentation**
   a) Many are incidentally identified on imaging for other reasons.
   b) Mucinous tumors can obstruct appendiceal lumen, causing the appendix to develop into a mucin-filled structure, mimicking acute appendicitis.
   c) If rupture occurs, mucin-secreting tumors can disseminate throughout the peritoneal cavity generating mucinous ascites called **pseudomyxoma peritonei (PMP)**.

iv. **Treatment**
   a) Surgical resection should be pursued for all appendiceal mucinous neoplasms to prevent rupture and to rule out concomitant malignancy.
   b) Additional treatment is determined by pathology.
      1) Unruptured appendices with LAMN or HAMN on histopathology do not require additional surgery.
      2) Mucinous adenocarcinomas require a formal oncologic resection.
      3) Ruptured mucinous neoplasms with the development of PMP are aggressively managed with **cytoreductive surgery (CRS)** and **hyperthermic intraperitoneal chemotherapy (HIPEC)**.

v. **CRS** involves resecting all visible tumor deposits within the peritoneal cavity, may include visceral and peritoneal resections.

vi. Once CRS is complete, **HIPEC** is instilled into the peritoneal cavity, commonly mitomycin and oxaliplatin, maximizing antitumor effects within the abdomen while limiting systemic adverse effects.

vii. Completeness of CRS is the most important procedure-associated predictor of survival; therefore, all visible tumor deposits should be excised if feasible, even if extensive organ resections are required.

c. **Adenocarcinoma**

i. Extremely rare, often discovered incidentally in appendectomy specimens

ii. Three types: Mucinous (described above), intestinal/colonic, and signet ring or goblet cell

iii. **Treatment**
   a) Colonic/Intestinal and signet ring/goblet cell types are treated like their colonic counterparts and, therefore, are resected with a formal right colectomy.
   b) Adjuvant chemotherapy regimens extrapolated from those of colonic adenocarcinoma (i.e., 5-fluorouracil based); however, given the rarity of appendiceal adenocarcinomas, the survival benefit has not been established.

Key References

Citation	Summary
Salminen P, Paajanen H, Rautio T, et al. Antibiotic therapy vs appendectomy for treatment of uncomplicated acute appendicitis: the APPAC randomized clinical trial. *JAMA.* 2015;313(23):2340-2348.	• Randomized control trial comparing antibiotic therapy alone vs. appendectomy for the treatment of uncomplicated acute appendicitis that found antibiotics alone as therapy for CT-proven, uncomplicated appendicitis was inferior to standard therapy with appendectomy.
Salminen P, Tuominen R, Paajanen H, et al. Five-year follow-up of antibiotic therapy for uncomplicated acute appendicitis in the APPAC randomized clinical trial. *JAMA.* 2018;320(12):1259-1265.	• Five-year observational follow-up of patients treated with antibiotics alone in the APPAC trial had rate of appendicitis recurrence of 39.1% after 5 years.
Hayes D, Reiter S, Hagen E, et al. Is interval appendectomy really needed? A closer look at neoplasm rates in adult patients undergoing interval appendectomy after complicated appendicitis. *Surg Endosc.* 2021;35(7):3855-3860.	• Retrospective chart review of 402 patients showing the risk of neoplasm in complicated appendicitis increases with age and recommended interval appendectomy in patients older than 30 y of age who present with complicated appendicitis.
Wei B, Qi CL, Chen TF, et al. Laparoscopic versus open appendectomy for acute appendicitis: a metaanalysis. *Surg Endosc.* 2011;25(4):1199-1208.	• Meta-analysis comparing laparoscopic vs. open appendectomy for acute appendicitis that recommend laparoscopic appendectomy as an effective and safe procedure for acute appendicitis after finding, despite the longer operative time, laparoscopic appendectomy results in less postoperative pain, faster postoperative rehabilitation, a shorter hospital stay, and fewer postoperative complications than open appendectomy.

CHAPTER 22: APPENDIX

Review Questions

1. Is the appendix a true or a false diverticulum?
2. What imaging modality should be used to diagnose appendicitis in children and pregnant women?

3. True/False: The presence of a fecalith on imaging predicts a high rate of failure of nonoperative management for acute appendicitis.
4. What is the preferred treatment for acute appendicitis in pregnancy, regardless of trimester?
5. What is the most common tumor of the appendix?
6. A 5-mm neuroendocrine tumor is discovered on pathologic evaluation of an appendix after appendectomy. What additional therapy is needed, if any?
7. A 2.5-mm neuroendocrine tumor is discovered on pathologic evaluation of an appendix after appendectomy. What additional therapy is needed, if any?

REFERENCES

1. Addiss DG, Shaffer N, Fowler BS, Tauxe RV. The epidemiology of appendicitis and appendectomy in the United States. *Am J Epidemiol.* 1990;132(5):910-925.
2. Di Saverio S, Podda M, De Simone B, et al. Diagnosis and treatment of acute appendicitis: 2020 update of the WSES Jerusalem guidelines. *World J Emerg Surg.* 2020;15(1):27.
3. Long SS, Long C, Lai H, Macura KJ. Imaging strategies for right lower quadrant pain in pregnancy. *AJR Am J Roentgenol.* 2011;196(1):4-12.
4. Sawyer RG, Claridge JA, Nathens AB, et al. Trial of short-course antimicrobial therapy for intraabdominal infection. *N Engl J Med.* 2015;372(21):1996-2005.
5. Mazuski JE, Tessier JM, May AK, et al. The surgical infection society revised guidelines on the management of intra-abdominal infection. *Surg Infect.* 2017;18(1):1-76.
6. Hayes D, Reiter S, Hagen E, et al. Is interval appendectomy really needed? A closer look at neoplasm rates in adult patients undergoing interval appendectomy after complicated appendicitis. *Surg Endosc.* 2021;35(7):3855-3860.
7. Mourad J, Elliott JP, Erickson L, Lisboa L. Appendicitis in pregnancy: new information that contradicts long-held clinical beliefs. *Am J Obstet Gynecol.* 2000;182(5):1027-1029.
8. Krishnamoorthi R, Ramarajan N, Wang NE, et al. Effectiveness of a staged US and CT protocol for the diagnosis of pediatric appendicitis: reducing radiation exposure in the age of ALARA. *Radiology.* 2011;259(1):231-239.
9. Shah SR, Sinclair KA, Theut SB, Johnson KM, Holcomb GW III, St Peter SD. Computed tomography utilization for the diagnosis of acute appendicitis in children decreases with a diagnostic algorithm. *Ann Surg.* 2016;264(3):474-481.
10. Mullen JT, Savarese DM. Carcinoid tumors of the appendix: a population-based study. *J Surg Oncol.* 2011;104(1):41-44.
11. Glasgow SC, Gaertner W, Stewart D, et al. The American society of colon and rectal surgeons, clinical practice guidelines for the management of appendiceal neoplasms. *Dis Colon Rectum.* 2019;62(12):1425-1438.
12. Carr NJ, Cecil TD, Mohamed F, et al. A consensus for classification and pathologic reporting of pseudomyxoma peritonei and associated appendiceal neoplasia: the results of the Peritoneal Surface Oncology Group International (PSOGI) modified delphi process. *Am J Surg Pathol.* 2016;40(1):14-26.

23 Colon and Rectum

Jorge G. Zarate Rodriguez and Steven R. Hunt

I. DISORDERS OF COLONIC PHYSIOLOGY

A. Normal physiology

1. The colon is responsible for the resorption of water and sodium, moving stool, and coordinating defecation.
   a. The colon resorbs 1 to 1.5 L of fluid daily but can reabsorb up to 5 to 6 L, primarily via passive means.
   b. Sodium and chloride are conserved by active transport in exchange for potassium and bicarbonate.
   c. The integrity and function of the colonic mucosa is heavily dependent on the intraluminal **microbiota**.
      i. Colonic bacteria participate in digestion via fermentation of complex carbohydrates, producing **short-chain fatty acids**, of which **butyrate** is the primary energy source for colonocytes.
   d. Normal colon motility is characterized by **segmental contractions** that mix stool and **mass movements** that move stool through the colon 3 to 4 times daily.

B. Functional constipation (see also Chapter 24).

1. Definition. Made by meeting two of the **Rome criteria**, in the absence of irritable bowel syndrome:
   a. Straining for >25% of defecations
   b. Lumpy or hard stools in >25% of defecations
   c. Sensation of incomplete evacuation for >25% of defecations
   d. Sensation of anorectal obstruction/blockage for >25% of defecations
   e. Manual maneuvers to facilitate for >25% of defecations (e.g., digital evacuation, support of the pelvic floor)
   f. <3 defecations per week
2. Etiologies
   a. Frequently due to medications, chronic laxative abuse, hypothyroidism, hypercalcemia, dietary factors, inactivity, and/or neurologic disorders.
   b. Differential should include mechanical obstruction (e.g., stricture, mass), pelvic floor dysfunction, rectal prolapse, or disorders of the colonic myenteric plexus (e.g., colonic inertia, Chagas disease, Hirschsprung disease).
3. Evaluation
   a. History and physical, including digital rectal examination (DRE)
   b. Laboratory evaluation of serum glucose, creatinine, calcium, and thyroid function.

c. Contrast enema or sigmoidoscopy/colonoscopy to rule out structural causes.
d. If tests are negative, trial of high-fiber diet (25-30 g/d) and increased fluid intake.
e. Next step is a **colonic transit study** with radiopaque markers, the stalling of which could warrant further evaluation based on the location and extent of the stalled markers.
f. Consider **defecography** to evaluate for obstructed defecation and/or **anal manometry** to evaluate for functional anorectal obstruction.

4. Treatment
   a. Increased water intake, osmotic laxatives, fiber, exercise, and avoidance of predisposing factors
   b. **Obstructed defecation/nonrelaxation of the puborectalis:** Pelvic floor physical therapy.
   c. **Colonic inertia**
      i. Medical therapy first (e.g., laxatives, lubiprostone, linaclotide).
      ii. **Total abdominal colectomy** (TAC) with **ileorectal anastomosis (IRA)** or **end ileostomy (EI)** for debilitating symptoms refractory to nonoperative measures.
         a) **Surgical approach: Total abdominal colectomy**
            1) Open or minimally invasive (laparoscopic or robotic) approach.
            2) Mobilize the right colon via medial or lateral approach, protecting retroperitoneal structures, including the duodenum; mobilize transverse colon taking down the attachments of the omentum and splenocolic ligaments; mobilize the descending and sigmoid colons while preserving the retroperitoneal structures including the left ureter and gonadal vessels.
            3) Control and ligate (with suture ligatures or energy device) the blood supply to the right, transverse, and left colons (can be at vessel origins or closer to the mesenteric border of the bowel since benign disease).
            4) Divide the terminal ileal mesentery and divide the terminal ileum just proximal to the ileocecal valve with a linear stapler; divide the rectosigmoid with a stapler just at or above where the taenia coli are noted to "splay" to the true rectum.
            5) Perform an IRA of the transected ends of ileum and rectosigmoid (surgeon preference as to anastomotic type and approach, e.g., **hand sewn** or stapled end-to-end or side-to-end, etc.) and air-leak test the anastomosis; or bring up an EI at preoperatively marked abdominal wall site where aperture is created.
            6) Abdomen is closed, and ileostomy, if present, is matured as a Brooke ileostomy.
         b) The determination of IRA versus EI is based on patient preference, continence, comorbidities, and pelvic floor

function/anatomy (patients with concomitant obstructed defecation should not have IRA).

c) Risk of persistent symptoms after colectomy for inertia is relatively high.

C. Colonic pseudo-obstruction (**Ogilvie syndrome**)

1. Marked colonic distention, the absence of intestinal contractility, and the absence of mechanical obstruction (must be excluded via imaging or colonoscopy, which carries higher risk of perforation)
2. Critically ill or institutionalized patients at increased risk
3. Initial management (without peritonitis/perforation): Nasogastric decompression, bowel rest, correction of contributing factors (e.g., shock, heart failure, metabolic derangements), and discontinuation of medications that decrease colonic motility
4. If symptoms persist after 24 to 48 hours: Consider **neostigmine**.
   a. A parasympathomimetic, should only be given in a monitored setting as it may cause significant bradycardia and bronchospasm.
   b. Contraindicated if significant cardiac disease or asthma
   c. Resolution occurs within 10 minutes of administration.
5. Second-line treatments: Repeat neostigmine dosing or continuous infusion, epidural anesthetic (sympathetic blockade), or colonoscopic decompression.
6. Failed medical treatment or evidence of perforation/peritonitis: Laparotomy with decompressing loop colostomy or resection of any ischemic or perforated segments with EI and mucous fistula

D. Volvulus

1. 10% to 15% of colonic obstruction in the US
2. **Sigmoid volvulus**
   a. Up to 60% of colonic volvulus cases
   b. Most common in elderly, institutionalized, and/or patients with neurologic disorders
   c. Acquired condition resulting from sigmoid redundancy with narrowing of the mesenteric pedicle leading to twisting at the mesenteric base.
   d. Diagnosis
      i. Abdominal pain, distention, cramping, obstipation
      ii. Abdominal radiograph shows a characteristic **inverted U,** or "**bent inner tube**" **sign** (**Figure 23.1A**).
      iii. If obtained, water-soluble contrast enema may show a **bird's beak deformity** at the obstructed rectosigmoid junction
      iv. CT may show the volvulus and characteristic **mesenteric whirl**.
   e. Treatment
      i. If stable, decompression via flexible or rigid sigmoidoscopy and placement of a rectal tube followed by elective sigmoid colectomy several days later to allow for colonic dilation to resolve, as risk of recurrence is as high as 40%.
      ii. Emergent resection is associated with higher mortality than elective operation.

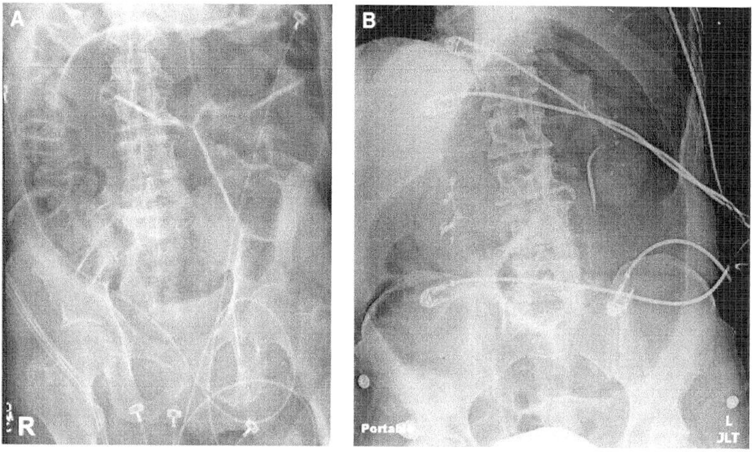

FIGURE 23.1 A, Supine abdominal radiograph showing sigmoid volvulus demonstrating a dilated loop of large bowel within the mid-abdomen with multiple folds pointing toward the right upper quadrant. Proximally, gas-filled loops of cecum and ascending colon are present. B, Supine abdominal radiograph showing cecal volvulus demonstrates dilated, gas-filled cecum within the left upper quadrant. Note that the large bowel emanates from the right lower quadrant, with gas seen distally in the sigmoid colon.

- **iii.** If peritonitis is present, sigmoidoscopy is unsuccessful, or if sigmoidoscopy reveals ischemia, the patient should undergo exploration and **Hartmann procedure** (sigmoidectomy and end-descending colostomy, blind rectal stump); consider primary anastomosis in select patients.

3. Cecal volvulus

- **a.** Up to 30% of colonic volvulus cases
- **b.** Occurs in younger patients, likely due to congenital failure of appropriate cecal tethering
- **c.** Occurs as true axially rotated volvulus (90%), or anterosuperior folding-in or "**cecal bascule**" (10%)
- **d.** Diagnosis
  - **i.** Presentation is similar to distal small bowel (SB) obstructions, with nausea, vomiting, abdominal pain, and distention.
  - **ii.** Abdominal radiograph shows **coffee bean–shaped**, air-filled cecum extending into the left upper quadrant (**Figure 23.1B**).
  - **iii.** Water-soluble contrast enema may be performed, but CT is more useful in the undifferentiated patient with abdominal pain.
- **e.** Treatment
  - **i.** Laparotomy and **ileocolectomy** with primary anastomosis or EI, depending on stability and patient factors
  - **ii.** **Cecopexy** alone has an unacceptably high rate of recurrence.

            iii. Colonoscopic decompression has limited utility, high risk for perforation.

4. **Transverse** and **splenic flexure volvulus**
    a. Extremely rare and present similarly to sigmoid volvulus
    b. Diagnosis based on abdominal radiography, contrast enema, or CT
    c. Operative resection is usually required.

II. DIVERTICULAR DISEASE

A. Definition and considerations

1. Outpouchings of colonic mucosa and submucosa through interruptions in the muscular layer and serosa (**"false diverticula"**) associated with weaknesses where the **vasa recta** penetrate the colonic wall
2. Formation related to high intraluminal pressures, commonly associated with low-fiber diets/constipation
3. The incidence increases with age (75% prevalence after age 80 years in the US).

B. Complications of diverticular disease

1. **Diverticulitis** occurs in 10% to 20% of patients with diverticulosis, and 95% occurs in the sigmoid colon.
    a. Abdominal pain the most common symptom, plus potential for constipation, diarrhea, fevers, and/or dysuria.
    b. Evaluation and staging using laboratory tests, examination, and CT
    c. Colonoscopy and contrast enemas are not recommended in the acute setting.
    d. Treatment
        i. **Uncomplicated diverticulitis** may involve fever and/or leukocytosis, localized (without gross perforation).
            a) Often treated with outpatient oral antibiotics and close follow-up.
            b) Supportive care without antibiotic therapy might be sufficient in select, healthy patients with early disease.[1]
        ii. **Complicated diverticulitis** involves perforation and is graded in severity using Hinchey classification to guide treatment (**Table 23.1**).
        iii. Radiologic-guided **percutaneous drainage** may be indicated in stable patients with accessible, localized abscess >3 cm in size and lack of diffuse peritonitis.
        iv. Surgical intervention for complicated diverticulitis can often be converted to elective operation in patients with localized abscesses using percutaneous drainage.
        v. Diffuse peritonitis generally requires urgent/emergent surgical intervention, usually a Hartmann procedure.
        vi. In stable patients with minimal contamination, resection and primary anastomosis (with or without **diverting loop ileostomy** [DLI]) can be considered.
        vii. Elective resection for diverticulitis usually consists of a sigmoid colectomy.

TABLE 23.1 Hinchey Classification of Complicated Diverticulitis

Grade	Description	Treatment
I	Localized pericolonic abscess or phlegmon	Conservative management with antibiotics, bowel rest, and monitoring Consider percutaneous drainage. Can be treated as outpatient in stable, reliable patients
II	Pelvic abscess	Bowel rest, IV antibiotics, monitoring, image-guided drainage, possible surgical intervention
III	Purulent peritonitis	Bowel rest, IV antibiotics, surgery
IV	Fecal peritonitis	Bowel rest, IV antibiotics, surgery

viii. Surgical approach: Laparoscopic sigmoid colectomy

a) Secure the patient to the operating room table in lithotomy position, arms tucked; consider rectal irrigation.

b) Port placement and entry technique varies by surgeon preference; some prefer a hand-assisted approach with a mini-Pfannenstiel incision and fewer laparoscopic ports. Consider: Periumbilical camera port (5 mm or 12 mm), two 5-mm ports on the left, one 5-mm port superiorly on the right, and one 12-mm port inferiorly.

c) Medial approach: In Trendelenburg position with patient's left side up, incise base of sigmoid mesentery from sacral promontory to and around the inferior mesenteric artery (IMA) and inferior mesenteric vein (IMV) in the avascular plane, protecting the hypogastric nerves, left ureter, gonadal vessels. Divide the IMA with clips, stapler, or energy device as well as the IMV, if needed for conduit mobility.

d) Free sigmoid and descending colon mesentery off the retroperitoneum superiorly and laterally, staying in the avascular plane of fusion, then divide the lateral colonic attachments toward and including, when needed, the splenic flexure, taking care not to tear the splenic capsule.

e) Identify the distal transection point (varies by pathologic indication), and divide the colon using a linear stapler; identify the proximal transection point in a location that will allow for a tension-free anastomosis, mark this location with clips or cautery.

f) Create a mini laparotomy by enlarging one of the port sites or through the Pfannenstiel to exteriorize the colon; transect the bowel at the previously marked transection point; purse-string suture the open bowel around the anvil of a circular stapler.

g) Return the bowel to the abdomen and close the mini laparotomy. Under laparoscopic visualization, insert the circular stapler and perform and end-to-end anastomosis, check for leaks by filling the pelvis with saline and insufflating transanally.
h) Place pelvic drain if preferred, then close the abdomen.

ix. Decision to perform elective colectomy is multifactorial, including
a) Identifying those at higher risk for complications from recurrent diverticulitis, including frequency, duration, and intensity of attacks, but not absolute indications
b) Patients who present with abscess should be considered for elective resection due to high risk of recurrence.
c) Diverticular disease complicated by stricture, obstruction, and/or fistula (see below) usually requires resection.
d) Immunocompromised patients are at increased risk for poor outcomes and should undergo elective resection.[2]
e) With increased use of CT, routine endoscopic evaluation after acute diverticulitis is not always necessary, but patients who are of appropriate age and/or have suspicious CT findings should undergo interval colonoscopy 4 to 6 weeks after resolution of symptoms, especially prior to elective resection.[3]

2. **Fistulization** secondary to diverticulitis may occur between colon and other organs (e.g., bladder, vagina, SB, skin).
   a. Diverticulitis is the most common etiology of **colovesical fistulas**.
   b. In women, **colovaginal** and colovesical fistulas usually occur in those who have previously undergone hysterectomy.
   c. **Colocutaneous fistulas** are uncommon and usually easy to diagnose; when they occur after percutaneous drainage of abscess, they are identified by drain studies after the abscess has resolved.
   d. **Coloenteric fistulas** uncommon, may be asymptomatic or result in diarrhea of varying severity.
   e. Fistula takedown and repair is usually performed at the time of resection.

III. LOWER GASTROINTESTINAL BLEEDING

A. Generally self-limiting, but up to 25% require surgical intervention.

B. Considered bleeding from the SB past ligament of Treitz, large bowel, or anus
   1. Colon is the most common location, with up to 15% located in the anorectal area and 5% in the SB.
   2. The most common cause is diverticular disease (30%), followed by anorectal disease (14%-20%), ischemia (12%), neoplasia (10%), colitides (9%), and angiodysplasia (3%).[4]

C. Management in acute setting depends on volume of bleeding.
   1. Patients with slow, intermittent bleeding often do not require hospitalization, but those with **massive lower gastrointestinal bleeding**

(LGIB) (requiring >2 units of red blood cells in a 24-hour period) and/or hemodynamic instability should be admitted and resuscitated (see Chapter 5).

2. Once resuscitation has been initiated, it is **critical to discern bleeding site before surgical intervention.**
   a. Without localization, operation should only be performed for refractory bleeding requiring large-volume transfusion.
   b. If anorectal source has been ruled out, an emergent **"blind" subtotal colectomy** may be performed but carries mortality of up to 30%.
3. History and physical are of some value to finding bleeding source.
   a. **Hematochezia** is usually associated with vigorous proximal bleeding or a more distal source, whereas **melena** is associated with an upper gastrointestinal (GI) or SB source, or slower, intermittent bleeding from proximal colon.
   b. Recent weight loss or anemia may be due to a chronic process, such as neoplasm or inflammatory bowel disease (IBD).
   c. **Stigmata of portal hypertension** may be evident on examination.
   d. DRE and anoscopy should be performed to rule out anorectal source.
   e. Nasogastric tube placement may help delineate upper GI source (i.e., bilious output without blood decreases, but does not eliminate, the likelihood of a gastric source).
   f. If on anticoagulation, this should be held and/or reversed.
4. Laboratory studies include complete blood count, coagulation profile, basic metabolic profile, and hepatic function panel to indicate the degree of anemia and coagulopathy as well as identify possible liver or renal dysfunction. Consider type and screen.
5. Diagnosing source/location
   a. Guides therapy and determines need for surgical intervention.
   b. **Endoscopy**
      i. **Esophagogastroduodenoscopy (EGD)** should be considered if massive LGIB or melena if an upper GI source has not been ruled out.
      ii. **Colonoscopy** can be diagnostic and therapeutic, as can EGD.
      iii. Actively bleeding lesions may be injected with epinephrine for vasoconstriction, cauterized, or clipped.
      iv. In stable patients without source found on endoscopy but with persistent transfusion requirement, **capsule endoscopy** or **SB "push" enteroscopy** should be considered.
   c. **CT angiogram** (**CTA**) has become the test of choice, quickly obtained and can detect continuous bleeding with a sensitivity of up to 90% at rates >0.35 mL/min and is more specific in identifying anatomic location compared with nuclear scans.
   d. **Nuclear scan** using Technetium-99m sulfur colloid or tagged red blood cells can identify bleeding with rates as low as 0.1 to 0.5 mL/min; the latter can identify bleeding up to 24 hours after isotope injection.
      i. Not specific in identifying the anatomic location of bleeding source (**Figure 23.2**)

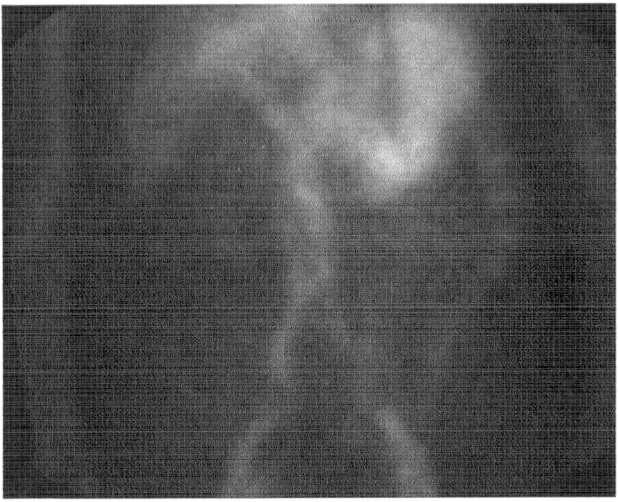

FIGURE 23.2 Technetium-99m tagged red blood cell scan demonstrating increased uptake within the distal transverse colon with antegrade propulsion of radiolabeled red blood cells. Findings are consistent with active extravasation (subsequent colonoscopy demonstrated a bleeding diverticulum).

e. **Mesenteric angiography** should be performed in patients with positive nuclear scan or CTA to localize (and potentially treat) source of bleeding.
   i. Angiography can localize bleeding exceeding 1 mL/min.
   ii. Allows for therapeutic interventions such as **vasopressin infusion** (0.2 unit/min) or selective **arterial embolization**, which together achieve hemostasis in 85% of cases but may result in ischemia of the treated bowel segment.

IV. COLITIDES

A. Introduction
1. **IBD** is a term that includes **ulcerative colitis (UC), Crohn's disease (CD)**, and **"indeterminate colitis."**
2. Etiology is not well understood; both environmental and genetic components are involved, as well as microbiome dysbiosis.
3. Extraintestinal manifestations include arthritis, primary sclerosing cholangitis (3%), pyoderma gangrenosum, erythema nodosum, iritis/uveitis (2%-8%), and stomatitis.
4. Patients with IBD have increased risk of thrombosis, including portal and mesenteric venous thrombosis, deep venous thrombosis (DVT), and pulmonary embolus.

B. Ulcerative colitis

1. Inflammatory process of colonic mucosa that **always involves the rectum** and **extends continuously** for a variable distance proximally **only in the colon**
2. Slight male predominance
3. Patients can present with bloody diarrhea, tenesmus, abdominal pain, fever, and weight loss.
4. As duration and intensity of inflammation increases, pathologic changes progress.
   a. Initially, mucosal ulcers and crypt abscesses are seen.
   b. Later, mucosal edema and pseudopolyps (islands of normal mucosa surrounded by deep ulcers) develop.
   c. End-stage pathologic changes show a flattened, dysplastic mucosa.
   d. Risk of colorectal cancer is increased in patients with UC related to the duration of disease, with risk increasing significantly after 20 years to almost 10%.
      i. Cancer must be considered in any colonic stricture in a patient with UC.
5. **Diagnosis**
   a. Constellation of symptoms as above
   b. Colonoscopy with biopsy
   c. Imaging studies can help determine if the patient has SB disease or fistulae indicative of CD.
   d. Laboratory work is nonspecific but may reveal anemia, low albumin, elevated erythrocyte sedimentation rate and C-reactive protein, and elevated stool inflammatory markers **(fecal calprotectin or lactoferrin)**.
6. **Medical management**
   a. Therapies that **induce and maintain remission** of colonic inflammation.
   b. Distal disease (**proctitis**) often responds to topical 5-aminosalicylic acid derivatives (5-ASA) as enemas or suppositories.
   c. For disease extending more proximally, oral 5-ASA or sulfasalazine (SSZ) may induce remission for mild or moderate disease.
   d. Oral or IV corticosteroids can be given to those unresponsive to 5-ASA or SSZ or are more systemically ill.
   e. Azathioprine and 6-mercaptopurine help wean off steroids and can be used as maintenance therapy.
   f. Biologic therapy with TNF-α inhibitors (e.g., infliximab, adalimumab, golimumab) has shown to decrease colectomy rates in the short term.[5] Long-term data show that patients with a good early response (within 3 months) are more likely to maintain this, resulting in lower long-term colectomy rates, too.[6]
7. Operation is indicated when UC is refractory to medical therapy (most common indication) and there is high risk of malignancy, **toxic colitis**, or intractable bleeding.
   a. For those acutely ill and with refractory UC, operation of choice is **TAC with EI.**

i. Once recovered, patients can be considered for **ileal pouch anal anastomosis (IPAA)** and DLI, followed by ostomy takedown at a later date (a **three-stage restorative proctocolectomy**).

b. For those subacutely ill or stable, a **two-stage approach** can be considered with initial **total proctocolectomy (TPC)** and IPAA with DLI, followed by subsequent DLI closure.

i. Some surgeons perform **one-stage approach** in optimal patients.

c. Regardless of approach, bowel function after restorative proctocolectomy is approximately six bowel movements daily, often with aid of bulking agents and/or antidiarrheals (>25%).

d. Complications after IPAA include leak, impaired continence, sexual dysfunction/infertility, pouchitis, and bowel obstruction.

e. IPAA is contraindicated in patients with poor baseline continence or low anorectal malignancy; older patients and obese patients have worse outcomes with IPAA.

f. CD and indeterminate colitis are relative contraindications for IPAA.

C. Crohn's disease

1. Introduction

a. **Transmural inflammatory process** that can affect **any area of the GI tract** from mouth to anus, often with a **segmental distribution** of normal mucosa interspersed between areas of diseased bowel.

i. Common pathologic changes include fissures, fistulae, transmural inflammation, and granulomas.

ii. **Terminal ileum** is involved in up to 45% of patients at presentation.

iii. Grossly, mucosa shows **aphthous ulcers** that deepen over time and are associated with **fat wrapping** and bowel wall thickening.

iv. As CD progresses, bowel lumen narrows and obstruction or perforation may result.

b. Female predominance

c. Common symptoms include diarrhea, abdominal pain, nausea, vomiting, weight loss, and/or fever.

d. Physical examination may show tender abdominal mass and/or perianal fistulas.

2. Diagnosis

a. Constellation of symptoms, examination, colonoscopy, imaging (CT, MRI, and/or contrast studies)

b. Patients with Crohn's colitis (CC) often present similarly to UC.

i. Up to one-third of patients with CC or UC will be diagnosed incorrectly prior to operative intervention.

ii. CC may be discerned from UC by the presence of perianal disease, "skip lesions," ileal inflammation, and presence of SB involvement on imaging.

c. Laboratory work is nonspecific but may reveal anemia, leukocytosis, iron and vitamin B12 deficiency, elevated erythrocyte sedimentation rate and C-reactive protein, and elevated stool inflammatory markers (fecal calprotectin or lactoferrin).

3. Medical management
   a. Immunosuppression used to induce and maintain remission.
   b. With acute flare and the presence of sepsis, source control should be obtained by drainage of any abscesses in addition to antibiotics.
   c. Steroids frequently used for induction of remission, then immunomodulators (as listed above for UC) used for remission as steroids weaned off.
   d. **Budesonide**, a topical oral corticosteroid with minimal systemic absorption, can be useful to minimize or avoid systemic steroids.
   e. Biologic therapy using **TNF-α inhibitors** has proven to decrease steroid use and prolong time to surgical intervention in CD.
4. Surgical intervention
   a. Indicated in patients with medically refractory disease, acute sepsis, perforation not amenable to percutaneous drainage, uncontrolled hemorrhage, failure to thrive/malnutrition, and dysplasia/malignancy.
   b. Segmental CD should be considered for limited resection.
   c. Colectomy with IRA can be considered for CC and rectal sparing with limited or no perianal disease.
   d. For CC with rectal involvement, TPC is the operation of choice, usually with EI, but some centers may perform IPAA for isolated CC with no perianal or SB disease.
   e. **Stricturoplasty** has a role in stricturing SB CD to decrease risks of **"short gut"** but plays no role in the treatment of stricturing CC due to 7% risk of malignancy over 20 years.

D. Indeterminate colitis
1. Term used for cases in which UC has not definitively been differentiated from CC (10%-15% of patients with IBD).
2. More than half of patients with initial diagnosis of indeterminate colitis will eventually be diagnosed with either UC or CD.
3. Medical and surgical approach for these patients is similar to those with UC, although higher rates of IPAA complications have been reported.

E. Ischemic colitis
1. Idiopathic in majority of patients, but due to colon malperfusion from global hypoperfusion, venous or arterial thrombosis or embolization, iatrogenic IMA ligation after abdominal aortic aneurysm repair, and/or vasculopathy.
2. Patients are usually elderly.
3. Present with lower abdominal pain, usually localizing to the left with melena or hematochezia
4. CT may show bowel wall thickening and inflammation that corresponds to submucosal hemorrhage and edema.
5. **Watershed areas** such as splenic flexure (**Griffith's point**) and sigmoid colon (**Sudeck's point**) more prone to ischemia, but ileocolic region can be impacted as well.
6. Ischemic colitis can be distinguished from **infectious colitis** by the appearance of the mucosa on endoscopy.

7. In presence of apparent full-thickness necrosis on endoscopy or peritonitis on examination, emergent resection with diversion is recommended.
8. Patients without peritonitis or free air, but with fever and/or an elevated white blood cell count, may be treated with bowel rest, close observation, and IV antibiotics.
9. Up to 50% of patients eventually develop focal strictures and may require resection.

F. Radiation proctocolitis

1. Results from intentional or incidental irradiation of colon or rectum for treatment of various malignancies (e.g., rectal, cervical, or prostate cancer)
2. Risk factors include doses >6000 cGy, vascular disease, diabetes mellitus, hypertension, prior low anterior resection (LAR), and advanced age.
3. Early phase occurs days to weeks from radiation and includes mucosal injury, edema, and ulceration with associated nausea, vomiting, diarrhea, and tenesmus.
4. Late phase occurs weeks to years from radiation with tenesmus, hematochezia, bowel thickening, and fibrosis, and ulceration with bleeding, stricture, and fistulae may occur.
5. Medical treatment may be successful in mild cases, with stool softeners, steroid enemas, sucralfate enemas, and/or topical 5-ASA products.
6. Endoscopic ablation or transanal application of **4% formalin** to affected mucosa may be effective in patients with transfusion-dependent rectal bleeding.[7]
7. Patients with stricture or fistula require proctoscopy and biopsy to rule out local recurrence or primary neoplasm.
8. Strictures may be treated by endoscopic dilation but often recur.
9. Surgical treatment consists of proximal diversion and is reserved for failure of medical therapy, recurrent strictures, and fistulae; resection of affected bowel may be indicated, including for recurrent/primary malignancy.

G. Infectious colitis

1. **Pseudomembranous colitis**
   a. Acute diarrheal illness resulting from toxins produced by overgrowth of ***Clostridioides difficile*** (formerly *Clostridium difficile*) after antibiotic treatment (especially clindamycin, ampicillin, or cephalosporins)
      i. Antibiotics already have been discontinued in one-fourth of the cases, and symptoms can occur up to 6 weeks after even a single dose.
   b. Diagnosis
      i. Made by detection of glutamate dehydrogenase or *C. difficile* **toxins** on enzyme immunoassays or nucleic acid amplification test
      ii. Proctoscopy/colonoscopy demonstrates sloughing colonic mucosa (**pseudomembranes**)
      iii. CT shows transmural colonic thickening.

c. Treatment
  i. Stop unnecessary antibiotics
  ii. Start oral vancomycin (125 mg qid) or fidaxomicin (200 mg bid) for nonsevere cases
  iii. Metronidazole alone is no longer considered first-line treatment.
  iv. For severe cases, treat with oral vancomycin (500 mg) and IV metronidazole, and consider vancomycin enemas for patients with ileus.
  v. Rarely, pseudomembranous colitis presents with severe sepsis and colonic distention with **toxic megacolon** or perforation and may require laparotomy with TAC and EI.
  vi. **Fecal microbiota transplantation** should be considered for patients with two recurrences of pseudomembranous colitis; delivery methods vary by institution, but studies report success rates of 60% to 90% regardless of method.[8]

H. Other causes of colitis include bacteria (Escherichia coli, Shigella), ameba, cytomegalovirus, and actinomycosis; however, these conditions are rare.
  1. Typically diagnosed by fecal testing or culture
  2. Treatment is dictated based on causative agent and clinical circumstances.

I. Neutropenic enterocolitis (typhlitis)
  1. Occurs most commonly in the setting of acute myelogenous leukemia after cytosine arabinoside therapy, but can occur after other chemotherapy regimens
  2. Present with abdominal pain, fever, bloody diarrhea, distention, and/or sepsis
  3. CT usually diagnostic, often involving right colon/cecum
  4. Treatment includes bowel rest, total parenteral nutrition, granulocyte colony-stimulating factor, and broad-spectrum IV antibiotics.
  5. Laparotomy with right colectomy or TAC and EI is required only if peritonitis develops.

V. NEOPLASTIC DISEASE

A. Introduction
  1. **Colorectal neoplasms** typically diagnosed incidentally on screening or with symptomatic presentation, including hematochezia, melena, anemia, abdominal pain, or constipation
  2. Colonoscopy is the gold standard screening test and has been shown to prevent cancer.
    a. The US Preventive Services Task Force recommends screening beginning at age 45 years until age 75 years with other details and screening options in **Table 23.2**.[9]
    b. Complications are rare, including perforation (0.04%), bleeding (0.1%), and mortality (0.2%).

B. Polyps
  1. **Nonadenomatous polyps**
    a. **Hyperplastic polyps**

i. Most common colorectal polyp (10 times more common than adenomas).
ii. Extremely limited malignant potential.
iii. Most are <0.5 cm in diameter, found in the distal colon, and rarely need treatment.
iv. Right-sided lesions or lesions >1 cm should be removed and may be a marker of increased risk of adenoma.

b. **Hamartomatous polyps**
i. <1% of all polyps
ii. Often associated with hereditary conditions including **Peutz–Jeghers syndrome, PTEN hamartoma tumor syndrome, multiple endocrine neoplasia 2B, familial juvenile polyposis syndrome**, and **neurofibromatosis type 1**
iii. Commonly pedunculated and >1 cm in size and have only rare malignant potential
iv. Isolated colonic hamartomas most often located in sigmoid colon or rectum and present with bleeding and/or prolapse
v. Less frequently, associated with anemia, diarrhea, obstruction, or mucoid stools.
vi. Treatment: Endoscopic resection, large polyps may require segmental colectomy.
vii. Rarely, total colectomy with IRA is required for colonic polyposis.

c. **Serrated polyps**
i. Have saw-tooth histologic configuration and are flat on endoscopy
ii. Previously thought to behave like hyperplastic polyps, now recognized as having an increased risk of colorectal cancer (CRC) and should be endoscopically removed

2. **Adenomas**
a. Dysplastic lesions with ability to progress to malignancy, thought to be **precursor of most CRC**
b. Risk of invasive malignancy is higher in villous adenomas than tubular; however, all adenomas are treated with endoscopic or surgical removal, and risk of malignancy increases with size.
c. Sessile polyps have a higher malignant risk than pedunculated polyps.
d. If polyp is not amenable to complete endoscopic removal, segmental colectomy should be considered.
e. **Subtypes**
i. **Tubular adenomas** usually sessile, account for roughly 85% of adenomas, can contain up to 25% villous features.
ii. **Tubulovillous adenomas** account for 10% to 15% of adenomas, contain 25% to 50% villous features.
iii. **Villous adenomas** usually sessile and account for 5% to 10% of adenomas, contain predominantly villous features.

3. **Malignant polyps**
a. Contain foci of invasion into the submucosa, considered T1 cancers
b. Level of invasion is an important factor in the treatment of malignant polyps, classified using **Haggitt (Table 23.3)** and **Kikuchi classifications (Table 23.4)**.

TABLE 23.2 Colorectal Cancer Screening Recommendations Based on Patient Risk

Risk	Description	Modality	Age at Initiation
Average (75% of newly diagnosed colorectal cancer, CRC)	Sporadic	**1.** Colonoscopy every 10 y **2.** Flexible sigmoidoscopy every 5 y **3.** CT colonography every 5 y **4.** High-sensitivity fecal occult blood test yearly **5.** Fecal immunochemical test yearly **6.** Multitarget stool DNA test every 3 y	45 y
Family history (15%-20%)	One first-degree relative with adenomatous polyps or CRC or two second-degree relatives with CRC	Colonoscopy every 10 y for second-degree relatives, or every 5 y for first degree relative	40 or 10 y prior to youngest relative's diagnosis (whichever is earliest)
Hereditary nonpolyposis colorectal cancer (HNPCC, 3%-8%), Lynch syndrome	Genetic or clinical diagnosis of HNPCC or individuals with high risk of HNPCC	Colonoscopy every 1-2 y, genetic counseling and consider genetic testing	Depends on family history (age of youngest cancer diagnosis) and genetic testing results, usually at 25-35 y
Familial adenomatous polyposis (FAP, 1%)	Genetic diagnosis of FAP or suspected FAP without diagnosis	Flexible sigmoidoscopy or colonoscopy every 1-2 y, genetic counseling, consider genetic testing	Puberty
Inflammatory bowel disease (1%)	Chronic Crohn's colitis or ulcerative colitis	Colonoscopy with random biopsies for dysplasia every 1-2 y, depending on personal risk	8 y after diagnosis, or at the time of primary sclerosing cholangitis

TABLE 23.3 Haggitt Classification of Malignant Polyps of the Colon and Rectum

Level	Description	Risk of Lymph Node Metastasis	Treatment
0	Noninvasive, high-grade dysplasia	<1%	Endoscopic removal with ≥2 mm margin
I	Focus of invasive cancer in head of pedunculated polyp	<3%	Endoscopic removal with ≥2 mm margin
II	Focus of invasive cancer in neck of pedunculated polyp	<3%	Endoscopic removal with ≥2 mm margin
III	Focus of invasive cancer in stalk of pedunculated polyp	<3%	Endoscopic removal with ≥2 mm margin
IV	Focus of invasive cancer in base of pedunculated polyp; all sessile polyps	Up to 25%	**See Kikuchi classification (Table 23.4)**

i. Classification systems stratify risk of lymph node (LN) metastasis.
ii. Those with low risk of LN involvement are treated with endoscopic removal.
iii. Those with high risk are treated with segmental colectomy.

TABLE 23.4 Kikuchi Classification of Submucosal Invasion of Malignant Polyps of the Colon and Rectum

Level	Description	Treatment
SM1	Invasion of the superficial one-third of submucosa	Endoscopic removal with ≥2 mm margin; in distal rectum transanal full-thickness removal
SM2	Invasion of the middle one-third of submucosa	Endoscopic removal with ≥2 mm margin; in distal rectum transanal full-thickness removal
SM3	Invasion of the deep one-third of submucosa	Segmental colectomy

iv. The Haggitt system classifies pedunculated polyps by depth and location of stalk invasion; sessile polyps are classified as Haggitt level 4.

v. Kikuchi classification further divides the submucosa into three levels from superficial to deep (SM1-3), used when considering local resection.

c. Lymphovascular invasion (LVI) and poor differentiation have been shown to increase likelihood of LN metastases.

d. Inadequate endoscopic resection margins (<2 mm), LVI, SM3 invasion, or poor differentiation should undergo segmental colectomy.

e. Surveillance after complete endoscopic removal of polyps with foci of invasive cancer without high-risk features involves repeat endoscopy at 1 year.[10]

f. Malignant polyps of the rectum

i. **Polyps of proximal two-thirds of rectum can be treated as colon polyps**

ii. Controversy regarding treatment of malignant polyps of distal one-third of rectum as they may have increased risk of LN metastasis.

iii. T1 lesions of distal rectum should be removed with full-thickness excision using traditional **transanal excision, transanal endoscopic microsurgery (TEM),** or **transanal minimally invasive surgery (TAMIS)** techniques, if not radical resection/proctectomy.

VI. COLON CANCER

A. Introduction

1. Approximately 150,000 new diagnoses of CRC each year in the US, of which 70% to 75% are colon cancer.
2. CRC is the fourth leading cause of cancer death worldwide, and one-third of patients will eventually die of their disease.
3. See **Table 23.5** for hereditary CRC syndromes.

B. Clinical presentation

1. Diagnosed via screening is usually asymptomatic and carries a very favorable prognosis.
2. If symptomatic, the most common symptoms are abdominal pain, hematochezia, change in bowel habits, or anemia.
3. Right-sided lesions more commonly present with anemia and abdominal pain, left-sided lesions with changes in bowel habits, rectal bleeding, and crampy abdominal pain with defecation.
4. Obstruction, weight loss, and perforation are uncommon due to effective screening programs and are associated with advanced disease.

C. Diagnosis and staging

1. Majority diagnosed based on biopsy results from a mass or polyp during colonoscopy, which can also be used to assess for **synchronous disease.**
2. Patients who are severely ill from obstruction or perforation and require urgent colectomy should undergo a completion colonoscopy within 3

TABLE 23.5 Hereditary Colorectal Cancer (CRC) Syndromes

Syndrome	Percent of Total CRC Burden	Genetic Basis	Phenotype	Extracolonic Manifestations	Treatment (in Addition to Genetic Counseling/ Testing)	Other Comments
Familial adenomatous polyposis (FAP)	<1%	Mutations in tumor suppressor gene *APC* (5q21)	>100 adenomatous polyps; near 100% with CRC by age 40 y	CHRPE, osteomas, epidermal cysts, periampullary neoplasms, thyroid cancer	TPC with end-ileostomy or IPAA or TAC with IRA and lifelong surveillance; upper GI and thyroid surveillance	Variants include Turcot (CNS tumors) and Gardener (desmoids, osteomas, etc.) syndromes
Hereditary nonpolyposis colorectal cancer (HNPCC); Lynch syndrome	3%-6%	Defective mismatch repair: *MSH2* and *MLH1* (85%), *MSH6* (10%), *PMS2* (5%)	Few polyps, predominantly right-sided CRC, lifetime risk of CRC depending on genotype	At risk for uterine, ovarian, small intestinal, pancreatic malignancies	Prophylactic resections, including TAH/BSO; extracolonic surveillance based on genotype and family history	Microsatellite instability high (MSI-H) tumors, better prognosis than sporadic CRC, immunotherapy responsive
Peutz–Jeghers syndrome (PJS)	<1%	Loss of tumor suppressor gene *LKB1/STK11* (19p13)	Hamartomas throughout GI tract	Mucocutaneous pigmentation, risk for pancreatic cancer	Surveillance EGD and colonoscopy q3yr; resect polyps >1.5 cm; small bowel surveillance	Majority present with bleeding or SBO due to intussuscepting polyp

(continued)

TABLE 23.5 Hereditary Colorectal Cancer (CRC) Syndromes (*Continued*)

Syndrome	Percent of Total CRC Burden	Genetic Basis	Phenotype	Extracolonic Manifestations	Treatment (in Addition to Genetic Counseling/ Testing)	Other Comments
Juvenile polyposis syndrome (JPS)	<1%	Mutations in *SMAD4* (18q21) or *BMPR1A* (10q22)	Hamartomas throughout GI tract starting in the first decade of life; 20% with CRC by age 35 y	Gastric, duodenal, and pancreatic neoplasms; pulmonary AVMs	Surveillance colonoscopy q1-3 y starting age 12-15 y or sooner if symptomatic; TAC with IRA if severe symptoms or concern for malignancy	Presents with anemia and rectal bleeding, intussusception, or diarrhea

AVM, arteriovenous malformation; CHRPE, congenital hypertrophy of retinal pigmented epithelium; CNS, central nervous system; EGD, esophagogastroduodenoscopy; GI, gastrointestinal; IPAA, ileal pouch–anal anastomosis; IRA, ileal–rectal anastomosis; SBO, small bowel obstruction; TAC, total abdominal colectomy; TAH/BSO, total abdominal hysterectomy and bilateral salpingo-oophorectomy; TPC, total proctocolectomy.

to 6 months after resection, taking into account completion of any adjuvant (postoperative) treatments.

3. Staging
   a. Chest and abdominopelvic CT scan to evaluate the primary tumor and lung and liver, most common sites of metastasis.
   b. **Routine positron emission tomography (PET)/CT** has no proven benefit for staging index disease but has role in detecting recurrent or metastatic disease.
   c. **MRI** may be useful if there are concerning hepatic lesions on CT.
   d. **Carcinoembryonic antigen (CEA)** ideally drawn prior to initiating therapy, can be used in follow-up, but not as useful for diagnosis or staging.
   e. Cancer stage is summarized using the American Joint Committee on Cancer (AJCC) **TNM staging system** (Chapter 20: Colon and rectum; *AJCC Cancer Staging Manual*, 8th ed.) based on tumor depth of invasion, number of lymph nodes with metastases, and presence or absence of distant metastases.[11]
      i. Five-year survival estimates
         a) Stage I: 90%
         b) Stage II: 60% to 80%
         c) Stage III: 40% to 60%
         d) Stage IV: 5% to 10%
      ii. Unfavorable characteristics include poor differentiation, pericolonic tumor deposits, multiple LN involvement, mucinous or signet-ring pathology, venous or perineural invasion, bowel perforation, aneuploid nuclei, and elevated CEA.
   f. Neoadjuvant chemotherapy and/or radiation may facilitate complete excision of locally advanced cancers or those with bulky nodal disease.

D. Treatment

1. **Surgical**
   a. Preoperative preparation focused on surgical site infection prevention, perioperative pain control, prevention of prolonged postoperative ileus, and DVT
      i. Preoperative oral antibiotics, mechanical bowel preparation, and prophylactic dose of IV antibiotics significantly decrease wound infections.
      ii. We employ multimodal pain management techniques including patient-controlled analgesia, scheduled NSAIDs, gabapentin, oral acetaminophen, and regional block techniques.
      iii. In opioid-naïve patients, alvimopan has been shown to decrease length of stay and speeds return of bowel function.[12]
      iv. All patients receive perioperative prophylactic doses of either enoxaparin or heparin to prevent DVT.
   b. **Colectomy may be approached laparoscopically, open, or robotically.**
      i. The laparoscopic approach has been found to be oncologically equal to open resection with the added benefit of shorter recovery.[13]
      ii. Lesions of cecum and ascending colon should be resected via right colectomy.

iii. Lesions of descending and sigmoid colon are removed via left colectomy.
iv. Transverse colon lesions are typically approached using an extended right or extended left colectomy based on tumor location.
v. Retrieval of **at least 12 LN** is required to ensure appropriate staging.
vi. In the emergent setting, surgical treatment may include tumor resection with or without anastomosis, or proximal diversion if tumor is unresectable.
vii. If resection is not performed in case of obstruction, distal obstructed limb should be vented via loop ostomy or mucous fistula.
viii. Endoscopic self-expanding metallic **stents** may be used for decompression of some obstructing lesions as bridge to surgery, to avoid risks of emergency operation and need for colostomy.
  a) Not all lesions are anatomically amenable to stenting, and these also carry relatively high risk of migration, occlusion, and perforation, which may compromise oncologic outcomes.[14]

2. **Medical treatment**
  a. **Adjuvant chemotherapy** currently recommended in patients with stage III-IV cancer
    i. Adjuvant therapy should be considered for patients with stage II disease with inadequate LN retrieval (<12) or high-risk features.
    ii. **High microsatellite instability (MSI-high)** cancers, suggestive of a defect in a **mismatch repair gene (MMR)**, tend to have better oncologic outcomes and have not been demonstrated to benefit from 5-fluorouracil-based adjuvant chemotherapy.
    iii. Current therapy involves the combination of 5-fluorouracil/leucovorin with either irinotecan (**FOLFIRI**) or oxaliplatin (**FOLFOX**).
    iv. Role of targeted therapy using vascular endothelial growth factor inhibitors (bevacizumab) or epidermal growth factor receptor (EGFR) inhibitors (cetuximab) has some benefit in treatment of stage IV disease.
      a) Mutation status for *KRAS* should be established before starting EGFR-directed therapy as the presence of *KRAS* mutation is associated with lack of response.
    v. **PD-1 blockade immunotherapy** by pembrolizumab and/or nivolumab is showing improved response to treatment and progression-free survival in treatment of patients with MSI-high disease.[15]
3. Follow-up is crucial in the first 2 years after resection as this is when 90% of recurrences occur, but surveillance thereafter is still indicated.
  a. Surveillance colonoscopy is recommended 1 year after resection, then every 3 years until negative, at which time, every 5 years is recommended.

b. Advanced CRC should undergo yearly CTs of the chest, abdomen, and pelvis for 3 years.
c. CEA should be followed, and rising levels should prompt a CT and colonoscopy if not recently performed.

VII. RECTAL CANCER

A. Introduction
1. Evaluation and treatment of rectal cancer differs from that of colon cancer due to anatomic factors:
   a. Bony confinement of pelvis and sphincters
   b. Proximity to urogenital structures and nerves
   c. Dual blood supply and lymphatic drainage
   d. Transanal accessibility
2. For treatment purposes, proximal extent of rectum is at approximately 12 to 15 cm from anal verge, above the third valve of Houston.

B. Diagnosis and staging
1. AJCC staging system for CRC with additional considerations regarding local staging
2. DRE can give information on size, height relative to anorectal ring/sphincters, fixation, ulceration, local invasion, and perhaps LN status.
3. Rigid or flexible sigmoidoscopy important for measuring tumor distance from anal verge to dentate line.
4. **Rectal cancer protocol MRI** is an integral part of staging to evaluate depth of invasion, **circumferential resection margin** (**CRM**), and LN status, which helps determine need for preoperative chemoradiation therapy (**Figure 23.3**).
5. **Endorectal ultrasound imaging** can be used when MRI is contraindicated or not available but does not assess CRM as well and susceptible to user error.
6. Chest and abdominopelvic CT evaluates distant spread.
7. Preoperative CEA may be used for follow-up.

C. Neoadjuvant chemoradiation
1. Improves local control, generating higher rates of **sphincter-sparing resections** and lower local recurrence rates, but does not prolong survival
2. Traditionally consists of 5-fluorouracil and leucovorin or capecitabine with concomitant radiation therapy over 5 to 6 weeks
   a. Currently the standard in the US for all with T3-T4 rectal lesions or node positive disease on imaging
3. Associated with similar results but significantly less toxicity than postoperative radiation[16]
4. Advancements in administration of radiation therapy such as **"short course" radiation** (25 Gy given in five fractions), chemotherapy regimens, and optimization of timing of surgery provide promising results with increased complete clinical and pathologic response rates.
5. Multiple centers now offer **total neoadjuvant therapy** (**TNT**) in which patients complete a course of radiation and receive systemic chemotherapy before surgical resection.

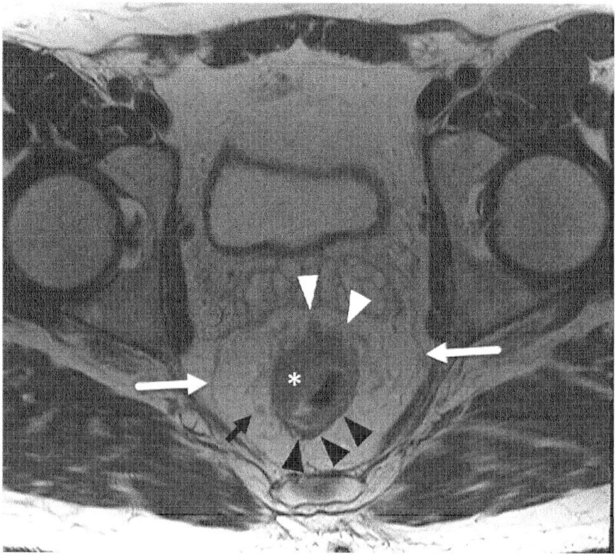

FIGURE 23.3 Pelvic MRI for rectal cancer: High-resolution, oblique axial, T2-weighted MRI image demonstrates a T2 hyperintense mass along the right and anterior aspect of the rectum (*), with nodular soft tissue extension (*white arrowheads*) through the T2 hypointense muscularis into the adjacent mesorectal fat. Normal T2 hypointense muscularis is seen along the posterior aspect of the rectum (*black arrowheads*). The findings are indicative of a T3 cancer. A small, indeterminate mesorectal lymph node is seen posteriorly and to the right of midline (*black arrow*). The circumferential resection margin is not involved (*white arrows*).

   a. Patients with complete clinical response after TNT may be managed with **"watch and wait" approach,** in which surgery is deferred in favor of close surveillance with examination/DRE and proctoscopy and laboratory tests (including CEA and some using circulating tumor DNA) every 3 to 4 months for 2 years, then 6 months for 5 years, as well as pelvic MRI every 6 months for 3 years to monitor for extraluminal recurrence.[17]

6. **Tenets of rectal cancer resection**
   a. Goal is to remove the cancer with adequate margins.
   b. Important surgical tenets of radical resection (vs. transanal excision) include **total mesorectal excision**, LN clearance with **high ligation of the arterial pedicle** (IMA), and consideration of future continence and urogenital function.
   c. Patients with clinical or imaging evidence of sphincter involvement, incontinence, or concern for distal margin involvement should undergo **abdominoperineal resection (APR)**.
   d. Proctectomy can be approached open, laparoscopically, or robotically, although there is ongoing discussion about the quality of

oncologic resection with minimally invasive approaches; there is no conclusive evidence that oncologic outcome is inferior.[18,19]

e. Distal margin can be <2 cm with distal tumors to preserve continence; however, it must be ensured that there is a negative margin.

f. Based on current data, a T2 rectal cancer should undergo radical excision with LAR (see below) or APR.

g. Possible ostomy sites including colostomy and proximal DLI should be marked preoperatively.

h. Preoperative **ureteral stents** should be considered with high risk of ureteral injury.

i. Optimal surgical treatment for T1 rectal cancers should be determined on a case-by-case basis.

- **i.** Lesions that are well/moderately differentiated, <3 cm in size, <30% of circumference of bowel wall, mobile, nonfixed, SM1-2, without LVI or perineural invasion, and without clinical evidence of nodal involvement are amenable to transanal full-thickness excision, TEM, or TAMIS as discussed above.

j. Rectal cancer with extension into local pelvic structures can possibly be resected en bloc with other involved organs for cure.

k. Infertility, sexual dysfunction, and continence are common complications.

l. **Anastomotic leak** is more common for colorectal (especially low pelvic) vs. colonic anastomoses, and leak testing of the anastomosis is recommended.

m. Proximal diversion is recommended for any low or tenuous anastomosis as leaks can have devastating consequences.

n. **Surgical approach: Low anterior resection**

- **i.** Position patient in lithotomy, irrigate the rectum with Betadine. Enter abdomen with open or minimally invasive approach.
- **ii.** Mobilize the sigmoid and descending colon (medial or lateral approach), protecting the retroperitoneal structures (e.g., ureter, gonadal vessels), ligate the IMA and IMV (suture ligature or energy device) at their origins, the latter to facilitate mobility of the colon conduit.
- **iii.** Mobilize the splenic flexure, releasing the splenocolic ligaments and omental attachments to the distal transverse colon.
- **iv.** Perform pelvic dissection and total mesorectal dissection via the avascular presacral space, extending this to the pelvic floor while preserving pelvic nerves; incise lateral peritoneal mesorectal attachments to the anterior peritoneal reflection and divide the lateral stalks, then incise anterior peritoneum and extend the dissection down to the pelvic floor circumferentially, retracting and protecting the prostate or cervix anteriorly.
- **v.** Identify the proximal point of colon transection that would allow for a tension-free low colorectal pelvic anastomosis and include the IMA mesenteric dissection with the specimen.
- **vi.** Transect the colon and purse-string suture the open end of the bowel around the anvil of a circular stapler, ensure

viability of the proximal conduit; divide the rectum with a stapler and the mesorectum appropriately to be removed with the specimen.

vii. Insert the circular stapler transanally and deploy the spike at or posterior to the staple line; perform the anastomosis and check for leaks.

viii. Consider a closed suction drain in the pelvis and consider a diverting loop ileostomy at the preoperatively marked site, depending on surgeon preference; close the abdomen.

7. **Obstructing rectal cancers**
   - **a.** Evaluate with Hypaque enema and/or colonoscopy in stable patient without peritonitis.
   - **b.** To facilitate preoperative chemoradiation therapy, a diverting loop colostomy should be fashioned, being thoughtful about an anticipated future colon conduit.
   - **c.** Endoluminal stents can sometimes be used as a bridge to operation for upper rectal/rectosigmoid tumors and/or in patients who are not candidates for neoadjuvant therapy.
8. Surveillance for rectal cancer is similar to that for colon cancer, although rectal surveillance with DRE, anoscopy, or proctoscopy may be warranted in addition to colonoscopy surveillance.[20]
9. **Rectal cancer recurrence**
   - **a.** Present with pain, rectal bleeding from local recurrence, or on routine follow-up testing for local or metastatic disease.
   - **b.** Diagnosis confirmed by examination, endoscopy, imaging, and ideally with biopsy
     - **i.** Local recurrence can be assessed with pelvic MRI (with or without PET) to evaluate CRM and involvement of other pelvic structures, and systemic recurrence should be evaluated with CT chest/abdomen/pelvis (with or without PET and/or liver MRI).
     - **ii.** Full colonoscopy should be considered.
   - **c.** If no systemic recurrence and favorable imaging characteristics, **reresection can be considered** if patients are fit.
     - **i.** Preoperative therapy can be considered if no prior radiation.
     - **ii.** Curative reresection can improve long-term survival.[21]
   - **d.** If metastatic disease found, chemotherapy can be initiated, and palliative vs. curative interventions considered for any areas of recurrence.

VIII. OTHER COLORECTAL TUMORS

A. Lymphoma

1. Most often metastatic to colorectum, but primary non-Hodgkin's colonic lymphoma accounts for 10% of all GI lymphomas.
   - **a.** GI tract is a common site of non-Hodgkin lymphoma associated with human immunodeficiency virus.
2. Most common symptoms include abdominal pain, altered bowel habits, weight loss, and hematochezia.

3. Biopsies are often not diagnostic because the lesion is submucosal.
4. Resection and/or chemotherapy should be considered as treatment options, with surgical intervention allowing for staging as well as to potentially be curative without chemotherapy.
5. Intestinal bypass/diversion, biopsy, and postoperative chemotherapy should be considered for locally advanced tumors.

B. Retrorectal tumors
1. Present with postural pain and a posterior rectal mass on examination and pelvic CT or MRI, or they are incidentally found on imaging.
2. Differential diagnosis includes congenital, neurogenic, osseous, and inflammatory masses.
3. The most common malignant retrorectal tumors are **chordomas**, typically slow growing but difficult to resect for cure.
4. Other retrorectal masses include dermoid and epidermoid cysts, teratomas, meningoceles and meningomyeloceles, neurofibromas, sarcomas, lipomas, leimomyomas, and desmoid tumors.[22]
5. Diagnosis based on examination findings and imaging
6. Biopsy should be performed selectively to assist in determining the need, and type, of neoadjuvant therapy.
   a. Should be **transcutaneous and not transrectal or transvaginal due to risk of seeding tumor.**
7. Formal resection should be performed, preferably from a perineal or transsacral approach, if symptomatic or concern for malignancy.

C. Neuroendocrine tumors (NETs)
1. **Colonic NETs** (formerly carcinoid) account for 2% of NETs of the GI tract, while **rectal NETs** account for 15%.
2. Colon lesions <2 cm in diameter rarely metastasize, but 80% of lesions >2 cm in diameter have local or distant metastases, with a median length of survival <12 months.
3. Colon lesions are treated with local excision if small and formal resection if >2 cm.
4. Rectal NET
   a. Tumors <1 cm in diameter have low malignant potential, can undergo local transanal or endoscopic resection.
   b. Tumors 1 to 2 cm should be considered for more extensive resection based on symptoms at diagnosis and characteristics including pathological findings, muscular invasion, or ulceration.
   c. Tumors >2 cm are treated with proctectomy.
5. Classic **"carcinoid syndrome"** is most commonly (90%) associated with **midgut tumors** (including the right colon and appendix).
   a. **Hindgut tumors** virtually always lack the ability to produce 5-hydroxytryptophan or serotonin, and therefore, even those with metastatic disease do not present with carcinoid syndrome.

IX. COLOSTOMY

A. Typically associated with fewer electrolyte and physiologic derangements than ileostomy (see Chapter 16)

B. Left-sided or sigmoid colostomies are preferred to right-sided or transverse colostomies due to output consistency and stoma care.
C. Colostomies can be created in loop, end, or end-loop configuration.
   1. If performed for an obstructing distal process, a mucous fistula or loop/end-loop should be created.
D. Colostomy complications include stenosis, retraction, prolapse, and parastomal hernia.
   1. Stenosis/retraction may require local revision if symptomatic or difficult to maintain appliance seal.
   2. Parastomal hernia repair (usually with mesh or relocation) is indicated for pain, obstruction, skin erosion, or pouching problems.
   3. Colostomy prolapse, usually treated with local revision, does not require repair unless there is an inability to reduce the prolapse/ischemia, obstruction, or pouching issues.
   4. Obstipation/constipation can be assessed with digital examination and treated with stoma irrigation and/or Hypaque enema, both diagnostic and possibly therapeutic.
E. End-colostomy takedown can be difficult, and all patients should undergo full colonoscopic evaluation including the distal defunctionalized colon/rectum to rule out stricture or mass prior to takedown.

Key References

Citation	Summary
Thillainadesan J, Yumol MF, Suen M, Hilmer S, Naganathan V. Enhanced recovery after surgery in older adults undergoing colorectal surgery: a systematic review and meta-analysis of randomized controlled trials. *Dis Colon Rectum.* 2021;64(8):1020-1028.	• Systematic review and meta-analysis of a total of seven studies comparing outcomes after the implementation of enhanced recovery protocols (ERPs) on geriatric patients undergoing elective colorectal surgery. ERPs are associated with decreased incidence of delirium and functional decline, as well as shorter hospitalizations and time to return of bowel function, mobilization, and pain control.
Dharmarajan S, Hunt SR, Birnbaum EH, Fleshman JW, Mutch MG. The efficacy of nonoperative management of acute complicated diverticulitis. *Dis Colon Rectum.* 2011;54(6):663-671.	• Retrospective review of patients with acute complicated diverticulitis (with abscess or free air). In this study, <4% required surgery on admission and 5% failed nonoperative management and had surgery while inpatient. Nonoperative management was successful in over 91% of patients, allowing for conversion from emergent surgery to the elective setting.

Citation	Summary
Aberra FN, Lewis JD, Hass D, Rombeau JL, Osborne B, Lichtenstein GR. Corticosteroids and immunomodulators: postoperative infectious complication risk in inflammatory bowel disease patients. *Gastroenterology.* 2003;125(2):320-327.	• Retrospective cohort study comparing outcomes after elective surgery in patients managed preoperatively with steroids, immunomodulators, both, or neither. Preoperative steroids were associated with increased infectious complications, whereas immunomodulators (alone or combined with steroids) were not.
Garcia-Aguilar J, Patil S, Gollub MJ, et al. Organ preservation in patients with rectal adenocarcinoma treated with total neoadjuvant therapy. *J Clin Oncol.* 2022;40(23):2546-2556.	• Prospective randomized controlled trial of patients with stage II-III rectal adenocarcinoma receiving total neoadjuvant therapy (TNT) and either surgical resection or watch-and-wait approach. No differences found in local disease-free survival, metastatic disease-free survival, or overall survival. Organ preservation is achievable in patients with rectal cancer with appropriate tumor response to TNT.
Fleshman J, Sargent DJ, Green E, et al; Clinical Outcomes of Surgical Therapy Study Group. Laparoscopic colectomy for cancer is not inferior to open surgery based on 5-year data from the COST Study Group trial. *Ann Surg.* 2007;246(4):655-662.	• Comparison of long-term outcomes for patients randomized to either laparoscopic or open colectomy. Short-term outcomes reported in the COST trial showed improved quality of life and decreased pain for patients undergoing laparoscopic surgery. After 5-y follow-up, data showed no difference in disease-free survival or overall recurrence rates.

CHAPTER 23: COLON AND RECTUM

Review Questions

1. What complications can be caused by neostigmine administration in the setting of Ogilvie syndrome?
2. What comprises definitive treatment of sigmoid volvulus?
3. Which Hinchey classes of acute diverticulitis demand operative therapy?
4. What features of Crohn's disease differentiate it from ulcerative colitis?
5. What is surgical treatment of medically refractory ulcerative colitis?
6. A patient presents to the ED with abdominal pain and hematochezia after endovascular aortic aneurysm repair; how would you confirm your clinical suspicion?
7. On pathologic examination after right colectomy, a patient is diagnosed with a T3 tumor with 0 of 9 lymph nodes negative. What do you tell this patient about their need for adjuvant therapy?
8. To appropriately stage rectal cancer, patients need what imaging studies for initial assessment?

REFERENCES

1. Hall J, Hardiman K, Lee S, et al. The American society of colon and rectal surgeons clinical practice guidelines for the treatment of left-sided colonic diverticulitis. *Dis Colon Rectum*. 2020;63(6):728-747.
2. Feingold D, Steele SR, Lee S, et al. Practice parameters for the treatment of sigmoid diverticulitis. *Dis Colon Rectum*. 2014;57(3):284-294.
3. Daniels L, Unlu C, de Wijkerslooth TR, Dekker E, Boermeester MA. Routine colonoscopy after left-sided acute uncomplicated diverticulitis: a systematic review. *Gastrointest Endosc*. 2014;79(3):378-389.
4. Feinman M, Haut ER. Lower gastrointestinal bleeding. *Surg Clin North Am*. 2014;94(1):55-63.
5. Sandborn WJ, Rutgeerts P, Feagan BG, et al. Colectomy rate comparison after treatment of ulcerative colitis with placebo or infliximab. *Gastroenterology*. 2009;137(4): 1250-1260.
6. Angelison L, Almer S, Eriksson A, et al. Long-term outcome of infliximab treatment in chronic active ulcerative colitis: a Swedish multicentre study of 250 patients. *Aliment Pharmacol Ther*. 2017;45(4):519-532.
7. Paquette IM, Vogel JD, Abbas MA, Feingold DL, Steele SR; Clinical Practice Guidelines Committee of The American Society of Colon and Rectal Surgeons. The American Society of colon and rectal surgeons clinical practice guidelines for the treatment of chronic radiation proctitis. *Dis Colon Rectum*. 2018;61(10):1135-1140.
8. Poylin V, Hawkins AT, Bhama AR, et al. The American Society of colon and rectal surgeons clinical practice guidelines for the management of clostridioides difficile infection. *Dis Colon Rectum*. 2021;64(6):650-668.
9. Wolf AMD, Fontham ETH, Church TR, et al. Colorectal cancer screening for average-risk adults: 2018 guideline update from the American Cancer Society. *CA Cancer J Clin*. 2018;68(4):250-281.
10. Kahi CJ, Boland CR, Dominitz JA, et al. Colonoscopy surveillance after colorectal cancer resection: recommendations of the US Multi-Society Task Force on Colorectal Cancer. *Gastroenterology*. 2016;150(3):758-768.e11.
11. Jessup JM, Goldberg RM, Asare EA, et al. Colon and rectum. In: Amin MB, ed. *AJCC Cancer Staging Manual*. 8th ed. Springer; 2017:251-274.
12. Delaney CP, Wolff BG, Viscusi ER, et al. Alvimopan, for postoperative ileus following bowel resection: a pooled analysis of phase III studies. *Ann Surg*. 2007;245(3):355-363.
13. Colon Cancer Laparoscopic or Open Resection Study Group; Buunen M, Veldkamp R, Hop WCJ, et al. Survival after laparoscopic surgery versus open surgery for colon cancer: long-term outcome of a randomised clinical trial. *Lancet Oncol*. 2009;10(1):44-52.
14. Hsu J, Sevak S. Management of malignant large bowel obstruction. *Dis Colon Rectum*. 2019;62(9):1028-1030.
15. Andre T, Shiu KK, Kim TW, et al. Pembrolizumab in microsatellite-instability-high advanced colorectal cancer. *N Engl J Med*. 2020;383(23):2207-2218.
16. van Gijn W, Marijnen CA, Nagtegaal ID, et al. Preoperative radiotherapy combined with total mesorectal excision for resectable rectal cancer: 12-year follow-up of the multicentre, randomised controlled TME trial. *Lancet Oncol*. 2011;12(6):575-582.
17. Glynne-Jones R, Wallace M, Livingstone JI, Meyrick-Thomas J. Complete clinical response after preoperative chemoradiation in rectal cancer: is a "wait and see" policy justified? *Dis Colon Rectum*. 2008;51(1):10-19; discussion 19-20.

18. Vennix S, Pelzers L, Bouvy N, et al. Laparoscopic versus open total mesorectal excision for rectal cancer. *Cochrane Database Syst Rev.* 2014;2014(4):CD005200.

19. Jones K, Qassem MG, Sains P, Baig MK, Sajid MS. Robotic total meso-rectal excision for rectal cancer: a systematic review following the publication of the ROLARR trial. *World J Gastrointest Oncol.* 2018;10(11):449-464.

20. Steele SR, Chang GJ, Hendren S, et al. Practice guideline for the surveillance of patients after curative treatment of colon and rectal cancer. *Dis Colon Rectum.* 2015;58(8):713-725.

21. Westberg K, Palmer G, Hjern F, Johansson H, Holm T, Martling A. Management and prognosis of locally recurrent rectal cancer: a national population-based study. *Eur J Surg Oncol.* 2018;44(1):100-107.

22. Neale JA. Retrorectal tumors. *Clin Colon Rectal Surg.* 2011;24(3):149-160.

24 Anorectal Disease

Julie M. Clanahan and Matthew G. Mutch

I. INTRODUCTION

Anorectal disease is commonly encountered within general surgery. This chapter aims to review the most common benign and malignant conditions with a focus on basic diagnosis and management.

A. Anatomy

1. The **anal canal** is the distalmost portion of the gastrointestinal (GI) tract and extends from the **anorectal ring**—or the convergence of the puborectalis with internal and external anal sphincter muscles—to the **anal verge**—the junction between the anoderm and perianal skin (**Figure 24.1**).
2. These three major muscles form the underlying structure of the anal canal and enable sphincter function.
   a. The **internal anal sphincter** is a continuation of circular smooth muscle of the distal rectum and is controlled by parasympathetic reflexes.
   b. The **external anal sphincter** is striated skeletal muscle that forms an elliptical tube around the internal sphincter and is under somatic control.
   c. The **puborectalis** arises from the pubic symphysis and forms a sling that encircles the bowel at the anorectal junction, creating the anorectal ring.
3. The **dentate line** in the anal canal marks the point of division between embryonic endoderm and ectoderm.
   a. Proximal to this line, nervous innervation is autonomically controlled and arteriovenous supply as well as lymphatic drainage is derived from the hypogastric system.
   b. Distal to this line, nervous innervation comes under somatic control and arteriovenous flow and lymphatic drainage is derived from the inferior hemorrhoidal system.

B. Histology

1. The proximal anal canal is lined by columnar epithelium that transitions to squamous epithelium in the **anal transition zone**. This zone begins just proximal to the dentate line.
2. **Anoderm** begins just distal to the dentate line as a modified squamous epithelium that becomes pigmented and thickened as it transitions to normal, hair-bearing skin at the anal verge.

C. Physiology

1. The rectum functions as a **reservoir organ** able to store between 650 and 1,200 mL of stool, with average daily stool output of 250 to 750 mL.
2. The **anal sphincter mechanism** allows control of defecation and maintains continence. The internal sphincter is under involuntary control

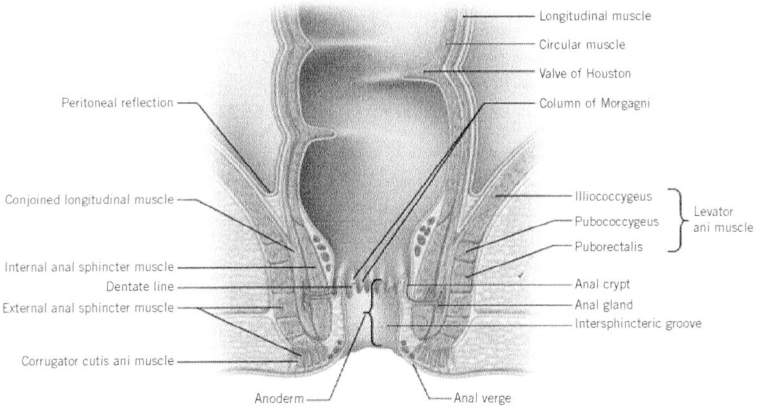

FIGURE 24.1 Coronal schematic of anal canal anatomy and key landmarks. *(Reprinted by permission from Springer: Carmichael JC, Mills S. Anatomy and embryology of the colon, rectum, and anus. In: Steele SR, Hull TL, Hyman N, Maykel JA, Read TE, Whitlow CB, eds. The ASCRS Textbook of Colon and Rectal Surgery. 4th ed. Springer International Publishing; 2022:3-27. Copyright 2022, Springer Nature Switzerland AG.)*

and accounts for the majority of resting pressure or sphincter tone. The external sphincter is under voluntary control and contributes primarily to squeeze pressure. The external anal sphincter normally contracts in response to increased rectal pressure to prevent incontinence, and it then relaxes during defecation.

3. **Continence** requires a combination of adequate rectal compliance, normal sensation at the anorectal transition zone, mechanically intact sphincter musculature, and coordinated neurogenic control of pelvic floor and sphincter complex mechanisms (in addition to appropriate stool consistency).
4. **Defecation** has several coordinated components (**Figure 24.2**).

II. FUNCTIONAL ABNORMALITIES OF THE RECTUM

A. Incontinence

1. Etiology: Inability to prevent elimination of rectal contents may occur from:
   a. **Mechanical defects** due to sphincter damage from obstetric trauma, previous operative injury (e.g., sphincterotomy, fistulotomy, hemorrhoidectomy), radiation (e.g., for cervical or prostate cancer), scleroderma, or poor rectal capacity, including from prior rectal resection.
   b. **Neurogenic defects** from spinal cord injuries, pudendal nerve injury due to birth trauma or lifelong straining, systemic neuropathies such as multiple sclerosis.
   c. **Stool content-related causes** such as high volume or liquid consistency.

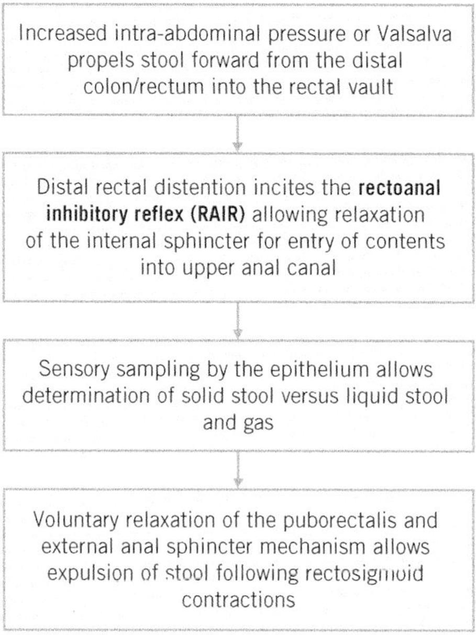

FIGURE 24.2 Coordinated defecation mechanism.

2. Symptoms: The spectrum of disease ranges as below. Differentiation becomes important when determining the aggressiveness of therapy for patients.
   a. **Anal seepage**—leakage of postdefecation mucus or stool
   b. **Fecal urgency**—inability to maintain continence for an extended period of time
   c. **Complete incontinence**—lack of any control of gas or stool
3. Evaluation
   a. Begins with thorough history including questions regarding any neurologic or medical disorders, prior anorectal surgery, vaginal deliveries (especially ones with forceps, vacuum, episiotomy), and medications.
      i. Degree of incontinence (gas, liquid, solid stool), frequency, need for wearing pads, impact to quality of life (QOL) and ability to work or leave the home are important to document.
      ii. Several scoring instruments are available to help clinicians grade the severity and impact of fecal incontinence symptoms.[1]
   b. Physical examination should include visual and digital examination of gross tone or squeeze abnormalities and a determination of muscle bulk.
   c. Testing should include consideration of multiple assessments as outlined in **Table 24.1**.

TABLE 24.1 Overview of Endoscopic and Physiologic Anorectal Testing Modalities

Modality	Description	Findings
Endoanal ultrasound (EAUS)	Allows for detailed evaluation of anal sphincter complex, pelvic floor (and local tumor staging for rectal cancers)	Highly sensitive and specific for locating sphincter defects
Anal manometry	Measures quantitative sphincter function such as resting tone, squeeze pressure, length of anal canal, RAIR presence, Valsalva reflex	Increased resting anal pressure or low anorectal pressure gradient during evacuation concerning for pelvic floor dysfunction; absent RAIR may suggest Hirschsprung's disease
Pudendal nerve terminal motor latency testing (PNTML)	Measures time between stimulation of pudendal nerve and external anal sphincter contraction	Prolonged times can represent neurogenic etiology or sphincter injury
Video or magnetic resonance (MR) defecography	Allows dynamic evaluation of defection mechanism to assess both anatomic or structural etiologies (e.g., rectocele, intussusception) and functional etiologies (e.g., non-relaxation of puborectalis)	Pelvic floor dysfunction suggested if contraction of puborectalis or increased anorectal angle during defecation
EMG testing	Assesses for issues with innervation or malfunction of pelvic floor muscle groups including puborectalis	Lack of reflexive contraction with muscle stimulation concerning for neurologic dysfunction, lack of relaxation with Valsalva suggestive of nonrelaxation of the puborectalis
Colonic transit study	Uses radiopaque markers to assess colonic motility and determine abnormal defection patterns	Concerning for slow transit if 20% or more of markers are retained in the colon at 5 d

EMG, Electromyography; RAIR, rectoanal inhibitory reflex.

4. Treatment: A nonoperative versus operative approach will typically depend on underlying cause and severity of disease.
   a. Nonoperative
      i. Neurogenic and minor mechanical anal sphincter defects are initially treated using **dietary fiber** to increase stool bulk and **pelvic floor** or **biofeedback therapy** to strengthen sphincter muscles and improve early sensation.
      ii. Trigger foods and medications should be avoided.
   b. Operative
      i. In patients with an intact sphincter complex or minimal defect, **sacral nerve stimulation** has emerged as a durable treatment.
         a) Patients keep an incontinence journal before and after temporary stimulation leads are embedded in the S2 to S4 nerve roots in stage 1.
         b) If there is a marked symptom improvement after 1 to 2 weeks, then a permanent device is placed in stage 2.
      ii. Patients with more severe sphincter defects may require **anal sphincter reconstruction** with sphincteroplasty.
      iii. **Colostomy** should be considered as a last resort but may improve the QOL of some patients.

B. Obstructive defection disorders
1. Etiology: Inability to evacuate rectal contents may arise from various forms of pelvic floor outlet obstruction, which requires careful history-taking and workup for correct diagnosis.
   a. Puborectalis pathology **(dyssynergic defection)** occurs with either nonrelaxation of the muscle or paradoxical contraction during attempted defection.
      i. Patients may describe symptoms of excessive straining or the feeling of incomplete evacuation.
   b. **Rectocele** occurs as a bulging of the anterior rectal wall or full-thickness herniation into the vagina often following pelvic floor injury (typically to the rectovaginal septum or pudendal nerve) and chronic straining.
      i. Patients typically exhibit stool trapping and may require manual reduction or vaginal splinting for defecation.
   c. Fecal impaction and stercoral ulceration (from pressure ischemia) are associated with both of these etiologies.
2. Evaluation: In addition to **anal manometry**, workup may include other physiologic and imaging tests (**Table 24.1**).
3. Treatment: The approach is often multimodal and starts nonoperatively.
   a. **Nonoperative:** This will typically start with combination of fiber diet/supplements, suppositories/enemas to facilitate evacuation, and laxatives/stool softeners, as well as pelvic floor physical therapy and biofeedback mechanisms, depending on the underlying etiology.
   b. Operative: Surgical correction (even fecal diversion with colostomy or ileostomy) is employed only as a last resort for dyssynergic defecation with or without colonic transit abnormalities.
      i. If persistently symptomatic, rectoceles may be treated typically through a transvaginal or transanal surgical approach.

C. Abnormal rectal fixation: These pathologies arise from defects in the ligamentous attachments of the distal colon and rectum that lead to partial (intussusception) or full-thickness rectal prolapse and can produce symptoms similar to obstructed defection.

1. **Internal intussusception (internal rectal prolapse)**
   - **a.** Etiology: This occurs as an invagination of the rectal wall or endoluminal intussusception during defecation in the setting of chronic straining from a nonrelaxing puborectalis muscle.
   - **b.** The degree of prolapse can be categorized by the Oxford grading system (**Figure 24.3**).
   - **c.** Repetitive chronic injury and trauma from straining may lead to the development of rectal ulceration.
   - **d.** Symptoms: Patients may present with rectal bleeding from the ulcer as well as ongoing symptoms of obstructive defection with constipation and incomplete evacuation, pelvic pressure, etc.
   - **e.** Evaluation
     - **i. Defecography** is typically performed to help distinguish the diagnosis from other obstructive pathologies.
     - **ii. Proctoscopy** or **flexible sigmoidoscopy** may demonstrate inflamed, irritated rectal mucosa and/or a **solitary rectal ulcer**.
     - **iii.** Biopsy of the lesion is recommended to rule out malignancy prior to any treatment for the underlying prolapse.
   - **f.** Treatment
     - **i.** Nonoperative: This typically starts with the same approach as other obstructed defecation syndromes to avoid straining (see above).
     - **ii.** Operative: Indications for operation include chronic bleeding and lifestyle-limiting symptoms.
       - **a)** Colostomy can be considered.
       - **b)** Surgical options are otherwise controversial and have evolved over the past decade, but **ventral mesh rectopexy** is now often being used to correct internal rectal prolapse (**Table 24.2**).[2]

Oxford rectal prolapse grade	Radiological characteristics of rectal prolapse
Internal rectal prolapse/intussusception	
I (low grade)	Descends no lower than proximal limit of the rectocele
II (low grade)	Descends into the level of the rectocele, but not into anal canal
III (high grade)	Descends into proximal anal canal
IV (high grade)	Descends into distal anal canal
External rectal prolapse	
V (overt rectal prolapse)	Protrudes from anus

FIGURE 24.3 Oxford rectal prolapse grading system. *(Reprinted by permission from Springer: Murphy M, Vogler SA. Rectal prolapse. In: Steele SR, Hull TL, Hyman N, Maykel JA, Read TE, Whitlow CB, eds. The ASCRS Textbook of Colon and Rectal Surgery. 4th ed. Springer International Publishing; 2022:1019-1033. Copyright 2022, Springer Nature Switzerland AG.)*

TABLE 24.2 Operative Procedures for Treatment of Rectal Prolapse

Procedure Name	Approach	Description	Characteristics
Suture rectopexy with or without mesh fixation	*Abdominal*	Posterior sacral fixation of rectum near level of sacral promontory	Recurrence rates are low (<10%) but risks include presacral bleeding or complications such as mesh infection or erosion if used in fixation
Sigmoid resection and rectopexy (Frykman–Goldberg)	*Abdominal*	Combines resection of redundant sigmoid with posterior sacral fixation	Used in patient who present with significant associated constipation pre-operatively, but adds risk of anastomosis to the rectopexy procedure
Ventral mesh rectopexy	*Abdominal*	Anterior rectal dissection with placement of anterior mesh anchor to sacral promontory to elevate pelvic floor	Can be used for correction of rectocele, prolapse and/or intussusception
Altemeier procedure	*Perineal*	Rectosigmoidectomy performed after delivery via anal canal with coloanal or low colorectal anastomosis	Overall lower morbidity and mortality for poor abdominal surgical candidates but still carries complication risk of anastomotic bleeding, leak; recurrence risk ~15%
Delorme procedure	*Perineal*	Circumferential mucosal resection of anal canal and distal roctum (mucosectomy) with muscular plication	Lower morbidity and mortality for patients who may be poor abdominal surgery candidates, low leak risk since not full thickness anastomosis, plicated muscle may help with continence, however recurrence rate generally around 20%

2. **External/full-thickness rectal prolapse**
   a. Etiology: This is full-thickness protrusion of the rectum through the anus (intermittent or persistent).
   b. Risk factors include increased age, female gender, institutionalization, antipsychotic medication, previous hysterectomy, and spinal cord injury.
   c. Symptoms: These typically progress as the prolapse does and include pain, bleeding, fecal incontinence, chronic mucous drainage.
   d. Evaluation: Physical examination should first confirm full-thickness rectal prolapse, which should appear as **concentric mucosal rings** and exclude prolapsing internal hemorrhoids with deep radial grooves and a rosebud appearance.
      i. Colonoscopy should be included in evaluation to rule out concomitant colonic pathology if age- or history-appropriate.
   e. Treatment
      i. **Acute prolapse** requires urgent bedside reduction.
         a) If unsuccessful, reduction or resection in the operating room may be needed, especially for bowel strangulation.
         b) Frequently, a perineal approach is necessary for operative approach to acute incarcerated prolapse.
      ii. Operative: Rectal prolapse can be treated with either **abdominal or perineal approaches**, a summary of options can be found in **Table 24.2**.
         a) In general, abdominal procedures trade higher operative morbidity with lower recurrence rates relative to perineal-only operations.
         b) Continence improves in almost all patients, regardless of procedure.

III. HEMORRHOIDS

The anal canal is lined by three columns of vascular cushions in the left lateral, right anterolateral, and right posterolateral locations that normally contribute to fecal continence.

A. Etiology: The causes of symptomatic hemorrhoidal disease are typically multifactorial and related to hard stools, prolonged straining and constipation, increased intra-abdominal pressure (e.g., pregnancy), and/or prolonged lack of support of the pelvic floor.

B. Symptoms
   1. When hemorrhoids cushions become engorged, they can cause symptoms of bleeding, stool or mucous leakage, and/or prolapse.
   2. Pain associated with internal or external hemorrhoids is typically rare and transient and should prompt investigation for other anorectal pathology, although **thrombosis of external hemorrhoids** or **incarceration of prolapsing internal hemorrhoids** can cause pain.

C. Evaluation
   1. It is critical to determine the hemorrhoidal location of origin either above or below the dentate line for appropriate therapy selection.

2. While history and physical examination may help to suggest the origin, true localization often requires full examination of the anal canal with anoscopy or proctoscopy.
3. **Internal hemorrhoids** that originate above the dentate line are covered with mucosa and devoid of noxious nervous innervation.
4. **External hemorrhoids** arise below the dentate line and are covered with squamous epithelium and innervated with somatic nerves, often resulting in pain as a primary symptom, especially related to thrombosis.

D. Treatment: A nonoperative versus operative treatment approach is based on grading and severity or persistence of patient symptoms (**Figure 24.4**), but a spectrum of options includes the following:

1. Nonoperative
    a. Medical treatment of grade 1,2, and 3 hemorrhoids includes increased **dietary fiber** and water to increase stool bulk, **stool softeners/laxatives**, and avoidance of straining during defecation.
    b. Additional medical treatments include over-the-counter topicals containing phenylephrine and sitz baths or tub soaks for symptom relief.
    c. **Elastic band ligation** may be used to treat refractory grade 2 and 3 hemorrhoids in the office but cannot be used for external hemorrhoids.
        i. Ligation must be done through an anoscope and applied 1 to 2 cm above the dentate line to avoid severe pain.
        ii. One to two quadrants are ligated every 2 to 8 weeks in the office, and the patient is warned that the necrotic hemorrhoid may slough in 4 to 10 days with potential bleeding occurring at that time.
        iii. Severe pain at the time of banding requires immediate removal, so testing of the mucosa for sensation prior to placement is required.
        iv. **Complications/risks of ligation**

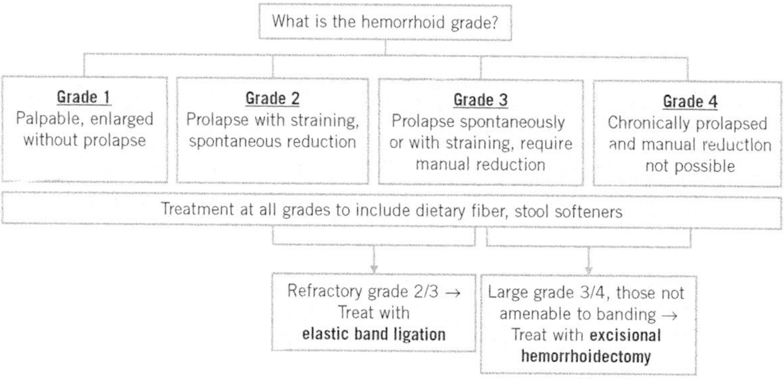

FIGURE 24.4 Classification and treatment of symptomatic internal hemorrhoids.

a) Patients on anticoagulation should stop it prior to banding, otherwise banding is contraindicated for the bleeding risks.
b) Other rare complications include local infection and **severe pelvic sepsis**, particularly in immunocompromised patients.
c) Overall, patients who undergo banding have a **30% recurrence rate**.
d) Accidental full-thickness ligation of the rectum in the prolapsed patient is rare but reported with typical presentation including **severe pain, fever, and urinary retention** within 12 hours of ligation.
e) These patients require examination under anesthesia, immediate removal of bands, debridement of any necrotic tissue, and broad-spectrum intravenous antibiotics to mitigate sepsis and infection progression risks.

2. Operative (approaches summarized in **Table 24.3**)
   a. **Excisional hemorrhoidectomy** is reserved for symptomatic hemorrhoids not amenable to banding, larger grade 3 to 4 hemorrhoids, mixed internal and external hemorrhoids, and thrombosed or incarcerated hemorrhoids with impending gangrene.

TABLE 24.3 Operative Procedures for Treatment of Hemorrhoids

Procedure Name	Description	Complications/Outcomes
Excisional hemorrhoidectomy	Hemorrhoids excised while protecting underlying sphincters; resulting elliptical defects can be completely closed with absorbable suture or left open, can be combined with hemorrhoid banding	10%-20% incidence of urinary retention (most common complication after pain), bleeding, infection, sphincter injury, and anal stenosis from excising excessive anoderm
Transanal hemorrhoidal dearterialization (THD)	Uses a proctoscope with Doppler transducer to selectively suture ligate branches of superior hemorrhoidal artery; can be combined with suture hemorrhoidopexy	Avoids tissue excision, produces less post-procedural pain; high recurrent for grade IV hemorrhoids
Thrombosed hemorrhoid excision	Elliptical dissection around hemorrhoid and clot, staying superficial to sphincter	Must include excision of entire clot and external hemorrhoid to minimize recurrence risk, especially vs. enucleation alone

i. **Surgical approach: Excisional hemorrhoidectomy**
   a) Place patient in prone jackknife position or lithotomy position (anesthesia options of conscious sedation with local vs. spinal vs. general anesthesia)
   b) Make elliptical incision in perianal skin and extend it to the anorectal ring to the hemorrhoid apex in the distal rectum, dissecting away from the sphincter complex, sparing as much anoderm as possible (to minimize stenosis risk)
   c) Continue dissection to the base of the internal hemorrhoid component, and suture ligate (or use other ligating device) the pedicle with subsequent amputation of hemorrhoid tissue; send to pathology
   d) Close the wound using absorbable suture in running, locking fashion for hemostasis (Ferguson technique); alternatively, the wounds may be left open for secondary intention wound healing (Milligan–Morgan technique)
   e) Dressing may be applied with or without antibiotic ointment or topical hemostatic agents per surgeon preference.

ii. Postoperative pain relief can include narcotics, nonnarcotics (e.g., NSAIDs), topical lidocaine, sitz baths/soaks, and bowel regimen with fiber diet/supplements, oral fluids, and laxatives/softeners as needed to avoid constipation and straining.

b. **Transanal hemorrhoidal dearterialization** is another alternative to elastic band ligation that can be used for grade 2 to 3 hemorrhoids with similar outcomes for bleeding, less so for prolapse symptoms.

c. **Thrombosed hemorrhoid excision** can be performed in the office or emergency department with local anesthesia but may require the operating room for patient comfort.
   i. **Clot evacuation alone** is simpler to perform than excision and is effective for acute pain relief but is associated with much higher recurrence rates.
   ii. If the thrombosis is more than 72 hours old (the time when the pain tends to peak), the patient is treated with nonsurgical management first, reserving excisional hemorrhoidectomy for persistence of symptoms.

IV. ANAL FISSURE AND STENOSIS

A. Anal fissure

1. Etiology
   a. Fissures occur as a tear in the anal mucosa, exposing the submucosa and underlying sphincter complex secondary to hypertrophy or spasm of the distal one-third of the internal anal sphincter and exaggerated constriction of this muscle in response to the rectoanal inhibitory reflex, which precludes spontaneous healing over time.
   b. Less common causes of atypical fissures include Crohn's disease, malignancy, abscess or fistula, and infections such as herpes, chancroid, and syphilis.

2. Symptoms: Patients may present with bleeding (usually streaking bright red blood on the paper when wiping), tearing pain, and severe anal spasm with defecation.
3. Evaluation
   a. Physical examination is typically sufficient for diagnosis and determination of the location and severity of the fissure.
   b. The vast majority of these (75%-90%) occur in the posterior midline, and 10% to 25% occur in the anterior midline.
   c. Any alternate location should raise suspicion of atypical etiology and consideration of infection assessment or biopsy.
   d. An external skin tag or **sentinel pile** and **hypertrophied anal papilla** are often associated with **chronic fissures**.
4. Treatment
   a. Nonoperative
      i. First-line therapy (90% of acute fissures will resolve with this approach) typically focuses on decreasing internal sphincter hypertonicity and is largely limited to medical therapies including fiber supplementation, stool softeners/laxatives, sitz baths, topical **calcium channel blockers** or **nitrates**, topical anesthetics, and oral nonnarcotic pain medications (to avoid constipating effects).
      ii. Second-line therapy can be pursued for those who fail to respond after 6 to 8 weeks of treatment, including use of **botulinum toxin injections** (performed in the office or operating room) that can be trialed with similar efficacy to topical agents but fewer side effects than operative options for chronic fissure (but less success than operative option below).
   b. Operative: **Lateral internal sphincterotomy (LIS)** is indicated for chronic fissures that have failed medical management.
      i. Surgical LIS is over 95% successful for long-term healing.
      ii. Although the rate of postoperative incontinence will depend on the degree of sphincter cut, the more recent literature suggests <5% rate of postoperative incontinence.[3]
      iii. **Surgical approach: Lateral internal sphincterotomy**
         a) Place patient in prone jackknife position or lithotomy position (anesthesia options of conscious sedation with local anesthetic vs. general anesthesia)
         b) Insert an anoscope or Hill–Ferguson retractor to inspect anal canal, confirm hypertonia in the internal sphincter, and locate intersphincteric groove distal to the dentate line between the internal and external sphincter muscles laterally (either side)
         c) Open technique: Small radial incision is made over this groove in the lateral position to expose fibers of internal anal sphincter; hypertonic band of internal sphincter muscle (usually width of the anal fissure itself) is then elevated and divided; wound is closed primarily with absorbable suture after hemostasis is confirmed

d) Closed technique: Scalpel (usually #11 blade) is introduced in groove in the lateral position and advanced to dentate line in submucosal plane; scalpel is directed medially to divide and release the hypertonic band of internal sphincter muscle; skin defect can be left open or closed with absorbable suture after hemostasis is confirmed

e) Dressing may be applied with or without antibiotic ointment per surgeon preference

B. Anal stenosis

1. Etiology: Abnormal narrowing of the anal canal most commonly occurs secondary to postsurgical scarring, radiation, chronic laxative abuse, recurrent anal ulcers, or trauma.
2. Symptoms: Patients typically present with pain during defecation, incomplete evacuation with fecal impaction, and thin stools.
3. Evaluation: This typically begins with a physical examination in the office; however, an examination under anesthesia with biopsy of any suspicious lesions may be required if the patient is unable to tolerate thorough examination in the office setting.
4. Treatment
   a. The approach will depend on etiology and severity of stenosis..
   b. Fiber supplementation and stool softeners/laxatives are used as an initial step followed by **serial mechanical dilations** (either home dilators or in the office or operating room, depending on degree of stenosis and patient tolerance) if symptoms are not improving.
   c. Operative correction with **internal sphincterotomy and cutaneous advancement flaps** is only pursued in severe, refractory cases.

V. INFECTIOUS PATHOLOGY OF THE ANORECTUM

A. Anorectal abscess

1. **Cryptoglandular abscess**
   a. Etiology
      i. These abscesses result from infection of the **anal glands** in the crypts at the dentate line.
      ii. The initial abscess develops in the intersphincteric space and extends into several surrounding spaces by which the abscesses are classified: **Perianal**, **ischiorectal**, **intersphincteric**, and **supralevator** (**Figure 24.5**).
   b. Symptoms: Patients primarily experience worsening perianal pain and may have associated symptoms of fever, swelling or induration, and difficulty urinating.
   c. Evaluation
      i. This starts with a physical examination to assess for areas of erythema and palpable fluctuance as well as a digital rectal examination to assess for fullness.
      ii. If diagnosis is not obvious on examination, contrast pelvic CT can be obtained.

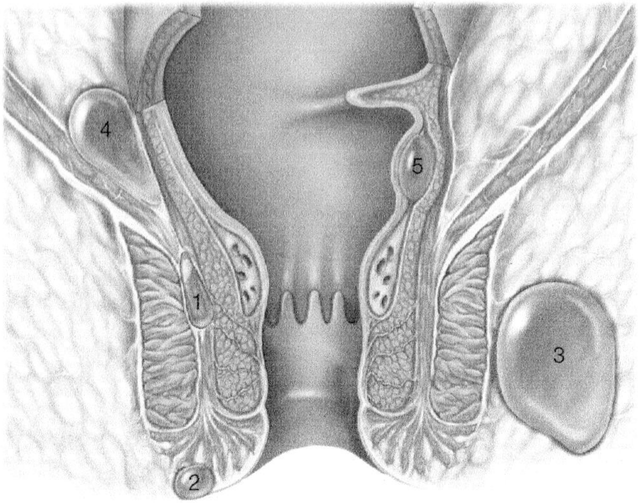

FIGURE 24.5 Common cryptoglandular perirectal abscess locations: 1. intersphincteric, 2. perianal, 3. ischiorectal, 4. supralevator, and less commonly, 5. submucosal/intermuscular. *(Reprinted with permission from Obias V, Abcarian H, Chen MY. Anorectal abscess and inflammatory processes. In: Britt LD, Peitzman AB, Barie PS, Jurkovich GJ, eds. Acute Care Surgery. 2nd ed. Wolters Kluwer; 2018:684-688. Figure 52.2.)*

- **d.** Treatment
  - **i.** Mainstay of treatment is **surgical drainage** and antibiotic therapy in specific cases only such as immunocompromised or diabetic patients, those with valvular heart disease, and those with extensive cellulitis or systemic symptoms concerning for sepsis.
  - **ii.** Drainage approaches depend on the abscess location (**Table 24.4**).
  - **iii.** Drainage alone is definitive therapy in over 60% of patients, the remainder typically have underlying acute fistula tracts present, which will develop into a chronic perianal fistula.
  - **iv.** It is not encouraged to search for a fistula tract in the acute setting given the potential risks of inappropriate instrumentation.

2. Fistula-in-ano

- **a. Etiology**
  - **i.** Also known as **perianal fistula**, this represents the chronic progression of a cryptoglandular abscess.
  - **ii.** Fistulas are classified based on their anatomic location and degree of sphincter involvement into four main types: **Intersphincteric**, **transsphincteric**, **suprasphincteric**, and **extrasphincteric** (**Figure 24.6**).
  - **iii.** In addition to initial abscess formation, etiology may also be related to trauma, Crohn's disease, radiation, or cancer.

TABLE 24.4 Drainage Approach for Anorectal Abscess by Location

Abscess Location	Approach	Notes
Perianal	Incision and drainage via perianal skin with or without mushroom catheter placement	Incision close to anal canal/dentate line to limit length of potential fistula
Ischiorectal	Incision and drainage over point of fluctuance in skin with or without mushroom catheter placement	Incision close to anal canal/dentate line to limit length of potential fistula
Intersphincteric	Internal sphincterotomy for drainage at dentate line over length of abscess	
Supralevator	May require transrectal vs. transcutaneous drainage depending on superior/inferior extension and source	May be from abdominal source (e.g., diverticulitis, appendicitis)
Horseshoe	Drainage of deep postanal space through incision via posterior midline and counterincisions over ischiorectal fossa	Penrose or mushroom catheter drain placement through tracts to ensure drainage

b. Symptoms: Patients present with persistent or intermittent purulent and/or feculent drainage from an external perianal opening(s) as well as perianal pain.

c. Evaluation

  i. Physical examination typically reveals one or more visible external openings.

  ii. The position of the corresponding internal opening can be visualized with anoscopy and predicted using **Goodsall's rule**: Fistulas with external openings anterior to a transverse plane through the anal canal typically penetrate toward the dentate line in a radial direction, whereas fistulas posterior to that plane often curve such that the internal opening is in the posterior midline (**Figure 24.7**).[4]

  iii. Although imaging adjuncts such as CT and/or magnetic resonance scans can be used to characterize a fistula tract, they are typically not needed in uncomplicated disease.

d. Treatment

  i. Approach will depend on the stability of the patient, the location of the fistula in relation to the sphincter, and baseline sphincter function.

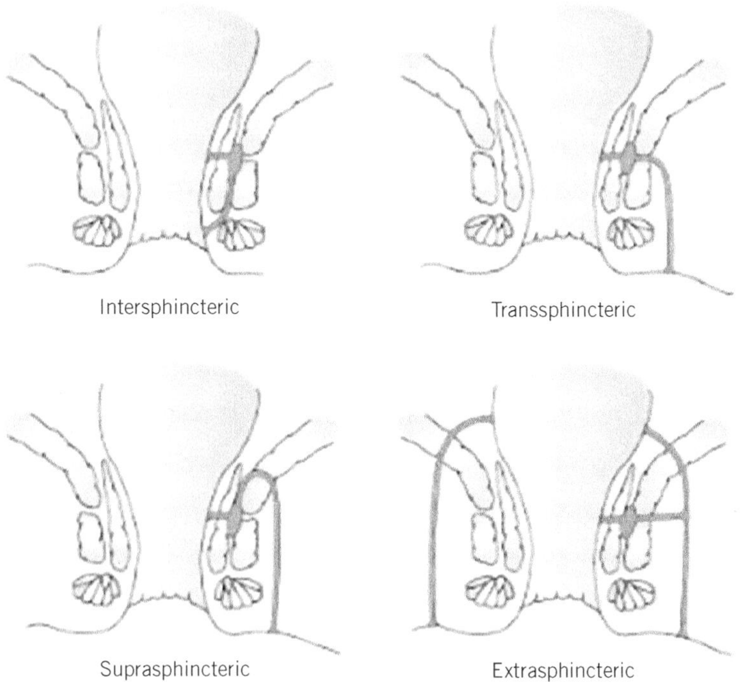

FIGURE 24.6 The four main anatomic types of anal fistula. *(Reprinted with permission from Maron DJ, Wexner SD. Anorectal disorders. In: Mulholland MW, Lillemoe KD, Doherty GM, et al., eds. Greenfield's Surgery: Scientific Principles and Practice. 6th ed. Wolters Kluwer; 2017: 1172-1198. Figure 70-18.)*

ii. The goals of treatment are to obtain source control of any underlying abscess, close the internal aspect of the fistula tract, and preserve the patient's continence.

iii. Options ranging from **fibrin glue** and **seton placement** to the more invasive **fistulotomy** as well as **ligation of intersphincteric fistula tract** and **endorectal advancement flaps** for complex fistulas are summarized in **Table 24.5**.

iv. Surgical approach: Anal fistulotomy

a) Place patient in prone jackknife position or lithotomy position (anesthesia options of conscious sedation with local anesthetic vs. general anesthesia)

b) Identify and connect the external and internal fistula openings with a probe; methylene blue or hydrogen peroxide through the external opening can be used if difficult to locate/confirm communications/find internal opening

c) Examine relationship of tract to sphincter complex in order to minimize the amount of internal and external sphincter that is divided

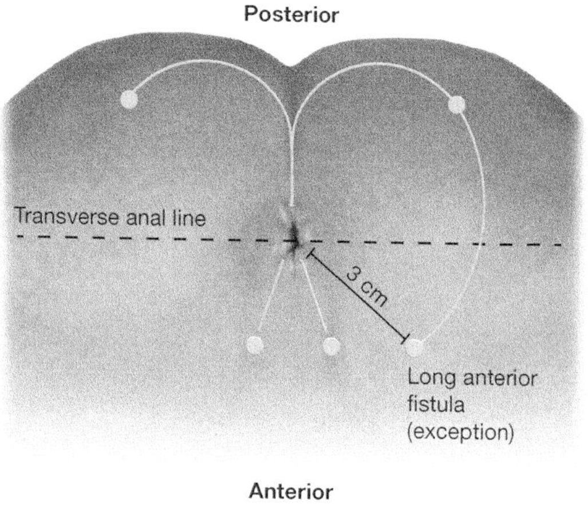

FIGURE 24.7 Goodsall's rule. The anterior -posterior location of the external opening of the fistula helps to identify the internal opening of the fistula, although there are exceptions to the rule, as noted. *(Reprinted with permission from Dhevan V, Galindo RM, Reinhart HA. Perirectal abscess and perianal fistula. In: Albo D, ed. Operative Techniques in Colon and Rectal Surgery. 2nd ed. Wolters Kluwer; 2023:455-459. Figure 49-6.)*

d) Divide tissue overlying fistula probe and subsequently debride the underlying fistula tract
e) Edges of wound can then be marsupialized with absorbable suture to promote wound healing

B. Necrotizing anorectal infection
1. Etiology
   a. Also known as **Fournier gangrene**, necrotizing perineal infections are deadly processes that require rapid intervention.
   b. Often originating with innocuous infections of synergistic GI flora (*Clostridia* and *Streptococcus*), patients will rapidly develop perianal pain and systemic toxicity.
2. Diagnosis
   a. On examination, **crepitus** or **pain out of proportion** to cutaneous findings should elicit concern.
   b. Hyponatremia may be found on diagnostic laboratory tests but is not always present.
3. Treatment
   a. Definitive therapy requires **wide excision** and **debridement** of all nonviable tissue as well as **IV antibiotics**, and multiple resections may be required in a staged fashion, but mortality approximates 50%.
   b. Definitive wound coverage often eventually requires skin grafting.
   c. Fecal diversion is rarely needed.

C. Pilonidal cyst
1. Etiology
   a. This infection usually occurs in hair-containing sinus tracts in the intergluteal cleft originating in midline visible "pits."

TABLE 24.5 Treatment Approaches for Anal Fistula

Treatment	Description	Complications/Outcomes
Seton placement	Placement of **draining seton** promotes source control and tract maturation prior to definitive repair Placement of **cutting seton** with serial tightening induces pressure necrosis of tissue and scar formation, like a slow fistulotomy with healing in behind as the seton cuts through	Preserves sphincter musculature Requires frequent visits for tightening; typically used in high complex anal fistula, but risks higher incontinence rates
Fibrin glue/anal plug	Placed into fistula tract to occlude it while sparing sphincter division	Low morbidity, but rarely used given low healing rates
Fistulotomy	Fistula tract laid opened and possible division of some internal sphincter; use for intersphincteric or low transsphincteric fistulas	High success rates (>90%) in patients with low intersphincteric or transsphincteric fistulas; avoid in high fistulas given incontinence risk
Ligation of intersphincteric fistula tract (LIFT)	Dissection in intersphincteric space allows proximal and distal ligation and division of fistula tract	Sphincter sparing but with variable healing rates (45%-95%)
Endorectal advancement flap	Rectal flap used to cover and close internal opening of fistula while external opening left for drainage	Sphincter-sparing, first-line approach for complex anal fistulas given high success rates (70%-90%)

b. Unless severe, these infections do not involve the anus or perianal tissue, separating them from anal fistulas.
c. They are most common in males in the second and third decades of life.

2. Diagnosis
   a. Patients often present with relapsing episodes of pain, drainage, and cellulitis in the cleft, and physical examination findings are often pathognomonic.
   b. Radiographic evaluation is not warranted except in severe or recurrent cases.

3. Treatment
   a. Approach involves incision, drainage, curettage, and **marsupialization** of the sinus tract(s).
   b. Care should be taken to treat all tracts and cysts.
   c. While secondary closure should be allowed in the setting of active inflammation (with recurrence rates up to 40%), primary closure with rotational flaps can be utilized electively for improved cosmesis and healing (e.g., **Bascom or Limberg flaps**).

D. Hidradenitis suppurativa
1. Etiology: **Apocrine sweat glands** of the groin and perineum serve as the nidus for the development of pustules, sinus tracts, scars, and nodules in this chronic, inflammatory skin disorder.
2. Diagnosis: Similar to fistula-in-ano, hidradenitis can by diagnosed on physical examination with evidence of superficial fistulous tracts external to the anal verge.
3. Treatment
   a. Nonoperative therapy involves chronic suppressive topical and/or oral antibiotics, retinoids, and even biologic agents such as TNF-α inhibitors in patients with moderate to severe disease.
   b. Definitive treatment involves excision of all involved tissue including areas of fibrosis and fistula.

E. Pruritus ani
1. Etiology: "Anal itching" is actually a symptom rather than a specific diagnosis that may arise from multiple etiologies such as hemorrhoids, fissure, prolapse, rectal polyps, anal warts, and intraepithelial dysplasia.
2. Evaluation/treatment
   a. The approach will depend on the underlying cause, and failure to determine an underlying cause should prompt investigation of dietary factors (e.g., coffee, alcohol).
   b. The most common cause is **overcleaning**.
   c. Treatment typically includes a high-fiber diet, minimizing wiping, avoiding the use of soaps and alcohol-containing products for cleaning, and using barrier creams and topical anesthetics.
   d. Children should be evaluated for pinworms; if found, these are treated with piperazine citrate.

F. Condyloma acuminatum
1. Etiology
   a. **Anorectal and urogenital warts** are caused by infection with **human papilloma virus (HPV)**.
   b. The virus is sexually transmitted, and lower-risk **subtypes 6 and 11** are typically associated with condyloma formation.
2. Presentation: Patients may present with visible perianal growth often accompanied by pruritus, anal discharge, bleeding, and pain.
3. Evaluation
   a. Physical examination should include visual inspection of the anus as well as digital examination for palpable lesions.
   b. Anoscopy and cytology should be considered in immunocompromised or high-risk patient populations for evaluation of anal dysplasia.

4. Treatment
    a. Both topical and surgical approaches may be pursued. Importantly, biopsies should be taken liberally to ensure invasive malignancy is not overlooked.
    b. Nonoperative: Topical therapies include application of **trichloroacetic acid** in the office and patient-administered **imiquimod** or **podofilox** for small lesions.
    c. Operative: Surgical **excision and fulguration** may be achieved with electrocautery or laser under local anesthesia depending on lesion size.
        i. Of note, HPV can be aerosolized during the fulguration process, so careful attention must be paid to proper ventilation and protective masks.

VI. ANAL NEOPLASIA

A. Anal intraepithelial neoplasia (AIN)
1. Etiology
    a. AIN is classified as **low-grade (LSIL)** vs. **high-grade squamous intraepithelial lesions (HSIL)**.
    b. HSIL—also known as **carcinoma in situ or Bowen's disease**—occurs as a premalignant stage of **anal squamous cell carcinoma (SCC)**.
    c. Risk factors for development include HPV and HIV infection, immunosuppression, smoking, and anal intercourse.
2. Evaluation
    a. At-risk patients should be evaluated with anal examination as well as cytology.
    b. If cytology screening reveals LSIL or HSIL, these patients are typically followed with **high-resolution anoscopy** using acetic acid to identify areas of dysplasia for biopsy.
3. Treatment
    a. Surgical approach to dysplastic lesions involves **local ablation** and **excision** with postoperative surveillance anoscopy and cytology to monitor for recurrence and/or disease progression (**Figure 24.8**).[5-9]
    b. For extensive lesions, skin grafting or flaps may be required.

B. SCC
1. Etiology
    a. This represents the vast majority of anal cancers.
    b. Risk factors for development are the same as mentioned previously for precursor AIN/HSIL lesions.
2. Symptoms: Patients may present with anal mass as well as associated bleeding and discharge, anal pain, anal itching, and changes in bowel habits.
3. Evaluation
    a. Anal and inguinal lymph node examination, anoscopy, and biopsy is necessary for diagnosis.
    b. Once histopathologic diagnosis is confirmed, workup proceeds with staging CT scan of the chest, abdomen, and pelvis (or MRI abdomen/pelvis with chest CT) and positron emission tomography scan in select patients to assess extent of locoregional involvement.

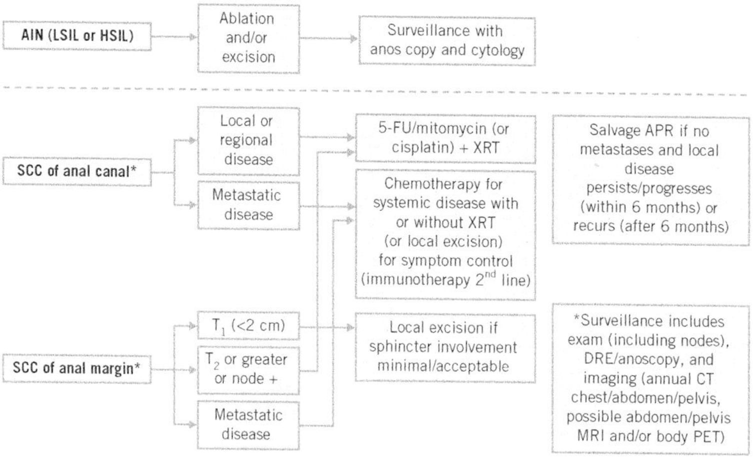

FIGURE 24.8 Treatment algorithm overview for anal squamous neoplasms. 5-FU, fluorouracil; AIN, anal intraepithelial neoplasia; APR, abdominoperineal resection; DRE, digital rectal examination; HSIL, high-grade squamous intraepithelial lesion; LSIL, low-grade squamous intraepithelial lesion; PET, positron emission tomography; SCC, squamous cell carcinoma; T, tumor category (in TNM staging) based on tumor size; XRT, radiation therapy.

c. Staging is based on the tumor size (T stage) and involvement of lymph nodes or distant metastasis, not depth of tumor invasion.

4. Treatment
   a. Based on cancer stage as well as location of primary lesion within anal canal vs. at the anal margin (**Figure 24.8**).
   b. Overall strategy has evolved based on **Nigro protocol** findings incorporating **chemoradiation** (80% cure rate) prior to the consideration of **salvage abdominoperineal resection** (APR) in instances of disease progression or persistence (within 6 months of treatment) or recurrence (after 6 months of treatment).

C. Other lesions of anal margin

1. **Paget disease** or intraepithelial adenocarcinoma is an in situ neoplasm originating in **apocrine sweat glands** that presents with pruritic, erythematous rash.
   a. Typically found in elderly patients
   b. Biopsy proves the diagnosis, and assessment must include colonic evaluation to rule out synchronous malignancy as the source of cancerous tissue.
   c. Up to 50% of patients will have a coexisting visceral carcinoma.
   d. **Wide local excision** is the treatment of choice, although radical resection and colostomy may be required for more invasive disease.
2. **Basal cell carcinoma** (BCC) is a rare, male-predominant disease similar to cutaneous BCC and is treated with wide local excision (see Chapter 28).

D. Other tumors of anal canal

1. **Primary anal adenocarcinoma**
   a. These rare lesions can arise from the anal glands or within chronic anal fistulas but are staged and treated similar to rectal adenocarcinomas.

b. Neoadjuvant chemoradiation followed by APR is the typical treatment approach.
2. Melanoma
a. **Anorectal melanoma** is a rare diagnosis, accounting for only 1% to 3% of anal malignancies, with a poor prognosis and 5-year survival <20%.
b. These are often misdiagnosed as thrombosed hemorrhoids given appearance of the mass with symptoms of bleeding and itching.
c. Surgical approach may include wide local incision or APR, the choice of which is controversial given comparable overall poor survival benefit in both groups.

Key References

Citation	Summary
Alonso-Coello P, Guyatt G, Heels-Ansdell D, et al. Laxatives for the treatment of hemorrhoids. *Cochrane Database Syst Rev.* 2005 ;2005(4):CD004649.	• Systematic review and meta-analysis of seven randomized controlled trials comparing fiber supplementation to nonfiber control that showed overall beneficial effect of fiber on hemorrhoid symptoms and bleeding; provides evidence for basis of medical management across hemorrhoid disease spectrum.
Brown CJ, Dubreuil D, Santoro L, et al. Lateral internal sphincterotomy is superior to topical nitroglycerin for healing chronic anal fissure and does not compromise long-term fecal continence: six-year follow-up of a multicenter, randomized, controlled trial. *Dis Colon Rectum.* 2007;50(4):442-448.	• Randomized controlled trial comparing nitroglycerin ointment to lateral internal sphincterotomy found decrease in post-treatment symptoms in sphincterotomy patients compared with nitroglycerin treatment and no difference in rates of fecal incontinence between groups.
Nigro ND, Vaitkevicius VK, Considine B Jr. Combined therapy for cancer of the anal canal: a preliminary report. *Dis Colon Rectum.* 1974;17(3):354-356.	• Original case report describing the use of neoadjuvant chemoradiation prior to abdominoperineal resection in patients with anal squamous cancers to improve survival rates of patients with primarily anal canal disease; observations transformed the direction of anal squamous cell cancer treatment for next 50 y.
Papaconstantinou HT, Bullard KM, Rothenberger DA, Madoff RD. Salvage abdominoperineal resection after failed Nigro protocol: modest success, major morbidity. *Colorectal Dis.* 2006;8(2):124-129.	• Retrospective review of patients who underwent abdominoperineal resection following failure of chemoradiation treatment found high rate of perineal wound complications (80%) with disease recurrence in up to half of patients at 2 y suggesting only modest success of procedure with high morbidity.

CHAPTER 24: ANORECTAL DISEASE

Review Questions

1. A 41-year-old woman has prolapsing hemorrhoidal tissue that requires manual reduction. What grade of internal hemorrhoids is this? What are available operative treatments for this patient?
2. What is the most common complication following hemorrhoidectomy?
3. A 26-year-old man has severe pain and some bright blood with defecation for the last week and a posterior midline tear in the anoderm on physical examination. What is the mainstay of treatment for this patient?
4. What should workup include for a patient who is at high risk for development of anal intraepithelial neoplasia (AIN)/HSIL?
5. A 54-year-old man is diagnosed on biopsy with a 3-cm squamous cell carcinoma of the anal canal without evidence of metastatic disease. What is the recommended first line of therapy for this patient?
6. A 78-year-old woman with multiple medical comorbidities and prior abdominal operations presents with refractory symptoms secondary to a grade V rectal prolapse. What perineal surgical approaches may be considered to correct this?
7. A 25-year-old woman with Crohn's disease presents with purulent perianal drainage with physical examination concerning for a recurrent transsphincteric fistula. What treatment can be pursued prior to definitive fistular repair?
8. Several years after a complicated vaginal delivery with third-degree perineal tear, a 36-year-old woman presents with ongoing fecal incontinence. What adjunct diagnostic test would be helpful to confirm and locate an anatomic sphincter defect?

REFERENCES

1. Hunt CW, Cavallaro PM, Bordeianou LG. Metrics used to quantify fecal incontinence and constipation. *Clin Colon Rectal Surg*. 2021;34(1):5-14.
2. Emile SH, Elfeki HA, Youssef M, Farid M, Wexner SD. Abdominal rectopexy for the treatment of internal rectal prolapse: a systematic review and meta-analysis. *Colorectal Dis*. 2017;19(1):O13-O24.
3. Liang J, Church JM. Lateral internal sphincterotomy for surgically recurrent chronic anal fissure. *Am J Surg*. 2015;210(4):715-719.
4. Yu Q, Zhi C, Jia L, Li H. Cutting seton versus decompression and drainage seton in the treatment of high complex anal fistula: a randomized controlled trial. *Sci Rep*. 2022;12(1):7838.
5. Ajani JA, Winter KA, Gunderson LL, et al. Fluorouracil, mitomycin, and radiotherapy vs fluorouracil, cisplatin, and radiotherapy for carcinoma of the anal canal: a randomized controlled trial. *JAMA*. 2008;299(16):1914-1921.
6. Rao S, Sclafani F, Eng C, et al. International rare cancers initiative multicenter randomized phase II trial of cisplatin and fluorouracil versus carboplatin and paclitaxel in advanced anal cancer: InterAAct. *J Clin Oncol*. 2020;38(22):2510-2518.

7. Chai CY, Tran Cao HS, Awad S, Massarweh NN. Management of stage I squamous cell carcinoma of the anal canal. *JAMA Surg*. 2018;153(3):209-215.
8. Richel O, de Vries HJ, van Noesel CJ, Dijkgraaf MG, Prins JM. Comparison of imiquimod, topical fluorouracil, and electrocautery for the treatment of anal intraepithelial neoplasia in HIV-positive men who have sex with men: an open-label, randomised controlled trial. *Lancet Oncol*. 2013;14(4):346-353.
9. Alam NN, White DA, Narang SK, Daniels IR, Smart NJ. Systematic review of guidelines for the assessment and management of high-grade anal intraepithelial neoplasia (AIN II/III). *Colorectal Dis*. 2016;18(2):135-146.

25 Hernias

Bradley S. Kushner and Jeffrey A. Blatnik

I. INGUINAL HERNIA

A. Incidence

1. A result of genetic and environmental factors combined with individual patient factors (e.g., immune status), comorbidities (i.e., chronic obstructive pulmonary disease), personal habits (e.g., smoking, obesity), and changes in body mass index.[1]
2. Contralateral defects are as high as 22%, with 28% of these becoming symptomatic during short-term follow-up.
3. Lifetime prevalence is estimated to be 25% in men and 2% in women.
4. Tends to be diagnosed at the extremes of age.
5. Male-to-female ratio > 10:1.

B. Classification

1. Two-thirds of inguinal hernias are indirect.
2. Nearly two-thirds of recurrent hernias are direct, especially after open repair.
3. Inguinal hernias are more common on the right side than left.[2]
4. Approximately 10% of inguinal hernias become incarcerated with a portion becoming strangulated.
5. Recurrence surgical repair is <1% in children and vary in adults depending on the method of repair (1%-3%).

C. Terminology and anatomy

1. **Inguinal canal (Figure 25.1)**
   a. A tunnel that traverses the layers of the abdominal wall musculature, bounded on the lateral deep aspect by an opening in the transversalis fascia/transversus abdominis muscle (**internal inguinal ring**).
   b. Travels along the fused edges of the transversus abdominis/internal oblique/inguinal ligament and iliopubic tract posteriorly and layers of the external oblique musculature anteriorly, ending on the medial superficial aspect at an opening in the external oblique aponeurosis (**external inguinal ring**).
   c. Contains the spermatic cord (males) or the round ligament (females).
   d. Subject to hernia formation primarily due to decreased mechanical integrity of the internal ring and/or transversalis fascia, allowing intra-abdominal contents to encroach into this space and form the characteristic bulge.
2. **Direct hernias**
   a. Weakness in the posterior wall of the inguinal canal due to attenuation of the transversalis fascia.

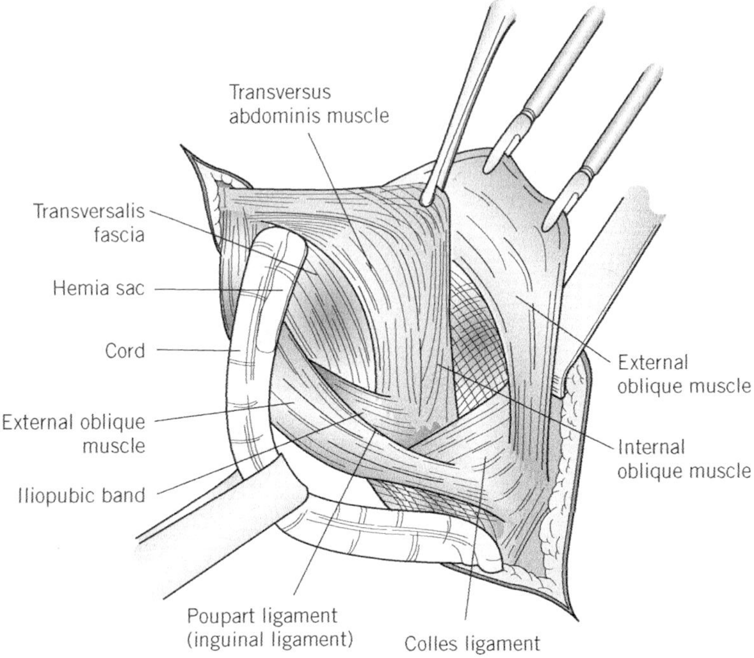

FIGURE 25.1 Inguinal hernia anatomy.

   b. The hernia sac protrudes through **Hesselbach triangle**, which is the **space bounded by the inferior epigastric artery, the lateral edge of the rectus sheath, and the inguinal ligament.**

3. **Indirect hernias**
   a. Pass through the internal inguinal ring lateral to the inferior epigastric vessels and follow the spermatic cord in males and the round ligament in females.
   b. Indirect hernia sac is typically found on the anteromedial aspect of the spermatic cord.
4. **Combined (pantaloon) hernias**
   a. Direct and indirect hernias coexist, and abdominal contents can protrude through both/either opening.
5. **Variants of inguinal hernias**
   a. **Sliding hernia:** (Usually indirect inguinal) denotes that a part of the wall of the hernia sac is formed by an intra-abdominal viscus (usually colon, sometimes bladder).
   b. **Richter hernia:** A portion of (rather than the entire circumference) of the bowel wall is incarcerated.
   c. **Littré hernia:** Contains a Meckel diverticulum.

d. **Amyand hernia:** An inguinal hernia that contains the appendix.
e. **Incarcerated inguinal hernias** cannot be reduced into the abdominal cavity and may or may not be symptomatic.
f. **Strangulated** hernias are incarcerated with vascular compromise of the herniated contents and warrant urgent surgical evaluation. Frequently, intense pain is caused by ischemia of the incarcerated segment.

D. Diagnosis

1. **Clinical presentation**
   a. Often presents as intermittent bulge in the groin.
   b. May extend into the scrotal sac in males.
   c. Symptoms are usually related to exertion or long periods of standing with unilateral discomfort and/or the presence of a bulge.
   d. In infants and children, a groin bulge is often noticed by caregivers during episodes of crying or defecation.
   e. Patients rarely present with bowel obstruction, but all patients presenting with small-bowel obstruction must be questioned and examined for all types of hernia (e.g., inguinal, umbilical, incisional, obturator)
2. **Physical examination**
   a. The main diagnostic maneuver for inguinal hernias is **palpation of the inguinal region**—best examined while standing and straining (cough or Valsalva).
   b. Hernias manifest as bulges with smooth, rounded surfaces that become more evident with straining.
   c. It may be necessary to invaginate the hemiscrotum to introduce an index finger through the external inguinal ring if the hernia is not apparent.
   d. Incarcerated inguinal hernias present with pain, abdominal distention, nausea, and vomiting due to intestinal obstruction.
   e. Strangulated hernias will present with severe pain and possibly with skin changes over the hernia.
3. **Radiographic evaluation**
   a. X-ray studies are rarely indicated.
   b. Ultrasonography or CT scan may occasionally be used to diagnose an occult groin hernia.
   c. Ultrasonography is often the preferred first-line imaging as it can be performed with the patient straining and without radiation exposure but is user-dependent.

E. Treatment

1. **Preoperative evaluation and preparation**
   a. Most patients with inguinal hernias should be treated surgically, although watchful waiting may be appropriate for individuals with asymptomatic hernias or for elderly patients with minimally symptomatic hernias as the risk for acute incarceration or strangulation is very low.[3]
   b. Associated conditions that lead to increased intra-abdominal pressure such as chronic cough, constipation, or bladder outlet obstruction should be evaluated and treated before elective hernia repair.

c. Incarcerated hernias with intestinal obstruction and/or strangulation, broad-spectrum antibiotics should be given, and nasogastric decompression may be necessary. Correction of volume status and electrolyte abnormalities is also important when there is associated small bowel obstruction (SBO).

2. **Reduction**
   a. In uncomplicated cases, the hernia should reduce with palpation over the inguinal canal while the patient is supine. Sedation and Trendelenburg positioning aide the reduction of an incarcerated hernia.
   b. When an incarcerated hernia is reduced nonsurgically, the patient should be observed for the potential development of peritonitis caused by perforation or ischemic necrosis of a loop of strangulated bowel. Strong suspicion of strangulation (e.g., erythema over hernia site, pain out of proportion to examination) is a surgical emergency and should be evaluated even if the bowel contents are reduced.

F. Surgical treatment (**Figure 25.2**)

1. **Choice of anesthetic**
   a. Local anesthesia with sedation and monitored anesthesia care
      i. Often preferred anesthetic for elective open repair of small to moderate-sized hernias.
      ii. Results in better postoperative analgesia, a shorter recovery room stay, and a negligible rate of postoperative urinary retention.
      iii. Lowest-risk anesthetic for patients with underlying cardiopulmonary disorders.
   b. General anesthesia
      i. Minimally invasive inguinal hernia repairs are performed under general anesthesia as pneumoperitoneum is required.

G. Primary tissue repairs (without mesh)

1. **Overview**
   a. Avoids placement of foreign prosthetic material but associated with **higher recurrence rates** (5% to 10% for primary repairs and 15% to 30% for repair of recurrent hernias).

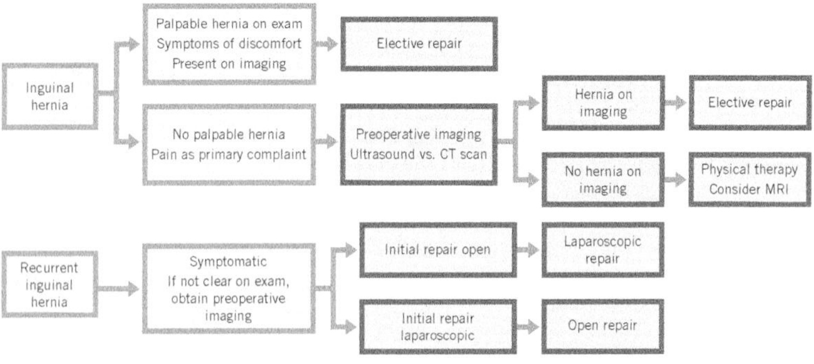

FIGURE 25.2 Considerations for inguinal hernia repair.

b. Although most inguinal hernias are now treated with a tension-free mesh repair, a primary tissue repair can be considered in contaminated wounds (e.g., bowel resection).

2. **Shouldice repair**
   a. The transversalis fascia is opened transversely from the internal ring toward the pubic tubercle (and partially excised if weakened).
   b. Retroperitoneal tissue, including fat, hernia sac, and peritoneum, is dissected off the posterior wall of the pelvic floor, and the cremasteric muscle is resected.
   c. Four imbricated layers of running nonabsorbable suture reapproximate a superior flap of the pelvic floor (containing the transversus abdominis and internal oblique) to an inferior flap (containing the transversalis fascia edge, shelving edge of the inguinal ligament, and external oblique aponeurosis).
   d. Closing the defect in multiple layers is thought to ensure that no one layer is under significant tension.
   e. The experience of the Shouldice Clinic (Thornhill, ON, Canada) with this repair has been excellent, with recurrence rates of <1%, but higher recurrence rates have been reported in nonspecialized centers.
3. **Bassini repair**
   a. The inferior arch of the transversalis fascia or conjoint tendon is approximated to the shelving portion of the inguinal ligament with interrupted, nonabsorbable sutures.
   b. Similar to the Shouldice repair but utilizes only one layer of sutures.
   c. Primarily for indirect hernias, including inguinal hernias in women.
4. **McVay repair**
   a. Transversalis fascia is sutured to Cooper ligament medial to the femoral vein and is then transitioned to the inguinal ligament at the level of, and lateral to, the femoral vein.
   b. Requires placement of a relaxing incision on the aponeuroses of the internal oblique muscle to avoid undue tension on the repair.
   c. Closes the femoral space and therefore, unlike the Bassini repair, is also effective for femoral hernias.

H. Open tension-free repairs (with mesh)

1. **Overview**
   a. Most common inguinal hernia repairs performed today are the tension-free mesh hernioplasty (**Lichtenstein repair**) and the patch-and-plug technique.
2. **Lichtenstein repair**
   a. **Surgical approach: Open Lichtenstein inguinal hernia repair**
      i. The patient is positioned supine, and arms are extended. Hair bearing area is clipped. The patient is given a dose of preoperative antibiotics.
      ii. A 4-cm incision is made overlying the inguinal ligament. The incision is carried down to the external oblique.
      iii. The external oblique aponeurosis is opened, and the spermatic cord and hernia sac are encircled.

iv. The hernia sac is teased free, opened to ensure all contents have been reduced, and ligated.
v. The inguinal floor is reconstructed using a piece of polypropylene mesh measuring approximately 6 × 3 in.
vi. The mesh is sutured to the transversalis fascia and conjoint tendon medially and to the inguinal ligament laterally.
vii. The mesh is slit at the level of the internal ring, and the two limbs are crossed around the spermatic cord and then tacked to the inguinal ligament, effectively creating a new internal ring.
viii. The incision is closed in several layers and hemostasis is ensured.

b. Recurrence rates have been consistently 1% or less.
c. Since the repair is without tension, patients are allowed to return to unrestricted physical activity in 2 weeks or fewer.

3. **Mesh plug**
   a. Placement of a preformed plug of mesh in the hernia defect (e.g., internal ring) that is then sutured to the rings of the fascial opening.
   b. An onlay piece of mesh is then placed over the inguinal floor, which may or may not be sutured to the fascia.
   c. Plug style repairs have fallen out of fashion due to potential complications attributed to the plug such as migration and pain.

I. Laparoscopic/minimally invasive inguinal hernia repair (**Figure 25.3**)

1. **Overview**
   a. Typically advocated in the elective setting, but with increased experience its use has been introduced for incarcerated and strangulated hernias.
   b. Contraindicated in those who cannot tolerate general anesthesia and/or pneumoperitoneum and previous cystectomy.
   c. Relatively contraindicated in patients who have previously undergone prostatectomy or other lower midline abdominal surgery due to scarring in the preperitoneal space.

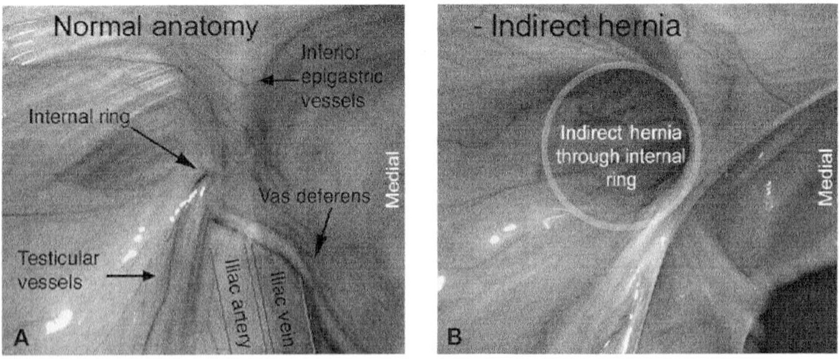

FIGURE 25.3 A, Laparoscopic view of normal inguinal anatomy (patient left). B, Laparoscopic view of indirect inguinal hernia.

2. **Transabdominal preperitoneal (TAPP) repair**
   a. After achieving abdominal access, the peritoneum overlying the inguinal floor is dissected away as a flap, the hernia is reduced, mesh is fixed over the internal ring opening in the preperitoneal space, and the peritoneum is reapproximated.
   b. The TAPP approach provides a large working space, familiar anatomic landmarks, and allows the contralateral groin to be examined for an occult hernia.
3. **Totally extraperitoneal repair (TEP)**
   a. The preperitoneal space is developed either with a dissecting balloon inserted between the posterior rectus sheath and the rectus abdominis or bluntly with the tip of the laparoscope and opened toward the pelvis inferior to the arcuate ligament (**Figure 25.4**).

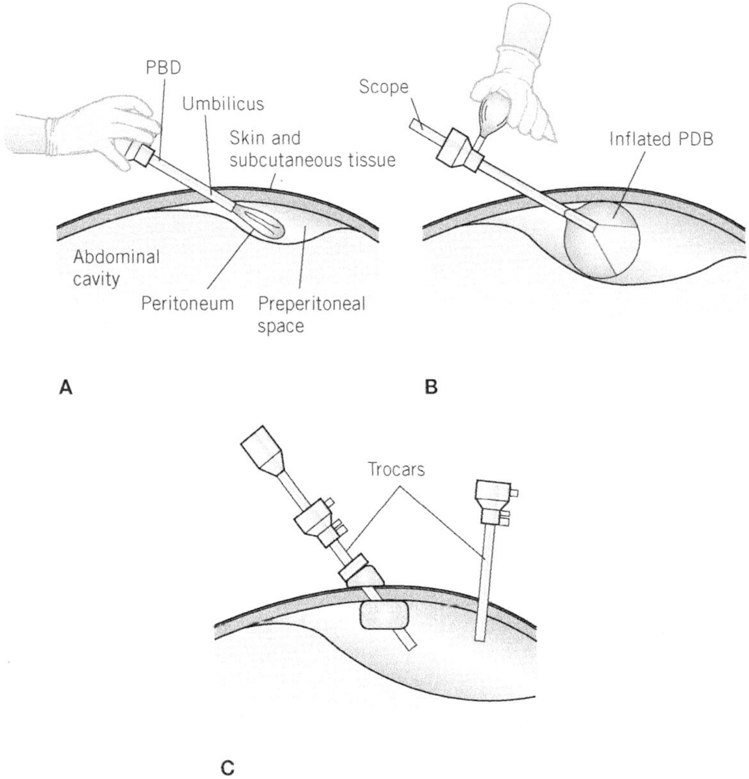

FIGURE 25.4 Laparoscopic total extraperitoneal approach with preperitoneal balloon dilation (PBD).

b. The other ports are inserted into this preperitoneal space without entering the peritoneal cavity.
c. Advantages: Peritoneum is not opened and, therefore, does not need to be closed, allowing for a shorter operative time.
d. Disadvantages: Smaller working space and potentially more challenging exposure.

4. **Mesh placement**
   a. In both the TAPP and TEP techniques, a large piece of mesh (6 × 4 in) is placed over the inguinal floor.
   b. Methods of fixation vary by surgeon and mesh choice, but traditionally fixation is performed
      i. superiorly to the posterior abdominal wall fascia on either side of the inferior epigastric vessels
      ii. inferiorly at the Cooper ligament
      iii. medially to the midline fascia
      iv. staples/tacks are **avoided** inferomedial to the internal ring or inferior to the iliopubic tract because of the risk of injury to the external iliac vessels ("**triangle of doom**") and ilioinguinal, genitofemoral, lateral femoral cutaneous, and femoral nerves ("**triangle of pain**").
5. **Outcomes**
   a. Laparoscopic repair is associated with less postoperative pain and faster recovery than open repair.
   b. Operative times, complications, and recurrence rates (<2%) are similar for both laparoscopic and open repairs.
   c. Special circumstances in which laparoscopic repair may also be favored include (1) recurrent hernias; (2) bilateral hernias, because both sides of the groin can be repaired with the same incisions; (3) in individuals with a unilateral hernia for whom a rapid recovery is critical (e.g., athletes and laborers); and (4) in obese patients.
6. **Complications:** Surgical complications include hematoma, infection, nerve injury (ilioinguinal, iliohypogastric, genital branch of the genitofemoral, lateral femoral cutaneous, femoral, chronic groin pain), vascular injury (femoral vessels, testicular artery, pampiniform venous plexus), vas deferens injury, ischemic orchitis, and testicular atrophy.
   a. **Recurrence rates** after tension-free mesh repairs for primary hernias are **<2%.**
      i. As mesh-based repairs have resulted in a decreased recurrence rate, chronic pain has emerged as one of the more prominent postoperative complications.
      ii. Management of postoperative pain requires a multidisciplinary team and evaluation for recurrent hernia.
7. **Recurrent inguinal hernias**
   a. More difficult to repair because scarring makes dissection difficult.
   b. Early recurrences within a few weeks or months of the initial repair suggest an inadequate initial repair and may reflect failure to identify an indirect hernia sac.

c. Recurrence after 1 or more years suggests progression of the disease process that caused the initial hernia.
d. Most surgeons advocate utilizing the alternate approach to the initial repair for management of recurrent hernias.

II. FEMORAL HERNIAS

A. Incidence
1. About 2% to 4% of all groin hernias, with >90% occurring in women.
2. Approximately 25% of femoral hernias become incarcerated or strangulated.

B. Anatomy
1. The abdominal viscera and peritoneum protrude through the femoral canal into the upper thigh.
2. The boundaries of the femoral canal are the lacunar ligament medially, the femoral vein laterally, the iliopubic tract anteriorly, and Cooper ligament posteriorly.
3. The rigid boundary of the femoral canal contributes to a higher rate of incarceration and strangulation in femoral hernias.

C. Clinical presentation
1. **Symptoms**
   a. Intermittent groin bulge or a groin mass felt below the inguinal ligament.
   b. Incarceration and/or obstruction may be a presenting feature.
   c. Elderly patients may not complain of groin pain even in the setting of incarceration; therefore, an occult femoral hernia should be considered in the differential diagnosis of any patient with SBO, especially if there is no history of abdominal surgery.
2. **Physical examination**
   a. Small, rounded bulge that appears in the upper thigh just below the inguinal ligament.
   b. An incarcerated femoral hernia usually presents as a firm, tender mass.
   c. The differential diagnosis is the same as that for inguinal hernia.
3. **Radiographic evaluation**
   a. Radiographic studies are rarely indicated. Occasionally, a femoral hernia is found on a CT scan performed to evaluate an SBO.

D. Treatment
1. **Inguinal approach—Cooper ligament repair** (McVay)
   a. Allows reduction of the hernia sac with visualization from above the inguinal ligament and closure of the femoral space.
   b. Occasionally, it may be necessary to divide the inguinal ligament to reduce the hernia.
   c. Repair can be performed with or without mesh.
2. **Preperitoneal approach**
   a. A transverse suprainguinal incision permits access to the extraperitoneal spaces of Bogros and Retzius.

b. Hernia is reduced from inside the femoral space, and the hernia defect is repaired preperitoneally, usually with mesh.
c. This approach is especially useful for incarcerated or strangulated femoral hernias.
d. Uncomplicated femoral hernias can also be repaired laparoscopically.

3. **Femoral approach**
   a. A horizontal incision is made over the hernia, inferior and parallel to the inguinal ligament. After the hernia sac is dissected free, it can be resected or invaginated.
   b. Femoral canal is closed by placing interrupted stitches to approximate Cooper ligament to the inguinal ligament or by using a plug of prosthetic material.

III. ABDOMINAL WALL HERNIA

A. Incidence and etiology

1. **Incisional hernias**
   a. Occur at sites of previous incisions where there was division of abdominal wall fascia.
   b. Contributing risk factors include obesity, diabetes mellitus, prior wound infection, malnutrition, smoking, and technical errors in wound closure.
   c. Hernias occur in up to 20% to 30% of patients undergoing abdominal operations and are most commonly seen with midline incisions.
   d. Multiple repair techniques have previously been described, and each have been met with varying success.
      i. Primary suture repair has unacceptably high failure rates of up to 50% and a long-lasting hernia repair requires a tension-free mesh reinforced herniorrhaphy.
   e. Patient optimization is critical for excellent clinical outcomes.
      i. Obesity, smoking, uncontrolled diabetes, malnutrition, and surgical site contamination can negatively affect surgical wound healing.
      ii. Perioperative wound complications greatly influence both the short- and long-term outcomes following hernia repair and can lead to hernia recurrence.
      iii. The surgeon must balance a patient's symptoms and their risk for having an acute event related to their hernia with preoptimization.
   f. **Surgical approach: Open abdominal wall reconstruction with transverses abdominis release**
      i. Patient is positioned supine with arms extended. Hair is clipped and the patient is given a dose of perioperative antibiotics.
      ii. Midline incision is made and carried through the layers of the abdominal wall to safely gain access to the peritoneal cavity.
      iii. Once abdominal adhesions are freed and the bowel is run to ensure no injury was made on entry, the posterior rectus space

is entered 1 cm medial to the linea alba. This is extended superiorly and inferiorly and then laterally to the linea semilunaris. Great care is ensured to protect the neurovascular perforators to the rectus complex.

iv. The posterior rectus sheath is entered, and the peritoneum is exposed. This plane is carried superiorly and inferiorly and connected bilaterally.

v. The posterior rectus sheath is closed with 2-0 absorbable braided suture.

vi. A large piece of mid-weight macroporous monofilament noncoated synthetic mesh is placed and transfascial sutures are not routinely used. Two drains are placed over the mesh.

vii. The anterior sheath is closed with a slowly absorbable monofilament suture.

viii. The incision is closed in several layers and hemostasis is ensured.

2. **Umbilical hernias**
   a. Congenital defects may enlarge over time and become protuberant and/or symptomatic.
   b. Most newborn umbilical hernias close spontaneously by the fifth year of life.
   c. Umbilical hernias are also common in adults, especially in the setting of obesity, prior pregnancy, and/or ascites.
   d. Small umbilical hernias can be present for years without causing symptoms and may even go unnoticed. Over time, these hernias can enlarge and become incarcerated, usually with preperitoneal fat or omentum.
   e. Small umbilical hernias can be closed primarily, but umbilical hernias >1 to 2 cm should be repaired with prosthetic mesh to reduce recurrence risk.
3. **Epigastric hernias**
   a. Hernias of the linea alba above the umbilicus.
   b. Occur more frequently in athletically active young men or women.
   c. When small or in obese individuals, epigastric hernias may be hard to palpate and difficult to diagnose.
   d. Usually, they produce epigastric pain that may be falsely attributed to other abdominal diagnoses.
   e. Most epigastric hernias occur within a few centimeters of the umbilicus and are associated with a small (1-2 cm) fascial defect and are filled with preperitoneal fat.
4. **Spigelian hernias**
   a. Protrude through the Spigelian fascia, near the termination of the transversus abdominis muscle along the lateral edge of the rectus abdominis near the junction of the linea semilunaris and linea semicircularis.
   b. These hernias can be difficult to diagnose because the herniated visceral contents are intraparietal (between the abdominal wall muscles).

c. Ultrasonography or CT scan can be useful in patients with focal symptoms in the appropriate region.
d. Laparoscopy can be utilized when there is a high level of suspicion and CT is negative.

5. **Lumbar hernia**
   a. Most commonly from an incisional hernia from a previous retroperitoneal or flank incision.
   b. Can also be seen spontaneously after blunt abdominal trauma.
   c. Lumbar hernias may also occur in two different triangles: The **Petit (inferior lumbar) triangle** and the **Grynfeltt–Lesshaft (superior lumbar) triangle**, although these hernias are quite rare.
6. **Obturator hernias**
   a. Rare hernias that occur predominantly in thin, older women and are difficult to diagnose.
   b. Classically present with bowel obstructions and focal tenderness on rectal examination.
   c. Pain along the medial aspect of the thigh with internal rotation of the thigh, known as the **Howship–Romberg sign**, results from **obturator nerve compression** and, when present, may aid in the clinical diagnosis.

B. Treatment and operative management

1. **Patient and hernia factors**
   a. There are numerous factors (both patient specific and hernia specific) to consider during repair (**Table 25.1**).
   b. Patient optimization including weight loss, smoking cessation, and nutrition optimization is key to ensuring a durable repair.
2. **Hernia factors**
   a. Small (<1.5 cm) epigastric, umbilical, obturator, and Spigelian hernias may be repaired primarily.
   b. Most incisional hernias as well as lumbar and obturator hernias require the use of a prosthetic mesh because of their size and high recurrence rates after primary repair.
3. **Prosthetic mesh in abdominal wall hernia repairs**
   a. The recurrence rate for ventral incisional hernia repair is 31% to 54% when primarily repaired.
   b. Long-term patient follow-up suggests that the use of mesh results in a lower recurrence rate and less abdominal pain than primary repairs.[4]
4. **Mesh choice**
   a. Complicated but should be based on location, mesh properties, and handling characteristics.
   b. Dozens of commercially available meshes with varying base materials, barrier materials, pore sizes, and mechanical properties.
   c. **Uncoated polypropylene mesh** should not be placed in an intraperitoneal position because it can form dense adhesions to the intestine and precipitate fistulization.

TABLE 25.1 Factors for Consideration in Ventral and Incisional Hernia Repair

Patient Factors	Hernia Factors	Imaging
Age	Size of hernia	Defect size
Body mass index	Location of hernia	Single hole vs. Swiss cheese defect
Diabetes	Previous repairs	Amount of bowel in hernia
Smoking	Loss of domain	Quality of surrounding muscle
Symptoms (obstruction, pain)		Evidence of previous repairs (tacks, old mesh)
Overlying skin		
Surgical history		
Abdominal wall compliance		

d. **Microporous polytetrafluoroethylene (PTFE) mesh** has a microporous architecture and hydrophobicity that prevent cellular penetration of intestine or abdominal viscera and may reduce the density of intraperitoneal adhesions.
   i. **Use of this has largely fallen out of favor due to higher infection rates.**

e. For intraperitoneal placement, either microporous PTFE mesh or a barrier-coated mesh should be used. There are several absorbable **barrier-coated meshes** with a polypropylene or polyester construction.

f. Different types of mesh are summarized in **Table 25.2**.

C. Operative approach

1. **Open repairs**
   a. Key principles include dissection and identification of all defects and repair with slowly absorbable sutures placed in healthy tissue.
   b. Incisional hernias should be repaired with mesh prosthesis with **at least 5 cm beyond the margins of the defect.**
   c. Numerous approaches that utilize separation of abdominal wall components and varying layers of mesh placement (e.g., onlay, see below) have been developed for the repair of large and complex abdominal wall hernias.

TABLE 25.2 Commonly Used Biomaterials for Incisional Hernia Repair

	Product Trade Name	Manufacturer	Components
Absorbable barrier composite meshes	Sepramesh	Genzyme Corp., Cambridge, MA	Polypropylene mesh on one side, absorbable sodium hyaluronate/carboxymethylcellulose on the other side
	C-Qur	Atrium Medical, Hudson, NH	Lightweight polypropylene mesh (Prolite) coated with omega-3 fatty acid
	Parietex	Covidien-Medtronic, Minneapolis, MN	Polyester mesh with bovine type I collagen coating covered with absorbable PEG/glycerol layer
	ProGrip	Covidien-Medtronic, Minneapolis, MN	Self-gripping Parietex
	Proceed	Ethicon, Inc, Somerville, NJ	Polypropylene mesh encapsulated with polydioxanone coated on one side with oxidized regenerated cellulose
	Ventralight ST	Bard-Davol, Warwick, RI	Polypropylene mesh with seprafilm barrier
Nonabsorbable barrier composite mesh	Bard Composix	Bard-Davol, Warwick, RI	Macroporous bilayer mesh; polypropylene and microporous PTFE
	Gore-Tex Dual Mesh	W.L. Gore & Associates, Flagstaff, AZ	PTFE with different architecture on the peritoneal (intra-abdominal) and parietal (abdominal wall) surfaces of the mesh

TABLE 25.2 Commonly Used Biomaterials for Incisional Hernia Repair (*Continued*)

	Product Trade Name	Manufacturer	Components
Nonabsorbable synthetic mesh	Bard Soft Mesh	C.R. Bard, Inc, Murray Hill, NJ	Large-pore monofilament polypropylene
Absorbable synthetic mesh	Phasix	Bard-Davol, Warwick, RI	Knitted monofilament mesh scaffold using poly-4-hydroxybutyrate (P4HB), a biologically derived, fully resorbable material
	BioA	W.L. Gore & Associates, Flagstaff, AZ	Polyglycolic acid and trimethylene carbonate
Bioremodelable materials (aka biologic meshes)	Surgisis	Cook Biotech, Inc, West Lafayette, IN	Acellular, extracellular matrix material derived from porcine small intestinal submucosa
	Alloderm	LifeCell Corp., Branchburg, NJ	Acellular dermal matrix harvested from cadaveric human dermis
	Flex HD	Musculoskeletal Transplant Foundation, Edison, NJ	Acellular dermal matrix harvested from cadaveric human dermis
	Strattice	LifeCell Corp., Branchburg, NJ	Acellular porcine dermal matrix
	Permacol	Tissue Science Laboratories, Covington, NJ	Acellular, cross-linked porcine dermal matrix

PEG, polyethylene glycol; PTFE, polytetrafluoroethylene.

i. **Onlay repair:** The mesh is secured on top of the anterior fascia that is closed below the mesh. This repair is technically easier to perform; however, it is also associated with a higher number of wound complications because it requires raising subcutaneous flaps.

ii. **Inlay repair:** The fascial defect is not closed. The mesh is placed in the hernia defect and the edges are secured to the surrounding fascia. The mesh can be exposed to bowel, and there is less mesh–tissue overlap than in other forms of repair, increasing the chances of hernia recurrence.

   a) **This technique is not recommended given its high recurrence rates.**

iii. **Sublay repair:** The mesh is placed in the retrorectus or preperitoneal space. This technique includes closure of the posterior rectus sheath beneath the mesh, **allowing for the use of uncoated mesh, as it is excluded from the peritoneal cavity.** The principles of this repair have been expanded to include transversus abdominis release for the repair of giant ventral/incisional hernias. Of the techniques described above, **sublay repairs often have lower rates of recurrence and surgical site infection.**

2. **Laparoscopic repairs**
   a. The repair traditionally involves the **intraperitoneal placement** of a mesh prosthesis to cover the hernia defect with or without primary defect closure.
   b. Broad steps include adhesiolysis of the entire prior incision, reduction of herniated abdominal contents, and broad coverage with a barrier-coated mesh. The mesh is anchored in place with sutures and tacks with a minimum 5-cm overlap past the edge of the hernia defect on all sides.
   c. For laparoscopic ventral hernia repairs, the mesh is routinely placed intraperitoneally (underlay or intraperitoneal onlay repair) with barrier-coated mesh.
3. **Open vs. minimally invasive approach**
   a. A pooled data analysis of 45 published series comparing open and laparoscopic ventral hernia repairs concluded that laparoscopic repair is associated with fewer wound-related (3.8% vs. 16.8%) and overall complications (22.7% vs. 41.7%) and has a lower rate of recurrence (4.3% vs. 12.1%) than open repairs.[5]
   b. Contraindications to laparoscopic ventral hernia repair include inability to establish pneumoperitoneum safely, peritonitis or an acute abdomen with strangulated or infarcted bowel, or loss of abdominal domain.

Key References

Citation	Summary
Fitzgibbons RJ Jr, Ramanan B, Arya S, et al. Long-term results of a randomized controlled trial of a nonoperative strategy (watchful waiting) for men with minimally symptomatic inguinal hernias. *Ann Surg*. 2013;258(3):508-515.	• Randomized control trial following male patients for 7-10 y with an inguinal hernia. Approximately 70% of male patients who elected for inguinal hernia observation underwent operative repair during the study period suggesting that surgical repair should be considered in patients with asymptomatic or minimally symptomatic inguinal hernia if they are an appropriate surgical candidate.
Petro CC, Zolin S, Krpata D, et al. Patient-reported outcomes of robotic vs laparoscopic ventral hernia repair with intraperitoneal mesh: the PROVE-IT randomized clinicAL TRIAL. *JAMA Surg*. 2021;156(1):22-29.	• Randomized control trial comparing laparoscopic and robotic ventral hernia repairs with intraperitoneal mesh suggesting that both approaches have similar patient-reported postoperative pain and hernia-specific quality-of-life scores.
Prabhu AS, Carbonell A, Hope W, et al. Robotic inguinal vs transabdominal laparoscopic inguinal hernia repair: the RIVAL randomized clinical trial. *JAMA Surg*. 2020;155(5):380-387.	• Randomized control trial comparing laparoscopic and robotic inguinal hernia repairs suggesting no significant difference in important postoperative hernia outcomes between the two approaches.
Rosen MJ, Krpata DM, Petro CC, et al. Biologic vs synthetic mesh for single-stage repair of contaminated ventral hernias: a randomized clinical trial. *JAMA Surg*. 2022;157(4):293-301.	• Randomized control trial comparing the use of synthetic mesh vs. biologic mesh in clean-contaminated and contaminated fields. Synthetic mesh demonstrated superior 2-y hernia recurrence risk compared with biologic mesh without increasing rates of wound infections.

CHAPTER 25: HERNIAS

Review Questions

1. What is the most common type of inguinal hernia?
2. What are the borders of Hesselbach's triangle?
3. An elderly female has pain with medial (internal) thigh rotation with no palpable hernia in the groin. What is the most likely diagnosis?
4. Which open inguinal repair can be used to fix a femoral hernia?

5. What location must be avoided when securing the mesh during a minimally invasive inguinal hernia repair?
6. What are the biggest patient risk factors for hernia recurrence after an open ventral hernia repair?
7. What is the minimal mesh overlap that must be achieved during a ventral hernia repair?

REFERENCES

1. Earle DB, Mark LA. Prosthetic material in inguinal hernia repair: how do I choose? *Surg Clin North Am.* 2008;88(1):179-201.
2. Fitzgibbons RJ Jr, Forse RA. Clinical practice. Groin hernias in adults. *N Engl J Med.* 2015;372(8):756-763.
3. Stroupe KT, Manheim LM, Luo P, et al. Tension-free repair versus watchful waiting for men with asymptomatic or minimally symptomatic inguinal hernias: a cost-effectiveness analysis. *J Am Coll Surg.* 2006;203(4):458-468.
4. Cobb WS, Kercher KW, Matthews BD, et al. Laparoscopic ventral hernia repair: a single center experience. *Hernia.* 2006;10(3):236-242.
5. Pierce RA, Spitler JA, Frisella MM, Matthews BD, Brunt LM. Pooled data analysis of laparoscopic vs. open ventral hernia repair: 14 years of patient data accrual. *Surg Endosc.* 2007;21(3):378-386.
6. Fitzgibbons RJ Jr, Ramanan B, Arya S, et al. Long-term results of a randomized controlled trial of a nonoperative strategy (watchful waiting) for men with minimally symptomatic inguinal hernias. *Ann Surg.* 2013;258(3):508-515.
7. Petro CC, Zolin S, Krpata D, et al. Patient-reported outcomes of robotic vs laparoscopic ventral hernia repair with intraperitoneal mesh: the PROVE-IT randomized clinical trial. *JAMA Surg.* 2021;156(1):22-29.
8. Prabhu AS, Carbonell A, Hope W, et al. Robotic inguinal vs transabdominal laparoscopic inguinal hernia repair: the RIVAL randomized clinical trial. *JAMA Surg.* 2020;155(5):380-387.
9. Rosen MJ, Krpata DM, Petro CC, et al. Biologic vs synthetic mesh for single-stage repair of contaminated ventral hernias: a randomized clinical trial. *JAMA Surg.* 2022;157(4):293-301.

26 Endoscopic, Laparoscopic, and Robotic Surgery

Leah Conant and Michael M. Awad

I. MINIMALLY INVASIVE TECHNIQUES

A. Minimally invasive surgical techniques are crucial to surgical care, and familiarity with basic principles of laparoscopic, robotic, and endoscopic surgery is critical for surgical trainees.

B. Benefits including
   1. Shorter length of hospital stays
   2. Less postoperative pain
   3. Lower rates of postoperative wound complications.

C. The use of robot-assisted laparoscopic surgery continues to expand in a variety of surgical fields, and diagnostic endoscopy has been instrumental in pioneering a variety of endoscopic surgical techniques.

D. Principles of flexible endoscopy and endoscopic surgery
   1. Performed using a flexible **fiberoptic endoscope**, connected to a source of water or saline, suction, and an air or gas insufflator
   2. Most endoscopes have a **working channel** allowing instruments to be passed through the scope for therapeutic and diagnostic interventions such as tissue biopsy.
   3. The most common endoscopes used by general surgeons are **gastroscopes** and **colonoscopes**. Gastroscopes are used for diagnostic **esophagogastroduodenoscopy** (**EGD**).
   4. Gastroscopes, compared with colonoscopes, are shorter and thinner but typically still have a working channel.

E. Principles of laparoscopic surgery
   1. **Basic principles**
      a. Laparoscopy is used to perform a vast assortment of operations with few contraindications to its use.
      b. Preoperative assessment for laparoscopic surgeries is comparable with that for open operations.
      c. By definition, laparoscopic surgery is the use of a fiberoptic camera to explore the abdominal cavity.
         i. Working space within the abdominal cavity is established through insufflation of carbon dioxide to create pneumoperitoneum.
         ii. Visualization is achieved using an endoscope connected to display monitors in the operating room.

d. The principle of **triangulation** dictates port placement in laparoscopic surgery.
   i. The camera port is placed centrally with working ports placed on either side in a triangulated fashion, thus allowing the laparoscopic instruments to converge at the surgical target without colliding with the laparoscope or the other working instruments.

2. **Limitations**
   a. Although the surgical field is a three-dimensional space, the image projected onto the monitor from the laparoscope is two-dimensional, often limiting the depth perception of the surgeon.
   b. While most laparoscopic instruments can rotate on their long axis and have some limited articulation at the instrument tip, there is limited dexterity compared with the human hand and wrist.
   c. In addition, haptic feedback with laparoscopy is limited, therefore, knowledge of tissue characteristics is imperative to safely operate laparoscopically.

3. **Patient selection**
   a. **Absolute contraindications:** Inability to tolerate general anesthesia; hemodynamic instability; uncorrected coagulopathy; no available experienced laparoscopic surgeons or staff
   b. **Relative contraindications:** Bowel obstruction; severe cardiopulmonary disease; peritonitis; loss of abdominal domain

4. **Equipment, troubleshooting, and techniques**
   a. **Room setup and positioning**
      i. Basic setup for laparoscopic surgery includes an insufflator, gas supply, light source, camera, laparoscope, display monitors, laparoscopic trocars, instruments, and instruments for conversion to open if necessary.
      ii. The patient, surgeon, and monitor should be positioned to place the operative field between the surgeon and the monitor.
      iii. Most abdominal operations have the patient in the supine position.
      iv. Standard patient securement should be employed in all operations.
      v. Monitors should be positioned to allow the operating surgeon to view them clearly without turning their head and with a 15° downward gaze, minimizing neck extension and postural fatigue.
      vi. The operating table height and port placement should allow the surgeon to keep both arms at their sides with their elbows flexed to 90° to 120°.
      vii. A preoperative safety and equipment checklist is essential prior to any laparoscopic operation.
   b. **Insufflation**
      i. Pressure-limited insufflation is typically used in laparoscopic surgery: the setup controls the flow of carbon dioxide into the abdominal cavity.

- **ii.** A commonly used target pressure is 15 mm Hg, which is then modulated throughout the surgery by gas flow.
    - **a)** Target pressure can be changed at the discretion of the surgeon: Often lowered in pediatric cases and raised in bariatric cases when necessary.
- **iii.** Loss of pneumoperitoneum or an increase in pressure can occur due to multiple factors, as described in the **Figure 26.1**.

c. Imaging system

- **i.** The imaging system consists of a laparoscope, a light source, a camera, and a monitor.
- **ii.** Surgeons should be familiar with troubleshooting issues that occur, as described in **Figure 26.1**.
- **iii.** Laparoscopes vary in diameter, but the most commonly used sizes in General Surgery are 10- and 5-mm scopes.
    - **a)** Advances in technology make it such that there is minimal difference in illumination and picture quality between scope diameters.
    - **b)** Laparoscopes can have a flat tip (0° scope) or an angled top (most commonly 30° scope or 45° scope) to allow for turning the view around the long axis of the scope.

5. Abdominal access

a. Safe access to the abdomen is the crucial first step to laparoscopic surgery.

- **i.** The two most common strategies are: The **Veress** needle, or closed technique, and the **Hasson** cannula, or open technique.

b. Closed technique with Veress needle

- **i.** This employs a Veress needle, which consists of a spring-loaded, beveled needle connected to a valve and stopcock allowing gas to insufflate through the needle.
- **ii.** Inserting the Veress needle into a safe location in the abdomen is imperative.
    - **a)** A commonly used site is at Palmer's point, which is two fingerbreadths below the left costal margin.
- **iii.** Once safely inserted into the peritoneal cavity, the gas insufflator is connected. The starting (i.e., "opening") pressure should be between 4 and 9 mm Hg, with obese patients being on the higher end of the spectrum due to the additional weight of the abdominal wall.

c. Open technique with Hasson

- **i.** Entry into the abdomen at the initial trocar site is completed under direct vision.
- **ii.** Often helpful when extensive intra-abdominal adhesions are anticipated.
- **iii.** Open port insertion is usually performed at the umbilicus; however, if the patient has had prior midline incisions, many will choose an alternative location such as the right-lower or left-upper quadrant.

Problem	Cause	Solution
1. Poor insufflation/loss of pneumoperitoneum	CO_2 tank empty	Change tank
	Accessory port stopcock(s) not properly adjusted	Inspect all accessory ports. Open or close stopcock(s) as needed
	Leak in sealing cap or stopcock	Change cap or cannula
	Excessive suctioning	Allow time to reinsufflate
	Loose connection of insufflator tubing at source or at port	Tighten connections
	Hasson stay sutures loose	Replace or secure sutures
	Tubing disconnection from insufflator	Connect tubing
	Flow rate set too low	Adjust flow rate
2. Excessive pressure required for insufflation (initial or subsequent)	Veress needle or cannula tip not in free peritoneal cavity	Reinsert needle or cannula
	Occlusion of tubing (kinking, table joint, etc.)	Inspect full length of tubing. Replace with proper size as necessary
	Port stopcock turned off	Fully open stopcock
	Patient is "light"	Give more muscle relaxant
	Cannula tip not in peritoneal space	Advance cannula under visual control
3. Inadequate lighting (partial/complete loss)	Loose connection at source or scope	Adjust connector
	Light is on "manual minimum"	Go to "automatic"
	Bulb is burned out	Replace bulb
	Fiber optics are damaged	Replace light cable
	Automatic iris adjusting to bright reflection from instrument	Reposition instruments, or switch to "manual"
	Monitor brightness turned down	Readjust setting
	Room brightness floods monitors	Dim room lights
4. Lighting too bright	Light is on "manual maximum"	Go to "automatic"
	"Boost" on light source is activated	Deactivate "boost"
	Monitor brightness turned up	Readjust setting

FIGURE 26.1 Troubleshooting algorithm for laparoscopic surgery.

iv. The open technique can be difficult in obese patients with thick abdominal walls; thus, the Veress technique is often preferred in bariatric surgery.

d. **Complications of abdominal access**
   i. Regardless of preferred technique, complications of abdominal access can ensue, including visceral and vascular injuries.
   ii. Careful inspection of the bowel and surrounding vasculature should take place if there is any suspicion of injury.

e. **Trocar insertion**
   i. Once the abdomen is insufflated to target pressure, the remaining trocars are inserted.
   ii. Even under direct visualization, bowel and other visceral injuries can occur.
   iii. If a rush of blood is encountered on trocar insertion, the surgeon must assume that a critical vascular injury occurred and conversion to open should be performed immediately, while keeping the inciting trocar in place as it may aid in partially tamponading the injury.

f. **Abdominal wall hemorrhage**
   i. Often related to injury to the epigastric arteries, veins, or their tributaries.
   ii. These injuries are often self-limited and cease with tamponade aided by the inserted port, but may require placement of a ligating suture.

6. **Port removal and closure**
   a. At the conclusion of the operation, instruments and ports are removed under direct visualization and the camera port is removed last.
   b. Incisions 5 mm or smaller do not require fascial closure. Any 10-mm or larger port sites may need fascial closure, especially if the fascia has been dilated or cut to remove a large specimen.
      i. Neglecting to close these fascial incisions can result in port site hernia.

7. **Physiologic effects of laparoscopy and pneumoperitoneum**
   a. Understanding the changes of pneumoperitoneum has on multiple physiologic changes to the body is imperative for the general surgeon.
      i. **Cardiovascular**
         a) Increased intra-abdominal pressure leads to increased systemic vascular resistance secondary to compression of venous and arterial structures.
         b) Decreased flow leads to renin–angiotensin–aldosterone axis activation.
         c) Compression of the inferior vena cava leads to reduced preload and lower cardiac output.
      ii. **Pulmonary**
         a) Increased intra-abdominal pressure decreases diaphragmatic excursion, resulting in decreased pulmonary compliance and increased thoracic pressure.
         b) Atelectasis is common following laparoscopy.

iii. **Renal**
a) Increased intra-abdominal pressure reduces afferent arterial renal flow, leading to decreased glomerular filtration rate and elevated renal venous pressure.
b) Transient decrease in urine output is common but usually resolves with the release of pneumoperitoneum.

iv. **Neurologic**
a) Increased intra-abdominal pressure leads to increased central venous pressure, which causes decreased venous return from the brain.
b) Often a transient increase in intracranial pressure ensues.

F. Principles of robotic surgery

1. Currently, the da Vinci Surgical System by Intuitive Surgical, Inc, is the main robotic surgical system in use. While other companies are developing other robotic platforms, Intuitive's da Vinci system was the first US Food and Drug Administration–approved system.
2. **Equipment and basic principles**
   a. Robotic surgery allows the surgeon to control robotic arms that use precision instruments to perform complex surgical tasks through small incisions.
   b. There are four key components to the robot system: Surgeon console, patient-side cart, EndoWrist instruments, and the vision cart.
      i. The **surgeon console** is used to manipulate the robotic arms and instruments. It consists of the display, the wrist support with master controls, and the foot pedal platform.
      ii. The **patient-side cart** supports the robotic arms (typically three to four) that carry out the surgeon's commands. Once the patient-side cart is in the proper position, the arms are docked to trocars that can then pivot around fixed points to decrease trauma to the patient's abdominal wall. One arm is used to hold the camera, and the other arms are used to control different instruments based on the operation performed.
      iii. The **EndoWrist instruments** allow the surgeon's hand and wrist movements to be replicated at the instrument tips.
      iv. The **vision cart** is equipped with a 3D-HD image-processing unit that transfers the image from the laparoscope to the surgeon console and to a viewing monitor for the assistant.

II. TRAINING PROGRAMS

A. Fundamentals of Laparoscopic Surgery (FLS)

1. FLS is a program developed by the Society of American Gastrointestinal and Endoscopic Surgeons (SAGES) for teaching and evaluation of knowledge and technical skills required for laparoscopy. The program is composed of a didactic curriculum, a written examination, and a skill-based examination. The web-based didactic modules cover basic preoperative considerations, intraoperative considerations, basic laparoscopic procedures, and postoperative care and complications.

2. The manual skills examination performed in a laparoscopic trainer box consists of five tasks: Peg transfer, precision cutting, ligating loop, extracorporeal knot tying, and intracorporeal knot tying.
3. Passing the FLS written and technical examinations is a **prerequisite for board eligibility in General Surgery in the US.**

B. Fundamentals of Endoscopic Surgery (FES)
1. A didactic curriculum and technical examination developed by SAGES to train surgical learners in the theory and technical skills necessary to perform diagnostic and interventional endoscopy. It includes a didactic web-based portion and a simulator-based curriculum. Passage of both the written and simulator portions of the FES examination are required for board eligibility in General Surgery in the US.

C. Safe use of surgical energy
1. For a full description of safe use of surgical energy, please refer to **FUSE (Fundamental Use of Surgical Energy)** modules from SAGES.
2. **Electrosurgery** is defined as using radiofrequency alternating current to increase intracellular temperature, resulting in cutting or coagulation of tissue.
   a. All advanced electrosurgery is **bipolar**, meaning there are two electrodes. Must create a circuit in order to perform electrosurgery. This is formed by the **electrosurgical unit**, the **electrodes** and **connecting wires**, and the **patient**. **Bipolar instruments** have both electrodes on the same device.
   b. **Monopolar instruments** have only one electrode mounted on the device, the other electrode in the circuit being the dispersive electrode. The current of electrons originates at an electrode at the surgical site and travels to a dispersive electrode elsewhere on the patient's body, usually a pad on their leg or back. The density of current at the site of the surgical electrode generates heat, leading to tissue disruption.
3. Temperature rise in the target tissue is affected by three properties: Current (I), voltage (V), and impedance or resistance (R) governed by **Ohm's law: $I = V/R$** [Current = Voltage/Resistance]. Resistance is most affected by tissue characteristics.
4. Surgeons must be aware of the possibility of thermal energy when using electrosurgical devices.
   a. Unintended radiofrequency burns can occur by inadvertent direct coupling, capacitive coupling, and/or insulation failures.
   b. Particularly with monopolar devices, direct coupling occurs when current passes from a monopolar instrument through another conductive instrument.
      i. While often used purposefully during surgery, direct coupling can inadvertently result in thermal injury.
   c. Bipolar devices usually do not have extensive spread around the operating tip. However, the longer the electrodes are activated, there is a greater chance for thermal spread.
5. **Ultrasonic energy** devices employ an active blade that vibrates at very high frequency, generating thermal energy.

III. KEY OPERATIVE STEPS

A. EGD

1. Diagnostic use: Insert endoscope into the gastrointestinal tract and meticulously examine the target mucosa while advancing or withdrawing the scope.
   a. **Air or carbon dioxide** is used to dilate and insufflate the gastrointestinal lumen to facilitate scope advancement and mucosal examination.
   b. **Irrigation** is used to clean the tip of the endoscope or wash debris from the mucosa.
2. All aspects of the endoscope are subject to malfunction; thus, general surgeons must be familiar with troubleshooting issues in a systematic fashion.
3. Average distance (in centimeters) from incisors of **important landmarks on upper endoscopy**
   a. Cricopharyngeal muscle: 16 cm
   b. Aortic constriction: 23 cm
   c. Lower esophageal sphincter and diaphragm: 38 cm
   d. Fundus of stomach: 40 cm

B. Colonoscopy

1. The most common indication for colonoscopy is for **screening of asymptomatic patients for neoplastic diseases**, such as polyps and cancer.
2. **Surgical approach: Colonoscopy**
   a. Inspect the perineum and perform a careful digital rectal examination.
   b. Insert a well-lubricated colonoscope into the rectum, keeping the lumen in view. Air insufflation is necessary to distend the lumen and obtain good visualization of the mucosal surfaces.
   c. Upon entering the rectum, the sigmoid colon is then encountered, followed by the descending colon, then the splenic flexure, the transverse colon, the hepatic flexure, the ascending colon, and finally the cecum.
   d. With ileocecal valve and appendiceal orifice in view, the end of the colon has been reached.
   e. After reaching the cecum, the colonoscope is gradually withdrawn, carefully inspecting the colonic mucosa circumferentially. **A withdrawal time of at least 6 minutes is recommended to ensure adequate detection of adenomas.**
   f. After visualization of the anal verge, the colonoscope is reinserted into the rectum and the scope is retroflexed. This allows for detection of low rectal malignant disease, internal hemorrhoids, and fissures.
3. While recommendations continue to evolve as younger individuals are being more frequently diagnosed with colorectal cancer, the current recommendations for screening colonoscopy in the average-risk patient is every 10 years, starting at age 45 years.
4. Patients with a family history of colon cancer, especially in a first-degree relative, should undergo screening colonoscopy at an earlier age (40 years or 10 years prior to the age of diagnosis of the affected family member).

5. Adequate bowel preparation is essential for a successful and complete examination.
   a. Residual stool in the colon prolongs examination, decreases visualization, and increases the risk of missing pathologic lesions.
6. Contraindications: Presence of peritonitis or suspected colorectal perforation, severe acute diverticulitis, and fulminant colitis.
7. Position: The most comfortable position for both patient and physician is left lateral decubitus.
8. Tips
   a. External rotation of the colonoscope to generate torque aids in the visualization of all aspects of the colonic mucosa.
   b. If a loop of colon is encountered, signaled by resistance or inability to advance the scope (loss of 1:1 motion), pulling back and rotating the scope to reduce the loop may allow for forward progress.

Key References

Citation	Summary
Gerull WD, Cho D, Kuo I, Arefanian S, Kushner BS, Awad MM. Robotic approach to paraesophageal hernia repair results in low long-term recurrence rate and beneficial patient-centered outcomes. *J Am Coll Surg*. 2020;231(5):520-526.	• Prospective longitudinal study demonstrating robotic paraesophageal hernia repairs are a both safe and effective alternative to laparoscopic repairs with excellent long-term outcomes and low recurrence rates.
Zárate Rodriguez JG, Zihni AM, Ohu I, Cavallo JA, Ray S, Cho S, Awad MM. Ergonomic analysis of laparoscopic and robotic surgical task performance at various experience levels. *Surg Endosc*. 2019;33(6):1938-1943.	• Study comparing muscle activation ("muscle strain") using surface electromyography between laparoscopy and robotic surgery. Muscle activation was higher during laparoscopy as compared with robotic surgery in all muscle groups except for the trapezius muscle.
Napolitano MA, Zebley JA, Wagner K, Holleran TJ, Werba G, Sparks AD, Trachiotis G, Brody F. Robotic foregut surgery in the veterans health administration: increasing prevalence, decreasing operative time, and improving outcomes. *J Am Coll Surg*. 20221;235(2):149-156.	• Retrospective study comparing 30-d outcomes between robotic-assisted foregut surgery and laparoscopic-assisted foregut surgery in the VA health system. The robotic approach was associated with shorter operative times and reduced complications.

CHAPTER 26: ENDOSCOPIC, LAPAROSCOPIC, AND ROBOTIC SURGERY

Review Questions

1. What are absolute contraindications to laparoscopic surgery?
2. What are the renal effects of pneumoperitoneum?
3. What are the cardiovascular effects of pneumoperitoneum?
4. What is the average distance from the incisors to the lower esophageal sphincter during an upper endoscopy?
5. What are contraindications to colonoscopy?
6. What is the recommended amount of time for withdrawal of the colonoscope from the cecum to the rectum for adequate adenoma detection?

27 Breast Disease

Faiz Gani and Julie A. Margenthaler

I. ANATOMY OF THE BREAST

A. Boundaries and attachments

1. The breast is located between the subcutaneous fat and the fascia of the pectoralis major and serratus anterior muscles (**Figure 27.1**).[1]
2. Bound superiorly by the clavicle, inferiorly by the inframammary fold, and medially by the lateral edge of the sternum, with its lateral border lying along the anterior border of the latissimus dorsi.[1]
3. Traditionally the breast is divided into **four quadrants:** The upper inner, the upper outer, the lower inner, and the lower outer.[1]
4. Suspensory ligaments **(Cooper's ligaments)** run through the breasts from the deep fascia to the skin and may cause skin dimpling when associated with a malignancy.[1]

B. Neurovascular and lymphatic anatomy

1. The arterial supply of the upper outer quadrant of the breast is via the lateral thoracic artery (from the axillary artery), while the central and medial portions of the breast are supplied by perforating branches of the internal thoracic artery (or internal mammary artery).[1]
2. Venous drainage is through the axillary vein, the internal mammary vein, and the intercostal veins.[1]
3. Superficial lymphatic drainage is via the subareolar **plexus of Sappey,** while deeper drainage is via the submammary plexus; these converge and drain into the axillary (75%) and internal mammary (25%) lymph nodes.[1]
4. Lateral and anterior cutaneous branches of the second to sixth intercostal nerves provide sensory innervation to the breast.[1]

C. Axillary anatomy

1. The borders of the axilla are defined superiorly by the axillary vein, the outer border of the first rib, and the posterior border of the clavicle.[1]
2. The lateral border is defined by the latissimus dorsi muscle, the medial border is defined by the serratus anterior muscle, the posterior border is defined by the subscapularis and teres major muscles, and the anterior border is defined by the pectoralis major and minor muscles.[1]
3. Contents of the axilla include the axillary artery and vein (and their branches/tributaries), which are the major vasculature for the upper limb.[1]

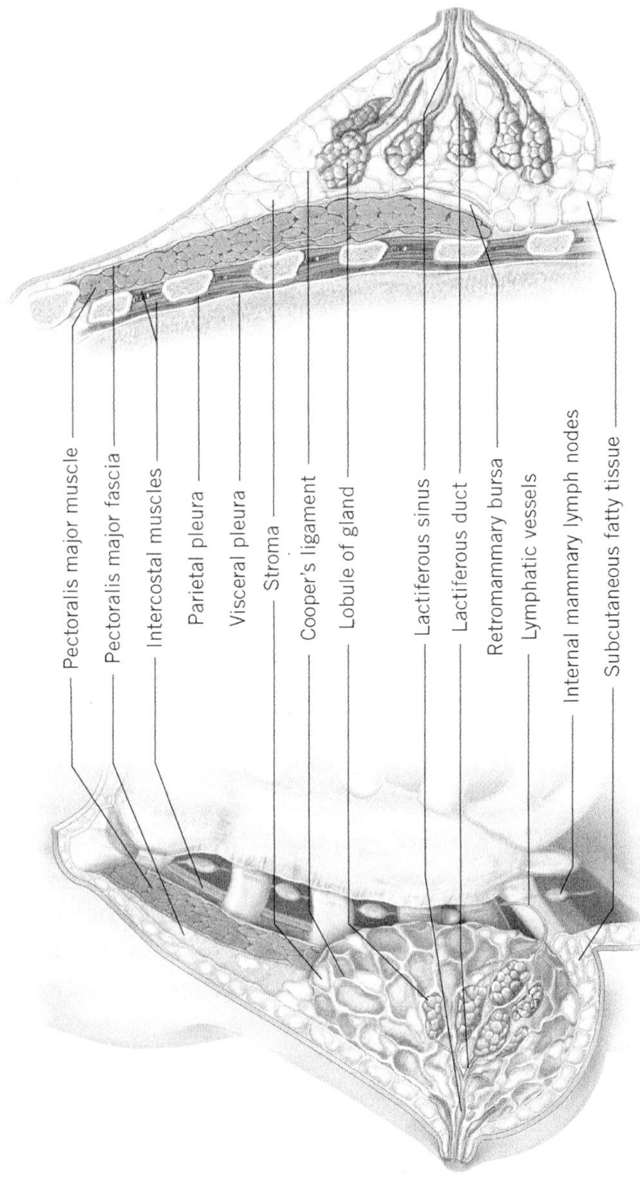

FIGURE 27.1 A tangential view of the breast on the chest wall and a sectional (sagittal) view of the breast and associated chest wall. *(Reprinted with permission from Bland KI. Embryology and anatomy of the breast. In: Fischer JE, ed. Fischer's Mastery of Surgery. 7th ed. Wolters Kluwer; 2019:594-603.)*

4. The axilla also contains important lymphatic structures and nerves relevant to operative decision-making (**Tables 27.1** and **27.2**), and preservation of all is preferred during an **axillary lymph node dissection** (ALND); however, direct tumor invasion may require resection along with the specimen.[1]

II. CLINICAL ASSESSMENT AND IMAGING

A. History: Patients seek medical attention most commonly for an abnormal mammogram, a breast mass, breast pain, nipple discharge, and/or skin changes.

1. Comprehensive medical history should include the following:
    a. Description and duration of signs and symptoms and their temporal relationship to pregnancy, menstrual cycle, or previous trauma, as appropriate
    b. Mammogram history
    c. Previous history (and outcomes) of breast biopsies and any previous breast operations
    d. History of oral contraceptive and/or hormone replacement therapy
    e. Date of last menstrual period and regularity of the menstrual cycle
    f. Age of menarche
    g. Number of pregnancies and age at first full-term pregnancy
    h. Lactation history
    i. Age at natural or surgical menopause (e.g., oophorectomy)
    j. Personal and family history of breast and gynecologic cancer, including age at diagnosis, and should include at least two generations as well as any associated cancers (e.g., ovarian, colon, prostate, gastric, pancreatic) to assess for hereditary cancer risk, as well as any genetic testing completed.
2. Assessment of cancer risks
    a. Hormonal and environmental exposures, genetics, and certain types of histology on previous breast biopsy that can all be associated with an increased risk for breast cancer (**Table 27.3**).

TABLE 27.1 Classification of Axillary Lymph Node Levels and Their Relation to the Pectoralis Minor Muscle

Level of Nodes	Anatomic Location
Level I	Lateral to the pectoralis minor muscle
Level II	Posterior to the pectoralis minor muscle
Level III	Medial to the pectoralis minor muscle and are most accessible with division of the muscle

TABLE 27.2 Sensory and Motor Nerves Located in the Axilla, and Associated Deficits Related to Injury to the Relevant Structure

Nerve	Anatomic Location	Function	Deficit Associated With Injury
Long thoracic nerve	Courses along the chest wall and medially within the axilla over the serratus anterior muscle	Innervates the serratus anterior muscle	Injury to the nerves causes a "winged" scapula
Thoracodorsal nerve	Courses along the posterior border of the axilla to the latissimus dorsi muscle	Innervates the latissimus dorsi muscle	Injury to this nerve causes weakness adduction at the shoulder joint and medial rotation
Medial pectoral nerve[a]	Courses from the posterior aspect of the pectoralis minor muscle around the lateral border of the pectoralis minor to the posterior aspect of the pectoralis major muscle	Innervates the lateral third of the pectoralis major	Injury to this nerve results in atrophy of the pectoralis major muscle
Lateral pectoral nerve[b]	Arises from the brachial plexus and courses below the clavipectoral fascia to enter the deep surface of the pectoralis major muscle	Innervates the pectoral major muscle Contributes to sensory supply of anterior chest wall	Injury to this nerve results in atrophy of the pectoralis major muscle
Intercostal brachial nerves	Course laterally in the axilla from the second intercostal space to the medial upper arm	Sensory innervation to the upper arm	Transection causes numbness in the posterior and medial surfaces of the upper arm

[a]The median pectoral nerve can be used as a donor nerve when reconstructing a damaged brachial plexus or used for reconstruction following axillary nerve injury.

[b]Given proprioceptive and nociceptive fibers, this nerve may be targeted for postoperative pain control via perioperative nerve blocks.

TABLE 27.3 Risk Factors for Breast Cancer and Approximate Strength of Association

Reproductive	Hormonal	Nutritional/Lifestyle/ Body Habitus	Other
Early menarche [+]	OC use (current vs. none) [+]	Obesity (>30 BMI vs. <25) Premenopausal [–] Postmenopausal [+]	Family history (mother and sister)[a] [+++]
Age at first delivery (>35 vs. <20) [++]	Estrogen replacement (10+ y vs. none) [+]	Adult weight gain (postmenopausal) [++]	Family history (first-degree relative)[b] [++]
No. of births (0 vs. 1 child) [+]	Estrogen plus progesterone replacement (>5 y vs. none) [++]	Alcohol (1 or more drink/day vs. none) [+]	Jewish heritage (yes vs. no) [+]
Age at menopause (5-y increment) [+]	High blood estrogens or androgens (post menopause) [+++]	Height (>5 ft 7 in) [+]	Ionizing radiation (yes vs. no) [+]
Breastfeeding (>1 y vs. none) [–]	High blood prolactin [++]	Physical activity (>3 h/wk) [–]	Benign breast disease (MD diagnosed)[d] [++]
		Monounsaturated fat[c] (vs. saturated fat) [–]	Mammographic density (highest category vs. lowest) [+++]
		Low intake of fruits and vegetables[c] (specifically for ER-breast cancer) [+]	

BMI, body mass index; ER, estrogen receptor; MD, medical doctor; OC, oral contraceptives.

[+] = relative risk (RR) 1.1-1.4; [++] = RR 1.5-2.9; [+++] = RR 3.0-6.9; [–] = RR 0.7-0.8.

[a]Two first-degree relatives who have a history of breast cancer before age 65 y vs. no relative.

[b]First-degree relative who has a history of breast cancer before age 65 y vs. no relative.

[c]Upper quartile (top 25%) vs. lower quartile (lowest 25%).

[d]Clinically recognized chronic cystic, fibrocystic, or other benign breast disease vs. none.

b. **Hereditary breast cancer** accounts for 5% to 10% of breast cancers, and approximately 80% of hereditary breast cancers are the result of mutations in ***BRCA1* and *BRCA2*.**

i. Women with *BRCA1* mutations have an estimated risk of 85% for breast cancer by the age of 70 years, a 50% chance of developing a second primary breast cancer, and a 20% to 40% chance of developing ovarian cancer (and increased risk of colon cancer as well).

ii. *BRCA2* mutations carry a slightly lower risk for breast and ovarian cancer and account for 4% to 6% of all male breast cancers.

iii. Genetic testing panels now include wider assessments for other less common "moderate penetrance" gene mutations, such as *CHEK2, PALB2, ATM*, and *PTEN*.

iv. Genetic counseling and testing should be considered for all newly diagnosed patients with breast cancer.

B. Physical examination: Complete examination of a patient requires inspection of the bilateral breasts and axillae.

1. Inspect the patient's breasts in both the upright and supine positions.

a. With the patient in the upright position, examine with the patient's arms relaxed and then raised, looking for shape asymmetry, deformity, skin changes (e.g., erythema, edema, dimpling), nipple changes or discharge, and lymphadenopathy (axillary, supraclavicular, and infraclavicular).

b. With the patient in the supine position, examine the entire breast systematically with the patient's ipsilateral arm raised above and behind the head. Clinical examination of the axilla is best completed with the arm positioned by the patient's side.

C. Breast imaging

1. **Screening mammograms** are performed in the asymptomatic patient and consist of two standard views, a mediolateral oblique view and a craniocaudal view.

a. **Tomosynthesis,** or **three-dimensional mammography,** improves the sensitivity and specificity of mammography, particularly for women with nonfatty breasts and in the assessment of noncalcified lesions.

b. The US Preventative Task Force recommends screening mammography annually for women beginning at age 50 years, while the National Cancer Institute, the American Congress of Obstetricians and Gynecologists, and the American Cancer Society recommend annual screening mammography for women starting at 45 years and older.[2]

2. **BI-RADS (Breast Imaging Reporting and Data System)** is used to classify breast lesions on mammography (**Table 27.4**).

a. **Malignant mammographic findings** include new or spiculated masses, clustered microcalcifications in linear or branching array, and/or architectural distortion.

b. **Benign mammographic findings** that might be mistaken for malignancy include radial scar (biopsy needed), fat necrosis (i.e., oil cysts; biopsy may be needed), and milk of calcium (no biopsy needed).

c. Cysts cannot be distinguished from solid masses by mammography, so ultrasound imaging is needed to make this distinction.

TABLE 27.4	BI-RADS (Breast Imaging Reporting and Data System)
0	Needs further imaging; assessment incomplete
1	Normal; continue annual follow-up (risk of malignancy: 1/2,000)
2	Benign lesion; no risk of malignancy; continue annual follow-up (risk of malignancy: 1/2,000)
3	Probably benign lesion; needs 4-6 mo follow-up (risk of malignancy: 1-2/100)
4	Suspicious for breast cancer; biopsy recommended. **A.** Low suspicion for malignancy (>2%-≤10%) **B.** Moderate suspicion for malignancy (>10%-≤50%) **C.** Finding of moderate concern of being cancer but not as high as category 5 (>50%-≤95%)
5	Highly suspicious for breast cancer; biopsy strongly recommended (≥95% are malignant)
6	Known biopsy-proven malignancy

3. Screening in high-risk patients

a. In patients with known genetic mutations, plan annual mammography and semiannual physical examinations beginning at 25 to 30 years.

b. In patients with a strong family history of breast cancer but undocumented genetic mutation, annual mammograms and semiannual physical examinations should begin 10 years earlier than the age at diagnosis of the youngest affected relative and no later than the age of 40 years.

c. MRI is recommended for screening in select high-risk patients including those with an elevated lifetime risk per a validated risk assessment model (e.g., Tyrer–Cuzick), a personal or family history of *BRCA* mutations or other predisposing genetic syndromes (e.g., Li–Fraumeni, Cowden, or Bannayan–Riley–Ruvalcaba), or a history of chest wall radiation between the ages of 10 and 30 years.

4. Diagnostic mammograms

a. Performed in the symptomatic patient or to follow-up an abnormality noted on a screening mammogram, and additional views (spot-compression views or magnification views) may be needed to further characterize any lesion(s).

b. A normal mammogram in the presence of a palpable mass does not exclude malignancy, and further workup should be performed with ultrasonography, MRI, and/or biopsy.

c. **Contrast-enhanced digital mammography** is being adopted in some centers as an adjunct in the diagnostic setting, and while data supporting this are currently limited, this adjunct is useful in patients who cannot tolerate an MRI due to the presence of medical devices or claustrophobia.

5. **Ultrasound imaging**
   a. Ultrasound imaging can determine whether a lesion is solid or cystic and can define the size, contour, or internal texture of the lesion.
   b. Not a useful screening modality by itself due to significant false-positive rates and significant time burden to accurately examine an entire breast
   c. When used as an adjunct with mammography, ultrasound imaging may improve diagnostic sensitivity of benign findings to >90%, especially among younger patients for whom mammographic sensitivity is lower due to denser breast tissue.
6. **MRI**
   a. Useful as an adjunct to mammography to determine extent of disease, to detect multicentric disease in the dense breast, to assess the contralateral breast, to evaluate patients with axillary metastases and an unknown primary (i.e., occult primary breast cancer), and in the diagnostic scenario where mammogram, ultrasound imaging, and clinical findings are inconclusive.
   b. Also useful for assessing chest wall involvement.
   c. Patients should be counseled about the relatively high false-positive rates associated with this modality.

D. Breast biopsy

1. **Fine-needle aspiration biopsy** (FNAB)
   a. Reliable and accurate, with sensitivity >90%
   b. Can determine the presence of malignant cells and **estrogen receptor** (ER) and **progesterone receptor** (PR) status but does not give information on tumor grade or the presence of invasion.
2. **Core needle biopsy** is preferred over FNAB as it can distinguish between invasive and noninvasive cancer and provides information on tumor grade as well as receptor status.
3. **Excisional biopsy** should primarily be used when a core biopsy cannot be done.
   a. Should be an infrequent diagnostic method.
   b. Performed in the operating room, and if feasible, incisions should be planned so that they can be incorporated into a future mastectomy incision.
   c. Masses should be excised as a single specimen and labeled to preserve three-dimensional orientations.
4. For **inflammatory breast cancer** with skin involvement, an incisional biopsy can consist of a **skin punch biopsy.**
5. Correlation between pathology results and imaging findings is mandatory.
   a. Patients with histologically benign findings on percutaneous biopsy do not require open biopsy if imaging and pathologic findings are concordant.
   b. Patients with high-risk lesions on image-guided biopsy (e.g., **atypical ductal hyperplasia** [ADH], **atypical lobular hyperplasia**

[ALH], **lobular carcinoma in situ** [LCIS], radial scar) may have malignancy at the same site and should undergo a surgical biopsy.

6. **Stereotactic core biopsy** is used for nonpalpable mammographically detected lesions, such as microcalcifications that cannot be seen with ultrasound imaging.
   a. A metallic marking clip is usually placed through the probe after sampling is complete to allow for identification of the biopsy site if excisional biopsy or partial mastectomy becomes necessary in the future.
   b. Contraindications include lesions close to the chest wall or in the axillary tail and thin breasts that may allow needle strikethrough into the thorax.
   c. Superficial lesions and lesions directly beneath the nipple–areolar complex are also often not approachable with stereotactic techniques.

III. BENIGN BREAST CONDITIONS

A. Fibrocystic breast change (FBC)

1. This refers to a variety of pathologic features including stromal fibrosis, macro- and microcysts, apocrine metaplasia, hyperplasia, and adenosis (which may be sclerosing, blunt duct, or florid).
2. FBC is common and may present as breast pain, a breast mass, nipple discharge, and/or abnormalities on mammography.
3. Patients presenting with suspected FBC should be reexamined in a short interval, preferably on day 10 of the menstrual cycle when hormonal influence is lowest and the mass may have diminished in size.
4. A persistent dominant mass must undergo further radiographic evaluation and tissue sampling, where indicated, to exclude cancer.

B. Breast cysts

1. Breast cysts frequently present as tender masses or as smooth, mobile, well-defined masses on palpation.
2. If discovered by mammography and confirmed as simple cysts by ultrasound imaging, asymptomatic cysts can be observed.
3. **Aspiration** can determine the nature of the mass (solid vs. cystic) but is not routinely necessary (see below), and cyst fluid color varies and can be clear, straw colored, or even dark green.
4. Symptomatic simple cysts should be aspirated.
   a. If no palpable mass is present after drainage, the patient should be evaluated in 3 to 4 weeks.
   b. If the cyst recurs, does not resolve completely with aspiration, or yields bloody fluid with aspiration, then mammography or ultrasound imaging should be performed to exclude intracystic tumor.
   c. Nonbloody clear fluid does not need to be sent for cytology.

C. Fibroadenoma

1. The most common discrete mass in women younger than 30 years
   a. Typically present as smooth, firm, mobile masses and can present as multiple lesions in 20% of cases.
   b. May enlarge during pregnancy and involute after menopause.

c. Have well-circumscribed borders on mammography and ultrasound imaging.
d. May be managed nonoperatively if clinical and radiographic appearance is consistent with a fibroadenoma, and it is <2 cm.
e. If the mass is symptomatic, >2 cm, or enlarges, it should be excised to rule out a malignant phyllodes tumor.

D. Mastalgia

1. Most women (70%) experience some form of breast pain or discomfort during their lifetime.
2. The pain may be cyclic (e.g., worse before a menstrual cycle) or noncyclical, which is more suspicious for malignancy, especially if focal and in association with a mass or bloody discharge.
3. In 15% of patients, the pain may be so disabling that it interferes with activities of daily living.
4. Etiology in most cases is benign disease; however, pain may be associated with cancer in up to 10% of patients.
5. Management
   a. Once cancer has been excluded, most patients can be managed successfully with symptomatic therapy and reassurance as it resolves in up to 30% of women, although it does recur in 60%.
   b. A well-fitting supportive bra is an important first step in pain relief.
   c. Topical NSAIDs (e.g., diclofenac gel) are considered first-line therapy.
   d. Low-dose Tamoxifen has been shown to provide good pain relief with tolerable side effects, although concerns over increased risks of endometrial cancer limit long-term use.
   e. Danazol, Bromocriptine, and Gonadorelin analogues treatment should be limited to refractory cases as they have significant side effects.
   f. Many patients also experience symptomatic relief by reducing caffeine intake or by taking vitamin E or evening primrose oil, although there is no scientific evidence supporting these lifestyle modifications.
6. Special circumstances
   a. Superficial thrombophlebitis of the veins overlying the breast (**Mondor disease**) may present as breast pain, and treatment is conservative with NSAIDs and hot compresses; antibiotics are not generally indicated.
   b. Breast pain in pregnancy and lactation can occur from engorgement, clogged ducts, trauma to the areola and nipple from pumping or nursing, or any of the aforementioned sources, and this is usually treated with warm compresses, soaks, and massage.

E. Nipple discharge

1. Lactation is the most common physiologic cause of nipple discharge.
   a. May continue for up to 2 years after cessation of breastfeeding.
   b. In parous nonlactating women, a small amount of milk may be expressed from multiple ducts and requires no treatment.

c. **Galactorrhea**
   i. Milky discharge unrelated to breastfeeding
   ii. Physiologic galactorrhea is the continued production of milk after lactation has ceased and menses has resumed, often caused by continued mechanical stimulation of the nipples.
   iii. Drug-related galactorrhea is generally bilateral and nonbloody and is caused by medications that affect the hypothalamic–pituitary axis by depleting dopamine (e.g., tricyclic antidepressants, reserpine, methyldopa, cimetidine, and benzodiazepines), blocking the dopamine receptor (e.g., phenothiazine, metoclopramide, and haloperidol), and/or having an estrogenic effect (e.g., digitalis).
   iv. Spontaneous galactorrhea in a nonlactating patient may be due to a pituitary prolactinoma and may be associated with amenorrhea.
      a) The diagnosis is established by measuring the serum prolactin level and performing a CT or MRI scan of the pituitary gland.
      b) Treatment is bromocriptine or resection of the prolactinoma.

d. Pathologic nipple discharge is usually bloody, spontaneous, unilateral, and/or originates from a single duct.
   i. Malignancy is the underlying cause in 10% of patients.
   ii. If not associated with a mass, the most likely etiologies are **benign intraductal papilloma** (peripheral papillomas put patients at slightly higher risk of malignancy), duct ectasia, and fibrocystic changes.
   iii. In lactating women, serosanguineous or bloody discharge can be associated with duct trauma, infection, or epithelial proliferation associated with breast enlargement.
   iv. Patients with persistent spontaneous discharge from a single duct require a surgical microdochectomy (i.e., excision of a single duct and its associated lobule) using a ductogram or ductoscopy or major duct excision (i.e., excision of all retroareolar ducts).

F. Breast infections
   1. **Lactational mastitis** is most commonly caused by *Staphylococcus aureus*.
   2. Presents as a swollen, erythematous, and tender breast.
   3. Purulent discharge from the nipple is uncommon.
   4. In the early cellulitic phase, the treatment is antibiotics, and the frequency of nursing or pumping should be *increased*.
   5. Approximately 25% of cellulitis progresses to abscess formation.
   6. Breast abscesses occur in the later stages and are often *not* fluctuant.
      a. The diagnosis is made by failure to improve on antibiotics, abscess cavity seen on ultrasound imaging, or aspiration of pus.
      b. Treatment is cessation of nursing and surgical drainage.

G. Granulomatous mastitis
   1. Presents as a painful breast mass that can mimic an abscess or malignancy with skin changes and ulceration.

2. Patients often present with repeated symptoms with slow resolution with nonoperative management.
3. Diagnosis is obtained via core needle biopsy of the mass, which demonstrates chronic necrotizing granulomatous lobulitis.
4. Management is with NSAIDs and antibiotics if a concomitant abscess develops, and immunosuppression with steroids or methotrexate is indicated in select circumstances.
5. Operative intervention is not generally recommended.

H. Nonpuerperal abscesses
1. Result from **duct ectasia** with periductal mastitis, infected cysts, infected hematoma, or hematogenous spread from another source.
2. Usually located in the peri/retroareolar area.
3. Anaerobes are the most common causative agent, although antibiotics should cover both anaerobic and aerobic organisms.
4. Treatment is surgical drainage.

I. Gynecomastia
1. Gynecomastia is hypertrophy of breast tissue in men that is usually secondary to an imbalance between the breast stimulatory effects of estrogen and the inhibitory effects of androgens.
2. Senescent gynecomastia is commonly seen after the age of 70 years as testosterone levels decrease.
3. Drugs that cause galactorrhea in women, including digoxin, spironolactone, methyldopa, cimetidine, tricyclic antidepressants, phenothiazine, reserpine, and marijuana, may result in gynecomastia in men.
4. Drugs used for androgen blockade, such as luteinizing hormone releasing hormone analogues for the treatment of prostate cancer and 5-alpha reductase inhibitors (e.g., finasteride) for the management of benign prostatic hypertrophy may also result in gynecomastia.
5. Tumors can cause gynecomastia secondary to excess secretion of estrogens (e.g., testicular teratomas and seminomas, bronchogenic carcinomas, adrenal tumors, and tumors of the pituitary and hypothalamus).
6. Gynecomastia may be a manifestation of systemic diseases such as hepatic cirrhosis, renal failure, hyperthyroidism, and malnutrition.
7. Cancer should be excluded by mammography and subsequently by biopsy if a mass is found, and if workup fails to reveal a medically treatable cause, or if the enlargement fails to regress, excision of breast tissue can be performed.
8. Pubertal hypertrophy occurs in adolescent boys, is usually bilateral, and resolves spontaneously in 6 to 12 months.

J. High-risk and premalignant conditions
1. ADH and ALH are proliferative lesions with cell atypia that arise within breast ducts and lobules, respectively.
2. ADH and ALH confer a 4 to 5 times increased relative risk of developing an invasive breast malignancy.

3. If atypia is found on needle biopsy, excisional biopsy is warranted to rule out associated malignancy.
   a. If no malignancy is found on postoperative pathology, patients with these conditions can simply undergo surveillance with imaging and physician examination at increased intervals as compared with low-risk patients.
   b. Chemoprevention with tamoxifen may also be considered.

K. LCIS
1. Not considered a preinvasive lesion but rather an indicator for increased breast cancer risk of approximately 1% per year.
2. It may be multifocal or bilateral.
3. Cancer that develops may be invasive ductal or lobular and may occur in either breast.
4. Treatment options include (1) lifelong close surveillance, (2) bilateral total mastectomies with immediate reconstruction for selected women with a strong family history after appropriate counseling, or (3) chemoprevention with tamoxifen, raloxifene, or an aromatase inhibitor.

IV. MALIGNANCY OF THE BREAST

A. Epidemiology
1. Breast cancer is the most common noncutaneous cancer in women, representing 30% of all female cancers in the US.
2. One in eight women will develop breast cancer during their lifetime.
3. Breast cancer is the second leading cause of cancer death in women, exceeded only by lung cancer.

B. Staging
1. Breast cancer stage is summarized using the American Joint Committee on Cancer (AJCC) **TNM staging system** (Chapter 48: Breast; *AJCC Cancer Staging Manual*, 8th ed.), which is both a clinical and pathologic staging system based on tumor size and chest wall involvement, level and/or number/extent of lymph nodes with metastases, and absence or presence and extent of distant metastases.[3]
   a. TNM staging is not applicable to breast sarcomas, lymphomas, or phyllodes tumors.
2. Workup should include the following in addition to breast-specific imaging:
   a. Complete blood cell count, complete metabolic panel including liver function tests (LFTs)
   b. A bone scan, if the alkaline phosphatase or calcium level is elevated, or if clinically symptomatic
   c. CT of the abdomen if LFTs are abnormal
   d. Patients with clinical stage III or IV disease should undergo bone scan and CT of the chest, abdomen, and pelvis due to a high probability of distant metastases.

C. Tumor biomarkers and prognostic factors

1. Tumor markers should be evaluated on all tumor specimens
   a. Expression of ER and PR should be evaluated by immunohistochemistry with ER and PR staining being a good prognostic factor.
   b. **Human epidermal growth factor receptor 2 (HER2)/neu** expression is measured by immunohistochemistry and, if equivocal, by fluorescence in situ hybridization.
      i. Overexpression of HER2/neu is a poor prognostic factor and is associated with increased rates of metastasis, decreased time to recurrence, and decreased overall survival.[4]
      ii. Patients with HER2/neu amplified tumors are treated with targeted monoclonal antibody therapies, such as Trastuzumab or Pertuzumab, which have demonstrated improvements in progression-free survival for these patients.
2. The presence or absence of disease in axillary lymph nodes is the single most important prognostic factor in breast cancer.[5]
3. Tumor size and grade are the most reliable pathologic predictors of outcome for patients without axillary nodal involvement.
4. Other adverse tumor characteristics include lack of expression of any tumor biomarkers, known as **triple-negative breast cancer**, lymphovascular invasion, and other indicators of a high proliferative rate (e.g., >20% Ki-67).
5. A number of **genome-based prediction tools** have also been developed to help predict patients who may be at risk for recurrent malignancy.[6]
   a. The most widely used currently being "Oncotype Dx," which analyzes specific genes to develop a recurrence score.
   b. In women with early-stage breast cancer, this helps determine which patients would benefit from adjuvant chemotherapy.

D. Ductal carcinoma in situ (DCIS).

1. Lesion with malignant cells that have not penetrated the basement membrane of the mammary ducts, and is treated as a malignancy because it has the potential to develop into an invasive breast cancer.
2. Physical examination is normal in the majority of patients.
3. Usually detected by mammography as clustered pleomorphic calcifications (**Figure 27.2**).
4. Can be **multifocal** (two or more lesions >5 mm apart within the same index quadrant) or **multicentric** (in different quadrants).
5. There are five main **architectural subtypes:** Papillary, micropapillary, solid, cribriform, and comedo (necrosis).
6. ER and PR expression levels should be assessed if hormone therapy is being considered.
   a. For patients with ER-positive DCIS, adjuvant antiestrogen therapy can reduce the risk of breast cancer recurrence and the risk of developing a new contralateral breast cancer but confers no survival benefit.
7. Surgical excision with negative margins >2 mm is recommended therapy when followed by whole breast irradiation.
   a. The addition of **adjuvant radiation** reduces the local recurrence rate but does not impact survival.
   b. Approximately half of DCIS recurrences present as invasive ductal carcinomas.

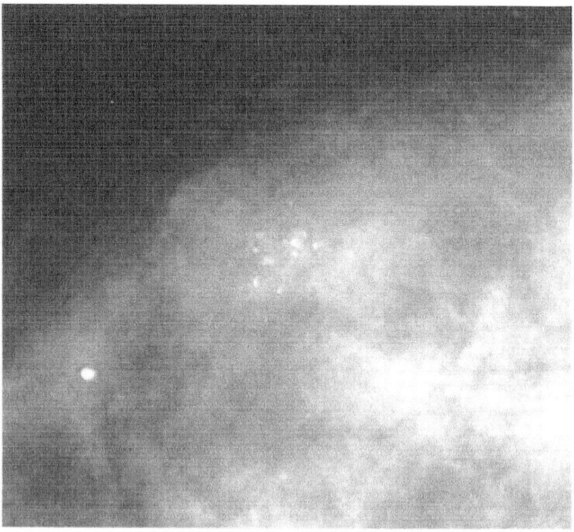

FIGURE 27.2 Mammogram of ductal carcinoma in situ. *(Reprinted with permission from Harris JR, Lippman ME, Osborne CK, et al., eds. Diseases of the breast. 5th ed. Wolters Kluwer Health; 2014.)*

8. **Partial mastectomy** is considered for unicentric lesions, whereas **total (simple) mastectomy** with or without immediate reconstruction is recommended for patients with multicentric lesions, extensive involvement of the breast (i.e., high tumor-to-breast-size ratio), or persistently positive margins with partial mastectomy.
9. Adjuvant radiation should be considered for all patients with DCIS treated with partial mastectomy to decrease the rate of local recurrence, particularly younger women with close margins or large tumors, although there is no survival benefit associated with adjuvant radiation therapy.
10. Axillary dissection should never be performed for pure DCIS.
11. **Sentinel lymph node biopsy** (SLNB)
    a. May be considered when there is a reasonable probability of finding invasive cancer on final pathologic examination (e.g., >4 cm, palpable, comedo subtype, or high grade); however, this is an area of ongoing controversy and research.
    b. A positive sentinel node indicates invasive breast cancer and changes the stage of the disease (see Management of the Axilla).

E. Invasive breast cancer

1. **Common histologies** include infiltrating ductal (75%-80%), infiltrating lobular (5%-10%), medullary (5%-7%), mucinous (3%), and tubular (1%-2%).
2. Surgical options for early-stage (T1–2, N1, or less clinical disease) breast cancer include **breast conservation therapy** (BCT) with adjuvant radiation therapy and mastectomy with or without reconstruction.

3. **Surgical approach: Simple mastectomy**
   a. The patient is positioned in the supine position, arms out, and the ipsilateral breast is prepped and draped in standard sterile fashion.
   b. A surgical time-out is completed, identifying the appropriate procedures, laterality, and indications being performed.
   c. A skin incision is made based on the location of the tumor and/or reconstruction to be pursued:
      i. If simple mastectomy without reconstruction is to be pursued, the skin incision is generally transverse and elliptical and surrounds the central breast and nipple–areolar complex so that this may be removed.
      ii. If a **nipple-sparing mastectomy** is to be pursued, an inframammary, periareolar incision is created.
      iii. If a **skin-sparing mastectomy** is to be pursued, a circumferential periareolar, periareolar ellipse, or circumferential periareolar with lateral or vertical incision is used.
      iv. In instances where the tumor invades the skin, the affected skin must be resected at the time of operation.
   d. Skin flaps are raised superiorly to the clavicle, inferiorly to the superior aspect of the rectus sheath, medially to the sternal border, and laterally to the edge of the latissimus dorsi muscle.
   e. Remove the breast tissue off the pectoralis fascia. The specimen is oriented for pathology and passed off the field.
   f. Hemostasis is ensured and a surgical drain is placed in the surgical bed over the pectoral fascia.
   g. The incision is closed in layers and skin approximated.
4. Breast conservation therapy (partial mastectomy) and SLNB with adjuvant radiation therapy has demonstrated survival and recurrence rates comparable with mastectomy.[7,8]
5. BCT is contraindicated in patients with unreliable follow-up, when the extent of disease prevents adequate negative margins, when there is a high tumor-to-breast-size ratio that prevents adequate resection without major deformity, with persistently positive margins on re-excision partial mastectomy and with the inability to receive adjuvant radiation (e.g., prior radiation to the chest wall, first- and second-trimester pregnancy in which the delay of radiation to the postpartum state is inappropriate, collagen vascular diseases such as scleroderma).[7,8]
   a. Neoadjuvant chemotherapy and/or neoadjuvant hormonal therapy should be administered to all patients with primary tumors measuring >2 cm, node-positive disease at presentation, triple-negative breast cancer, or HER2-positive disease.[9,10]
   b. Adjuvant radiotherapy decreases the breast cancer recurrence rate from approximately 35% to <10% at 12 years and is a required component of BCT.
   c. Follow-up after BCT includes annual physical examinations and annual bilateral mammography.
   d. Total (simple) mastectomy with SLNB is considered for patients with a clinically negative axilla.

i. A skin-sparing mastectomy (preserves skin envelope and inframammary ridge) may be performed with immediate reconstruction, resulting in improved cosmesis.

ii. The nipple–areolar complex, a rim of periareolar breast skin, and any previous excisional biopsy or partial mastectomy scars are excised.

iii. Nipple-sparing mastectomy, in which all of the skin including the nipple–areolar complex is left in place, may also be an option for select patients presenting with primary lesions 2 cm or more from the nipple base and lack of severe ptosis.

iv. Patients undergoing nipple-sparing mastectomy must be counseled that the preserved nipple is often insensate and that nipple necrosis is not an infrequent complication of the procedure, occurring in an estimated 10% to 15% of patients.

v. Follow-up after mastectomy includes physical examination at 6 months, 12 months, and then annually.

vi. Mammography of the contralateral breast should continue yearly.

vii. **Modified radical mastectomy** (MRM) involves total mastectomy, and ALND and is indicated for patients with clinically positive lymph nodes or a positive (i.e., with macrometastases) axillary node based on previous SLNB or FNAB.

viii. **Radical (Halsted) mastectomy,** which is largely historical and is rarely, if ever, performed in modern practice, involves total mastectomy, complete ALND (levels I, II, and III), removal of the pectoralis major and minor muscles, and removal of all overlying skin.

ix. Immediate reconstruction at the time of mastectomy should be offered to eligible patients.

a) Options include latissimus dorsi myocutaneous flaps, transverse rectus abdominis myocutaneous flaps, and inflatable tissue expanders followed by exchange for saline or silicone implants.

b) Immediate reconstruction has been shown not to affect patient outcome adversely or delay chemotherapy, and the detection of subsequent recurrence is also not delayed.

F. Management of the axilla

1. **SLNB**

a. Justification

i. Approximately 30% of patients with clinically negative examinations will have positive lymph nodes in an ALND specimen.

ii. Given the associated morbidity with ALNB, SLNB was developed to provide effective sampling of axillary lymph nodes with less morbidity.

iii. The use of SLNB was furthered by data from ACOSOG Z0011 and ACOSOG Z1071 clinical trials, which demonstrated equivalent disease recurrence between ALNB and SLNB.[11,12]

b. Requires a multidisciplinary approach, often including nuclear medicine, pathology, and radiology.

c. **Surgical approach: SLNB**

   i. The patient is positioned in the supine position, arms out, and the ipsilateral axilla is prepped and draped in standard sterile fashion, and a surgical time-out is completed identifying the appropriate procedures, laterality, and indications being performed.

   ii. If **blue dye** (either Lymphazurin or methylene blue) is to be used, this should be injected, and if previously a **technetium-labeled sulfur colloid** was injected in the nuclear medicine department, relevant counts can be measured to guide the extent of surgical resection/biopsy.

      a) The combination of blue dye and radioisotope provides higher node identification rates and increases the sensitivity of the procedure relative to using either agent alone.

      b) **Indocyanine green** may also be used as an alternative to the blue dye; however, the efficacy of this is yet to be completely studied.

   iii. A skin incision is made below the axillary hairline (if using a separate incision from the mastectomy incision). This can be performed along the pectoralis muscle and along the latissimus dorsi muscle.

   iv. The incision is carried down to the clavipectoral fascia, which is divided to expose the axillary tissue.

   v. Lymphatic tissue is identified by its blue color, by high activity detected by a hand-held gamma probe, and/or by a blue lymphatic seen to enter a nonblue node and is removed. Palpable nodes are also considered sentinel nodes even if not blue or radioactive and are also sampled.

   vi. Care is taken to ensure hemostasis and to ensure ligation of relevant lymphatic structures. If being used, the hand-held gamma probe is used to measure activity following removal of sentinel lymph nodes to ensure radiation values measuring <10% of the removed nodes is obtained.

   vii. The clavipectoral fascia is reapproximated, and surgical incision **closed with layers** and skin approximated.

d. All node-positive patients should be considered for adjuvant chemotherapy.

e. Patients with early T stage breast cancer with positive SLN may benefit from adjuvant radiation therapy to the axilla as an alternative to ALND as evidenced from the AMAROS noninferiority study.

2. ALND

   a. Patients with clinically positive lymph nodes should undergo ALND for local control.

   b. Includes removal of level I and level II nodes and, if grossly involved, level III nodes while motor and sensory nerves are preserved unless there is direct tumor involvement.

   c. Patients with four or more positive lymph nodes should undergo adjuvant radiation to the axilla, and selective patients with one to three positive nodes may benefit from radiation therapy to the axilla.

d. **Surgical approach: ALND**
   i. The patient is positioned in the supine position, arms out, and the ipsilateral axilla is prepped and draped in standard sterile fashion, and a surgical time-out is completed identifying the appropriate procedures, laterality, and indications being performed.
   ii. A skin incision is made below the axillary hairline (if using a separate incision from the mastectomy incision). This can be performed along the pectoralis muscle and along the latissimus dorsi muscle.
   iii. The incision is carried down to the clavipectoral fascia, which is divided to expose the axillary tissue.
   iv. Additional dissection is completed to define the pectoral muscles and preserve the median pectoral neurovascular bundle.
   v. The latissimus dorsi muscle is identified and further dissection is performed superiorly along the latissimus dorsi muscle to visualize the axillary vein and the thoracodorsal neurovascular bundle along the latissimus dorsi muscle. The long thoracic nerve is identified along the serratus anterior muscle and preserved.
   vi. Nodal tissue from levels I and II is identified and removed with careful hemostasis and ensuring ligation of relevant lymphatics. Relevant specimens are labeled and appropriately oriented/identified for pathology.
   vii. The clavipectoral fascia is reapproximated, and surgical incision closed with layers and skin approximated (a closed suction drain may be placed in the axillary space through a separate stab incision in the low axilla above the bra line).

e. Complications
   i. The most frequent postoperative complications are wound infections and seromas, and persistent seroma may be treated with repeated aspirations or reinsertion of a drain.
   ii. Other complications include pain and numbness in the axilla and upper arm, as well as impaired shoulder mobility.
   iii. **Lymphedema** occurs in approximately 10% to 40% of women undergoing ALND, and radiation to the axilla increases the risk of lymphedema.
      a) The most effective therapy is early intervention with intense occupational therapy with massage.
      b) Graded pneumatic compression devices and a professionally fitted compression sleeve can also provide relief and prevent worsening lymphedema.
      c) Blood draws, blood pressure cuffs, and intravenous lines should be avoided in the affected arm, mainly to avoid infection, and infections of the hand or arm should be treated promptly and aggressively with antibiotics and arm elevation because infection can further damage lymphatics leading to irreversible lymphedema.
      d) Lymphedema increases the risk of developing **angiosarcoma.**
   iv. All node-positive patients should be considered for adjuvant chemotherapy.
   v. Node-negative patients may have increased disease-free survival from adjuvant chemotherapy and/or hormonal therapy.

G. Locally advanced breast cancer (LABC)

1. Definition: Includes AJCC cT3, cT4, cN2, and/or cN3 clinical disease.
2. As up to 10% to 20% of patients have distant metastasis at the time of presentation with LABC, all should receive a bone scan and CT of the chest and abdomen before treatment.
3. Patients presenting with noninflammatory LABC should receive neoadjuvant chemotherapy (which also provides information regarding tumor response to treatment that may aid to guide further adjuvant therapy) followed by surgery and radiation.[9,10]
4. **Inflammatory LABC** (AJCC cT4d) represents 1% to 6% of all breast cancers and is characterized by erythema, warmth, tenderness, and edema (**Figure 27.3**), which can be misdiagnosed initially as mastitis.
   a. Skin punch biopsy confirms the diagnosis, and in two-thirds of cases, tumor emboli are seen in dermal lymphatics. An underlying mass is present in 70% of cases, and axillary adenopathy is noted in 50% of cases.
   b. Approximately 30% of patients have distant metastasis at the time of diagnosis.
   c. Despite aggressive multimodal therapy, median survival is approximately 2 years with a 5-year survival of only 5%.
5. Owing to the high risk for local and distant recurrence, patients should be examined every 3 months by all specialists involved in their care.
6. Patients with locoregional recurrence should complete a metastatic workup to exclude visceral or bony disease and should be considered for systemic chemotherapy or hormonal therapy.

V. SPECIAL CONSIDERATIONS

A. Breast conditions during pregnancy

1. Bloody nipple discharge may occur in the second or third trimester, typically resulting from epithelial proliferation under hormonal influences and usually resolves by 2 months postpartum.
   a. If it does not resolve, standard evaluation of pathologic nipple discharge should be undertaken (see above).

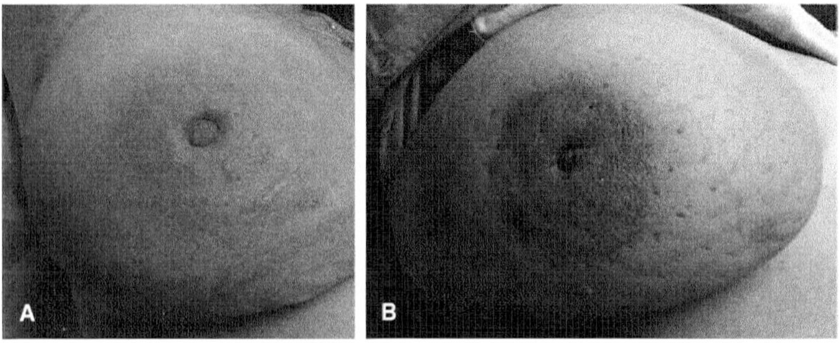

FIGURE 27.3 Classic clinical features of inflammatory breast cancer, including (A) erythema and (B) peau d'orange. *(Reprinted with permission from Harris JR, Lippman ME, Osborne CK, et al., eds. Diseases of the breast. 5th ed. Wolters Kluwer Health; 2014.)*

2. Breast masses occurring during pregnancy include galactoceles, lactating adenoma, simple cysts, breast infarcts, fibroadenomas, *and* carcinoma.
   a. **Fibroadenomas** may grow during pregnancy due to hormonal stimulation.
   b. Masses should be evaluated by ultrasound imaging, and a core needle biopsy should be performed for any suspicious lesion.
   c. Mammography can be performed with uterine shielding but is rarely helpful due to increased breast density.

B. Breast cancer during pregnancy
   1. May be difficult to diagnose due to low levels of suspicion and increased breast nodularity and density.
   2. If a breast lesion is diagnosed as malignant, the patient should be given the same surgical treatment options, stage for stage, as a nonpregnant woman, and the treatment should not be delayed because of the pregnancy.
   3. Therapeutic decisions are influenced by the clinical cancer stage and the trimester of pregnancy and must be individualized.
   4. For advanced-stage disease, MRI scan or ultrasound imaging may be used in lieu of CT for staging.
   5. Excisional biopsy can be safely performed under local anesthesia if there is some contraindication to the preferred core needle biopsy.
   6. The radiation component of BCT cannot be applied during pregnancy, and delaying radiation therapy is not ideal; thus BCT is usually not recommended to patients in their first or second trimester, but for patients in the third trimester, radiation can begin after delivery.
   7. Chemotherapy may be given by the mid-second trimester.

C. Paget disease of the nipple
   1. Characterized by eczematoid changes of the nipple–areolar complex, and burning, pruritus, and hypersensitivity may be prominent symptoms.
   2. Almost always accompanied by malignancy, and in 60% of cases is associated with a palpable mass.
   3. Mammography should be performed to identify other areas of involvement.
   4. If clinical suspicion is high, a pathologic diagnosis should be obtained by wedge biopsy of the nipple and underlying breast tissue.
   5. Treatment should include excision of the nipple–areolar complex (i.e., a central lumpectomy) but is otherwise dictated by the underlying malignancy.

D. Breast cancer in men
   1. This accounts for <1% of male cancers and <1% of all breast cancers.
   2. *BRCA2* mutations are associated with approximately 4% to 6% of these cancers.
   3. Mammography can be helpful in distinguishing gynecomastia from malignancy.
   4. Eighty-five percent of malignancies are infiltrating ductal carcinoma.
   5. MRM was traditionally the surgical procedure of choice; however, SLNB has been shown to be effective in men.
   6. Adjuvant hormonal, chemotherapeutic, and radiation treatment criteria are the same as in women.
   7. Overall survival per stage is comparable with that observed in women, although men tend to present in later stages.

E. Phyllodes tumors
   1. Phyllodes tumors account for 1% of breast neoplasms.
   2. Present as large, smooth, lobulated masses and may be difficult to distinguish from fibroadenomas on physical examination.
   3. Diagnosis is confirmed via a core needle biopsy.
   4. Ninety percent are benign, and thus 10% are malignant with biologic behavior similar to that of sarcomas.
   5. Treatment is wide local excision to tumor-free margins or total mastectomy.
   6. Axillary assessment is not needed in clinically node-negative patients.
   7. Tumors >5 cm in diameter and with evidence of stromal overgrowth may benefit from adjuvant chemotherapy.
   8. Patients should be followed with semiannual physical examinations and annual mammograms and chest radiographs.

Key References

Citation	Summary
– Veronesi U, Cascinelli N, Mariani L et al. Twenty-year follow-up of a randomized study comparing breast-conserving surgery with radical mastectomy for early breast cancer. *N Engl J Med.* 2002;347(16):1227-1232 – Fisher B, Bauer M, Margolese R et al. Five-year results of a randomized clinical trial comparing total mastectomy and segmental mastectomy with or without radiation in the treatment of breast cancer. *N Engl J Med.* 1985;312(11):665-673. – Fisher B, Anderson S, Bryant J et al. Twenty-year follow-up of a randomized trial comparing total mastectomy, lumpectomy, and lumpectomy plus irradiation for the treatment of invasive breast cancer. *N Engl J Med.* 2002;347(16):1233-1241	• Studies supporting use of breast conservation therapies with adjuvant radiation therapy.
– Fisher B, Brown A, Mamounas E et al. Effect of preoperative chemotherapy on local-regional disease in women with operable breast cancer: findings from National Surgical Adjuvant Breast and Bowel Project B-18. *J Clin Oncol.* 1997;15(7):2483-2493. – von Minckwitz G, Raab G, Caputo A et al. Doxorubicin with cyclophosphamide followed by docetaxel every 21 days compared with doxorubicin and docetaxel every 14 days as preoperative treatment in operable breast cancer: the GEPARDUO study of the German Breast Group. *J Clin Oncol.* 2005;23(12):2676-2685. – Rastogi P, Anderson SJ, Bear HD et al. Preoperative chemotherapy: updates of National Surgical Adjuvant Breast and Bowel Project Protocols B-18 and B-27. J Clin Oncol. 2008 Feb 10;26(5):778-85.	• Studies supporting the use of neoadjuvant chemotherapy in breast cancer.

Citation	Summary
– Giuliano AE, Ballman KV, McCall L et al. Effect of axillary dissection vs no axillary dissection on 10-year overall survival among women with invasive breast cancer and sentinel node metastasis: the ACOSOG Z0011 (Alliance) Randomized Clinical Trial. *J Am Med Assoc.* 2017;318(10):918-926. – Giuliano AE, Hunt KK, Ballman KV et al. Axillary dissection vs no axillary dissection in women with invasive breast cancer and sentinel node metastasis: a randomized clinical trial. *J Am Med Assoc.* 2011;305(6):569-575. – Boughey JC, Suman VJ, Mittendorf EA et al. Alliance for clinical trials in oncology. Sentinel lymph node surgery after neoadjuvant chemotherapy in patients with node-positive breast cancer: the ACOSOG Z1071 (Alliance) clinical trial. *J Am Med Assoc.* 2013;310(14):1455-1461.	• Studies supporting the use of sentinel lymph node biopsy over routine axillary lymph node biopsy in clinically node-negative patients.

CHAPTER 27: BENIGN AND MALIGNANT DISEASES OF THE BREAST

Review Questions

1. What are the boundaries of the breast?
2. What are the boundaries of the axilla?
3. What group of women should undergo routine screening mammography?
4. What is the overall utility of administering adjuvant radiation therapy to patients undergoing breast conservation therapy (BCT)?
5. Among patients diagnosed with breast cancer, who should be considered for neoadjuvant chemotherapy?
6. What is a modified radical mastectomy?
7. What is a radical mastectomy?

REFERENCES

1. Klimberg VS, Hunt KK. Diseases of the breast. In: Townsend C, ed. *Sabiston Textbook of Surgery: The Biological Basis of Modern Surgical Practice*. 21st ed. Elselvier; 2021.
2. US Preventative Services Taskforce. *Breast Cancer: Screening*. 2016. Accessed 2023. https://www.uspreventiveservicestaskforce.org/uspstf/recommendation/breast-cancer-screening
3. Hortobagyi GN, Connolly JL, D'Orsi CJ, et al. Breast. In: Amin MB, ed. *AJCC Cancer Staging Manual*, 8th ed. Springer; 2017:589-628.
4. Burstein HJ. The distinctive nature of HER2-positive breast cancers. *N Engl J Med.* 2005;353(16):1652-1654.
5. Tonellotto F, Bergmann A, de Souza Abrahao K, de Aguiar SS, Bello MA, Thuler LCS. Impact of number of positive lymph nodes and lymph node ratio on survival of women with node-positive breast cancer. *Eur J Breast Health.* 2019;15(2):76-84.

6. Gluz O, Nitz UA, Christgen M, et al. West German study group phase III PlanB trial: first prospective outcome data for the 21-gene recurrence score assay and concordance of prognostic markers by central and local pathology assessment. *J Clin Oncol.* 2016;34(20):2341-2349.
7. Veronesi U, Cascinelli N, Mariani L, et al. Twenty-year follow-up of a randomized study comparing breast-conserving surgery with radical mastectomy for early breast cancer. *N Engl J Med.* 2002;347(16):1227-1232.
8. Fisher B, Anderson S, Bryant J, et al. Twenty-year follow-up of a randomized trial comparing total mastectomy, lumpectomy, and lumpectomy plus irradiation for the treatment of invasive breast cancer. *N Engl J Med.* 2002;347(16):1233-1241.
9. Rastogi P, Anderson SJ, Bear HD, et al. Preoperative chemotherapy: updates of national surgical adjuvant breast and bowel project protocols B-18 and B-27. *J Clin Oncol.* 2008;26(5):778-785.
10. Korde LA, Somerfield MR, Carey LA, et al. Neoadjuvant chemotherapy, endocrine therapy, and targeted therapy for breast cancer: ASCO guideline. *J Clin Oncol.* 2021;39(13):1485-1505.
11. Giuliano AE, Ballman KV, McCall L, et al. Effect of axillary dissection vs No axillary dissection on 10-year overall survival among women with invasive breast cancer and sentinel node metastasis: the ACOSOG Z0011 (alliance) randomized clinical trial. *J Am Med Assoc.* 2017;318(10):918-926.
12. Boughey JC, Suman VJ, Mittendorf EA, et al. Sentinel lymph node surgery after neoadjuvant chemotherapy in patients with node-positive breast cancer: the ACOSOG Z1071 (Alliance) clinical trial. *J Am Med Assoc.* 2013;310(14):1455-1461.

28 Skin and Soft Tissue Tumors

Ken Newcomer and Ryan C. Fields

I. SKIN LESIONS

A. Diagnosis
1. Physical examination is the mainstay of diagnosis.
   a. Melanoma is not limited to cutaneous surfaces, and examination for subungual, uveal, and mucosal lesions is essential.
2. Color, size, shape, borders, elevation, location, firmness, and surface characteristics should be documented.
   a. Uniformly colored, small, round, circumscribed lesions are more likely to be benign while irregularly colored, larger, asymmetric lesions with indistinct borders and ulceration are worrisome for malignancy.
   b. Melanoma may present with nonpigmented macules/papules, or classically as pigmented skin lesions.
3. Consider ABCDE: Asymmetry, Borders, Color variation, Diameter, and Evolution (**Figure 28.1**).

B. Biopsy
1. Warranted for lesions with worrisome features or that change over time.
2. Full-thickness tissue biopsy is preferred, including the entire lesion with clinically negative margins.
   a. Deep shave, punch, or excisional biopsy.
   b. Biopsy should include the thickest portion of the lesion, avoiding areas of crusting, ulceration, or necrosis.
3. Incisional biopsies should be oriented parallel to **Langer's lines** to facilitate subsequent wide resection and closure.
4. For pigmented lesions, it is essential that the specimen allows for assessment of the **Breslow depth** (thickness of the melanoma from the surface of the skin to the deepest point of the tumor) of invasion (**Figure 28.2**).
5. Superficial shave biopsies should be avoided, but deep shave biopsies are usually adequate.[1]
6. **Fine-needle aspiration** (FNA) biopsy is the modality of choice for clinically positive lymph nodes.

II. MELANOMA

A. Etiology and epidemiology
1. The incidence of melanoma continues to rise at an epidemic rate and is currently the fifth-most common cancer in the US.[2]

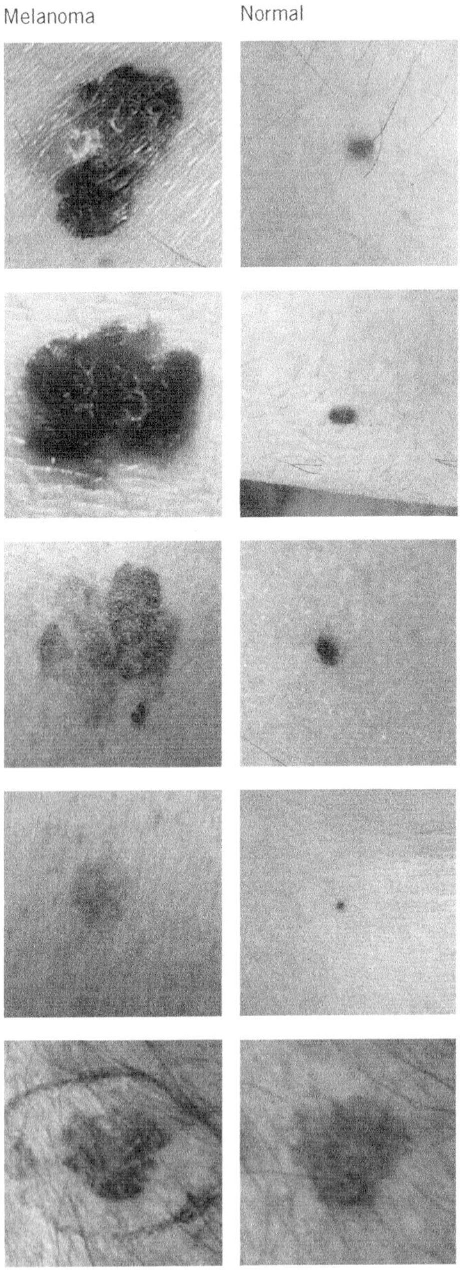

ASYMMETRY:

Melanomas tend to lack symmetry, unlike benign nevi

BORDER:

The borders of melanomas are typically indistinct, with blurred or jagged edges

COLOR:

The color of a melanoma is often heterogeneous with tan, brown, black, red, blue, or white areas

DIAMETER:

Lesions larger than 6 mm are more concerning than smaller lesions

EVOLUTION:

A nevus that changes in shape, size, or color could represent a melanoma. The lesion pictured evolved from a red-tan lesion (right) to a darker brown lesion (left) over the course of 28 mo.

FIGURE 28.1 ABCDE of melanoma.

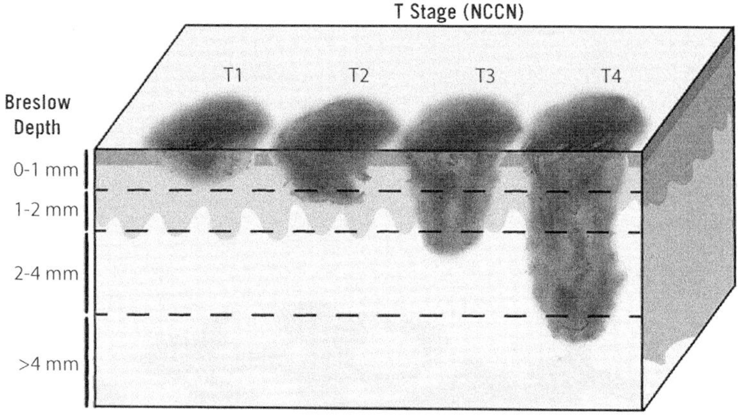

FIGURE 28.2 Depiction of Breslow depth. *(Courtesy of Erica K. Barnell.)*

2. Most pigmented skin lesions are benign, but most melanomas arise from pigmented nevi.
3. Breslow thickness is the most important factor in overall survival, nodal, and distal metastatic risk.[3]
   a. Lesions <1 mm thick have a 10-year survival of 92%.
   b. Lesions >4 mm thick have a 10-year survival of ~50%.
4. The presence of ulceration at the primary tumor is a negative prognostic factor.
5. Regional node metastasis severely worsens prognosis with 5-year survival, from 93% to 32%.
6. Distant metastases portend a dismal prognosis with 5-year survival, <10%.

B. Diagnosis
1. Risk factors
   a. Phenotypic factors (**Table 28.1**)
   b. Environmental risk largely related to prolonged or severe sun exposure.
      i. A history of peeling sunburn or tanning bed usage conveys a considerably increased risk.[4]
   c. Medical history
      i. Genetic conditions (e.g., xeroderma pigmentosum)
      ii. Immunosuppression (e.g., transplant, HIV)
      iii. History of prior cancer
      iv. Hereditary factors
   d. Family history
      i. About 5% to 12% of melanomas occur in a familial pattern.
      ii. **Familial atypical multiple-mole melanoma syndrome** conveys a substantial lifetime risk for melanoma.

TABLE 28.1 Relative Risk for Melanoma Associated With Phenotypic Factors

Phenotypic Factor	Relative Risk for Melanoma (95% Confidence Interval)
Family history	RR = 1.74, 1.41-2.14
Fitzpatrick skin type (I vs IV)	RR = 2.09, 1.67-2.58
High density of freckles	RR = 2.10, 1.80-2.45
Skin color (fair vs dark)	RR = 2.06, 1.68-2.52
Eye color (blue vs dark)	RR = 1.47, 1.28-1.69
Hair color (red vs dark)	RR = 3.64, 2.56-5.37

Reprinted from Newcomer K, Robbins KJ, Perone J, et al. Malignant melanoma: evolving practice management in an era of increasingly effective systemic therapies. *Curr Probl Surg.* 2022;59(1):101030. Copyright 2022, Elsevier. With permission.

a) Results from germline loss-of-function mutation in *CDKN2A* or, less commonly, an oncogenic *CDK4* mutation.

iii. Patients with a personal or family history of multiple melanomas or pancreatic cancer should be referred to genetic counseling based on available screening criteria (**Table 28.2**).

C. Imaging and laboratory studies

1. CT or positron emission tomography (PET) should be obtained for patients with an advanced (T4b) primary tumor, patients with stage III disease, or patients with symptoms concerning for advanced disease.
2. Brain MRI should be considered for stage IIIC or above.
3. **Lactate dehydrogenase** levels are not routinely obtained for initial staging.

D. Staging

1. Melanoma staging is summarized using the American Joint Committee on Cancer (AJCC) **TNM staging system** (Chapter 47: Melanoma of the Skin; *AJCC Cancer Staging Manual*, 8th ed.) based on tumor depth

TABLE 28.2 Rule of Two's and Three's for Familial Melanoma

- Any patient with three primary melanomas
- A patient with one primary melanoma and two 1st- or 2nd-degree relatives (same side) with a diagnosis of melanoma or pancreatic cancer

in the skin, number of lymph nodes with metastases (or local lymphatic spread, see below), and presence or absence of distant metastases.[5]

2. Histologic subtype is not a factor for staging, but some subtypes have differential sensitivity to adjuvant treatment and should be considered in treatment selection (e.g., nodular and pure desmoplastic).[6,7]
3. Breslow depth (or tumor thickness), measuring the depth of invasion of the primary tumor, is used to classify the tumor ("T classification").
4. Stage III melanomas are defined by the T stage and number of lymph nodes involved to reflect changing prognostic outcomes, especially with the development of systemic therapies (See AJCC guidelines for details).
5. **In-transit metastases** or **satellite lesions** (**Figure 28.3**) result from regional spread of tumor via dermal or subcutaneous lymphatic vessels, and are included, in part, as part of the AJCC nodal staging.
   a. Signifies poor prognosis with a high risk of local recurrence and distant metastasis.

E. Treatment

1. Surgical management
   a. Surgical decision making relies on many factors (**Figure 28.4**).
   b. Disagreement remains about best management for 1- to 2-mm melanomas, which is currently being addressed in the randomized **MelMarT trial** (enrollment in 2022).
2. **Surgical approach: Wide local excision (WLE)**
   a. Minimum appropriate margins are identified (**Figure 28.4**), and an elliptical incision is made around the lesion or biopsy site, including dermis and subcutaneous tissue.
   b. Incisions should be oriented longitudinally to facilitate wound closure along Langer's lines.

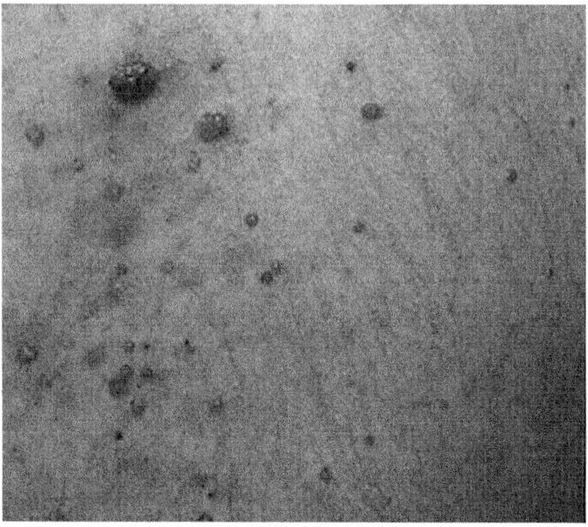

FIGURE 28.3 Cutaneous melanoma of the thigh with satellitosis.

   c. The soft tissue is completely excised. Deep fascia is typically spared unless visually involved.
   d. Specimen is oriented and passed off the field for permanent pathology.
   e. Hemostasis is obtained, and wounds are closed primarily in multiple layers, with flaps or skin grafts reserved for large defects.
3. **Surgical approach: Sentinel lymph node biopsy** (SLNB, **Figure 28.4** summarizes the indications)
   a. Preoperatively, the sentinel lymph node (SLN) is identified by scintigraphy. At the time of operation, dye is injected for visual identification (details below).
   b. Incision is made over lymph node bed, allowing for gentle exploration of the area with the assistance of gamma counter and visual feedback from blue dye.
   c. Excellent hemostasis must be obtained.
   d. Wound is closed in layers.
4. Detection of **sentinel nodes**
   a. Preoperative injection of both radiotracer and blue dye has led to SLN identification rate of 99%.[8] Based on these results, both radiotracer and dye are typically used for SLN detection unless contraindicated (see below).
   b. All lymph nodes with an intraoperative gamma count >10% of the most radioactive node should be resected.
   c. Blue dye (e.g., isosulfan blue or methylene blue) is injected into the subdermal tissue at the tumor site.
      i. **Methylene blue** can cause soft tissue necrosis if injected intradermally, and it is typically used only at sites that will be excised.
      ii. **Isosulfan blue** may cause anaphylaxis in patients with sulfa allergy.
      iii. All dyes are contraindicated in pregnant patients.
   d. SLNB is a nontherapeutic intervention, but it remains the strongest prognostic factor with respect to overall and melanoma-specific survival.
5. **Completion lymph node dissection** (CLND)
   a. Does not improve overall or melanoma-specific survival in large international RCTs.
      i. The "MSLT-II trial" compared patients with positive SLNB treated with CLND or nodal basin ultrasound surveillance. CLND increased the rate of regional disease control but did not improve melanoma-specific survival.[9]
      ii. The "DeCOG trial" showed no survival difference in patients treated with CLND compared with surveillance only.[10]
      iii. For patients with one to two occult positive SLN, active nodal basin surveillance with ultrasound is an acceptable treatment option.
6. **Therapeutic lymph node dissection** (TLND)
   a. Recommended for clinically positive or biopsy-proven axillary and superficial inguinal lymph nodes unless unresectable distant metastases are present.
   b. Pelvic TLND can achieve 5-year survival rates >40%.[11]

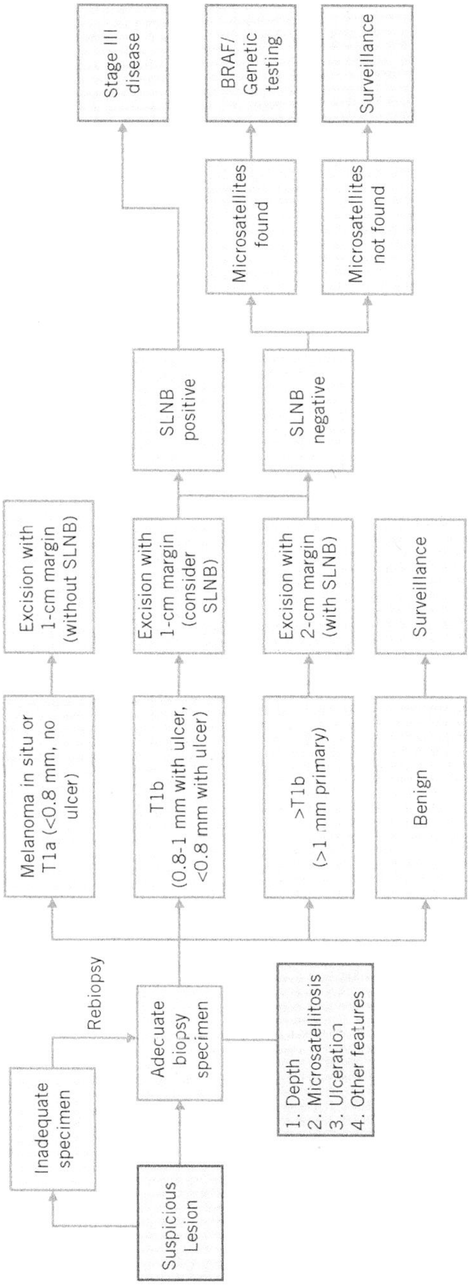

FIGURE 28.4 Treatment paradigm for operable melanoma.

c. For inguinal nodes, dissection is extended to the deep ilioinguinal region (including iliac and obturator lymph nodes) if there is radiographic evidence of lymph node involvement or if **Cloquet's node** is positive (most superior deep inguinal lymph node in the femoral canal).

7. Complications of melanoma excision
   a. Functional disability, infection, and difficulty with wound healing due to hematoma or lymph leak.
   b. For patients who have undergone CLND/TLND, **lymphedema** is a substantial problem.
      i. In MSLT-II, 24% of the patients in the CLND group reported lymphedema, which is treated with compression garments and physiotherapy.
8. Resection of metastases
   a. Curative or palliative resection is possible.
   b. Favorable factors for curative surgery include long disease-free intervals, fewer metastatic sites, responsiveness to targeted and/or systemic therapy, and good functional status.
   c. With the advent of effective systemic therapy, curative-intent surgery for metastatic disease is becoming more common.

F. Perioperative systemic therapy

1. Immunotherapy
   a. **Immune checkpoint proteins** such as programmed cell death 1 (PD-1) and cytotoxic T-lymphocyte associated protein 4 (CTLA-4) are associated with T-lymphocyte exhaustion and attenuated immune responses over time.
   b. Monoclonal antibodies that inactivate these checkpoints result in augmented antitumor immunity and are currently being used in single agent and combination therapy for patients with melanoma.
   c. Combination regimens have greater efficacy at the expense of increased adverse events.
      i. In patients with advanced melanoma, 5-year survival rate was higher with nivolumab (anti-PD1) and ipilimumab (anti-CTLA4) combined (52%) than with either nivolumab alone (44%) or ipilimumab alone (26%).[12]
   d. New checkpoint inhibitors are under investigation. Anti-PD1 and anti-Leukocyte Activation Gene 3 (LAG3) combination therapy recently received US Food and Drug Administration approval and may have a more favorable toxicity profile compared with PD-1/CTLA4 blockade.[13]
   e. Adverse events
      i. More often seen in combination regimens.
      ii. Common immune-related adverse events: Mucositis, skin lesions, fatigue, hepatotoxicity, endocrinopathy, pneumonitis.
      iii. Severe (grade III/IV) adverse events occur in up to 59% of patients with combination PD-1/CTLA-4 regimens.
2. **Kinase inhibitors**
   a. *BRAF* proto-oncogene encodes a protein kinase normally activated by Ras in response to extracellular cues.

b. An activating driver mutation in *BRAF* (typically at the V600 codon) is present in ~50% of patients with a new melanoma diagnosis. Testing for *BRAF* mutations is now standard of care for patients with advanced melanoma.
c. Targeted small molecule kinase inhibitors have been developed against the BRAF kinase (e.g., vemurafenib and dabrafenib) and one of its downstream effectors, MAP-Erk Kinase (MEK) (e.g., trametinib and cobimetinib).
d. Combination therapies with BRAF and MEK inhibitors have demonstrated improved efficacy over BRAF monotherapy for patients with *V600 BRAF* mutations.[14,15]
e. Adverse events of kinase inhibition
   i. Most common toxicities are cutaneous (nonspecific rash, phototoxicity, alopecia, petechiae, and easy bruising).
   ii. Fewer adverse events than immune checkpoint blockade.
3. Other systemic therapy
   a. Immunostimulatory molecules such as IFN-α and IL-2 have been historically used but are no longer first line.
4. Neoadjuvant treatment
   a. Currently under investigation.
   b. Most cases are considered as part of a clinical trial (**Figure 28.5**).
   c. Recent trials of combination immunotherapy in patients with confirmed nodal metastasis (e.g., OpACIN-neo trial) have demonstrated that resection of the primary tumor and "index" lymph nodes has equivalent clinical outcomes compared with CLND in patients who show major pathologic response to neoadjuvant treatment.[16]
   d. Neoadjuvant treatment of patients with clinical stage III disease is an area of active research.

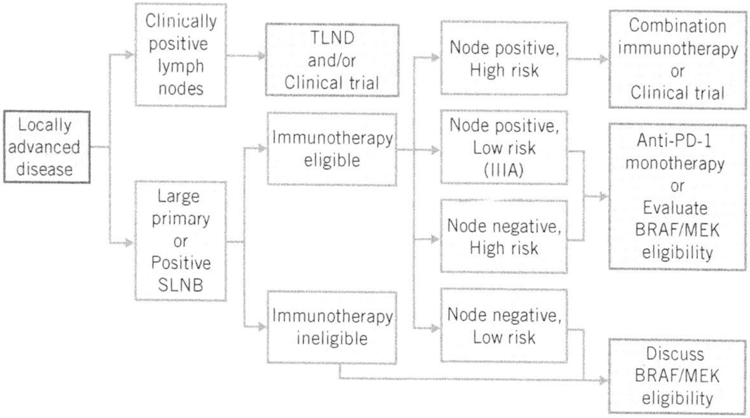

FIGURE 28.5 Management of locally advanced melanoma.

G. Regional therapies for melanoma

1. **Isolated limb perfusion** (ILP) or **isolated limb infusion** (ILI)
    a. Used for locally advanced and/or unresectable disease.
    b. Delivers high-dose regional chemotherapy to the affected extremity while minimizing systemic toxicity.
    c. ILI is simpler and less toxic than ILP, but its response rates are lower.[17,18]
2. **Intralesional therapy**
    a. Potentially a first-line treatment for select patients with unresectable disease, especially with in-transit metastases or small (<3 cm) visceral metastases.
    b. **Talimogene laherparepvec** (T-VEC) is an HSV-derived oncolytic agent designed to selectively replicate within tumors and produce granulocyte macrophage colony-stimulating factor, which enhances systemic antitumor immune responses.
        i. T-VEC has produced durable antitumor responses in advanced melanoma and may result in **abscopal effects** (i.e., shrinking of nontargeted remote tumor metastases).[19]
    c. Other historical agents include Coley's toxins (1890s), intralesional IL-2, bacillus Calmette–Guerin, and IFN-a. None of these are first-line treatments in modern melanoma therapy.

III. NONMELANOMA SKIN CANCERS

A. Basal cell carcinoma (BCC)

1. Etiology and epidemiology
    a. The most common skin cancer
    b. Slow growing, may be large, disfiguring, and locally invasive.
    c. Rarely metastasize (<0.1%)
    d. Sun exposure is the most significant epidemiologic factor.
    e. More common in patients >40 years old
2. Diagnosis
    a. Appearance
        i. Sun-exposed areas
        ii. Flat lesion with smooth, whitish, waxy surface and indistinct borders.
        iii. Most common is the noduloulcerative form—shiny translucent nodules with central umbilication and pearly, rolled edges.
    b. Skin biopsy
3. Treatment
    a. Recurrence risk determines treatment plan (**Table 28.3**).
    b. Surgical excision
        i. Generally with margin ≥4 mm
        ii. High-risk lesions require larger margins.
        iii. **Mohs micrographic surgery** is the gold standard for resection of high-risk tumors in cosmetically sensitive areas. It may also be used for re-excision of positive margins.
    c. Other treatments
        i. **Curettage with electrodesiccation** (CED)
            a) Used in low-risk areas without hair growth.

TABLE 28.3 High-Risk Factors for Local Recurrence or Metastases for Basal Cell Skin Cancer
Area L ≥ 20 mm
Area M ≥ 10 mm
Area H, any size
Aggressive growth pattern
Poorly defined borders
Immunosuppression
Site of prior RT
Recurrent BCC
Perineural involvement

Area H, "mask areas" of face (central face, eyelids, eyebrows, periorbital, nose, lips, chin, mandible, preauricular and postauricular skin, temple, ear), genitalia, hands, feet; area M, cheeks, forehead, scalp, neck, and pretibial; area L, trunk and extremities.

BCC, basal cell carcinoma; RT, radiation therapy.

b) Not recommended for high-risk lesions, because no specimen is available for margin evaluation.

ii. Radiation therapy
 a) For nonsurgical candidates, or as adjuvant therapy following resection of tumors with extensive perineural involvement

iii. Topical agents
 a) Cryotherapy, topical 5-fluorouracil (5-FU), topical imiquimod, and/or photodynamic therapy
 b) Generally reserved for low-risk lesions where resection and radiation are not options.

iv. Systemic agents
 a) Vismodegib and sonidegib **(hedgchog pathway inhibitors)** are therapies that have shown efficacy in patients with inoperable and metastatic BCC.[20,21]

B. Squamous cell carcinoma (SCC)

1. Etiology and epidemiology
 a. Second most common skin cancer
 b. Most common for patients with impaired immunity
 c. Most common risk factor—ultraviolet radiation
2. Diagnosis
 a. Appearance
  i. Sun-exposed areas

ii. May also develop in draining sinuses, radiation, chronic ulcers, scars, and burns (a.k.a., **Marjolin ulcers**).
iii. Firm, erythematous plaque with smooth or verrucous surface and indistinct margins.
iv. May be preceded by actinic keratosis.
v. Nodal metastasis is present in <1%.

3. Treatment
   a. Recurrence risk determines treatment plan (**Table 28.4**).
   b. Surgical treatment
      i. Low-risk lesions require surgical margin of at least 4 to 6 mm.
      ii. High-risk patients require larger margins.
   c. Nonsurgical treatment
      i. CED
         a) Can be used for low-risk lesions.
      ii. Radiation therapy
         a) Definitive therapy for nonsurgical candidates

TABLE 28.4 High-Risk Factors for Local Recurrence or Metastases for Squamous Cell Skin Cancer
Area L ≥ 20 mm
Area M ≥ 10 mm
Area H, any size
Poorly defined borders
Recurrent SCC
Immunosuppression
Site of prior RT
Rapidly growing tumor
Neurologic symptoms
Poorly differentiated
Acantholytic, adenosquamous, desmoplastic, or metaplastic subtypes
≥2 mm depth
Perineural, lymphatic, or vascular involvement

Area H, "mask areas" of face (central face, eyelids, eyebrows, periorbital, nose, lips, chin, mandible, preauricular and postauricular skin, temple, ear), genitalia, hands, feet; area M, cheeks, forehead, scalp, neck, and pretibial; area L, trunk and extremities.

SCC, squamous cell carcinoma; RT, radiation therapy.

b) Adjuvant treatment after resection for patients with extensive perineural involvement

c) Adjuvant therapy for patients with close or positive margins that are unresectable

d) Adjuvant therapy for patients with T3 or T4 tumors

iii. Topical therapies: Cryotherapy, topical 5-FU, imiquimod, or photodynamic therapy can be used for SCC in situ.

d. Systemic treatment

i. Cisplatin, cisplatin +5-FU, EGFR inhibitors (cetuximab), or checkpoint inhibitors may all be used for patients with metastatic disease.

C. Merkel cell carcinoma

1. Etiology and epidemiology

a. Rare

b. Derived from **neural crest cells** in basal epidermis

c. Risk factors

i. Immunosuppression

ii. Infection with oncovirus **Merkel cell polyoma virus** (MCPyV)

a) Eighty percent of new cases have MCPyV-mediated oncogenic transformation and detection of MCPyV oncoproteins.

iii. Virus-positive patients generally have better outcomes and can be serologically surveilled for recurrent disease.[22]

d. Aggressive with frequent local recurrence as well as nodal and metastatic disease.

2. Treatment

a. WLE of all superficial tissue with 1 to 2 cm margin

b. SLNB should be performed for all patients.

c. CLND or TLND with or without radiation therapy is performed for positive SLNB or for biopsy-proven regional disease.

d. Adjuvant radiation is used for patients at high risk for local recurrence.

i. Primary tumor size >1 cm

ii. Positive margins

iii. Lymphovascular invasion

e. Immunotherapy is used for patients with advanced disease.

i. Response rate to PD-L1 inhibitor (avelumab) in advanced lesions was 32% during 10-month median follow-up.[23]

ii. Pembrolizumab has been shown to be an effective first-line therapy for advanced lesions with response rate of 56%.[24]

IV. BENIGN SKIN LESIONS

A. Seborrheic keratoses

1. Irregularly rounded lesions with verrucous, friable, and waxy surface

2. Found in older people

3. No treatment required

4. If resection is desired, can have surgical excision, shave biopsy, CED, topical trichloroacetic acid, or cryotherapy.

5. Eruptive development of seborrheic keratoses (**sign of Leser–Trélat**) is a paraneoplastic syndrome most commonly associated with adenocarcinomas of the stomach and colon.

B. **Actinic keratosis**

1. Due to sun exposure
2. Small, flat, multiple reddish or black lesions
3. Have malignant potential—20% develop into well-differentiated SCC.
4. Treatment options include excision, cryotherapy, dermabrasion, laser therapy, chemical peel, photodynamic therapy, or topical agents.

C. **Dysplastic nevi**

1. Variegated color (tan to brown on pink base)
2. Large (5-12 mm) with irregular edges
3. Can have macular or papular components.
4. Patients with multiple dysplastic nevi should undergo frequent skin examinations to monitor for the ABCDE features of melanoma.
5. Changing or symptomatic lesions that are clinically suspicious for melanoma should be excised and sent for evaluation.

D. **Congenital nevi** ("birthmarks")

1. Increased risk of melanoma development particularly for giant congenital nevi (>20 cm).
2. Biopsied nevi with moderate or severe atypia should be excised.
3. **Spitz nevi** are pink-red papules that are benign melanocytic lesions seen in childhood.
   a. Histologically similar to melanoma leading to frequent misdiagnosis.
4. Treatment
   a. Small or medium-sized lesions can be observed or excised depending on the ability for follow-up and cosmetic effect.
   b. Large lesions are very rare, and observation vs. surgical approaches should be discussed with a multidisciplinary team.

V. SOFT TISSUE MASSES

A. Workup

1. History including location, duration, change in size, and associated symptoms
2. Physical examination including size, anatomic relationships, borders, and mobility as well as neurovascular and nodal examination of the affected area and region
3. Imaging
   a. MRI—best to determine relationship to large nerves and other structures.
      i. Main choice in pelvis, extremities, and trunk
      ii. T2-weighted and gadolinium enhancement can help distinguish normal edematous tissue and tumors.
   b. CT—best to determine relationship to vascular structures
      i. CT-guided core needle biopsy (CNBx) is used for tumors that are difficult to access.
   c. PET/CT—utilized for pathologically confirmed lesions for staging and prognosis as well as response to therapy
      i. Maximum standardized uptake value (SUVmax) is used to differentiate necrotic tumor or scar vs. metabolically active disease.

B. Biopsy
1. CNBx is preferred as it does not impact future surgical plans.
   a. Indeterminate results should be confirmed by repeat CNBx.
2. Incisional biopsy can be performed for masses >3 cm.
   a. Incision oriented parallel to long axis of extremity to allow for scar excision at next operation.
   b. Meticulous hemostasis is critical to prevent hemorrhage from spreading tumor.
   c. Drains should be avoided, but if needed, drain sites should be placed in excisable locations.
3. Excisional biopsy is reserved for tumors <3 cm or after failed attempts by other methods.
4. FNA is frequently only used to confirm recurrence or metastasis as it can determine the presence of malignancy and histologic type but cannot determine grade.

VI. SOFT TISSUE SARCOMA AND RELATED MALIGNANCIES

A. Epidemiology and etiology
1. Very rare (<1% of all new adult malignancies)
2. Very diverse set of cancers (>100 subtypes)
   a. Most common: **Undifferentiated pleomorphic sarcoma** (40%) and **liposarcoma** (25%)
3. Derived from connective tissue (typically mesoderm) vs. carcinoma, which arises from epithelial tissue (ectoderm).
4. Most commonly de novo but can be associated with congenital cancer syndromes (e.g., Li–Fraumeni or exposure [e.g., toxins or radiation]).
5. Hematologic spread is most common with rare lymph node metastasis (excluding rhabdomyosarcoma, epithelioid sarcoma, synovial sarcoma, clear cell sarcoma, angiosarcoma).[25]

B. Diagnosis
1. Should be evaluated by multidisciplinary team.
2. Presentation
   a. Extremities (thigh, buttock, groin, arm) are the most common sites (60%).
   b. Grow and expand along tissue planes.
   c. Tissues in body cavities (i.e., retroperitoneal sarcomas) may be asymptomatic until very large.
3. Diagnosis
   a. CNBx is the preferred method for diagnosis.
   b. MRI is the preferred imaging modality for soft tissue sarcoma (STS) of the extremities, head, and neck.
   c. CT scan is the most commonly used imaging technique for retroperitoneal and visceral sarcomas.
   d. Preoperative imaging of the tumor defines its relation to surrounding structures to determine feasibility of resection.

C. Classification/staging
1. Generally sarcomas are described by tissue of origin, histologic grade, and maximum diameter.

2. Tumor grade is the most important prognostic factor, but size is also directly related to prognosis.
3. Staging with chest CT
   a. Eighty percent of metastasis are to the lungs.
   b. Less aggressive tumors (e.g., well-differentiated liposarcoma) may not require chest CT.
4. Size, depth, grade, and presence of local or remote metastases are used to stage STS.

D. Treatment
1. Extremity sarcoma
   a. Limb-sparing treatment has equivalent outcomes compared with amputation and is now standard of care.
   b. Local excision and adjuvant radiation are the most common treatment.
      i. Low-grade tumors <5 cm that are superficial to the deep fascia may be treated with surgery alone.
      ii. **Myxofibrosarcoma and dermatofibrosarcoma protuberans** (DFSP; see below) require wider margins of resection as they have wide invasion along fibrous septae.
   c. Amputation may be required for advanced, recurrent, or extremely large tumors.
2. Retroperitoneal sarcoma: Should be resected en bloc with all involved tissue and viscera to negative margins.
3. Neoadjuvant radiation: May be used for large tumors where a negative surgical resection margin is anticipated to not be feasible.
4. Chemotherapy
   a. There are mixed data regarding the use of cytotoxic chemotherapy in the adjuvant and neoadjuvant setting.
   b. Specific agents vary based on tumor subtype, but anthracyclines (e.g., doxorubicin, epirubicin) and alkylating agents (e.g., ifosfamide, dacarbazine) are the most common chemotherapeutics used for sarcoma.
   c. Trabectedin (a small molecule inhibitor of DNA nucleotide excision repair), pazopanib (tyrosine kinase inhibitor), eribulin (a microtubule-inhibiting agent), and olaratumab (a monoclonal antibody against platelet-derived growth factor α[PDGFRα]) are new therapies with some efficacy in select histologic STS subtypes for patients with advanced disease.
   d. Anlotinib (cataquetinib), a promiscuous tyrosine kinase inhibitor, increased median progression-free survival in patients with advanced STS and intolerance or failure to anthracycline-based chemotherapy.[26]
5. Regional therapy
   a. ILP and ILI with melphalan has been described for patients with unresectable or recurrent in-transit disease.[27]

E. Sarcoma-like tumors
1. DFSP
   a. Fibroblastic origin
   b. Locally aggressive with rare metastasis
   c. Wide and irregular subcutaneous extensions

d. Requires excision with generous margins or Mohs surgery in areas of cosmetic sensitivity.
e. Patients with positive margins may benefit from radiation therapy if additional resection is not feasible.
f. Targeted therapy is recommended for unresectable, recurrent, or metastatic disease, and most commonly, imatinib is used for advanced or unresectable DFSP tumors with activating mutations in the platelet-derived growth factor β (PDGFRB) gene.

2. **Desmoid tumor**
   a. Locally aggressive
   b. Do not metastasize
   c. Often observed in the abdomen or extremities. They can present at the site of a healed wound.
   d. Associated with familial adenomatous polyposis, pregnancy, and use of oral contraceptives.
   e. Small, asymptomatic tumors can be observed.
   f. Large or symptomatic tumors may require excision with margin of normal tissue.
   g. Adjuvant radiation therapy is generally indicated.
   h. Estrogen receptor modulators (e.g., tamoxifen), NSAIDs (e.g., sulindac), cytotoxic chemotherapy, and tyrosine kinase inhibitors (e.g., imatinib and sorafenib) may be used for advanced tumors.
      i. Sorafenib for desmoid tumors in patients with unresectable, progressive, or symptomatic disease and for those with unacceptable surgical risk.[28]
   i. Patients may require colonoscopy and/or genetic assessment due to potential association with familial polyposis syndromes.

VII. BENIGN SOFT TISSUE LESIONS

A. **Cutaneous cysts**
   1. Epidermal, dermal, trichilemmal, or sebaceous
   2. Treatment
      a. Symptomatic cysts—excision
      b. Infected cysts—drainage
      c. Asymptomatic cysts can be removed for diagnosis, prevention of infection, or cosmesis.
   3. Excision should include the entire cyst, its lining, and any skin tract or drainage site.
   4. All excised cysts should be sent for pathology review to exclude the rare case of cystic malignancy (e.g., porocarcinoma).

B. **Neurofibromas**
   1. Benign **Schwann cell nerve sheath tumors**
   2. Soft, pendulous, and sometimes lobulated subcutaneous masses of variable size
   3. If multiple, consider **neurofibromatosis type 1.**
   4. Indications for removal
      a. Pain

b. Increase in size
c. Concern for malignant degeneration
d. Cosmesis

C. Ganglion cysts
1. Subcutaneous cysts that communicate with a joint capsule or tendon sheath
2. Firm, round masses of hands and wrists
3. Most common among young and middle-aged women
4. Indications for removal
a. Pain
b. Limitation of movement
c. Nerve palsies
5. Treatment
a. Aspiration (40% recurrence rate)
b. Surgical excision of capsular attachment and joint capsule.

D. Lipomas
1. Benign proliferations of adipocytes
2. Soft, encapsulated, and mobile subcutaneous masses of variable size
3. Malignant potential is near zero
4. Treatment
a. Asymptomatic and small tumors are observed.
b. Symptomatic/enlarging tumors should undergo biopsy and/or removal.
c. When excised, a complete gross resection should be performed to rule out malignancy and prevent recurrence.

Key References

Citation	Summary
Larkin J, Chiarion-Sileni V, Gonzalez R, et al. Five-year survival with combined nivolumab and ipilimumab in advanced melanoma. *N Engl J Med.* 2019;381(16):1535-1546.	• In a randomized controlled trial, previously untreated patients with advanced melanoma were assigned to receive nivolumab (PD-1) monotherapy, ipilimumab (CTLA-4) monotherapy, or nivolumab plus ipilimumab. Median survival in the nivolumab-plus-ipilimumab group was >60 mo, compared with 36.9 mo in the group receiving PD-1 monotherapy and 19.9 mo in patients receiving CTLA-4 monotherapy. Overall survival at 5 y was 52% in the nivolumab-plus-ipilimumab group and 44% in the nivolumab group, as compared with 26% in the ipilimumab group. No sustained deterioration of health-related quality of life was observed in the combination group. • **Conclusion:** Combination immunotherapy is effective for advanced melanoma and can achieve >50% 5-y survival in a population that previously had dismal prognosis.

Citation	Summary
Larkin J, Ascierto PA, Dréno B, et al. Combined vemurafenib and cobimetinib in BRAF-mutated melanoma. *N Engl J Med*. 2014;371(20):1867-1876.	• In a randomized controlled trial, patients with unresectable melanoma with *BRAF* V600 mutation were treated with either vemurafenib (BRAF V600E inhibitor) or vemurafenib plus cobimetinib (MEK inhibitor). The median progression-free survival was 9.9 mo in the combination group and 6.2 mo in the control group (hazard ratio for death or disease progression, 0.51; 95% confidence interval, 0.39-0.68; $P < .001$). The combination was associated with a nonsignificantly higher incidence of adverse events of grade 3 or higher, as compared with vemurafenib and placebo (65% vs. 59%), but there was no significant difference in the rate of study-drug discontinuation. • **Conclusion:** The addition of cobimetinib to vemurafenib was associated with a significant improvement in progression-free survival among patients with unresectable melanoma that bears a *BRAF V600* mutation, providing an important systemic treatment option for at least half of all patients with melanoma.
Faries MB, Thompson JF, Cochran AJ, et al. Completion dissection or observation for sentinel-node metastasis in melanoma. *N Engl J Med*. 2017;376(23):2211-2222.	• Patients with sentinel node metastasis detected by pathology or multiplex molecular assay were randomly assigned to undergo immediate CLND or node basin surveillance by ultrasound imaging. In the per-protocol analysis, the mean (±SE) 3-y rate of melanoma-specific survival was similar in the dissection group and the observation group (86 ± 1.3% and 86 ± 1.2%, respectively; $P = .42$ by the log-rank test) at a median follow-up of 43 mo. Lymphedema was observed in 24.1% of the patients in the dissection group and in 6.3% of those in the observation group. • **Conclusion:** Nodal basin ultrasound imaging is an acceptable option for patients with melanoma with occult lymph node metastasis. Aside, if patients have clinically positive nodes, they can be evaluated for candidacy for neoadjuvant clinical trials such as *OPACIN-Neo*.

CHAPTER 28: SKIN AND SOFT TISSUE TUMORS

Review Questions

1. A 55-year-old man presents after deep shave biopsy with a 0.9-mm deep melanoma. There is no ulceration or palpable lymphadenopathy. What is the best surgical plan?
2. For an elderly man with fair skin and a slowly growing, smooth, pearly, hypopigmented lesion of the face, what would you recommend? And what is your suspected diagnosis?
3. A 58-year-old, healthy firefighter has a nonhealing wound at the periphery of a previous burn injury sustained 20 years ago. A biopsy is obtained. What is the pathologist likely to discover on histology?
4. A healthy young patient referred to your clinic after punch biopsy of a lesion on his shoulder reveals a 2.1-mm superficial spreading melanoma. There is no clinical adenopathy. What is the next step in management?
5. What is the most appropriate management of a suspicious pigmented skin lesion?
6. A patient presents with a superficial, painless, subcutaneous mass of the posterior neck. The mass is soft, mobile, and feels encapsulated. What is the most likely diagnosis?
7. A young, healthy patient underwent curative resection of melanoma and negative SLNB. Three months later, they present with multiple mass lesions in the right hemiliver. Biopsy confirms malignant melanoma that is negative for *BRAF* mutation. PET/CT shows no other lesions. What is the best treatment option for this patient?
8. A 63-year-old woman presents with new painless axillary mass. Mammography is negative. How would you proceed with evaluation of this mass?
9. What is the most important prognostic factor for soft tissue sarcoma?
10. What is the most common treatment paradigm for an >5 cm extremity sarcoma in an otherwise healthy patient?
11. How would you manage a high-grade retroperitoneal liposarcoma with isolated invasion of the right renal vein and no distal metastasis?

REFERENCES

1. Zager JS, Hochwald SN, Marzban SS, et al. Shave biopsy is a safe and accurate method for the initial evaluation of melanoma. *J Am Coll Surg.* 2011;212(4):454-460; discussion 460-462.
2. Siegel RL, Miller KD, Fuchs HE, Jemal A. Cancer statistics, 2021. *CA Cancer J Clin.* 2021;71(1):7-33.
3. Balch CM, Soong SJ, Gershenwald JE, et al. Prognostic factors analysis of 17,600 melanoma patients: validation of the American Joint Committee on Cancer melanoma staging system. *J Clin Oncol.* 2001;19(16):3622-3634.
4. Newcomer K, Robbins KJ, Perone J, et al. Malignant melanoma: evolving practice management in an era of increasingly effective systemic therapies. *Curr Probl Surg.* 2022;59(1):101030.

5. Gershenwald JE, Scolyer RA, Hess KR, et al. Melanoma of the skin. In: Amin MB, ed. *AJCC Cancer Staging Manual*. 8th ed. Springer; 2017:563-588.

6. Hawkins WG, Busam KJ, Ben-Porat L, et al. Desmoplastic melanoma: a pathologically and clinically distinct form of cutaneous melanoma. *Ann Surg Oncol*. 2005;12(3):207-213.

7. Lattanzi M, Lee Y, Simpson D, et al. Primary melanoma histologic subtype: impact on survival and response to therapy. *J Natl Cancer Inst*. 2019;111(2):180-188.

8. Faries MB, Morton DL. Surgery and sentinel lymph node biopsy. *Semin Oncol*. 2007;34(6):498-508.

9. Faries MB, Thompson JF, Cochran AJ, et al. Completion dissection or observation for sentinel-node metastasis in melanoma. *N Engl J Med*. 2017;376(23):2211-2222.

10. Leiter U, Stadler R, Mauch C, et al. Complete lymph node dissection versus no dissection in patients with sentinel lymph node biopsy positive melanoma (DeCOG-SLT): a multicentre, randomised, phase 3 trial. *Lancet Oncol*. 2016;17(6):757-767.

11. Badgwell B, Xing Y, Gershenwald JE, et al. Pelvic lymph node dissection is beneficial in subsets of patients with node-positive melanoma. *Ann Surg Oncol*. 2007;14(10):2867-2875.

12. Larkin J, Chiarion-Sileni V, Gonzalez R, et al. Five-year survival with combined nivolumab and ipilimumab in advanced melanoma. *N Engl J Med*. 2019;381(16):1535-1546.

13. Tawbi HA, Schadendorf D, Lipson EJ, et al. Relatlimab and nivolumab versus nivolumab in untreated advanced melanoma. *N Engl J Med*. 2022;386(1):24-34.

14. Long GV, Stroyakovskiy D, Gogas H, et al. Combined BRAF and MEK inhibition versus BRAF inhibition alone in melanoma. *N Engl J Med*. 2014;371(20):1877-1888.

15. Larkin J, Ascierto PA, Dréno B, et al. Combined vemurafenib and cobimetinib in BRAF-mutated melanoma. *N Engl J Med*. 2014;371(20):1867-1876.

16. Rozeman EA, Menzies AM, van Akkooi ACJ, et al. Identification of the optimal combination dosing schedule of neoadjuvant ipilimumab plus nivolumab in macroscopic stage III melanoma (OpACIN-neo): a multicentre, phase 2, randomised, controlled trial. *Lancet Oncol*. 2019;20(7):948-960.

17. Beasley GM, Caudle A, Petersen RP, et al. A multi-institutional experience of isolated limb infusion: defining response and toxicity in the US. *J Am Coll Surg*. 2009;208(5):706-715; discussion 715-717.

18. Turley RS, Raymond AK, Tyler DS. Regional treatment strategies for in-transit melanoma metastasis. *Surg Oncol Clin N Am*. 2011;20(1):79-103.

19. Andtbacka RHI, Collichio F, Harrington KJ, et al. Final analyses of OPTiM: a randomized phase III trial of talimogene laherparepvec versus granulocyte-macrophage colony-stimulating factor in unresectable stage III-IV melanoma. *J Immunother Cancer*. 2019;7(1):145.

20. Sekulic A, Migden MR, Oro AE, et al. Efficacy and safety of vismodegib in advanced basal-cell carcinoma. *N Engl J Med*. 2012;366(23):2171-2179.

21. Migden MR, Guminski A, Gutzmer R, et al. Treatment with two different doses of sonidegib in patients with locally advanced or metastatic basal cell carcinoma (BOLT): a multicentre, randomised, double-blind phase 2 trial. *Lancet Oncol*. 2015;16(6): 716-728.

22. Helmink BA, Ansstas G, Fields RC. Biomarker-driven prognostication in Merkel cell carcinoma: a paradigm for personalized therapy. *Ann Surg Oncol*. 2022;29(3):1498-1501.

23. Kaufman HL, Russell J, Hamid O, et al. Avelumab in patients with chemotherapy-refractory metastatic Merkel cell carcinoma: a multicentre, single-group, open-label, phase 2 trial. *Lancet Oncol*. 2016;17(10):1374-1385.

24. Nghiem PT, Bhatia S, Lipson EJ, et al. PD-1 blockade with pembrolizumab in advanced Merkel-cell carcinoma. *N Engl J Med.* 2016;374(26):2542-2552.

25. Basile G, Mattei JC, Alshaygy I, et al. Curability of patients with lymph node metastases from extremity soft-tissue sarcoma. *Cancer.* 2020;126(23):5098-5108.

26. Chi Y, Fang Z, Hong X, et al. Safety and efficacy of anlotinib, a multikinase angiogenesis inhibitor, in patients with refractory metastatic soft-tissue sarcoma. *Clin Cancer Res.* 2018;24(21):5233-5238.

27. Hayes AJ, Neuhaus SJ, Clark MA, Thomas JM. Isolated limb perfusion with melphalan and tumor necrosis factor alpha for advanced melanoma and soft-tissue sarcoma. *Ann Surg Oncol.* 2007;14(1):230-238.

28. Gounder MM, Mahoney MR, Van Tine BA, et al. Sorafenib for advanced and refractory desmoid tumors. *N Engl J Med.* 2018;379(25):2417-2428.

29 Adrenal Gland and Hereditary Endocrine Syndromes

C. Corbin Frye and L. Michael Brunt

I. DISEASES OF THE ADRENAL GLAND

A. Introduction/anatomy/physiology

1. **Embryology**
   a. The **adrenal cortex** arises from the coelomic mesoderm around the fifth week of gestation.
   b. The **adrenal medulla** is populated by the neural crest cells originating from the neural ectoderm that migrate ventrally, resulting in the potential for adrenal **pheochromocytomas** and **paragangliomas** along the paraspinal axis.
2. **Anatomy**
   a. The adrenal glands are retroperitoneal structures that lie along the superior border of each kidney and are adjacent to the inferior vena cava (IVC) on the right and the renal vessels on the left.
   b. Arterial supply is from three sources: The superior adrenal artery (from the inferior phrenic artery), the middle adrenal artery (from the aorta), and the inferior adrenal artery (from the renal artery).
   c. Each adrenal has only one vein, with the right adrenal vein draining directly into the IVC and the left adrenal vein draining into the left renal vein (**Figure 29.1**).[1]
3. **Histology and physiology.** The adrenal gland is histologically composed of four layers, each with its own biosynthetic products.
   a. **Adrenal cortex**
      i. The **zona glomerulosa** is the exclusive site for the synthesis of the mineralocorticoid **aldosterone.**
         a) Aldosterone production is stimulated via the **renin–angiotensin** pathway in response to decreased pressure in the afferent renal arterioles and decreased sodium.
         b) Aldosterone acts to increase circulating blood volume by increasing sodium and chloride reabsorption in the distal tubule of the kidney.
      ii. The **zona fasciculata** produces the glucocorticoids, of which cortisol is the primary product.
         a) Cortisol secretion occurs in response to the secretion of **corticotropin-releasing hormone (CRH)** from

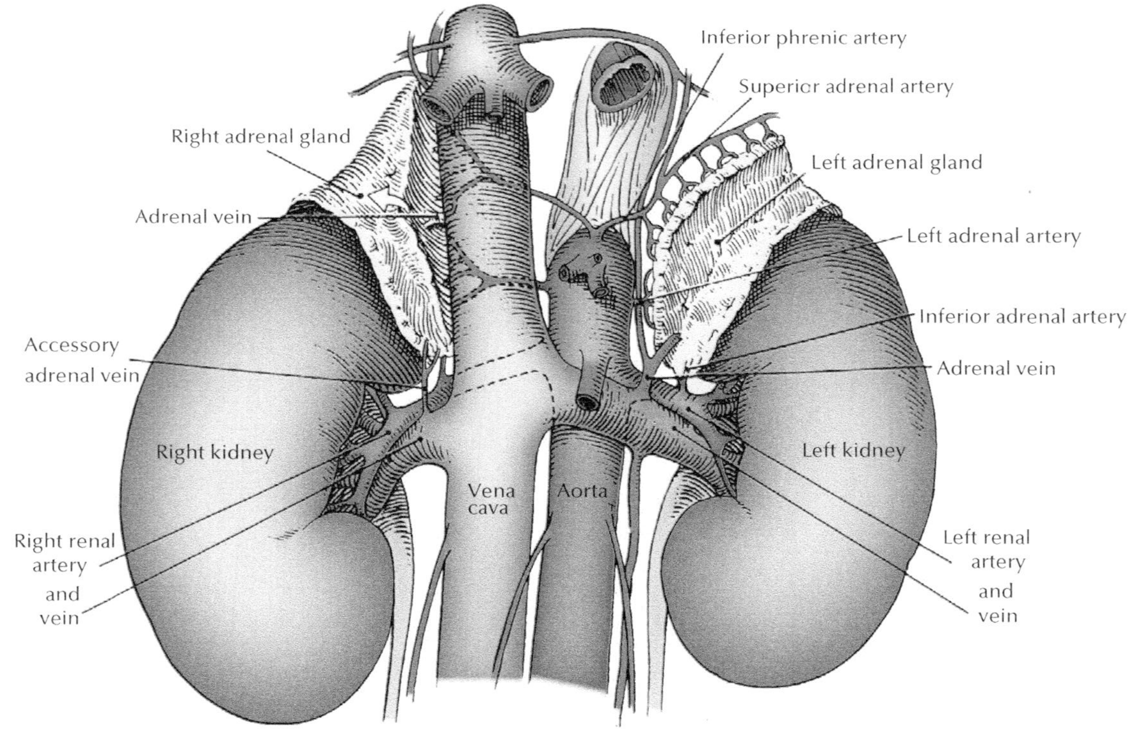

FIGURE 29.1 Anatomy of the adrenal glands. Note that the right adrenal vein is short and generally exits the central medial portion of the adrenal to drain directly into the inferior vena cava. *(Reprinted with permission from Brunt LM. Laparoscopic adrenalectomy. In: Eubanks WS, Swanström LL, Soper NJ, eds.*

the hypothalamus and **adrenocorticotropic hormone (ACTH)** from the anterior pituitary gland.

b) As cortisol levels increase, CRH and ACTH secretion are suppressed (classic negative feedback loop).

c) The overall effect of glucocorticoids is the induction of a catabolic state and a bodily stress response by increasing blood glucose concentration, stimulating lipolysis, enhancing adrenergic stimulation of the cardiovascular system, and reducing the inflammatory response of the immune system.

iii. The **zona reticularis** produces the adrenal sex hormones androstenedione and dehydroepiandrosterone that support the gonadal production of testosterone and estrogen.

b. **Adrenal medulla**

i. The **medulla** produces the catecholamines **norepinephrine** and **epinephrine** that act on peripheral α- and β-adrenergic receptors.

ii. α-Receptor stimulation produces peripheral vasoconstriction.

iii. β_1-Receptor stimulation results in increased heart rate and myocardial contractility.

iv. β_2-Receptor stimulation produces peripheral vasodilation.

B. Adrenal incidentaloma (**Figure 29.2**)

1. Presentation: An adrenal incidentaloma is a >1 cm adrenal lesion(s) discovered in patients who undergo cross-sectional imaging for an unrelated cause, such as during workup for abdominal pain or trauma.

2. Epidemiology: They are the most commonly identified adrenal lesions with incidence between 1% to 4% of all abdominal CT scans, increasing to 7% in patients over 70 years old.[2]

3. Diagnosis

a. Patients presenting with an adrenal incidentaloma should undergo a complete biochemical workup that includes[3,4]

i. **Plasma metanephrines** and **normetanephrines** and/or 24-hour urinary catecholamines and metanephrines to evaluate for a pheochromocytoma.

ii. **Overnight low-dose dexamethasone suppression test** to screen for hypercortisolism (see below in Cushing syndrome diagnosis).

iii. Plasma aldosterone and plasma renin activity in hypertensive or hypokalemic patients to evaluate for an aldosteronoma.

b. Certain characteristic radiologic features increase the suspicion of malignancy in an incidental adrenal mass (**Table 29.1**).[5]

i. Size >4-5 cm (note that adrenal myelolipomas are benign lesions that can be very large)

ii. Irregular borders or local invasiveness

iii. CT attenuation >10 Hounsfield units. (Note: Pheochromocytomas have higher attenuation values.)

iv. Slower washout on contrast-enhanced CT

v. No loss of signal on opposed-phase chemical shift imaging

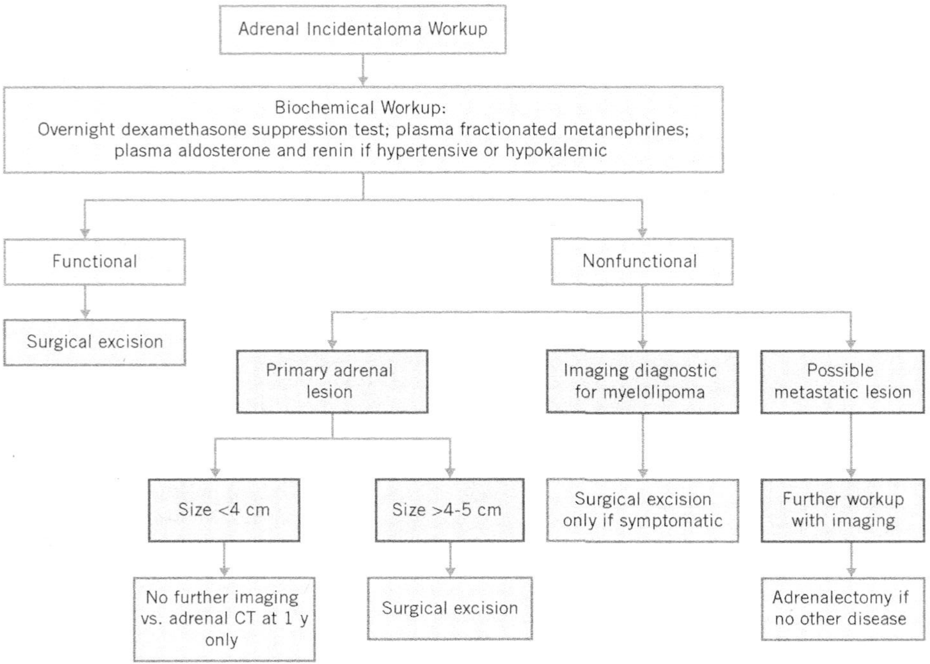

FIGURE 29.2 Algorithm for evaluation and treatment of adrenal incidentaloma.

TABLE 29.1 Imaging Characteristics of Adrenal Masses

Adrenal Mass	Typical Imaging Characteristics
Adrenocortical adenoma	Unilateral, <4-5 cm in diameter Round, homogeneous density with smooth border Low attenuation on CT scan (<10 HU) Rapid, intense contrast enhancement followed by early contrast washout (absolute percent washout >60%, relative percent washout >40%) Intracellular fat with signal loss on opposed-phase MRI images
Myelolipoma	Macroscopic fat on CT Calcification Hyperintense signal on T1 MRI
Pheochromocytoma	Hypervascularity with cystic areas in larger lesions Rapid, intense contrast enhancement with variable delayed washout High T2 MRI signal intensity (light-bulb sign)
Adrenocortical carcinoma	Unilateral, >4-5 cm Irregular shape, heterogeneous, central tumor necrosis, local invasion Calcification Increased attenuation on CT (>10 HU) Delay in contrast washout No loss of signal on opposed-phase MRI Elevated SUV on PET
Adrenal metastasis	Irregular shape, heterogeneous May be bilateral or with other metastatic disease Increased attenuation on CT (>10 HU) Delay in contrast washout No loss of signal on MRI Elevated SUV on PET

HU, Hounsfield units; PET, positron emission tomography; SUV, standardized uptake values.

c. Adrenal biopsy is rarely indicated for an adrenal incidentaloma and should never be done unless a pheochromocytoma has been excluded biochemically, as biopsy has the potential to precipitate a hypertensive crisis.
   i. The main indication for adrenal biopsy is an unresectable suspected malignancy.

4. Treatment
   a. Treatment of adrenal incidentalomas is based primarily on size, functionality, and malignant potential.

b. Adrenalectomy should generally be performed if the mass is larger than 4 to 5 cm (excluding asymptomatic myelolipomas), is functional (i.e., biochemically active), and/or is radiologically suspicious for malignancy.

C. Cushing syndrome and hypercortisolism

1. Definition/etiology

a. **Cushing syndrome** refers to the clinical manifestations of hypercortisolism. There are multiple causes of Cushing syndrome, all of which involve excess circulating glucocorticoids.

i. **Iatrogenic.** The most common cause of Cushing syndrome is from administration of exogenous glucocorticoids.

ii. **Cushing disease.** Hypersecretion of ACTH from the anterior pituitary gland is the most common pathologic cause (65%-70% of cases) of endogenous hypercortisolism.

a) Elevated ACTH results in bilateral adrenal hyperplasia.

b) Cushing disease is almost always caused by a pituitary microadenoma.

c) Transsphenoidal resection is the treatment of choice.

d) Excessive release of CRH by the hypothalamus is a rare cause of hypercortisolism.

iii. **Cortisol-producing adrenal tumor.** Abnormal secretion of cortisol from a primary adrenal adenoma accounts for 10% to 20% of cases of Cushing syndrome, and the high cortisol levels result in suppressed plasma ACTH and atrophy of the adjacent and contralateral adrenocortical tissue.

iv. **Ectopic ACTH production.** Ectopic ACTH production from tumors such as small cell lung carcinoma, neuroendocrine tumors, thymic carcinoma, and medullary thyroid carcinoma accounts for approximately 10% to 15% of cases.

a) Patients with ectopic ACTH-secreting neoplasms can present primarily with hypokalemia, glucose intolerance, and hyperpigmentation and with few other chronic signs of Cushing syndrome.

b) Bilateral adrenalectomy may be occasionally indicated for control of excess hypercortisolism in the setting of an unresectable primary tumor.

b. **Mild autonomous cortisol secretion** (MACS)

i. MACS, also known as subclinical hypercortisolism, occurs when there is biochemical evidence of autonomous cortisol secretion in patients with an adrenal tumor but an absence of the features classically associated with Cushing syndrome.

ii. Although asymptomatic, these patients may share many of the same risk of comorbidities as those with Cushing syndrome, including cardiovascular disease, obesity, diabetes mellitus type 2, and hypertension.

2. Presentation

a. Clinical manifestations of Cushing syndrome include hypertension, central obesity (e.g., moon facies, prominent supraclavicular fat pads, buffalo hump), facial plethora, edema, muscle weakness, glucose intolerance, mood swings, irregular menses, osteoporosis, easy bruising, and purplish striae.

b. Women may develop acne, hirsutism, and amenorrhea as a result of adrenal androgen excess.

3. Diagnosis (**Figure 29.3**)

   a. Diagnostic evaluation sequentially includes (1) establishing the presence of hypercortisolism; (2) differentiation of ACTH dependence or independence; and (3) anatomic localization of the source.

   b. Establishing the presence of hypercortisolism. While controversial, many practitioners advocate that two abnormal results from the following tests are generally required to make the diagnosis:

      i. **Twenty-four-hour urinary excretion of free cortisol** measures total daily cortisol secretion to mitigate variations in the diurnal circadian rhythms that affect cortisol.

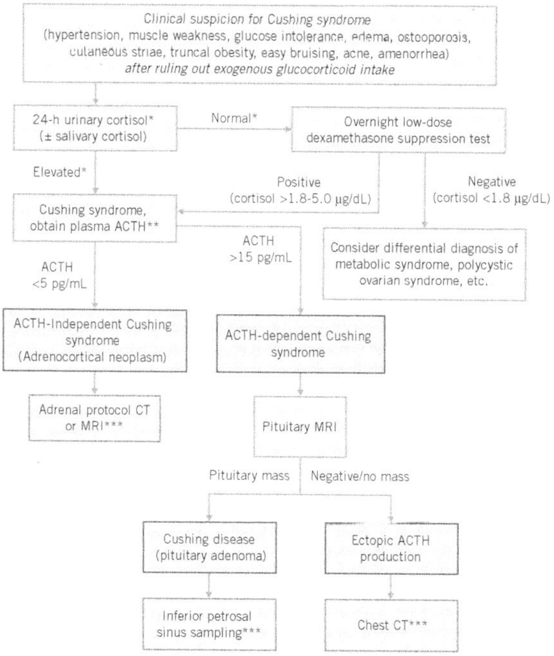

*"Normal" and "Elevated" based on individual lab; at least two measurements of urinary and/or salivary cortisol are recommended to ensure reliability of result due to cortisol level variability.
**ACTH levels between 5-15 pg/mL are indeterminate and may require CRH stimulation testing
***if etiology not confirmed, more extensive imaging or subsequent studies over time may be needed to reveal source

FIGURE 29.3 Algorithm for diagnosing Cushing syndrome and localizing etiology/source.

a) Values >62 μg/d in the setting of clinically suspected Cushing syndrome is highly correlated with a positive diagnosis, and no further confirmatory tests are needed.[6]

ii. **Late-night salivary cortisol testing** (samples are taken near 11 PM over 3 days) is based on the normal evening nadir of plasma cortisol that is lost in patients with Cushing syndrome.

iii. **Low-dose overnight dexamethasone suppression test**

a) Performed by administering oral dexamethasone 1 mg at 11 PM and measuring plasma cortisol and dexamethasone levels at 8 AM

b) Patients with autonomous hypercortisolism have lost the normal adrenal–pituitary feedback and have elevated cortisol levels of 1.8 to 5.0 μg/dL (exact cutoff is controversial).

c. **Differentiation of ACTH-dependent from ACTH-independent causes**

i. Once hypercortisolism is diagnosed, plasma ACTH should be measured.

ii. Suppression of plasma ACTH to <5 pg/mL is indicative of an ACTH-independent source of hypercortisolism due to an adrenocortical neoplasm.

iii. ACTH levels >15 pg/mL demonstrate ACTH-dependent hypercortisolism.

iv. Values of 15 to 500 pg/mL suggest Cushing disease caused by pituitary adenoma, while ACTH levels >1,000 pg/mL may indicate ectopic ACTH production.

v. The high-dose dexamethasone test is no longer widely used to differentiate causes of ACTH-dependent Cushing syndrome.

d. **Localization of the hypercortisolism source**

i. **ACTH-dependent Cushing syndrome**

a) Pituitary MRI is generally the first step in distinguishing between pituitary and ectopic sources.

b) In patients with tumors >6 mm in the anterior pituitary, further testing can be foregone.

c) In those with smaller tumors or no abnormalities on MRI, **inferior petrosal sinus sampling** is often performed to confirm ACTH secretion from the pituitary.

d) Patients with suspected ectopic ACTH release should have a CT scan of the chest to identify possible small cell lung cancers.

ii. Patients with ACTH-independent hypercortisolism (adrenal source) require thin-section CT or MRI imaging of the adrenals, both of which identify adrenal abnormalities with more than 95% sensitivity.

4. Treatment

a. **Transsphenoidal resection** of an ACTH-producing pituitary tumor is successful in ≥80% of cases of Cushing disease, but in patients who fail surgical treatment, bilateral adrenalectomy may occasionally be indicated.

b. Treatment of ectopic ACTH syndrome involves resection of the primary lesion, if possible, and less often bilateral adrenalectomy.
c. Primary adrenal Cushing syndrome is treated by adrenalectomy
   i. Rarely, the cause may be adrenal hyperplasia, which is treated with **bilateral adrenalectomy.**
   ii. All patients who undergo adrenalectomy for primary adrenal causes of Cushing syndrome require perioperative glucocorticoid replacement, while the suppressed pituitary–adrenal axis recovers over 3 to 6 months.
d. For cases of MACS, the rate of progression to overt Cushing syndrome is low, but MACS also infrequently resolves spontaneously.
   i. Options for management include observation vs. adrenalectomy—the latter because studies suggest (but are not conclusive) that adrenalectomy for MACS may improve cardiovascular risk, glucose control, hypertension, and dyslipidemia.[7,8]

D. Primary hyperaldosteronism
1. Epidemiology and etiology
   a. Primary hyperaldosteronism has a prevalence as high as 8% to 12% in hypertensive populations.
      i. Secondary hyperaldosteronism is a physiologic response of the renin–angiotensin system to renal artery stenosis, congestive heart failure, cirrhosis, or even normal pregnancy.
   b. There are **four subtypes of primary hyperaldosteronism** that all result in elevated mineralocorticoid levels:
      i. **Aldosterone-producing adrenal adenoma**, also known as **Conn syndrome**, is the cause of primary hyperaldosteronism in up to two-thirds of cases and is one of the few surgically correctable causes of hypertension.
      ii. **Idiopathic hyperaldosteronism** from bilateral cortical hyperplasia accounts for 30% to 40% of cases of primary aldosteronism and is best managed medically.
      iii. **Aldosterone-producing adrenal carcinoma** is very rare.
      iv. **Glucocorticoid-suppressible aldosteronism** may be familial, is rare, is due to ACTH control of aldosterone secretion, and responds to administration of exogenous corticosteroids.
2. Presentation
   a. Patients present with hypertension and hypokalemia related to how aldosterone acts on the kidneys to stimulate salt and water resorption (hypertension) and potassium excretion (hypokalemia).
   b. Patients can also present with insulin resistance and hyperglycemia.
3. Diagnosis
   a. Screening for primary hyperaldosteronism should be carried out in patients with hypertension that is characterized as early onset, poorly controlled, requiring multiple medications, predominantly diastolic, and/or associated with hypokalemia.
   b. Laboratory diagnosis
      i. Screening for hyperaldosteronism consists of measurement of upright **plasma aldosterone concentration** (PAC) and **plasma renin activity** (PRA).

ii. A PAC:PRA ratio of >25 to 30 in conjunction with a primary aldosterone level >15 ng/dL and plasma renin <0.5 ng/mL/h is diagnostic of primary hyperaldosteronism.

iii. Primary hyperaldosteronism is confirmed by demonstration of lack of aldosterone suppression (>10-12 ng/dL) on 24-hour urine aldosterone measurements after salt loading with 5 to 6 g salt/d for 3 days or 2 L intravenous normal saline infusion over 4 hours.[9]

c. Localization of hyperaldosteronism source

i. Thin-cut (3-mm) adrenal CT may show a unilateral adenoma with better spatial resolution than MRI.

ii. For patients under 40 to 45 years with a unilateral macroadenoma >1 cm, adrenalectomy may be performed without further testing.

iii. In patients with bilateral adenomas, normal adrenals, and age older than 40 to 45 years, **adrenal vein sampling** (AVS) should be performed to confirm the laterality of aldosterone production before proceeding to operation.

iv. In AVS, simultaneous blood samples for aldosterone and cortisol are taken from both adrenal veins and the IVC, and an aldosterone to cortisol ratio >4:1 between sides supports a lateralizing source and management with adrenalectomy.

4. Treatment

a. Adrenalectomy should be performed in patients with a unilateral source of increased aldosterone production and results in cure or substantial improvement in hypertension and hypokalemia in >90% of patients.

i. Preoperatively, patients should have hypertension controlled and electrolytes corrected.

ii. Postoperatively, it is *critical to stop any potassium sparing diuretics after adrenalectomy* to avoid severe hyperkalemia.

iii. Normal aldosterone and renin levels postoperatively suggest biochemical cure.

b. Patients with bilateral adrenal hyperplasia are best treated pharmacologically with potassium-sparing diuretics, such as spironolactone, amiloride, or eplerenone.

E. Pheochromocytoma and paraganglioma

1. Epidemiology and etiology

a. Pheochromocytomas are neoplasms derived from **chromaffin cells** of the sympathoadrenal system that engage in unregulated, episodic oversecretion of catecholamines.

b. Approximately 85% to 90% of pheochromocytomas in adults arise in the adrenal medulla, whereas 10% to 15% are paragangliomas that arise in the **extra-adrenal chromaffin tissue**, including near the renal hilum, paravertebral ganglia, posterior mediastinum, **organ of Zuckerkandl**, and urinary bladder.

c. Pheochromocytomas can occur in association with several hereditary syndromes, including **multiple endocrine neoplasia** (MEN) types 2A and 2B, von Hippel–Lindau syndrome, neurofibromatosis type 1, and succinate dehydrogenase mutations.

   i. Pheochromocytomas that are bilateral, occur in young patients, or are extra-adrenal should undergo genetic testing (although recent recommendations suggest all patients with pheochromocytoma might benefit from genetic assessment).

2. Presentation: Clinical manifestations include symptoms like paroxysms of frontal headache, diaphoresis, palpitations, flushing, and/or anxiety related to the excess sympathetic stimulation from catecholamines, and the most common sign is episodic or sustained hypertension.

3. Diagnosis

  a. Biochemical testing. The biochemical diagnosis is made by demonstrating elevated levels of plasma metanephrines or 24-hour urinary catecholamines and metanephrines. Urine vanillylmandelic acid is no longer utilized due to lack of specificity of this test.

  b. Localization

   i. CT identifies 90% to 95% of pheochromocytomas >1 cm.

   ii. Up to 30% to 40% of pheochromocytomas present as an incidental mass found on imaging done for other reasons (see adrenal incidentaloma above).

   iii. MRI scan can be useful because T2-weighted images have a characteristic high intensity in patients with pheochromocytoma compared with those with adenomas (**Figure 29.4**).

   iv. In patients with biochemical evidence of pheochromocytoma and negative CT and MRI, functional imaging can help identify occult tumors and metastatic pheochromocytoma.

    a) **68-Ga DOTATATE positron emission tomography** scanning has the highest sensitivity and can be helpful in identifying occult tumors or suspected metastatic disease.

    b) **Scintigraphic scanning** after the administration of ^{123}I-meta-iodobenzylguanidine provides a functional and anatomic test of hyperfunctioning chromaffin tissue that is very specific for both intra- and extra-adrenal pheochromocytomas but is expensive and less frequently utilized.

4. Treatment

  a. The treatment of benign and malignant pheochromocytomas is surgical excision.

  b. Preoperative preparation for adrenalectomy for pheochromocytomas includes:

   i. Administration of **α-adrenergic blockade** to control hypertension and to permit re-expansion of intravascular volume.

    a) Phenoxybenzamine is a nonspecific α-blocker that has classically been used, although its use today is limited by the high cost of the medication.

    b) Consequently, selective α-blockers such as doxazosin and calcium channel blockers are preferred given their lower cost and more favorable side-effect profiles.

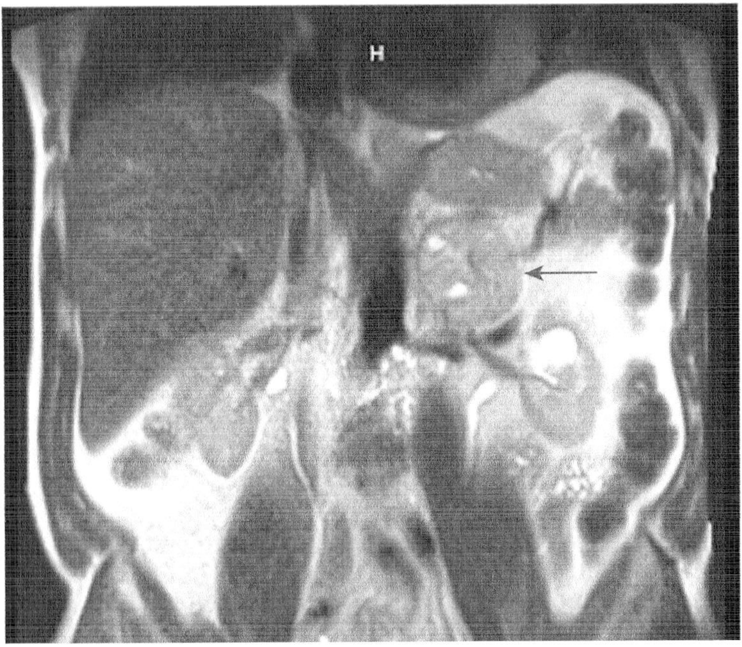

FIGURE 29.4 MRI T2-weighted image showing typical appearance for pheochromocytoma. The arrow points to the tumor seen on MRI.

c) The goal of therapy is to control hypertension, and tachycardia with some degree of postural hypotension is expected.

ii. **β-Adrenergic blockade** (e.g., metoprolol) may be added for patients with persistent tachycardia or arrhythmias but should only be initiated after complete α-adrenergic blockade to avoid unopposed α-effect and precipitation of a hypertensive crisis.

c. Intraoperative considerations

i. All patients should be monitored intraoperatively with an arterial line and selectively with central line placement.

ii. Intraoperative labile hypertension can occur during resection of pheochromocytoma, which can be managed by minimizing manipulation of the tumor and with IV vasodilators (sodium nitroprusside or nitroglycerin).

iii. After the adrenal has been disconnected from its blood supply, many patients require transient pressor support for up to a few hours.

d. Technical considerations

i. The vast majority of pheochromocytomas can be removed with minimally invasive techniques, either the lateral transabdominal approach (most commonly used) or a posterior retroperitoneal endoscopic approach for smaller tumors in nonobese patients.

ii. In patients with MEN type 2A or 2B and bilateral tumors, preservation of adrenal cortical function may be considered by carrying out **cortical-sparing adrenalectomy.**

e. Postoperative considerations and follow-up

i. The majority of patients can be monitored on a regular nursing unit postoperatively while surgical intensive care unit monitoring is reserved for patients who require ongoing vasopressor support.

ii. Most patients can be discharged on the first postoperative day; blood pressure medications should be adjusted appropriately and, in many cases, can be stopped altogether.

iii. α-Blockade is no longer needed postoperatively.

iv. Annual follow-up with measurement of plasma fractionated metanephrines is recommended for at least 5 years after adrenalectomy because of the risk of recurrence, even after resection of an apparently benign lesion.

v. Genetic testing should be discussed and referral made to a medical geneticist for interested patients.

F. Adrenocortical carcinoma (ACC)

1. Epidemiology and etiology

a. ACC is a rare but aggressive malignancy with a reported annual incidence of 0.5 to 2 cases per million people and accounts for 2% to 4% of adrenal incidentalomas.

b. Overall, the prognosis for patients with ACC is poor with survival rates of 15% to 20%.

2. Presentation: More common in females; most patients present with some evidence of adrenal hormone excess, such as hypercortisolism or virilizing features (**Figure 29.5**); as well as the majority present with locally advanced or metastatic disease.

3. Diagnosis

a. Made via cross-sectional imaging.

b. Any large adrenal cortical tumor >4 to 5 cm or with irregular features or invasiveness on imaging should raise suspicion for an adrenal cancer.

c. Many adrenal cancers are 10 cm or larger and may extend to surrounding structures, and associated tumor thrombi in the adrenal or renal veins may occur.

4. Nonoperative treatment

a. Chemotherapy with **mitotane** can be used as stand-alone treatment or as adjuvant therapy after complete resection.

b. In patients with metastatic ACC (most often involving the lung, lymph nodes, liver, or bone), palliative surgical debulking may provide symptomatic relief from some hormone-producing cancers.

5. Operative treatment

a. Complete surgical resection is the only chance for cure.

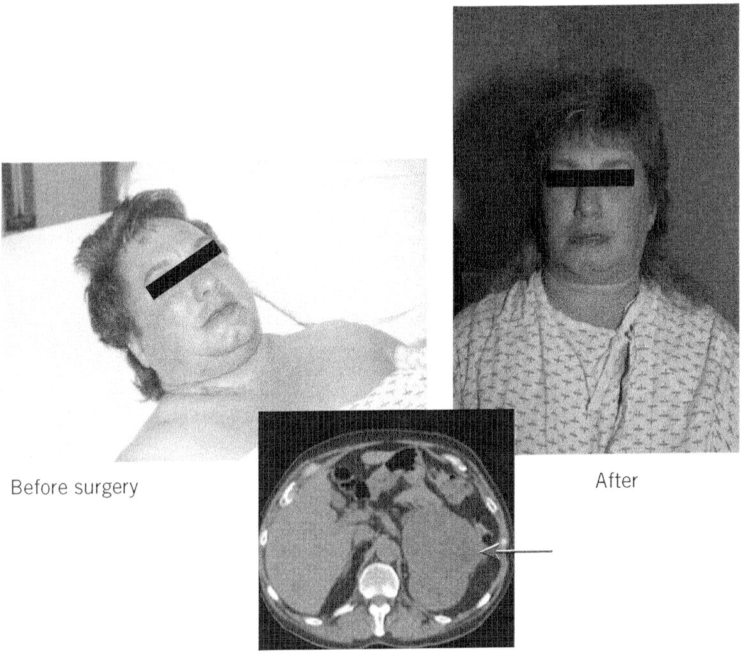

FIGURE 29.5 Adrenocortical carcinoma (ACC). The arrow points to an ACC seen on CT scan.

b. Classically, ACC is resected with an open approach to avoid tumor capsule violation and peritoneal dissemination.
c. Definitive staging requires operative and pathologic demonstration of nodal or distant metastases.
d. A number of histologic criteria (e.g., **Weiss criteria**) are used for the histologic diagnosis of ACC and include presence of necrosis, increased mitotic rate, high nuclear grade, and invasion of vessels or adrenal capsule.

G. Miscellaneous nonfunctional adrenal masses

1. **Nonfunctional adrenocortical adenoma**
   a. Benign tumors that are not hormonally active, these comprise the majority of adrenal incidentalomas and many have no clinical significance.
   b. Resection should be performed in patients with nonfunctional adrenal adenomas >4 to 5 cm in diameter, if atypical features are present, or if there is significant growth during follow-up.[4]
   c. Tumors <4 cm with clearly benign features on imaging may require no further imaging or, if done, only a one-time follow-up noncontrast CT scan at 1 year.

d. For indeterminate <4 cm nonfunctioning adrenal masses, options include imaging with a different modality, follow-up imaging at 6 to 12 months, or surgical excision depending on clinical assessment of risk.[3,10]
e. Any tumor that enlarges by >1 cm during the follow-up period should be removed.
f. Biochemical testing for cortisol function may be optionally repeated at 1 year.

2. **Adrenal myelolipoma**
   a. Benign tumors composed of mature fat and hematopoietic elements.
   b. Identified radiographically by the characteristic macroscopic fat on CT imaging.
   c. May enlarge over time, but routine follow-up imaging is not necessary except for large lesions.
   d. Surgical excision is only indicated for masses causing local mass-effect symptoms, and only 4% will require adrenalectomy.[11]
   e. Spontaneous retroperitoneal hemorrhage may occur rarely with very large masses.
3. **Adrenal metastases**
   a. The most common malignant lesions involving the adrenal gland and are frequently bilateral.
   b. Lung, breast, melanoma, colorectal, pancreatic, hepatocellular, and renal cell cancers all may metastasize to the adrenal glands.
   c. Diagnosis of metastatic disease can often be made from the imaging appearance and a history of cancer.
   d. A need for pathologic confirmation of metastatic disease is rare and should mainly be done for unresectable primary tumors in order to direct therapy.
   e. *Biochemical testing for pheochromocytoma should always be performed prior to biopsy.*
   f. Patients with bilateral metastatic disease should be evaluated for adrenal insufficiency.
   g. Adrenalectomy for metastatic disease may be considered for an isolated adrenal lesion.

H. Acute adrenal insufficiency

1. Epidemiology and etiology
   a. An emergency that should be suspected in physiologically stressed patients with a history of either adrenal insufficiency or exogenous steroid use.
   b. **Adrenocortical insufficiency** is most often caused by acute withdrawal of chronic corticosteroid therapy but can occur in the postoperative setting following adrenal surgery or from autoimmune destruction of the adrenal cortex, adrenal hemorrhage (**Waterhouse–Friderichsen syndrome**), or, rarely, infiltration with metastatic carcinoma.
   c. The diagnosis and treatment in patients in septic shock is controversial, but Surviving Sepsis Guidelines call for the use of corticosteroids

only in cases of septic shock where the blood pressure is not responsive to fluid administration or vasopressor therapy.[12]

2. Presentation: Signs and symptoms include fever, nausea, vomiting, severe hypotension, and lethargy, and characteristic laboratory findings of adrenal insufficiency include hyponatremia, hyperkalemia, azotemia, and hypoglycemia.
3. Diagnosis is through a **rapid ACTH stimulation test** with IV **cosyntropin** administration (i.e., synthetic ACTH, 250 μg), and then plasma cortisol levels are measured on completion of the administration and then 30 and 60 minutes later—normal peak cortisol response should exceed 20 μg/dL.
4. Treatment
   a. **Adrenal crisis** must be immediately addressed based on clinical suspicion before laboratory confirmation is available.
      i. IV volume replacement with dextrose is essential, as is immediate IV steroid replacement therapy with 4 mg of dexamethasone followed by 50 mg of IV hydrocortisone every 8 hours and then tapered to standard replacement doses as the patient's condition stabilizes.
      ii. Mineralocorticoid replacement is not required until IV fluids are discontinued and oral intake resumes.
5. Prevention: Patients who have known adrenal insufficiency or have received supraphysiologic doses of steroid for at least 1 week in the year preceding surgery should receive 100 mg of hydrocortisone the evening before and the morning of major surgery, followed by 50 to 100 mg of hydrocortisone every 8 hours during the first postoperative 24 hours, then reduced to their preoperative doses in a slow or fast taper, depending on the clinical circumstances.

I. Adrenalectomy
1. **Laparoscopic adrenalectomy** has become the standard of care for the vast majority of patients with adrenal tumors.
2. The only absolute contraindication to laparoscopy is local tumor invasion, but suspected adrenal cortical carcinomas >6 to 7 cm should also be approached in an open fashion because of an increased risk of local recurrence when done laparoscopically.
3. Both laparoscopic transperitoneal adrenalectomy and retroperitoneoscopic adrenalectomy have been described with similar outcomes in terms of operative time, blood loss, length of hospitalization, time to oral intake, morbidity, and mortality.[13]
4. The retroperitoneal approach is commonly used for smaller tumors in nonobese patients, especially if there is a history of previous abdominal surgery.
5. **Surgical approach: Laparoscopic transabdominal right adrenalectomy**
   a. The patient is placed on a well-padded mattress bean bag in the left lateral decubitus position (slightly less than fully lateral) with the bed flexed at the midpoint of the patient's costal margin and anterior superior iliac spine (**Figure 29.6**). The patient's arm is brought over

the chest and supported, and a pad is placed under the chest wall to protect the axilla.

b. Abdominal entry with 5-mm port for initial access, then two other 5-mm ports are placed and one 12-mm port in the subcostal/flank region spaced 5 cm apart (**Figure 29.7**).
c. Mobilize the right lobe of the liver by dividing the triangular ligament.
d. Identify the IVC and dissect the medial border of adrenal (with monopolar electrosurgical instrument and/or advanced energy device); isolate and ligate the right adrenal vein as it enters the IVC with clips.
e. Mobilize the inferior adrenal from the IVC and superior kidney, then dissect the adrenal gland from surrounding retroperitoneal fat and superior kidney, taking care to ligate the arterial branches.
f. Remove the specimen using a retrieval bag by enlarging the incision somewhat and close the fascia in layers.
g. Consider a transversus abdominus plane (TAP) block under laparoscopic visualization for postoperative pain control

6. **Surgical approach: Laparoscopic transabdominal left adrenalectomy**
   a. Position the patient on a padded bean bag in the right lateral decubitus position (slightly less than fully lateral) similar to the right side above.
   b. Abdominal entry with 5-mm port for initial access, then two other 5-mm ports are placed and one 12-mm port in the subcostal/flank region spaced 5 cm apart.
   c. Mobilize the splenic flexure of the colon laterally to the inferior aspect of the spleen and divide the splenorenal ligament to the diaphragm to allow the spleen to roll medially.
   d. Develop the plane between the tail of the pancreas and the kidney and positively identify the tail of the pancreas and splenic vessels in order to avoid injuring them. Gently retract the spleen and pancreatic tail medially.
   e. Define the medial and inferior-lateral borders of the adrenal and mobilize them with an electrosurgical and/or advanced energy device.
   f. Identify the left adrenal vein at the medial-inferior edge of the adrenal gland and ligate it just prior to where it is joined by the left inferior phrenic vein. Identify the renal vein at the inferior edge of the adrenal (the renal artery is just cephalad and deep to the renal vein).
   g. Circumferentially dissect the adrenal gland, ligating all small vessels using electrosurgical energy.
   h. Remove the specimen using a retrieval bag by enlarging the incision as needed and close the fascia in layers.
   i. Consider a TAP block under laparoscopic visualization for postoperative pain control.

7. **Surgical approach: Retroperitoneal endoscopic adrenalectomy**
   a. Patient position is prone with padding at the lower chest and pelvis and the legs flexed (**Figure 29.8**).
   b. Access is via an open 2.5-cm incision below the right 12th rib, and the space is bluntly dissected with a finger, the two additional ports are placed by palpation on either side (**Figure 29.9**). The space is insufflated to a pressure of 20 to 25 mmHg+, and blunt dissection with the laparoscope is used to develop the retroperitoneal space further.
   c. The kidney is pushed anteriorly, and an advanced energy device is used to divide attachments. Peritoneal entry should be avoided as this will compromise the working space.
   d. The adrenal borders are defined, and the adrenal vein is taken medially with advanced energy usually with no clips.
   e. For right adrenalectomy, the IVC should be identified medially, and the vein will be entering it on the posterior-lateral aspect and medial border of the adrenal.
   f. For left adrenalectomy, the adrenal vein is medial/inferior just above the renal vein.
   g. The adrenal is disconnected from the kidney and placed in an entrapment bag and removed, after which the abdomen is closed.

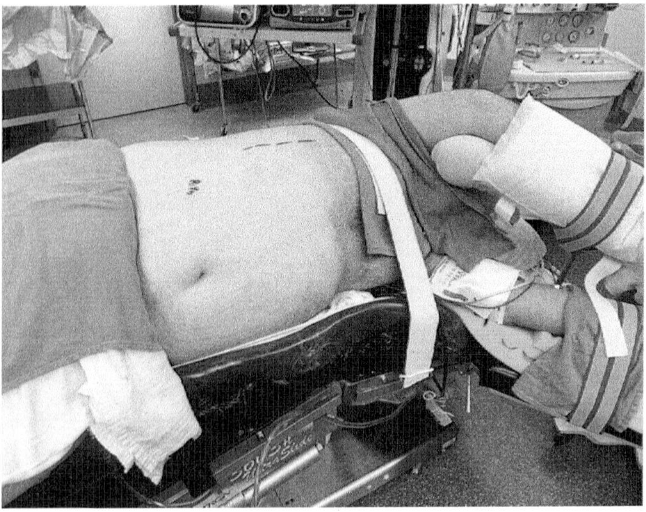

FIGURE 29.6 Patient positioning for a right-sided transabdominal adrenalectomy.

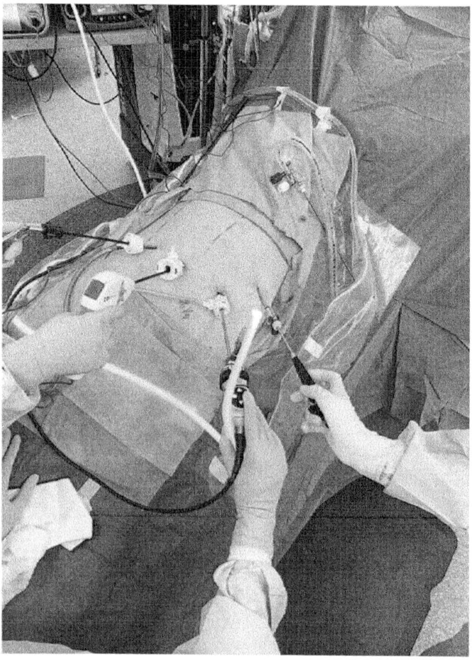

FIGURE 29.7 Port placement for a right-sided transabdominal adrenalectomy. The dashed lines represent location of anterior and posterior axillary lines.

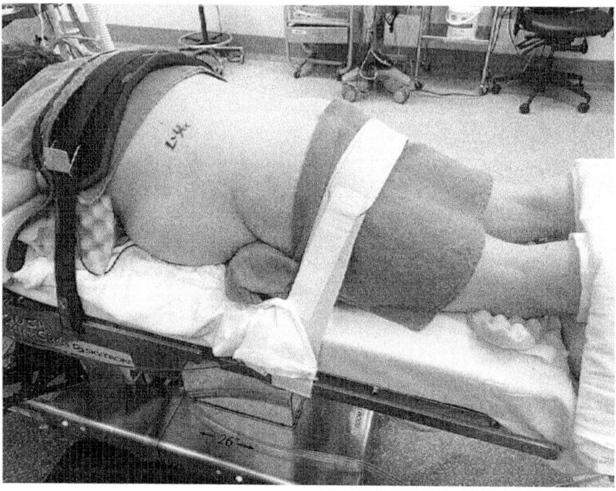

FIGURE 29.8 Patient positioning for a left-sided retroperitoneoscopic adrenalectomy.

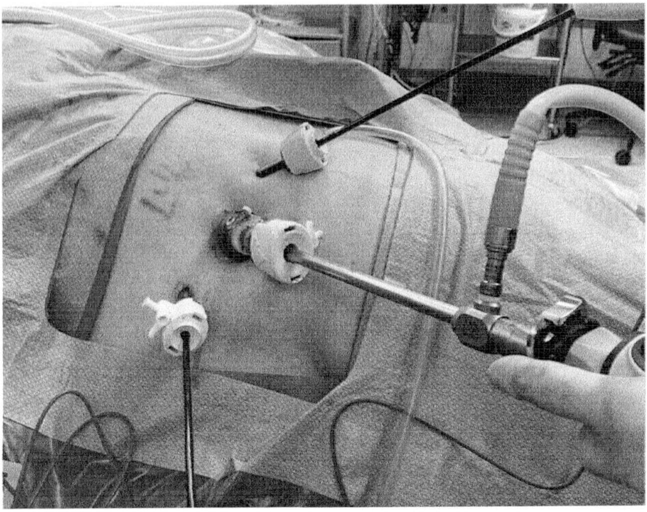

FIGURE 29.9 Port positioning for a left-sided retroperitoneoscopic adrenalectomy.

II. HEREDITARY ENDOCRINE TUMOR SYNDROMES (TABLE 29.2)

A. Multiple endocrine neoplasia type 1 (MEN-1)

1. MEN-1 is an autosomal-dominant syndrome characterized by tumors of the parathyroid glands, pancreatic islet cells, and pituitary gland.
2. The gene responsible for MEN-1, ***MENIN***, is located on chromosome 11q13 and appears to act through transcription factors.
3. Patients with MEN-1 should begin screening for the below disease processes in their early teens.
   a. **Hyperparathyroidism**
      i. Patients with hyperparathyroidism and MEN-1 usually have generalized (4-gland) parathyroid enlargement.

TABLE 29.2 Multiple Endocrine Neoplasia (MEN) Syndromes

	MEN-1	MEN-2A	MEN-2B
Gene mutation	*MENIN*	*RET*	*RET*
Endocrinopathy (approximate % penetrance)	HPT (100%) Pituitary (25%) Pancreatic endocrine tumors (50%)	MTC (100%) Pheo (45%) HPT (30%)	MTC (100%) Pheo (variable)

HPT, hyperparathyroidism; MTC, medullary thyroid carcinoma; Pheo, pheochromocytoma.

ii. Surgical treatment should consist of **3.5-gland parathyroidectomy** or a **total parathyroidectomy with autotransplantation** of parathyroid tissue to the sternocleidomastoid muscle or forearm, which achieves cure in more than 90% of cases and results in hypoparathyroidism in <5%.

iii. Graft-dependent recurrent hyperparathyroidism, however, is seen in up to 50% of cases and is managed by debulking of the autografted material.

iv. Family members of patients with MEN-1 should undergo annual screening with calcium levels.

b. **Pituitary tumors**

i. These tumors in patients with MEN-1 are most commonly benign prolactin-producing adenomas.

ii. Patients may present with headache, diplopia, or symptoms referable to hormone overproduction.

iii. **Bromocriptine** inhibits prolactin production and may reduce tumor bulk.

iv. **Transsphenoidal hypophysectomy** may be necessary if medical treatment fails.

c. **Pancreatic islet cell tumors**

i. These pose the most difficult clinical challenge in MEN-1 and account for most of the morbidity and mortality of the syndrome.

ii. **Gastrinomas (i.e., Zollinger–Ellison syndrome)** are most common, but vasoactive intestine peptide (VIP)-secreting tumors, insulinomas, glucagonomas, and somatostatinomas are also encountered.

iii. Treatment goal is relief of symptoms related to excessive hormone production and cure or palliation of any malignant process.

iv. Patients frequently require medical and surgical therapy.

B. Multiple endocrine neoplasia type 2 (MEN-2)

1. MEN-2 is characterized by **medullary thyroid carcinoma** (MTC) and includes MEN-2A and MEN-2B.

   a. **Familial MTC** was previously recognized as a distinct syndrome but is now considered a variant of MEN-2A.

2. These autosomal-dominant syndromes are caused by gain-of-function mutations in the ***RET* proto-oncogene**, which encodes a transmembrane tyrosine kinase receptor.

3. Because MTC occurs universally in all MEN-2 variants, thyroidectomy is indicated for all *RET*-mutation carriers, and current guidelines call for **prophylactic thyroidectomy** in the first months to year of life for MEN-2B and codon M918T mutation, thyroidectomy before age 5 years for patients with mutations defined as high risk, and thyroidectomy beginning after 5 years of age for patients with elevated serum calcitonin levels and mutations defined as moderate risk.[14]

4. **Calcitonin** serves as a tumor marker for MTC and can be used to guide timing of thyroidectomy as well as postoperative monitoring for disease recurrence.

5. **MEN-2A**
   a. Patients with MEN-2A will develop MTC starting from the mid-teens up to the third decade of life, depending on the codon mutation.
   b. These patients also can develop pheochromocytomas and hyperplasia of the parathyroid glands, which typically occur after MTC has developed, although pheochromocytoma in children as young as 8 years has been reported.[15]
   c. Biochemical testing to exclude pheochromocytoma is mandatory in all patients with either MEN-2 or MTC prior to any elective surgical operation.
6. **MEN-2B**
   a. MTC in patients with MEN-2B is particularly aggressive, even presenting at birth, and invasive disease with lymph node metastasis can occur at an early age.
   b. Pheochromocytoma penetrance is variable.
   c. Patients also develop ganglioneuromatosis and a characteristic physical appearance, with hypergnathism of the midface, marfanoid body habitus, and multiple mucosal neuromas.
   d. Patients with MEN-2B may also demonstrate multiple gastrointestinal symptoms and megacolon.

Key References

Citation	Summary
Yip L, Duh QY, Wachtel H, et al. American Association of Endocrine Surgeons guidelines for adrenalectomy: executive summary. *JAMA Surg.* 2022;157(10):870-877.	• This up-to-date set of guidelines provides evidence-based recommendations for safe and effective adrenalectomy.
Kebebew E. Adrenal incidentaloma. *N Engl J Med.* 2021;384(16):1542-1551.	• This case-based review provides a detailed summary of adrenal incidentaloma evaluation and assessment.
Bancos I, Alahdab F, Crowley RK, et al. THERAPY OF ENDOCRINE DISEASE: Improvement of cardiovascular risk factors after adrenalectomy in patients with adrenal tumors and subclinical Cushing's syndrome: a systematic review and meta-analysis. *Eur J Endocrinol.* 2016;175(6):R283-R295.	• This systematic review demonstrates that, compared with surveillance, surgical treatment of patients with subclinical Cushing's syndrome improves cardiometabolic risk factors such as hypertension and diabetes.
Nölting S, Bechmann N, Taieb D, et al. Personalized management of pheochromocytoma and paraganglioma. *Endocr Rev.* 2022;43(2):199-239.	• This review describes the pathophysiology, workup, and management of pheochromocytomas and paragangliomas.

CHAPTER 29

Review Questions

1. Into which structure does the left adrenal vein directly drain?
2. What is the embryologic origin of the adrenal medulla?
3. What is the most common type of tumor of an adrenal incidentaloma?
4. What laboratory tests comprise the workup for an adrenal incidentaloma?
5. Which adrenal incidentalomas should be resected?
6. What is the most common cause of Cushing syndrome?
7. What study can be useful in determining which adrenal gland is the source for primary hyperaldosteronism?
8. Preoperative preparation for adrenalectomy for patients with pheochromocytoma begins with what kind of pharmacologic agent?
9. Which chemotherapy agent has been shown to be effective in the adjuvant setting after resection of adrenocortical adenocarcinoma?
10. What are the gene mutations associated with MEN-1, MEN-2A, and MEN-2B, respectively?

REFERENCES

1. Brunt LM, Moley JF. The pituitary and adrenal glands. In: Townsend CM, ed. *Sabiston's Biologic Basis of Modern Surgical Practice*. 17th ed. WB Saunders Co; 2004:1023-1070.
2. Davenport C, Liew A, Doherty B, et al. The prevalence of adrenal incidentaloma in routine clinical practice. *Endocrine*. 2011;40(1):80-83.
3. Fassnacht M, Arlt W, Bancos I, et al. Management of adrenal incidentalomas: European society of endocrinology clinical practice guideline in collaboration with the European network for the study of adrenal tumors. *Eur J Endocrinol*. 2016;175(2):G1-G34.
4. Zeiger MA, Thompson GB, Duh QY, et al. American Association of Clinical Endocrinologists and American Association of Endocrine Surgeons Medical guidelines for the management of adrenal incidentalomas: executive summary of recommendations. *Endocr Pract*. 2009;15(5):450-453.
5. Schieda N, Siegelman ES. Update on CT and MRI of adrenal nodules. *AJR Am J Roentgenol*. 2017;208(6):1206-1217.
6. Loriaux DL. Diagnosis and differential diagnosis of cushing's syndrome. *N Engl J Med*. 2017;376(15):1451-1459.
7. Toniato A, Merante-Boschin I, Opocher G, Pelizzo MR, Schiavi F, Ballotta E. Surgical versus conservative management for subclinical Cushing syndrome in adrenal incidentalomas: a prospective randomized study. *Ann Surg*. 2009;249(3):388-391.
8. Bancos I, Alahdab F, Crowley RK, et al. Therapy of endocrine disease: improvement of cardiovascular risk factors after adrenalectomy in patients with adrenal tumors and subclinical Cushing's syndrome. A systematic review and meta-analysis. *Eur J Endocrinol*. 2016;175(6):R283-R295.
9. Funder JW, Carey RM, Mantero F, et al. The management of primary aldosteronism: case detection, diagnosis, and treatment. An endocrine society clinical practice guideline. *J Clin Endocrinol Metab*. 2016;101(5):1889-1916.

10. Chomsky-Higgins K, Seib C, Rochefort H, et al. Less is more: cost-effectiveness analysis of surveillance strategies for small, nonfunctional, radiographically benign adrenal incidentalomas. *Surgery*. 2018;163(1):197-204.

11. Bittner JG., Brunt LM. Evaluation and management of adrenal incidentaloma. *J Surg Oncol*. 2012;106(5):557-564.

12. Dellinger RP, Levy MM, Rhodes A, et al. Surviving sepsis campaign. International guidelines for management of severe sepsis and septic shock: 2012. *Crit Care Med*. 2013;39(2):165-228.

13. Nigri G, Rosman AS, Petrucciani N, et al. Meta-analysis of trials comparing laparoscopic transperitoneal and retroperitoneal adrenalectomy. *Surgery*. 2013;153(1):111-119.

14. Wells SA Jr, Asa SL, Dralle H, et al. Revised American Thyroid Association guidelines for the management of medullary thyroid carcinoma. *Thyroid*. 2015;25(6):567-610.

15. Rowland KJ, Chernock RD, Moley JF. Pheochromocytoma in an 8-year-old patient with multiple endocrine neoplasia type 2A: implications for screening. *Surg Oncol*. 2013;108(4):203-206.

30 Parathyroid and Thyroid Glands

Eileen R. Smith and William E. Gillanders

I. INTRODUCTION

A. Anatomy

1. **Parathyroid**
   a. **Superior glands**
      i. Derived from the fourth pharyngeal pouches
      ii. Less variable in position
      iii. Usually found at the posterolateral aspect of superior thyroid lobe, posterior to **recurrent laryngeal nerve** (RLN) and superior to inferior thyroid artery
   b. **Inferior glands**
      i. Derived from the third pharyngeal pouches
      ii. Intimately associated with **thymus**, which also develops from the third pharyngeal pouch
      iii. Ectopic inferior glands may be found anywhere along the thymus descent tract into the chest that becomes the thyrothymic ligament.
      iv. Usually found inferior to inferior thyroid artery and anterior to RLN
   c. Inferior thyroid artery is the main blood supply for all parathyroids (**Figure 30.1**).
2. **Thyroid**
   a. Develops from endoderm of primitive foregut and arises in the ventral pharynx near base of the tongue, which ultimately becomes the foramen cecum.
   b. Thyroid then descends in the midline of the neck anterior to the hyoid and laryngeal cartilages.
      i. Congenital anomalies such as ectopic thyroid tissue or **thyroglossal duct cysts** are related to variations in this process.
   c. The thyroid is a bilobar structure connected by an isthmus that lies anterior to the trachea.
   d. Blood supply is from superior and inferior thyroid arteries, branches of the external carotid artery, and thyrocervical trunk.
   e. The thyroid is in close proximity to the parathyroid glands, trachea, esophagus, external branch of the **superior laryngeal nerve** (SLN, located near the superior pole of the thyroid), and the RLN (located just anterior or posterior to the inferior thyroid artery in the tracheoesophageal groove) (**Figure 30.1**).

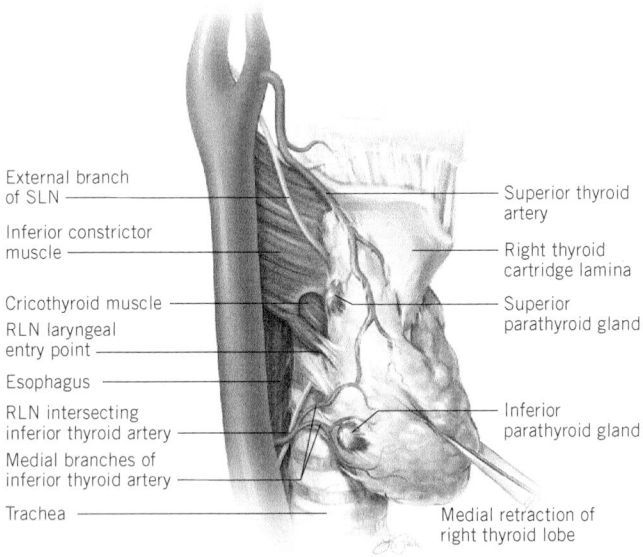

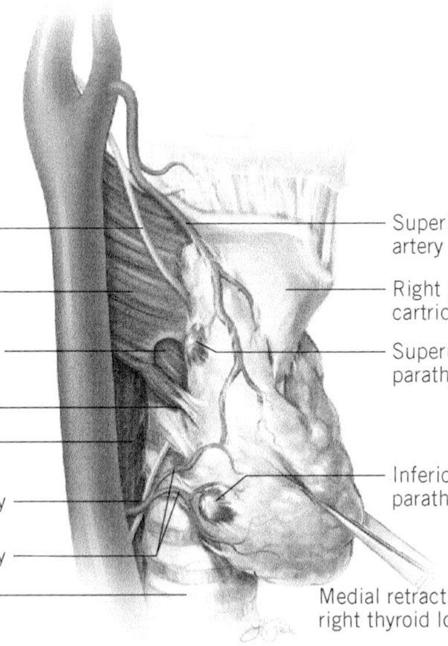

FIGURE 30.1 Thyroid and parathyroid anatomy and blood supply. *(Reprinted with permission from Hunt KK, Katz MH; American College of Surgeons Cancer Research Program; Alliance for Clinical Trials in Oncology. Operative Standards for Cancer Surgery. Vol 2. Thyroid, Gastric, Rectum, Esophagus, Melanoma. Wolters Kluwer; 2019.)*

B. Physiology

1. **Parathyroid**
   a. Serum calcium levels are maintained within normal range by the interplay of **parathyroid hormone** (PTH) and vitamin D.
   b. Low calcium levels stimulate chief cells of the parathyroid glands to secrete PTH, which
      i. Stimulates calcium and phosphate release from bone
      ii. Increases calcium reabsorption and inhibits phosphate reabsorption in the kidneys
      iii. Enhances intestinal absorption of calcium through increased renal activation of vitamin D
   c. Vitamin D is initially absorbed through the small intestine, undergoes hydroxylation in the liver to 25(OH)D_3, and then undergoes a second hydroxylation in the kidney under the influence of PTH to its active form, 1,25(OH)D_3.
   d. **Calcitonin** antagonizes the effect of PTH in the bones and kidneys.
2. **Thyroid**
   a. Hypothalamus secretes **thyrotropin-releasing hormone**, which stimulates anterior pituitary gland to secrete **thyroid-stimulating hormone** (TSH).

b. TSH stimulates thyroid gland to secrete thyroid hormone.
c. **Thyroid hormone** synthesis
   i. Begins when dietary iodide is ingested, actively transported into the thyroid, and oxidized by thyroid peroxidase into iodine
   ii. Iodination of tyrosine residues in thyroglobulin creates monoiodotyrosine and diiodotyrosine.
   iii. Coupling reactions of monoiodotyrosine and diiodotyrosine result in the formation of **triiodothyronine** (T_3) and **thyroxine** (T_4), both of which are bound to thyroglobulin and stored in thyroid follicles.
d. In the plasma, more than 99% of T_3 and T_4 are bound to carrier proteins, including thyroxine-binding globulin, thyroxine-binding prealbumin, and albumin.
   i. Only unbound hormones are active, and T_4 is converted to T_3 by deiodinases in the peripheral tissues.
   ii. Compared with T_3, T_4 has a 20-fold higher circulating concentration but is 3 to 5 times less potent.
e. Measurement of TSH is the most useful biochemical test in the assessment of thyroid function.
   i. In most patients without hypothalamic or pituitary disease, TSH and free T_4 (FT_4) vary inversely around a euthyroid state:
      a) Increased TSH and low FT_4 signify **hypothyroidism**
      b) Suppressed TSH and high FT_4 signify **hyperthyroidism**

C. Histology
1. **Parathyroid**
   a. **Chief cells** secrete PTH.
   b. Function of **oxyphil cells** is not fully understood.
2. **Thyroid**
   a. The **follicular cells** secrete iodine-containing thyroid hormones.
   b. The parafollicular cells, or **C cells**, are derived from the neural crest and migrate to the thyroid to produce calcitonin.

II. HYPERPARATHYROIDISM

A. Epidemiology/etiology/classification
1. **Primary hyperparathyroidism (HPT)**
   a. Incidence of 0.25 to 1 per 1,000 in the US
   b. Especially common in postmenopausal women
   c. Usually sporadic but can be inherited alone or as a component of familial endocrinopathies, including **multiple endocrine neoplasia** (MEN) types 1 and 2A
   d. PTH and calcium levels are high.
2. **Secondary HPT**
   a. Most commonly caused by renal failure
   b. Decreased serum calcium is a terminal feature of kidney dysfunction, which becomes evident through phosphate retention, decreased vitamin D activation, and poor calcium absorption.
   c. Intestinal malabsorption of calcium or vitamin D can also result in elevated PTH levels and secondary HPT.
   d. Patients with secondary HPT have high PTH levels and low calcium levels.

3. **Tertiary HPT**
   a. Seen in patients who have undergone prior kidney transplant for renal failure
   b. Typically, parathyroid gland function returns to normal within 1 year after kidney transplant, but in patients with tertiary HPT, the parathyroids fail to respond to normal signals for PTH secretion.
   c. Both PTH and calcium levels are high.

B. Presentation/symptoms
1. The most common presentation of HPT is incidental elevation of calcium.
2. Elevated calcium levels may be found incidentally, or patients can present with symptomatic hypercalcemia.
3. Other presentations of HPT include nephrolithiasis, osteoporosis or pathologic fracture, severe hypercalcemia, and emotional disturbances.
4. Patients may also have subtle symptoms such as muscle weakness, polyuria, anorexia, fatigue, bone/joint pain, poor sleep, reflux, and nausea.

C. Diagnosis/testing
1. Laboratory studies
   a. Serum or ionized calcium
   b. PTH immunoassay
   c. Twenty-four-hour urine calcium or renal calcium/creatinine clearance ratio
      i. Helpful in distinguishing primary HPT from **familial hypocalciuric hypercalcemia** (FHH), which presents with mild hypercalcemia and low urine calcium.
      ii. FHH is caused by loss-of-function mutations in renal and parathyroid calcium sensing receptors.
      iii. About 15% to 20% of patients with FHH will have elevated PTH.
      iv. A UrCa < 100 mg/24 hours and a Ca/Cr excretion ratio < 0.01 suggests FHH.
2. Imaging
   a. Technetium-99m sestamibi scintigraphy has been used historically to localize hyperfunctioning parathyroid tissue.
   b. Ultrasound with color Doppler examination complements the sestamibi scan and can assist in precise localization of adenomas, assessment of concomitant thyroid pathology, or fine needle aspiration (FNA) of equivocal/concerning lesion.
   c. Newer scintigraphy modalities in combination with single-photon emission computed tomography (SPECT), SPECT with CT, and four-dimensional (4D) CT have demonstrated higher sensitivity and positive predictive values.[1]

D. Nonoperative treatment
1. Only surgical intervention offers curative therapy for HPT.
2. Medical management is largely related to management of hypercalcemia, which is described further in Section III.
3. There are additionally various medical agents available for treatment of osteoporosis including bisphosphonates, denosumab, and raloxifene.

4. Hypercalcemia from secondary and tertiary HPT can be treated initially with dietary phosphate restriction, phosphate binders, vitamin D supplementation, and cinacalcet (a "calcimimetic").

E. Operative treatment
   1. Surgery is recommended for all patients with symptomatic disease.
   2. Indications for surgical intervention in asymptomatic patients are detailed in **Table 30.1**.[2]
   3. Minimally invasive parathyroidectomy
      a. Preoperative localization with rapid intraoperative PTH measurement enables minimally invasive techniques, including open, radioguided, video-assisted, and endoscopic methods.
      b. Successful preoperative localization allows for directed unilateral neck exploration and normal parathyroids do not need to be identified.
      c. Following adenoma removal, a 50% decrease in PTH levels at 10 minutes is highly indicative of cure from HPT per the Miami criterion.
         i. This can be used in conjunction with the "Normal Range" or "Dual" criteria in which cure is determined by both 50% drop and return of PTH to normal (or near normal) range.
   4. **Surgical approach: minimally invasive parathyroidectomy**
      a. Position patient with arms at sides and neck in extension.
      b. Make a **Kocher incision** approximately 3 cm superior to the sternal notch (or over the isthmus of the thyroid) and raise subplatysmal flaps.
      c. Incise the median raphe and dissect the strap muscles off the underlying thyroid gland.
      d. Identify and resect abnormal parathyroid gland taking care to identify and protect the RLN.
      e. Using intraoperative PTH monitoring, ensure a 50% drop in PTH levels in accordance with **Miami criterion**.
         i. If intraoperative PTH does not confirm appropriate drops, proceed to explore the other parathyroid glands, starting with the ipsilateral gland to identify additional abnormal glands (see conventional neck exploration below).
      f. Obtain meticulous hemostasis and close in layers.

TABLE 30.1 Indications for Operation in Asymptomatic Patients With Primary Hyperparathyroidism

Age < 50 y
Unable to participate in appropriate follow-up
Serum calcium level < 1 mg/dL above normal range
Urine calcium > 400 mg/24h
Creatinine clearance < 60 mL/min
Complications of hyperparathyroidism

5. **Conventional neck exploration**
   a. Bilateral neck exploration and identification of all four parathyroids was traditionally the cornerstone of surgical management in HPT.
   b. If an abnormally enlarged parathyroid or all four parathyroids cannot be found, exploration for ectopic or supernumerary glands should be performed.
      i. Ectopic superior glands may be found posterior and deep to the thyroid, in the tracheoesophageal groove, or between the carotid artery and the esophagus.
      ii. Ectopic inferior glands are most likely found embedded in the thymus in the anterior mediastinum
   c. Four-gland parathyroid hyperplasia is less common, and acceptable management options include total parathyroidectomy with parathyroid autotransplantation (below) or **3.5-gland parathyroidectomy**
   d. When multiple adenomas are found, they should be excised, leaving at least one normal parathyroid behind
6. **Parathyroid autotransplantation**
   a. Total parathyroidectomy with heterotopic parathyroid autotransplantation should be considered in patients with renal failure and secondary HPT, four-gland parathyroid hyperplasia, and those undergoing neck reexploration in which the adenoma is the only remaining parathyroid gland.
   b. The sternocleidomastoid or the brachioradialis muscles of the patient's nondominant forearm are common sites for autotransplantation
   c. To autotransplant
      i. After excision, mince parathyroid tissue finely and place in sterile iced saline.
      ii. Create separate intramuscular beds in muscle fibers of the brachioradialis or sternocleidomastoid with a fine forceps.
      iii. Several pieces of parathyroid tissue are placed in each site for a total transplant volume of approximately 100 mg.
      iv. Nonabsorbable suture is used to close the beds and to mark the site.
   d. Transplanted parathyroid tissue begins to function within 14 to 21 days of surgery.
   e. **Cryopreservation** of parathyroid glands can be performed in patients who are at risk for permanent hypoparathyroidism after repeat exploration allowing for future autotransplantation in patients with failure of the initial graft.

F. Outcomes/complications
1. Outcomes
   a. Cure rates for sporadic primary HPT approach 95% to 99%, with cure defined as the reestablishment of normal calcium homeostasis lasting at least 6 months postoperatively.[3]
2. Complications
   a. **Hypocalcemia**
      i. Transient hypocalcemia commonly occurs after total thyroidectomy or parathyroidectomy.
      ii. Treat if severe (total serum calcium < 7.5 mg/dL) or symptomatic.

iii. Symptoms may involve numbness/paresthesia in the distal extremities, perioral numbness, hyperactive tendon reflexes, facial twitching with tapping of the cheek (**Chvostek sign**), flexing of the wrist and hand joints when a blood pressure cuff is inflated (**Trousseau's sign**).

iv. Patients typically require supplementation for 2 weeks and are given oral calcium carbonate (500-1000 mg tid).

a) Calcitriol (0.25 μg/d) may also be helpful.

v. IV calcium supplementation of calcium gluconate or calcium chloride may be necessary in persistently symptomatic patients or in emergent situations such as hypocalcemic tetany.

a) About 10 to 20 mL of 10% calcium gluconate is given IV over 10 minutes and may be repeated every 15-20 minutes as required until symptom resolution.

b) Subsequently, a continuous infusion of calcium gluconate in D5W is initiated at a rate of 1 g/h with correction of any concurrent hypomagnesemia.

b. Persistent disease or missed glands

i. Surgical reexploration should be considered for persistent and/or recurrent disease after thorough biochemical evaluation and imaging localization.

ii. Missed parathyroid glands can be found in normal anatomic locations or ectopic sites.

a) May occasionally be intrathyroidal, and thyroid lobectomy can be performed if an exhaustive search fails to identify a parathyroid adenoma.

b) If four normal glands have been located, a supernumerary gland is likely responsible.

c) Mediastinal adenomas in the thymus are managed by resecting the cranial portion via gentle traction on the thyrothymic ligament or by a complete transcervical thymectomy.

d) Median sternotomy is rarely indicated to excise a retrosternal adenoma.

iii. Intraoperative ultrasound and/or venous sampling from the internal jugular veins can sometimes be useful in localizing adenomas.

c. Rates of nerve injury and hemorrhage are similar to those in thyroid surgery (see Section V).

III. PARATHYROID CANCER

A. Epidemiology/etiology/classification

1. Rare disease accounting for <1% of patients with primary HPT
2. Incidence similar in men and women
3. Mostly sporadic but some cases may be associated with syndromes such as hyperparathyroidism–jaw tumor syndrome or MEN-1 and -2A

B. Presentation/symptoms

1. Most (>90%) of parathyroid carcinomas are biochemically functional.
2. In contrast to benign disease, patients with carcinoma are more likely to present with a palpable neck mass.

3. May present with signs of mass effect and symptoms of severe hypercalcemia, including profound muscular weakness, nausea and vomiting, drowsiness, and confusion.

C. Diagnosis/testing
   1. Laboratory studies
      a. PTH levels are often 5 times the upper limit of normal (300 pg/mL or more).
      b. Serum calcium levels may exceed 15 mg/dL.
   2. Imaging
      a. Ultrasound and ^{99m}Tc sestamibi imaging can be used to localize disease, but diagnosis depends on histologic findings of vascular or capsular invasion, metastases, or gross invasion of local structures.

D. Nonoperative treatment
   1. Only surgical therapy is curative, but medical management of associated hypercalcemia may be required preoperatively or in patients with unresectable disease.
      a. First-line therapy is fluid resuscitation with infusion of normal saline.
      b. In patients with severe hypercalcemia (serum calcium > 14 mg/dL), concurrent use of both calcitonin and bisphosphonates is recommended.
      c. Other strategies include the use of loop diuretics, glucocorticoids, calcimimetics, denosumab, or hemodialysis.

E. Operative treatment
   1. Surgery is the only known curative therapy and entails radical local excision of the tumor en bloc with surrounding soft tissue, lymph nodes, and ipsilateral thyroid lobe.
   2. In instances where malignancy is not suspected prior to operation, a grayish-white, hard mass with adherence to or invasion of surrounding structures should raise suspicion.
   3. Reoperation should be considered for local and distant recurrences to control malignant hypercalcemia

F. Outcomes/complications
   1. Outcomes
      a. Recurrence rates are as high as 50%, but survival rates at 10 years are 60% to 70%.
      b. Mortality is more often related to complications of severe hypercalcemia rather than tumor burden.
      c. Patient should be followed with close monitoring of serum calcium and PTH as well as annual neck ultrasound.
   2. Complications
      a. Similar to parathyroidectomy for benign disease and include nerve injury, postoperative hypocalcemia, and hemorrhage.

IV. THYROID NODULES

A. Epidemiology/etiology/classification
   1. A **thyroid nodule** is defined as a discrete lesion distinct from surrounding thyroid tissue.
   2. Very common with up to 7% of adults having palpable nodules and as many as 68% of adults on ultrasound imaging.

3. Evaluation is recommended to distinguish patients with underlying malignancy from the majority with benign nodules. **Figure 30.2** illustrates the algorithm for the workup of a newly diagnosed thyroid nodule.[4]

B. Presentation/symptoms
1. May be incidentally found on imaging or present with palpable neck mass.
2. Rapid growth, pain, or compressive symptoms as well as a firm nodule with irregular texture should raise suspicion for malignancy.
3. Functional nodules may present with symptoms of hyperthyroidism.

C. Diagnosis/testing
1. Laboratory studies
   a. TSH, T3, and T4 levels
      i. Should be measured during initial evaluation of thyroid nodule.

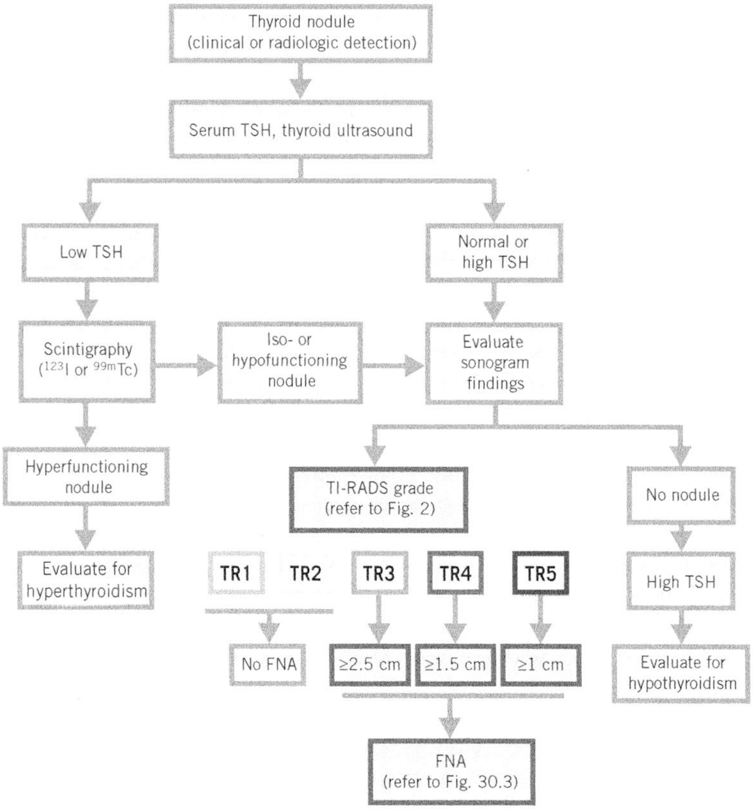

FIGURE 30.2 Thyroid nodule initial evaluation algorithm. FNA, fine-needle aspiration; TI-RADS, Thyroid Imaging, Reporting and Data System; TSH, thyroid-stimulating hormone.

ii. Suppressed TSH level: Thyroid scan should be performed.
iii. Normal or elevated TSH level: Thyroid ultrasound imaging should be performed.

2. **FNA biopsy**
   a. An accurate and cost-effective method for evaluating thyroid nodules after ultrasound imaging is completed as indicated by imaging features (see below).
      i. Ultrasound imaging is performed prior to FNA to stratify risk and identify high-risk nodules that meet criteria for biopsy.
   b. The **Bethesda System** for Reporting Thyroid Cytopathology (**Table 30.2** and **Figure 30.3**) can be used to guide further management based on biopsy results.[5]
3. **Molecular testing**
   a. Multiple tests are available and can be useful in risk-stratifying Bethesda type III/IV nodules to avoid operation for diagnostic purposes.[4]
   b. New RNA and DNA sequencing tests may allow up to 50% of patients with indeterminate thyroid nodules to avoid operation.[6]

TABLE 30.2 Bethesda System for Reporting Thyroid Cytopathology

Diagnostic Category	Risk for Malignancy (%)[a]	Recommendation
(I) Nondiagnostic or unsatisfactory	5-10	Repeat FNA with US guidance
(II) Benign	0-3	Clinical follow-up, repeat US (12-24 mo)
(III) Atypia of undetermined significance Follicular lesion of undetermined significance	6-18	Molecular testing, repeat FNA (3 mo), or lobectomy
(IV) Follicular neoplasm Suspicious for follicular neoplasm	10-40	Molecular testing or lobectomy
(V) Suspicious for malignancy	45-60	Near-total thyroidectomy or lobectomy
(VI) Malignant	94-96	Near-total thyroidectomy or lobectomy

FNA, fine-needle aspiration; NIFTP, noninvasive follicular thyroid neoplasm with papillary-like nuclear features; US, ultrasound.

Adapted by permission from Springer: Baloch ZW, Cooper DS, Gharib H, Alexander EK. Overview of diagnostic terminology and reporting. In: Ali S, Cibas E, eds. *The Bethesda System for Reporting Thyroid Cytopathology: Definitions, Criteria and Explanatory Notes*. 2nd ed. Springer International Publishing; 2018:1-6. Copyright 2018, Springer International Publishing AG.

[a]NIFTP is no longer considered malignancy.

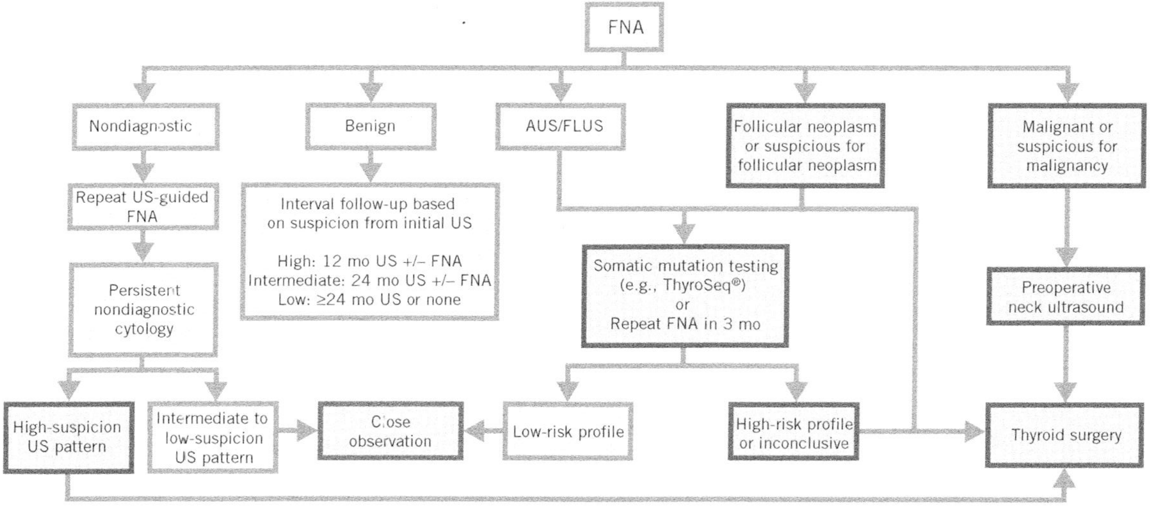

FIGURE 30.3 Thyroid nodule management following fine-needle aspiration (FNA) biopsy. AUS, atypia of undetermined significance; FLUS, follicular lesion of undetermined significance; US, ultrasound.

4. Imaging
   a. **Thyroid ultrasound imaging**
      i. Imaging study of choice to evaluate thyroid nodules
      ii. Nodules with low risk for malignancy are cystic and anechoic with smooth margins and either with no echogenic foci or with large comet-tail artifact.
      iii. Nodules with elevated risk of malignancy are solid, hypoechoic, taller than wide, with irregular margins and small punctate echogenic foci.
      iv. The ACR **TI-RADS** (Thyroid Imaging, Reporting and Data System) is commonly used to risk stratify nodules based on ultrasound imaging features and identify those appropriate for biopsy[7] (**Figure 30.4**).
   b. Thyroid scan
      i. ^{123}**I thyroid scanning** can be helpful to distinguish solitary functioning nodules from **multinodular goiter** or **Graves' disease** in patients with suppressed TSH.
      ii. Hypofunctioning areas are "cold" while hyperfunctioning areas are "hot" demonstrating increased uptake.
      iii. Cold nodules are more likely than hot nodules to be malignant.
   c. CT or MRI
      i. Reserved for evaluation of substernal or retrosternal masses, evaluating local invasion, or for staging known malignancy

D. Nonoperative treatment

1. **Radioactive iodine (RAI) ablation**
   a. Can be used to treat hyperthyroid symptoms due to functional nodules in the case of toxic adenoma or toxic multinodular goiter
2. **Thionamides** to inhibit thyroid hormone synthesis
   a. Methimazole
   b. Propylthiouracil
      i. Utilized during the first trimester of pregnancy due to teratogenic effects of methimazole
3. **Radiofrequency ablation**
   a. Can be used for treatment of confirmed benign, predominantly solid nodules as an alternative to surgery

E. Operative treatment

1. Indications
   a. Confirmed or suspected malignancy (Bethesda V/VI)
   b. Bethesda III/IV nodules in which molecular testing reveals a high-risk profile or subsequent FNA is inconclusive
   c. Persistently nondiagnostic FNA in a nodule with suspicious ultrasound imaging features
   d. Multiple large nodules
   e. Obstructive symptoms
   f. **Thyrotoxicosis** or hyperthyroidism refractory to medical management
   g. Failure of RAI therapy

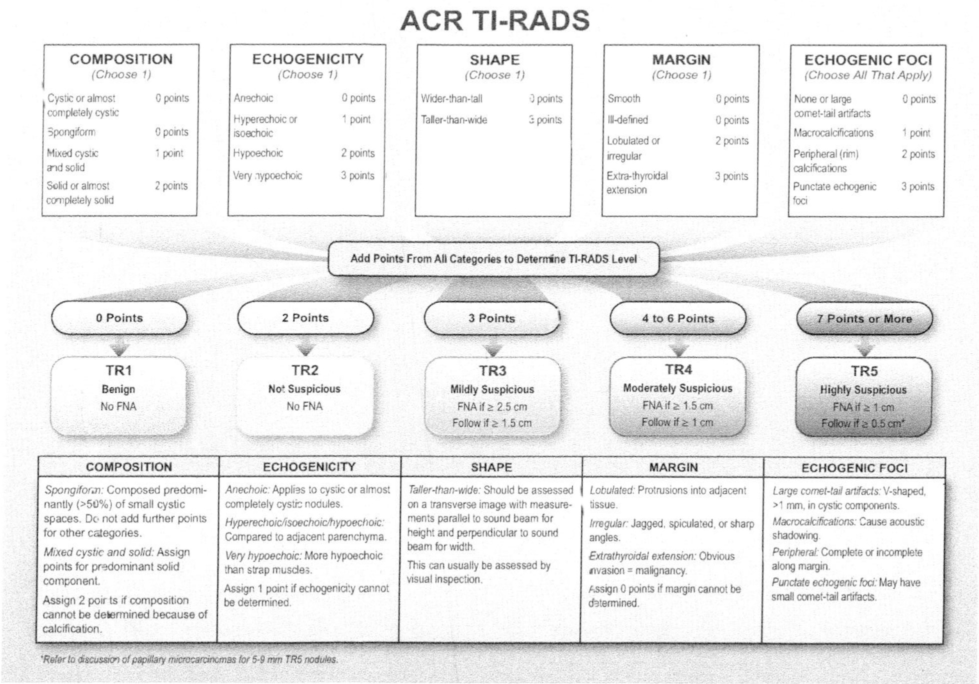

FIGURE 30.4 ACR Thyroid Imaging, Reporting and Data System. FNA, fine-needle aspiration. *(From Tessler FN, Middleton WD, Grant EG, et al. ACR thyroid imaging, reporting and data system (TI-RADS): white paper of the ACR TI-RADS committee. J Am Coll Radiol. 2017;14(5):587-595. Reprinted with permission from American College of Radiology.)*

2. Resection
   a. For benign disease, total thyroidectomy or lobectomy can be selected based on location and extent of disease.
   b. For malignancy, total thyroidectomy vs. lobectomy is determined based on diagnosis.

F. Outcomes/complications
1. Outcomes
   a. The vast majority of thyroid nodules are benign (95%) and can be managed without resection.
   b. Outcomes related to thyroid malignancy are described in the section on thyroid cancers.
2. Complications
   a. Surgical complications include nerve injury, postoperative hypocalcemia, and hemorrhage (and are discussed further below).

V. THYROID CANCER

A. Epidemiology/etiology/classification
1. **Papillary thyroid cancer** (PTC)
   a. Accounts for 85% of thyroid carcinomas
   b. Often multifocal and metastasizes to lymph nodes
   c. Features associated with worse prognosis
      i. Male gender
      ii. Primary tumor > 4 cm
      iii. Gross local invasion or extrathyroidal extension
      iv. Age > 45 years
      v. Lymphovascular invasion
      vi. Certain histologic subtypes: Tall cell, follicular, insular, columnar, diffuse sclerosis, hobnail
      vii. Known metastatic disease
2. **Follicular thyroid cancer** (FTC)
   a. Rare before age 30 years
   b. More common in women
   c. Slightly worse prognosis than PTC
   d. Hematogenous spread to bone, lung, or liver
3. **Medullary thyroid cancer** (MTC)
   a. Arises from parafollicular C cells
   b. May occur sporadically or as part of MEN types 2A and 2B or familial medullary thyroid carcinoma syndrome
   c. Can spread early to cervical lymph nodes and metastasize to liver, lung, or bone
4. **Anaplastic** or undifferentiated thyroid carcinoma
   a. Accounts for 1% to 2% of thyroid cancers
   b. Poor prognosis
   c. Typically > age 50 years
   d. Over 90% of patients have invasive disease either locoregional or metastasis at time of diagnosis.
5. **Primary thyroid lymphoma**
   a. Typically non-Hodgkin type
   b. Often associated with **Hashimoto thyroiditis**

6. An overview of the major categories of malignancies is seen in **Table 30.3**.

B. Presentation/symptoms

1. Many thyroid malignancies may be asymptomatic and discovered incidentally on imaging or workup of thyroid nodules.
2. Patients with anaplastic thyroid carcinoma often present with compressive symptoms including dysphagia, respiratory compromise, or hoarseness.

C. Diagnosis/testing

1. Laboratory studies
   a. FNA biopsy
   b. Genetic testing in patients with MTC to test for MEN syndrome by evaluation of germline mutations of ***RET*** **proto-oncogene**
   c. For patients with MEN syndrome, screening for **pheochromocytoma** should occur in patients with MTC with serum or urine metanephrines.
   d. Carcinoembryonic antigen and calcitonin are important tumor markers for MTC.
2. Imaging
   a. Thyroid ultrasound imaging including the neck to evaluate lymph nodes
   b. Neck CT can be useful for surgical planning in patients with compressive symptoms.

D. Treatment

1. The vast majority of patients with thyroid cancer will be treated with resection. However, alternatives for nonoperative candidates or patients with recurrent disease include RFA and ablation via injection with sclerosing agents (ethanol).
2. **Surgical approach: partial and total thyroidectomy**
   a. Position patient with arms at sides and neck in extension. Consider the use of intraoperative nerve monitoring especially in patients with known unilateral RLN dysfunction or prior neck operations.[8]
   b. Make a low cervical incision approximately 3 cm superior to the sternal notch and raise subplatysmal flaps.
   c. Incise the median raphe and dissect the strap muscles off the underlying thyroid gland.
   d. Ligate the middle thyroid vein and isolate and divide the superior thyroid vessels. The superior pole vessels should be divided as close as possible to the thyroid gland to avoid injury to SLN.
   e. Retract the superior pole medially and superiorly to facilitate dissection of the rest of the thyroid lobe. Take care to identify and protect the RLN and preserve the parathyroid glands and their blood supply.
   f. Once the lobe is fully mobilized, dissect the isthmus off the trachea posteriorly. At this point, divide the thyroid at the isthmus if performing a lobectomy or proceed to repeat the dissection of the contralateral lobe in the same method for a total.
   g. Obtain meticulous hemostasis and close in layers.

TABLE 30.3 Categories, Features, and Management of Thyroid Malignancies

Category	Percent of All Thyroid Malignancies	Clinical Features	Management
Papillary carcinoma	70-80	Indolent, often multifocal Frequently metastatic to cervical lymph nodes	Surgery with or without RAI ablation therapy With or without thyroid hormone suppression therapy Follow-up: Serum thyroglobulin, neck ultrasound imaging
Follicular carcinoma	10-15	More common in women, age ≥ 30 y Hematogenous spread to bone, lung, liver	Surgery with or without RAI ablation therapy with or without thyroid hormone suppression therapy. Follow-up: Serum thyroglobulin, neck ultrasound imaging
Medullary carcinoma	5-10	Sporadic (75%) vs. familial (25%) Familial forms: MEN syndromes type 2A and 2B Frequent early nodal metastasis Elevated calcitonin and CEA levels	Genetic testing (*RET* proto-oncogene) for all patients Screening for pheochromocytoma Total thyroidectomy with lymph node dissection
Anaplastic carcinoma	1-2	Frequently presents at advanced stage May be highly symptomatic with local invasion Nearly 100% disease-specific mortality	Palliative surgery Chemotherapy with or without external beam radiation
Lymphoma	2-8	Often non-Hodgkin type Associated with Hashimoto thyroiditis	External beam radiation vs. chemotherapy

CEA, carcinoembryonic antigen; MEN, multiple endocrine neoplasia; RAI, radioactive iodine.

3. **Operative options for PTC**
   a. Total thyroidectomy for
      i. Tumors > 4 cm
      ii. Bilateral nodules
      iii. Regional or metastatic disease
      iv. Personal history of head/neck radiation exposure
      v. First-degree relatives with PTC
   b. Thyroid lobectomy for
      i. Low-risk patients with <1 cm, intrathyroidal unifocal tumors
      ii. Low-risk patients with tumor size 1 to 4 cm, either lobectomy or total thyroidectomy can be considered
   c. **Lymph node dissection** (LND)
      i. Therapeutic: LND of the central compartment (level VI) and/or ipsilateral lateral neck (levels II, III, IV) performed in all patients with nodal disease
      ii. Prophylactic: LND of level VI nodes considered for high-risk patients (T3/4, radiation exposure, involved lateral nodes)
      iii. Ultrasound imaging can be used preoperatively to mark suspicious lymph nodes.
4. **Operative options for FTC**
   a. Lobectomy for unilateral tumors < 1 cm with limited invasion of the tumor capsule
   b. Total thyroidectomy
      i. Tumors > 1 cm
      ii. Tumors with extensive capsular or vascular invasion
      iii. Distant metastases
5. **Operative options for MTC**
   a. Total thyroidectomy
      i. Patients with MEN 2 with thyroid nodules < 5 mm and calcitonin levels < 40 pg/mL.
      ii. Patients with MEN 2 can be considered for prophylactic thyroidectomy as young as age 3 years in MEN2A and in infancy in MEN2B.
   b. Total thyroidectomy with central neck (level VI) LND
      i. All other cases of sporadic and non-MEN-related familial MTC require central LND.
      ii. Additional dissection of ipsilateral lateral compartment nodes should be performed in patients with palpable primary tumors
   c. Surgical excision for residual or recurrent disease
6. **Operative option for anaplastic thyroid carcinoma** is focused on palliative procedure(s) to relieve compressive symptoms and decrease tumor burden
7. **Adjuvant therapies**
   a. Adjuvant treatment and follow-up after PTC resection:
      i. RAI after resection recommended for
         a) Primary tumor size > 4 cm
         b) Gross local invasion
         c) Select patients with tumor size 1 to 4 cm with high-risk features

d) For patients with low-risk differentiated thyroid cancer, RAI was not superior to observation alone.[9] (*N Engl J Med.* 2022;386(10):923-932.)

ii. Thyroid hormone suppression therapy
   a) Suppressing TSH with hormone replacement can decrease recurrence and improve survival.

iii. Follow-up
   a) Monitoring serum thyroglobulin at least every 6 to 12 months
   b) Neck ultrasound imaging at least every 12 months

iv. Small molecule inhibitors
   a) For patients with radioactive iodine–resistant refractory differentiated thyroid cancer, cabozantinib (a tyrosine kinase inhibitor) has been shown to improve disease-free survival.[10]
   b) Other small molecule inhibitors may be appropriate based on genomic profile.

b. Adjuvant treatment after FTC resection
   i. RAI
   ii. Thyroid hormone suppression therapy
   iii. Follow-up
      a) Thyroglobulin serum levels every 6 to 12 months for at least 5 years

c. Adjuvant treatment after MTC
   i. No role for RAI
   ii. Can consider tyrosine kinase inhibitors of *RET* and *VEGF*
   iii. Follow-up
      a) Calcitonin levels every 6 to 12 months

8. Nonoperative treatment
   a. Radiation and chemotherapy can be used for palliation of undifferentiated thyroid carcinoma or primary thyroid lymphoma

E. Outcomes/complications

1. Hemorrhage
   a. Occurs in 0.3% to 1% of operations
   b. Typically occurs within 6 hours of operation
   c. Must secure airway and then proceed to operating room to control bleeding
      i. In rare circumstances, respiratory difficulty can necessitate opening the incision at bedside prior to proceeding to the operation.

2. Hypocalcemia
   a. Typically transient and occurs 24 to 48 hours after surgery
   b. Supplementation
      i. Calcium carbonate 1 g tid for 2 weeks postoperatively
      ii. Additional calcium carbonate and calcitriol can be added if symptomatic.
      iii. Postoperative PTH levels can be used to guide decision making on additional supplementation.
      iv. IV calcium gluconate infusion can be utilized in severe cases
   c. Permanent hypoparathyroidism is rare, and autotransplantation of devitalized parathyroid glands can decrease this risk (see autotransplantation above).

3. **Nerve injury**
   a. RLN
      i. Injury occurs in <1% of cases
      ii. Unilateral: Presents as hoarseness
      iii. Bilateral: Can result in airway compromise potentially requiring tracheostomy
      iv. May be transient (improving over 1-6 weeks postoperatively) or permanent, in which case cord medialization procedure can be considered
   b. SLN
      i. The external branch of the SLN can be injured when taking down the superior pole.
      ii. Can present as difficulty with vocal pitch control

VI. GRAVES' DISEASE (AUTOIMMUNE DIFFUSE TOXIC GOITER)

A. Epidemiology/etiology/classification
   1. The most common cause of hyperthyroidism
   2. Occurs up to 7 times more commonly in women
   3. Typically presents in the 2nd to 4th decade of life
   4. Hyperthyroid symptoms occur due to excess hormone as a result of constitutive activation of the TSH receptor by simulating immunoglobulins.

B. Presentation/symptoms
   1. Symptoms of hyperthyroidism include weight loss, heat intolerance, excessive perspiration, anxiety, irritability, palpitations, fatigue, and oligomenorrhea.
   2. Signs of hyperthyroidism include goiter, sinus tachycardia and atrial fibrillation, tremor, hyperreflexia, fine or thinning hair, eyelid lag or retraction, thyroid bruit, muscle wasting, and proximal muscle weakness
   3. Infiltrative ophthalmopathy
   4. Pretibial myxedema

C. Diagnosis/testing
   1. Laboratory studies
      a. TSH levels: Typically suppressed
      b. Anti-TSH-R antibodies
   2. Imaging
      a. Thyroid ultrasound imaging
         i. Imaging study of choice to evaluate thyroid nodules as described above
         ii. Can be useful to assess any concurrent nodules for need to biopsy
      b. Thyroid scan
         i. ^{123}I thyroid scanning can be helpful to distinguish solitary functioning nodules from multinodular goiter or Graves' disease in patients with suppressed TSH.
      c. CT or MRI
         i. Reserved for evaluation of substernal or retrosternal masses

D. Nonoperative treatment
   1. RAI ablation
      a. Cure rates approach 90%.
      b. Hypothyroidism will develop in the majority of patients.

c. Contraindications include pregnancy or lactation, newborns, patient refusal or inability to comply with radiation safety recommendations, and low RAI uptake <20%.
d. **Exophthalmos** is a relative contraindication.
2. Thionamides to inhibit thyroid hormone synthesis
a. Notably long-term remission is achieved in <20% to 30% with pharmacologic therapy alone.
b. Agents include
i. Methimazole: Preferred agent, used to prepare thyrotoxic patients for resection or ablative therapy
ii. Propylthiouracil: Utilized during first trimester of pregnancy due to teratogenic effects of methimazole
3. Monoclonal antibody inhibitors of IGF-IR have recently been approved to treat Graves'-associated moderate to severe ophthalmopathy.[11]

E. Operative treatment
1. Surgical therapy with near-total or total thyroidectomy indicated for patients with contraindications to RAI, obstructive goiter, and/or exophthalmos
2. Near-total or total thyroidectomy is recommended due to high recurrence rates in subtotal (8%-15%) and risk of occult malignancy (5%-20%).
3. Patients should be treated with preoperative antithyroid medical therapy to ensure that they are euthyroid prior to operation.
4. Iodine drops can be used preoperatively to decrease thyroid vascularity and reduce operative blood loss

F. Outcomes/complications
1. Surgical complications are similar to thyroidectomy and include nerve injury, postoperative hypocalcemia, and hemorrhage
2. Patients with recurrent disease after operation can be considered for RAI

VII. THYROIDITIS

A. Epidemiology/etiology/classification
1. Painless thyroiditis
a. **Hashimoto thyroiditis**
i. Chronic autoimmune disorder involving destructive lymphocytic infiltration of the thyroid
ii. Most common cause of hypothyroidism in the US
iii. More common in women
iv. Patients may have circulating antimicrosomal, antithyroglobulin, and TSH receptor antibodies
v. Increased risk of thyroid lymphoma
b. **Postpartum thyroiditis**
i. Autoimmune thyroiditis within 1 year of pregnancy
ii. Course often progresses serially through hyperthyroidism, euthyroidism, and hypothyroidism.
c. **Reidel thyroiditis**
i. Rare invasive fibrous thyroiditis characterized by replacement of the thyroid with dense fibrous tissue

2. Painful thyroiditis
   a. **Acute suppurative thyroiditis**
      i. Most often caused by *Streptococcus* or *Staphylococcus* infection
   b. **Subacute (de Quervain) thyroiditis**
      i. Painful self-limited inflammation of the thyroid associated with viral infection
      ii. Typically presents with thyrotoxicosis followed by euthyroidism, hypothyroidism, and subsequent return of normal function

B. Diagnosis/testing
1. Laboratory studies
   a. Antimicrosomal, antithyroglobulin, anti-thyroid peroxidase and anti-TSH receptor antibodies
   b. TSH level and T4 level to evaluate thyroid function
2. Imaging
   a. Thyroid ultrasound imaging can be used to assess for nodules and malignancy.
   b. Neck CT can be used to evaluate patients with compressive symptoms to aid in operative planning.

C. Nonoperative treatment
1. Thyroid hormone replacement indicated in patients with subclinical and overt hypothyroidism
2. Antibiotic therapy can be useful in acute suppurative thyroiditis, and anti-inflammatory medications such as NSAIDs and/or steroids can be useful for subacute thyroiditis.

D. Operative treatment
1. Thyroidectomy may be indicated to exclude malignancy or relieve compressive symptoms, particularly in the care of Riedel thyroiditis. Operation can also be considered for patients with thyrotoxicosis refractory to medical management.

E. Outcomes/complications
1. Many patients do well with medical management.
2. Following an episode of thyroiditis, 30% to 50% of patients will develop permanent hypothyroidism.
3. Operative complications of thyroidectomy are described in Section V.F. above

Key References

Citation	Summary
Nikiforova MN, Mercurio S, Wald AI, et al. Analytical performance of the ThyroSeq v3 genomic classifier for cancer diagnosis in thyroid nodules. *Cancer.* 2018;124(8):1682-1690.	• ThyroSeq genomic classifier was able to distinguish cancer from benign nodules with 93.9% sensitivity, 89.4% specificity, and 92.1% accuracy.

Citation	Summary
Wilhelm SM, Wang TS, Ruan DT, et al. The American Association of endocrine surgeons guidelines for definitive management of primary hyperparathyroidism. *JAMA Surg.* 2016;151(10):959-968.	• American Association of Endocrine Surgeons guidelines for treatment of primary hyperparathyroidism including preoperative workup, indications for surgery, and management of persistent disease.
Haugen BR, Alexander EK, Bible KC, et al. 2015 American Thyroid Association management guidelines for adult patients with thyroid nodules and differentiated thyroid cancer: the American Thyroid Association guidelines task force on thyroid nodules and differentiated thyroid cancer. *Thyroid.* 2016;26(1):1-133.	• Evidenced-based clinical guidelines for management of thyroid nodules and cancers, which includes a shift toward lobectomy alone as definitive treatment for certain lower-risk thyroid malignancies.
Hoang JK, Middleton WD, Farjat AE, et al. reduction in thyroid nodule biopsies and improved accuracy with American College of radiology thyroid imaging reporting and data system. *Radiology.* 2018;287(1):185-193.	• A retrospective study in which the evaluation of thyroid nodules by radiologists with their own individual approach was compared with those radiologists utilizing TI-RADS criteria demonstrating that ACR TI-RADS criteria offer a meaningful reduction in the number of thyroid nodules recommended for biopsy and significantly improved the accuracy of the recommendations for nodule management.

CHAPTER 30: PARATHYROID AND THYROID GLANDS

Review Questions

1. What provides the blood supply to the superior and inferior parathyroid glands?
2. What is the initial treatment in patients presenting with severe hypercalcemia?
3. What percentage drop in PTH levels at 10 minutes is considered suggestive of cure in minimally invasive parathyroid surgery according to the Miami criterion?
4. What is the imaging study of choice to evaluate thyroid nodules?
5. Radioactive iodine ablation after resection is recommended for which type(s) of thyroid carcinoma?
6. All patients with medullary thyroid cancer should be screened for what prior to undergoing surgery?
7. Thyroid lymphoma is associated with which benign pathology of the thyroid?

REFERENCES

1. Lavely WC, Goetze S, Friedman KP, et al. Comparison of SPECT/CT, SPECT, and planar imaging with single- and dual-phase (99m)Tc-sestamibi parathyroid scintigraphy. *J Nucl Med.* 2007;48(7):1084-1089.
2. Bilezikian JP, Brandi ML, Eastell R, et al. Guidelines for the management of asymptomatic primary hyperparathyroidism: summary statement from the Fourth International Workshop. *J Clin Endocrinol Metab.* 2014;99(10):3561-3569.
3. Wilhelm SM, Wang TS, Ruan DT, et al. The American Association of endocrine surgeons guidelines for definitive management of primary hyperparathyroidism. *JAMA Surg.* 2016;151(10):959-968.
4. Haugen BR, Alexander EK, Bible KC, et al. 2015 American Thyroid Association management guidelines for adult patients with thyroid nodules and differentiated thyroid cancer: the American Thyroid Association guidelines task force on thyroid nodules and differentiated thyroid cancer. *Thyroid.* 2016;26(1):1-133.
5. Cibas ES, Ali SZ. The 2017 Bethesda system for reporting thyroid cytopathology. *Thyroid.* 2017;27(11):1341-1346.
6. Livhits MJ, Zhu CY, Kuo EJ, et al. Effectiveness of molecular testing techniques for diagnosis of indeterminate thyroid nodules: a randomized clinical trial. *JAMA Oncol.* 2021;7(1):70-77.
7. Tessler FN, Middleton WD, Grant EG, et al. ACR Thyroid Imaging, Reporting and Data System (TI-RADS): white paper of the ACR TI-RADS committee. *J Am Coll Radiol.* 2017;14(5):587-595.
8. Cirocchi R, Arezzo A, D'Andrea V, et al. Intraoperative neuromonitoring versus visual nerve identification for prevention of recurrent laryngeal nerve injury in adults undergoing thyroid surgery. *Cochrane Database Syst Rev.* 2019;1(1):CD012483.
9. Leboulleux S, Bournaud C, Chougnet CN, et al. Thyroidectomy without radioiodine in patients with low-risk thyroid cancer. *N Engl J Med.* 2022;386(10):923-932.
10. Brose MS, Robinson B, Sherman SI, et al. Cabozantinib for radioiodine-refractory differentiated thyroid cancer (COSMIC-311): a randomised, double-blind, placebo-controlled, phase 3 trial. *Lancet Oncol.* 2021;22(8):1126-1138.
11. Smith TJ, Kahaly GJ, Ezra DG, et al. Teprotumumab for thyroid-Associated ophthalmopathy. *N Engl J Med.* 2017;376(18):1748-1761.
12. Nikiforova MN, Mercurio S, Wald AI, et al.. Analytical performance of the ThyroSeq v3 genomic classifier for cancer diagnosis in thyroid nodules. *Cancer.* 2018;124(8):1682-1690.
13. Hoang JK, Middleton WD, Farjat AE, et al. Reduction in thyroid nodule biopsies and improved accuracy with American College of radiology thyroid imaging reporting and data system. *Radiology.* 2018;287(1):185-193.

31

Lung and Mediastinal Diseases

Louisa Yun Zhu Bai, Brendan T. Heiden, and Varun Puri

I. ANATOMY

A. Lung anatomy

1. The right lung has 3 lobes (upper, middle, lower) and 10 segments; the left lung has 2 lobes (upper, lower) and 8 segments (**Figure 31.1**).
2. The **major (oblique) fissure** divides lower lobes from remaining lobes on both sides.
3. The **minor (horizontal) fissure** is only present on the right and divides the upper and middle lobes.
4. The relative locations of the pulmonary artery, pulmonary veins, and mainstem bronchi differ between the left and right hilum (**Figure 31.2**).
5. It is important to know the mediastinal and hilar lymph node stations as these are typically sampled during lung cancer resection (**Figure 31.3**).
6. There are two circulatory systems: pulmonary and bronchial.
   a. **Pulmonary system**
      i. Deoxygenated blood from superior and inferior vena cavae → right atrium → right ventricle → bilateral pulmonary arteries → bilateral lungs for gas exchange
      ii. Oxygenated blood from lungs → pulmonary veins → left atrium → left ventricle → systemic circulation
   b. **Bronchial system**
      i. Left and right bronchial arteries supply oxygenated blood directly from the aorta to the hilum and larger airways, as well as some adjacent mediastinal structures.
      ii. Drainage of the bronchial system is largely into the pulmonary circulation via the pulmonary veins; however, some blood is drained via the bronchial veins into the **azygous vein** on the right and the **hemiazygous vein** on the left.[2]
7. The respiratory system can be divided into a conducting portion and a respiratory portion.
   a. The conducting portion includes nasopharynx, larynx, trachea, bronchi (main, lobar, and segmental), and smaller bronchioles.
   b. The respiratory portion includes terminal bronchioles, alveolar ducts, alveolar sacs, and alveoli.

B. Mediastinal anatomy

1. Borders of the anterior mediastinum: sternum anteriorly, pericardium posteriorly, T4 vertebral plane superiorly, T9 vertebral plane inferiorly
2. Borders of the middle mediastinum: pericardial sac anteriorly and posteriorly, pleural sacs bilaterally, sternal angle superiorly, diaphragm inferiorly

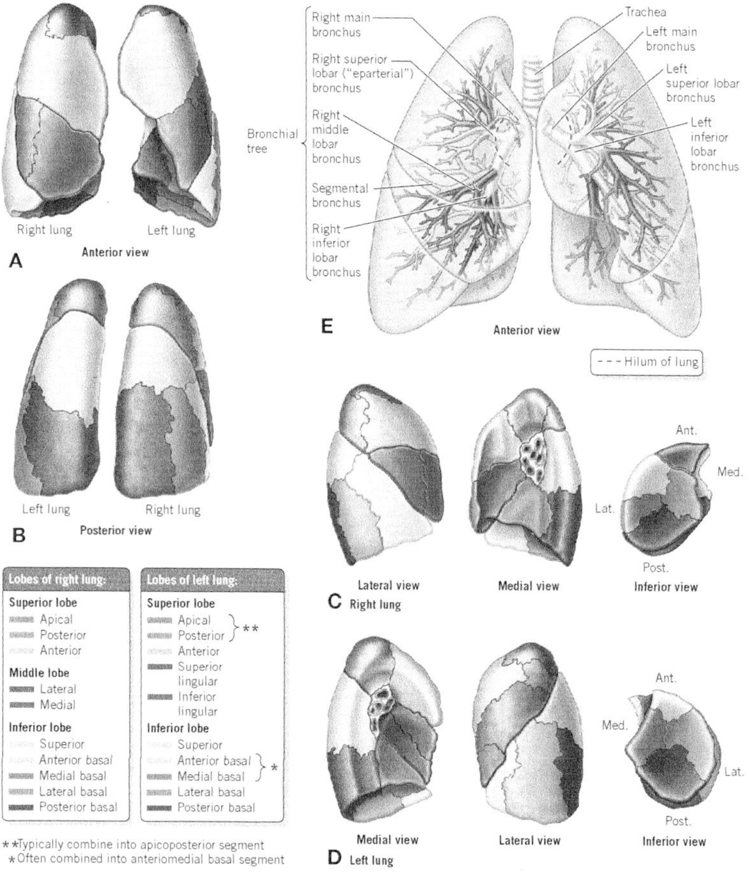

FIGURE 31.1 Pulmonary anatomy and bronchopulmonary segments (A-E views as noted). *(Reprinted with permission from Dalley AF II, Agur AMR, eds. Thorax. In: Moore's Clinically Oriented Anatomy. 9th ed. Wolters Kluwer; 2023:296-409. Figure 4.35.)*

3. Borders of the posterior mediastinum: pericardium anteriorly, T4-12 vertebral bodies posteriorly, pleural sacs bilaterally, sternal angle superiorly, diaphragm inferiorly

C. Physiology

1. Normal respiratory physiology is a negative pressure system
    a. This becomes a positive pressure system during mechanical ventilation.
2. **Oxygenation** is defined as diffusion of oxygen across alveoli into pulmonary capillaries, binding of oxygen to hemoglobin in red blood cells

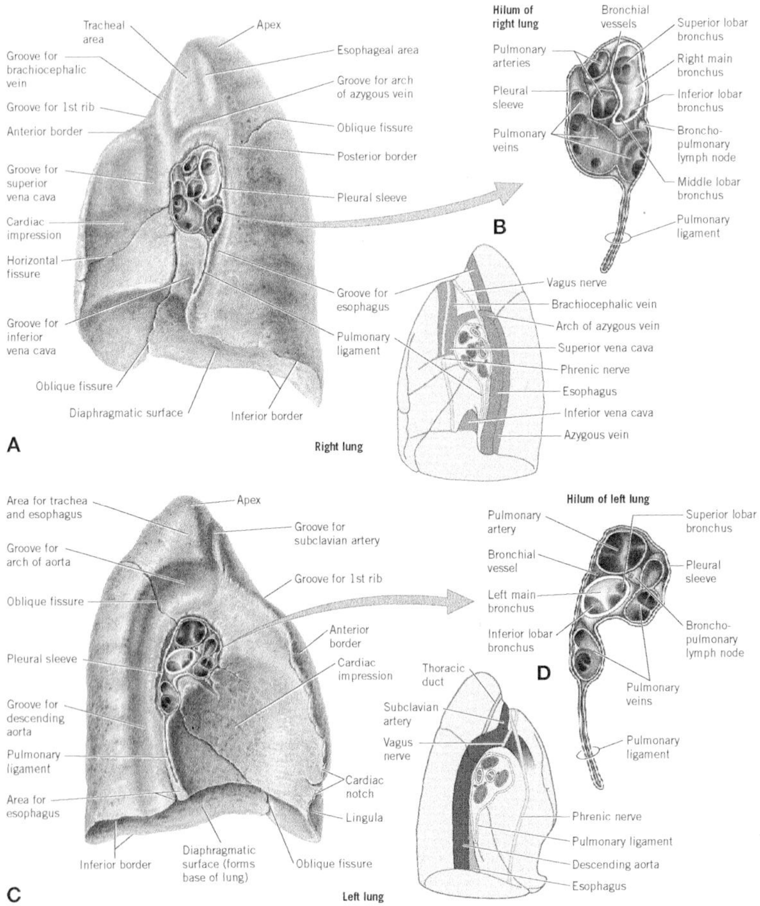

FIGURE 31.2 Right (A, B) and left (C, D) lung and hilar medial view anatomy, respectively. *(Reprinted with permission from Dalley AF II, Agur AMR, eds. Thorax. In: Moore's Clinically Oriented Anatomy. 9th ed. Wolters Kluwer; 2023:296-409. Figure 4.34.)*

and diffusion into blood, so that oxygen can be delivered to organs and peripheral tissues.

   a. Can be altered by the fraction of **inspired oxygen (FiO_2)** and **positive end-expiratory pressure**.

3. **Ventilation** refers to the exchange of air between the lungs and the environment and thus removal of carbon dioxide from the body.
   a. Can be altered by the **respiratory rate** and **tidal volume**.
4. Respiratory mechanics depend on lung and chest wall compliance.
5. Pulmonary function tests are noninvasive assessments that can be used in preoperative evaluation prior to lung resection (**Figure 31.4**).

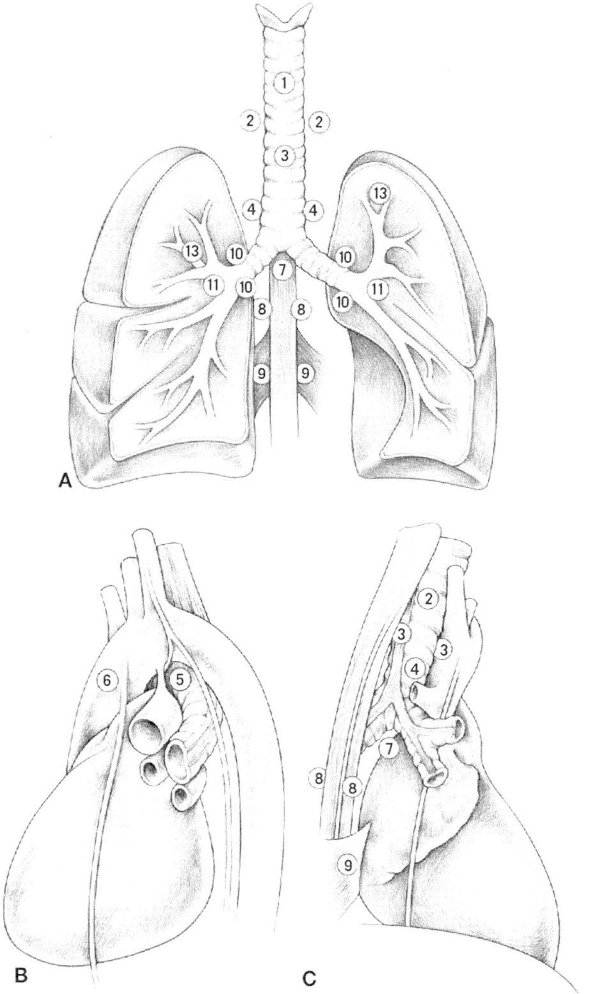

FIGURE 31.3 Thoracic lymph node stations. Anterior (A), left (B), and right (C) chest views. *(Reprinted with permission from Jensen MO. Surgical Anatomy for Mastery of Open Operations: A Multimedia Curriculum for Training Surgery Residents. Wolters Kluwer; 2019.)*

Fraction of total resected lung can be obtained by counting segments or by radionuclide perfusion scan.

a. **FEV1** = forced expiratory volume in 1 second
b. **DLCO** = diffusing capacity for carbon monoxide
c. **Predicted postoperative FEV1** (ppoFEV1) = preoperative FEV1 × (1 – fraction of total resected lung)

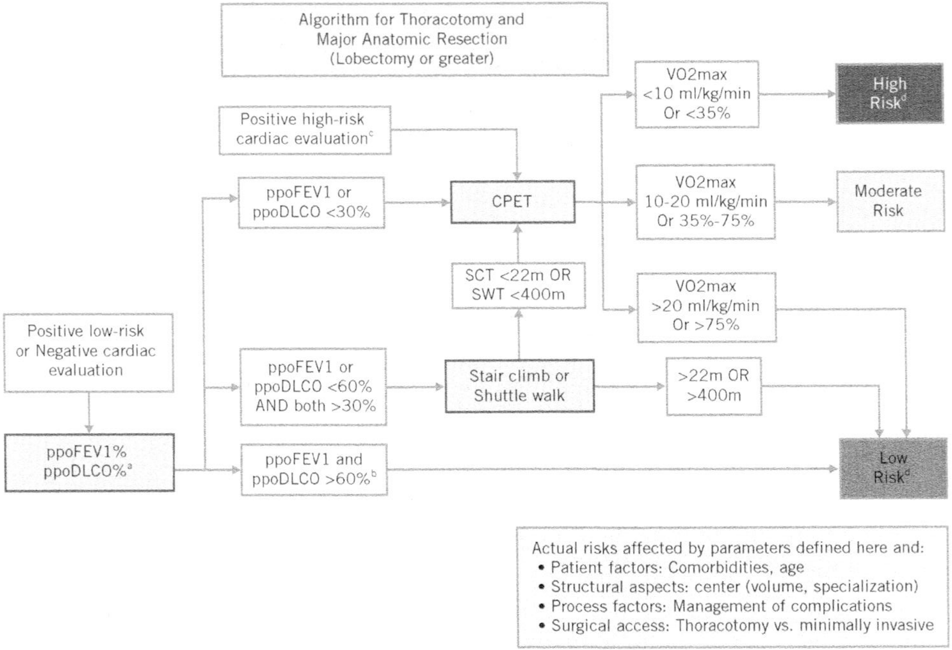

FIGURE 31.4 Preoperative lung function assessment algorithm. CPET, cardiopulmonary exercise test; ppoDLCO, predicted postoperative diffusing capacity for carbon monoxide; ppoFEV1, predicted postoperative forced expiratory volume in 1 second; SCT, stair climb test; SWT, shuttle walk test; VO2max, maximal oxygen consumption (volume). *(Reprinted from Brunelli A, Kim AW, Berger KI, et al. Physiologic evaluation of the patient with lung cancer being considered for resectional surgery: diagnosis and management of lung cancer, 3rd ed: American College of Chest Physicians evidence-based clinical practice guidelines. Chest. 2013;143(5 suppl):e166S-e190S. Copyright 2013, The American College of Chest Physicians. With permission.)*

   d. **Predicted postoperative DLCO** (ppoDLCO) = preoperative DLCO × (1 − fraction of total resected lung)
   e. If both ppoFEV1 and ppoDLCO ≥60%, then proceed with lung resection; otherwise, additional testing is required.

D. Histology
   1. **Respiratory epithelium** covers almost the entire tracheobronchial tree.
      a. Comprises ciliated pseudostratified columnar epithelium
      b. Includes cell types such as ciliated cells, goblet cells, basal cells, brush cells, neuroendocrine cells
   2. **Alveolar epithelium** makes up the alveoli
      a. Composed of type I pneumocytes, type II pneumocytes, club cells, and alveolar macrophages
      b. **Type I pneumocytes**—majority of the epithelial cells (90%-95%), flat, squamous epithelial cells that allow for gas exchange, very susceptible to injury
      c. **Type II pneumocytes**—fewer in number, secrete pulmonary surfactant to prevent alveolar collapse, regenerate both type I and type II pneumocytes

II. PNEUMOTHORAX

A. Subtype definitions
   1. **Simple pneumothorax**—air within pleural cavity, leading to separation of visceral and parietal pleura (**Figure 31.5**)
   2. **Tension pneumothorax**—pressure in pleural cavity builds up enough to compromise venous return, usually due to a one-way valve mechanism by which air enters but cannot exit pleural space.

B. Etiology
   1. Spontaneous (apical blebs, emphysema-related bullae, cystic fibrosis, tuberculosis)
   2. Traumatic (discussed in Chapter 7)
   3. Iatrogenic (central venous catheter placement, pacemaker placement, transthoracic biopsy, transbronchial lung biopsy)

C. Presentation
   1. Shortness of breath, tachypnea, respiratory distress
   2. Chest pain
   3. Cyanosis, hypoxia
   4. Decreased breath sounds and hyperresonance to percussion on involved side
   5. Tension pneumothorax is a clinical diagnosis and is characterized by
      a. Tracheal deviation to contralateral side
      b. Distended neck veins
      c. Hypotension

D. Diagnosis/testing
   1. Laboratory studies: Arterial blood gas (ABG)
   2. Imaging
      a. Upright chest Xray (CXR)
      b. CT scan—can identify smaller pneumothoraces not otherwise visible on CXR

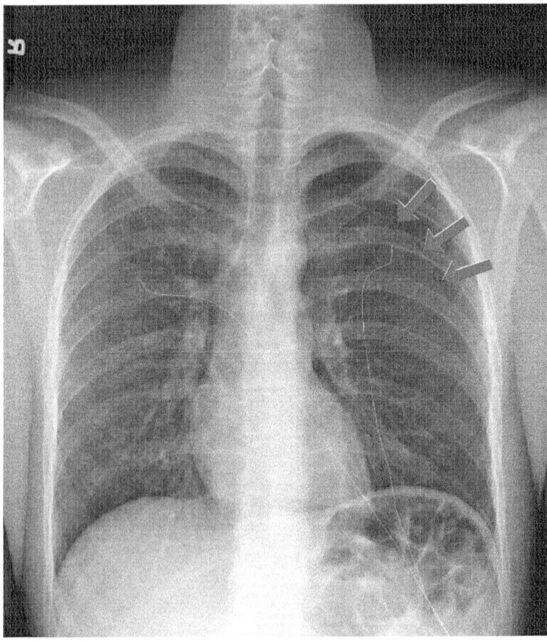

FIGURE 31.5 Spontaneous simple left-sided pneumothorax (red arrows).

E. Nonoperative management
  1. Observation
    a. Appropriate for asymptomatic patients with a small pneumothorax
    b. Supplemental oxygen
    c. Interval CXR to assess for change
  2. Aspiration
    a. Appropriate for small to moderate pneumothorax with low risk for ongoing air leak
    b. Using small catheter attached to a three-way stopcock
  3. **Needle thoracostomy**
    a. Appropriate if there is hemodynamic compromise suspected due to tension pneumothorax
    b. This is a temporizing measure and *must* be followed by tube thoracostomy.
    c. **Surgical approach: Needle thoracostomy**
      i. A large-bore IV catheter (14 or 16 gauge; with needle introducer and syringe) is placed in the second intercostal space in the midclavicular line on the affected side (ipsilateral to absent breath sounds, contralateral to direction of mediastinal shift/tracheal deviation).

ii. The needle is advanced into the pleural space until air is freely aspirated into the syringe.
iii. The needle is then removed, and the catheter is kept open and in place until a formal chest tube can be placed.

4. **Percutaneous catheter**
 a. Small-caliber chest tubes (20 Fr or smaller) placed using the Seldinger technique for moderate pneumothoraces
 b. Contraindications
  i. Concern for lung adhesions leading to greater risk of parenchymal injury
  ii. Significant component of hydro- or hemothorax. A small-bore catheter is likely unable to adequately drain a large fluid collection; a larger-bore chest tube is indicated.
 c. Persistent air leak present if the water-seal chamber has bubbles with expiration
 d. Air leak and CXRs should be assessed daily to determine duration of pleural catheter.
5. **Bedside pleurodesis**
 a. Appropriate for persistent pneumothoraces for poor surgical candidates and selected patients with malignant pleural effusion
 b. Involves administration of sclerosing agents (such as povidone-iodine, bleomycin, talc) through the tube thoracostomy
 c. Leads to fusion of parietal and visceral pleura and therefore obliteration of the potential pleural space
 d. Requires appropriate analgesia as procedure is often painful
 e. Can be associated with inflammatory pneumonitis and lead to hypoxia, particularly in patients with limited pulmonary reserve

F. Operative management
1. Indicated for
 a. Recurrent spontaneous ipsilateral pneumothoraces
 b. Persistent air leaks in chest tube (usually >3–5 days)
 c. First spontaneous pneumothorax in patients with high-risk occupations (e.g., pilots, divers)
 d. Large, obvious offending target such as bleb or bullae on CT scan
2. Surgical approach depends on the etiology of the pneumothorax:
 a. Obvious cause (bleb/bulla): Wedge resection
 b. No obvious cause/no easily resected target: Pleurodesis
  i. Pleurodesis causes the pleura to adhere to the chest wall, eliminating the potential space for extrapulmonary air collection.
3. **Surgical approach: Video-assisted thoracoscopic surgery (VATS) wedge resection/pleurodesis**
 a. Intubation with a double-lumen endotracheal tube or bronchial blocker for single lung ventilation
 b. Patient positioning: Lateral decubitus with operative side facing up and bed flexed at the hip to allow for expansion of rib spaces on the operative side
 c. If a wedge resection is planned, place a 3-cm utility port: Anterior axillary line at 4th intercostal space for upper lobe resection/5th intercostal space for lower lobe resection

d. A 1-cm camera port is placed in the anterior axillary line two interspaces below the utility port.
e. A 2-cm assistant port is placed in the posterior axillary line, along the same interspace as the camera port.
f. Using a 30° thoracoscope, the lung and pleural cavity can be visually inspected. Next steps depend on the etiology of the pneumothorax (as described above):
   i. Wedge resection: Can be performed with a stapler using ringed forceps to hold the lung (typically apex of the upper lobe or superior segment of the lower lobe; ringed forceps can be inserted via the assistant port).
   ii. Pleurodesis
      a) **Mechanical**—scratch entire pleural surface with a Bovie scratch pad or similar rough surface held by ringed forceps
      b) **Talc**—insufflate talc powder into pleural cavity, taking care to cover the entire pleural surface
g. Placement of a 20 to 28 French chest tube at the end of the case (required for virtually all intrathoracic procedures) (see also "Surgical approach: Tube thoracostomy")

III. PLEURAL EFFUSION

A. Epidemiology/etiology/classification
1. Fluid accumulation in pleural space (**Figure 31.6**)
2. Transudative vs. exudative
   a. Determined using **Light's criteria**
      i. Ratio of pleural fluid protein to serum protein >0.5
      ii. Ratio of pleural fluid lactate dehydrogenase (LDH) to serum LDH > 0.6
      iii. Pleural fluid LDH > two-thirds of upper normal limit of serum LDH
   b. **Transudative**—protein-poor fluid from increased intravascular pressure
      i. Diagnosed if <u>none</u> of Light's criteria are met
      ii. Typically, thin yellow or clear fluid
      iii. Underlying causes include congestive heart failure, cirrhosis, nephrotic syndrome.
   c. **Exudative**—protein- or cell-rich fluid resulting from increased vascular permeability
      i. Diagnosed if <u>at least one</u> of Light's criteria is met
      ii. Underlying causes include
         a) Pneumonia → parapneumonic effusion
         b) Empyema
         c) Chyle leak → chylous effusion/chylothorax
         d) Inflammatory/reactive (e.g., from pancreatitis)
         e) Malignancy (e.g., breast, lung, or ovarian cancers; lymphoma)

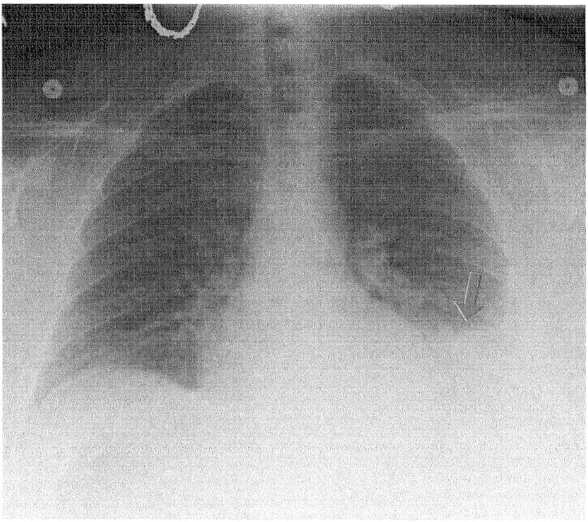

FIGURE 31.6 Left-sided moderate pleural effusion (red arrow).

B. Presentation
  1. Asymptomatic
  2. Dyspnea, cough, pleuritic chest pain

C. Diagnosis/testing
  1. Imaging
     a. Upright CXR—blunting of costophrenic angle (**Figure 31.6**)
     b. Ultrasound imaging
     c. CT scan
  2. Thoracentesis with laboratory studies on pleural fluid
     a. pH, glucose, amylase
     b. Pleural and serum protein and LDH
     c. Gram stain, bacterial and fungal culture
     d. Differential cell count
     e. Cytology
  3. Pleural biopsy if pleural fluid studies are nondiagnostic

D. Nonoperative management
  1. Underlying cause of pleural effusion should be identified and treated.
  2. **Thoracentesis**
     a. Initial thoracentesis should be done to diagnose etiology of pleural effusion (see **Figure 31.7**).
     b. If recurs, repeated thoracentesis can be done; however, may ultimately need more definitive management.
  3. **Tube thoracostomy**
     a. Often initial management strategy in large-volume recurring effusions of unknown etiology

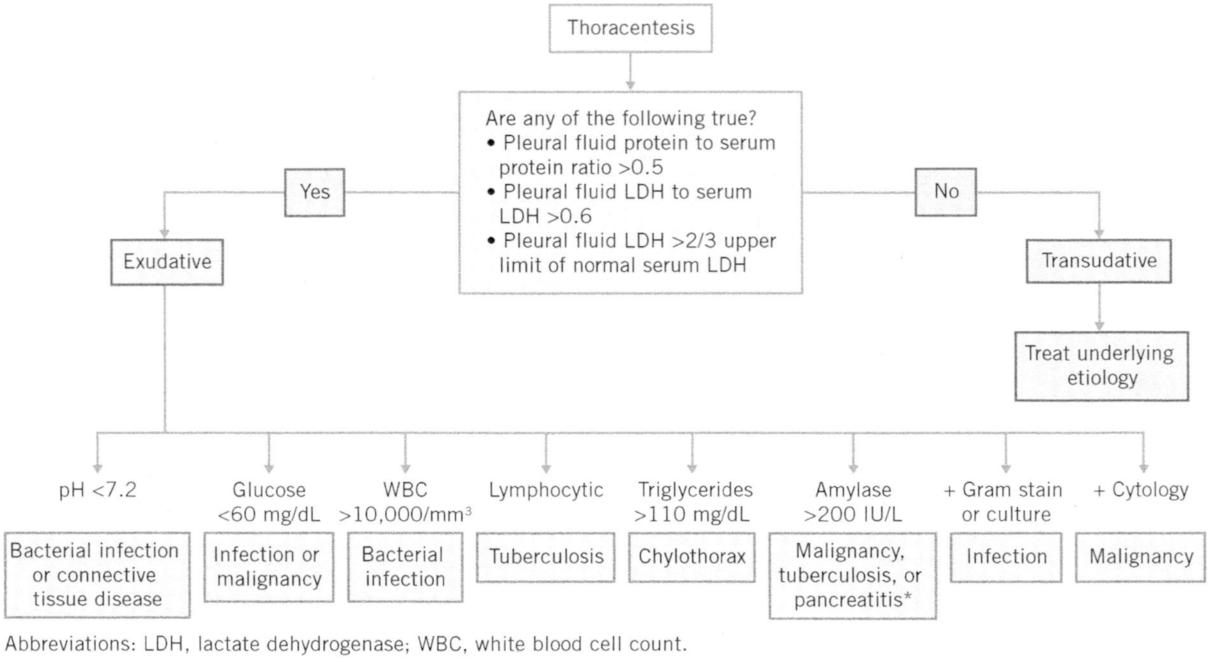

FIGURE 31.7 Interpreting laboratory results from a thoracentesis.[4] LDH, lactate dehydrogenase; WBC, white blood cell count. *(Modified from Villena V, Pérez V, Pozo F, et al. Amylase levels in pleural effusions: a consecutive unselected series of 841 patients. Chest. 2002;121:470-474.)*

b. **Surgical approach: Tube thoracostomy**
   i. A 2- to 3-cm incision is made at the 5th intercostal space in the mid-axillary line using the following landmarks—the nipple in men and the inframammary crease in women.
   ii. Dissection of subcutaneous tissue is performed sharply down to the level of the 5th and 6th ribs.
   iii. A Kelly clamp is used to puncture the pleura just cranial to the lower rib and spread open to widen this defect. A finger can be used to sweep away the lung and any adhesions that may be present.
   iv. A Kelly clamp is used to guide an appropriately sized chest tube into the pleural space, angling the tube posteriorly and superiorly.
   v. The tube is secured at the skin with heavy suture (0 or 1-0 silk).
   vi. Chest tubes can be connected to a one-way Heimlich valve, a simple underwater-seal system, or vacuum suction at 10 to 20 cmH_2O.

4. Tunneled indwelling pleural catheter (e.g., PleurX, Aspira) with intermittent drainage
   a. Generally reserved for recurrent and formally diagnosed malignant effusions

E. Operative management
   1. VATS pleurodesis (described above)

IV. EMPYEMA

A. Epidemiology/etiology/classification
   1. Purulent collection in pleural space
   2. Most are secondary to pneumonia, but can be iatrogenic after esophageal, pulmonary, or mediastinal surgery or due to retained hemothorax or extension from subphrenic abscesses.
   3. Most common organisms are *Staphylococcus aureus, Streptococci* species, *Escherichia coli, Pseudomonas, Klebsiella,* and anaerobic bacteria (*Bacteroides* species).
   4. **Phases**
      a. Early or exudative (day 1-5) —simple infected fluid
      b. Fibropurulent or fibroproliferative (day 5-10)—loculated fluid with fibrin
      c. Advanced or organizing phase (day 10-14)—thicker fluid and fibrous peel entrapping lung, limiting its expansion

B. Presentation/symptoms
   1. Pleuritic chest pain, fever, cough, dyspnea, sepsis

C. Diagnosis/testing
   1. Imaging
      a. CXR
      b. CT scan with IV contrast
   2. Laboratory studies
      a. Complete blood count with differential

b. Pleural fluid analysis (abundant white blood cells, low glucose, low pH, positive Gram stain and culture)

D. Nonoperative management

1. Antibiotics (based on suspected organisms and, ideally, sensitivities)[5]
2. Tube drainage of pleural space (20-32 Fr chest tube)
3. Intrapleural fibrinolytic therapy (tissue plasminogen activator with DNase) for advanced or organizing empyema

E. Operative management

1. **Thoracoscopic decortication** for early empyema
2. **Open decortication** may be needed for fibropurulent or organizing empyemas.
3. **Surgical approach: Posterolateral thoracotomy with decortication**
   a. Intubation with a double-lumen endotracheal tube or bronchial blocker for single lung ventilation.
   b. Patient positioning: Lateral decubitus with operative side facing up and bed flexed at the hip to allow for expansion of rib spaces on the operative side.
   c. A curved infrascapular incision is made and the latissimus dorsi muscle is divided and the serratus anterior retracted.
   d. The pleural cavity is entered above the lower rib in the 5th intercostal space.
   e. A rib spreader is placed and opened slowly to the extent needed for adequate visualization. A small section of the posterior 6th rib is often resected to improve exposure.
   f. Loculations in the pleural space are broken up by blunt dissection.
   g. The rind overlying the visceral pleura is meticulously removed to allow for adequate lung expansion.
   h. A chest tube is placed, and the chest closed.
4. **Clagett window** involves resection of posterolateral rib with creation of an open intrapleural window to allow for repeated bedside/nonoperative debridement, drainage, and irrigation of pleural space with antibiotic solution.

F. Associated complications

1. **Lung abscess**
   a. Can be associated with empyema, both often secondary to necrotizing pneumonia
   b. Initial management with antibiotics and pulmonary toilet
   c. If medical management fails, surgical intervention involves resection of involved lung parenchyma.

V. THORACIC EMERGENCIES

A. Massive hemoptysis

1. Defined as >600 mL of blood loss from the lungs in 24 hours
2. Surgical emergency; delayed intervention can lead to fatal asphyxiation.
3. Etiology can be infectious, malignant, or cardiac (e.g., bronchitis or tuberculosis, bronchogenic carcinoma, mitral stenosis).
4. Bronchial circulation is almost always the source of bleeding.

5. Bleeding from pulmonary circulation is only seen in patients with pulmonary hypertension and some lung cancers.
6. Management
   a. Secure the airway (using double-lumen endotracheal tube if available)
   b. Urgent bronchoscopy—can identify side of bleeding and allow for prompt protection by either controlling the bleeding or selective ventilation
      i. Bleeding can be controlled using topical or injected vasoconstrictors (epinephrine or vasopressin) or by placement of a balloon-tipped catheter in the lobar orifice.
      ii. Selective ventilation can be achieved with a double-lumen tube or by direct intubation of contralateral mainstem bronchus.
   c. Angiographic embolization—after temporizing the bleed and particularly if unable to identify the source of bleeding on bronchoscopy, angiographic embolization of a bronchial arterial source may allow for lung salvage without the need for resection.
   d. Surgical resection—rarely needed, only if the above efforts fail, definitive therapy may require thoracotomy with lobar resection (or more).
      i. It is important to consider the etiology of the bleeding and pulmonary reserve of the patient as the degree of resection necessary may not be tolerated.

B. Emergency **cricothyroidotomy** is covered in Chapter 5.

VI. LUNG CANCER

A. Epidemiology/etiology[6]
1. Leading cause of cancer-related mortality (US and worldwide)
2. Second most common nonskin malignancy (following prostate cancer in men and breast cancer in women)
3. Estimated 236,740 new cases and 130,180 deaths in the US in 2022
4. Incidence rates for male to female patients are about equal; mortality rates for males are about 10% higher
5. Incidence rates are highest in black males
6. Leading risk factor: Cigarette smoking

B. Screening
1. US Preventative Services Taskforce recommends annual screening for lung cancer via low-dose CT scan for high-risk adults[7]
2. Eligibility criteria (expanded in 2021[8])
   a. Adults 50 to 80 years old
   b. Smoking history of 20 pack-year
   c. Currently smoking or quit within the past 15 years

C. Pathology
1. **Small cell lung carcinoma** (SCLC)
   a. Accounts for <15% of all lung cancers
   b. Often centrally located near the hilum
   c. Occurs almost exclusively in smokers

d. May be initially responsive to chemotherapy; surgical treatment is rare because often widely metastatic at diagnosis
e. Poor prognosis (5-year overall survival <10%)

2. **Non–small cell lung carcinoma** (NSCLC)
   a. Approximately 85% of all lung cancers
   b. Less aggressive than SCLC, often diagnosed at earlier stage
   c. Three main subtypes
      i. **Adenocarcinoma** (30%-50% of cases)
         a) Bronchioalveolar carcinoma is a variant of adenocarcinoma that produces mucin and can be multifocal.
      ii. **Squamous cell** (20%-35%)
      iii. **Large cell** (4%-15%), typically carries a relatively poor prognosis
3. Lung **neuroendocrine tumor** subgroups include SCLC, some NSCLCs, and carcinoids. Carcinoids are further divided into typical and atypical types.

D. Presentation
1. Can be incidentally diagnosed or based on symptoms, with symptomatic presentation implying more advanced stage and worse prognosis
2. Bronchopulmonary symptoms
   a. Worsening cough, increased sputum production, dyspnea, and wheezing
   b. Hemoptysis (minor hemoptysis in smokers >40 years old should be evaluated with bronchoscopy)
   c. May also present with postobstructive pneumonia
3. Extrapulmonary thoracic symptoms
   a. Chest pain (secondary to local tumor invasion of chest wall)
   b. Hoarseness (from invasion of left recurrent laryngeal nerve near aortopulmonary window)
   c. Shortness of breath (secondary to malignant pleural effusion or phrenic nerve invasion)
   d. **Superior vena cava syndrome** causing facial, neck, and upper extremity swelling
   e. Ipsilateral **Horner syndrome** (ptosis, miosis, anhidrosis) from **Pancoast tumor** (superior sulcus), due to invasion of cervical sympathetic ganglia
   f. Dysphagia (less common) secondary to compression or invasion of esophagus by bulky mediastinal lymph nodes or by primary tumor
   g. Venous thromboembolism associated with malignancy
4. Distant metastases
   a. Most common: Liver, bone, brain, adrenal glands, contralateral lung
   b. Pathologic fractures from bony metastases
   c. Headaches, cranial neuropathies, changes in mental status from brain metastases
   d. Adrenal insufficiency from adrenal invasion (lung cancer is the most common tumor causing adrenal dysfunction)
5. **Paraneoplastic syndromes**
   a. Due to ectopic release of endocrine substances by tumor
   b. **Ectopic Cushing syndrome**—adrenocorticotropic hormone secretion from SCLC

c. Syndrome of inappropriate ADH secretion—ADH secretion from SCLC
d. Hypercalcemia—parathyroid hormone-related protein secretion from squamous cell carcinoma
e. Hypertrophic pulmonary osteoarthropathy—from adenocarcinoma
    i. Characterized by clubbed fingers, joint stiffness, periosteal thickening on radiography
f. Neurologic sequelae of **Lambert–Eaton syndrome** (autoimmune destruction of neuromuscular junctions)—from SCLC

6. Solitary pulmonary nodules
    a. Often discovered during lung cancer screening or incidentally on imaging for other reasons
    b. Small (<3 cm), circumscribed, asymptomatic lesion
        i. If > 3 cm, then called a lung mass
    c. First step to evaluation is to compare with prior imaging (**Figure 31.8**).
    d. Specific guidelines exist for following suspicious pulmonary nodules (**Figure 31.9**).

E. Diagnosis
1. **CT chest** including upper abdomen
    a. Ideal to assess and follow pulmonary nodules.
    b. IV contrast should be used, when possible, to identify mediastinal lymphadenopathy and to evaluate for liver or adrenal metastases.
    c. Allows assessment of the tumor's size, location, and degree of local invasion.
    d. Factors favoring a benign lesion include stable size, lesion diameter <6 mm, and certain patterns of calcification such as diffuse, centrally located, laminar, or popcorn-like calcifications.
    e. Factors favoring malignancy include intravenous contrast enhancement, irregular borders, lobulations, and eccentric or stippled calcifications.
    f. Mediastinal lymph node assessment by CT is generally inadequate, with a sensitivity of approximately 55% and a specificity of about 81%.[10]

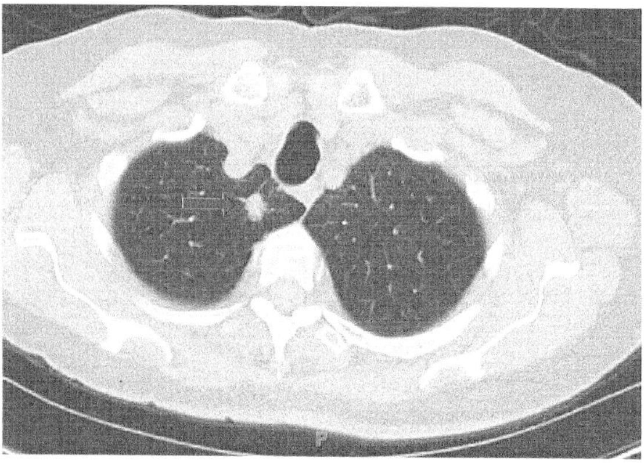

FIGURE 31.8 Solitary pulmonary nodule in right upper lobe (red arrow).

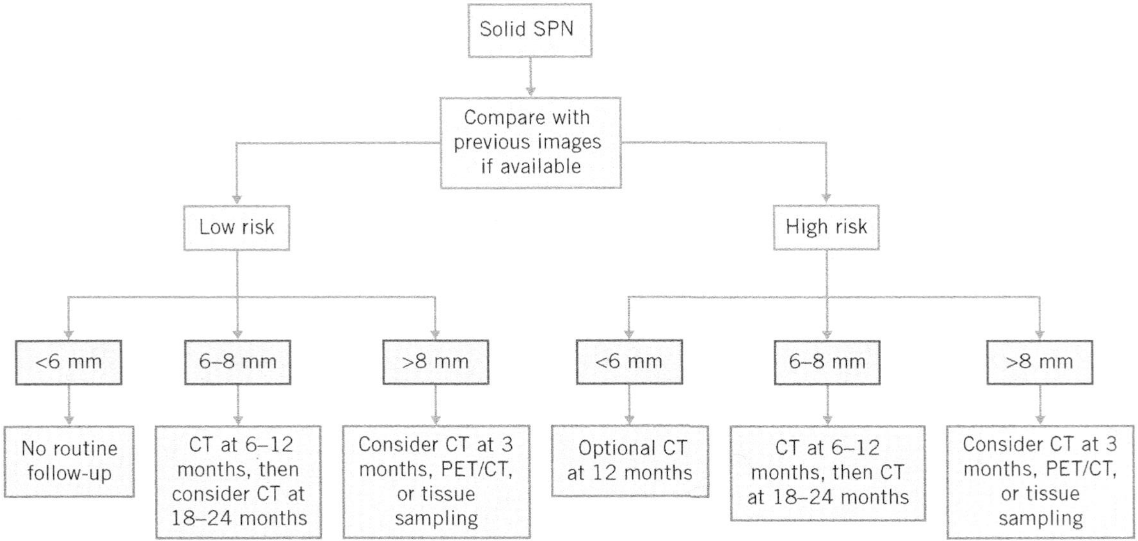

Abbreviations: CT, computed tomography; PET/CT, positron emission tomography with computed tomography.

FIGURE 31.9 Management of solid solitary pulmonary nodule (SPN) based on Fleischner Society 2017 Guidelines.[9] High-risk features include older age, heavy smoking history, irregular or spiculated border, and upper lobe location, as well as other pertinent factors like family history and environmental exposures. PET, positron emission tomography.

2. **Positron emission tomography** (PET) scan
   a. Used to further assess suspicious nodules for metabolic activity and is the standard method for staging patients with NSCLC
   b. Degree of PET avidity in the primary tumor can help to differentiate benign from malignant processes.
   c. Whole-body nature of the scan can also identify occult nodal disease and sites of distant metastasis.
   d. However, it is somewhat limited by false positives (e.g., inflammatory/infectious processes, granulomatous disease) and false negatives (e.g., bronchoalveolar carcinoma, carcinoid tumor).
   e. Therefore, PET imaging must be considered in the context of known risk factors (e.g., negative PET scan in high-risk, elderly smokers may be discordant and needs further evaluation).
3. **Tissue biopsy** (gold standard)
   a. May be obtained by bronchoscopy in patients with central lung lesions or by CT-guided biopsy for peripheral lesions
   b. **Endobronchial ultrasound** (EBUS) can also access select lesions.
   c. Surgical biopsy via video thoracoscopy can provide a definitive diagnosis, often as a prelude to therapeutic resection during the same operation.

F. Staging
1. Accurate clinical and pathologic staging is critical for understanding prognosis and planning treatment.
2. Resection is preferred treatment for functionally fit patients with early-stage (stage I-II) disease.
3. Resection is increasingly employed for select patients with stage III disease, especially since the introduction of immune checkpoint inhibitors.
4. Lung cancer stage is summarized using the American Joint Committee on Cancer (AJCC) **TNM staging system**[11] (Chapter 36: Lung; *AJCC Cancer Staging Manual*, 8th ed.) based on tumor size and local structure invasion, location of lymph nodes with metastases, and presence/extent of distant metastases.
5. Appropriate staging includes
   a. Chest and abdominal CT and PET/CT imaging (as described above)
   b. Lymph node staging
      i. EBUS-guided fine-needle aspiration or (rarely) **mediastinoscopy** can be used to access pretracheal, paratracheal, and subcarinal lymph nodes.
      ii. Aortopulmonary nodes can be sampled via endoscopic (transesophageal) ultrasound imaging, VATS, or, less commonly, anterior mediastinoscopy (**Chamberlain procedure**).
      iii. Routine use of either of these techniques in the staging of patients with NSCLC should be favored, except for select patients with clinical stage I lung cancer with no lymphadenopathy by PET/CT.[12]
   c. CT or MRI of the brain
      i. To evaluate for brain metastases
      ii. Mandatory for patients with neurologic symptoms, stage III-IV disease, SCLC, or **superior sulcus tumors** (given the higher probability for occult brain metastasis)

d. **Fiberoptic bronchoscopy**
   i. Important in diagnosing and assessing the extent of endobronchial lesions
   ii. Preoperative bronchoscopy is important for excluding synchronous lung cancers (found in approximately 1% of patients) prior to resection and can help rule out suspicious mediastinal nodal metastasis.

G. Principles of management by stage

1. **Stage I**
   a. Generally treated with surgical resection alone
   b. Certain high-risk stage I tumors (based on grade, genetic profiling, etc.) may benefit from adjuvant therapy
2. **Stage II**
   a. Also treated with resection, but additional therapeutic interventions, including neoadjuvant immunotherapy and/or neoadjuvant/adjuvant/induction + adjuvant chemotherapy, have been associated with improved outcomes
   b. Adjuvant radiation therapy is considered in patients with close surgical margins or central lymph node metastasis.
3. **Stage IIIA**
   a. Patients appear to benefit from neoadjuvant immunotherapy and chemotherapy followed by surgical resection.[13]
   b. Selected patients with mediastinal lymph node metastasis (N2 disease) may be candidates for surgical resection after neoadjuvant chemoradiation therapy (or immunotherapy) with good clinical response.
4. **Stage IIIB**
   a. Patients with bulky, diffuse mediastinal lymphadenopathy or stage IIIB tumors are typically treated using definitive chemoradiation
5. **Stage IV**
   a. Patients have distant metastases and are generally considered unresectable
   b. Some patients with node-negative lung cancer and a solitary brain metastasis have achieved long-term survival with combined resection and adjuvant chemotherapy

H. Nonoperative management

1. Can include a combination of chemotherapy, immunotherapy, and/or radiation therapy
2. Detailed discussion of specific agents is outside the scope of this chapter; however, recent advances in adjuvant and neoadjuvant immunotherapies and other targeted therapies are likely to change the treatment paradigm for both early- and late-stage cancers.[14]
3. **Stereotactic body radiation therapy** (SBRT)
   a. External beam radiation therapy that precisely delivers high-dose radiation to a target in the body over one or more treatments
   b. SBRT has been shown to be effective for early-stage lung cancer in patients who are poor candidates for surgical resection.
   c. Prospective studies comparing outcomes between surgery and SBRT are limited—at least four trials have been closed early due to issues

with patient accrual/treatment preference—but one such study is currently ongoing (VALOR: Veterans Affairs Lung cancer surgery Or stereotactic Radiotherapy trial).[15-17]

I. Operative management

1. **Anatomic resection**
   a. In patients eligible for operation, the extent of resection is usually an anatomic lobectomy, although select patients may benefit from segmental resection.[18]
   b. **Surgical approach: Lobectomy with lymph node sampling**
      i. Exposure of the hilum is accomplished via thoracotomy or via video- or robot-assisted thoracoscopic surgery (see above).
      ii. The pulmonary vein and arterial branches of the involved lobe are dissected.
      iii. Mediastinal and hilar lymph nodes are removed (see **Figure 31.3**, station map).
      iv. The pulmonary vein and arterial branches are ligated with a vascular stapler.
      v. The lobar bronchus is divided, using either a stapler or cut-and-sew technique.
      vi. A chest tube is placed, and the chest closed.
   c. Most centers report operative mortality of <1% to 2% with lobectomy.
   d. More recently, video- and robotic-assisted thoracoscopic surgical techniques have become widely adopted, associated with less postoperative pain and faster recovery.
   e. Open thoracotomy can be performed when there is local invasion that requires en bloc resection.
   f. Routine intraoperative lymph node sampling remains critical in all patients[19]
   g. The timing of mediastinal assessment, whether before or during a planned resection, depends on surgeon preference and the availability of accurate pathologic evaluation of mediastinal lymph node frozen sections.
2. **Nonanatomic resection**
   a. Nonanatomic wedge resection remains suboptimal due to higher rates of cancer recurrence and diminished overall survival.[20]
   b. However, segmental or wedge resection may be used in patients with limited pulmonary reserve.

J. Complications after lung resection

1. Atrial fibrillation (AF)/flutter[21]
   a. Occurs in 10% to 20% of patients following pulmonary resection and typically arises within 1 to 4 postoperative days
   b. Initiate/continue continuous ECG telemetry, obtain ABG and serum electrolyte panel.
   c. Assess for possible triggers: Pneumothorax, pulmonary embolism, pericarditis, bleeding, myocardial ischemia, infection/sepsis.
   d. Minimize catecholaminergic inotropes if possible (epinephrine, norepinephrine, dopamine, dobutamine).

e. Patients' fluid status should be examined, and efforts should be made to achieve euvolemia.
f. Correct any electrolyte imbalances.
g. AF management depends on the patient's clinical stability.
   i. Unstable
      a) Immediate direct current cardioversion, with IV heparin if AF duration >48 hours and no contraindication
      b) Consider rate/rhythm control and consult cardiology.
   ii. Stable
      a) Frequently, rate control can be achieved with β-blockers or calcium channel blockers.
      b) Chemical (e.g., amiodarone) or electrical cardioversion can be considered if patient fails to achieve normal sinus rhythm spontaneously.
         1) Anticoagulation and echocardiographic assessment of possible intracardiac thrombus depend on duration of AF and patient factors (risk of stroke/embolization, any contraindications).

2. Prolonged postoperative air leak
   a. Defined as air leak lasting >5 days
   b. Risk factors include severely emphysematous lungs, male sex, steroid use.
   c. Patients can be discharged with a one-way Heimlich valve for 1 to 2 weeks, which typically resolves the air leak.
3. Bronchopleural fistula
   a. Most commonly occurs following major anatomic resection with incidence of 0.5% to 1% following lobectomy, 1.5% to 4.5% following pneumonectomy
   b. Initially managed with chest tube drainage of pleural space, minimizing suction (5-10 mm Hg)
   c. Surgical revision with bronchial stump debridement and revision if nonoperative management fails

K. Surveillance
   1. Patients should undergo routine surveillance via chest CT following definitive treatment of lung cancer to monitor for disease recurrence and secondary lung cancers.[22]

VII. TUMORS OF THE PLEURA

A. Mesothelioma
   1. The most common tumor of the pleura
   2. Rare and aggressive cancer that has been linked to asbestos exposure with a latency period of decades
   3. Classified into different subtypes: Epithelioid (50%), sarcomatoid (20%), mixed, and desmoplastic
   4. Presentation
      a. Chest pain, malaise, cough, weakness, weight loss, shortness of breath with pleural effusions

b. One-third of patients report paraneoplastic symptoms of osteoarthropathy, hypoglycemia, and fever
5. Diagnosis
a. Cytology of pleural fluid
b. Core needle biopsy or thoracoscopic biopsy of suspicious pleural nodules
c. CT scans can differentiate pleural from parenchymal disease.
d. PET scan to identify distant metastatic disease
6. Treatment
a. Multimodal therapy comprising operation, chemotherapy, and radiation
b. Surgical options include **extrapleural pneumonectomy** (EPP) or **pleurectomy/decortication**, but not all patients with mesothelioma are candidates for these.
c. For early-stage cases, EPP may offer the best chance of cure—the reported 5-year survival following completion of multimodal therapy in patients without nodal metastasis may be as high as 50% but is typically much lower.[23]
d. Median survival of patients with untreated malignant mesothelioma is 8 to 10 months.

B. Less common tumors of the pleura include lipomas, angiomas, soft tissue sarcomas, and fibrous histiocytomas

VIII. TUMORS OF THE MEDIASTINUM

A. Epidemiology/etiology
1. Location of mediastinal masses relative to other structures in the mediastinum can help to form a differential diagnosis (**Table 31.1**).
2. Mediastinum can be divided into anterior, middle, and posterior compartments.

TABLE 31.1 Differential Diagnosis of Tumors Located in the Mediastinum[24]

Anterior		Middle	Posterior
Thymoma	Lymphoma	Congenital enteric cyst	Neurogenic
Germ cell	Parathyroid	Lymphoma	Lymphoma
Teratoma	Lipoma	Primary cardiac cyst	Mesenchymal
Seminoma	Fibroma	Neural crest	
Nonseminoma	Lymphangioma	Bronchogenic cyst	
Aberrant thyroid			

Modified from Young RM, Kernstine KH, Corson JD. Miscellaneous cardiopulmonary conditions. In: Corson JD, Williamson RCN, eds. *Surgery*. Mosby; 2001. Copyright 2001, Elsevier. With permission.

3. Lymphoma is the most common mediastinal tumor.
4. Neurogenic tumors are more likely in children.

B. Presentation
1. Symptoms vary and are only present in one-third of patients.
2. Often nonspecific and include dyspnea, cough, hoarseness, weight loss, vague chest pain, and fever.

C. Radiographic evaluation
1. Initially CXR
2. Typically followed by chest CT scan to further delineate surrounding anatomic structures
3. Malignant germ cell tumors are further evaluated with abdominal CT and scrotal ultrasound imaging.

D. Anterior mediastinal masses
1. Represented by the "**Four Ts**": Thymoma, teratomas/germ cell tumors, "terrible" lymphoma, or thyroid tumors
2. **Thymomas**
   a. Approximately 20% of mediastinal neoplasms
   b. Malignant in roughly 15% of cases (**thymic carcinoma**), which are staged according to the AJCC TNM classification system[11]
   c. Presence of capsular invasion associated with decreased survival
   d. Approximately 50% of patients with a thymoma have paraneoplastic syndromes, including myasthenia gravis, hypogammaglobulinemia, and red cell aplasia.
   e. **Myasthenia gravis** (MG)
      i. Thymomas can lead to development of MG, but MG can also lead to development of thymomas.
      ii. Thymus contributes to pathophysiology by generating autoreactive antibodies against acetylcholinesterase receptors.
      iii. Roughly 10% of patients with MG develop thymomas.
      iv. Thymectomy has been shown to improve outcomes in patients with nonthymomatous MG.[25]
      v. Thymectomy is now recommended for patients with MG.
      vi. Preoperative preparation for patients with MG includes weaning corticosteroids and anticholinesterases. This can be supplemented by preoperative plasmapheresis. Muscle relaxants and atropine should be avoided during anesthesia.
   f. Treatment: Often involves en bloc resection via a transcervical, transsternal, or minimally invasive (VATS or robot-assisted) approach. For more advanced stages of thymoma, neoadjuvant chemotherapy (such as cyclophosphamide, doxorubicin, and cisplatin [CAP]) may be indicated.
3. **Germ cell tumors:** Should be biochemically evaluated with β-human chorionic gonadotropin (β-HCG) and α-fetoprotein (AFP).
   a. **Teratomas**
      i. Elevation of both β-HCG and AFP is very rare and suggests a malignant teratoma
      ii. Usually benign and often contain ectodermal components such as hair, teeth, and bone
      iii. Treatment is surgical resection

b. **Seminomas**
   i. No elevation of AFP; fewer than 10% of patients have an elevated β-HCG
   ii. CT scan of the abdomen and pelvis should be obtained to rule out advanced disease.
   iii. Treatment is primarily nonsurgical (with radiation and chemotherapy), except in the case of localized disease.

c. **Nonseminomatous germ cell tumors**
   i. Elevation of both β-HCG and AFP
   ii. Treatment is with platinum-based chemotherapy, followed by resection of residual masses.

4. **Lymphomas**
   a. Often present as irregular masses on CT scan
   b. Diagnosed with core needle biopsy, which helps to guide treatment
   c. Treatment is primarily nonsurgical and involves chemoimmunotherapy.

E. Middle mediastinal masses
   1. Include bronchogenic and enteric cysts
   2. Resection is indicated for symptomatic or enlarging masses, or if the diagnosis is unclear.

F. Posterior mediastinal masses
   1. Most commonly neurogenic tumors and typically present as paravertebral masses.
   2. Serum catecholamine levels should be measured to rule out pheochromocytomas.

IX. LUNG TRANSPLANTATION

A. The number of lung transplants performed in the US has been steadily increasing over the past 3 decades, with over 2,500 lung transplants performed annually.

B. Both single and bilateral lung transplants are performed, with the majority being bilateral.

C. Common indications
   1. Chronic obstructive pulmonary disease
   2. Interstitial pulmonary fibrosis
   3. Cystic fibrosis
   4. α-1 Antitrypsin deficiency
   5. Pulmonary artery hypertension

D. Donor selection detailed in **Table 31.2**

E. **Surgical approach: Lung transplantation**
   1. **Donor operation**
      a. A median sternotomy is performed.
      b. The lungs are inspected for gross pathology and compliance.
      c. The ascending aorta, pulmonary artery (PA), and superior vena cava (SVC) are dissected and exposed. A PA cannula is placed and secured.

d. Once all organ procurement teams have completed their dissections and systemic heparin has been administered, the SVC is ligated, the inferior vena cava is transected, the left heart is vented (via an incision in either the left atrium or the left atrial appendage), and the aorta is cross-clamped.
e. Lung preservation solution (extracellular, low-potassium, dextran-based electrolyte solution) is administered via the PA cannula.
f. The heart is excised leaving a generous left atrial cuff, and the double lung-block is procured.

2. **Recipient operation**
a. A clamshell sternothoracotomy is performed.
b. Hilar dissection is performed with isolation of the PA and pulmonary veins.
c. Back-table dissection and preparation of the donor lung block is performed.
d. A single-lung recipient pneumonectomy is performed, followed by donor lung implantation with bronchial, PA, and pulmonary vein cuff anastomoses.
e. An identical contralateral pneumonectomy and donor lung implantation is performed.
f. Chest tubes are placed, and the chest is closed.

F. Ex vivo lung perfusion (EVLP)
1. Involves procurement and preservation of marginally acceptable donor lungs ex vivo to improve their utilization rate
2. Benefits include potentially increasing the pool of organs available for transplant
3. Donor lungs initially cold preserved in lung-preservation solution and brought to a lung rehabilitation facility, where they are flushed with perfusate and slowly rewarmed to body temperature and ventilated with 7 mL/kg of ideal body weight at 7 breaths/min, which can be maintained for up to 12 hours.

TABLE 31.2 Ideal Lung Donor Selection Criteria

1. Age < 55 years
2. No history of pulmonary disease
3. PaO_2 > 300 mm Hg, FiO_2 = 1.0, PEEP = 5 cm H_2O
4. Negative serologic screening for hepatitis B and HIV
5. Normal CXR
6. Normal bronchoscopic examination
7. ABO compatibility
8. Size matching

FiO_2, fractional inspired oxygen; PaO_2, arterial oxygen partial pressure; PEEP, positive end-expiratory pressure.

a. Can potentially improve oxygen exchange, airway pressures, pulmonary compliance, and pulmonary vascular resistance
b. Improvements in the above parameters are assessed in order to determine adequacy for transplantation.
c. Assessment of lungs varies by provider/center—currently there is no standard criteria that these lungs must meet.

4. The effects of EVLP on rehabilitation of marginal donor lungs are still under investigation.

G. Outcomes and complications

1. The International Society for Heart and Lung Transplantation (ISHLT) reports 1-year survival of 85% and 5-year survival of 59% for adult lung transplant recipients since 2010.[26]
2. **Primary graft dysfunction (PGD)**
   a. Acute lung injury with multifactorial etiology
   b. A severity grading system was created by the ISHLT taking into account the ratio of arterial oxygen partial pressure to fractional inspired oxygen (PaO_2/FiO_2) at times 0, 24, 48, and 72 hours post transplant and presence of pulmonary edema on CXR.[27]
   c. PGD predisposes to chronic rejection, **bronchiolitis obliterans syndrome** (BOS), and late mortality.
3. **Chronic lung allograft dysfunction (CLAD)**
   a. Defined as ≥20% decline in FEV1 compared with posttransplant baseline
   b. Develops in about 50% of lung transplant recipients at 5 years post transplant
   c. Commonly presents with dyspnea and chronic nonproductive cough
   d. Risk factors include PGD, acute rejection, viral and bacterial infections.
   e. BOS is a phenotype of CLAD that is characterized by fibrosis of small airways associated with obstructive physiology
   f. Treatment initially involves addition of azithromycin and optimization of immunosuppressive regimen; however, disease is often progressive and refractory to treatment.

Key References

Citation	Summary
Saji H, Okada M, Tsuboi M, et al. Segmentectomy versus lobectomy in small-sized peripheral non-small-cell lung cancer (JCOG0802/WJOG4607L): a multicentre, open-label, phase 3, randomised, controlled, non-inferiority trial. *Lancet.* 2022;399(10335):1607-1617.	• Multicenter randomized controlled noninferiority trial comparing overall survival between segmentectomy and lobectomy for stage IA NSCLC • There was equivalent 5-y survival in these two populations for small peripheral NSCLC.

Citation	Summary
Forde PM, Spicer J, Lu S, et al. Neoadjuvant nivolumab plus chemotherapy in resectable lung cancer. *N Engl J Med.* 2022;386(21):1973-1985.	• Open-label, phase 3, randomized trial comparing event-free survival between neoadjuvant nivolumab plus platinum-based chemotherapy and platinum-based chemotherapy alone for stage IB to IIIA resectable NSCLC • Neoadjuvant nivolumab plus chemotherapy in resectable stage IB to IIIA) NSCLC resulted in longer event-free survival and higher rates of complete pathologic response than neoadjuvant chemotherapy alone
Altorki NK, Wang X, Wigle D, et al. Perioperative mortality and morbidity after sublobar versus lobar resection for early-stage non-small-cell lung cancer: post-hoc analysis of an international, randomised, phase 3 trial (CALGB/Alliance 140503). *Lancet Respir Med.* 2018;6(12):915-924.	• Multicenter international randomized noninferiority trial comparing disease-free survival and perioperative morbidity and mortality between lobar and sublobar (including wedge) resection for clinical stage T1aN0 NSCLC • Primary endpoint of disease-free survival is not yet mature. • Post hoc comparative analysis of 30-d and 90-d mortality and perioperative morbidity (graded using the Common Terminology Criteria for Adverse Events 4.0) was equivalent for both groups.
Darling GE, Allen MS, Decker PA, et al. Randomized trial of mediastinal lymph node sampling versus complete lymphadenectomy during pulmonary resection in the patient with N0 or N1 (less than hilar) non-small cell carcinoma: results of the American College of Surgery Oncology Group Z0030 Trial. *J Thorac Cardiovasc Surg.* 2011;141(3):662-670.	• Randomized trial comparing survival between mediastinal lymph node sampling and complete lymphadenectomy during pulmonary resection in nonhilar N1 or lower and T2 or lower NSLSC • The 5-y disease-free survival was equivalent between the two treatment groups, suggesting that complete mediastinal lymphadenectomy does not improve survival over mediastinal lymph node sampling in patients with early-stage NSCLC.

Citation	Summary
Wolfe GI, Kaminski HJ, Aban IB, et al. Randomized trial of thymectomy in myasthenia gravis. *N Engl J Med.* 2016;375(6):511-522.	• Multicenter randomized trial comparing myasthenia gravis (MG) disease severity at 3 y between thymectomy plus prednisone and prednisone alone in patients with nonthymomatous MG • Disease severity was measured by time-weighted average Quantitative Myasthenia Gravis score (scale 0-39, higher being more severe). • In patients with nonthymomatous MG, thymectomy improved clinical disease severity at 3 y compared with medical management alone.

CHAPTER 31: LUNG AND MEDIASTINAL DISEASES

Review Questions

1. From which major vessel do the bronchial arteries originate?
2. What is the cell type that produces pulmonary surfactant?
3. What is the most commonly used substance for chemical pleurodesis?
4. What is the treatment for advanced organizing empyema with a trapped lung?
5. What population should get annual screening for lung cancer with a low-dose CT scan?
6. What is the most common primary pleural malignancy?
7. What are the different types of anterior mediastinal masses?
8. What are the most common indications for lung transplantation?

REFERENCES

1. Dalley AF II, Agur AMR. *Moore's Clinically Oriented Anatomy*. 9th ed. Lippincott Williams & Wilkins; 2021.
2. Kotoulas C, Panagiotou I, Tsipas P, Melachrinou M, Alexopoulos D, Dougenis D. Experimental studies in the bronchial circulation. Which is the ideal animal model? *J Thorac Dis.* 2014;6(10):1506-1512.
3. Brunelli A, Kim AW, Berger KI, Addrizzo-Harris DJ. Physiologic evaluation of the patient with lung cancer being considered for resectional surgery: diagnosis and management of lung cancer, 3rd ed—American College of Chest Physicians evidence-based clinical practice guidelines. *Chest.* 2013;143(5 suppl):e166S-e190S.
4. Villena V, Pérez V, Pozo F, et al. Amylase levels in pleural effusions: a consecutive unselected series of 841 patients. *Chest.* 2002;121(2):470-474.

5. Shen KR, Bribriesco A, Crabtree T, et al. The American Association for thoracic surgery consensus guidelines for the management of empyema. *J Thorac Cardiovasc Surg.* 2017;153(6):e129-e146.
6. *Lung Cancer Statistics.* Accessed January 5, 2023. https://www.cancer.org/cancer/lung-cancer/about/key-statistics.html
7. National Lung Screening Trial Research Team; Aberle DR, Adams AM, et al. Reduced lung-cancer mortality with low-dose computed tomographic screening. *N Engl J Med.* 2011;365(5):395-409.
8. US Preventive Services Task Force, Krist AH, Davidson KW, Mangione CM, et al. Screening for lung cancer: US preventive services task force recommendation statement. *JAMA.* 2021;325(10):962-970.
9. MacMahon H, Naidich DP, Goo JM, et al. Guidelines for management of incidental pulmonary nodules detected on CT images: from the Fleischner Society 2017. *Radiology.* 2017;284(1):228-243.
10. Silvestri GA, Gonzalez AV, Jantz MA, et al. Methods for staging non-small cell lung cancer: diagnosis and management of lung cancer, 3rd ed—American College of Chest Physicians evidence-based clinical practice guidelines. *Chest.* 2013;143(5 suppl):e211S-e250S.
11. Amin M, Edge SB, Greene FL, et al, eds. *AJCC Cancer Staging Manual.* 8th ed. American Joint Committee on Cancer, Springer; 2017.
12. Meyers BF, Haddad F, Siegel BA, et al. Cost-effectiveness of routine mediastinoscopy in computed tomography- and positron emission tomography-screened patients with stage I lung cancer. *J Thorac Cardiovasc Surg.* 2006;131(4):822-829; discussion 822-829.
13. Forde PM, Spicer J, Lu S, et al. Neoadjuvant Nivolumab plus chemotherapy in resectable lung cancer. *N Engl J Med.* 2022;386(21):1973-1985.
14. Wu YL, Tsuboi M, He J, et al. Osimertinib in resected EGFR-mutated non–small-cell lung cancer. *N Engl J Med.* 2020;383(18):1711-1723.
15. Hamaji M. Surgery and stereotactic body radiotherapy for early-stage non-small cell lung cancer: prospective clinical trials of the past, the present, and the future. *Gen Thorac Cardiovasc Surg.* 2020;68(7):692-696.
16. Ijsseldijk MA, Shoni M, Siegert C, et al. Oncologic outcomes of surgery versus SBRT for non–small-cell lung carcinoma: a Systematic review and meta-analysis. *Clin Lung Cancer.* 2021;22(3):e235-e292.
17. Franks KN, McParland L, Webster J, et al. SABRTooth: a randomised controlled feasibility study of stereotactic ablative radiotherapy (SABR) with surgery in patients with peripheral stage I nonsmall cell lung cancer considered to be at higher risk of complications from surgical resection. *Eur Respir J.* 2020;56(5):2000118.
18. Saji H, Okada M, Tsuboi M, et al. Segmentectomy versus lobectomy in small-sized peripheral non-small-cell lung cancer (JCOG0802/WJOG4607L): a multicentre, open-label, phase 3, randomised, controlled, non-inferiority trial. *Lancet.* 2022;399(10335):1607-1617.
19. Heiden BT, Eaton DB Jr, Chang SH, et al. Assessment of updated commission on cancer guidelines for intraoperative lymph node sampling in early stage NSCLC. *J Thorac Oncol.* 2022;17(11):1287-1296.
20. Wang P, Wang S, Liu Z, et al. Segmentectomy and wedge resection for elderly patients with stage I non-small cell lung cancer: a Systematic review and meta-analysis. *J Clin Med.* 2022;11(2):294.

21. Frendl G, Sodickson AC, Chung MK, et al. 2014 AATS guidelines for the prevention and management of perioperative atrial fibrillation and flutter for thoracic surgical procedures. *J Thorac Cardiovasc Surg.* 2014;148(3):e153-e193.

22. Westeel V, Foucher P, Scherpereel A, et al. Chest CT scan plus x-ray versus chest x-ray for the follow-up of completely resected non-small-cell lung cancer (IFCT-0302): a multicentre, open-label, randomised, phase 3 trial. *Lancet Oncol.* 2022;23(9): 1180-1188.

23. de Perrot M, Feld R, Cho BCJ, et al. Trimodality therapy with induction chemotherapy followed by extrapleural pneumonectomy and adjuvant high-dose hemithoracic radiation for malignant pleural mesothelioma. *J Clin Oncol.* 2009;27(9):1413-1418.

24. Young RM, Kernstine KH, Corson JD. Miscellaneous cardiopulmonary conditions. In: Corson JD, Williamson RCN, eds. *Surgery.* Mosby; 2001.

25. Wolfe GI, Kaminski HJ, Aban IB, et al. Randomized trial of thymectomy in myasthenia gravis. *N Engl J Med.* 2016;375(6):511-522.

26. Bos S, Vos R, Van Raemdonck DE, Verleden GM. Survival in adult lung transplantation: where are we in 2020? *Curr Opin Organ Transplant.* 2020;25(3):268-273.

27. Snell GI, Yusen RD, Weill D, et al. Report of the ISHLT Working Group on primary lung graft dysfunction, part I: definition and grading-A 2016 Consensus Group statement of the International Society for Heart and Lung transplantation. *J Heart Lung Transplant.* 2017;36(10):1097-1103.

28. Altorki NK, Wang X, Wigle D, et al. Perioperative mortality and morbidity after sublobar versus lobar resection for early-stage non-small-cell lung cancer: post-hoc analysis of an international, randomised, phase 3 trial (CALGB/Alliance 140503). *Lancet Respir Med.* 2018;6(12):915-924.

29. Darling GE, Allen MS, Decker PA, et al. Randomized trial of mediastinal lymph node sampling versus complete lymphadenectomy during pulmonary resection in the patient with N0 or N1 (less than hilar) non-small cell carcinoma: results of the American College of Surgery Oncology Group Z0030 Trial. *J Thorac Cardiovasc Surg.* 2011;141(3):662-670.

30. Jensen MO. *Surgical Anatomy for Mastery of Open Operations: A Multimedia Curriculum for Training Surgery Residents.* 5th ed. Wolters Kluwer; 2018.

32 Cardiac Surgery

Meghan O. Kelly and Matthew R. Schill

I. ANATOMY

A. Circulatory pathways of oxygenated and deoxygenated blood
   1. Oxygenated pulmonary venous blood → pulmonary veins → left atrium (LA) → through the mitral valve (bicuspid) → left ventricle (LV) → through the aortic valve → systemic circulation
   2. Deoxygenated systemic venous blood → superior and inferior venae cavae (SVC, IVC) → right atrium (RA) → through the tricuspid valve (TV) → right ventricle (RV) → through the pulmonary valve (PV) → pulmonary circulation

B. Coronary arteries (**Figure 32.1**)
   1. Arise from **sinuses of Valsalva** just above left and right coronary cusps of the aortic valve
      a. The **aortic valve** has three cusps: Left coronary cusp, right coronary cusp, and noncoronary cusp.
   2. The **left main coronary artery** has two main branches:
      a. **Left anterior descending artery** (LAD)
      b. **Left circumflex artery** (LCx)
   3. The **right coronary artery** (RCA) descends in the atrioventricular (AV) groove.
      a. Left vs. right coronary dominance determined by which coronary artery gives rise to **posterior descending artery** (PDA):
         i. Right dominant (80%-85%)—PDA from the RCA
         ii. Left dominant (10%-15%)—PDA from the LCx
      b. *Clinical correlation:* Dominance is important in selecting targets during **coronary artery bypass grafting** (CABG) and in predicting culprit vessels in post–myocardial infarction (MI) **ventricular septal defect** (VSD).

C. Coronary sinus
   1. Venous drainage of the heart
   2. Runs in the AV groove, empties into RA near IVC

D. Electrical anatomy
   1. Activation begins in **sinoatrial node** located at the junction of the anteromedial aspect of the SVC and the RA and then travels to the AV node.
   2. The AV node is located in the **triangle of Koch** (defined by the coronary sinus, tendon of Todaro, and the septal leaflet of the tricuspid valve; **Figure 32.2**) and protects the ventricle from atrial tachyarrhythmias.
   3. From the AV node, conduction travels to the right and left **bundles of His**.

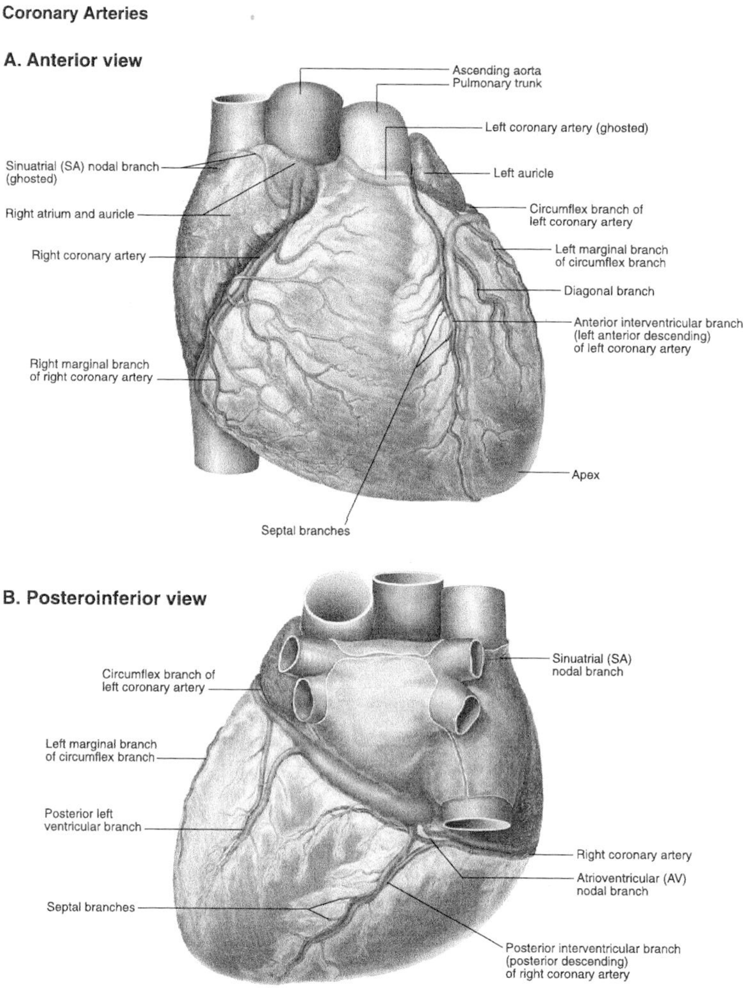

FIGURE 32.1 Coronary artery anatomy. A, Anterior view. B, Posteroinferior view. *(Reprinted with permission. Tank PW, Gest TR. Lippincott Williams & Wilkins Atlas of Anatomy. Lippincott Williams and Wilkins; 2008.)*

II. PREOPERATIVE EVALUATION

A. Commonly used preoperative assessment tools

1. Society of Thoracic Surgeons Risk Score (http://riskcalc.sts.org)
2. *Euro*SCORE II (http://www.euroscore.org)

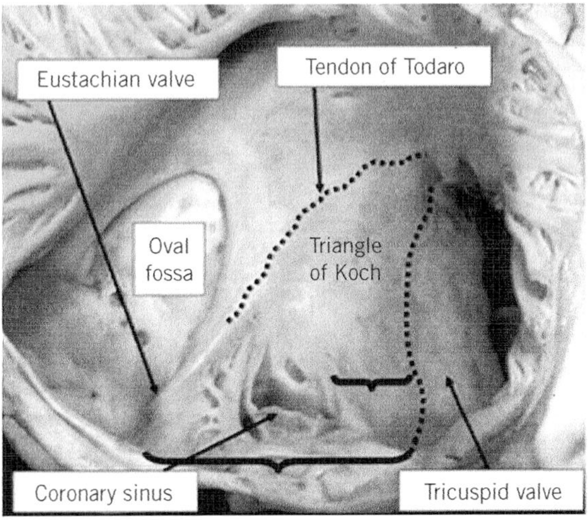

FIGURE 32.2 Triangle of Koch viewed from the inside of the right atrium. Patient head at top and feet at bottom of page. *(From Anderson RH, Cook AC. The structure and components of the atrial chambers. Europace. 2007; 9(suppl 6):vi3-vi9. Reproduced by permission of The European Society of Cardiology.)*

B. History and physical examination
  1. **Table 32.1** highlights impact on outcomes.

C. CXR can show the following:
  1. Aortic calcification that would influence cannulation, cross clamp, and proximal coronary anastomosis strategies (**Figure 32.3**)
  2. Significant lung disease
  3. Mediastinal pathology

D. CT
  1. Chest/abdomen CT scan can assess
     a. Aortic calcifications (**Figure 32.4**)
        i. Significant calcification increases risk of embolization/stroke and indicates potential need for alternate cannulation sites or even inoperability.
     b. Reoperative surgery: Extent of adhesions between the heart and the sternum, how to avoid injury upon reentry/dissection
     c. Lung pathology

E. Cardiac catheterization
  1. Nearly all adult cardiac patients will undergo cardiac catheterization to determine the presence of coronary artery disease (CAD) and to delineate coronary anatomy for bypass planning.
  2. Prior to contrast injection, calcified valve annuli and coronary arteries may be visualized.
  3. Significantly stenotic coronary arteries must be of sufficient size and have a patent, anatomically accessible target in order to accept a bypass graft.

TABLE 32.1 Preoperative Risk Assessment

History	Potential Complication and Evaluation
• Diabetes mellitus (DM) • Immunosuppression • Abnormal body mass index	Increased risk of infection and poor wound healing
• Poorly controlled DM • Increased age • Sex (female)	Increased mortality
• Hypertension	Increased risk of stroke
• Recent cardiac catheterization	Increased risk of renal failure
• Home oxygen use/lung disease • Tobacco use • Previous tracheostomy	Increased risk of prolonged ventilation → Consider pulmonary function tests
• Liver disease • Recent antiplatelet agent use (Plavix, IIb–IIIa inhibitors, thrombin inhibitors) • Thrombocytopenia	Increased risk of bleeding → Consider hematology or hepatology consults
• Previous sternotomy • Chest wall radiation • Pericarditis	Anticipate difficult dissection
• Poor social support • Neurologic dysfunction	Increased risk of difficult rehabilitation
• Exercise tolerance	Good indicator of outcome
• Pulsatile abdominal mass	Concern for abdominal aortic aneurysm → Obtain abdominal ultrasound
• Carotid bruit • Transient ischemic attack symptoms • History of stroke • History of carotid endarterectomy	Concern for carotid stenosis, increasing risk of stroke → Obtain carotid Doppler
• Poor dental hygiene	Concern for dental infection that could potentially seed a prosthetic valve/valve repair materials → Obtain panorex prior to valve procedure

Adapted with permission of John Wiley & Sons from Lawton JS, Gay WA Jr. On-pump coronary artery bypass grafting. In: Little AG, Merrill WH, eds. *Complications in Cardiothoracic Surgery: Avoidance and Treatment.* 2nd ed. Blackwell Publishing; 2010:334-335; permission conveyed through Copyright Clearance Center, Inc.

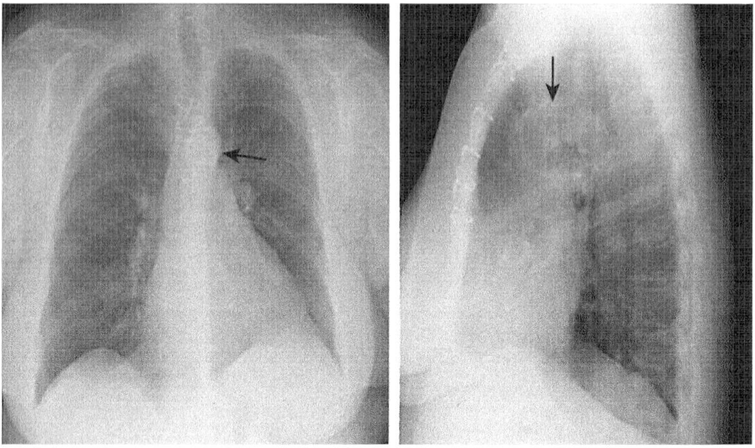

FIGURE 32.3 Anteroposterior (left) and lateral (right) CXR demonstrating a calcified aorta (*black arrows*).

4. **Left ventriculogram** is particularly valuable as it provides an estimation of wall motion and ejection fraction (EF), as well as the size of the ascending aorta and a visual estimation of **mitral valve** (MV) competence.

F. Echocardiography
1. Assesses ventricular function and valvular pathology
2. **Transthoracic echocardiogram** (TTE)
   a. Noninvasive, does not require sedation
   b. Images limited by intervening skin/soft tissue/lung/bone between the probe and the heart

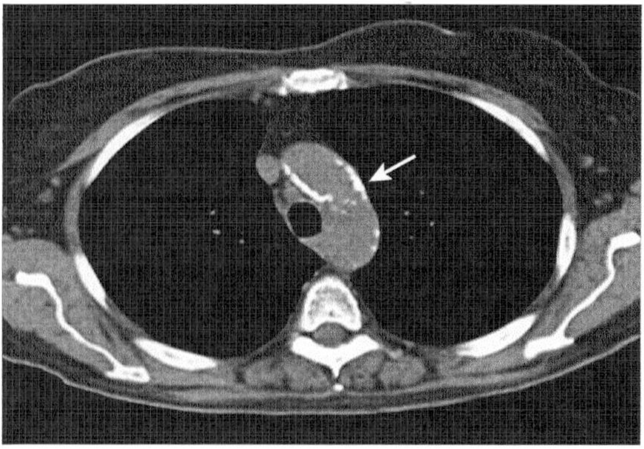

FIGURE 32.4 CT scan demonstrating a calcified aorta (*white arrow*).

3. **Transesophageal echocardiogram** (TEE)
   a. Requires sedation
   b. Superior imaging to TTE because of the esophagus' close proximity to the posterior aspect of the heart without intervening structures
      i. Visualization of posterior cardiac structures (e.g., the MV) is especially superior.

G. Viability studies
1. If EF is significantly reduced on echocardiography, then consider assessment of myocardial viability.
   a. Revascularization of nonviable myocardium has no benefit.
   b. **Viability study** may reveal that a patient will not benefit from CABG or that only some of their coronaries can/should be bypassed.
2. Types: Dobutamine stress echocardiography, single-photon emission computed tomography, positron emission tomography, MRI

III. CARDIOPULMONARY BYPASS (CPB)

A. Benefits
1. Facilitates a quiet, motionless, bloodless operative field

B. Drawbacks
1. Requires systemic anticoagulation
2. Exposure of blood to nonendothelialized surfaces provokes a systemic inflammatory response.
3. Nonpulsatile flow can precipitate renal hypoperfusion
4. Risk of air and particulate embolism to cerebral and systemic circulations (especially with a calcified aorta)
5. Prolonged CPB time (e.g., >3 hours) is a significant risk factor for postoperative complications
6. **Arresting the heart**
   a. Not required for CPB, but often done given safer and technically easier dissection while arrested
   b. Accomplished via administration of **cardioplegia** (high potassium concentration solution) to the coronary vasculature
   c. Cardioplegia can be antegrade and/or retrograde.
      i. Antegrade: Flows in the normal direction of flow in the coronary circulation, usually instilled via aortic root cannula (proximal to a clamp occluding the ascending aorta)
      ii. Retrograde: Opposite to normal physiologic flow, usually instilled via coronary sinus
   d. Cardioplegia complications: Electrolyte imbalances, pH abnormalities, myocardial stunning
7. **CPB circuit:** Venous cannula, venous line (tubing), reservoir, heat exchanger, pump, membrane oxygenator, air vent, arterial line (tubing), arterial cannula (**Figure 32.5**)
   a. Venous reservoir
      i. Stores the blood volume that drains by gravity
      ii. Allows for the escape of air
      iii. All pump suction devices also drain to this reservoir, to return operative blood loss to the patient.

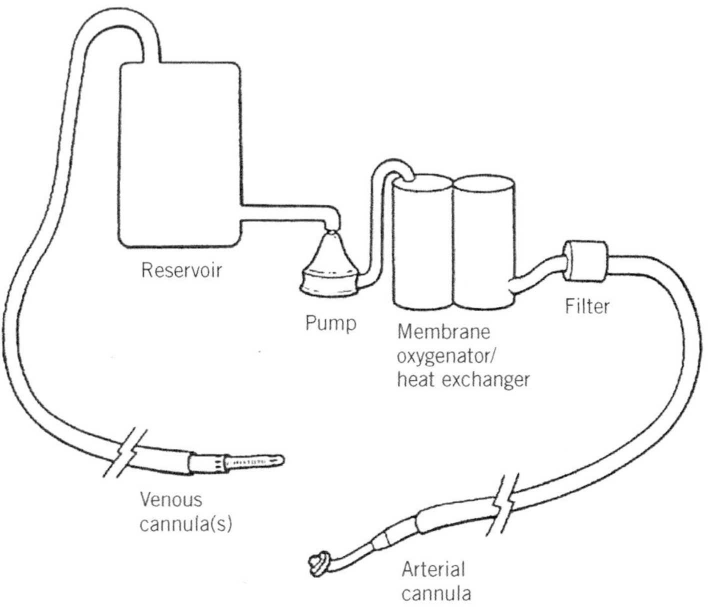

FIGURE 32.5 Cardiopulmonary bypass circuit. *(Reprinted from Punjabi PP, Taylor KM. The science and practice of cardiopulmonary bypass: from cross circulation to ECMO and SIRS. Glob Cardiol Sci Pract. 2013;2013(3):249-260. https://creativecommons.org/licenses/by/3.0.)*

- **b.** Membrane oxygenator performs gas exchange
- **c.** Heat exchanger regulates blood temperature
- **d.** Arterial pump returns warm, oxygenated blood back to the patient via the arterial cannula

8. Surgical approach: CPB with cardiac arrest

- **a.** (With chest already open) place arterial cannula in the ascending aorta and venous cannula in the RA.
- **b.** Place the antegrade cardioplegia cannula and aortic root vent into the ascending aorta and retrograde cardioplegia cannula into the coronary sinus.
- **c.** Confirm activated clotting time > 470 s, begin CPB
- **d.** Cool the patient; 34 °C is often sufficient. Place a thermistor in the intraventricular septum to measure myocardial temperature.
- **e.** Place the aortic cross-clamp between the arterial cannula and the antegrade cannula, infuse cold cardioplegia into the aortic root.
- **f.** Cool the heart (myocardium) to ~15 °C and achieve electromechanical arrest. This is primarily accomplished by the cold cardioplegia, but iced saline can be used if needed.
- **g.** An LV vent may be placed via the right superior pulmonary vein.
- **h.** Give retrograde cardioplegia

IV. CORONARY ARTERY DISEASE

A. Classification and associated conditions

1. Leading cause of death in the US
2. **Angina pectoris**
   a. Occurs when there is reversible myocardial ischemia without cellular necrosis
   b. May manifest as pain/pressure that radiates to the left shoulder and down the left arm or into the jaw/neck
   c. Anginal equivalent: Epigastric discomfort or shortness of breath
      i. Such presentations, without "classic" chest pain, are commonly seen in female patients and patients with diabetes.
   d. Angina occurs during increased myocardial oxygen demand (exercise) and typically resolves with rest/nitrates.
   e. **Unstable angina:** Chest pain that occurs at rest/with increasing frequency/duration/severity.
3. **MI**
   a. Irreversible muscle injury and cell death from lack of myocardial oxygen supply
   b. Increases in cardiac-specific enzymes and ECG changes (ST-segment elevation, T-wave inversions, and new Q waves)
   c. Early and late sequelae: Arrhythmias, VSD, papillary muscle rupture, LV rupture/aneurysm, congestive heart failure (CHF), and/or ischemic cardiomyopathy
   d. Continued angina following MI warrants consideration for urgent/emergent revascularization.
   e. Medical optimization includes aspirin, oxygen, nitrates, IV heparin, and placement of an **intra-aortic balloon pump** (IABP).
4. Acute complications
   a. Arrhythmias
      i. Common during the first 24 hours
      ii. Include potentially fatal ventricular arrhythmias, atrial fibrillation (AF), atrial flutter, heart block, junctional rhythm
   b. In any patient with sudden hemodynamic instability after MI, once arrhythmia is treated/ruled out, suspect mechanical complications
      i. A new holosystolic murmur may reflect VSD/papillary muscle rupture
         a) Treatment is emergent **mechanical circulatory support** (MCS; IABP or **extracorporeal membrane oxygenation** [ECMO]) followed by urgent surgery.
   c. **VSD**
      i. Acute post-MI VSDs
         a) Occur in ~2% of patients with MI
         b) Usually between 5 and 14 days post MI
      ii. Location within the septum depends on location of the coronary artery occlusion and coronary artery dominance: 60% anterior septal wall, 40% inferior septal wall

iii. Diagnosis made by cardiac catheterization (oxygen saturation step-up in the right side of the heart and left-to-right shunt noted on left ventriculogram) and by TEE

d. **Papillary muscle rupture** with severe **mitral regurgitation** (MR)
   i. Results when MI involves a papillary muscle and often the adjacent myocardial wall

e. **LV rupture**
   i. Results when blood dissects through a transmural MI and enters the pericardial space
   ii. Causes tamponade and shock
   iii. Requires emergent surgical repair

5. Chronic complications
   a. **LV aneurysm**
      i. Develops in 5% to 10% of patients
      ii. Well-defined fibrous scar that is dyskinetic
      iii. Large LV aneurysms: Reduce LV EF leading to CHF, serve as substrate for ischemic reentrant ventricular arrhythmias, and create an area of stagnant blood that may lead to thrombus/peripheral emboli
      iv. LV aneurysmectomy (Dor procedure) indicated in patients who may benefit from restoration of ventricular geometry
   b. **CHF**
      i. May result when a large portion of the LV is infarcted
      ii. CHF is graded according to the **New York Heart Association classification** and reflects the extent to which the patient's activity is limited:
         a) Class I—no symptoms
         b) Class II—symptoms (fatigue, palpitation, dyspnea) with heavy exertion
         c) Class III—symptoms with mild exertion
         d) Class IV—symptoms at rest
   c. **Ischemic cardiomyopathy**
      i. May develop after multiple MIs
      ii. Associated with signs/symptoms of CHF
      iii. Treatment is optimal medical management, placement of an automatic implantable cardioverter defibrillator for sudden-cardiac-death prevention in patients with significantly reduced EF, and consideration of other support (see section on heart failure).

B. Operative management

1. Myocardial revascularization via **percutaneous coronary intervention** (PCI) or CABG.
   a. Goals are to relieve angina, prevent repeat MI, avoid need for repeat revascularization, and prolong survival.
   b. The American Heart Association (AHA) and American College of Cardiology (ACC) have established guidelines for coronary artery revascularization.[1]

2. Treatment depends on acuity of presentation, anatomy, predicted operative risk, and patient values/preferences. The associated literature is complex and incrementally changing.
   a. Acute (<12 hours) ST-segment elevation myocardial infarction (**STEMI**)
      i. Emergent PCI
      ii. Urgent CABG indicated if
         a) PCI is not feasible.
         b) Presence of mechanical complications of STEMI
         c) PCI is unsuccessful and ischemia persists.
   b. Non-ST segment elevation myocardial infarction (**NSTEMI**) or stable ischemic heart disease (SIHD)
      i. CABG is indicated to improve survival for appropriate candidates with EF < 35% or significant (≥50%) left main stenosis.
      ii. CABG (including a **left internal mammary artery** [LIMA] to LAD graft) is reasonable to improve survival for select patients with multivessel CAD and EF 35% to 50%.
3. SIHD and EF > 50%
   a. Proximal LAD stenosis (≥70%) and three-vessel disease, formerly generally accepted indications for CABG, have been downgraded to class 2b indications in current guidelines based on the ISCHEMIA trial.[2]
      i. These indications for surgery are still used in most centers and are an area of active debate.[3]
      ii. CABG is preferred over PCI to improve survival for patients with diabetes and multivessel CAD with LAD involvement.
      iii. Revascularization (CABG or PCI) is indicated for symptom relief for patients with SIHD with refractory angina, significant coronary artery stenoses, and physiological evidence of ischemia.
4. In a patient with three-vessel disease, it is reasonable to choose CABG over PCI based on the results of the SYNTAX trial.[4]
5. CABG is also routinely performed for significant coronary artery stenoses in patients undergoing other cardiac operations.
6. **Surgical approach: Median sternotomy**
   a. Identify landmarks: Sternal notch (between strap muscles), sternal angle (insertion of 2nd costal cartilage), xiphoid process. Mark the midline (equidistant between palpable medial margins of intercostal spaces)
   b. Skin incision: From midway between sternal notch and sternal angle to just above the xiphoid
   c. Dissect through the subcutaneous tissue to the periosteum using electrocautery. Palpate and mark the midline with electrocautery.
   d. Divide the interclavicular ligament at the sternal notch with electrocautery.
   e. Sweep the left brachiocephalic vein posteriorly using a gloved finger.
   f. Divide the sternum with sternal saw used either top-down (right-handed surgeon standing on patient's right) or bottom-up (left-handed surgeon standing on patient's right).

g. Obtain hemostasis of the periosteum on anterior and posterior tables using electrocautery, and apply a topical hemostatic agent (e.g., 2 g vancomycin mixed with saline to form a paste) to exposed cancellous bone.

7. **Surgical approach: CABG**
   a. Perform a median sternotomy (see above) and harvest conduits: LIMA, radial artery, and/or saphenous vein.
   b. Cannulate for CPB (see above). Identify target vessels, measure conduits to ensure adequate length. Go on CPB. Arrest with antegrade and retrograde cardioplegia.
   c. Open target vessels and perform distal anastomoses then punch small arteriotomies in the ascending aorta and perform proximal anastomoses, all with fine polypropylene suture.
   d. Ensure hemostasis, de-air the aortic root, reperfuse the heart, and place temporary atrial and ventricular pacing wires (placed in almost all adult cardiac surgery patients in case of life-threatening postoperative arrhythmias).
   e. Separate from CPB, verify cardiac function, remove venous cannula and vents, administer protamine (reverse heparinization), and remove aortic cannula.
   f. Obtain hemostasis. Place chest tubes. Close the chest with sternal wires. Close the subcutaneous tissue and skin in layers.
8. **Conduit selection** for CABG
   a. Common conduits include single or bilateral internal mammary arteries (BIMAs), radial artery, and saphenous vein.
   b. LIMA to the LAD
      i. Patency of 96% at 10 years, prolongs patient survival[5]
      ii. Considered a quality metric by the Centers for Medicare and Medicaid Services
   c. **Saphenous vein grafts** (SVGs) are used in most CABG operations to graft additional target vessels. Preoperative *venous mapping* can determine presence and size of bilateral greater and lesser saphenous veins.
   d. Current ACC/AHA guidelines on conduit selection are controversial.[3] Multiple arterial grafting is becoming more common as more data are published on its use:
      i. In a pooled analysis of six randomized trials, **radial artery** as a second conduit compared with SVG was associated with higher patency and fewer major adverse cardiac events at 5 years, but without a survival benefit.[6]
      ii. BIMA use is associated with improved survival in observational studies[7]; not supported by a randomized controlled trial.[8]
   e. In real-world practice, conduit selection is influenced by several factors:
      i. BIMAs generally contraindicated in patients with conditions that increase risk of sternal wound complications (BIMAs are the main sternal blood supply): Smoking, diabetes, obesity, prior chest wall radiation
      ii. BIMAs contraindicated in subclavian artery stenosis, as subclavian supplies blood to ipsilateral IMA

iii. Radial artery use is influenced by **Allen testing** (test for radial- vs. ulnar-dominant hand circulation), anticipated patient life span (arterial grafts generally last longer than venous grafts), severe diabetes, peripheral vascular disease, chronic kidney disease, and emergency surgery.

V. AORTIC VALVE DISEASE

A. Aortic stenosis (AS)
1. Etiologies: Senile degeneration and calcification, congenitally bicuspid valve, rheumatic disease
2. Pathophysiology: Stenotic valve decreases LV outflow → LV *pressure* overload → LV hypertrophy
   a. *Clinical correlation:* Because of LV hypertrophy, hypotension after aortic valve replacement should first be treated with volume instead of vasoconstrictors
3. Symptoms: Chest pain/angina, shortness of breath, CHF
   a. Syncope indicates severe AS
4. Examination findings: Loud systolic murmur across the precordium, radiates to the carotid arteries
5. Grading based on echocardiography (aortic valve area, pressure gradient across the valve, maximum blood velocity through the valve)
6. Operative management
   a. **Surgical aortic valve replacement** (SAVR; see below) or **transcatheter aortic valve replacement** (TAVR)
   b. Indications
      i. Symptomatic severe AS, as aortic valve replacement improves survival and relieves symptoms compared with medical management alone.[9]
      ii. Asymptomatic severe AS plus either planned concomitant cardiac surgery or LV EF $< 50\%$

B. Aortic insufficiency (AI)
1. Etiologies
   a. Senile degeneration or rheumatic heart disease leading to leaflet thickening, calcification, and fixation
   b. Myxomatous degeneration (noninflammatory progressive impaired synthesis/remodeling of type VI collagen) leading to leaflet redundancy/destruction
   c. Aortic root dilation or dissection leading to poor leaflet coaptation
   d. Inflammatory disease (e.g., ankylosing spondylitis)
   e. Trauma (blunt, iatrogenic)
   f. Endocarditis
2. Pathophysiology
   a. Chronic insufficiency → chronic LV *volume* overload → LV enlargement and wall thickening, pulmonary congestion
   b. Acute AI → acute LV *volume* overload → fulminant pulmonary edema, myocardial ischemia, cardiovascular collapse

c. *Clinical correlation:* IABP is contraindicated with severe AI as the balloon inflates during diastole, increasing AI.

3. Symptoms: Exertional dyspnea, angina, CHF
4. Examination findings: Widened pulse pressure, decrescendo diastolic murmur best heard at left sternal border 3rd/4th intercostal space
5. Grading based on echocardiography (regurgitant jet dimensions/velocity, flow reversal in the proximal aorta, LV dilation)
6. Operative management
   a. SAVR/TAVR
   b. Indications
      i. Symptomatic severe AI
      ii. Asymptomatic severe/moderate AI plus either planned concomitant cardiac/aortic surgery or LV EF < 50%
      iii. Relative indication for asymptomatic patients with severe AI and severe LV dilatation but preserved EF

C. SAVR/TAVR

1. TAVR originally restricted to patients prohibitively high risk for open surgery, but now more common than SAVR for AS[10]
   a. TAVR adoption accelerated after PARTNER 3 trial showed superior 1-year outcomes (stroke, death, readmission) relative to SAVR.[11]
2. Current ACC/AHA guidelines recommend[12]
   a. SAVR in patients <65 year old or with >20 years life expectancy
   b. TAVR in patients >80 year old or with <10 years life expectancy
   c. Shared decision-making for patients in-between
3. TAVR usually transfemoral but can be via ascending aorta, LV apex, subclavian or carotid artery
4. **Surgical approach: Aortic valve replacement (SAVR)**
   a. Median sternotomy (see above); administer heparin and go on CPB; arrest the heart with antegrade cardioplegia (with or without retrograde depending on presence of CAD)
   b. Make a transverse aortotomy and expose the aortic valve with retraction sutures or self-retaining retractor, and resect the native aortic valve. An assistant *must* collect any displaced calcific debris using open-tip wall suction to prevent embolization.
   c. Place horizontal mattress sutures in a radial orientation—one at each commissure (where the cusps meet) and at least three sutures along each cusp, pass the sutures through an aortic valve prosthesis, then secure it in place.
   d. Close the aorta with two layers of polypropylene suture. De-air the heart before tying the suture.
   e. Ensure hemostasis, de-air the aortic root, reperfuse the heart, place temporary atrial and ventricular pacing wires.
   f. Separate from CPB, verify cardiac and valve function (intraoperative TEE), remove venous cannula and vents, administer protamine (reverse heparin), remove aortic cannula.
   g. Obtain hemostasis. Place chest tubes. Close the chest with sternal wires. Close the subcutaneous tissue and skin in layers.

VI. MITRAL VALVE DISEASE

A. Mitral stenosis (MS)
   1. Etiologies
      a. Valve leaflet thickening/calcification (senile degeneration, rheumatic heart disease, collagen vascular diseases, amyloidosis)
      b. Congenital stenosis
      c. Mitral inflow obstruction from tumors/masses
   2. Pathophysiology: Valve stenosis → LA *pressure* overload → LA dilation
   3. Symptoms: Usually develop late and reflect downstream effects:
      a. Dyspnea from pulmonary congestion
      b. Low cardiac output (CO) syndrome from reduced LV preload
      c. Thromboembolism from AF (especially if LA dilation >45 mm)
   4. Examination findings: Apical diastolic murmur, loud S1
   5. Grading: Based on echocardiographic assessment of valve area
      a. Critical MS: Valve area ≤ 1.5 cm^2
   6. Operative management
      a. **Mitral valve repair or replacement**
      b. Indications
         i. Severe MS with severe symptoms
         ii. Moderate MS and planned concomitant cardiac surgery
         iii. Recurrent embolic events while adequately anticoagulated
            a) Surgery should include left atrial appendage exclusion in these patients.
      c. High-risk patients
         i. Nonrheumatic calcific MS
         ii. Severe mitral annular calcification (ring of calcium around the valve) makes valve replacement technically challenging.

B. MR
   1. Etiologies
      a. Primary/degenerative: Pathology intrinsic to the valvular apparatus
         i. Leaflet: Prolapse, fibroelastic deficiency/connective tissue disorders, rheumatic disease, radiation injury, trauma (e.g., iatrogenic, endocarditis)
         ii. **Chordae tendinae** (anchor the valve leaflets to the papillary muscles): Rupture from endocarditis or MI, degenerative fusion/elongation
         iii. Papillary muscle: Ischemic dysfunction after MI
      b. Secondary/functional: Chronic ischemic or idiopathic cardiomyopathy leads to secondary dilation of the valve annulus.
   2. Pathophysiology
      a. Chronically regurgitant valve → chronic LA and later LV *volume* overload → LA and LV dilation and wall thickening, pulmonary congestion
         i. LA dilation can lead to AF.
         ii. LV dilation can lead to LV dysfunction/CHF.
      b. Acute severe MR results in pulmonary congestion and low CO and necessitates urgent operative intervention

i. *Clinical correlation:* IABP beneficial because it decreases afterload, thereby increasing forward flow and decreasing regurgitant volume

3. Symptoms: Dyspnea, CHF
4. Examination findings: Systolic murmur loudest at the apex of the heart
5. Grading based on echocardiography (specific valvular pathology, regurgitant jet morphology/dimensions/velocity, ventricular dilation/dysfunction, reversal of pulmonary venous flow)
6. Management based on etiology and/or severity of concomitant disease[12]
   a. **Primary MR**
      i. Operative management (mitral valve repair[13]/replacement) for
         a) Symptomatic chronic severe MR
         b) Asymptomatic chronic severe MR with EF < 60%
      ii. Repair vs replacement
         a) For degenerative MR in elective setting, repair is standard of care. Guidelines recommend such cases be done at centers of excellence with 95% repair rate and <1% operative mortality
         b) Replacement acceptable for urgent/emergent, failed repair, mixed regurgitation/stenosis, severe mitral annular calcification
   b. **Secondary MR**
      i. First line is guideline-directed medical therapy (GDMT) for heart failure.
      ii. Operative management considered for nonischemic secondary MR refractory to GDMT
      iii. Operation for chronic ischemic MR is challenging with increased operative risk. Results of randomized controlled trials so far have not shown survival benefit from repair vs replacement, but replacement so far has shown better freedom from recurrent regurgitation.[14,15]
   c. **Transcatheter (transfemoral) mitral valve therapies**
      i. Percutaneous transcatheter edge-to-edge repair (TEER; MitraClip [Abbott Laboratories, Abbott Park, IL] procedure)
         a) Clips the two valve leaflets together
         b) Survival advantage in severe MR with advanced heart failure on GDMT[16]
         c) Reasonable for severely symptomatic patients with severe primary MR, high/prohibitive surgical risk, favorable anatomy, and life expectancy >1 year[12]
      ii. Transcatheter mitral valve replacement

VII. OTHER VALVULAR DISEASES

A. Tricuspid stenosis (TS)

1. Most commonly secondary to rheumatic disease or infective endocarditis
2. May be associated with regurgitation
3. May not be detectable on bedside examination

4. Operative management
   a. Mainly repair, can be replaced
   b. Indications
      i. Severe TS already planned for left-sided valve (aortic/mitral) procedure
      ii. Isolated symptomatic severe TS

B. Tricuspid regurgitation (TR)
   1. Etiologies
      a. Primary: Rheumatic disease, infective endocarditis (often in IV drug abuse [IVDA]), carcinoid tumors, **Ebstein anomaly** (TV malformed and malpositioned), blunt trauma
      b. Secondary/functional (most common): Dilation of valve annulus due to pulmonary hypertension, usually secondary to intrinsic mitral/aortic valve disease
      c. Mild to moderate TR usually well tolerated
   2. Examination findings: Systolic murmur, prominent jugular venous pulse, pulsatile liver
   3. Operative management
      a. Indication: Moderate to severe TR and planned concomitant cardiac surgery
      b. Generally repair via **annuloplasty**, can also be replaced
      c. Adaptations to surgical technique to avoid damage to the AV node resulting in heart block:
         i. Annuloplasty repair: Use an incomplete ring prosthesis
         ii. Replacement: Place annular sutures in the leaflet tissue only (**tendon of Todaro**, **Figure 32.2**).

C. Pulmonary insufficiency
   1. Etiologies: Status-post childhood repair of **tetralogy of Fallot** (most common indication for surgical repair in adults), endocarditis, tumors, radiation
   2. Does not require intervention if: Mild to moderate, asymptomatic, and normal RV size/function

D. Pulmonary stenosis
   1. Rarely seen in adults

E. Infective endocarditis
   1. Etiology: Bacteremia seeds native or prosthetic valve (secondary to dental infections/procedures, IVDA, nosocomial infection, indwelling IV/dialysis catheters)
   2. Management
      a. Appropriate antibiotics (empiric based on suspected source, then narrowed based on blood cultures)
         i. Risk of embolization of valve vegetations reduced significantly following antibiotic initiation
      b. Surgical treatment associated with increased survival compared with antibiotics alone; debridement should be aggressive to eradicate all infected tissue.[17,18]
      c. Indications for urgent surgery[19]
         i. Mobile vegetations >10 mm with evidence of embolization despite antibiotics

ii. Aortic root abscess

d. Other surgical indications[19]

i. Valve dysfunction resulting in symptomatic heart failure

ii. Left-sided with *Staphylococcus aureus*, fungi, or resistant microorganisms

iii. Heart block

iv. Destructive lesions/abscess

v. Persistent (>5-7 days) bacteremia despite appropriate antibiotics

vi. Relapsed prosthetic valve endocarditis (after antibiotic therapy)

3. The risk for reoperation for recurrent infective endocarditis is about 17% in IVDA and 5% for non-IVDA.[20]

VIII. ADDITIONAL NOTES ON VALVULAR DISEASE

A. Prosthetic valve selection

1. **Tissue bioprostheses**
   a. Porcine aortic valves, bovine pericardial valves
   b. Benefit: Low rate of thromboembolism, even without long-term anticoagulation (daily aspirin recommended)
   c. Downside: Less durable than mechanical valves (mean time to failure ~10-15 years)
   d. Preferred for patients >65 years or with contraindication to anticoagulation
2. **Mechanical valves**
   a. Benefit: Excellent long-term durability
   b. Downside: Require lifelong anticoagulation, with cumulative rate of thromboembolic complications (0.5%-3% per year)
   c. Preferred for most patients under age 50 years who can take warfarin. In women of childbearing age, issue of anticoagulation in pregnancy must be considered.
3. **Homograft and autograft valved conduits**
   a. Homograft: Human cadaveric valve
   b. Autograft: Patient's own valve (pulmonary) reimplanted in another location
   c. Useful in special circumstances, such as endocarditis or for the Ross procedure (reimplantation of the PV in the aortic valve position, performed for severe aortic valve disease in children).[21]

IX. HYPERTROPHIC CARDIOMYOPATHY

A. Pathophysiology: Asymmetric myocardial hypertrophy and fibrosis, causing obstruction of the **LV outflow tract** (LVOT)

B. Management

1. Medical therapy
   a. First line: β-Blockade or calcium channel blockade
   b. Avoid vasodilators that can exacerbate LVOT obstruction: Nifedipine, nitroglycerin, angiotensin-converting enzyme inhibitors, angiotensin II blockers.

2. Transcatheter therapy: **Septal ablation** (alcohol injected to infarct part of the intraventricular septum)
3. Surgical therapy is **septal myectomy**.
   a. Recommended for symptomatic patients with documented at-rest LVOT gradient of ≥30 mmHg who have failed medical therapy/transcatheter ablation

X. ATRIAL FIBRILLATION

A. Epidemiology: Affects 1% to 2% of the general population; affects nearly 10% of individuals >80 years of age
B. Pathophysiology
   1. Fibrillation/stagnant blood flow leads to thromboembolism, thus risk of stroke, acute mesenteric/limb ischemia.
   2. Loss of LA "kick" decreases left-sided heart pump function, can lead to heart failure/hemodynamic compromise.
C. Symptoms: Palpitations, CHF, thromboembolic complications
D. Nonoperative management
   1. Medical rate control (e.g., β-blockade)
   2. Transcatheter ablation (using radiofrequency/cryoablation)
E. Operative management
   1. Indications
      a. Symptomatic AF and planned concomitant cardiac surgery
      b. Low-risk patients with asymptomatic AF and planned concomitant cardiac surgery
      c. Patients with symptomatic AF who prefer a surgical approach, who have failed one or more attempts at catheter ablation, or are not catheter ablation candidates[22,23]
   2. Gold standard: **Cox–Maze IV procedure** (CMP-IV)
      a. Uses both cryoablation and bipolar radiofrequency ablation
      b. CMP-IV at Washington University in St. Louis postoperative freedom from AF: 92% at 1 year, 84% at 5 years, and 77% at 10 years, substantially higher than catheter ablation (at best about 50% at 1 year)[24]

XI. SURGICAL TREATMENT OF HEART FAILURE

A. Epidemiology: ~250,000 people suffer from advanced heart failure in the US[25]
B. General concepts
   1. First line: GDMT
   2. Patients who fail GDMT can be considered for MCS that can act as a bridge to **heart transplantation** or as **destination therapy**.
C. MCS
   1. **IABP**
      a. Catheter-mounted balloon, positioned in the descending thoracic aorta
      b. Physiology

   i. Functions by counterpulsation, inflating during diastole and rapidly deflating during systole
   ii. Augments coronary perfusion (which occurs primarily during diastole)
   iii. Reduces afterload, providing an additional 500 mL/min of CO
  c. Indications
   i. First line in *acute* heart failure
   ii. In the perioperative period, can be used for: Perioperative low CO, preoperative unstable angina refractory to medical therapy, and/or difficulty weaning from CPB
  d. Contraindications: AI, aortic dissection, severe peripheral vascular disease
  e. Potential complications: Abdominal organ/lower extremity malperfusion, perforation of the aorta, femoral artery injury
2. **ECMO**
  a. Similar to a simplified CPB circuit (no venous reservoir)
  b. Can provide full support of CO for up to ~6 L/min and can provide cardiac, pulmonary, or cardiopulmonary support
  c. Indications
   i. Postoperative myocardial stunning
   ii. Acute heart failure as bridge to recovery or a durable device
   iii. Respiratory failure
  d. Contraindications
   i. Nonreversible process
    a) ECMO is not destination therapy, so it should only be employed for patients expected to recover from their primary process with ECMO support.
  e. Complications: Bleeding/clotting, low-flow/malperfusion
3. Temporary **ventricular assist devices** (VADs)
  a. Small, catheter-mounted devices: e.g., Impella (Abiomed, Danvers, MA), TandemHeart (TandemLife, Pittsburgh, PA)
  b. Placement via femoral or axillary artery
  c. Provides 1 to 5.5 L/min of flow
  d. Indications: Short-term support in acute heart failure
4. **Durable VADs**
  a. Mechanical heart pump used for long-term ventricular support either as destination therapy or bridge to transplant
  b. Requires long-term anticoagulation
  c. Blood flow through device: LV → inflow graft → pump → outflow graft → ascending aorta
  d. Drive line from the pump traverses the skin via a permanent port and is attached to external battery pack. Batteries must be frequently charged and replaced.
   i. Only model currently marketed in the US is HeartMate 3 (Abbott, Abbott Park, IL).
  e. Can provide up to 7 L/min of flow
  f. Indications

i. In adults, only approved for long-term support as LV assist devices
ii. Can be used temporarily as RV assist devices in the postoperative period

g. Contraindications: Patients must be able to manage the external battery pack and tolerate long-term anticoagulation.
h. Complications: Bleeding, thromboembolic, drive line infection

D. Heart transplantation

1. Estimated survival of 90% at 1 year and 79% at 5 years[26]
2. Indications: End-stage cardiomyopathy refractory to GDMT
3. Contraindications[27]
   a. Age > 70 years
   b. Irreversible pulmonary hypertension
   c. Active infection/malignancy
   d. Recent pulmonary embolus
   e. Excessive comorbidity (renal or hepatic dysfunction, systemic disease [amyloidosis], significant peripheral vascular disease, active peptic ulcer disease, uncontrolled diabetes, morbid obesity, severe/refractory mental illness, active tobacco/substance abuse)
   f. Inadequate social support
4. Complications: acute and chronic rejection
   a. Diagnosed by endomyocardial biopsy or echocardiography
   b. **Coronary artery vasculopathy**
      i. Major long-term source of morbidity after cardiac transplantation
         a) Responsible for 30% of deaths after 5 years[28]
      ii. **Chronic vascular rejection:** Diffuse small-vessel disease
         a) Usually not amenable to conventional revascularization
         b) May require retransplantation

XII. POSTOPERATIVE MANAGEMENT AND COMPLICATIONS

A. Hemodynamic monitoring

1. Typically via a combination of pulmonary artery catheter, arterial line, and central venous catheter (normal values and formulas are listed in **Table 32.2**). Key values:
   a. **Cardiac index** (CI): 2 L/min/m^2 is generally the minimum acceptable value
      i. CI = CO/(patient's estimated body surface area)
   b. **Mixed venous oxygen saturation** <60% suggests inadequate peripheral tissue perfusion and increased peripheral oxygen extraction.

B. Postoperative complications

1. Low CO = **shock**
   a. Etiologies include myocardial stunning/ischemia and cardiac tamponade.
   b. **Myocardial stunning**
      i. Transient postischemic myocardial dysfunction that persists despite adequate reperfusion and without irreversible damage

TABLE 32.2 Hemodynamic Formulas and Normal Parameters

Parameter	Formula	Normal Values	
Cardiac output (CO)	CO = SV·HR	4-8	L/min
Cardiac index (CI)	CI = CO/BSA	2.2-4.0	L/min/m^2
Stroke volume (SV)	SV = (CO/HR)·(1,000 mL/L)	60-100 1	mL/beat mL/kg/beat
Stroke volume index (SVI)	SVI = SV/BSA	33-47	mL/beat/m^2
Mean arterial pressure (MAP)	MAP = DP + ([SP-DP]/3)	70-100	mm Hg
Systemic vascular resistance (SVR)	SVR = ([MAP-CVP]/CO)·80	800-1,200	dynes·s/cm^5
Pulmonary vascular resistance (PVR)	PVR = ([PAP-PCWP]/CO)·80	50-250	dynes·s/cm^5
Left ventricular stroke work index (LVSWI)	LVSWI = SVI·(MAP-PCWP)·0.0136	45-75	g/M/m^2/beat

BSA, body surface area; CVP, central venous pressure; DP, diastolic pressure; HR, heart rate; PAP, mean pulmonary artery pressure; PCWP, pulmonary capillary wedge pressure; SP, systolic pressure.

Adapted from Bojar RM, ed. Cardiovascular management. In: *Manual of Perioperative Care in Adult Cardiac Surgery*. 6th ed. Wiley-Blackwell; 2021:513-671. Copyright 2021, John Wiley & Sons Ltd. Reprinted by permission of John Wiley & Sons, Inc.

c. **Myocardial ischemia**
   i. Perioperative MI occurs in approximately 1% to 2% of patients.
   ii. Thrombosis or spasm can occlude new bypass grafts.
   iii. Cardiac catheterization can guide treatment, including return to the operating room or PCI.

d. **Cardiac tamponade**
   i. Potentially fatal
   ii. Clinical diagnosis: Narrowed pulse pressure, increased jugular venous distention, rising central venous pressure, muffled heart sounds, pulsus paradoxus
   iii. Confirm via echocardiography
   iv. Treatment: Emergent drainage

e. **Figure 32.6**: Treatment algorithm for low CO
   i. Aggressively correct via manipulation of heart rate, preload, afterload, and/or contractility

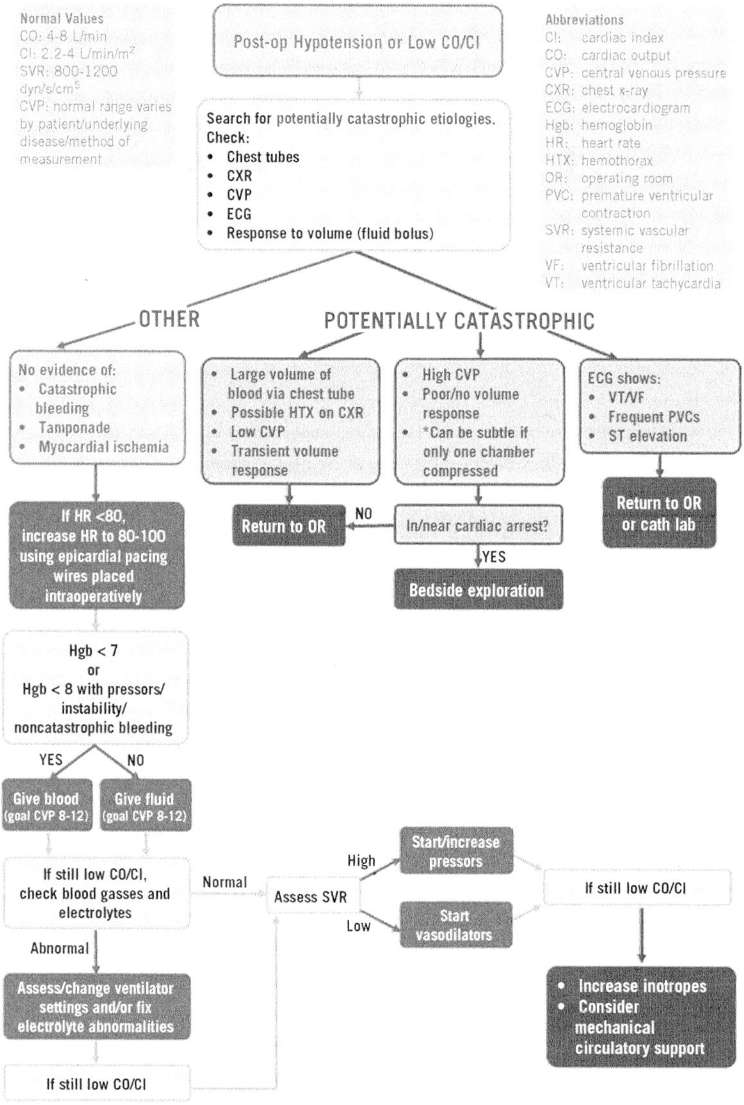

FIGURE 32.6 Postoperative evaluation and treatment of low cardiac output state.

ii. One of the easiest methods to increase CO is to increase heart rate (to 80-100 beats/min) using temporary epicardial pacing electrodes placed intraoperatively

2. Bleeding
   a. Necessitates re-exploration in up to 5% of patients.
   b. Acceptable levels of postoperative bleeding (as monitored by chest-tube output) vary by the procedure performed and patient factors (e.g., on multiple chronic anticoagulants/antiplatelet agents). Generally
      i. <100 mL/h is excellent/nonconcerning.
      ii. 100 to 250 mL/h is acceptable.
      iii. >250 mL/h is concerning and necessitates close monitoring/consideration of return to operating room (OR) depending on patient status/timing.
         a) If >1 L bleeding over the first 4 hours postoperatively, strong indicator of need to return to OR
      iv. >400 mL/h is a strong indicator of need to return to OR.
      v. Make sure the chest tube is not clotted/blocked; can also check CXR for possible hemothorax.
   c. If there is concern for bleeding, other parameters to check/intervene upon:
      i. Hypothermia
      ii. Cardiac surgery–induced coagulopathy
         a) International normalized ratio (INR): Give fresh frozen plasma if INR < 2
         b) Platelet count: Transfuse platelets if level <100,000/mm^3
         c) Consider desmopressin (DDAVP), particularly in patients with likely poor platelet function secondary to chronic renal disease
         d) Consider factor VIIa administration
3. Arrhythmias
   a. Supraventricular arrhythmias (AF/atrial flutter/atrial tachycardia) are most common.
   b. Postoperative AF occurs in 30% of patients with peak incidence on postoperative day 2.[29]
   c. Treatment depends on arrhythmia and hemodynamics.
      i. Supraventricular arrhythmias with hemodynamic compromise require rapid electrical cardioversion
      ii. Hemodynamically stable atrial flutter: Overdrive pacing can be used
      iii. Hemodynamically stable AF/flutter
         a) Ventricular rate control with β-blockade and amiodarone
         b) If persists >12 hours, anticoagulation should be considered to reduce stroke risk.
      iv. Sustained *ventricular arrhythmias* other than premature ventricular contractions suggest underlying ischemia and require investigation

4. Respiratory failure
   a. Postoperative mechanical ventilation >24 hours associated with increased rates of morbidity including pneumonia
   b. Early extubation preferred if patient is hemodynamically stable and bleeding is minor (as bleeding is a common cause for return to the operating room).
5. Renal dysfunction
   a. Significantly increases mortality
   b. Prevention
      i. Maintain adequate CI and mean arterial pressure.
      ii. Avoid/limit nephrotoxic agents, dose-adjust any renally excreted medications.
6. Cerebrovascular accident
   a. Signs range from delirium to obvious focal neurologic deficits.
   b. With a new focal neurologic deficit, immediately obtain a head CT and CT angiogram head/neck with perfusion imaging to assess for intracranial hemorrhage or large vessel occlusion amenable to thrombectomy.[30]
      i. Immediately post cardiac surgery patients are not candidates for IV tissue plasminogen activator.
      ii. Without a focal examination, imaging is of limited utility.[31]
7. Deep sternal wound infection
   a. Treatment
      i. Operative debridement of devitalized sternal and soft tissue
      ii. Administration of broad-spectrum IV antibiotics
      iii. Muscle flap closure of soft tissue defects often needed
   b. Prophylaxis
      i. Perioperative IV antibiotics
      ii. Aggressive blood sugar management

Key References

Citation	Summary
Lawton JS, Tamis-Holland JE, Bangalore S, et al. 2021 ACC/AHA/SCAI guideline for coronary artery revascularization: executive summary: a report of the American College of Cardiology/American Heart Association Joint Committee on Clinical Practice Guidelines. *Circulation.* 2022;145(3):e4-e17.	• Multispecialty clinical practice guidelines for coronary artery disease • Standard reference for clinical decision-making
Sabik JF III, Bakaeen FG, Ruel M, et al. The American Association for thoracic surgery and The Society of Thoracic Surgeons reasoning for not endorsing the 2021 ACC/AHA/SCAI coronary revascularization guidelines. *Ann Thorac Surg.* 2022;113(4):1065-1068.	• Surgical perspective regarding the contemporary evidence for coronary artery bypass grafting

Citation	Summary
Otto CM, Nishimura RA, Bonow RO, et al. 2020 ACC/AHA guideline for the management of patients with valvular heart disease: A report of the American College of Cardiology/American Heart Association Joint Committee on Clinical Practice Guidelines. *Circulation.* 2021;143(5):e72-e227.	• Multispecialty clinical practice guidelines for valvular heart disease • Standard reference for clinical decision-making
Carpentier A. Cardiac valve surgery: the "French correction." *J Thorac Cardiovasc Surg.* 1983;86(3):323-337.	• A technical tour de force. Describes the paradigm for mitral valve repair; similar techniques were later applied to the tricuspid valve, and the thought process has been extended to the aortic valve
Leon MB, Mack MJ, Hahn RT, et al. Outcomes 2 years after transcatheter aortic valve replacement in patients at low surgical risk. *J Am Coll Cardiol.* 2021;77(9):1149-1161.	• Multicenter randomized controlled trial for TAVR compared with SAVR in an appropriately selected population (cited paper is the 2-y report) • TAVR had equivalent mortality and superior composite outcome (death/stroke/hospitalization) compared with SAVR at 2 y post procedure
Maron DJ, Hochman JS, Reynolds HR, et al. Initial invasive or conservative strategy for stable coronary disease. *N Engl J Med.* 2020;382(15):1395-1407.	• Multicenter randomized controlled trial comparing invasive vs conservative management strategy for stable ischemic heart disease • Invasive revascularization defined as either percutaneous coronary intervention or coronary artery bypass grafting • Conservative defined as medical management only • Found equivalent risk of ischemic cardiovascular events or death from any cause over a median of 3.2 y for invasive vs conservative management • Highly controversial, principal topic in revised coronary guidelines

CHAPTER 32: CARDIAC SURGERY

Review Questions

1. What is the most durable conduit for coronary artery bypass grafting?
2. What factors guide shared decision making between bioprosthetic and mechanical valves?
3. What are surgical options for acute stabilization of cardiogenic shock?
4. What are surgical options for durable treatment of end-stage heart failure?
5. What is the differential diagnosis for hemodynamic instability a few hours after open heart surgery?
6. What are contraindications to IABP and VA ECMO support?
7. When a patient with acute myocardial infarction (MI) has decompensation, what diagnoses should be considered?

REFERENCES

1. Lawton JS, Tamis-Holland JE, Bangalore S, et al. 2021 ACC/AHA/SCAI guideline for coronary artery revascularization: executive summary—a report of the American College of Cardiology/American Heart association joint committee on clinical practice guidelines. *Circulation*. 2022;145(3):e4-e17.
2. Maron DJ, Hochman JS, Reynolds HR, et al. Initial invasive or conservative strategy for stable coronary disease. *N Engl J Med*. 2020;382(15):1395-1407.
3. Sabik JF III, Bakaeen FG, Ruel M, et al. The American Association for thoracic surgery and the society of thoracic surgeons reasoning for not endorsing the 2021 ACC/AHA/SCAI coronary revascularization guidelines. *Ann Thorac Surg*. 2022;113(4):1065-1068.
4. Thuijs DJFM, Kappetein AP, Serruys PW, et al. Percutaneous coronary intervention versus coronary artery bypass grafting in patients with three-vessel or left main coronary artery disease: 10-year follow-up of the multicentre randomised controlled SYNTAX trial. *Lancet*. 2019;394(10206):1325-1334.
5. Loop FD, Lytle BW, Cosgrove DM, et al. Influence of the internal-mammary-artery graft on 10-year survival and other cardiac events. *N Engl J Med*. 1986;314(1):1-6.
6. Gaudino M, Benedetto U, Fremes S, et al. Radial-artery or saphenous-vein grafts in coronary-artery bypass surgery. *N Engl J Med*. 2018;378(22):2069-2077.
7. Lytle BW, Blackstone EH, Loop FD, et al. Two internal thoracic artery grafts are better than one. *J Thorac Cardiovasc Surg*. 1999;117(5):855-872.
8. Taggart DP, Benedetto U, Gerry S, et al. Bilateral versus single internal-thoracic-artery grafts at 10 years. *N Engl J Med*. 2019;380(5):437-446.
9. Schwarz F, Baumann P, Manthey J, et al. The effect of aortic valve replacement on survival. *Circulation*. 1982;66(5):1105-1110.
10. Bowdish ME, D'Agostino RS, Thourani VH, et al. STS adult cardiac surgery database: 2021 update on outcomes, quality, and research. *Ann Thorac Surg*. 2021;111(6):1770-1780.
11. Mack MJ, Leon MB, Thourani VH, et al. Transcatheter aortic-valve replacement with a balloon-expandable valve in low-risk patients. *N Engl J Med*. 2019;380(18):1695-1705.
12. Otto CM, Nishimura RA, Bonow RO, et al. 2020 ACC/AHA guideline for the management of patients with valvular heart disease: a report of the American College of Cardiology/American Heart Association joint committee on clinical practice guidelines. *Circulation*. 2021;143(5):e72-e227.

13. Carpentier A. Cardiac valve surgery: the "French correction." *J Thorac Cardiovasc Surg.* 1983;86(3):323-337.
14. Acker MA, Parides MK, Perrault LP, et al. Mitral-valve repair versus replacement for severe ischemic mitral regurgitation. *N Engl J Med.* 2014;370(1):23-32.
15. Goldstein D, Moskowitz AJ, Gelijns AC, et al. Two-year outcomes of surgical treatment of severe ischemic mitral regurgitation. *N Engl J Med.* 2016;374(4):344-353.
16. Stone GW, Lindenfeld J, Abraham WT, et al. Transcatheter mitral-valve repair in patients with Heart failure. *N Engl J Med.* 2018;379(24):2307-2318.
17. Akowuah EF, Davies W, Oliver S, et al. Prosthetic valve endocarditis: early and late outcome following medical or surgical treatment. *Heart.* 2003;89(3):269-272.
18. Netzer ROM, Altwegg SC, Zollinger E, Täuber M, Carrel T, Seiler C. Infective endocarditis: determinants of long term outcome. *Heart.* 2002;88(1):61-66.
19. AATS Surgical Treatment of Infective Endocarditis Consensus Guidelines Writing Committee Chairs; Pettersson GB, Coselli JS, Hussain ST, et al. 2016 the American Association for Thoracic Surgery (AATS) consensus guidelines: surgical treatment of infective endocarditis—executive summary. *J Thorac Cardiovasc Surg.* 2017;153(6):1241-1258.e29.
20. Kaiser SP, Melby SJ, Zierer A, et al. Long-term outcomes in valve replacement surgery for infective endocarditis. *Ann Thorac Surg.* 2007;83(1):30-35.
21. Oswalt J. Management of aortic infective endocarditis by autograft valve replacement. *J Heart Valve Dis.* 1994;3(4):377-379.
22. Calkins H, Hindricks G, Cappato R, et al. 2017 HRS/EHRA/ECAS/APHRS/SOLAECE expert consensus statement on catheter and surgical ablation of atrial fibrillation. *Heart Rhythm.* 2017;14(10):e275-e444.
23. Badhwar V, Rankin JS, Damiano RJ Jr, et al. The society of thoracic surgeons 2017 clinical practice guidelines for the surgical treatment of atrial fibrillation. *Ann Thorac Surg.* 2017;103(1):329-341.
24. Khiabani AJ, MacGregor RM, Bakir NH, et al. The long-term outcomes and durability of the Cox-Maze IV procedure for atrial fibrillation. *J Thorac Cardiovasc Surg.* 2022;163(2):629-641.e7.
25. Goldfinger JZ, Adler ED. End-of-life options for patients with advanced heart failure. *Curr Heart Fail Rep.* 2010;7(3):140-147.
26. Colvin M, Smith JM, Hadley N, et al. OPTN/SRTR 2018 annual data report: Heart. *Am J Transplant.* 2020;20:340-426.
27. Mehra MR, Canter CE, Hannan MM, et al. The 2016 International Society for Heart Lung Transplantation listing criteria for heart transplantation: a 10-year update. *J Heart Lung Transplant.* 2016;35(1):1-23.
28. Taylor DO, Edwards LB, Boucek MM, et al. Registry of the International Society for Heart and Lung Transplantation: twenty-fourth official adult heart transplant report—2007. *J Heart Lung Transplant.* 2007;26(8):769-781.
29. Melby SJ, George JF, Picone DJ, et al. A time-related parametric risk factor analysis for postoperative atrial fibrillation after heart surgery. *J Thorac Cardiovasc Surg.* 2015;149(3):886-892.
30. Wilkinson DA, Koduri S, Anand SK, et al. Mechanical thrombectomy improves outcome for large vessel occlusion stroke after cardiac surgery. *J Stroke Cerebrovasc Dis.* 2021;30(8):105851.
31. Beaty CA, Arnaoutakis GJ, Grega MA, et al. The role of head computed tomography imaging in the evaluation of postoperative neurologic deficits in cardiac surgery patients. *Ann Thorac Surg.* 2013;95(2):548-554.

32. Tank PW, Gest TR. *Lippincott Williams & Wilkins Atlas of Anatomy*. Lippincott Williams and Wilkins; 2008.

33. Anderson RH, Cook AC. The structure and components of the atrial chambers. *Europace*. 2007;9(suppl 6):vi3-vi9.

34. Lawton JS, Gay WA Jr. *On-pump coronary artery bypass grafting. Complications in Cardiothoracic Surgery*. Wiley-Blackwell; 2009:333-350.

35. Bojar RM. *Manual of Perioperative Care in Adult Cardiac Surgery*. Wiley-Blackwell; 2021.

33 Endovascular Basics

Martha M. O. McGilvray and J. Westley Ohman

I. CHAPTER GOALS

A. Provide trainees with a ***Tool Box*** of general concepts, common terms, and commonly used tools in endovascular intervention.
B. Focus on safe arterial access.
C. *Not* intended to be a comprehensive compendium of endovascular techniques (see other Vascular chapters for more details).

II. BASIC CONCEPTS

A. **General steps in an endovascular case:**
   1. Preoperative imaging and planning (angiography, e.g., CT angiography)
   2. Vascular access
   3. Heparinize, monitor activated clotting time
   4. Establish platform for intervention (e.g., wire across the lesion/working sheath just proximal to the lesion)
   5. Decision-making for intervention, and intervention as indicated
   6. Safely remove all instrumentation, close, and ensure hemostasis (including heparin reversal, if used)

B. A powerful tool, but not a universal solution as endovascular repairs:
   1. Involve less access-related trauma and a lower wound-healing burden compared with open operations
   2. May not have the same longevity as open repairs
   3. Can entail significant risk (e.g., spinal cord ischemia after thoracic endovascular aortic repair)

III. ACCESS

A. *Tool Box* → Initial vascular access site depends on target location (**Table 33.1**).
   1. Retrograde femoral access is most common (i.e., accessing the common femoral artery [CFA] opposite to the direction of blood flow).

B. Generally percutaneous, with cut-down as a back-up option
   1. Percutaneous access generally associated with lower rates of complications and less postoperative pain[1]
   2. Closure considerations
      a. Previously, large-diameter devices (e.g., endovascular [abdominal aortic] aneurysm repair stent grafts) required open access to enable adequate closure of the accessed artery as holding pressure would be insufficient.

TABLE 33.1 Toolbox: Common Endovascular Access Sites by Target Lesion Location

Target Lesion Location	Vascular Access Site	Additional Details
Majority of lesions, including:	Retrograde CFA	
Contralateral iliac/femoral/popliteal/distal lower extremity (anterior tibial/posterior tibial/peroneal)	Retrograde CFA	Pathway to the lesion is "up and over" the aortic bifurcation
Abdominal/thoracic aorta	Retrograde CFA	Usually obtain bilateral retrograde CFA access for EVAR/TEVAR
Bilateral Subclavian/carotid/axillary/brachial	Retrograde CFA	e.g., TF-CAS
Ipsilateral femoral/popliteal/distal lower extremity	Antegrade CFA	Option when contraindication to traversing the aortic bifurcation from the contralateral side (e.g., heavy calcification, prior aortic endograft)
Ipsilateral distal site	Specific distal arteries, including:	Useful when femoral access is not possible (e.g., small caliber/tortuous) or when traversing the aorta is high risk (e.g., heavy calcification)
Ipsilateral brachial/radial/ulnar arteries	Antegrade brachial artery	
Ipsilateral distal lower extremity	Retrograde tibial artery	e.g., secondary access for complex tibial/pedal revascularization

CFA, common femoral artery; EVAR, endovascular (abdominal aortic) aneurysm repair; TEVAR, thoracic endovascular aortic repair; TF-CAS, transfemoral carotid artery stenting.

b. **Percutaneous closure devices** now more commonly available, allowing most endovascular procedures to be accomplished percutaneously
3. Access considerations
   a. Difficult/tortuous anatomy or a reoperative access site may increase the risk of percutaneous access failure or favor open access as initial attempt.
4. *Key concept:* ability to ensure **hemostasis**
   a. A key tenet of open vascular surgery—obtaining direct proximal and distal control—is not possible with percutaneous access.
   b. Before percutaneously accessing a vessel, you must ensure you can *effectively hold pressure* over the access site to prevent hemorrhage or pseudoaneurysm formation.
      i. Requires that the vessel to be accessed lies over a bony prominence to enable adequate compression
         a) The CFA should be accessed where it runs over the medial half of the femoral head (**Figure 33.1**).

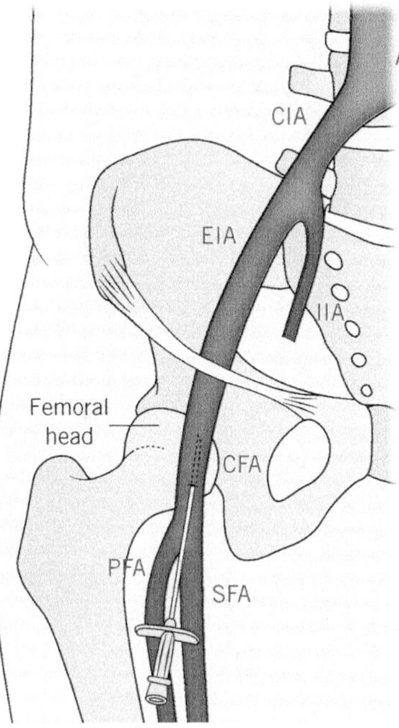

FIGURE 33.1 Access site visualization for percutaneous retrograde common femoral artery (CFA) access. CIA, common iliac artery; EIA, external iliac artery; IIA, internal iliac artery; PFA, profunda femoris artery; SFA, superficial femoral artery. *(Modified from Phillips DA, Kandarpa K. Complications of femoral artery access. In: Ouriel K, Katzen BT, Rosenfield K, eds. Complications in Endovascular Therapy. CRC Press; 2006:101-112. Figure 4. Copyright 2006, by Taylor & Francis Group, LLC. Reproduced by permission of Taylor & Francis Group.)*

5. **Surgical approach: Percutaneous retrograde CFA access**
   a. Use ultrasound to visualize the CFA, superficial femoral artery, and profunda femoris artery (aka deep femoral artery).
   b. Place the tip of a radio-opaque instrument (e.g., a mosquito/Kelly clamp) over the CFA at planned access site, just proximal to its bifurcation, and take a single-frame radiograph with the C-arm (*jargon: "spot"*) to confirm location over medial aspect of femoral head.
   c. Under ultrasound guidance, puncture the anterior wall of the CFA using a needle at a 45° angle to the skin and in-line with the course of the CFA.
   d. Inject contrast while acquiring fluoroscopic (continuous radiographic) images (*jargon: "fluoro"*) to confirm placement.
   e. Gently insert and advance a guidewire—do not force a wire against resistance; stop and reassess (e.g., via ultrasound), or if this fails or lose back-bleeding from the needle, remove the needle, hold pressure, and try again (*maintain control over the needle and guidewire at all times*).
   f. Use the wire to exchange the needle for a sheath (Seldinger's technique) with a flush port and a working hemostasis valve; every sheath exchange should be aspirated and flushed through the flush port to remove air and particulates (keep syringe plunger toward the ceiling to avoid injecting bubbles/air).
   g. Inject contrast through the flush port while acquiring fluoroscopic images to confirm no access-related issues.

IV. GETTING TO THE VASCULAR "LESION"

A. Goal: to place a wire from the access point to/across the target lesion
B. Multiple different wires/catheters/sheaths may be needed to advance through the various arteries between the access site and the target, depending on:
   1. Anatomy (e.g., angulation of arterial branch points, diameter of the target vessel)
   2. Burden and nature of disease (e.g., different wire stiffness/coating used to traverse a healthy artery vs. a heavily calcified one)
   3. Planned intervention, since various devices may require different diameter or rigidity of the wire
C. *Tool Box* → Commonly used wires (**Table 33.2**)
D. *Tool Box* → Catheters and sheaths (**Table 33.3**)
   1. Catheters are defined by their *outer* diameter, measured in French (Fr) units
      a. 1 Fr = 0.33 mm
   2. Sheaths are defined by their *inner* diameter
      a. A 5Fr sheath should accommodate a 5Fr catheter

V. TREATING THE LESION

A. *Tool Box* → General techniques (**Table 33.4**)

TABLE 33.2 Toolbox: Features and Descriptions of Commonly Used Wires

	Bentson	Glidewire	Amplatz	Lunderquist
Dimensions				
• Diameter in *inches*	0.035 (*jargon: "oh-three-five"*)	0.014, 0.018, 0.035	0.035, 0.038	0.035, 0.038
• Length in *centimeters*	145, 180	150, 180, 260	180, 260	260
Coating				
As coefficient of friction ↓: • ↑ ease of passing wire through difficult lesions/anatomy • ↓ tactile-feedback	PTFE: • Hydrophobic • Medium coefficient of friction	Polyurethane: • Hydrophilic • Low coefficient of friction	PTFE	PTFE
Stiffness/support				
Determined by core composition/thickness. As stiffness ↑: • ↑ support • risk endothelial injury	Medium	Low/medium	High	Extremely high

(*continued*)

TABLE 33.2 Toolbox: Features and Descriptions of Commonly Used Wires (*Continued*)

	Bentson	Glidewire	Amplatz	Lunderquist
Special features				
• Tip shape • Core tapering (tapered areas more flexible)	• Floppy tip (no core) • Long tapered segment	• Straight or angled tip • Short tapered segment	• Straight, J-tip, curved tip • Short/medium tapered segment	• Straight or curved tip • Floppy tip • Long tapered segment
Typical use	• General use • Beginning of case	• Cross lesions • Select branches	• Exchange (support over-the-wire devices)	• Exchange • Maximum support needed

PTFE, polytetrafluoroethylene.

TABLE 33.3 Toolbox: Catheters and Sheaths

Catheter Types			
	Flush	**Exchange**	**Selective**
Special features	• Multiple side holes for contrast ejection • Typically have a rounded/curved tip to *avoid* selective catheterization	• Straight tip	• Single hole in tip for wire egress • Various tip shapes designed for specific arterial anatomy
Typical use	• Angiography (aortography)	• Exchange guidewires	• Selective catheterization (directs a wire into a specific branch vessel)
Examples	• Pigtail • Tennis racquet • Universal/omni flush	• Straight	• Multipurpose • RIM
Sheath Types			
	Introducer	**Guide**	**Implant delivery system**
Special features	• Usually short (6-10 cm)	• Often consist of braided material to increase support • Often long	• Specialized sheaths designed for delivery of specific devices
Typical use	• Access	• Stabilize platform in a deep vessel/difficult area (e.g., aortic arch)	• Stent-graft delivery/deployment

RIM, Roche Inferior Mesenteric.

TABLE 33.4 Toolbox: General Endovascular Treatment Techniques

Technique	Mechanism & Important Concepts	Options & Key Definitions
Balloon angioplasty	• Blunt dehiscence of atherosclerotic lesions • Fracture and separation of media from intima • Stretching of media and adventitia	• "Plain old" balloon (no coating) • Drug coated • *Nominal pressure* = pressure at which balloon reaches its intended diameter • *Rated burst pressure* = pressure at which 99.9% of balloons will not rupture with 95% confidence

Stenting	• Improved longevity (reduced risk of restenosis) but at the cost of permanent device placement
	• Can be used to treat balloon-angioplasty failures (elastic recoil, dissection)
		• Bare-metal
		• Covered ("stent graft", "endograft")
		• Balloon-expandable
		  ◦ Appropriate sizing: diameter 1:1 with vessel; based on rigidity of stent
		• Self-expandable
		  ◦ Appropriate sizing: stent diameter > vessel diameter; based on elasticity of stent
		• Drug-eluting

Atherectomy	• Mechanically remove/reduce heavy plaque burden • Prepare a vessel for balloon angioplasty and/or stenting • Use where stents are contraindicated (e.g., popliteal fossa, where physiologic knee bending increases chance of stent fracture/occlusion)	• *Directional* = cutting blade shaves plaque • *Rotational/orbital* = small metallic drill coated with diamond chips abrades plaque • *Laser* = plaque ablated by direct application of kinetic and thermal energy

Key References

Citation	Summary
Schneider P. *Endovascular Skills: Guidewire and Catheter Skills for Endovascular Surgery*. CRC Press; 2019.	• How-to guide to endovascular therapy aimed at trainees
Stone PA, AbuRahma AF, Campbell JE, ed. *Vascular/Endovascular Surgery Combat Manual*. W. L. Gore & Associates, Inc; 2013.	• Manual with brief high-yield entries on a broad spectrum of vascular topics
Sidawy AP, Perler BA. *Rutherford's Vascular Surgery and Endovascular Therapy, 2-Volume Set*. Elsevier Health Sciences; 2022.	• The reference for vascular surgery
Valentine RJ, Wind GG. *Anatomic Exposures in Vascular Surgery*. 4th ed. LWW; 2020.	• Atlas of common anatomic surgical exposures
Jimenez JC, Wilson SE, eds. *50 Landmark Papers Every Vascular and Endovascular Surgeon Should Know*. 1st ed. CRC Press; 2020.	• Good reference for landmark trials grouped by subject matter

CHAPTER 33: ENDOVASCULAR BASICS

Review Questions

1. When obtaining percutaneous femoral arterial access, where should you access the common femoral artery (CFA)?
2. What criteria defines the size of a catheter? Of a sheath?
3. What is the conversion from French sizes to millimeters?
4. What is the main risk of using a wire with high stiffness/support?
5. What are the three histological effects of balloon angioplasty treatment of atherosclerotic arterial lesions?
6. What are three (lesion-specific) indications for use of atherectomy during endovascular treatment of atherosclerotic arterial lesions?

REFERENCES

1. Uhlmann ME, Walter C, Taher F, Plimon M, Falkensammer J, Assadian A. Successful percutaneous access for endovascular aneurysm repair is significantly cheaper than femoral cutdown in a prospective randomized trial. *J Vasc Surg*. 2018;68(2):384-391.
2. Schneider P. *Endovascular Skills: Guidewire and Catheter Skills for Endovascular Surgery*. CRC Press; 2019.

3. Stone PA, AbuRahma AF, Campbell JE, eds. *Vascular/Endovascular Surgery Combat Manual.* W. L. Gore & Associates, Inc.; 2013.

4. Sidawy AP, Perler BA. *Rutherford's Vascular Surgery and Endovascular Therapy, 2-Volume Set.* Elsevier Health Sciences; 2022.

5. Valentine RJ, Wind GG. *Anatomic Exposures in Vascular Surgery*. ed. LWW; 2020.

6. Jimenez JC, Wilson SE, eds. *50 Landmark Papers Every Vascular and Endovascular Surgeon Should Know*. 1st ed. CRC Press; 2020.

7. Ouriel K, Katzen BT, Rosenfield K, eds. *Complications in Endovascular Therapy*. CRC Press; 2006.

34 Cerebrovascular Disease

Momodou L. Jammeh and Mohamed A. Zayed

I. ANATOMY

A. Carotid artery
   1. Branches of the aortic arch, from right to left: **Brachiocephalic trunk** also known as **innominate artery**, left common carotid artery (CCA), left subclavian artery (**Figure 34.1**)
      a. The right subclavian and right CCA branch off the innominate.
      b. Arch branch anatomy varies, but the above configuration is the most common (~65%).
   2. Both CCAs branch into an external carotid artery (ECA) and an internal carotid artery (ICA) just below the angle of the mandible.
      a. Important ECA branches: Superior thyroid, ascending pharyngeal, lingual, occipital
      b. The ICA has no branches in the neck.

B. Juxtacarotid structures
   1. Veins
      a. The **internal jugular** vein lies lateral to the CCA and ICA.
         i. One or more branches (common facial vein) travel medially directly anterior to the carotid, often requiring ligation during open carotid artery procedures (**Figure 34.2**).
   2. Nerves (**Figure 34.3**)
      a. **Superior laryngeal nerve**
         i. Runs along the ascending pharyngeal artery
         ii. Innervates the cricothyroid muscle of the larynx
         iii. Injury can lead to voice hoarseness and loss of higher pitches.
         iv. See Chapter 30 for information about the **recurrent laryngeal nerve (RLN)**.
      b. **Hypoglossal nerve**
         i. Runs just anterior to the ECA, ICA, and lingual artery; runs just posterior to the occipital artery
            a) Joined by the superior root of the **ansa cervicalis**, which is often cut in open approach to the carotid (**Figure 34.2**)
         ii. Innervates the muscles of the tongue
         iii. Injury can lead to unilateral tongue paralysis.
      c. **Vagus nerve**
         i. Runs posterolateral to the CCA and ICA
      d. **Carotid sinus/bulb:** Baroreceptor (sensitive to changes in blood pressure) located at the carotid bifurcation/most inferior portion of the ICA, seen as a dilation/widening of the arteries at this point.

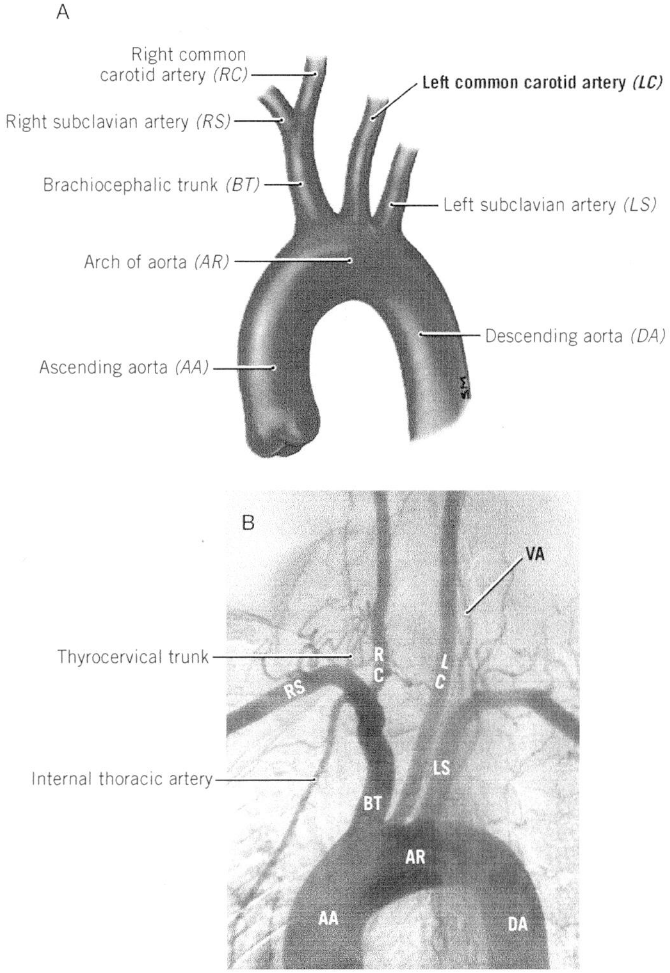

FIGURE 34.1 Aortic arch anatomy. A, Branches of the aortic arch; B, aortic angiogram, left anterior oblique view. VA, left vertebral artery. *(Modified with permission from Agur AMR, Dalley AF II, eds. Thorax. In: Grant's Atlas of Anatomy. 15th ed. Wolters Kluwer; 2021:193-289. Figures 3.64A-B.)*

e. **Carotid body:** A small cluster of chemoreceptors (sensitive to low oxygen/high carbon dioxide levels in the blood) located in the adventitia of the carotid bifurcation
f. Both the carotid sinus and body are innervated by the carotid sinus nerve, a branch of the glossopharyngeal nerve.

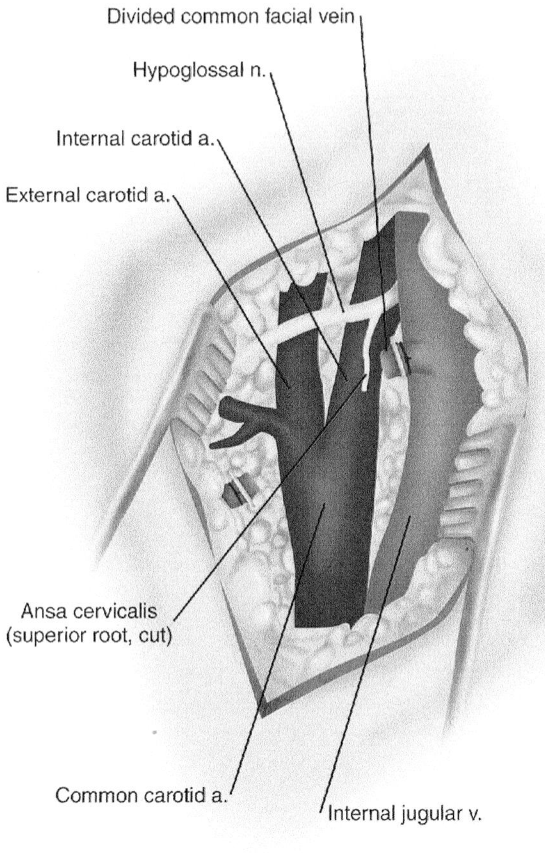

FIGURE 34.2 Traditional (left) carotid exposure. *(Reprinted from AbuRahma AF, AbuRahma Z. Cerebrovascular exposure. In: Sidawy AP, Perler BA, eds. Rutherford's Vascular Surgery and Endovascular Therapy. 10th ed. Elsevier; 2023:721-733. Figure 57.3. Copyright 2023, Elsevier. With permission.)*

II. STROKE AND EXTRACRANIAL CAROTID ARTERY ATHEROSCLEROSIS

A. Epidemiology[1]

1. Stroke is the most common cause of disability and the fifth leading cause of death in the US.
   a. Each year, over 795,000 people suffer from a stroke.
   b. Annual associated cost is approximately $50 billion in healthcare-related expenses and lost productivity.

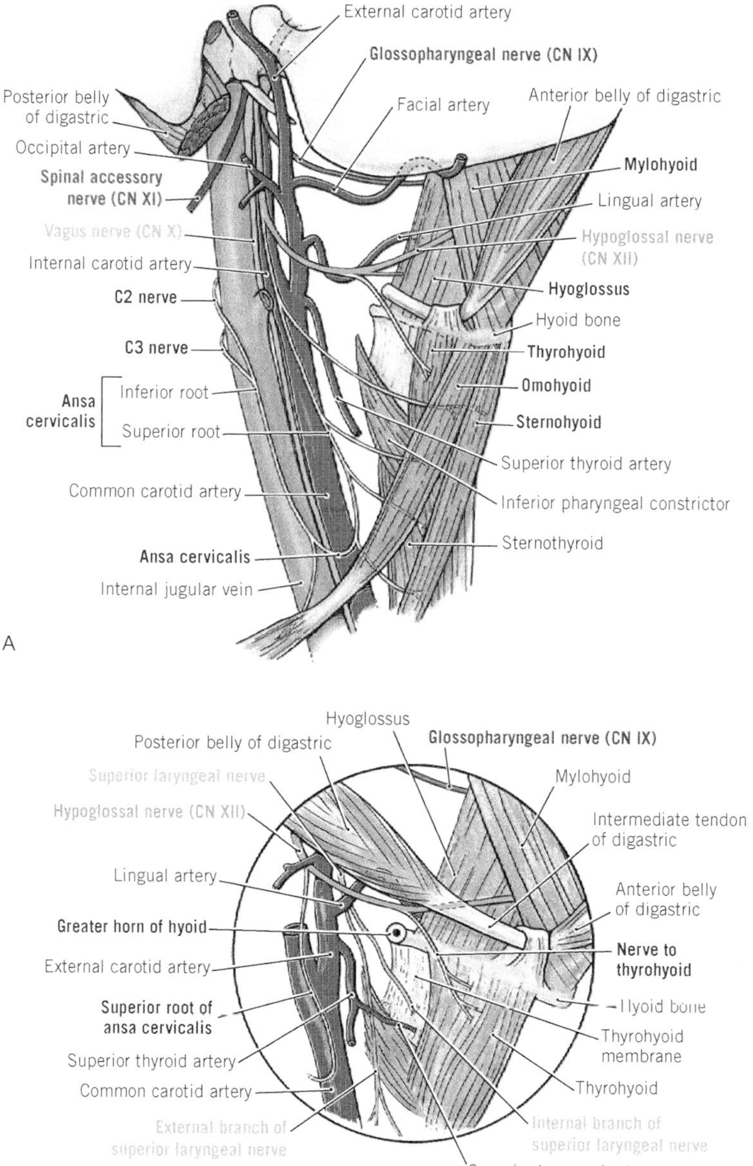

FIGURE 34.3 Relationship of nerves and vessels in the carotid triangle. *(Reprinted with permission from Agur AMR, Dalley AF II, eds. Neck. In: Grant's Atlas of Anatomy. 15th ed. Wolters Kluwer; 2021:725-786. Figure 8.16A-B.)*

B. Pathophysiology

1. Multiple stroke etiologies[1]
   a. Hemorrhagic (~13%): Intracranial hemorrhage, subarachnoid hemorrhage
   b. Ischemic (~87%): Cardioembolic (e.g., embolism from the heart), extracranial carotid artery stenosis, intracranial/small artery occlusion[2]
      i. Approximately 20% of ischemic strokes are result of arterial embolization from an extracranial carotid artery.
      ii. Intracranial carotid artery disease is typically managed by Neurosurgery and/or Interventional Radiology and therefore will not be covered in this chapter.
2. Extracranial carotid artery stenosis is caused by atherosclerotic plaque.
   a. Risk factors: Increasing age, cigarette smoking, hypertension, hyperlipidemia, peripheral vascular disease, diabetes
3. Carotid plaque can cause cerebral ischemia either by thromboembolization or by hypoperfusion through narrowing of the lumen limiting flow.
   a. Risk of cerebral ischemia correlates with degree of stenosis (see section on management) and presence of symptoms.
   b. Risk of stroke with asymptomatic carotid artery stenosis is ≤1%.
   c. In symptomatic patients, there is a 20% to 30% risk of recurrent stroke or transient ischemic attack (TIA) within 1 year of symptom onset/ischemic event.

C. Presentation

1. Asymptomatic carotid artery stenosis: Often identified through auscultation of a carotid bruit on examination or as an incidental finding on head/neck imaging.
2. Symptomatic carotid artery stenosis: Hemispheric ischemic events within the last 6 months that may result in expressive or receptive aphasia, contralateral sensory and/or motor deficits, or ipsilateral visual disturbances.
   a. **TIAs:** Temporary neurologic deficits that may last from several seconds to hours but no longer than 24 hours
      i. Crescendo TIAs occur in rapid succession with increased frequency and carry high risk for progression to stroke.
   b. **Stroke:** Neurological deficits that persist beyond 24 hours
      i. "Stroke in evolution": Fluctuating or gradually worsening deficits over a period of hours or days without a return to baseline
   c. **Amaurosis fugax:** Temporary ipsilateral monocular blindness resulting from embolization to the ophthalmic artery.
      i. Funduscopic examination may reveal **Hollenhorst plaques** (yellow plaques/crystals, generally seen at retinal artery bifurcations). However, this finding alone does not necessarily indicate arterial embolization from carotid disease.
   d. Global ischemic events such as vertigo, ataxia, or syncope are rarely associated with carotid disease and more likely a consequence of vertebrobasilar insufficiency or hypoperfusion from heart disease.
   e. Nonspecific symptoms are common.

D. Diagnosis

1. A patient suspected of having carotid artery disease requires a careful history and physical examination before obtaining any diagnostic studies.
   a. History: Assessment of symptoms should include timing of onset, duration, and extent of recovery. History of neck dissection or radiation should be considered.
   b. Physical examination: Should include blood pressure, heart rhythm, and a complete neurological examination and neck auscultation for bruits.
2. Imaging
   a. Any concern for acute neurological changes/stroke should prompt noncontrast brain CT to rule out cerebral hemorrhage.
   b. **Carotid duplex ultrasonography:** Utilizes B-mode imaging with color-flow Doppler measurements to quantify the degree of stenosis and extent of disease.
   c. **CT angiography** assesses
      i. Burden of disease: Extent of stenosis in the carotid artery system, severity of calcification
      ii. Impactful anatomic features like eccentric plaque, tandem lesions, intracranial arterial disease
   d. **Magnetic resonance angiography:** More sensitive for acute stroke but often overestimates the degree of stenosis
   e. **Catheter-based angiography**
      i. Remains the "gold standard" for evaluating the extra- and intracranial arterial system, but only provides luminagrams (only reliably shows the lumen of a vessel as opposed to the vessel itself) and limited information on the surrounding anatomy
      ii. Invasive with potential risks including contrast nephropathy or allergy, arterial access site complications, and procedure-related strokes in <1% patients
   f. Grading of carotid artery stenosis: Methodologies vary, but generally grouped into four categories: Mild (<50%), moderate (50%-69%), severe (70%-99%), and occluded (100%).

E. Nonoperative management

1. Indicated for
   a. Patients with asymptomatic <50% carotid artery stenosis and almost all patients with asymptomatic 50% to 70% stenosis
   b. Symptomatic patients with severe disability after stroke without a reasonable expectation of recovery
2. Best medical therapy
   a. Summarized in **Table 34.1**. Focused on risk modification, comorbidity optimization, and smoking cessation
   b. Recommended in asymptomatic patients with moderate carotid artery stenosis

F. Operative management

1. Recommended for[3]
   a. Asymptomatic patients with >70% carotid artery stenosis with a life expectancy of at least 3 to 5 years

TABLE 34.1 Summary of Effect of Best Medical Therapy for Prevention of Stroke and Cardiovascular Events

Treatment	Target	Evidence
Antiplatelet therapy	**1.** Either single or dual antiplatelet therapy acceptable **2.** Aspirin 81 mg/d is recommended **3.** Plavix 75 mg equivalent to aspirin **4.** Ticlopidine 250 mg twice daily similar to aspirin in effectiveness	Reduces both stroke risk and overall cardiovascular morbidity
Antihypertensive therapy	Variable depending on age and comorbidities	Reduces stroke recurrence—wait at least 24 hours after acute stroke to implement regimen; No definitive benefit of one class of antihypertensive agents over another
Diabetes mellitus	Target Hgb A1C < 7	Reduce overall stroke rate No definitive benefit of tight control (i.e., Hgb A1C ≤ 6)
Smoking cessation	Complete abstinence	Reduces risk of stroke and major adverse cardiovascular events
Statin therapy	**1.** Reduce LDL by 50% **2.** Target LDL < 70 mg/dL **3.** Atorvastatin 80 mg, Rosuvastatin 20 mg most common	Reduces risk of stroke and major adverse cardiovascular events, particularly among patients with a history of cardiovascular disease

Hgb, hemoglobin; LDL, low-density lipoprotein.

b. Symptomatic patients with >50% carotid artery stenosis
   i. In the setting of stroke, intervention should be performed after 48 hours but within 2 weeks of the initial event.

c. Surgery is rare for patients with totally occlusive disease but can be considered for

- **i.** Thrombosis after recent endarterectomy
- **ii.** Recent carotid obstruction with fluctuating symptoms
- **iii.** There is no role for revascularization in asymptomatic patients with a chronic total ICA occlusion.

2. Carotid endarterectomy (CEA)

- **a.** Considered the gold standard for carotid revascularization with proven outcomes as summarized in the trials section below
- **b.** To ensure potential benefit outweighs potential risk, CEA should be performed by surgeons who have a perioperative rate of stroke/death of <3% for asymptomatic patients and <6% symptomatic patients.[4,5]
- **c.** Anesthesia can be general or regional. Prophylactic antibiotics (e.g., cefazolin) should be given, and arterial line access should be obtained for close hemodynamic monitoring.
  - **i.** Mean arterial pressure of 80 to 100 or systolic pressures >150 mm Hg should be maintained intraoperatively.
- **d. Surgical approach: CEA**
  - **i.** Position the patient with their head up and turned to the contralateral side. A shoulder roll can be placed to help flex and extend the ipsilateral neck.
  - **ii.** Make an incision centered over the carotid bifurcation along the anterior border of the sternocleidomastoid muscle (SCM) or transversely in the mid-neck skin crease; divide the subcutaneous tissues, platysma muscle, and deep cervical fascia; reflect the SCM laterally.
  - **iii.** Ligate and divide the facial vein. Expose and encircle the proximal CCA, distal ICA, ECA, and superior thyroid artery with vessel loops. Visualize and protect the vagus and hypoglossal nerves. Avoid manipulation of the carotid bulb.
  - **iv.** Administer systemic anticoagulation (e.g., heparin 80-100 U/kg for activated clotting time >250) then clamp the arteries in the following order: ICA, CCA, ECA.
  - **v.** Make a longitudinal arteriotomy. Perform the endarterectomy, tack down intimal flaps in the proximal ICA with interrupted fine Prolene sutures. Flush with heparinized saline.
  - **vi.** Close the arteriotomy with a fashioned patch of bovine pericardium, Dacron, or autogenous vein, using fine Prolene sutures. Prior to completion of the patch repair, flush the ICA retrograde, then flush the CCA and ECA antegrade.
  - **vii.** Remove clamps in the following order: CCA, ECA, after a few seconds ICA and confirm carotid artery flow with Doppler.
  - **viii.** Reverse anticoagulation (0.5-1 mg Protamine sulfate per 100 units heparin). Reapproximate the platysma and close in layers.
- **e.** Additional operative details
  - **i.** The omohyoid muscle can be divided if needed for additional proximal exposure of the CCA.
  - **ii.** A small volume of 1% lidocaine can be infiltrated into the adventitia of the carotid bulb to help mitigate intraoperative reflex bradycardia.
  - **iii.** Endarterectomy is performed by lifting the plaque off the vessel wall in the submedial plane. The plaque is transected in the

distal CCA and everted toward the ECA. The remainder of the plaque is then removed from the proximal ICA lumen.

iv. **Shunting** may be performed after the arteriotomy is made to prevent cerebral arterial malperfusion during clamping.

a) For surgeons who do not shunt routinely, a stump pressure <40 mm Hg, intraoperative cerebral oximetry, or somatosensory evoked potentials and transcranial Doppler ultrasonography may be used for cerebral monitoring and to facilitate the decision of whether or not to shunt.

f. Complications

i. Perioperative stroke risk of <3% for asymptomatic patients, and <6% for symptomatic patients, is expected.

ii. Cranial nerve injury occurs in 5% of patients with <1% persisting at postoperative follow-up.

iii. **Cerebral hyperperfusion syndrome**

a) Presents with severe ipsilateral headache

b) Can result in cerebral hemorrhage in severe cases

c) Strict blood pressure control is the mainstay for prevention and treatment.

d) There is a lack of definitive data to guide pressure thresholds, but generally it is reasonable to target a systolic blood pressure of <160 mm Hg or within 20% of preoperative pressure.[6]

iv. Myocardial infarction is the most common cause of death in the postoperative period.

3. **Transfemoral carotid artery stenting (TF-CAS)**

a. An alternative option for patients considered "high risk" for CEA due to severe cardiac disease, prior radiation or neck dissection, contralateral permanent cranial nerve injury, or a surgically inaccessible lesion (above the level of the C2 vertebra).

b. Performed under local anesthesia with slight sedation.

c. **Surgical approach: TF-CAS**

i. Obtain retrograde common femoral artery access under ultrasound guidance with a micropuncture needle and sheath.

ii. Using appropriate wires and catheters, traverse the arterial system from the femoral artery and selectively catheterize the CCA.

iii. Perform an arteriogram with the fluoroscopy C-arm positioned in an obliquity that best visualizes the carotid bifurcation, the segment of high-grade stenosis, and the distal ICA.

iv. Advance the working sheath into the CCA, a few centimeters below the bifurcation. Administer a full dose of heparin (see CEA).

v. Gently cross the lesion with a fine wire (0.014"). Deploy a distal embolic protection device over the wire in the distal ICA.

vi. Pretreat the lesion with a 2- to 3-mm angioplasty balloon (particularly for severely stenosed segments); stent across the lesion with an appropriately sized bare-metal stent; dilate the stented segment with a 5-mm angioplasty balloon

vii. Carefully remove the embolic protection device through a sheath and perform a completion arteriogram, then close the femoral access site with either a percutaneous closure device or by holding direct pressure

d. Dual antiplatelet therapy is administered perioperatively and continued for at least 6 weeks postoperatively.
   i. Dual therapy with aspirin and clopidogrel remains the mainstay of therapy.
e. Complications
   i. Embolic stroke can occur in ~4% of patients and can be difficult to manage if the embolus comprises atheroma or chronic thrombus.[7]
   ii. Hemodynamic instability may occur with balloon angioplasty of the carotid bifurcation.
   iii. Reflex bradycardia can be prevented or treated with atropine or glycopyrrolate.
   iv. Femoral access-related complications such as hematoma or pseudoaneurysm are possible but rare.
   v. Carotid injury can be prevented by careful positioning and removal of the distal embolic protection device.

4. **Transcarotid artery revascularization (TCAR)**
   a. A hybrid technique that involves carotid stenting via open proximal CCA exposure and cannulation
   b. Like TF-CAS, indicated in patients considered high-risk for CEA
   c. **Carotid flow reversal** is used for distal embolic protection.
      i. This is accomplished via an external shunt that pulls blood retrograde from the CCA, filters it, and returns it (antegrade) to the femoral vein (**Figure 34.4**).
      ii. This avoids the need for traversing the descending aorta and the arch, which may have significant atherosclerotic disease.
         a) Also avoids the need to pass a distal embolic protection device through the area of stenosis
   d. Performed under general or regional/local anesthesia

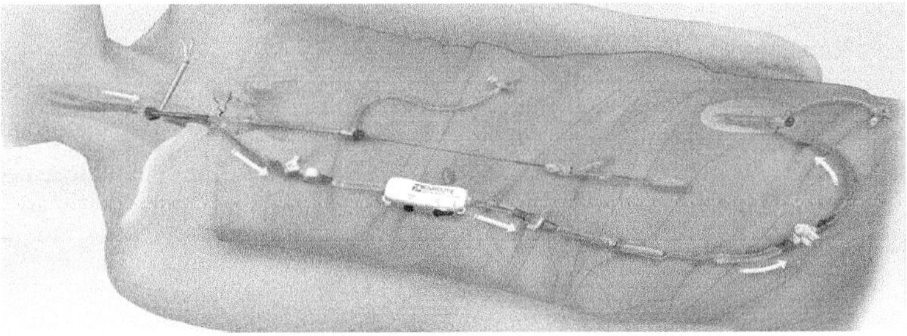

FIGURE 34.4 Flow reversal for distal embolic protection used in transcarotid artery revascularization. *(Reprinted from Deery SE, Hicks CW. Carotid artery stenting. In: Sidawy AP, Perler BA, eds. Rutherford's Vascular Surgery and Endovascular Therapy. 10th ed. Elsevier; 2023:1241-1257. Figure 94.8A. Copyright 2023, Elsevier. With permission.)*

e. **Surgical approach: TCAR**
   i. Make a 2- to 3-cm incision one fingerbreadth above the clavicle.
   ii. Expose the CCA between the two heads of the SCM at the base of the neck. Protect the RLN. Place a Rumel tourniquet as proximally as possible.
   iii. Place a cannulation stitch in the CCA (fine Prolene suture), and obtain antegrade CCA access using a specialized micropuncture kit and sheath. Perform an arteriogram with the fluoroscopy C-arm positioned in an obliquity that best visualizes the carotid bifurcation, the segment of high-grade stenosis, and the distal ICA.
   iv. Access the contralateral femoral vein under ultrasound guidance using a micropuncture needle and sheath. Attach and prime the flow reversal system.
   v. Administer systemic anticoagulation (see CEA) then clamp the CCA and initiate flow reversal. Systolic blood pressure should be maintained at 140 to 160 mm Hg to optimize flow reversal.
   vi. Gently cross the lesion with a fine wire (0.014″). Stent across the lesion with an appropriately sized bare-metal stent.
   vii. Stop flow reversal. Perform a completion arteriogram. Remove the external flow reversal shunt device. Close the CCA with the previously placed cannulation stitch, and close the skin and soft tissue in layers.
   viii. Remove all instrumentation from the femoral access site, and obtain hemostasis via holding direct pressure.

f. Dual antiplatelet therapy must be maintained throughout the perioperative period similar to TF-CAS.

g. Complications
   i. Perioperative stroke risk is ~1%[8]
      a) Distal embolization is less frequent than TF-CAS.
   ii. Access site complications (bleeding, pseudoaneurysm, nerve injury)

Key References

Citation	Summary
Asymptomatic Carotid Atherosclerosis Study (ACAS) Walker MD, Marler JR, Goldstein M, et al. Endarterectomy for asymptomatic carotid artery stenosis. *JAMA*. 1995;273(18):1421-1428.	• Randomized prospective multicenter trial evaluating daily aspirin vs. CEA in 1,662 patients with >60% carotid artery stenosis. • The 5-y aggregate risk of ipsilateral stroke, any perioperative stroke, or death was significantly lower in the CEA group at 5.1% vs. 11.0% in the medical therapy group (*P* < .004), with an aggregate 53% risk reduction.

Citation	Summary
North American Symptomatic Carotid Endarterectomy Trial (NASCET) Barnett HJM, Taylor DW, Eliasziw M, et al. Benefit of carotid endarterectomy in patients with symptomatic moderate or severe stenosis. *N Engl J Med.* 1998;339(20):1415-1425. North American Symptomatic Carotid Endarterectomy Trial Collaborators; Barnett HJM, Taylor DW, et al. Beneficial effect of carotid endarterectomy in symptomatic patients with high-grade carotid stenosis. *N Engl J Med.* 1991;325(7):445-453.	• A multicenter, parallel group, randomized controlled trial in patients with symptomatic mild (<50%), moderate (50%-69%), and severe (70%-99%) carotid artery stenosis comparing CEA to medical management. • Randomization was halted in the severe stenosis group due to early significant benefit from CEA. All patients in this group originally randomized to medical management were recommended to undergo CEA. • In patients with severe stenosis, CEA resulted in a 65% relative risk reduction for any ipsilateral stroke and 81% relative risk reduction in major/fatal ipsilateral stroke at 2 y. • In the moderate stenosis group, CEA resulted in a 29% relative risk reduction for ipsilateral stroke within 5 y. • No benefit from CEA was seen in the mild stenosis group.
Carotid Revascularization Endarterectomy vs. Stenting Trial (CREST) Brott TG, Hobson RW II, Howard G, et al. Stenting versus endarterectomy for treatment of carotid-artery stenosis. *N Engl J Med.* 2010;363(1):11-23.	• A multicenter, parallel group, randomized, superiority trial of TF-CAS vs. CEA in 2,502 patients with asymptomatic and symptomatic carotid stenosis. • There was no significant difference between stenting and CEA in rate of the composite primary outcome—stroke, myocardial infarction (MI), or death—at 4 y • Four-year rate of stroke or death was significantly higher in the stenting group. • Periprocedural rate of stroke was higher in the stent group; periprocedural rate of MI was higher in the CEA group.
Reverse Flow Used During Carotid Artery Stenting Procedure (ROADSTER) trial Kwolek CJ, Jaff MR, Leal JI, et al. Results of the ROADSTER multicenter trial of transcarotid stenting with dynamic flow reversal. *J Vasc Surg.* 2015;62(5):1227-1234.	• A 30-d safety and efficacy prospective, single-arm, multicenter trial of TCAR with the ENROUTE® flow-reversal system in 208 patients considered high-risk for CEA with asymptomatic stenosis ≥70% or symptomatic stenosis ≥50% (25% of the trial population had symptomatic disease). • Reported a periprocedural stroke rate of 1.4% and composite stroke, death, and MI risk of 3.5%.

CHAPTER 34: CEREBROVASCULAR DISEASE

Review Questions

1. What constitutes best medical management in asymptomatic carotid atherosclerotic disease?
2. What is the recommended timing for carotid intervention in symptomatic patients with carotid atherosclerosis?
3. When is operative intervention recommended in asymptomatic carotid atherosclerotic disease?
4. What are two major nerves that one must be careful to protect during carotid endarterectomy?
5. What is one rare but major complication of carotid endarterectomy associated with restoration of normal flow, and what is its main presenting symptom?
6. What are two common approaches for carotid artery stenting?
7. What are four modalities for evaluating cerebral perfusion in selective shunting during carotid endarterectomy?
8. What are the target hemoglobin A1C and low-density lipoprotein (LDL) levels for optimal medical management of carotid atherosclerosis?

REFERENCES

1. Tsao CW, Aday AW, Almarzooq ZI, et al. Heart disease and stroke statistics—2022 update: a report from the American Heart Association. *Circulation*. 2022;145(8):e153-e639.
2. Adams HP Jr, Bendixen BH, Kappelle LJ, et al. Classification of subtype of acute ischemic stroke. Definitions for use in a multicenter clinical trial. TOAST. Trial of Org 10172 in Acute Stroke Treatment. *Stroke*. 1993;24(1):35-41.
3. AbuRahma AF, Avgerinos ED, Chang RW, et al. Society for Vascular Surgery clinical practice guidelines for management of extracranial cerebrovascular disease. *J Vasc Surg*. 2022;75(1S):4S-22S.
4. Kernan WN, Ovbiagele B, Black HR, et al. Guidelines for the prevention of stroke in patients with stroke and transient ischemic attack: a guideline for healthcare professionals from the American Heart Association/American Stroke Association. *Stroke*. 2014;45(7):2160-2236.
5. Meschia JF, Bushnell C, Boden-Albala B, et al. Guidelines for the primary prevention of stroke: a statement for healthcare professionals from the American Heart Association/American Stroke Association. *Stroke*. 2014;45(12):3754-3832.
6. Stoneham MD, Thompson JP. Arterial pressure management and carotid endarterectomy. *Br J Anaesth*. 2009;102(4):442-452.
7. Brott TG, Hobson RW II, Howard G, et al. Stenting versus endarterectomy for treatment of carotid-artery stenosis. *N Engl J Med*. 2010;363(1):11-23.
8. Kwolek CJ, Jaff MR, Leal JI, et al. Results of the ROADSTER multicenter trial of transcarotid stenting with dynamic flow reversal. *J Vasc Surg*. 2015;62(5):1227-1234.
9. Walker MD, Marler JR, Goldstein M, et al. Endarterectomy for asymptomatic carotid artery stenosis. *JAMA*. 1995;273(18):1421-1428.
10. Barnett HJM, Taylor DW, Eliasziw M, et al. Benefit of carotid endarterectomy in patients with symptomatic moderate or severe stenosis. *N Engl J Med*. 1998;339(20):1415-1425.

11. North American Symptomatic Carotid Endarterectomy Trial Collaborators; Barnett HJM, Taylor DW, Haynes RB, et al. Beneficial effect of carotid endarterectomy in symptomatic patients with high-grade carotid stenosis. *N Engl J Med.* 1991;325(7):445-453.

12. Agur AMR, Dalley AF II. *Grant's Atlas of Anatomy*. Wolters Kluwer; 2021.

13. Sidawy AP, Perler BA. *Rutherford's Vascular Surgery and Endovascular Therapy, 2-Volume Set.* Elsevier Health Sciences; 2022.

35 Thoracoabdominal Vascular Disease

Martha M. O. McGilvray, J. Westley Ohman, and
Luis A. Sanchez

I. ANATOMY AND HISTOLOGY

A. Aorta
1. Divided into three segments: Ascending, arch, descending
2. Descending divided into two segments: Thoracic and abdominal
3. Ascending aorta: Left ventricular outflow tract → aortic valve → aortic root → ascending aorta → aortic arch

B. Aortic arch and thoracic aorta (**Figure 35.1**)
1. **Aortic arch**
   a. Branches (in order): Right brachiocephalic (a.k.a. innominate), left common carotid artery (LCCA), left subclavian artery
      i. Right brachiocephalic branches into right subclavian and right common carotid arteries.
   b. Nearby structures
      i. **Left brachiocephalic vein**
         a) Drains into the superior vena cava (SVC)
         b) Lays diagonally across aortic arch branches
            1) Needs to be identified and protected/ligated during median sternotomy approach to the aortic arch
      ii. **Left vagus nerve** (**Figure 35.2**)
         a) Runs in the neck and into the chest between the LCCA and the left internal jugular vein
         b) Runs across the anterior aspect of the arch and branches into the left recurrent laryngeal nerve (LRLN) at its inferior aspect
         c) LRLN wraps around the inferior aspect of the arch from lateral to medial, then ascends cranially in the tracheoesophageal groove.
2. **Descending thoracic aorta**
   a. Major branches: Bronchial, esophageal, mediastinal, pericardial, superior phrenic, posterior intercostal arteries
      i. Posterior intercostal arteries (**Figure 35.2**)
         a) Paired arteries arising from the posterior thoracic aorta at the level of each thoracic vertebra
         b) Contribute to the anterior spinal circulation
   b. Crosses the diaphragm into the abdomen via the aortic hiatus at the level of the T12 vertebra

C. Abdominal aorta (**Figure 35.3**)
1. Abdominal branches, in order from superior to inferior
   a. **Inferior phrenic arteries** (paired)
   b. **Celiac trunk**

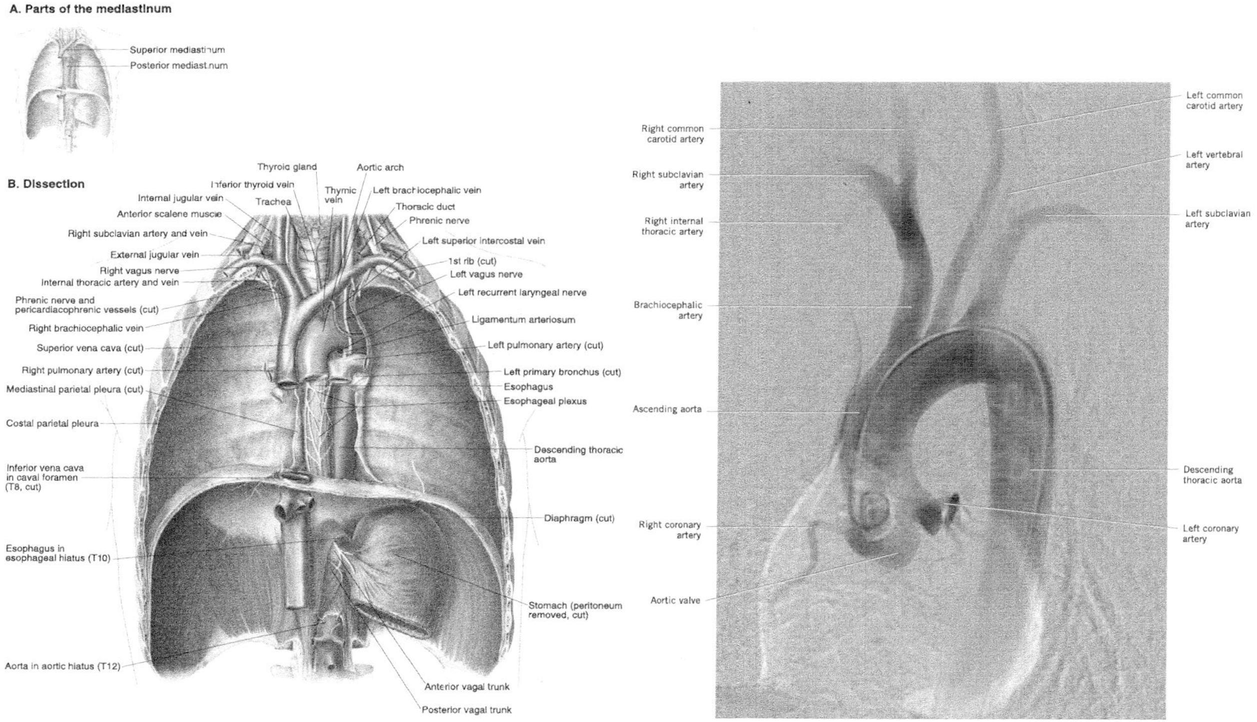

FIGURE 35.1 Thoracic aorta, anatomic diagram (left) and aortogram (right). *(Left panel reprinted with permission from Gest TR, ed. The thorax. In: Lippincott® Atlas of Anatomy. 2nd ed. Wolters Kluwer; 2020:176-229. Plate 4-38. Right panel reprinted with permission from Uflacker A, Guimaraes M, eds. Thoracic aorta and arteries of the trunk. In: Uflacker's Atlas of Vascular Anatomy: An Angiographic Approach. 3rd ed. Wolters Kluwer; 2021:176-246. Figure 7.2A.)*

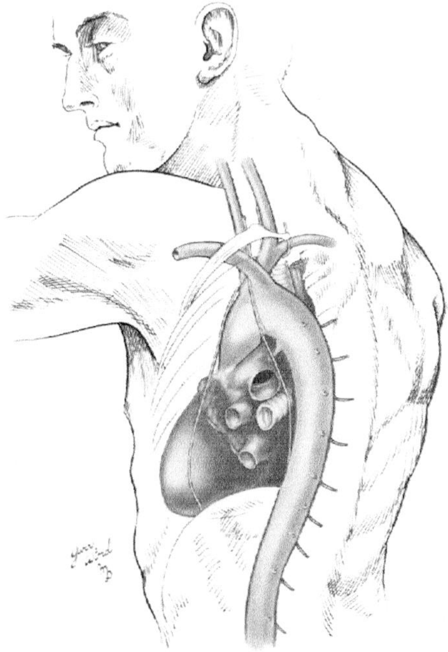

FIGURE 35.2 Left lateral view of the thoracic aorta. *(Reprinted with permission from Valentine RJ, Wind GG, eds. Thoracic aorta. In: Anatomic Exposures in Vascular Surgery. 4th ed. Wolters Kluwer; 2021:65-98. Figure 3-14.)*

i. Take off is very close to the **aortic hiatus**, such that the celiac can be impinged upon by the **median arcuate ligament** (which runs just anterior to the aorta and unites the left and right diaphragmatic crura at the hiatus; rare)

ii. Multiple branch variations, but most typical has left gastric artery as the first branch, then bifurcates into the common hepatic (to the right) and the splenic (to the left) arteries

c. **Superior mesenteric artery (SMA)**

d. **Renal arteries** (paired)

e. **Gonadal arteries** (paired; a.k.a. ovarian/testicular arteries)

f. **Inferior mesenteric artery (IMA)**

2. Bifurcates into the left and right **common iliac arteries** (CIAs)
   a. CIA bifurcates into internal iliac artery (IIA; a.k.a. hypogastric artery) and external iliac artery (EIA).
   b. Right CIA lies anterolateral to the left common iliac vein (CIV) and can cause left CIV compression (May–Thurner physiology; rare).

D. Histology (**Figure 35.4**)

1. Layers of the arterial wall
   a. **Intima:** Lined by endothelium

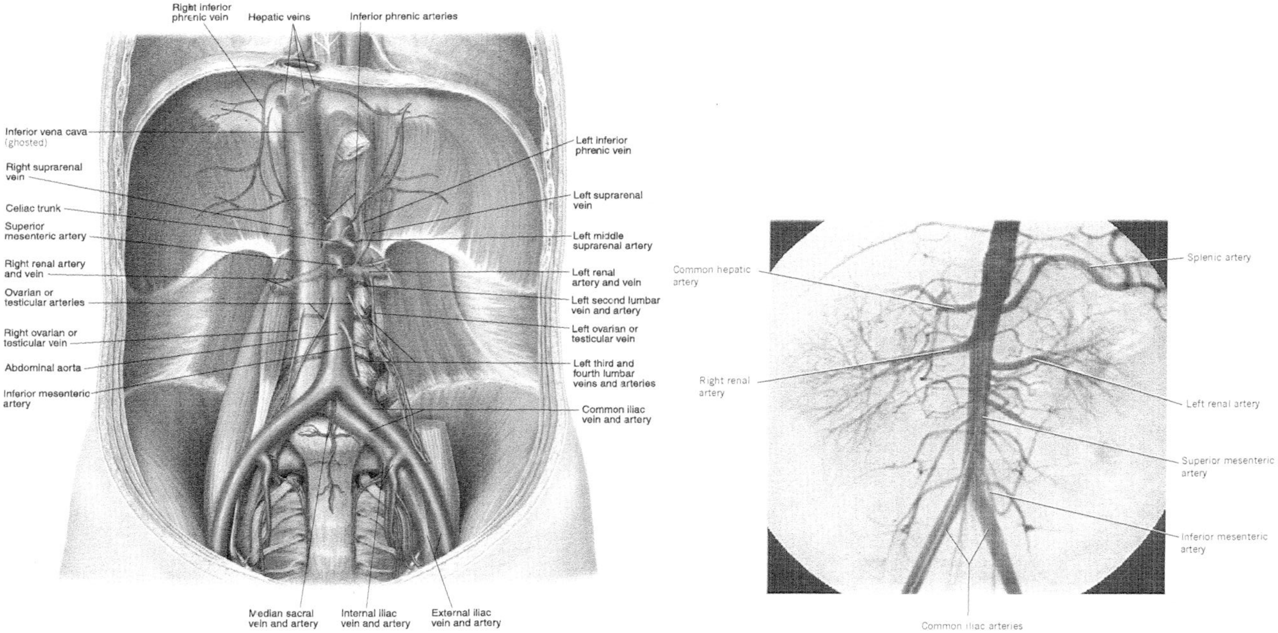

FIGURE 35.3 Abdominal aorta, anatomic diagram (left) and aortogram (right). *(Left panel reprinted with permission from Gest TR, ed. The abdomen. In: Lippincott® Atlas of Anatomy. 2nd ed. Wolters Kluwer; 2020:230-279. Plate 5-36. Right panel reprinted with permission from Uflacker A, Guimaraes M, eds. Abdominal aorta and branches. In: Uflacker's Atlas of Vascular Anatomy: An Angiographic Approach. 3rd ed. Wolters Kluwer; 2021:560-758. Figure 18.6.)*

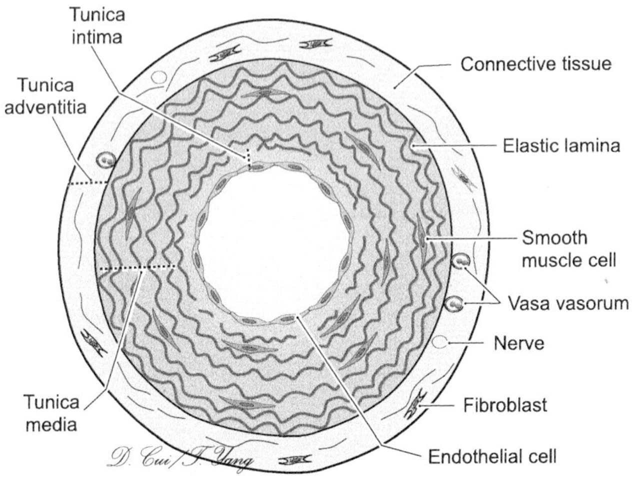

FIGURE 35.4 Histologic cross section of a large artery. *(Reprinted with permission from Cui D, Daley WP, eds. Circulatory system. In: Histology From a Clinical Perspective. 2nd ed. Wolters Kluwer; 2023:207-234. Figure 9.8A.)*

b. **Media:** Comprises smooth muscle cells and extracellular matrix (ECM) proteins
c. **Adventitia:** Includes loose connective tissue and fibroblasts

II. ABDOMINAL AORTIC ANEURYSMS

A. Epidemiology and screening recommendations
1. The most common type of aortic aneurysmal disease
2. Prevalence increases with age and male vs. female sex.[1]
3. More common in high-income nations[2]
   a. Estimated prevalence of abdominal aortic aneurysms (AAAs) in males 65 to 80 years old in these populations is 4% to 8%.[3]
   b. In the US, prevalence of AAA by sex and race[4]: 3:1 males to females and 2:1 white to black
4. Other nonmodifiable risk factors:
   a. Family history
   b. Presence of other aneurysms
      i. Fourteen percent of patients with AAA have peripheral aneurysms (e.g., femoral, popliteal).[5]
      ii. About 26% to 62% of patients with popliteal aneurysms have AAA.[6–9]
      iii. Up to 82% of patients with femoral aneurysms may have AAA[10]
5. The only modifiable risk factor consistently strongly associated with AAA development, expansion, and rupture is cigarette smoking.[3,11]

6. **Screening recommendations** (from the most recent [2018] Society for Vascular Surgery [SVS] guidelines):
   a. Preferred imaging modality: Ultrasound imaging
   b. The presence of a peripheral aneurysm mandates screening for AAA.
   c. One-time ultrasound screening is recommended for
      i. Individuals 65 to 75 years old with a history of tobacco use, or >75 and in good health
      ii. First-degree relatives of patients with AAA who are 65 to 75 years old, or >75 and in good health
   d. Rescreening after 10 years is indicated if initial screening identified aortic diameter between 2.5 and 3 cm.
   e. SVS guidelines differ from US Preventive Services Task Force recommendations.[12]
      i. No recommendation for screening after 75 years old
      ii. No recommendation for screening of women who have ever smoked or who have family history (recommends no screening for women who have never smoked *and* do not have family history)
7. The most dreaded outcome of AAA is rupture as this is immediately life-threatening and carries a high mortality rate.
   a. In the US, ruptured AAAs are the 13th leading cause of death overall and the 10th leading cause of death in men >55 years old, a rate that has held steady for the past 2 decades despite improvements in operative technique/perioperative management.[13]
   b. For patients who survive until hospital presentation, mortality rate has been estimated at 36%.[14]
   c. Risk factors for rupture:[15]
      i. Female sex
      ii. Increasing diameter
         a) Annual rupture risk estimates[15,16]
            1) 5.5 to 7.0 cm: 5.3% per year
            2) >7.0 cm: 6.3% per year
      iii. Current cigarette smoking
      iv. High mean blood pressure

B. Pathophysiology/etiology
1. Definition of a **true aneurysm** (vs. **pseudoaneurysm** [PSA]): A permanent localized dilation of all three layers of the arterial wall >50% of the normal or adjacent vessel diameter (e.g., AAA: >50% dilation *or* diameter >3 cm)
2. Anatomic distribution[17]
   a. 85% infrarenal
   b. 25% involve the iliac arteries.
   c. 2% involve the renal or other visceral arteries.
3. Aortic dilation is a degenerative process in which
   a. Vascular smooth muscle cells (VSMCs) of the media undergo apoptosis or become dysfunctional in terms of ECM production/maintenance.
   b. Microfibrils in the media are broken down by aberrantly released proteases.
   c. Wall thinning and loss of elasticity

4. Research into the pathogenesis of AAA is ongoing. Candidate inciting mechanisms for VSMC dysfunction/ECM remodeling[18]
   a. Inflammation: Innate (neutrophils, macrophages) and adaptive immune cells (T and B lymphocytes) invade the aortic wall
   b. Atherothrombosis: Atherosclerotic plaque in the intima causes abnormal blood flow and sheer stress.
      i. The vast majority of AAAs are associated with atherosclerotic disease, but a causative relationship has not been firmly established.
   c. Inherited factors: Gene variants including single nucleotide polymorphisms, epigenetic factors

C. Presentation
1. Most commonly asymptomatic and found incidentally/on screening
2. Expansion/rupture presents with shock, severe back/flank/abdominal pain.
   a. Hemodynamically stable patients may also present with abdominal or back pain (less severe and subacute/chronic).
3. Rarely with thrombosis (including aortic thrombosis and distal embolization of mural thrombus), can lead to limb ischemia.

D. Diagnosis
1. Physical examination
   a. Abdominal palpation is approximately 68% sensitive and 75% specific[19] for (nonruptured) AAA.
   b. When nonurgent/emergent, should include palpation of the femoral and popliteal arteries for associated peripheral aneurysms.
2. Imaging
   a. **Ultrasound imaging:** Study of choice for screening/surveillance
   b. **CT angiography (CTA):** Study of choice for operative planning
   c. **MRI/magnetic resonance angiography (MRA):** Good sensitivity for AAA, but not for aortic wall calcification, can be performed without contrast (e.g., in patients with chronic kidney disease)
   d. **Aortography** (angiography of the aorta) is not sensitive for the diagnosis of AAA because the study is a luminogram and will therefore underestimate the total aortic size (especially in the presence of mural thrombus).

E. Elective management
1. Management of asymptomatic AAA is primarily based on aneurysm morphology, diameter, and sex in the most recent SVS guidelines[15]:
   a. **Saccular aneurysms (Figure 35.5)**: Operative management (in acceptable surgical candidates)[20,21]
   b. **Fusiform aneurysms**
      i. 3.0 to 4.9 cm: Medical management and ultrasonography surveillance at the following intervals:
         a) 3.0 to 3.9 cm—every 3 years
         b) 4.0 to 4.9 cm—every 12 months
      ii. 5.0 to 5.4 cm: Management depends on sex
         a) Female: Operative management
         b) Male: Ultrasonography surveillance every 6 months

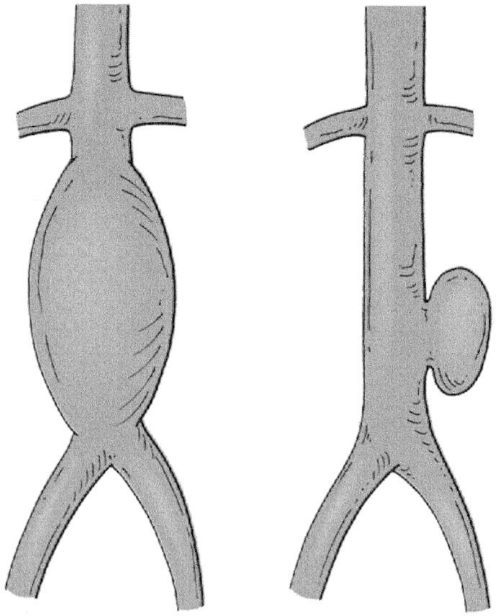

FIGURE 35.5 Fusiform vs. saccular aneurysm morphology. *(Modified from Lawrence PF, Rigberg DA. Arterial aneurysms: etiology, epidemiology and natural history. In: Sidawy AP, Perler BA, eds. Rutherford's Vascular Surgery and Endovascular Therapy. 10th ed. Elsevier; 2023:905-913. Figure 71.3. Copyright 2023, Elsevier. With permission.)*

   iii. ≥5.5 cm: Operative management
   iv. Any size, with increase in diameter by >0.5 cm/6 months or 1 cm/y: Operative management
2. Relative contraindications to elective repair: Recent myocardial infarction, intractable congestive heart failure, coronary artery disease not amenable to revascularization, life expectancy <2 years, stroke with incapacitating neurologic deficits
3. Medical management
   a. Risk-factor modification—most importantly smoking cessation
   b. Optimization of comorbidities, particularly other cardiovascular diseases (e.g., hypertension, hyperlipidemia) and chronic obstructive pulmonary disease (COPD)
   c. No medications have proven efficacy in the direct prevention of AAA progression/dilation1.[18]
4. Operative management
   a. Open or endovascular techniques (see Chapter 33 for endovascular basics)
   b. **Endovascular aortic aneurysm repair (EVAR)** has become the treatment of choice for elective AAA repair (and for emergent repair, see below) when it is anatomically feasible.[15,22]

i. Several multicenter randomized controlled trials (RCTs) have shown that 30-day and in-hospital mortality is significantly lower in EVAR (1.4%-1.6%) than in open AAA repair (4.2%-5.2%).[23–27]
   a) However, further pooled analyses of these studies showed that this survival benefit was not seen in patients with moderate renal dysfunction or previous coronary artery disease.

ii. In addition, analyses of the longer-term results of these trials show that this survival advantage is mostly limited to the perioperative period[27]:
   a) Survival curves for EVAR and open repair converge within 3 years of the index operation and remain so through 8 years postoperatively.
   b) Aneurysm-related mortality is higher in EVAR patients after 3 years.
   c) Patients with peripheral arterial disease have lower mortality with open repair between about 6 months to 4 years.
   d) For elective EVAR, perioperative mortality is lowest at centers that perform ≥30 EVARs per year.[28]

iii. Therefore, open AAA repair may be indicated as the primary approach for highly selected patients (who would otherwise be eligible for EVAR).

c. EVAR prostheses (**endografts/stentgrafts**)

i. Consist of a metal stent (e.g., stainless steel, nitinol) and a polyester or polytetrafluoroethylene graft

ii. Are usually bifurcated, with two distal limbs placed in each iliac system
   a) A common configuration is two parts, with a main body that consists of the aortic portion narrowing into one iliac limb and with a hole surrounded by a radio-opaque ring ("**gate**") for the other limb, and a second part that consists of the remaining iliac limb (**Figure 35.6**).
   b) **Fenestrated (FEVAR) repair** allows for a more proximal seal across the renal or visceral orifices, with the fenestration allowing continued blood flow into said vessels.

d. Requirements for EVAR can generally be conceptualized as ensuring the following:

i. Good seal of the device to the aortic wall, meaning that the stentgraft adequately excludes the weakened aneurysmal section and does not leak/migrate after deployment.

ii. Essential branches are not covered.

iii. The device (and its deployment system) can physically get to the aneurysm.

e. Requirements to ensure good seal

i. Adequate landing zones
   a) Adequate length of healthy aorta to form a good seal with the two ends of the endograft

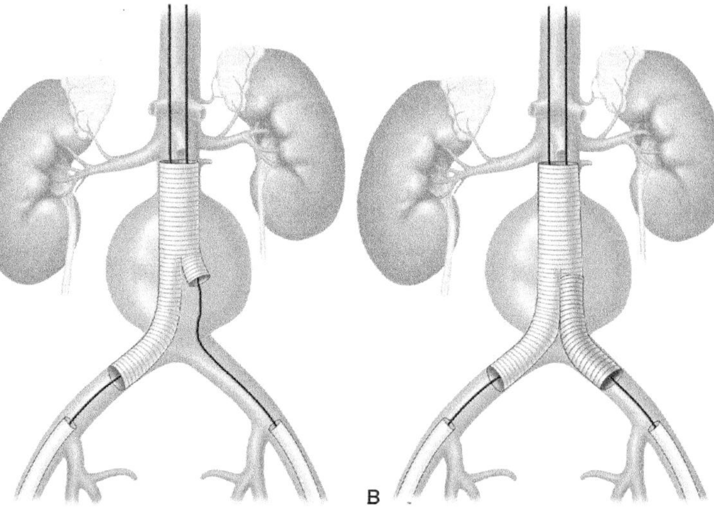

FIGURE 35.6 Anatomic diagram of bifurcated infrarenal aortic endograft deployment. A, main body deployed and contralateral gate cannulated; B, contralateral limb deployed. *(Reprinted with permission from Hnath JC. EVAR for infrarenal abdominal aortic aneurysm repair. In: Darling RC III, Ozaki CK, eds. Master Techniques in Surgery: Vascular Surgery: Arterial Procedures. Wolters Kluwer; 2016:343-350. Panel A: Figure 32.2, Panel B: Figure 32.3.)*

1) Proximal landing zone area also referred to as the "**neck**" (**Figure 35.7**).
2) In the US the majority of commercially available endografts require 15-mm landing zones.
3) Endografts that require only 10 mm have more recently become available.

b) Diameter of landing zones: Typically available stentgrafts can be used with aortic landing zones of 16 to 32 mm diameter

c) Stentgrafts can extend into the CIA/EIA (most stentgrafts are bifurcated, i.e., designed to extend into the CIA), in which case iliac landing zones also need to be assessed.

ii. Angle of the neck and body of the AAA

a) Extreme angulation between the wall of the aorta that is healthy vs. portion that is aneurysmal precludes good seal

b) This angle is measured when viewing the aorta coronally/sagittally (not axially) from the external aspect.

c) Most devices can only tolerate angulation of <60°.

iii. Relative contraindications (depending on device availability and surgeon preference/experience):

a) Intraluminal thrombus in the proximal neck

b) More complicated neck morphology (cone shaped, reverse taper [widens more distally])

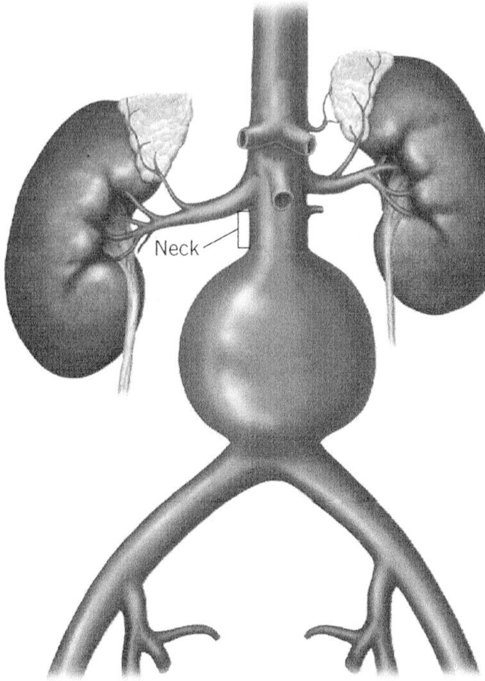

FIGURE 35.7 Aortic aneurysm neck angulation measurement. *(Reprinted with permission from Hnath JC. EVAR for infrarenal abdominal aortic aneurysm repair. In: Darling RC III, Ozaki CK, eds. Master Techniques in Surgery: Vascular Surgery: Arterial Procedures. Wolters Kluwer; 2016:343-350. Figure 32.1.)*

f. Requirements to maintain major branches

i. In most patients, the SMA can adequately perfuse the intestines without the IMA, so the IMA is often covered (or ligated in open repair).

a) A large patent IMA suggests abnormal mesenteric blood supply (i.e., IMA dependent) and therefore that the visceral collateralization should be evaluated (may necessitate keeping the IMA uncovered).

b) Patients with prior colonic resection are more likely to be dependent on the IMA.

ii. Similarly, large accessory renal arteries or the presence of a horseshoe kidney with multiple renal arteries is often a contraindication.

iii. The distal end of the iliac limbs is typically positioned proximal to the IIA orifice to maintain pelvic perfusion and collateral supply to the spinal artery.

iv. Patent lumbar arteries arising from the aneurysm *do not* preclude EVAR.

g. Requirements that allow for device delivery
  i. Iliac arteries cannot be prohibitively tortuous or calcified
  ii. Femoral and iliac arteries must be large enough to accommodate advancing the device
    a) Iliofemoral adjuncts have been described to overcome this (e.g., femoral endarterectomy, open chimney graft, endochimney)

h. Surgical approach: EVAR for infrarenal AAA with iliac extension
  i. Access bilateral femoral arteries; can be done percutaneously (retrograde) under ultrasonography guidance using a micropuncture kit and percutaneous closure devices or in an open fashion.
    a) Establishing which side the main body will be advanced through ("ipsilateral") is determined by a variety of considerations, including:
      1) Relative tortuosity of the femoral/iliac arteries
      2) Relative degree of atherosclerotic disease
      3) Prior iliac stent
  ii. Systemically heparinize (e.g., bolus of 100 U/kg), then advance a small (e.g., 5Fr) pigtail marker catheter over-the-wire through the contralateral common femoral artery (CFA), and obtain aortogram and pelvic angiogram. Measure the length of the aorta from the lowest renal artery to the ipsilateral CIA bifurcation to confirm the length of stentgraft needed. Mark the lowest renal artery (on the fluoroscopy screen).
  iii. Insert the main body of the stentgraft into the ipsilateral femoral sheath and position it in the infrarenal aorta over-the-wire using fluoroscopy, ensuring proper orientation (not yet deployed) and that the proximal marker is just under the lowest renal artery. Locating the contralateral gate slightly anteriorly will allow for easier cannulation. Pull the ipsilateral sheath back, exposing the stentgraft; deploy the main body of the stentgraft.
  iv. Using the appropriate catheters and wires via the contralateral sheath, cannulate the contralateral gate. Insert a pigtail catheter over-the-wire and obtain a retrograde angiogram allowing for measurement from the gate to the contralateral CIA bifurcation, to confirm length needed for the contralateral limb of the stentgraft.
  v. Exchange the short contralateral sheath for a longer sheath (e.g., 30 cm, 12Fr), and advance the sheath through the contralateral gate over-the-wire.
  vi. Insert the contralateral stentgraft limb via the contralateral sheath and over the wire until its proximal marker is about 3 cm cephalad to the gate marker. Pull the sheath back, exposing the contralateral limb; deploy the contralateral limb of the stentgraft.
  vii. Balloon angioplasty the proximal aortic and distal iliac landing zones and the zone of overlap between the main body and

contralateral limb of the stentgraft. Obtain a completion angiogram; confirm good position and no endoleaks (see below).

viii. Remove all instrumentation, reverse heparinization with protamine, and close (either using previously placed percutaneous closure devices or with fine sutures/patch angioplasty if needed and closure of skin and subcutaneous tissue in layers).

i. Open operative technique

i. Increased perioperative morbidity and mortality compared with EVAR is likely secondary to need for aortic cross-clamping during repair. The more proximally the aorta needs to be clamped (e.g., **infrarenal, suprarenal, supraceliac**), the more organs are at risk for complications secondary to transient ischemia.

a) Management of resuscitation, electrolytes, and pressors critically important during aortic unclamping given the risk of sudden hypotension from a decrease in systemic vascular resistance and introduction of previously sequestered metabolites

ii. Two approaches—transabdominal and retroperitoneal

a) Transabdominal: Technically less difficult than a retroperitoneal approach, but violates the peritoneum and may therefore be more difficult in a reoperative abdomen and less well tolerated. More prone to postoperative ileus

b) Left retroperitoneal: Particularly useful in patients with obesity (avoiding intraperitoneal fat allows for better exposure/visualization), COPD (better respiratory recovery), and previous abdominal operations

1) The anterolateral aspect of the aorta is exposed and increases the ease of either suprarenal or supraceliac control.

2) Does increase the difficulty of controlling the right renal artery, which has to be controlled from within the aneurysm sac

j. Surgical approach: Open transabdominal AAA repair

i. Perform a midline laparotomy, mobilize the transverse colon cephalad, and eviscerate the small bowel to the patient's right. Incise the retroperitoneum to expose the aorta and mobilize the duodenum and the left renal vein from its anterior aspect.

ii. Systemically heparinize for a goal activated clotting time >250. Control aortic branches that will be below the aortic clamp with vessel loops to prevent back-bleeding; clamp the aorta proximally and distally. Care should be taken to avoid areas of heavy calcification if possible, as it will not be possible to adequately clamp in these areas and clamping may lead to fracturing of plaque and possible dissection.

iii. Make an aortotomy and extend it longitudinally through the aneurysm neck; "T" off the proximal end of the incision to facilitate the proximal anastomosis. Once the aneurysm is opened, retrograde bleeding from lumbar arteries must be controlled rapidly with silk ligation. Blood should be salvaged and autotransfused. Remove any mural thrombus and oversew involved lumbar arteries from within the aneurysm sac.

iv. Perform the proximal anastomosis, anastomosing the proximal (healthy) aortic cuff to a conduit graft (e.g., Dacron, cryopreserved artery, vein composite). Flush the graft and move the clamp as distally as possible given the anatomy and conduit choice (clamping of cryopreserved grafts should be avoided, as this can lead to delayed PSA development).

v. Perform the distal anastomosis at the aortic bifurcation ("tube" graft, i.e., no limbs/branches) or at the iliac arteries (bifurcated graft), depending on aneurysmal involvement of the iliacs.

vi. Remove aortic clamps, check for good flow through the graft and in the distal extremities (compared with preoperative extremity perfusion). Trim the aneurysm sac and close it over the graft to reduce risk of enteroaortic fistula development.

vii. Ensure hemostasis and replace the abdominal viscera ensuring no twisting of the mesentery. Close the fascia; close the skin and subcutaneous tissue in layers

F. Urgent/emergent management

1. Emergent operative repair is required for ruptured AAAs with a goal of 90 minutes from door to intervention.[15]
2. Patients with symptomatic AAA but without hemodynamic instability and without rupture on CT can be admitted to the intensive care unit for medical optimization prior to proceeding to the operating room (OR).[15]
3. Preoperative management of the unstable patient with presumed ruptured AAA (hypotension, abdominal/back pain, and pulsatile abdominal mass/known AAA):
   a. Permissive hypotensive resuscitation
      i. Essential not to overresuscitate, as significant increases in blood pressure (BP) may lead to worsened hemorrhage/destabilization of any tamponade
         a) Aggressive preoperative fluid resuscitation is associated with higher postoperative mortality.[29,30]
      ii. Fluids (blood preferred over crystalloid) should only be given as needed to maintain end-organ perfusion (e.g., maintain consciousness, prevent ST elevation) and systolic BP 70 to 90 mm Hg.[15,22]
   b. Other strategies to avoid hemodynamic collapse prior to aortic control
      i. Avoid elective intubation/intubation prior to transport to OR
      ii. Use local/regional anesthesia as possible (over general anesthesia; only relevant for EVAR)
      iii. When general endotracheal anesthesia is required, delay induction until just before the initial incision is made.

4. Key concepts of operative management
   a. Can be achieved endovascularly or open.
      i. In the US, EVAR has become the more common technique.[31] The most recent SVS recommendation is for use of EVAR over open repair for ruptured AAAs when anatomically feasible.[15]
         a) RCTs have so far not shown a 30-day or 1-year mortality benefit, but results may be confounded by intention-to-treat analysis.[15,32]
         b) Limited data have shown no significant difference between percutaneous and open femoral access for EVAR in the setting of rupture.[33]
   b. The primary goal is rapid control of the supraceliac aorta.
      i. Can be accomplished with aortic balloon occlusion (endovascularly) or via clamp (open)
      ii. Open approach
         a) A midline laparotomy is performed, the **pars flaccida** is divided at the diaphragmatic hiatus, the left lateral segment of the liver is mobilized to patient's right, the aortic crus is divided, the aorta is isolated from the adjacent esophagus and controlled with either a clamp or via direct manual pressure against the spine.
         b) The retroperitoneal hematoma is then opened and the proximal neck of the aneurysm identified, allowing for the cross-clamp to be moved distally if possible.
   c. Heparin should be used judiciously as the coagulopathy of the patient allows.

G. Complications in the postoperative period after AAA repair
1. Postoperative morbidity mainly secondary to ischemia, whether it be from
   a. Rupture/pre- or intraoperative hypotension
   b. Intraoperative aortic occlusion (e.g., cross-clamping)
   c. Intra-/postoperative thromboembolization
   d. Arterial dissection (more common in EVAR)
2. Ischemic complications are generally more common in elective open AAA repair vs. elective EVAR but are most common in the setting of rupture. They include:
   a. Myocardial ischemia/infarction, arrhythmias (can also be due to electrolyte abnormalities)
   b. **Ischemic colitis** of the left colon
      i. Secondary to ligation/coverage of the IMA
      ii. Signs include: Leukocytosis, significant fluid requirement in the first 8 to 12 postoperative hours, hematochezia, and/or peritonitis
      iii. Diagnosis: Flexible sigmoidoscopy to 20 cm above the anal verge
      iv. Management depends on extent of colonic necrosis
         a) Limited to the mucosa: Can treat expectantly with IV antibiotics and bowel rest
         b) Involves the muscularis: Can also manage expectantly as long as hemodynamically stable and not worsening. May

cause segmental strictures necessitating delayed segmental resection

c) Transmural: Requires immediate resection with end colostomy

c. Renal insufficiency
   i. In elective open suprarenal AAA repair, can administer cold perfusate to the renal arteries with Pruitt catheters to reduce the risk of ischemic renal dysfunction
   ii. Can also be due to contrast nephrotoxicity in EVAR
d. Lower extremity ischemia
   i. Important to check distal perfusion preoperatively and after repair while still in the OR for early identification and treatment of possible intraoperative thromboembolism/dissection
   ii. Microemboli can also cause cutaneous ischemia in the lower extremities, presenting with mottled skin in areas of local necrosis. Typically treated expectantly in the setting of patent major vessels.
e. Paraplegia due to anterior spinal cord ischemia is rare, particularly in infrarenal AAA repair.

3. Complications secondary to open operative dissection/exposure include ureteral injury, serosal injury, and sexual dysfunction resulting from damage to the sympathetic plexus over the left CIA or in the pelvis ("**nervi erigentes**").

H. Late graft-specific complications

1. Generally much less common in open vs. endovascular repair (open grafts have transmural [suture] fixation)
   a. Reflected by recommended postoperative EVAR surveillance: Repeated CTs within 30 days, at 6 months, and at 1 year and every year thereafter[15]
   b. Surveillance after open repair less codified. May consist of a single surveillance CT 3 to 5 years postoperatively or diagnostic CT for symptom development
2. Open repairs
   a. Stenosis/occlusion or PSA at the anastomotic sites, more commonly at distal iliac/femoral anastomoses
   b. Dilation of the aorta just proximal to the proximal anastomosis
   c. May be less rare than currently appreciated, given lack of rigorous surveillance guidelines[34]
3. Endograft (EVAR) complications
   a. **Primarily endoleak**, but also limb occlusion, graft thrombosis or fracture, and/or graft migration
   b. **Graft migration** usually occurs in a caudal direction and is due to failure of fixation of the proximal end of the endograft
      i. Reports of significant migration (>5-10 mm) vary, with rates from 2% to 5% at 1 year to 45% at 5 years[35,36]
      ii. Associated with challenging arterial anatomy
      iii. Does not necessarily need to be treated
         a) Treatment indicated when leads to type I endoleak (see below), usually with secondary endovascular procedures (e.g., extension with an additional graft segment)

c. Endoleaks
  i. Failure of aneurysmal sac exclusion, potential predisposition for rupture
  ii. Aneurysm expansion is an indication for reoperation to prevent rupture.
  iii. Without expansion, management varies by type (**Figure 35.8**).[15]
    a) **Type I:** Leak from the **proximal (Ia) or distal (Ib)** attachment sites
      1) Operative repair indicated regardless of aneurysm expansion due to direct flow into the aneurysm sac
      2) Repair with proximal or distal extension graft
    b) **Type II:** Due to collateral flow from covered branches (e.g., IMA, lumbar arteries)
      1) Can be observed if no expansion
      2) Repair entails embolization/ligation of collaterals
    c) **Type III:** Leak between graft components or through an erosion in the graft fabric
      1) Like type I, operative repair always indicated due to direct flow into sac
      2) Repair: Bridging stent between separated components or "relining" (deploying another stent within the old stent) to cover erosion

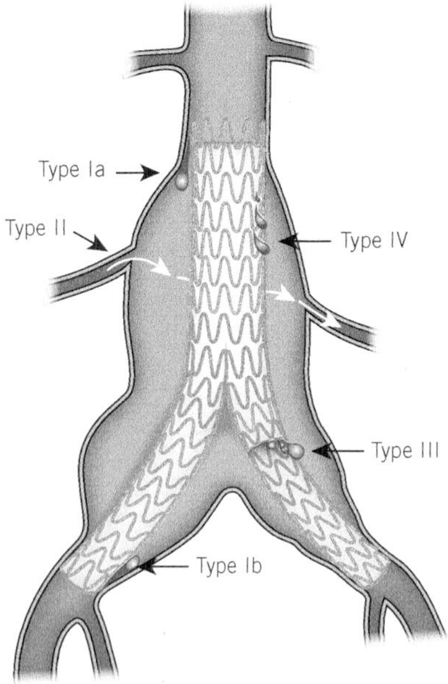

FIGURE 35.8 Endoleak types, see text for descriptions.

d) **Type IV:** Leak through intact graft material due to fabric porosity (visualized as a generalized weak contrast blush within the aneurysm sac)
   1) Usually resolves spontaneously; observe if no expansion
   2) Repair entails relining
e) **Type V**/"endotension": Sac enlargement *without* a visible endoleak
   1) Mechanism unknown, possibly secondary to leak too small to be visualized, or transmission of systemic pressure through sac thrombus (**endotension**)
   2) By definition associated with aneurysm expansion, and therefore requires operative management (relining with proximal and/or distal extension)

III. THORACIC AORTIC ANEURYSMS

A. Epidemiology
   1. Compared with AAA, fewer high-quality and recently performed studies, leading to fewer widely accepted guidelines for screening/management/surveillance, and a less robust understanding of the underlying pathophysiology[37,38]
   2. A recent metanalysis[39] estimated a global prevalence of 0.16% and incidence of 5.3 per 100,000 individuals per year, with an incidence of rupture of 1.6 per 100,000 per year
      a. Relative rates of thoracic aorta areas involvement: Ascending 46%, arch 21%, descending 35%
      b. In North America: Prevalence 0.12%, incidence 7.3 per 100,000 individuals/y; incidence of rupture 1.8 per 100,000/y
   3. Given lack of screening programs and that most thoracic aortic aneurysms (TAAs) are incidentally found, these are most likely underestimations of the true incidence/prevalence.

B. Classification and pathophysiology
   1. TAAs are typically classified by their location—ascending, transverse (arch), descending, thoracoabdominal—with a fifth classification of traumatic TAA.
   2. Thoracic aortic pathophysiology is complex, with multiple possible disease processes. The most common histopathology associated with TAA is **medial degeneration.**[22,37]
      a. Elastic tissue fragmentation, loss of smooth muscle cells, accumulation of mucopolysaccharide cysts between muscle fibers
      b. Inflammation may also play important role.
   3. Risk factors/associated diseases include advanced age, hypertension, connective tissue disorders, congenital defects (bicuspid aortic valve, coarctation), and vasculitis.[37,38]
   4. Female sex appears to be associated with a faster rate of TAA dilation/enlargement, up to twice as fast.[40]

C. Presentation
   1. Typically asymptomatic and discovered incidentally
      a. Screening with axial imaging may be indicated for select high-risk populations (e.g., patients with connective tissue disorders)

2. Symptoms secondary to aneurysm expansion may include chest pain and/or compressive symptoms from impingement upon nearby structures (e.g., recurrent laryngeal nerve, left mainstem bronchus, esophagus, SVC).
3. Symptoms can be secondary to TAA sequelae, including aortic valve insufficiency, congestive heart failure, erosion into adjacent structures (e.g., hemoptysis from airway/pulmonary erosion, hematemesis from esophageal erosion), or distal embolization leading to end-organ/limb ischemia

D. Diagnosis
1. CXR
   a. May show widened mediastinum or, less likely, an enlarged calcific aortic shadow
   b. May be more useful in excluding other diagnoses
   c. In the setting of trauma, may show associated bony injury
2. Axial imaging with CTA (or MRA) best for diagnosis and necessary for operative planning

E. Management
1. Depends on acuity of presentation, underlying etiology, and aortic location
2. Majority of patients with known TAA are managed medically with hypertension management, smoking cessation, and management of underlying associated diseases (if present)
3. Surgical management is indicated for[37,41,42]:
   a. Symptomatic patients
   b. Asymptomatic patients with any of the following:
      i. Ascending aortic diameter ≥5.0 cm
      ii. Ascending aortic diameter ≥4.5 cm and planned for aortic valve repair/replacement
      iii. Ascending aortic diameter ≥4.5 cm with high-risk features
         a) Rapidly expanding aneurysms (≥0.5 cm/y or ≥0.3 cm/y over 2 consecutive years)
         b) Family history of aortic dissection at aortic diameter <5.0 cm
         c) Family history of unexplained sudden death at age <50 years
      iv. Descending thoracic aortic diameter ≥5.5 cm in males
      v. Descending thoracic aortic diameter <5.5 cm in patients with risk factors for rupture
         a) Female sex
         b) Rapidly expanding aneurysms (≥0.5 cm/y)
         c) Infectious aneurysm (requires open resection and repair)
         d) Saccular aneurysm (high likelihood of mycotic/infectious etiology)
   c. Intervention for asymptomatic disease may be indicated at smaller aortic diameters than those listed above for female patients and for specific populations (e.g., patients with **Marfan syndrome**).
   d. May be reasonable to use slightly higher size thresholds for patients with asymptomatic descending thoracic aneurysms with increased risk of perioperative morbidity and mortality, including patients with advanced age (≥75 years), pulmonary disease, renal insufficiency, previous stroke, and/or functional dependence
   e. Size alone is not used as an indication for arch repair given the complexity of managing the arch and its branches.

4. Surgical management can be open or endovascular depending on the area of involvement and arterial anatomy (and etiology, particularly infectious).
   a. General concepts of open vs. endovascular repair
      i. **Thoracic endovascular aortic repair (TEVAR)** generally preferred (when anatomically feasible) given the relatively high morbidity associated with open repair
      ii. Open approaches preferred for younger patients with connective tissue/other genetic disorders due to greater graft longevity and possibility of later endovascular reintervention over their lifetime
      iii. A totally endovascular approach to extensive thoracoabdominal disease carries high risk of **spinal cord ischemia**, with coverage of the entire descending thoracic aorta through to aortic bifurcation without the possibility of intercostal artery reimplantation (available via open approach).
         a) Particularly important to preserve the left subclavian and bilateral IIA
   b. General requirements for TEVAR[22]
      i. Adequate femoral access with diameter >7 to 8 mm (depending on device to be used) and without overly tortuous or calcified femoral and iliac anatomy
      ii. Lack of extreme thoracic aortic tortuosity
      iii. Adequate landing zones (typically ≥20 mm in a relatively straight aorta, 25-30 mm when landing zone in an angled area)
   c. Endovascular ascending and arch management
      i. Historically, TEVAR use limited to the descending thoracic aorta
      ii. Newer devices/hybrid approaches have expanded TEVAR use into the arch.
      iii. In-depth discussion of endovascular arch repair is beyond the scope of this chapter, but briefly
         a) Hybrid approaches involve open debranching of one to three of the arch vessels to allow for use of the arch as a landing zone while maintaining perfusion to the territory of said branches.
            1) Debranching entails a bypass (e.g., carotid-subclavian bypass).
         b) Devices with multiple branches/fenestrations can be used to treat the arch totally endovascularly.
   d. Highlights of open management by TAA type
      i. Ascending and proximal arch repairs are performed through median sternotomy and require cardiopulmonary bypass (CPB) and circulatory arrest (see Chapter 32).
      ii. Descending TAAs and thoracoabdominal aneurysms
         a) Can be performed via left posterolateral thoracotomy or thoracoabdominal incision (with extension from the thoracotomy to the umbilicus), and may be facilitated by single lung ventilation (right lung, requires appropriate endotracheal tube [see Chapter 31])

b) **Left-sided heart (atriofemoral) bypass** can be used to protect the heart from overdistention (during clamping, with the forward flow of the aorta totally occluded within the thorax) and to provide distal blood flow to the intra-abdominal aorta/mesentery/pelvis and spine (with distal thoracic aorta clamping).
c) CPB via distal cannulation (CFA and common femoral vein) can be used to facilitate deep hypothermic circulatory arrest for difficult proximal anastomoses.
d) Thoracoabdominal aneurysms require reanastomosis of the major visceral branches of the aorta (e.g., celiac, SMA, renals) directly to the tube graft, or with additional interposition grafts.
1) Temporary perfusion to branches can be maintained during aneurysm repair by using balloon catheters connected to the bypass circuit.

e. **Traumatic aortic injuries**
i. For patients who survive to hospital presentation, typically secondary to blunt trauma with acceleration–deceleration injury (restrained person in a motor vehicle collision)
a) The aorta is relatively fixed at the level of the **ligamentum arteriosum** between the aortic arch and the pulmonary artery (remnant of the fetal **ductus arteriosus**) and is therefore prone to tear at that location.
ii. Classified into four grades
a) **I: Intimal tear**
b) **II: Intramural hematoma (IMH)**
c) **III: PSA**
d) **IV: Rupture**
iii. Management by grade[42]
a) Grades I and II: Most can be observed with serial imaging.
b) Grades III and IV: Urgent repair, except when repair precluded by more immediately life-threatening injuries/major central nervous system trauma
iv. Endovascular repair preferred when possible given relative expediency and lower morbidity/less associated bleeding
a) Advanced age is not a contraindication.[43]

F. Complications
1. Postoperative complications similar to AAA, with the notable exception of higher rates of postoperative paralysis
a. Older estimates placed paraplegia incidence for open repair of various TAAs between 2% and 30%,[44,45] with significant reductions in risk associated with multimodal therapies used to minimize spinal cord ischemia (SCI)
b. More recent national estimates place rates of permanent SCI after TEVAR at just 2.1%, but with notable associated 1-year mortality of 46%[46]
i. Some estimates place 1-year mortality with permanent SCI without functional improvement as high as 75%.[47]
ii. Preoperative planning and patient discussion of this potentially devastating complication is essential.

c. No specific guidelines for optimal spinal protection for TAA repair/TEVAR, but generally best practice is to have a standard institutional protocol for multimodal therapies including distal aortic perfusion, pre- or intraoperative localization of spinal cord blood supply, hypothermia, cerebrospinal fluid drainage (prophylactic or rescue), and pharmacotherapy.[37]

IV. ACUTE AORTIC SYNDROME: AORTIC DISSECTION AND RELATED AORTOPATHIES

A. Epidemiology

1. Despite the relatively nonspecific terminology, "**acute aortic syndrome**" (AAS) refers specifically to aortic dissection, **penetrating aortic ulcer** (PAU), and IMH, and all three can be acute or chronic in nature.
2. Like TAA, epidemiologic data are limited.[48]
3. The most recent data from the US (Minnesota, 1995-2015) estimates a relatively stable AAS incidence of 7.7 per 100,000 person-years.[49]
   a. Incidence by specific entity
      i. Dissection 4.4/100,000 person-years
      ii. PAU 2.1/100,000 person-years
      iii. IMH 1.2/100,000 person-years
   b. Higher incidence with increased age and male sex[48]
   c. Mortality rate more than twice that of population-based controls: 39% at 5 years and 57% at 10 years[49]

B. Pathophysiology and classification

1. Risk factors include long-standing uncontrolled hypertension, tobacco abuse, family history, and connective tissue/collagen vascular diseases such as Marfan syndrome.
2. Dissection, PAU, and IMH are classified along a spectrum of underlying pathophysiology, distinct from aneurysmal disease[37,48] (although some TAAs may be secondary to chronic degeneration of dissection):
   a. Dissection: An intimal tear allowing blood to flow between the intima and media, resulting in the creation of a new flow channel ("false lumen") in addition to the physiologic "true lumen"
   b. IMH: Focal hemorrhage in the aortic wall between the intima and media due to rupture of the vasa vasorum, without intimal tear
   c. PAU: Ulceration/intimal tear with bleeding into an isolated segment of media
3. There are multiple **dissection classification systems** according to ascending/arch involvement:
   a. The Stanford classification system simplified the previous DeBakey classification (**Figure 35.9**); type A involves the proximal ascending aorta with or without arch, type B is limited to the descending aorta
   b. The SVS and Society of Thoracic Surgeons released a joint classification system, based on location of the intimal tear (A vs. B) and distal extent of dissection (**Figure 35.10**).[50]
      i. Distal extent/involvement of aortic branches dictates risk of end-organ ischemia and therefore need for surgical management
4. Presentation/diagnosis/management similar across AAS; the remainder of this section will focus on dissection.

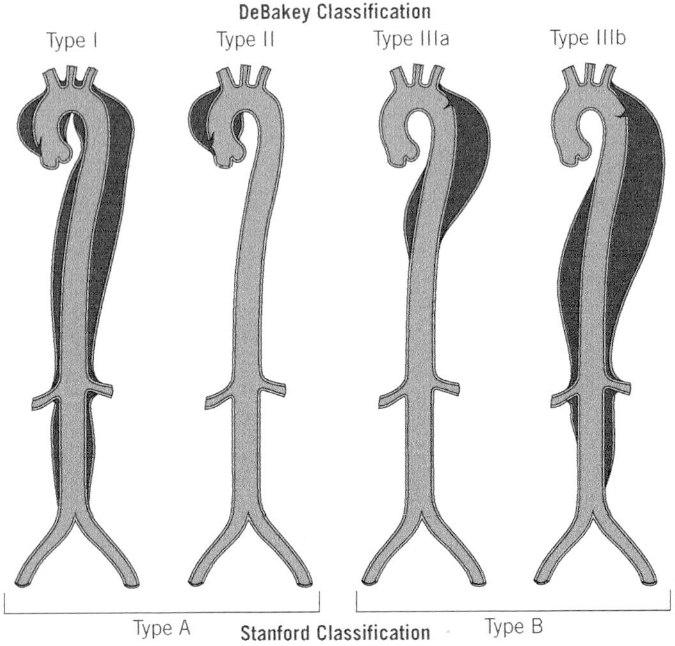

FIGURE 35.9 DeBakey and Stanford classification of aortic dissection.

C. Presentation

1. Depends on acuity/chronicity; symptoms typically associated with acute disease progression
2. Hallmark symptom: Sudden-onset, ripping chest/abdominal pain, radiating to the back
3. Other possible signs and symptoms: Blood pressure discrepancy between upper extremities, new-onset heart murmur, renovisceral ischemia, and/or paraplegia/paresthesias (less common)

D. Diagnosis

1. CTA is the gold standard for diagnosis and operative planning.
2. MRA often used for surveillance imaging given decreased cumulative radiation exposure and contrast administration

E. Management

1. Depends on classification (A vs. B)
2. **Type A**
   a. Surgical emergency given high associated mortality rate secondary to myocardial ischemia (from retrograde dissection into/compromised perfusion of coronary arteries) and cardiac tamponade
   b. Repair typically entails graft replacement of the proximal ascending aorta and arch with or without aortic valve replacement.

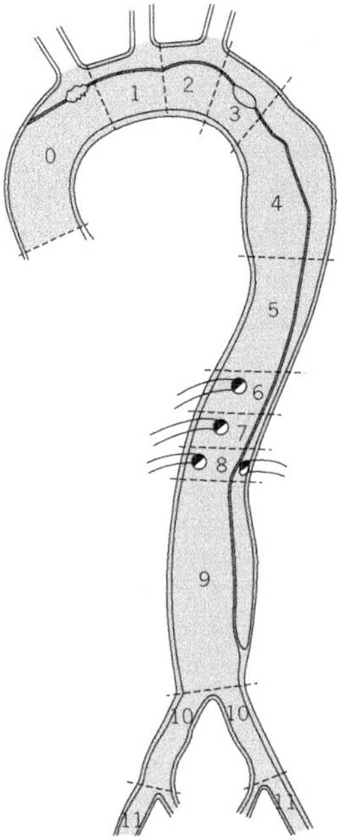

Type	Proximal Extent	Distal Extent
A_D	0	0
Entry tear: **Zone 0**	1	1
	2	2
	3	3
B_{PD}	4	4
Entry tear: **≥Zone 1**	5	5
	6	6
	7	7
	8	8
I_D	9	9
Unidentified entry tear involving **Zone 0**	10	10
	11	11
	12	12

FIGURE 35.10 Society for vascular surgery/Society of thoracic surgeons aortic dissection classification system.

3. **Type B**
   a. Management depends on characterization as uncomplicated or complicated, with complicated defined as associated with end-organ dysfunction (e.g., refractory pain, visceral malperfusion, SCI).
   b. Uncomplicated: Generally medical management, with strict BP monitoring and goal systolic BP 100 to 120 mm Hg
      i. Approximately 25% will progress to complicated and require intervention within 4 years.[51]
      ii. A multicenter European RCT showed improved long-term survival with TEVAR plus optimal medical management vs. medical management alone.[52]
   c. Complicated: Requires urgent/emergent operative repair with two main goals:
      i. Primary goal is revascularization of the affected segment/ischemic territories in order to save the patient's life/limb(s).
         a) Techniques depend on what branches are involved and their origin in the true vs. false lumen. They include interposition graft replacement of the affected segment via thoracotomy, removal of the flap via aortotomy, or endovascular fenestration with or without stenting.

ii. Secondary goal is elimination of the intimal tear, typically via endovascular coverage.
  a) Promotes favorable aortic remodeling to decrease risk of long-term complications/progression of disease and therefore reduce mortality[52]

V. MESENTERIC ISCHEMIA

A. Acute mesenteric ischemia (AMI)
  1. Pathophysiology
    a. Most commonly due to **embolization** to the SMA, often secondary to atrial fibrillation (can also be secondary to deep vein thrombosis/pulmonary embolism in a patient with a patent foramen ovale)
      i. Other etiologies include SMA thrombosis, portomesenteric venous thrombosis, and **nonocclusive mesenteric ischemia** (NOMI).
      ii. Arterial ischemia is often seen in patients with severe atherosclerotic disease of nonmesenteric vessels.
    b. Acute NOMI is secondary to globally reduced perfusion, usually in the setting of low cardiac output/cardiovascular collapse.
  2. Presentation
    a. Arterial ischemia typically presents with acute-onset abdominal pain progressing from intermittent to continuous, with severe pain out of proportion to examination; may also present with hematochezia/bloody diarrhea.
    b. Presentation of venous ischemia more varied, from asymptomatic to profound shock
      i. Pain typically more generalized, with more gradual progression
      ii. May have occult gastrointestinal bleeding without frank hemorrhage
  3. Diagnosis
    a. Laboratory findings are nonspecific and insensitive (e.g., leukocytosis, metabolic acidosis, lactic acidosis), so may be more useful in predicting severity/prognosis than diagnosis.
    b. Primarily diagnosed via CTA, which can also show signs of intestinal ischemia (decreased enhancement in bowel wall, pneumatosis, perforation [late sign])
  4. Management
    a. Depends on etiology and associated processes
    b. Arterial (occlusive) AMI is a surgical emergency with high associated morbidity and mortality.
      i. Revascularization typically in an open fashion given need for assessment of bowel viability and likelihood of need for bowel resection
      ii. In select hemodynamically stable patients, bowel viability can be assessed via diagnostic laparoscopy.
      iii. In the setting of questionable bowel viability or bowel resection, the abdomen should be left open with a temporary closure device to facilitate second-look procedures within 24 to 72 hours.

a) Important both in order to manage questionable bowel that may worsen after the index operation and to allow for possible bowel salvage in cases of extensive bowel involvement

c. Venous mesenteric ischemia portends a high mortality, with laparotomy reserved for evidence of perforation despite anticoagulation.
   i. In the absence of compromised bowel and/or shock, management typically consists of anticoagulation and bowel rest.
   ii. Percutaneous, transhepatic portal or superior mesenteric venous thrombectomy should be reserved for experienced centers.
d. Acute NOMI has very high mortality. The primary goal of management is improved global perfusion by increasing cardiac output and addressing the underlying disease process.

B. Chronic mesenteric ischemia
1. Pathophysiology: Secondary to atherosclerotic occlusive disease of multiple mesenteric vessels
2. Presentation: Includes postprandial pain (abdominal pain that starts within 1 hour of eating and stops within 4 hours), "**food fear**" (decreased oral intake to avoid anginal pain), and unintentional weight loss
3. Diagnosis
   a. Primarily via CTA
   b. Requires a high index of suspicion as presentation can be nonspecific and may have been previously misdiagnosed
4. Management
   a. Operative management is reserved for symptomatic patients.
      i. SVS guidelines recommend endovascular revascularization with balloon-expandable covered stent, with open repair reserved for select younger patients and patients with prohibitive anatomy. However, these recommendations are only grade 2 (weak) given paucity of supporting data.[53]
      ii. Open techniques include endarterectomy and bypass.
      iii. Nutritional status must be assessed and optimized prior to operative intervention.
   b. Long-term surveillance required for postoperative patients and for asymptomatic patients with severe atherosclerotic disease (given the risk of progression to symptomatic chronic ischemia/acute ischemia)

Key References

Citation	Summary
Endovascular or open repair strategy for ruptured abdominal aortic aneurysm: 30 d outcomes (IMPROVE trial) IMPROVE Trial Investigators. Endovascular or open repair strategy for ruptured abdominal aortic aneurysm: 30 day outcomes from IMPROVE randomised trial. *Br Med J.* 2014;348.	• Multicenter international (UK and Canada) RCT of 613 patients with clinical diagnosis of AAA rupture, randomized to endovascular vs. open repair. Primary outcome was 30-d mortality. • No difference in 30-d mortality between the endovascular and open repair groups.

Citation	Summary
Long-term comparison of endovascular and open repair of abdominal aortic aneurysm (OVER trial) Lederle FA, Freischlag JA, Kyriakides TC, et al. Long-term comparison of endovascular and open repair of abdominal aortic aneurysm. *N Engl J Med.* 2012;367(21):1988-1997.	• Multicenter RCT in US Veterans Administration centers of 881 patients 49 y or older with asymptomatic AAA who were candidates for either endovascular or open repair, randomized to endovascular or open repair and followed for a mean of 5 y. Primary outcome was all-cause mortality. • No difference in all-cause mortality between the endovascular and open repair groups over the entire follow-up period. • Endovascular repair was associated with a significantly smaller hazard ratio of mortality within the first 2 postoperative years.
Meta-analysis of individual-patient data from EVAR-1, DREAM, OVER, and ACE trials comparing outcomes of endovascular or open repair for abdominal aortic aneurysm over 5 y Powell JT, Sweeting MJ, Ulug P, et al. Meta-analysis of individual-patient data from EVAR-1, DREAM, OVER and ACE trials comparing outcomes of endovascular or open repair for abdominal aortic aneurysm over 5 years. *Br J Surg.* 2017;104(3):166-178.	• Meta-analysis combining results of four RCTs of elective EVAR vs. open AAA repair, with a total of 2783 patients from France, the Netherlands, the UK, and the US. • Thirty-day survival was superior in patients who underwent EVAR. • Survival curves converged at 3 y and remained so through to 8 y, indicating no survival benefit from EVAR over this period.
Endovascular repair of type B aortic dissection: Long-term results of the randomized investigation of stent grafts in aortic dissection trial (INSTEAD-XL trial) Nienaber CA, Kische S, Rousseau H, et al. Endovascular repair of type B aortic dissection: long-term results of the randomized investigation of stent grafts in aortic dissection trial. *Circ Cardiovasc Interv.* 2013;6(4):407-416.	• Multicenter RCT (France, Germany, Italy) of 140 patients with uncomplicated type B aortic dissections randomized to TEVAR with optimal medical management vs. medical management alone. Long-term retrospective analysis of 2- and 5-y outcomes. • All-cause mortality, aorta-specific mortality, and dissection progression were significantly better at 2 and 5 y in the TEVAR group.

CHAPTER 35: THORACOABDOMINAL VASCULAR DISEASE

Review Questions

1. What is the only modifiable risk factor consistently strongly associated with AAA development, expansion, and rupture?
2. What are the current screening recommendations for asymptomatic AAA?
3. What are the aortic diameter thresholds for operative AAA intervention for fusiform aneurysms?
4. If a patient is discovered to have a popliteal artery aneurysm, what other disease processes do they need to be screened for?
5. What is the main survival difference seen for endovascular vs. open AAA repair?
6. When do endoleaks need to be operatively managed?
7. What are three key concepts guiding preoperative management of the patient with a ruptured AAA?
8. What is the most important factor in preventing postoperative SCI after TAA repair?
9. Describe Stanford type A vs. B aortic dissections
10. What are three key components of operative management of acute (arterial) mesenteric ischemia?

REFERENCES

1. Heart Association Council on Epidemiology. Heart disease and stroke statistics—2022 update: a report from the American Heart Association. *Circulation*. 2022;145(8):e153-e639.
2. Sampson UKA, Norman PE, Fowkes FGR, et al. Estimation of global and regional incidence and prevalence of abdominal aortic aneurysms 1990 to 2010. *Glob Heart*. 2014;9(1):159-170.
3. Nordon IM, Hinchliffe RJ, Loftus IM, Thompson MM. Pathophysiology and epidemiology of abdominal aortic aneurysms. *Nat Rev Cardiol*. 2011;8(2):92-102.
4. Marcaccio CL, Schermerhorn ML. Epidemiology of abdominal aortic aneurysms. *Semin Vasc Surg*. 2021;34(1):29-37.
5. Diwan A, Sarkar R, Stanley JC, Zelenock GB, Wakefield TW. Incidence of femoral and popliteal artery aneurysms in patients with abdominal aortic aneurysms. *J Vasc Surg*. 2000;31(5):863-869.
6. Ramesh S, Michaels JA, Galland RB. Popliteal aneurysm: morphology and management. *Br J Surg*. 1993;80(12):1531-1533.
7. Whitehouse WM Jr, Wakefield TW, Graham LM, et al. Limb-threatening potential of arteriosclerotic popliteal artery aneurysms. *Surgery*. 1983;93(5):694-699.
8. Szilagyi DE, Schwartz RL, Reddy DJ. Popliteal arterial aneurysms. Their natural history and management. *Arch Surg*. 1981;116(5):724-728.
9. Dawson I, Sie RB, van Bockel JH. Atherosclerotic popliteal aneurysm. *Br J Surg*. 1997;84(3):293-299.
10. Graham LM, Zelenock GB, Whitehouse WM Jr, et al. Clinical significance of arteriosclerotic femoral artery aneurysms. *Arch Surg*. 1980;115(4):502-507.

11. Sweeting MJ, Thompson SG, Brown LC, Powell JT; RESCAN collaborators. Meta-analysis of individual patient data to examine factors affecting growth and rupture of small abdominal aortic aneurysms. *Br J Surg.* 2012;99(5):655-665.
12. Guirguis-Blake JM, Beil TL, Senger CA, Coppola EL. *Primary Care Screening for Abdominal Aortic Aneurysm: A Systematic Evidence Review for the U.S. Preventive Services Task Force.* Agency for Healthcare Research and Quality (US); 2019.
13. Wang LJ, Prabhakar AM, Kwolek CJ. Current status of the treatment of infrarenal abdominal aortic aneurysms. *Cardiovasc Diagn Ther.* 2018;8(suppl 1):S191-S199.
14. IMPROVE Trial Investigators, Anjum A, Thompson L, et al. The effect of aortic morphology on peri-operative mortality of ruptured abdominal aortic aneurysm. *Eur Heart J.* 2015;36(21):1328-1334.
15. Chaikof EL, Dalman RL, Eskandari MK, et al. The society for vascular surgery practice guidelines on the care of patients with an abdominal aortic aneurysm. *J Vasc Surg.* 2018;67(1):2-77.e2.
16. Parkinson F, Ferguson S, Lewis P, Williams IM, Twine CP; South East Wales Vascular Network. Rupture rates of untreated large abdominal aortic aneurysms in patients unfit for elective repair. *J Vasc Surg.* 2015;61(6):1606-1612.
17. Aggarwal S, Qamar A, Sharma V, Sharma A. Abdominal aortic aneurysm: a comprehensive review. *Exp Clin Cardiol.* 2011;16(1):11-15.
18. Golledge J. Abdominal aortic aneurysm: update on pathogenesis and medical treatments. *Nat Rev Cardiol.* 2019;16(4):225-242.
19. Fink HA, Lederle FA, Roth CS, Bowles CA, Nelson DB, Haas MA. The accuracy of physical examination to detect abdominal aortic aneurysm. *Arch Intern Med.* 2000;160(6):833-836.
20. Kristmundsson T, Dias N, Resch T, Sonesson B. Morphology of small abdominal aortic aneurysms should be considered before continued ultrasound surveillance. *Ann Vasc Surg.* 2016;31:18-22.
21. Nathan DP, Xu C, Pouch AM, et al. Increased wall stress of saccular versus fusiform aneurysms of the descending thoracic aorta. *Ann Vasc Surg.* 2011;25(8):1129-1137.
22. Sidawy AP, Perler BA. *Rutherford's Vascular Surgery and Endovascular Therapy, 2-Volume Set.* Elsevier Health Sciences; 2022.
23. De Bruin JL, Baas AF, Buth J, et al; DREAM Study Group. Long-term outcome of open or endovascular repair of abdominal aortic aneurysm. *N Engl J Med.* 2010;362(20):1881-1889.
24. United Kingdom EVAR Trial Investigators, Greenhalgh RM, Brown LC, et al. Endovascular versus open repair of abdominal aortic aneurysm. *N Engl J Med.* 2010;362(20):1863-1871.
25. Lederle FA, Freischlag JA, Kyriakides TC, et al. Long-term comparison of endovascular and open repair of abdominal aortic aneurysm. *N Engl J Med.* 2012;367(21):1988-1997.
26. Becquemin JP, Pillet JC, Lescalie F, et al. A randomized controlled trial of endovascular aneurysm repair versus open surgery for abdominal aortic aneurysms in low- to moderate-risk patients. *J Vasc Surg.* 2011;53(5):1167-1173.e1.
27. Powell JT, Sweeting MJ, Ulug P, et al. Meta-analysis of individual-patient data from EVAR-1, DREAM, OVER and ACE trials comparing outcomes of endovascular or open repair for abdominal aortic aneurysm over 5 years. *Br J Surg.* 2017;104(3):166-178.
28. Zettervall SL, Schermerhorn ML, Soden PA, et al. The effect of surgeon and hospital volume on mortality after open and endovascular repair of abdominal aortic aneurysms. *J Vasc Surg.* 2017;65(3):626-634.

29. Roberts K, Revell M, Youssef H, Bradbury AW, Adam DJ. Hypotensive resuscitation in patients with ruptured abdominal aortic aneurysm. *Eur J Vasc Endovasc Surg.* 2006;31(4):339-344.

30. Dick F, Erdoes G, Opfermann P, Eberle B, Schmidli J, von Allmen RS. Delayed volume resuscitation during initial management of ruptured abdominal aortic aneurysm. *J Vasc Surg.* 2013;57(4):943-950.

31. Bath J, Hartwig J, Dombrovskiy VY, Vogel TR. Trends in management and outcomes of vascular emergencies in the nationwide inpatient sample. *Vasa.* 2020;49(2):99-105.

32. IMPROVE Trial Investigators, Powell JT, Sweeting MJ, et al. Endovascular or open repair strategy for ruptured abdominal aortic aneurysm: 30 day outcomes from IMPROVE randomised trial. *Br Med J.* 2014;348:f7661.

33. Chen SL, Kabutey NK, Whealon MD, Kuo IJ, Fujitani RM. Comparison of percutaneous versus open femoral cutdown access for endovascular repair of ruptured abdominal aortic aneurysms. *J Vasc Surg.* 2017;66(5):1364-1370.

34. Coscas R, Greenberg RK, Mastracci TM, et al. Associated factors, timing, and technical aspects of late failure following open surgical aneurysm repairs. *J Vasc Surg.* 2010;52(2):272-281.

35. Sternbergh WC III, Money SR, Greenberg RK, Chuter TAM; Zenith Investigators. Influence of endograft oversizing on device migration, endoleak, aneurysm shrinkage, and aortic neck dilation: results from the Zenith Multicenter Trial. *J Vasc Surg.* 2004;39(1):20-26.

36. Asenbaum U, Schoder M, Schwartz E, et al. Stent-graft surface movement after endovascular aneurysm repair: baseline parameters for prediction, and association with migration and stent-graft-related endoleaks. *Eur Radiol.* 2019;29(12):6385-6395.

37. Upchurch GR Jr, Escobar GA, Azizzadeh A, et al. Society for Vascular Surgery clinical practice guidelines of thoracic endovascular aortic repair for descending thoracic aortic aneurysms. *J Vasc Surg.* 2021;73(1S):55S-83S.

38. Cebull HL, Rayz VL, Goergen CJ. Recent advances in biomechanical characterization of thoracic aortic aneurysms. *Front Cardiovasc Med.* 2020;7:75.

39. Gouveia E Melo R, Silva Duarte G, Lopes A, et al. Incidence and prevalence of thoracic aortic aneurysms: a systematic review and meta-analysis of population-based studies. *Semin Thorac Cardiovasc Surg.* 2022;34(1):1-16.

40. Cheung K, Boodhwani M, Chan KL, Beauchesne L, Dick A, Coutinho T. Thoracic aortic aneurysm growth: role of sex and aneurysm etiology. *J Am Heart Assoc.* 2017;6(2):e003792.

41. Hiratzka LF, Bakris GL, Beckman JA, et al. 2010 ACCF/AHA/AATS/ACR/ASA/SCA/SCAI/SIR/STS/SVM guidelines for the diagnosis and management of patients with thoracic aortic disease: a report of the American College of Cardiology Foundation/American Heart Association Task Force on practice guidelines, American Association for Thoracic Surgery, American College of Radiology, American Stroke Association, Society of Cardiovascular Anesthesiologists, Society for Cardiovascular Angiography and Interventions, Society of Interventional Radiology, Society of Thoracic Surgeons, and Society for Vascular Medicine. *Circulation.* 2010;121(13):e266-e369.

42. Isselbacher EM, Preventza O, Hamilton Black J, et al. 2022 ACC/AHA guideline for the diagnosis and management of aortic disease: a report of the American Heart Association/American College of Cardiology joint committee on clinical practice guidelines. *Circulation.* 2022;146(24):e334-e482.

43. Lee WA, Matsumura JS, Mitchell RS, et al. Endovascular repair of traumatic thoracic aortic injury: clinical practice guidelines of the society for vascular surgery. *J Vasc Surg.* 2011;53(1):187-192.

44. Conrad MF, Crawford RS, Davison JK, Cambria RP. Thoracoabdominal aneurysm repair: a 20-year perspective. *Ann Thorac Surg.* 2007;83(2):S856-S861; discussion S890-S892.

45. Safi HJ, Estrera AL, Azizzadeh A, Coogan S, Miller CC III. Progress and future challenges in thoracoabdominal aortic aneurysm management. *World J Surg.* 2008;32(3):355-360.

46. Scali ST, Giles KA, Wang GJ, et al. National incidence, mortality outcomes, and predictors of spinal cord ischemia after thoracic endovascular aortic repair. *J Vasc Surg.* 2020;72(1):92-104.

47. DeSart K, Scali ST, Feezor RJ, et al. Fate of patients with spinal cord ischemia complicating thoracic endovascular aortic repair. *J Vasc Surg.* 2013;58(3):635.e2-642.e2.

48. Sen I, Erben YM, Franco-Mesa C, DeMartino RR. Epidemiology of aortic dissection. *Semin Vasc Surg.* 2021;34(1):10-17.

49. DeMartino RR, Sen I, Huang Y, et al. Population-based assessment of the incidence of aortic dissection, intramural hematoma, and penetrating ulcer, and its associated mortality from 1995 to 2015. *Circ Cardiovasc Qual Outcomes.* 2018;11(8):e004689.

50. Lombardi JV, Hughes GC, Appoo JJ, et al. Society for vascular surgery (SVS) and society of thoracic surgeons (STS) reporting standards for type B aortic dissections. *J Vasc Surg.* 2020;71(3):723-747.

51. Brunkwall J, Kasprzak P, Verhoeven E, et al. Endovascular repair of acute uncomplicated aortic type B dissection promotes aortic remodelling: 1 Year results of the ADSORB trial. *Eur J Vasc Endovasc Surg.* 2014;48(3):285-291.

52. Nienaber CA, Kische S, Rousseau H, et al. Endovascular repair of type B aortic dissection: long-term results of the randomized investigation of stent grafts in aortic dissection trial. *Circ Cardiovasc Interv.* 2013;6(4):407-416.

53. Huber TS, Björck M, Chandra A, et al. Chronic mesenteric ischemia: clinical practice guidelines from the society for vascular surgery. *J Vasc Surg.* 2021;73(1S):87S-115S.

54. Gest TR. *Lippincott® Atlas of Anatomy.* 2nd ed. Wolters Kluwer; 2020.

55. Uflacker A, Guimaraes M, Uflacker R. *Uflacker's Atlas of Vascular Anatomy: An Angiographic Approach.* Wolters Kluwer; 2021.

56. Valentine RJ, Wind GG. *Anatomic Exposures in Vascular Surgery.* 4th ed. LWW; 2020.

57. Cui D, Daley WP. *Histology from a Clinical Perspective.* Lippincott Williams & Wilkins; 2021.

36 Peripheral Arterial Disease

María del Pilar Martínez Santos and Vipul Khetarpaul

I. VASCULAR ANATOMY OF THE LOWER EXTREMITY

A. Arterial anatomy and closely related structures

1. The **external iliac artery** (EIA) becomes the **common femoral artery** (CFA) as it passes under the inguinal ligament (**Figures 36.1** and **36.2**).
2. The same is true of the **external iliac vein** and the **common femoral vein** (CFV), immediately medial to EIA/CFA.
3. The last anterior branch off the EIA just proximal to the inguinal ligament is the inferior epigastric artery; the first medial and lateral branches off the CFA just distal to the inguinal ligament are the superficial epigastric and superficial circumflex iliac arteries, respectively.
4. The CFA branches into the **superficial femoral artery** (SFA) and **deep femoral/profunda femoris artery** (PFA), and the CFV branches into the superficial and deep femoral veins (SFV and DFV). The saphenous vein branches off the CFV just before the SFV/DFV bifurcation.
5. The lateral femoral circumflex artery branches off the PFA shortly after its SFA takeoff. The lateral femoral circumflex vein (LFCV) branches off the DFV and crosses the PFA anteriorly and the SFA posteriorly. The LFCV can be divided in order to facilitate PFA exposure (**Figure 36.3**).
6. PFA provides the main blood supply to the thigh; SFA has no major thigh branches.
7. SFA and SFV run down the anteromedial thigh within the adductor canal, which makes a 90° twist around the medial thigh to end at the adductor hiatus in the posteromedial thigh just superior to the knee. SFA runs superficial to the SFV in the canal and becomes the popliteal artery when it exits the hiatus, now medial and deep to the popliteal vein, which is just medial to the tibial nerve within the **popliteal fossa** (**Figure 36.4**).
8. Below the knee, the **anterior tibial artery** (AT) branches laterally off of the popliteal artery, which is then referred to as the **tibioperoneal** (TP) trunk.
   a. The TP trunk branches into the **posterior tibial artery** (PT) and peroneal artery.
   b. The PT runs posteromedially and wraps posteroinferiorly around the medial malleolus.
9. The **greater saphenous vein** (GSV) and saphenous nerve run superficially on the medial aspect of the tibia.

B. Lower leg compartments and their vascular/nerve contents (**Figure 36.5**)

1. **Anterior compartment**

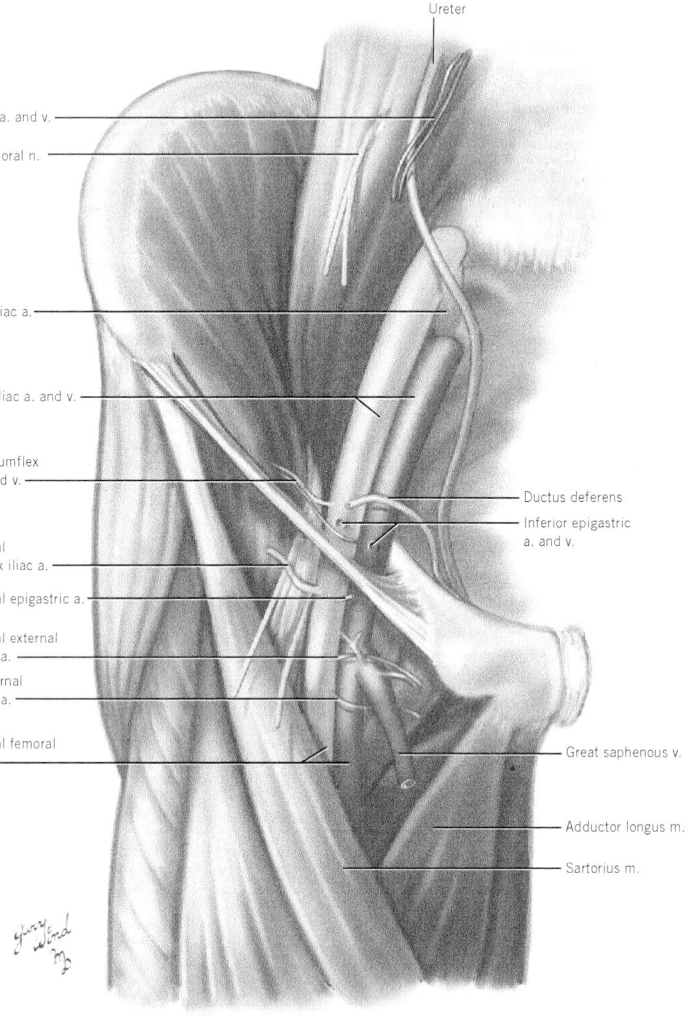

FIGURE 36.1 Vascular anatomy in the inguinal region. *(Reprinted with permission from Valentine RJ, Wind GG, eds. Common femoral artery. In: Anatomic Exposures in Vascular Surgery. 4th ed. Wolters Kluwer; 2021:375-411. Figure 16-4.)*

   a. AT and paired veins
   b. Deep fibular (peroneal) nerve
2. Lateral compartment
   a. Superficial fibular (peroneal) nerve

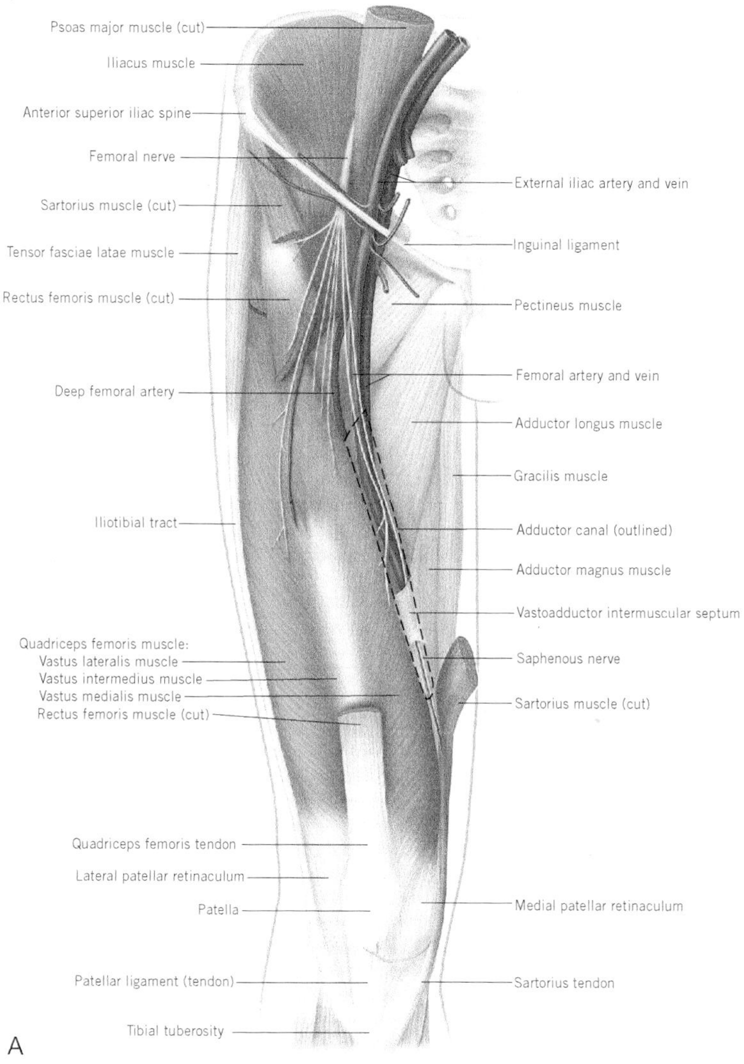

FIGURE 36.2 Anatomy of the (right) thigh. A, Anatomical diagram; B, angiography. *(Panel A reprinted with permission from Gest TR, ed. The lower limb. In: Lippincott® Atlas of Anatomy. 2nd ed. Wolters Kluwer; 2020:96-175. Plate 3-17. Panel B reprinted with permission from Uflacker A, Guimaraes M, eds. Arteries of the lower extremity. In: Uflacker's Atlas of Vascular Anatomy: An Angiographic Approach. 3rd ed. Wolters Kluwer; 2021:966-1039. Figure 22.9.)*

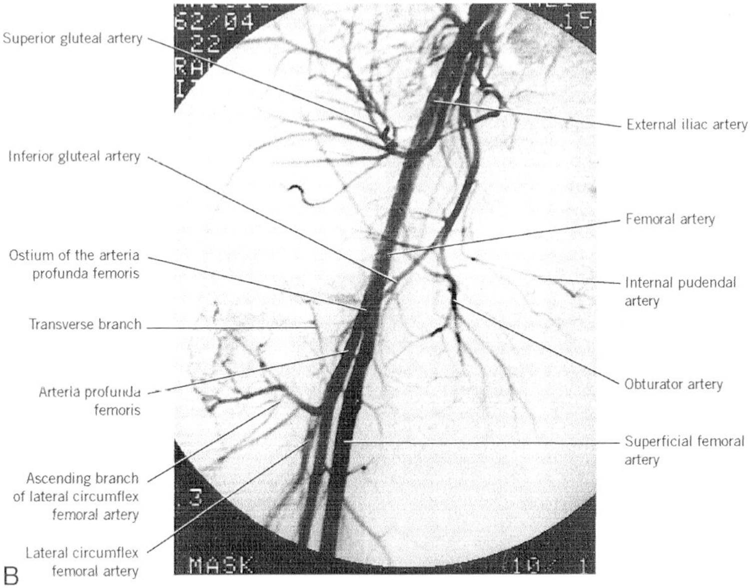

FIGURE 36.2 (*Continued*)

3. **Deep posterior compartment**
   a. PT and paired veins
   b. Tibial nerve
   c. Fibular artery and paired veins
4. **Superficial posterior compartment**
   a. None (has both soleus and gastrocnemius muscles)
5. Of note, the GSV and nerve run superficially under the skin and soft tissue along the posterior border of the tibia.

II. PERIPHERAL ARTERIAL DISEASE

A. Epidemiology
   1. The most recently reported international data (2010) estimated 202 million people globally with **peripheral arterial disease** (PAD).[4]
   2. In high-income countries, prevalence by sex is approximately 1:1 and increases continuously with age from 5.3% to 5.4% between ages 45 and 49 years to 13.7% to 14.1% between ages 75 and 79 years.

B. Pathophysiology/etiology
   1. Most commonly a chronic inflammatory condition due to atherosclerotic change of the arterial intima and media that predominantly affects the lower (vs upper) extremities.
      a. Leads to luminal narrowing in the affected vessel.

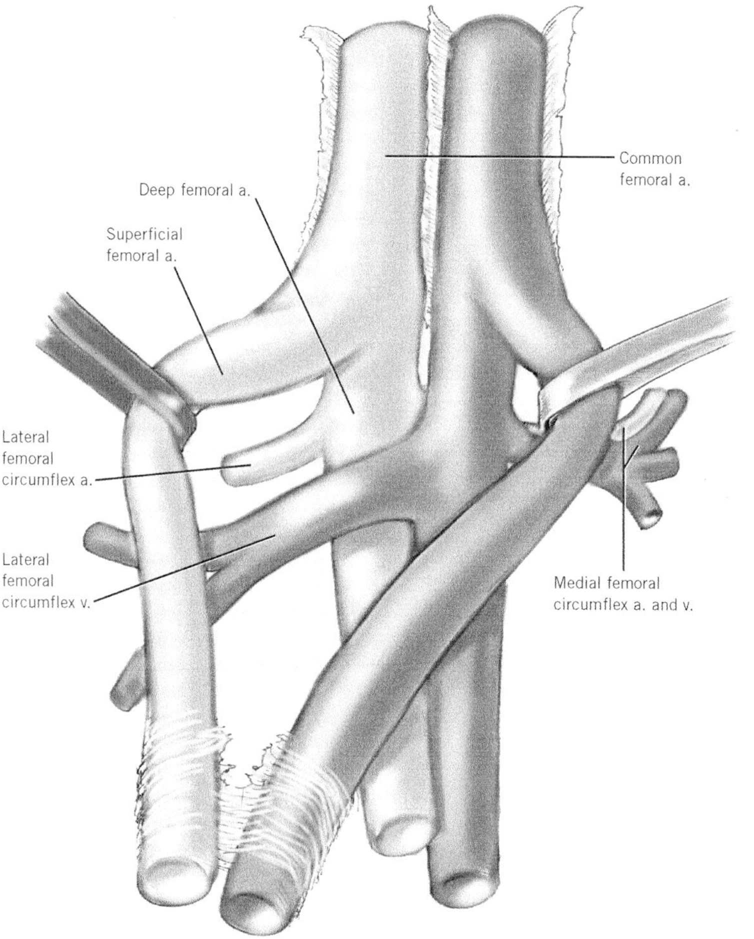

FIGURE 36.3 Profunda femoris exposure (right leg). *(Reprinted with permission from Valentine RJ, Wind GG, eds. Common femoral artery. In: Anatomic Exposures in Vascular Surgery. 4th ed. Wolters Kluwer; 2021:375-411. Figure 16-14.)*

b. Symptoms arise when tissue demand for oxygen/nutrients exceeds the delivery capacity of the involved vessel.

2. **Atherosclerosis** itself is a systemic illness; patients with PAD often have disease in other arterial beds, particularly the coronary arteries.
   a. A large percentage of postoperative mortality for peripheral arterial reconstructions for atherosclerotic disease is cardiac in nature.

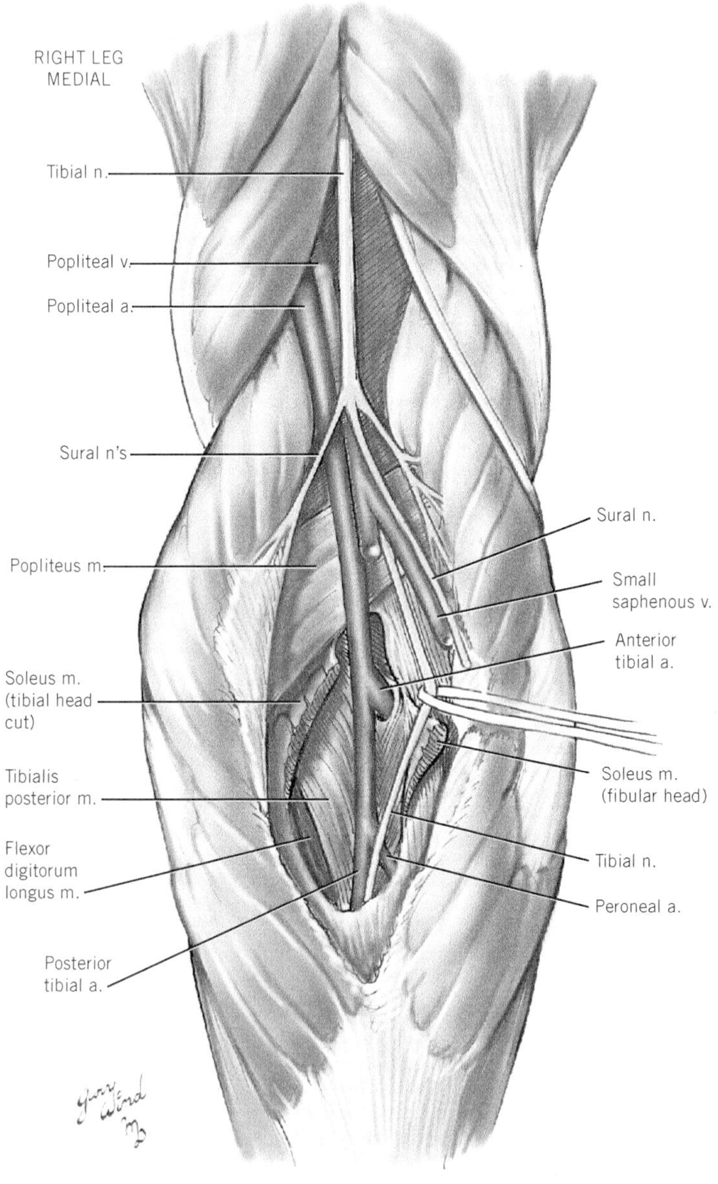

FIGURE 36.4 Posterior view of the (right) popliteal fossa and its contents. *(Reprinted with permission from Valentine RJ, Wind GG, eds. Vessels of the leg. In: Anatomic Exposures in Vascular Surgery. 4th ed. Wolters Kluwer; 2021:469-524. Figure 19-20.)*

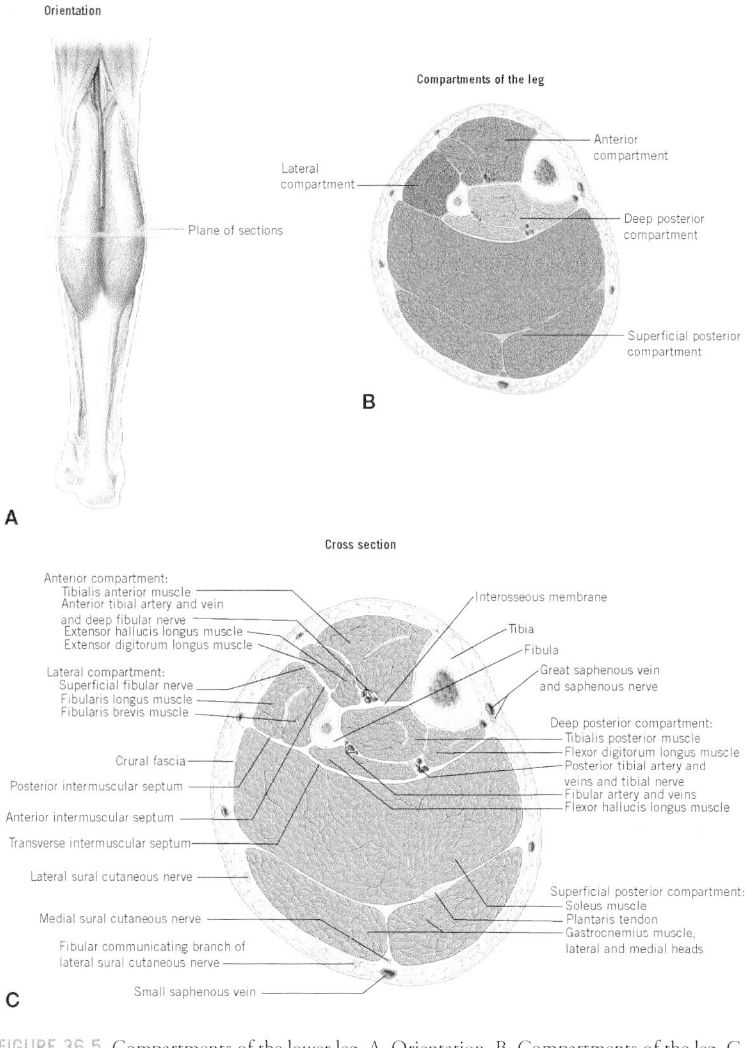

FIGURE 36.5 Compartments of the lower leg. A, Orientation. B, Compartments of the leg. C, Cross section. *(Reprinted with permission from Gest TR, ed. The lower limb. In: Lippincott® Atlas of Anatomy. 2nd ed. Wolters Kluwer; 2020:96-175. Plate 3-32.)*

b. Patients with PAD need preoperative assessment and (in nonemergent situations) optimization of cardiac disease.

3. The most important risk factors for atherosclerotic PAD are current or former cigarette smoking, history of other cardiovascular disease (e.g., coronary artery disease [CAD], congestive heart failure, stroke), diabetes

mellitus, dyslipidemia, hypertension, and/or hyperhomocystinemia (serum homocysteine >15 μM/L).

a. Current smoking and cardiovascular disease are estimated to each approximately triple the odds of having PAD.[4]

b. Diabetes doubles the odds of PAD.[4]

4. Other less common etiologies of PAD include fibromuscular dysplasia, radiation-induced vascular injury, and vasculitis (e.g., Takayasu arteritis and Buerger disease [thromboangiitis obliterans]).

5. PAD is a chronic disease that can progress to being limb-threatening both in the acute and chronic setting.

III. ACUTE ARTERIAL OCCLUSION OF THE EXTREMITY

A. Etiology

1. The most common cause of acute arterial insufficiency is **embolization**.

a. Cardiac sources account for >70% of emboli.

i. Usually the result of mural thrombi that develop due to arrhythmias such as **atrial fibrillation**

ii. Other cardiac sources include cardiac aneurysms following myocardial infarction (MI), valvular heart disease, prosthetic heart valves (particularly mechanical), bacterial endocarditis, and atrial myxoma.

b. Arterial emboli

i. Can result from ulcerated atheroma or aneurysms, rarely from abdominal aortic aneurysms

ii. Can also be iatrogenic secondary to plaque disruption by catheter-based intervention

iii. Upper extremity ischemia can be secondary to arterial thoracic outlet syndrome, in which the first rib or an anomalous cervical rib or band causes compression of the subclavian artery with subsequent poststenotic dilation and mural thrombus formation.

c. Venous emboli (**paradoxical emboli**) can reach the arterial system via an **intracardiac shunt** (e.g., patent foramen ovale) or **intrapulmonary arteriovenous malformations** (e.g., Osler–Weber–Rendu syndrome).

2. Other causes of acute ischemia include arterial thrombosis, aortic dissection, venous outflow obstruction, a low-flow state (i.e., low cardiac output/hypovolemia), and trauma.

3. Acute arterial insufficiency secondary to trauma may be direct or indirect.

a. **Direct arterial trauma:** Frequently obvious but may initially be occult (e.g., an intimal flap or arterial wall hematoma may later progress to arterial stenosis or occlusion).

b. **Indirect trauma:** Due to compression by joint dislocations (e.g., popliteal artery due to posterior knee dislocation), bone fragments (e.g., tibial plateau fracture), or compartment syndrome.

B. Presentation

1. Presentation of acute arterial ischemia includes the "**six Ps**": Pain, pallor, pulselessness, paresthesias, poikilothermia (cold extremity), and paralysis.

a. Pulselessness, paresthesias, and paralysis are late findings, the latter two particularly indicating the window for possible revascularization has been missed.
b. Irreversible changes may appear as early as 4 to 6 hours after onset of ischemia, although patients with chronic PAD may have developed collateral circulation, in which case it may take somewhat longer for progression to irreversible damage.

2. Occasionally difficult to discern etiology of ischemia symptoms, between acute embolus of a relatively healthy artery and acute thrombosis of an already compromised vessel.
   a. Palpable contralateral pulses and absence of claudication history suggest the former.
3. **Blue toe syndrome** occurs in patients with microemboli from unstable proximal arterial plaques, characterized by intact pulses and painful ischemic lesions in the distal lower extremity.

C. Diagnosis

1. **Nontraumatic acute arterial ischemia**
   a. Clinical categorization as determined via the **Rutherford classification** directs options and timing for management (**Table 36.1**).
   b. **CT angiography** (CTA): Provides rapid diagnostic confirmation and anatomic details critical for operative planning.
      i. Delayed sequences needed to visualize arteries beyond the level of occlusion
      ii. Distinguishing features of embolic (vs thrombotic) occlusions
         a) More likely seen at arterial bifurcations
         b) Concave shadow formed at interface with contrast
         c) Important distinction as embolic patients will need systemic anticoagulation and, if no known embolic source/risk factor, workup for source/hypercoagulable state
   c. Intraoperative angiography can be used to verify occlusion clearance.
2. **Traumatic acute arterial ischemia**
   a. Associated with penetrating trauma, long bone fractures, and/or joint dislocations.
   b. Presence of hard vs soft signs of vascular injury determines need for further evaluation and urgency of intervention.
      i. Hard signs
         a) Include diminished/absent pulses distal to injury, ischemia distal to injury, visible arterial (pulsatile) bleeding, bruit at or distal to the injury, large/expanding/pulsatile hematomas.
         b) Require proceeding directly to operative intervention.
      ii. Soft signs
         a) Anatomic proximity of a wound to a major vessel, injury to an anatomically related nerve, unexplained hemorrhagic shock, moderately sized/nonexpanding hematoma
         b) Require continued evaluation with physical and Doppler examination of pulses and blood pressure (BP) comparison with contralateral limb (i.e., **ankle-brachial index** [ABI])

TABLE 36.1 Rutherford Classification: Clinical Categories of Acute Limb Ischemia

			Clinical Findings		Doppler Signals	
	Category	Prognosis	Sensory Loss	Muscle Weakness	Arterial	Venous
I	**Viable**	Not immediately threatened	None	None	Audible	Audible
II	**Threatened**					
a	**Marginally**	Salvageable if promptly treated	Minimal (toes) or none	None	Inaudible	Audible
b	**Immediately**	Salvageable with immediate revascularization	More than toes, associated with rest pain	Mild, moderate	Inaudible	Audible
III	**Irreversible**	Major tissue loss or permanent nerve damage inevitable	Profound, anesthetic	Profound, paralysis (rigor)	Inaudible	Inaudible

Adapted from Rutherford RB, Baker JD, Ernst C, et al. Recommended standards for reports dealing with lower extremity ischemia: revised version. *J Vasc Surg.* 1997;26(3):517-538. Copyright 1997, Society for Vascular Surgery and International Society for Cardiovascular Surgery, North American Chapter. With permission

c. Check ABIs for lower extremity trauma, brachial-brachial index (BBI) for upper extremity, making sure to measure BP in the affected limb *distal* to the injury.
   i. Calculate individual leg ABI by dividing the ankle BP by uninjured arm brachial BP and then compare ABIs of the affected and nonaffected limbs.
   ii. BBI: Divide the BP of the affected arm by the unaffected arm brachial BP.
   iii. Indicates need for arterial imaging (CTA/angiography) or operative exploration:
      a) >10% to 20% difference in ABIs
      b) BBI < 0.8 to 0.9
d. Ultrasound duplex scan of the injured area can be useful in the diagnosis of intimal flap, pseudoaneurysm (PSA), and/or arterial or venous thrombi.

D. Management
1. Management of acute arterial ischemia is uniformly operative (unless the patient is not expected to survive).
2. Once the diagnosis of acute arterial ischemia is made in the nontraumatic setting, **intravenous heparin** should be administered immediately.
   a. Goal is to maintain partial thromboplastin time between 60 and 80 seconds. Bolus of 80 U/kg followed by infusion of 18 U/kg/h is usually sufficient.
   b. If associated with trauma, risk of bleeding from other traumatic injuries (e.g., intercranial bleed) must be taken into account when making decision to anticoagulate.
3. Operative management of nontraumatic acute arterial ischemia
   a. **Surgical approach: Femoral cut-down**
      i. Longitudinal or horizontal incision can be made in the groin, usually longitudinal (better facilitates exposure of both the CFA and the PFA/SFA, especially with extensive extent of atherosclerosis).
      ii. Dissect soft tissue until femoral sheath is encountered, being careful to ligate lymphatics to avoid postoperative lymphocele.
      iii. Open the femoral sheath longitudinally.
      iv. Circumferentially dissect the CFA, with dissection extending proximally to the superficial epigastric artery medially and the superficial circumflex iliac artery laterally, and extending distally to the CFA bifurcation into the SFA/PFA.
      v. Control the CFA proximally and distally with vessel loops.
   b. **Surgical approach: Femoral thromboembolectomy**
      i. Check distal (PT and dorsalis pedis) and popliteal Doppler signals for a baseline comparator.
      ii. Perform femoral cut-down (see above). Circumferentially dissect the proximal segments of the SFA and PFA and obtain distal control via vessel loops (proximal control already obtained via vessel loop around proximal CFA).

iii. Patient should already be heparinized, but can give an additional bolus of intravenous heparin (100 U/kg) as needed. Make an arteriotomy in the CFA—transverse for an artery with little to no atherosclerotic burden, longitudinal for a diseased artery (femoral endarterectomy or femoral to distal bypass may be required in a heavily diseased artery, not described here).

iv. Use an appropriately sized (#3 or 4) **Fogarty (balloon) catheter** to remove thromboembolus from the PFA and SFA, with multiple passes as needed to ensure good back-bleeding.

v. Pass a Fogarty catheter retrograde into the EIA and remove thromboembolus from the EIA and CFA, with multiple passes as needed to ensure good pulsatile flow.

vi. Close the arteriotomy—primarily with fine Prolene sutures for a transverse arteriotomy and with patch angioplasty for longitudinal arteriotomy.

vii. Check distal and popliteal Doppler signals.

a) If triphasic/significantly improved, complete the operation (ensure hemostasis, close skin and soft tissue in layers, perform four-compartment fasciotomy if indicated by duration of ischemia/examination).

b) If absent/weak, an attempt can be made to resolve possible postembolectomy vasospasm with intra-arterial infusion of 200 μg nitroglycerin. If this is not successful, perform antegrade angiography via the CFA. If a distal occlusion is identified (e.g., distal popliteal), perform the anatomically appropriate distal cut-down incision/dissection and perform catheter-thromboembolectomy (as above). Once triphasic/significantly improved Doppler signals are achieved, complete the operation as described above.

c. Due to the irreversible tissue damage, the only treatment option for Rutherford class III acute arterial ischemia is **amputation** (or palliative care; see section on chronic PAD for more information on amputation).

d. Thrombolytic therapy and **pharmacomechanical thrombectomy** may be useful in patients with clearly viable extremities and in whom thrombosis is the likely etiology.

i. Thrombolysis and follow-up angiography frequently can identify an underlying stenosis that may be treated by balloon angioplasty/stent or by open surgical intervention.

ii. Commonly used thrombolytic agents, such as alteplase, are instilled through an intra-arterial perfusion catheter positioned within the thrombosed vessel; these agents are also commonly used in conjunction with percutaneous mechanical thrombectomy for large clot burdens.

e. Follow-up care after reperfusion of nontraumatic acute ischemia is usually directed at treating the underlying cause of the obstruction.

i. Patients with mural thrombi or arrhythmias will require long-term anticoagulation.

   ii. The in-hospital mortality rate associated with embolectomy is as high as 30%.

4. Operative management of traumatic acute arterial ischemia
   a. Vascular management in the setting of multiple associated injuries
      i. Traumatic extremity arterial injuries often seen in the context of other acute (orthopedic/neurologic) injuries, so management timing and approach have to take management of these other injuries into account.
      ii. If associated with **joint dislocation**, should be reduced and the involved artery and distal perfusion reassessed (pulse examination, ABI, CTA), as reduction may resolve extrinsic arterial compression/obstruction and therefore alleviate the need for arterial reconstruction.
         a) Frequent vascular examinations are needed within the first 24 hours to ensure operative arterial repair is not required.
      iii. In the presence of coexistent operative orthopedic injuries, operative steps should proceed as follows:
         a) First, reestablish arterial flow by direct repair, bypass grafting, or temporary shunting.
            1) For temporary shunting, Doppler examination to assess shunt patency needs to be repeatedly performed throughout the case.
         b) Once orthopedic repair is complete, arterial repair should be reexamined to ensure that it has not been disrupted and that it is correctly fashioned to the final bone length (i.e., not on undue tension).
   b. Key steps of repair
      i. The uninjured leg or other potential vein harvest site should be prepared and included in the sterile field in case a conduit is required.
      ii. Essential to obtain proximal and distal control of the injured artery before exploring the hematoma/wound.
      iii. After debridement of devitalized arterial tissue, end-to-end reanastomosis is preferred over use of a conduit if there is adequate length to create an anastomosis without tension. Proximal and distal arteries can be mobilized to increase available length.
      iv. When an interposition graft is necessary, **autologous vein** is preferred over **cryopreserved cadaveric vein** (e.g., CryoVein) or **polytetrafluoroethylene** (PTFE).
      v. Significant vasospasm is often seen and may result in diminished/absent distal pulses or inadequate Doppler signals even after adequate arterial repair. If this is suspected, a completion angiogram should be performed to interrogate/document distal flow.
   c. Artery-specific concepts
      i. Arteries that should be repaired: Subclavian, axillary, brachial, CFA, SFA, PFA, popliteal
      ii. Arteries that can be ligated

a) Radial <u>or</u> ulnar artery, only if the other vessel is intact and the hand is well perfused
b) A single tibial artery (PT, AT, peroneal) can be ligated if *at least* one other tibial artery is intact and the foot is well perfused.

E. Complications

1. Reperfusion injury
   a. Results from the formation of oxygen-free radicals that directly damage tissue and cause white blood cell accumulation and sequestration in the microcirculation.
   b. Can lead to significant swelling and, particularly in the extremities, can lead to compartment syndrome as muscle swells within relatively limited fascial compartments.
   c. Should be low threshold to perform fasciotomies at the time of revascularization.
2. **Compartment syndrome**
   a. Results when prolonged ischemia and delayed reperfusion cause cell membrane damage and leakage of fluid into the interstitium.
   b. Additional muscle and nerve necrosis occurs when the intracompartmental pressures exceed **capillary perfusion pressure** (generally >30 mm Hg), leading to ischemia.
   c. Compartment syndrome is more common in the distal extremity, i.e., lower leg and forearm.
      i. In these areas, **fasciotomies** should be performed prophylactically when there is concern for the *possibility* of developing compartment syndrome, given the high morbidity of delayed treatment.
      ii. *Fasciotomy should be routinely considered in any patient with >6 hours of acute extremity ischemia, or in the presence of combined arterial and venous injuries.*
   d. Thigh compartment syndrome is rare and thigh fasciotomies are less commonly indicated, likely given that the larger size of these compartments are able to accommodate more swelling prior to development of compressive ischemia.
   e. **Surgical approach: Lower leg two-incision four-compartment fasciotomy (Figure 36.6)**
      i. Lateral incision: Anterior and lateral compartments
         a) On the lateral aspect of the lower leg, make a longitudinal skin incision parallel and 3 cm lateral to the tibia, starting two finger breadths inferior to the fibular head (being careful to avoid the superficial fibular nerve) and ending at the level of the ankle.
         b) Deepen the incision to the level of the fascia and develop skin flaps anteriorly and laterally.
         c) Create a horizontal incision in the fascia to ensure accurate identification of the anterior intermuscular septum (between anterior and lateral compartments)—this is important to ensure *both* compartments are opened.

d) Create longitudinal incisions the length of the skin incision in the fascia overlying both compartments, 1 cm anterior and 1 cm posterior to the intermuscular septum, creating an "H" with the previous horizontal incision.

ii. Medial incision: Superficial and deep posterior compartments

a) On the medial aspect of the lower leg, make a longitudinal skin incision parallel and one finger breadth posterior to the posterior border of the tibia—being careful to avoid the GSV and nerve—starting a few centimeters below the knee and ending 5 cm above the ankle (avoiding injury to the PT).

b) Deepen the incision until the fascia is identified.

c) Develop skin flaps anteriorly and posteriorly; create a longitudinal incision in the superficial fascia over the gastrocnemius muscle to release the superficial posterior compartment.

d) Divide soleus muscle attachments from the posterior tibia to release the deep posterior compartment.

1) Deep posterior is the most common compartment missed/incompletely opened during fasciotomy.

2) Adequate fasciotomy should expose the posterior tibial neurovascular bundle.

iii. Ensure hemostasis, cover exposed muscle with nonadherent dressing, plan for second-stage skin-closure when appropriate.

3. **Rhabdomyolysis**

a. Reperfusion releases the by-products of ischemic muscle, including potassium, lactic acid, myoglobin, and creatine phosphokinase.

b. The electrolyte and pH changes that occur can trigger dangerous arrhythmias, and precipitation of myoglobin in the renal tubules can cause pigment nephropathy and acute renal failure.

c. The likelihood of developing these complications relates to the duration of ischemia and the muscle mass at risk.

d. Management of rhabdomyolysis is generally supportive and aimed at mitigating renal impairment and consists of aggressive hydration, diuresis, and IV infusion of bicarbonate to alkalinize the urine.

IV. CHRONIC ARTERIAL AND ATHERO-OCCLUSIVE DISEASE

A. Distribution

1. Lower extremities are most frequently affected by chronic occlusive disease, although upper extremity disease can occur.

2. Lower extremity disease is subdivided into three anatomic sections with differences in presentation and management, although all levels of disease can be present in a single patient:

a. "Inflow"/**aortoiliac occlusive disease**: Affects the infrarenal aorta, CIA, and EIA.

b. "Outflow"/**femoral–popliteal occlusive disease**: Affects the CFA, SFA, and popliteal artery.

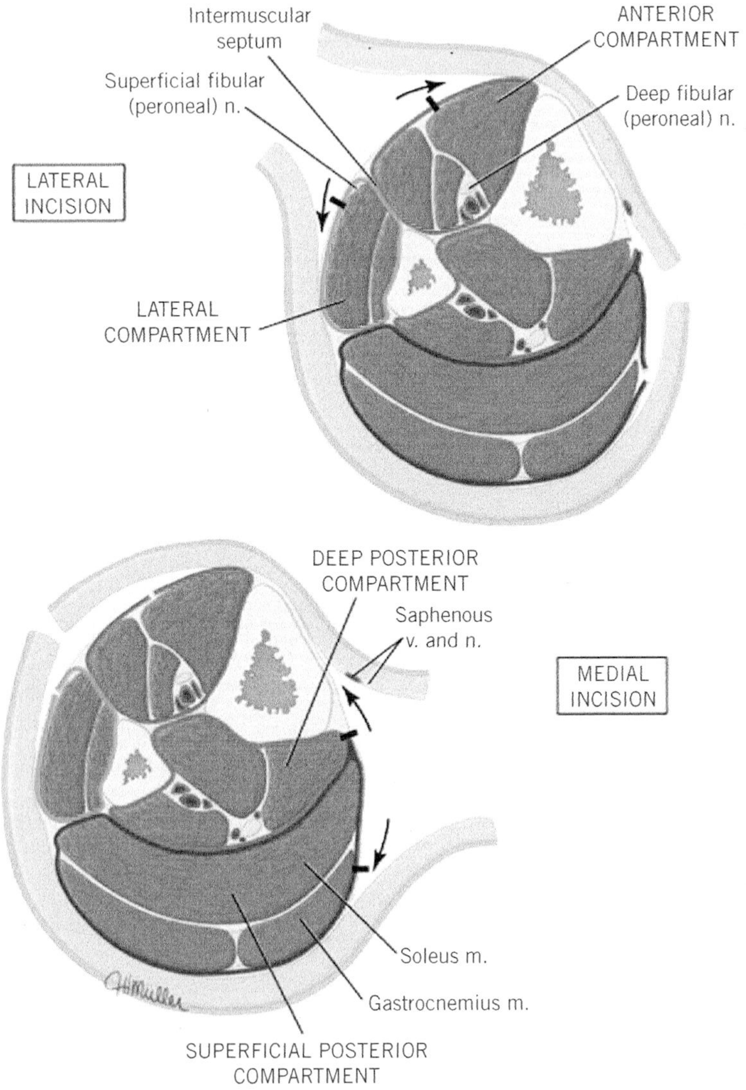

FIGURE 36.6 Anatomical diagram of two-incision four-compartment fasciotomy of the lower leg. The four compartments are outlined in color; arrows represent subcutaneous flaps developed to gain access to the compartments; thick black lines indicate approximate locations of the fascial incisions for each compartment. *(Reproduced with permission from Hammerberg EM. Acute Compartment Syndrome of the Extremities. In: UpToDate, Post TW (ed.), UpToDate. Accessed March 20, 2023. Copyright 2023, UpToDate, Inc. and its affiliates and/or licensors. All rights reserved.)*

c. "Run-off"/**tibial–peroneal disease**: Affects the vessels distal to the popliteal artery.

3. Upper extremity disease most commonly affects the proximal subclavian artery, followed by the axillary and brachial arteries.

B. Presentation

1. Variable and depends on the degree and location of disease.
   a. Asymptomatic in early stages.
   b. In intermediate stages, commonly presents with **intermittent claudication**: Pain related to activity, occurs after a predictable/reproducible amount of exercise (e.g., pain when walking three or more blocks), and resolves with rest.
   c. **Chronic limb-threatening ischemia** (CLTI): Advanced disease leads to rest pain, nonhealing wounds, and tissue loss.
2. Aortoiliac disease
   a. Claudication of the hip, thigh, or buttock. May coexist with femoral–popliteal disease, contributing to more distal symptoms as well.
   b. Symptoms usually develop gradually; sudden worsening suggests acute thrombosis of a diseased vessel.
   c. Patients ultimately develop incapacitating claudication, but not rest pain unless distal disease is also present.
   d. **Leriche syndrome**: Constellation of symptoms (sexual impotence, buttock and leg claudication, leg musculature atrophy, trophic changes of the feet, and leg pallor) that results from the gradual occlusion of the terminal aorta
3. Femoral–popliteal and tibial–peroneal disease
   a. Claudication of the lower extremity, usually most prominent in the calf
   b. In femoral–popliteal or tibial–peroneal CLTI, rest pain is a burning pain in the distal foot, exacerbated by limb elevation, and is often relieved by placing the leg in a dependent position.
   c. Common examination findings
      i. Decreased or absent distal pulses
      ii. **Dependent rubor**
      iii. **Trophic changes** that include thickening of the nails, loss of leg hair, shiny skin, and ulceration at the tips of the toes
4. Upper extremity
   a. Symptomatic arterial occlusive disease of the upper extremity is relatively rare.
   b. Typical presentation: Arm claudication or finger-hand ischemia/necrosis
   c. **Subclavian steal**
      i. Can result when an occlusive subclavian artery lesion is located proximal to the origin of the vertebral artery.
      ii. With exercise of the affected limb, the arm's demand for blood is supplied by retrograde flow in the ipsilateral vertebral artery, shunting blood from the posterior cerebral circulation.
      iii. Results in drop attacks (sudden fall while walking/standing *without* loss of consciousness), ataxia, sensory loss, and/or diplopia.

C. Diagnosis
1. Goal is to determine presence of significant flow-limiting lesions and distinguish chronic arterial occlusive disease from other mimicking conditions.
2. Key examination findings
   a. Proximal and distal pulses must be examined at rest and after exercise.
      i. Stenosis may manifest as palpable pulses at rest that are absent after exercise.
   b. Absence of femoral pulses is indicative of aortoiliac disease.
   c. Bruits may be heard over lower abdomen or femoral vessels.
   d. Tissue loss/ulcers
      i. **Arterial insufficiency ulcers** are usually painful and have a pale appearance.
      ii. **Neuropathic ulcers** are painless and usually occur over bony prominences, particularly the plantar aspect of the metatarsophalangeal joints.
      iii. **Venous stasis ulcers** are located on the distal calves and perimalleolar region ("gaiter" distribution) and are dark and irregular in shape (see Chapter 37).
3. Doppler waveforms and ABI
   a. Segmental arterial Doppler readings with waveforms help to localize the level of disease and the severity of obstruction.
   b. ABI allows quantification of the degree of peripheral arterial flow:
      i. No vascular disease (normal ABI): 1.0
      ii. ABI < 0.8 is consistent with claudication
      iii. ABI < 0.4 is typically seen in patients with rest pain
   c. Patients with history of claudication and normal resting waveforms require postexercise ABI measurements.
   d. In patients with diabetes and/or renal insufficiency, calcified vessels can result in a falsely elevated ABI measurement.
      i. Digit pressures are less affected by calcification and thus often provide a more accurate representation of arterial perfusion.
      ii. Toe pressures < 50 mm Hg consistent with CLTI
4. Imaging
   a. Digital subtraction arteriography
      i. Gold standard for evaluating the arterial tree before planned revascularization
      ii. Typical digital subtraction arteriography of the lower extremities extends from the proximal abdomen to the toes.
      iii. Can be performed with carbon dioxide contrast when iodinated contrast will not be tolerated (requires a specialized injection system).
   b. CTA and magnetic resonance angiography (MRA) have also gained widespread use.
      i. CTA requires iodinated contrast.
      ii. Diffuse calcifications may make CTA interpretation difficult.

iii. MRA is especially useful for evaluating distal tibial patency but may overestimate the degree of stenosis, cannot assess degree of calcification, and is inaccurate in previously stented arteries.

D. Nonoperative management

1. **Risk factor modification** is the most important intervention to reduce progression of PAD via optimal medical management of diabetes, hypertension, and hyperlipidemia, in addition to smoking cessation, weight management, and involvement with an exercise program.[6]
   a. Blood pressure goals are <140/90 mm Hg generally and <130/80 mm Hg in patients with diabetes or renal insufficiency.[7]
   b. Treatment of hyperlipidemia is largely aimed at prevention of cardiac morbidity/mortality given association of PAD and CAD.
      i. High-intensity statin is indicated for symptomatic PAD.[8]
      ii. Recommended LDL levels[9] are <100 mg/dL generally and <70 mg/dL in those with atherosclerotic disease in two or more vascular beds.
   c. **Dual antiplatelet therapy** to reduce the risk of MI or stroke:
      i. Daily **aspirin** therapy (81 mg or 325 mg; inhibits platelet aggregation) recommended for all patients
      ii. **Clopidogrel**[10] (inhibits platelet aggregation)
      iii. **Cilostazol**
         a) A type III phosphodiesterase inhibitor that inhibits platelet aggregation and causes vasodilation.
         b) Associated with improved amputation-free survival, limb salvage rate, decreased repeat revascularization, and restenosis.[11]
         c) Contraindicated in New York Heart Association class III or IV heart failure.
      iv. **Rivaroxaban** (2.5 mg)
         a) A factor Xa inhibitor
         b) Low-dose rivaroxaban and aspirin have been shown to reduce composite outcome of acute limb ischemia, amputations, MI, stroke, and death.[12]

E. Operative management

1. Indicated for
   a. CLTI
   b. Incapacitating claudication that jeopardizes a patient's livelihood, daily activities, or quality of life and that has not adequately improved with risk factor modification and exercise therapy
2. Society for Vascular Surgery (SVS) Lower Extremity Threatened Limb Classification System **WIfI (Wound, Ischemia, and foot Infection) classification** uses the severity of limb ischemia, wound complexity, and foot infection to estimate the likelihood of limb salvage in patients with CLTI.[13]
3. SVS, European Society of Vascular Surgery, and World Federation of Vascular Societies issued joint Global Vascular Guidelines on the Management of CLTI, including the **Global Limb Anatomic Staging System** (GLASS).[14]
   a. Based on level and extent of disease (as assessed by angiography)

   b. Serves as a tool for defining the preferred target artery path (selected on the basis of the least diseased artery) and choosing a revascularization strategy.
4. Endovascular options are particularly useful in treating short-segment stenoses, while long-segment occlusions are better addressed by open techniques.[7]
5. The Bypass versus Angioplasty in Severe Ischemia of the Leg (BASIL) trial showed that outcomes were worse for patients who underwent angioplasty followed by salvage bypass surgery rather than a bypass-first approach.[15]
   a. Good surgical candidates with complex anatomic lesions—in particular, those possessing good venous conduit—should be considered for open reconstruction.
   b. Endovascular intervention is the preferred approach for the medically compromised patient, particularly those lacking autologous venous conduit.
6. Hybrid open/endovascular procedures are frequently utilized in the treatment of CLTI with excellent results and combine best aspects of both approaches to tailor a plan best suited for the unique needs of an individual patient (**Figure 36.7**).
7. Preoperative management must include cardiac assessment and optimization and should also include a multidisciplinary evaluation for the goal of limb preservation (e.g., podiatry, vascular surgery, plastic surgery).
8. Open surgical therapy
   a. Intraoperative anticoagulation: Generally, unfractionated heparin (80-100 U/kg) is administered shortly before cross-clamping and supplemented as necessary until cross-clamps are removed.
      i. Goal: Activated clotting time >250 seconds
      ii. Can be reversed with **protamine** at the end of the case.
      iii. For patients with history of heparin-induced thrombocytopenia, use a **direct thrombin inhibitor** such as bivalirudin.
   b. Aortoiliac disease
      i. **Aortobifemoral bypass grafting**
         a) Treatment of choice in low-risk patients with diffuse aortoiliac stenoses/occlusions
         b) May be performed via transperitoneal or retroperitoneal approach.
         c) Distal endarterectomy and/or profundaplasty may be performed in conjunction with a bypass to improve outflow.
         d) Results are excellent, with reported patency rates of up to 95% at 5 years.
      ii. **Axillobifemoral bypass**
         a) A less-invasive alternative for high-risk patients, in whom bilateral lower extremity revascularization is needed.
         b) Shorter procedure time, avoids need for intra-abdominal (peritoneal/retroperitoneal) dissection or aortic cross-clamping.

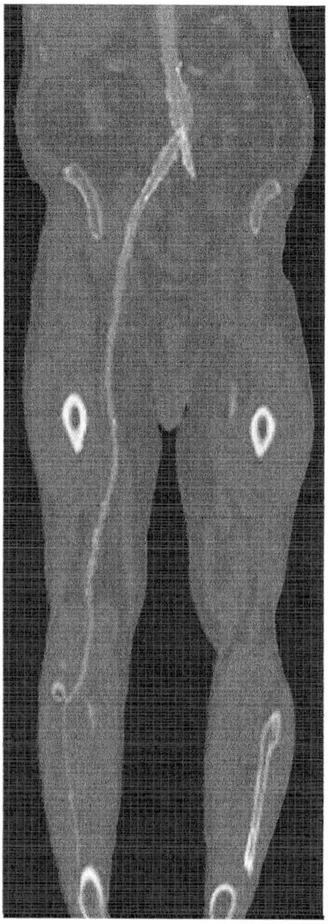

FIGURE 36.7 Extensive PAD, with left iliac chronic total occlusion (CTO). Aortoiliac GLASS classification IIB (CTO of the CIA and EIA, significant CFA disease) and infrainguinal GLASS stage III (SFA CTO > 20 cm, popliteal CTO). This patient underwent hybrid approach with shockwave lithotripsy, patch angioplasty, and balloon angioplasty with stent placement.

c) Can also be used in the setting of an infected field, where an extra-anatomic bypass is required.

iii. Femorofemoral bypass

a) Alternative in high-risk patients with unilateral iliac disease

b) Patency rates lower than aortounifemoral bypass, but better tolerated

iv. Aortoiliac endarterectomy

a) Use is now uncommon; considered for patients who have disease localized to the distal aorta and CIAs.

b) Advantages include avoidance of prosthetic material and preservation of antegrade flow into the internal iliac arteries.

c. Femoral, popliteal, and tibial occlusive disease
   i. **Femoral-above-knee-popliteal bypass** used for patients with SFA occlusion
   ii. **Femoral-distal bypass** used for patients with disease below the knee, with the distal anastomosis to the below-knee popliteal, PT, AT, or peroneal arteries
   iii. Pedal arteries can be used as a distal target if all tibial arteries are occluded.
   iv. The proximal anastomosis of the above grafts is generally at the CFA, but more distal sites can be used provided they receive unobstructed flow (e.g., SFA, above-knee-popliteal).
   v. **Graft material options**
      a) Best is autologous vein.
         1) Single-segment GSV is the conduit of choice.
         2) Lesser saphenous vein or arm veins can also be used (may need multiple segments).
         3) GSV can be used either in situ or in reversed orientation. *In situ* advantages are that (1) the vein's nutrient supply is left intact and (2) the vein orientation allows for a better size match. The disadvantage of in situ is that mechanical valve lysis (and resultant endothelial trauma) is necessary to allow for reversed flow.
      b) If autologous vein is not available, PTFE or cryopreserved vein can be used.
         1) PTFE patency rates for above-knee grafts approach those of autogenous vein but are substantially lower than those of below-the-knee grafts.
         2) PTFE is only used for below-the-knee grafts in patients with CLTI with no autogenous option.
         3) Use of a small cuff of vein (**Miller cuff**) or patch angioplasty (**Taylor patch**) at the distal anastomosis with a PTFE graft may improve patency.
         4) Cryopreserved vein is typically reserved for infected fields.
   vi. Endarterectomy is most commonly used for severe stenosis/occlusion of the CFA and PFA.

d. **Deep venous arterialization**
   i. Used for patients with CLTI with "**desert foot**" (all main pedal arteries occluded, with only collateral flow to the foot) with limited tissue loss/rest pain.
   ii. Involves connection between a proximal artery and a distal vein with disruption of vein valves in the foot.
   iii. Recent analyses have shown success in limb salvage.[16]

e. **Amputation**
   i. Reserved for patients with gangrene or persistent painful ischemia not amenable to vascular reconstruction. These patients often have severe coexistent vascular and cardiovascular disease,

and the survival rate for patients undergoing major amputations is approximately 50% at 3 years and 30% at 5 years.

ii. Level of amputation is determined clinically, with the goals of
- **a)** Ensuring adequate blood supply for healing
- **b)** Removing all infected tissue
- **c)** Preserving as much length of the extremity as possible to improve the patient's opportunity for rehabilitation

iii. Digital amputations are performed for isolated gangrene and/or recalcitrant osteomyelitis.

iv. **Transmetatarsal amputation** is usually performed when several toes are involved or after previous single-digit amputations.

v. **Below-knee amputation** (BKA) is the most common type of amputation performed for patients with severe occlusive disease.

vi. **Above-knee amputation** heals more easily than BKA and is useful in nonambulatory patients.

vii. **Hip disarticulation** is rarely performed for vascular disease.

f. Surgical approach: BKA

i. Mark the planned incision: Transversely across the anterior lower leg 10 to 12 cm below the tibial tuberosity and extending medially and laterally for half to two-thirds of the circumference of the leg, then for the posterior flap mark longitudinally and distally for 13 to 15 cm on the medial and lateral aspects of the leg, connecting the two lines with a soft curve. Perform the skin incision.

ii. Divide the fascia and muscle in the anterior and lateral compartments; ligate and divide the AT vascular bundle and the deep and superficial fibular nerves.

iii. Transect the tibia at the level of the anterior skin incision, and the fibula 1 to 2 cm proximally.

iv. Detach the posterior muscular tissue from the bone to form the posterior muscle flap. Divide the fascia and muscle in the posterior compartments at the level of the posterior flap incision, ligating the PT and peroneal vascular bundles and the tibial and sural nerves. Remove the specimen from the field (send to pathology).

v. Irrigate, obtain hemostasis, smooth the transected bone, particularly rounding the anterior aspect of the tibial transection.

vi. Approximate the fascia of the anterior/lateral compartments and the posterior muscle flap with interrupted absorbable sutures. Close the skin with staples or interrupted nylon sutures.

vii. Dress and wrap the amputation site and place the leg in a well-padded splint/knee immobilizer to prevent flexion contracture at the knee, which will limit subsequent mobility/ability to fit a prosthesis.

g. Proximal subclavian disease
   i. Choice of bypass depends primarily on the patency of the ipsilateral common carotid artery (CCA; see Figure 34.1).
   ii. If ipsilateral CCA is patent
      a) **Carotid–subclavian bypass** is performed through a supraclavicular approach using a prosthetic graft (vein grafts are avoided).
      b) **Subclavian artery transposition** to ipsilateral CCA is an excellent alternative if anatomically feasible.
   iii. If ipsilateral CCA is occluded
      a) **Subclavian–subclavian bypass** is an extra-anatomic approach that uses a longer-segment prosthetic graft with reduced patency.

h. Postoperative complications
   i. Most early complications are secondary to preoperative comorbid disease (e.g., CAD/MI, congestive heart failure, pulmonary insufficiency, renal insufficiency).
   ii. Aortic revascularization
      a) Early complications occur in approximately 5% to 10% of patients, mainly due to comorbidities.
      b) Complications related directly to reconstruction include hemorrhage, embolization/thrombosis of the distal arterial tree, microembolization, ischemic colitis (see Chapter 35), ureteral injuries, impotence, paraplegia, and wound infection.
      c) Late complications include anastomotic PSA or graft dilation, graft limb occlusion, aortoenteric erosion or fistula, and graft infections.
   iii. Distal revascularizations
      a) Early graft thrombosis (within 30 days) most often results from technical errors, hypercoagulability, inadequate distal runoff, and/or postoperative hypotension.
      b) Technical errors include graft kinks, retained valve leaflets, valvulotome trauma, intimal flaps, significant residual arteriovenous fistulas, and/or the use of a poor-quality conduit.
   iv. Postoperative management and follow-up
      a) Distal pulses assessed regularly
      b) Twenty-four hours of perioperative antibiotics, longer with infected ulcers
      c) Perioperative antithrombotic therapy including aspirin (81-325 mg/d) for all infrainguinal reconstructions. If intolerant of aspirin, clopidogrel (75 mg/d) may be substituted.
      d) Anticoagulation is generally limited to grafts considered to be at a high risk for thrombosis.
      e) Early ambulation is encouraged; physical therapy is needed for patients who cannot immediately ambulate in order to gain strength and prevent contractures.

f) Any patient with a femoral anastomosis should avoid sitting with the hips flexed ≥90°.
g) Elevation of the leg while resting
h) Following major amputations (above the ankle), weight bearing is delayed for 4 to 6 weeks. Early consultation with a physical therapist and prosthetist is highly recommended.
i) Surveillance of bypass grafts
   1) Distal bypass grafts should undergo serial evaluations of patency by clinical examination and duplex ultrasound imaging.
   2) Less frequent follow-up is necessary for aortoiliac bypasses.
   3) Detection of severe stenosis predicts impending graft failure, and such grafts should undergo arteriography and correction.

9. Endovascular management
  a. See Chapter 33 for endovascular basics.
  b. Aortoiliac occlusive disease
    i. Short-segment stenoses (<3 cm) of the CIA and EIA have excellent long-term patency rates when treated with angioplasty alone or with stent placement. CIA patency is generally better than that of EIA.
    ii. Immediate angioplasty failure (defined as residual stenosis of ≥30%, residual mean translesional pressure gradient of ≥10 mm Hg, or flow-limiting dissection) is an indication for stent deployment.
  c. Infrainguinal occlusive disease
    i. Bare nitinol stents, drug-eluting stents, covered stents, and drug-coated balloons have been shown to improve long-term patency after angioplasty of femoral and popliteal arteries.
    ii. Paclitaxel-eluting and paclitaxel-coated balloons offer the best long-term results.[17]
    iii. The ZILVER PTX randomized controlled trial (RCT) of paclitaxel-eluting nitinol stents for femoropopliteal disease has shown superior 5-year patency rates compared with angioplasty alone or bare metal stent deployment.[18]
    iv. Plaque modification tools like atherectomy and lithotripsy are useful in select cases.
  d. Complications
    i. Include arterial dissection, vessel occlusion, arterial rupture, and distal embolization, which may result in the need for open intervention or amputation.
    ii. Complications at the puncture site include hematoma, PSA, or retroperitoneal bleed.
    iii. In infrainguinal repair, bleeding and arteriovenous fistula can also be seen.
    iv. Early postoperative failure is usually due to **intimal hyperplasia**, whereas late failure may also be caused by progressive atherosclerosis.

Key References

Citation	Summary
BASIL Trial: Bradbury AW, Adam DJ, Bell J, et al. Bypass versus Angioplasty in Severe Ischaemia of the Leg (BASIL) trial: a survival prediction model to facilitate clinical decision making. *J Vasc Surg.* 2010;51(5 suppl):52S-68S.	• Multicenter (UK) RCT of 452 patients with CLTI randomized to either open revascularization or balloon angioplasty (with intention to treat analysis). • Showed long-term follow-up has an advantage in both overall survival and amputation-free survival in those patients who underwent bypass surgery and survived beyond 2 y. • Outcomes were worse for patients who underwent angioplasty followed by salvage bypass surgery, rather than bypass-first approach.
Zilver PTX Trial: Dake MD, Ansel GM, Jaff MR, et al. Durable clinical effectiveness with paclitaxel-eluting stents in the femoropopliteal artery: 5-year results of the zilver PTX randomized trial. *Circulation.* 2016;133(15):1472-1483.	• Multicenter international (Germany, Japan, US) RCT of 474 patients with symptomatic chronic femoral–popliteal arterial-occlusive disease were randomized to balloon angioplasty vs Zilver PTX paclitaxel-coated drug-eluting stent placement. Patients who had immediate balloon angioplasty failure were secondarily randomized to Zilver vs bare metal stent placement. • Paclitaxel-coated drug-eluting stent had superior 5-y patency rates compared with angioplasty alone or bare metal stent deployment.
VOYAGER PAD Trial: Bonaca MP, Bauersachs RM, Anand SS, et al. Rivaroxaban in peripheral artery disease after revascularization. *N Engl J Med.* 2020;382(21):1994-2004.	• Multicenter international (34 countries) double blind RCT of 6,564 patients with PAD who were randomized to aspirin plus placebo vs aspirin plus rivaroxaban within 10 d of revascularization • The rivaroxaban group had lower incidence of major amputation for vascular causes, MI, ischemic stroke, or death from cardiovascular causes.

CHAPTER 36: PERIPHERAL ARTERIAL DISEASE

Review Questions

1. A 47-year-old man with medical history of smoking, diabetes, hypertension, and hyperlipidemia presents with right calf claudication at six blocks of ambulation. He states that the symptoms do not hinder his desired activities. He has no skin breakdown/ulcers. ABIs are 0.6 on the right and 1.1 on the left. What is the appropriate initial management?
2. A patient who presented with an 18-hour history of acute-onset left leg pain and Rutherford class IIB ischemia underwent femoral embolectomy and now has palpable pedal pulses but tense calf muscles. What should you do next?
3. In a patient with posterior knee dislocation after a motor vehicle collision and concern for lower leg ischemia, what should initial management consist of?
4. At what duration of acute extremity ischemia should fasciotomy be routinely considered/performed?
5. What must you obtain before exploring a hematoma/wound associated with traumatic vascular injury?
6. Which Rutherford acute ischemia class requires emergent revascularization? Which can only be managed with amputation?
7. Which compartment is most commonly missed/incompletely opened during lower leg four-compartment fasciotomy?
8. What is the clinical definition of chronic limb-threatening ischemia (CLTI)?
9. What ABI is consistent with claudication? With rest pain?
10. What are the seven components of medical management for chronic PAD?

REFERENCES

1. Valentine RJ, Wind GG. *Anatomic Exposures in Vascular Surgery*. 4th ed. LWW; 2020.
2. Gest TR. *Lippincott Atlas of Anatomy*. 2nd ed. Wolters Kluwer; 2020.
3. Uflacker A, Guimaraes M, Uflacker R. *Uflacker's Atlas of Vascular Anatomy: An Angiographic Approach*. Wolters Kluwer; 2021.
4. Fowkes FGR, Rudan D, Rudan I, et al. Comparison of global estimates of prevalence and risk factors for peripheral artery disease in 2000 and 2010: a systematic review and analysis. *Lancet*. 2013;382(9901):1329-1340.
5. Hammerberg ME. Acute compartment syndrome of the extremities. In: Moreira ME, Grayzel J, eds. *UpToDate*. UpToDate; 2022.
6. Parvar SL, Fitridge R, Dawson J, Nicholls SJ. Medical and lifestyle management of peripheral arterial disease. *J Vasc Surg*. 2018;68(5):1595-1606.
7. Norgren L, Hiatt WR, Dormandy JA, et al. Inter-Society Consensus for the management of peripheral arterial disease (TASC II). *Eur J Vasc Endovasc Surg*. 2007;33(suppl 1):S1-S75.
8. Foley TR, Singh GD, Kokkinidis DG, et al. High-intensity statin therapy is associated with improved survival in patients with peripheral artery disease. *J Am Heart Assoc*. 2017;6(7):e005699.

9. Heart Protection Study Collaborative Group. Randomized trial of the effects of cholesterol-lowering with simvastatin on peripheral vascular and other major vascular outcomes in 20,536 people with peripheral arterial disease and other high-risk conditions. *J Vasc Surg.* 2007;45(4):645-654; discussion 653-654.
10. De Carlo M, Di Minno G, Sayre T, Fazeli MS, Siliman G, Cimminiello C. Efficacy and safety of antiplatelet therapies in symptomatic peripheral artery disease: a systematic review and network meta-analysis. *Curr Vasc Pharmacol.* 2021;19(5):542-555.
11. Desai K, Han B, Kuziez L, Yan Y, Zayed MA. Literature review and meta-analysis of the efficacy of cilostazol on limb salvage rates after infrainguinal endovascular and open revascularization. *J Vasc Surg.* 2021;73(2):711-721.e3.
12. Bonaca MP, Bauersachs RM, Anand SS, et al. Rivaroxaban in peripheral artery disease after revascularization. *N Engl J Med.* 2020;382(21):1994-2004.
13. Mills JL Sr, Conte MS, Armstrong DG, et al. The society for vascular surgery lower extremity threatened limb classification system: risk stratification based on wound, ischemia, and foot infection (WIfI). *J Vasc Surg.* 2014;59(1):220-234.e1-2.
14. Conte MS, Bradbury AW, Kolh P, et al. Global vascular guidelines on the management of chronic limb-threatening ischemia. *J Vasc Surg.* 2019;69(6S):3S-125S.e40.
15. Bradbury AW, Adam DJ, Bell J, et al. Bypass versus Angioplasty in Severe Ischaemia of the Leg (BASIL) trial: a survival prediction model to facilitate clinical decision making. *J Vasc Surg.* 2010;51(5 suppl):52S-68S.
16. Miranda JA, Pallister Z, Sharath S, et al. Early experience with venous arterialization for limb salvage in no-option patients with chronic limb-threatening ischemia. *J Vasc Surg.* 2022;76(4):987-996.e3.
17. Katsanos K, Spiliopoulos S, Karunanithy N, Krokidis M, Sabharwal T, Taylor P. Bayesian network meta-analysis of nitinol stents, covered stents, drug-eluting stents, and drug-coated balloons in the femoropopliteal artery. *J Vasc Surg.* 2014;59(4):1123-1133.e8.
18. Dake MD, Ansel GM, Jaff MR, et al. Durable clinical effectiveness with paclitaxel-eluting stents in the femoropopliteal artery: 5-year results of the zilver PTX randomized trial. *Circulation.* 2016;133(15):1472-1483.

37 Venous and Lymphatic Disease

Julia Suggs and Nanette R. Reed

I. ANATOMY

A. Lower extremity venous anatomy (**Figure 37.1**)
   1. Divided into three compartments: **superficial**, **perforating**, and **deep**.
      a. Blood flows from the superficial to the deep veins through the perforating system.
   2. Major superficial veins
      a. **Greater saphenous vein** (GSV) formed from the union of the dorsal vein of the great toe and the dorsal venous arch
   3. Small saphenous vein formed from the joining of the dorsal vein of the fifth toe and the dorsal venous arch
   4. Posterior arch vein
      a. Also called "**Leonardo vein**"
      b. Beginning in the medial ankle and joining the GSV below the knee
   5. Deep veins
      a. Named according to their paired arteries
      b. Deep veins of the calf
         i. Typically duplicated as **venae comitantes** with numerous communicating branches
         ii. The posterior tibial and peroneal veins also communicate with the soleal sinusoids.
      c. Deep veins of the thigh
         i. The **common femoral vein** is formed by the joining of the femoral and deep femoral veins approximately 4 cm below the inguinal ligament.
   6. Perforating veins connect the superficial and deep systems through both direct and indirect mechanisms.
   7. Venous return from the lower extremities depends largely on compression of the deep veins by the muscles during ambulation.
   8. Venous blood flow is unidirectional due to a series of one-way valves, which prevent reflux, and failure of these valves to close leads to pooling, stasis, and congestion of veins in the lower extremities.

B. Lymphatic anatomy (**Figure 37.2**)
   1. Lymphatics generally parallel venous drainage and have similar mechanics (maintain unidirectional flow via one-way valves with forward flow facilitated by muscle contractions).
   2. Lymph capillaries have thin endothelial walls, allowing interstitial fluid to enter.

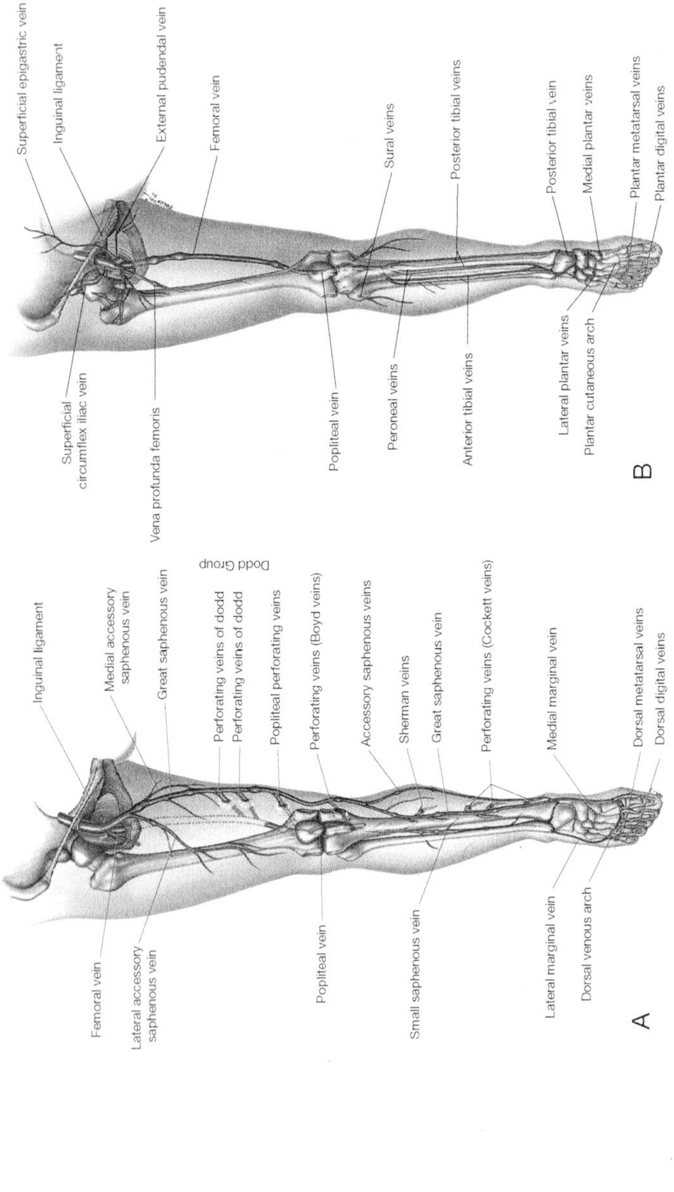

FIGURE 37.1 Venous anatomy of the lower extremity. A, Superficial veins, B, deep veins. *(Reprinted with permission from Uflacker A, Guimardes M, eds. Veins of the lower extremity. In: Uflacker's Atlas of Vascular Anatomy: An Angiographic Approach. 3rd ed. Wolters Kluwer; 2021:1040-1060. Figures 23.2 and 23.7.)*

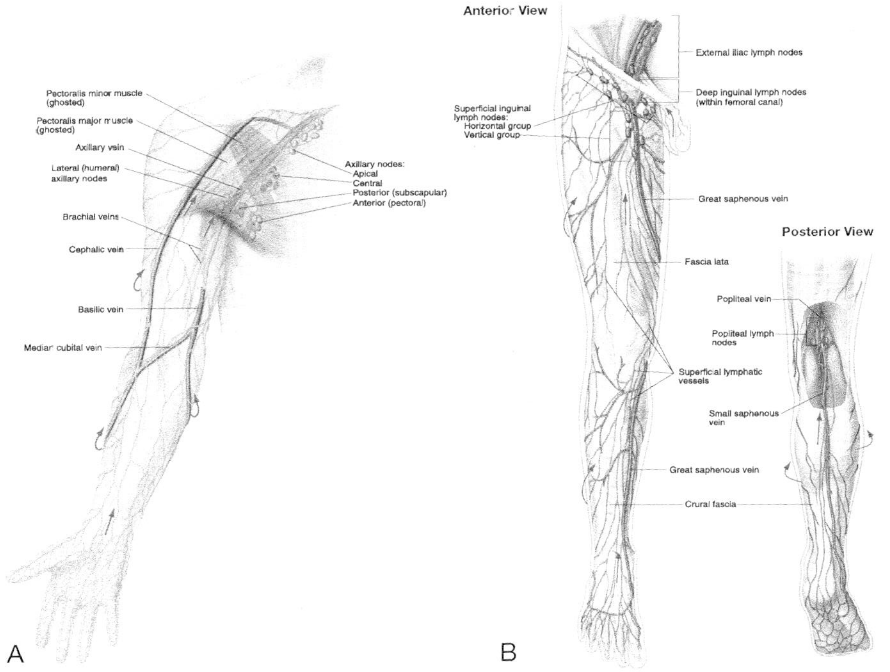

FIGURE 37.2 Lymphatic anatomy of the upper (A) and lower (B) extremities. Lymphatics are shown in green, veins in blue. *(A, reprinted with permission from Gest TR, ed. The upper limb. In: Lippincott® Atlas of Anatomy. 2nd ed. Wolters Kluwer; 2020:32-95. Plate 2-55. B, reprinted with permission from Gest TR, ed. The lower limb. In: Lippincott® Atlas of Anatomy. 2nd ed. Wolters Kluwer; 2020:96-175. Plate 3-71.)*

3. Lymphatic vessels run through lymph nodes (located at the confluence of major blood vessels) that filter the fluid, particularly removing dead or dying cells, and allow monocytes and lymphocytes to enter the fluid.
4. Lymphatic vessels form superficial and deep systems and eventually drain into either the **right lymphatic duct** or the **thoracic duct**, which in turn drain into the right and left subclavian arteries, respectively.
   a. The right arm/upper quadrant of the body is drained via the right lymphatic duct, while the thoracic duct receives drainage from the rest of the body.
5. Superficial and deep lymphatics of the upper extremity drain through the lateral axillary lymph nodes, and then onto the central nodes, then apical nodes.
   a. The anterior and posterior axillary nodes drain the chest wall, breast, and scapula.
6. Lymphatics of the lower extremity drain through the inguinal lymph nodes.
   a. **Deep inguinal:** Drain deep lymph of the leg.
   b. **Superficial vertical group:** Drain superficial lymph of the leg.
   c. **Superficial horizontal group:** Drain the perineum/genitals, gluteal region, part of the abdominal wall.

II. CHRONIC VENOUS INSUFFICIENCY

A. A spectrum of pathology, which includes telangiectasias, varicose veins, venous ulceration, and venous claudication.

B. Epidemiology
1. Published data on epidemiology in the US are lacking over the last 20 years, but the most recent reports (from 1999) estimate that there are over 25 million people in the US with chronic venous insufficiency (CVI), with about 6 million suffering from venous stasis ulcers.
2. CVI is seen more commonly in females, with a ratio of 3:1 female to male.

C. Pathophysiology
1. Etiology: Congenital, primary (i.e., cause undetermined), and secondary (e.g., postthrombotic, posttraumatic) with postthrombotic being the most common etiology.
2. Risk factors: Obesity, tobacco use, multiparity, genetics, hormone therapy, obstruction (e.g., from adenopathy, compression, pregnancy), and history of **deep venous thrombosis** (DVT).
3. Venous valvular incompetence
   a. Reflux from venous valvular incompetence accounts for >80% of chronic venous disease.
   b. Valve malfunction can be inherited or acquired through sclerosis, elongation of valve cusps, or dilation of the valve annulus despite normal valve cusps.
   c. **Varicose veins** can be due to
      i. Superficial venous insufficiency in the presence of competent deep and perforator systems

ii. Perforator or deep venous disease

d. Valvular disease below the knee appears to be more critical in the pathophysiology of severe venous disease as opposed to valvular disease above the knee.

e. **Venous ulcers**

i. Often secondary to incompetent perforator veins

ii. Can be secondary to incompetence in any component of the venous system, either alone or in combination

D. Nomenclature: The **CEAP classification** serves as the standardized nomenclature of chronic venous disease, based on Clinical signs, Etiology, Anatomic distribution, and Pathophysiology (**Table 37.1**).[1,2]

E. Symptoms

1. Signs and symptoms include lower extremity edema, pain, skin irritation, and varicose veins.
2. Pain is typically dull and achy and worsens at the end of the day.
3. Symptoms are often improved with elevation and compression and improve over time with moderate exercise.
4. **Venous claudication** is rare; causes acute, bursting pain with ambulation; and tends to be improved with rest and leg elevation.

F. Physical examination

1. Findings may include ankle edema, subcutaneous fibrosis, hyperpigmentation, lipodermatosclerosis, venous eczema, subcutaneous vein dilation, and ulcers.

a. **Hyperpigmentation:** Brownish discoloration secondary to hemosiderin deposition

b. **Lipodermatosclerosis:** Painful inflammation of the fat layer leading to fibrosis and thickening of the skin

c. **Subcutaneous vein dilation** includes telangiectasias (0.1-1 mm), reticular veins (1-4 mm), and varicose veins (>4 mm).

d. **Ulcers:** Typically proximal to the medial malleolus in the **gaiter distribution** (**Figure 37.3**)

2. Signs of infection should be noted.
3. Pulse examination should be performed.

G. Imaging

1. **Duplex scanning**

a. B-mode ultrasound imaging combined with Doppler frequency shift display is used to assess venous valvular competence, obstruction, and presence of acute or chronic DVT.

b. Diagnosis of reflux is made based on the duration of retrograde or reversed flow in the particular vein (>500 ms is considered pathologic).

H. Nonoperative management

1. **Compression therapy**

a. Stockings do not correct the abnormal venous hemodynamics and must be worn consistently to prevent a recurrence of symptoms.

i. Should be worn from awakening and removed at bedtime.

ii. Patient adherence is the principal limiting factor.

2. **Venous ulcer management**

TABLE 37.1 Classification of Chronic Lower Extremity Venous Disease

Classification	Definition
C	**Clinical classification**
	C_0: No visible or palpable signs of venous disease
	C_1: Telangiectasias or reticular veins
	C_2: Varicose veins; distinguished from reticular veins by a diameter of 3 mm or more
	C_3: Edema
	C_4: Changes in skin and subcutaneous tissue secondary to CVD
	C_{4a}: Pigmentation or eczema
	C_{4b}: Lipodermatosclerosis or atrophie blanche
	C_5: Healed venous ulcer
	C_6: Active venous ulcer
	S: Symptomatic (includes aching, pain, tightness, skin irritation, heaviness, muscle cramps, and other complaints attributable to venous dysfunction)
	A: Asymptomatic
E	**Etiologic classification**
	E_c: Congenital
	E_p: Primary
	E_s: Secondary (i.e., postthrombotic)
	E_n: No venous cause identified
A	**Anatomic distribution**
	A_s: Superficial veins involved
	A_p: Perforator veins involved
	A_d: Deep veins involved
	A_n: No venous location identified

TABLE 37.1 Classification of Chronic Lower Extremity Venous Disease (*Continued*)

Classification	Definition
P	**Pathophysiologic dysfunction**
	P_r: Reflux
	P_o: Obstruction
	$P_{r,o}$: Reflux and obstruction
	P_n: No venous pathophysiology identified

CVD, chronic venous disease.

a. Infected ulcers require treatment of infection first with local wound care and antibiotics.
   i. *Streptococcus pyogenes* and *Pseudomonas* species are responsible for most infections.
b. Specialized compression therapy
   i. Ulcer healing may take weeks to months, and compression is required long term to prevent recurrent ulceration.
   ii. **Unna boots** combine compression therapy with a zinc oxide paste to assist in wound healing and prevent further skin breakdown and are changed once or twice a week.
   iii. **Pneumatic compression devices** provide dynamic sequential compression and are used primarily in the prevention of DVT

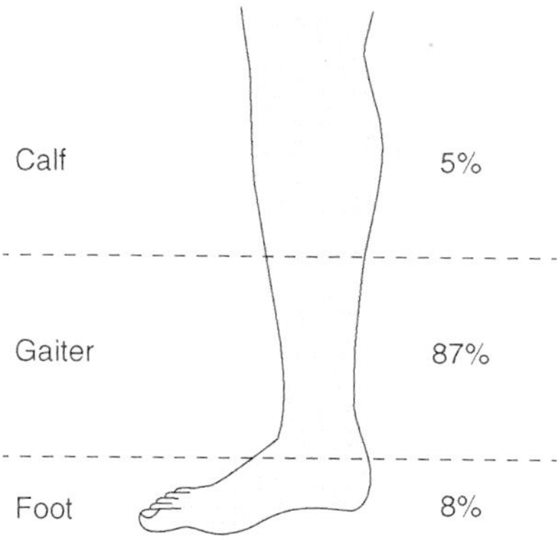

FIGURE 37.3 Lower extremity distribution of venous ulcers. *(Modified from London NJ, Donnelly R. ABC of arterial and venous disease. Ulcerated lower limb. BMJ. 2000;320(7249):1589-1591, with permission from BMJ Publishing Group Ltd.)*

in hospitalized patients but can be used successfully to treat venous insufficiency.

c. Early **ablation** of incompetent superficial veins results in faster healing of venous leg ulcers and more time free from ulcers than deferred intervention (see operative management below).[3]

I. Operative management

1. Indicated for severe disease refractory to medical treatment or in the setting of venous ulceration.
2. Open varicose vein surgery
   a. **Ligation** and **stripping** of the GSV removes this vein from the deep system.
   b. In current surgical practice in the US, has mostly been replaced by endovenous approaches.
3. **Sclerotherapy**
   a. Injection of a chemical sclerosant directly into the vein that disrupts the vein endothelium and leads to vein spasm, further leading to occlusion and subsequent fibrosis.
   b. Can be used for a variety of vein sizes including telangiectasias.
      i. Liquid sclerotherapy is reserved for veins <3 mm in diameter.
      ii. Foam sclerotherapy can be used in larger veins.
      iii. Approach depends on the size/depth of the vein(s) being treated (e.g., direct syringe injection, endovenous).
4. **Endovenous techniques**
   a. Disruption of venous flow via
      i. Thermal ablation (radiofrequency ablation, laser ablation)
      ii. Cyanoacrylate (glue) embolization
      iii. Ultrasound-guided foam sclerotherapy
      iv. Mechanochemical ablation
   b. Endovenous treatment modalities for the saphenous vein are superior to traditional GSV stripping in terms of reduced pain and faster recovery.
   c. In the setting of current or healed ulcers, associated incompetent perforators should be treated with endovascular techniques.
5. **Ambulatory phlebectomy:** Treats superficial varicosities via small incisions.

III. VENOUS THROMBOEMBOLISM

A. Epidemiology

1. The most recently reported US national data show that in 2018 there were[4]
   a. Over one million cases of **DVT/pulmonary embolism** (PE)
   b. Approximately 276,000 hospitalizations for DVT/PE
2. Approximately 50% to 60% of DVT episodes are asymptomatic.
3. In patients with DVTs, 30% will have a symptomatic PE with a mortality of 17.5% if untreated.
4. DVT and PE can occur in approximately 10% to 40% of general surgical patients without perioperative prophylaxis and 40% to 60% following major orthopedic operations.[5,6]

5. **Venous thromboembolism** (VTE) is the fifth most common cause for postoperative hospital readmissions.[7]

B. Pathophysiology

1. DVT starts as a platelet nidus, usually on the venous valves of the calf.
2. The thrombogenic nature of the nidus activates the clotting cascade, leading to platelet and fibrin accumulation.
3. The fibrinolytic system is subsequently activated leading to thrombus propagation.
   a. A thrombus can detach from the endothelium and migrate into the pulmonary system, becoming a PE.
   b. Alternatively, it can also organize and grow into the endothelium, resulting in venous incompetency and **phlebitis**.
4. Thrombi localized to the calf have lesser tendency to embolize than thrombi that extend into the thigh veins.[8]
   a. Approximately 20% of cases of calf DVT propagate to the thigh, and 50% of cases of proximal DVT embolize.
5. Risk factors are identified in 80% of patients with VTE and include
   a. Personal or family history of VTE, advanced age, malignancy and cancer therapy, pregnancy and postpartum state, endothelial injury, venous stasis, perioperative status, oral contraceptives (OCPs) or hormonal therapy, and (other) hypercoagulable states.
      i. Patients using OCPs or hormonal therapy have 3 to 5 times higher odds of DVT when compared with non-OCP-using patients.
      ii. Smoking and increased age increase the risk of DVT formation for patients taking OCPs.
      iii. **Hypercoagulable states** are present in 25% of patients with VTE.
         a) Primary hypercoagulable states are inherited conditions that can lead to abnormal endothelial cell thromboregulation.
         b) Secondary hypercoagulable states are acquired disorders in which endothelial activation by cytokines leads to an inflammatory, thrombogenic vessel wall.

C. DVT diagnosis and management

1. General findings: Unilateral leg swelling and/or pain associated with warmth and/or discoloration, dilation of superficial veins of the suspected extremity only, and/or calf pain on dorsiflexion of the ankle.
2. Specific presentations
   a. **Phlegmasia alba dolens**
      i. A more severe manifestation of DVT in which the deep venous channels of the extremity are affected while sparing collateral veins and therefore maintaining some degree of venous return.
      ii. Patients present with edema, pain, and white appearance (alba) of the affected limb.
      iii. Commonly seen in pregnancy or just after birth secondary to compression of the left common iliac vein.
   b. **Phlegmasia cerulea dolens**
      i. Occurs with extension of thrombus into the collateral venous system, resulting in limb pain and swelling, accompanied by cyanosis, a sign of arterial ischemia.

ii. This can be acutely limb threatening, and often requires aggressive management (see below).

3. Imaging
   a. Duplex ultrasound imaging of the femoral, popliteal, and calf trifurcation veins is highly sensitive (>90%) in detecting thrombosis of the proximal veins (femoral and popliteal) but less sensitive in detecting calf vein thrombosis.
   b. DVT can be detected on CT with venous phase; usually obtained concomitantly with chest CT in the setting of concern for PE.
4. Management reflects the **CHEST Guideline** for Antithrombotic Therapy for VTE Disease, most recently updated in 2021.[9]
5. Nonoperative management
   a. Acute isolated distal lower extremity DVT
      i. Distal lower extremity is limited to calf veins such as anterior tibial, posterior tibial, or peroneal veins but does not extend into the popliteal vein.
      ii. Management depends on severity of symptoms, risk factors for extension, risk of bleeding, and patient preference.
         a) Risk factors for extension include extensive thrombosis, no reversible provoking factor for DVT, active cancer, prior history of VTE, inpatient status, COVID-19.
         b) For patients without severe symptoms or risk factors
            1) Serial imaging of the deep veins for 2 weeks (e.g., ultrasound imaging at 1 and 2 weeks)
            2) If thrombus is found to extend into proximal veins on serial imaging, start therapeutic anticoagulation.
         c) For patients with severe symptoms and/or risk factors for extension, start therapeutic anticoagulation.
   b. Acute proximal lower extremity DVT: Therapeutic anticoagulation
   c. Choice and duration of anticoagulation for VTE
      i. **Direct oral anticoagulants** (e.g., apixaban, dabigatran, rivaroxaban) preferred over **vitamin K antagonists** (e.g., warfarin), given improved safety (particularly for bleeding or life-threatening bleeding) and no need for frequent monitoring.
      ii. All patients in whom anticoagulation is indicated should start with a 3-month course, with assessment for possible extended-phase therapy at the completion of 3 months.
      iii. Generally, extended-phase treatment is not indicated for patients in whom the initial VTE was associated with a transient risk factor that has resolved.
      iv. **Extended-phase treatment**
         a) Indicated for patients with unprovoked VTE or with VTE provoked by persistent risk factor (e.g., active malignancy/malignancy undergoing treatment, active inflammatory bowel disease).
            1) Decision should also take into account patient preference, predicted risk of recurrent VTE, and bleeding risk.
            2) Reassess on an annual basis.

d. DVT associated with a long-term catheter[6]
   i. Catheter does not need to be removed if it is functional and necessary.
   ii. Anticoagulation is started and continued for 3 months after removal of the catheter (i.e., indefinitely if the catheter is never removed).

6. Operative management
   a. Indicated in patients with severe symptoms, in which the affected limb is acutely threatened, and/or in which there is a high risk of adverse sequelae of DVT.
      i. In particular, phlegmasia cerulea dolens and phlegmasia alba dolens require therapeutic anticoagulation but may require more aggressive treatment if the limb is threatened, such as systemic thrombolytic therapy or invasive strategies including **endovascular mechanical thrombectomy** or **catheter-directed thrombolysis**.
      ii. Catheter-directed thrombolysis and mechanical thrombectomy of acute DVT has been advocated to avoid adverse sequelae of iliofemoral DVT with the goal to restore venous flow, preserve venous valve function, and eliminate the possibility of post-thrombotic syndrome.
      iii. The ATTRACT trial (multicenter randomized controlled trial [RCT] comparing anticoagulation alone with pharmacomechanical thrombolysis in patients with proximal acute DVT) showed no difference in the incidence of postthrombotic syndrome between patients treated with thrombolysis and those treated with anticoagulation alone. Those treated with thrombolysis had higher risk of major bleeding.[10]
      iv. In patients with migration of DVT resulting in severe PE and hemodynamic instability, potentially life-saving thrombolysis should be considered (see PE management below).[6,9,11]

7. **Inferior vena cava (IVC) filter**
   a. Recommended only in patients with proven VTE with a contraindication for anticoagulation, a complication of anticoagulation, or recurrent VTE despite adequate anticoagulation.
   b. There is no role for an IVC filter in the setting of ongoing anticoagulation.
   c. Most patients have a temporary contraindication to anticoagulation. Temporary filters should be removed as soon as possible once anticoagulation can be restarted.
   d. Prophylactic IVC filters (i.e., without a proven VTE) are not recommended for PE prevention.
   e. **Surgical approach: IVC filter placement**
      i. Either the transfemoral or transjugular approach can be utilized, with dedicated filters designed for each site. Before the operative site is prepped, use ultrasound imaging to assess the planned access site vein to ensure no clot is present.
      ii. Access the vein under ultrasound guidance with a micropuncture needle and sheath.

iii. Advance a guide-wire through the access sheath into the IVC under fluoroscopic guidance, then advance a flush catheter (e.g., pigtail) over the wire into the IVC, remove the wire.
iv. Obtain a venogram to verify location of the renal veins and the IVC bifurcation, and mark this location on the fluoroscopy viewing screen.
v. Over a guide-wire, exchange the flush catheter with a sheath with the filter device, and verify that the hook on the filter is distal to the renal veins.
vi. Deploy the filter, then perform a completion venogram to verify good positioning.
vii. Remove all instrumentation and hold pressure at the access site (15 min).

f. **Surgical approach: IVC filter removal**
i. IVC filters must be removed via a transjugular approach (because of the design of the filter, with the retrieval hook facing cranially and the tines/basket facing caudally).
ii. Access the internal jugular vein under ultrasound guidance with a micropuncture needle and access sheath.
iii. Use over-the-wire technique to advance a large sheath through the SVC and the right atrium into the IVC, just proximal to the filter.
iv. Obtain a venogram to ensure there is no large clot burden in the IVC filter.
v. Use a filter retrieval hook/snare to hook the IVC filter. Advance the sheath over the filter to swallow the entire filter (including all tines).
vi. Remove the filter and inspect it to confirm that it is intact.
vii. Perform a completion venogram to ensure there is no perforation/active bleeding from the IVC.
viii. Remove all instrumentation, hold pressure over the access site (15 min).

g. Complications related to IVC filters occur in 4% to 11% of patients.
i. The most common complications are thrombotic, including insertion site thrombosis (2%-28%), IVC thrombosis (3%-11%), and recurrent DVT (6%-35%).
ii. Other complications include filter migration, penetration/perforation of the IVC, and filter fracture.
iii. Use of retrievable filters can reduce the incidence of thrombotic complications.[12]

D. PE diagnosis and management

1. Symptoms: Shortness of breath, chest pain, cough, palpitations, lightheadedness/dizziness, diaphoresis
2. Physical examination: Tachypnea, signs of DVT, tachycardia, jugular venous distention, hypoxia, more rarely fever (mimicking pneumonia)
3. Laboratory tests: Assess for cardiac strain/ischemia with troponin, brain natriuretic peptide.

a. A high-sensitivity assay for plasma **D-dimer** levels can be useful in the diagnosis of PE in patients who are unlikely to have PE/have low clinical probability for PE.

4. Imaging: Establish diagnosis of PE and assess for right-sided heart strain.
   a. **Contrast-enhanced spiral chest CT** is standard of care.
      i. Preferable to pulmonary angiography as it is less invasive, more readily available, and has sensitivity of 94%.[13]
      ii. Can also assess for right ventricular (RV) dilation.
   b. **Radionucleotide ventilation and perfusion lung imaging** (V/Q scan)
      i. Used in nonemergent situations in which CT is not feasible, such as in hemodynamically stable pregnant patients or in patients who cannot receive IV contrast dye.
      ii. Scans classified as high, intermediate, low probability, with a V/Q scan result of "high probability" strongly suggestive of the presence of PE.
   c. **Pulmonary angiography** is primarily a historic reference diagnostic test reserved for patients in whom PE diagnosis is still uncertain. Can also be performed as part of an intervention.
   d. Echocardiography with indicators of right-sided heart strain include RV > left ventricular (LV) end-diastolic volume, rightward bowing of the interventricular septum, reduced tricuspid annular plane systolic excursion, and/or RV hypokinesis.
   e. ECG is useful primarily in assessing for alternate diagnoses, i.e., acute myocardial infarction.
      i. The ECG changes classically associated with PE are the same as those seen with any cause of pulmonary hypertension/RV strain and are seen in <20% of patients with PE.
      ii. RV strain is better assessed via echocardiography.
5. Management is primarily determined by patients' hemodynamic stability, clot burden, and presence/absence of right-sided heart strain as well as markers of myocardial damage (troponin elevation). Patients with PE can be divided into high, intermediate, and low risk.[14,15]
   a. High risk (may also be referred to as "**massive PE**")
      i. Hemodynamic instability or inability to maintain oxygenation
      ii. Clot-in-transit (clot in the heart) is also considered a high-risk feature.
      iii. ≥30% predicted 30-day adverse event rate
   b. Intermediate risk (may also be referred to as "**submassive PE**")
      i. No hemodynamic instability, but laboratory tests indicate end organ damage (e.g., renal or hepatic dysfunction).
      ii. Other independent risk factors for adverse events/poor outcome: Age > 80 years, presence of other underlying illness such as cancer or chronic cardiopulmonary disease.
      iii. ~10% 30-day in-hospital mortality rate
   c. **Low risk**
      i. No hemodynamic changes or end-organ damage
      ii. ~1% 30-day in-hospital mortality rate

6. Nonoperative management
   a. Patients with high- and intermediate-risk PE are preload dependent, so interventions to increase preload (e.g., fluid bolus) may be helpful.
   b. Anticoagulation is recommended for majority of patients per CHEST guidelines[9]; choice and duration of anticoagulation same as listed for DVT above.
   c. **Thrombolysis** (e.g., recombinant tissue plasminogen activator [alteplase]) is indicated if the patient is high risk and does not have a contraindication (e.g., high risk of bleeding/high risk for intracranial bleeding).
      i. Systematic review of 15 RCTs including >2,000 patients showed that thrombolytic therapy is associated with absolute 30-day mortality reduction of 1.6%, although patients had a 1.4% increased risk of fatal hemorrhage or intracranial bleed.[16]
7. Operative management
   a. Indicated for hemodynamically unstable patients and those with right-sided heart dysfunction or respiratory deterioration in whom thrombolysis is contraindicated or has failed.
   b. Approaches include transcatheter **mechanical thrombolysis/ thrombectomy** and **open surgical thrombectomy**.
      i. Open thrombectomy requires cardiopulmonary bypass, is rarely performed, and is reserved for patients with refractory cardiogenic shock who are not candidates for catheter-directed therapy.
      ii. Studies are ongoing as to which intermediate-risk patients benefit most from percutaneous catheter-directed mechanical thrombectomy.
   c. In cases of refractory/profound shock, **extracorporeal membrane oxygenation** support may be indicated (see Chapter 32).

E. Prevention of venous thromboembolism in surgical patients
1. **Low-dose unfractionated heparin** (LDUH)
   a. Standard dose is 5,000 units administered subcutaneously 1 to 2 hours preoperatively and every 8 to 12 hours postoperatively; higher doses may be required in patients with higher body mass index.[17]
   b. Reduces the risk of VTE by 50% to 70%[17] and does not require laboratory monitoring.
   c. Should not be used for patients undergoing cerebral, ocular, or spinal surgery given potential for minor bleeding.
2. **Low-molecular-weight heparin** (LMWH; e.g., enoxaparin)
   a. Several studies have shown reduced bleeding risks for surgical patients treated with prophylactic dosing of LMWH vs LDUH.
   b. LMWH has been shown to be more effective than LDUH in preventing VTE in trauma patients.[18]
3. Other medications
   a. Direct thrombin inhibitors and fondaparinux
   b. Commonly reserved for patients with history of heparin allergy or heparin-induced thrombocytopenia

4. Recommendations for anticoagulation following specific procedures can be found in the CHEST guidelines.[6,9]
5. **Intermittent pneumatic compression** of the extremities
   a. Enhances blood flow in the deep veins and increases blood fibrinolytic activity through upregulation of thrombomodulin, fibrinolysin, tissue plasminogen activator, and endothelial nitric oxide synthase expression.[19]
   b. Compression devices should not be placed on an extremity with known DVT. In the case of known bilateral lower extremity DVTs, devices can be placed on the upper extremity as the upregulated agents have systemic effects.

IV. LYMPHEDEMA

A. Epidemiology
1. Estimated 30,000 to 35,000 inpatient admissions in the US annually, with vast majority in the setting of superimposed cellulitis.[20]

B. Pathophysiology and classification
1. **Primary lymphedema**
   a. Due to congenital aplasia, hypoplasia, or hyperplasia of lymphatic vessels and nodes that causes the accumulation of protein-rich lymph fluid in the interstitial space.
   b. Swelling of the patient's leg initially produces pitting edema, which progresses to a nonpitting form and may lead to dermal fibrosis and disfigurement.
   c. Classified according to age at presentation
      i. **Congenital primary lymphedema** (present at birth)
         a) About 10% to 15% of primary lymphedema cases
         b) Can be hereditary (**Milroy disease**) or sporadic
      ii. **Praecox** (early in life) or **Meige disease**
         a) About 70% to 80% of primary lymphedema cases
         b) Presents during second and third decades of life.
         c) About 80% to 90% of patients are female.
         d) Seventy percent of patients have a single affected lower extremity.
         e) Typically presents with localized swelling of the foot and ankle that is worsened by prolonged standing.
      iii. **Tarda** (late in life)
         a) About 10% to 15% of primary lymphedema cases
         b) Presents after the third or fourth decade of life.
         c) Seen equally in men and women.
2. **Secondary lymphedema**
   a. Due to impaired lymphatic drainage secondary to a known cause, including surgical/traumatic interruption of lymphatic vessels (often from an axillary or groin lymph node dissection), carcinoma, infection, VTE, radiation, or filariasis.
      i. Nonfilarial secondary lymphedema is the most common etiology of lymphedema in the US.

ii. Filarial secondary lymphedema is the most common global etiology, caused by the parasite *Wuchereria bancrofti*.

C. Symptoms

1. Early: Unilateral/bilateral arm or pedal swelling that resolves overnight
2. Intermediate: Swelling increases and extends up the extremity, producing discomfort and thickened skin.
3. Late: Swelling not relieved with elevation.
4. Significant pain is unusual.
5. Patients with secondary lymphedema commonly present with repeated episodes of cellulitis secondary to high interstitial protein content.
   a. Cellulitis and lymphangitis should be suspected when sudden onset of pain, increased swelling, or erythema of the leg occurs.

D. Physical examination

1. When a lower extremity is involved, the toes are often spared.
2. With advanced disease, the extremity becomes tense with nonpitting edema and dermal fibrosis results in skin thickening, hair loss, and generalized keratosis.

E. Differential diagnosis

1. Broad, given that the primary sign/symptom is a swollen extremity and can be unilateral or bilateral.
2. Includes trauma, infection, arterial disease, CVI, lipedema (excessive subcutaneous fat and fluid), neoplasm, radiation effects, and systemic diseases (e.g., heart failure, myxedema, nephrosis, nephritis, protein deficiency).

F. Imaging

1. **Lymphoscintigraphy**
   a. Injection of radiolabeled (technetium-99m) colloid into the web space between the patient's second and third digits.
   b. Limb is exercised periodically, and images are taken of the involved extremity and the whole body.
   c. Lymphedema is seen as an abnormal accumulation of tracer or as slow tracer clearance along with the presence of lymphatic collaterals.
   d. Shows 92% sensitivity, 100% specificity for lymphedema.[21]
2. CT or MRI
   a. Can detect a mass obstructing the lymphatic system.
   b. MRI may be able to differentiate lymphedema from chronic venous edema and lipedema.

G. Nonoperative management

1. Objectives: Control edema, maintain healthy skin, and avoid cellulitis and lymphangitis.
2. Limited by the physiologic and anatomic nature of the disease:
   a. Diuretics are ineffective because of the high interstitial protein concentration.
   b. Development of fibrosis and irreversible changes in the subcutaneous tissue further limit options.

3. Primary approach: Combination of physical therapies[22,23]
   a. Two-stage treatment program of skin care followed by the application of compression bandages.
   b. Topical hydrocortisone cream may be needed for eczema.
   c. Sequential pneumatic compression has been shown to improve lymphedema.
4. Cellulitis and **lymphangitis**
   a. Antibiotics to cover staphylococci and β-hemolytic streptococci
      i. Topical antifungal cream may be needed for chronic infections.
   b. Limb elevation and immobilization
   c. Warm compresses can be used for symptomatic relief.

H. Operative management
1. Objective: Reduce limb size and improve function
   a. Cosmetic deformities persist postoperatively, and functional results are best when performed for severely impaired movement and recurrent cellulitis.
   b. Therefore, only 10% of patients with lymphedema are surgical candidates.
2. **Lymphatic transposition**
   a. Includes direct (e.g., lymphovenous bypass, lymphatic grafting) and indirect (e.g., mesenteric bridge, omental flap) procedures.
      i. Lymphatic grafting is performed for upper extremity or unilateral lower extremity lymphedema, with good results reported in 80% of patients.[24]
3. **Reductive techniques**
   a. Resection of the skin and subcutaneous tissues with potential closure by a split- or full-thickness skin graft from the resected specimen or a split-thickness skin graft from an involved site.
   b. Liposuction may also be attempted.

Key References

Citation	Summary
EVRA Trial: Gohel MS, Heatley F, Liu X, et al. A randomized trial of early endovenous ablation in venous ulceration. *N Engl J Med.* 2018;378(22):2105-2114.	• RCT in 450 patients with venous leg ulcers comparing early endovenous ablation of superficial venous reflux (within 2 wk of randomization) and compression plus deferred ablation (after ulcer had healed or after 6 mo, whichever occurred first), with the primary outcome of time to ulcer healing. • Patients in the early ablation group had a shorter median ulcer healing time, a higher rate of ulcer healing, and a longer ulcer-free period.

Citation	Summary
ATTRACT Trial: Vedantham S, Goldhaber SZ, Julian JA, et al. Pharmacomechanical catheter-directed thrombolysis for deep-vein thrombosis. *N Engl J Med.* 2017;377(23):2240-2252.	• RCT in 692 patients with acute proximal DVT comparing anticoagulation alone versus anticoagulation plus transcatheter pharmacomechanical thrombolysis (device-delivery of tissue plasminogen activator and thrombus maceration/aspiration), with primary outcome of postthrombotic syndrome (severe chronic venous insufficiency) 6-24 mo post intervention. • There was no difference between groups in the rate of postthrombotic syndrome, recurrent thrombosis, or quality of life, but the pharmacomechanical group did have higher rates of major bleeding.
Preventing VTE after major trauma: Geerts WH, Jay RM, Code KI, et al. A comparison of low-dose heparin with low-molecular-weight heparin as prophylaxis against venous thromboembolism after major trauma. *N Engl J Med.* 1996;335(10):701-707.	• RCT in 344 trauma patients without intracranial bleeding comparing thromboprophylaxis with low-dose heparin (5,000 units) vs low-molecular-weight heparin (enoxaparin; 30 mg), each given subcutaneously every 12 h. Primary outcome was development of DVT diagnosed by contrast venography performed on or before day 14 of randomization, and secondary outcomes were rate of proximal DVT and major bleeding. • Of the 265 patients with adequate venograms, the enoxaparin group had lower rates of DVT and proximal DVT. Both interventions were safe (full cohort).
Reducing fatal postoperative VTE/PE: Collins R, Scrimgeour A, Yusuf S, Peto R. Reduction in fatal pulmonary embolism and venous thrombosis by perioperative administration of subcutaneous heparin. *N Engl J Med.* 1988;318(18):1162-1173.	• Systematic review and meta-analysis of 74 RCTs (15,598 total patients) of prophylactic perioperative subcutaneous heparin administration for patients undergoing general, urologic, or orthopedic surgery, evaluating rates of DVT, pulmonary embolism (PE), fatal PE, and bleeding. • Apparent odds of DVT, PE, and fatal PE were lower in groups that received heparin prophylaxis compared with controls. Bleeding events were also more frequent in the heparin groups. • Estimated that perioperative use of prophylactic heparin can prevent about half of all PEs and about two-thirds of all DVTs.

Citation	Summary
PREPIC2 Trial: Mismetti P, Laporte S, Pellerin O, et al. Effect of a retrievable inferior vena cava filter plus anticoagulation vs anticoagulation alone on risk of recurrent pulmonary embolism: a randomized clinical trial. *JAMA*. 2015;313(16):1627-1635.	• RCT in 399 patients with acute, symptomatic PE associated with acute lower-limb vein thrombosis and at least one additional criterion for severity. Randomized to anticoagulation alone or anticoagulation with retrievable IVC filter placement (filter retrieval planned at 3 mo). Primary outcome was symptomatic recurrent PE at 3 mo. • Use of retrievable IVC filter plus anticoagulation compared with anticoagulation alone did not reduce the risk of symptomatic recurrent PE at 3 mo. These findings do not support the use of retrievable filters in patients who can be treated with therapeutic anticoagulation.

CHAPTER 37: VENOUS AND LYMPHATIC DISEASE

Review Questions

1. A 35-year-old female patient presents to your clinic with isolated right calf swelling and tenderness. She has no personal history of DVT but is actively using OCPs. What test should you order?
2. You are consulted for IVC filter placement in a 45-year-old male who is 2 weeks post motor vehicle accident with multiple fractures, now found to have a left common femoral DVT. All teams have cleared the patient for anticoagulation. What management is indicated by the CHEST guidelines?
3. You are consulted for IVC filter placement in a patient prior to spine surgery who has no evidence of DVT on venous duplex but will be nonambulatory for 7 days postoperatively. Is there a role for prophylactic IVC filter placement in this patient?
4. A 43-year-old female is incidentally noted to have a right peroneal DVT while undergoing vein mapping. She has no symptoms associated with this DVT and is ambulatory. What is your recommended management course?
5. A 52-year-old man presents to your clinic with a history of DVT 6 months ago following spine surgery, which was initially managed with IVC filter placement due to high risk of bleeding. He has now been on anticoagulation for 3 months. What is your recommendation for his IVC filter at this time?
6. A 37-year-old female patient presents to the emergency department (ED) with left leg swelling a few days after an international flight and denies other symptoms. She is found on venous duplex to have a left popliteal vein DVT. What is the recommended management for this patient?

7. A 47-year-old female patient presents to clinic with swelling and heaviness of her right lower extremity. Her venous duplex is negative for DVT and her ankle-brachial indexes (ABIs) are normal. She has no associated wounds, but does have significant venous reflux in the affected limb. What nonsurgical treatment recommendations do you make?

REFERENCES

1. Eklöf B, Rutherford RB, Bergan JJ, et al. Revision of the CEAP classification for chronic venous disorders: consensus statement. *J Vasc Surg.* 2004;40(6):1248-1252.
2. Beebe HG, Bergan JJ, Bergqvist D, et al. Classification and grading of chronic venous disease in the lower limbs. A consensus statement. *Eur J Vasc Endovasc Surg.* 1996;12(4):487-491; discussion 491-492.
3. Gohel MS, Heatley F, Liu X, et al. A randomized trial of early endovenous ablation in venous ulceration. *N Engl J Med.* 2018;378(22):2105-2114.
4. Tsao CW, Aday AW, Almarzooq ZI, et al. Heart disease and stroke statistics—2022 update: a report from the American Heart Association. *Circulation.* 2022;145(8):e153-e639.
5. Geerts WH, Bergqvist D, Pineo GF, et al. Prevention of venous thromboembolism: American College of chest physicians evidence-based clinical practice guidelines (8th Edition). *Chest.* 2008;133(6 suppl l):381S-453S.
6. Kearon C, Akl EA, Ornelas J, et al. Antithrombotic therapyor VTE disease: CHEST guideline and expert panel report. *Chest.* 2016;149(2):315-352.
7. Merkow RP, Ju MH, Chung JW, et al. Underlying reasons associated with hospital readmission following surgery in the United States. *JAMA.* 2015;313(5):483-495.
8. Moser KM. Venous thromboembolism. *Am Rev Respir Dis.* 1990;141(1):235-249.
9. Stevens SM, Woller SC, Kreuziger LB, et al. Antithrombotic therapy for VTE disease: second update of the CHEST guideline and Expert panel report. *Chest.* 2021;160(6):e54 5-e608.
10. Vedantham S, Goldhaber SZ, Julian JA, et al. Pharmacomechanical catheter-directed thrombolysis for deep-vein thrombosis. *N Engl J Med.* 2017;377(23):2240-2252.
11. Motsch J, Walther A, Bock M, Böttiger BW. Update in the prevention and treatment of deep vein thrombosis and pulmonary embolism. *Curr Opin Anaesthesiol.* 2006;19(1):52-58.
12. Crowther MA. Inferior vena cava filters in the management of venous thromboembolism. *Am J Med.* 2007;120(10 suppl 2):S13-S17.
13. Patel P, Patel P, Bhatt M, et al. Systematic review and meta-analysis of test accuracy for the diagnosis of suspected pulmonary embolism. *Blood Adv.* 2020;4(18):4296-4311.
14. Jiménez D, Aujesky D, Moores L, et al. Simplification of the pulmonary embolism severity index for prognostication in patients with acute symptomatic pulmonary embolism. *Arch Intern Med.* 2010;170(15):1383-1389.
15. Sanchez O, Trinquart L, Caille V, et al. Prognostic factors for pulmonary embolism: the prep study, a prospective multicenter cohort study. *Am J Respir Crit Care Med.* 2010;181(2):168-173.
16. Marti C, John G, Konstantinides S, et al. Systemic thrombolytic therapy for acute pulmonary embolism: a systematic review and meta-analysis. *Eur Heart J.* 2015;36(10):605-614.
17. Collins R, Scrimgeour A, Yusuf S, Peto R. Reduction in fatal pulmonary embolism and venous thrombosis by perioperative administration of subcutaneous heparin. Overview of results of randomized trials in general, orthopedic, and urologic surgery. *N Engl J Med.* 1988;318(18):1162-1173.

18. Geerts WH, Jay RM, Code KI, et al. A comparison of low-dose heparin with low-molecular-weight heparin as prophylaxis against venous thromboembolism after major trauma. *N Engl J Med.* 1996;335(10):701-707.

19. Kohro S, Yamakage M, Sato K, Sato JI, Namiki A. Intermittent pneumatic foot compression can activate blood fibrinolysis without changes in blood coagulability and platelet activation. *Acta Anaesthesiol Scand.* 2005;49(5):660-664.

20. Lopez M, Roberson ML, Strassle PD, Ogunleye A. Epidemiology of lymphedema-related admissions in the United States: 2012-2017. *Surg Oncol.* 2020;35:249-253.

21. Gloviczki P, Calcagno D, Schirger A, et al. Noninvasive evaluation of the swollen extremity: experiences with 190 lymphoscintigraphic examinations. *J Vasc Surg.* 1989;9(5):683-689; discussion 690.

22. International Society of Lymphology. The diagnosis and treatment of peripheral lymphedema. 2009 Consensus document of the International Society of Lymphology. *Lymphology.* 2009;42(2):51-60.

23. International Society of Lymphology. The diagnosis and treatment of peripheral lymphedema: 2013 consensus document of the International Society of Lymphology. *Lymphology.* 2013;46(1):1-11.

24. Baumeister RG, Siuda S. Treatment of lymphedemas by microsurgical lymphatic grafting: what is proved? *Plast Reconstr Surg.* 1990;85(1):64-74; discussion 75-76.

25. Mismetti P, Laporte S, Pellerin O, et al. Effect of a retrievable inferior vena cava filter plus anticoagulation vs anticoagulation alone on risk of recurrent pulmonary embolism: a randomized clinical trial. *JAMA.* 2015;313(16):1627-1635.

26. Uflacker A, Guimaraes M, Uflacker R. *Uflacker's Atlas of Vascular Anatomy: An Angiographic Approach.* Wolters Kluwer; 2021.

27. Gest TR. *Lippincott® Atlas of Anatomy.* 2nd ed. Wolters Kluwer; 2020.

28. London NJ, Donnelly R. ABC of arterial and venous disease. Ulcerated lower limb. *BMJ.* 2000;320(7249):1589-1591.

38 Dialysis Access

Brian Sullivan and Surendra Shenoy

I. CHRONIC KIDNEY DISEASE

A. Epidemiology
   1. The 10th most common cause of death in the US (~13% of all annual deaths)
   2. Increasingly common given rising prevalence of diabetes, hypertension, obesity, and sedentary lifestyle
   3. Chronic kidney disease (CKD) is staged as in **Table 38.1**.
   4. Without proper monitoring/management, patients with CKD rapidly progress to **end-stage kidney disease** (ESKD), which is fatal without renal replacement (i.e:, dialysis/renal transplantation).
   5. Approximately 807,920 patients with ESKD in the US in 2020: 61.0% receive **hemodialysis** (HD); 8.1% **peritoneal dialysis** (PD); 30.0% preemptive renal transplant.[1]

B. Planning for/initiation of dialysis
   1. Education regarding renal replacement should start at CKD stage 4.
      a. Approximately 40% to 60% of patients start dialysis unplanned (requiring hospitalization).
   2. Dialysis modalities: HD and PD
      a. Choice should be shared decision between patients and providers.

TABLE 38.1 Stages of Chronic Kidney Disease (>3 mo Duration)

Stage	Kidney Function	eGFR (mL/min/1.73 m^2)
1	Normal to high	>90
2	Mildly decreased	60-89
3a	Mildly moderately decreased	45-59
3b	Moderately severely decreased	30-44
4	Severely decreased	15-29
5	Kidney failure	<15 (or requiring dialysis)

eGFR, estimated glomerular filtration rate.

b. Both can be used for urgent and nonurgent dialysis; however, PD is not a good option for patients requiring urgent dialysis for hyperkalemia, volume overload, or marked uremia.

II. PERITONEAL DIALYSIS

A. Physiology
   1. Utilizes the semipermeability of the peritoneal lining to exchange fluid and electrolytes and correct acid–base balance.
   2. Exchanges slow and gradual, making PD gentler than HD and better tolerated by the cardiovascular system.
   3. Fluid (dialysate) instilled into the peritoneal cavity, then time is given (dwell) for exchange of fluid/electrolytes and then draining.

B. Indications/contraindications are noted in **Table 38.2**.

C. Catheter placement
   1. Techniques: Open or laparoscopic and percutaneous image-guided

TABLE 38.2 Indications and Contraindications for Peritoneal Dialysis (PD)

Indications for PD	
Absolute	***Relative***
Vascular access failure	Needle anxiety
Intolerance of HD (severe PVD, severe cardiac disease)	Bleeding diathesis
Children 0-5 years old	Multiple myeloma
Patient preference	
Contraindications for PD	
Absolute	***Relative***
Intra-abdominal infection	Severe obesity
Inflammatory bowel disease	Abdominal wall defect/hernia
Severe/refractory psychiatric disorders	Proteinuria
Unstable housing conditions	Intra-abdominal adhesive disease
Women in 3rd trimester of pregnancy	Stoma and/or feeding tube
	Proteinuria >10 g/d

HD, hemodialysis; PVD, peripheral vascular disease.

2. Percutaneous and immediate use catheters are usually single-cuff, placed at bedside.
3. Long-term catheters usually have ≥2 cuffs.
4. **Surgical approach: Laparoscopic PD catheter placement**
   a. Abdominal access
      i. Open Hassan: Enter the abdomen via an infraumbilical incision under direct vision, insert a 5-mm trocar, and insufflate the abdomen with CO_2.
      ii. Veress entry: Use a Veress needle to access the abdomen in the left upper quadrant (LUQ), insufflate the abdomen with CO_2, remove the needle, and use a 5-mm optical access trocar to enter the abdomen in the LUQ.
   b. Place the patient head down (Trendelenburg position), insert a 5-mm 0° or 30° laparoscope, and visually examine the peritoneum.
   c. Place a second 5-mm port. Lyse adhesions as needed.
   d. Place a double-cuffed PD catheter into the abdomen, with the distal tip in the pouch of Douglas (most caudal portion of the peritoneum).
   e. Create a rectus sheath tunnel: Using an 8-mm laparoscopic trocar, penetrate the anterior rectus fascia, bluntly and caudally create a several centimeter tunnel through the rectus muscle, penetrate the posterior rectus sheath, and enter the peritoneal space under direct visualization.
   f. Position the catheter through the tunnel, with the deep cuff in the rectus muscle and the superficial cuff in subcutaneous tissue.
   g. Check catheter flow/gravity drainage.
   h. Ensure hemostasis, remove ports, and close fascia and skin.

D. Complications
1. Early/postoperative
   a. Injury to intraperitoneal structures, perforation, bleeding
   b. Idiopathic pain, hernia exacerbation, scrotal swelling, hydrothorax
   c. Catheter dysfunction due to malposition/kink, fibrin sheath/coagulum, constipation
2. Late (after the postoperative period)
   a. Catheter related: Leakage from fractures, catheter obstructions, intra-abdominal bleeding, intestinal obstruction, intestinal perforations from erosions, hernia at catheter tunnel site.
   b. Inadequate dialysis from peritoneal membrane failure, usually secondary to recurrent/chronic infections.
3. Infections
   a. Intraperitoneal sepsis is a major cause of hospitalization, PD failure, and mortality (35 deaths per 1,000 years at risk).
   b. Management
      i. Infection limited to exit site and/or cuff may be treated with appropriate antibiotics or cuff removal in multicuff catheters.
      ii. Peritonitis[2]
         a) Empiric intraperitoneal vancomycin/cephalosporin to cover gram-positive bacteria and third-/fourth-generation cephalosporin or aminoglycoside to cover gram-negative bacteria.

b) Regimen is then narrowed based on blood/peritoneal-fluid cultures/sensitivities.
c) Catheter removal for severe, recurrent, or resistant infections.

III. HEMODIALYSIS

A. Physiology
1. Dialyzing machine clears toxins/metabolism end-products via diffusion, osmosis, ultrafiltration.
2. Requires 100 to 500 mL/min blood flow.

B. Types of vascular access (**Figure 38.1**)
1. **Catheters**
a. Indication: Urgent HD, can be placed bedside and used immediately.
b. Design
i. Two lumens (one for blood withdrawal, one for return)
ii. Inserted through large veins (e.g., internal jugular vein [IJV]); tip positioned in the right atrium (RA).
iii. Short term
a) Insert by skin puncture directly over the vein.
b) Due to associated risk of complications, only recommended for ≤10 days.
iv. Intermediate/long-term catheters
a) Tunneled, less prone to complications.
b) Cuff in subcutaneous tissue between vein entry and skin exit where tissue in-growth fixates the catheter and is a barrier to cutaneous flora.
c) Can be used for weeks to months.

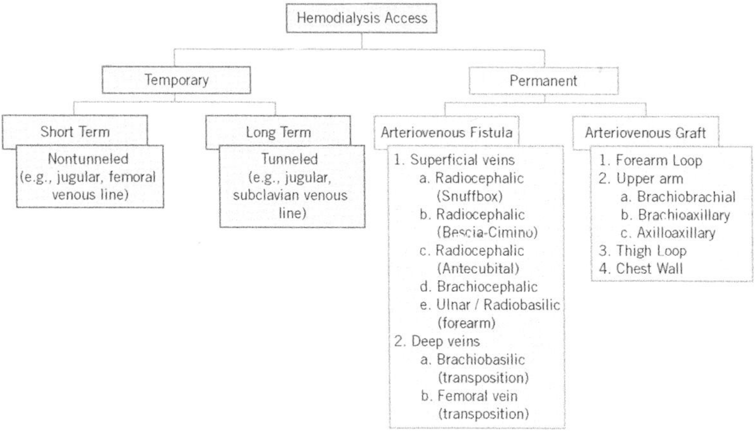

FIGURE 38.1 Choice of hemodialysis access flow chart.

c. Location
  i. Right IJV preferred given straight path to RA, left IJV less ideal given curved path and therefore increased risk of central vein stenosis.
  ii. Subclavian veins should *not* be used due to high rate of stenosis.

d. Procedural approach: HD catheter placement
  i. Place the patient in Trendelenburg position to reduce risk of air embolization.
  ii. Under ultrasound guidance, access the vein and place the guidewire, confirm position by ultrasound and/or column equilibration (maintain control over the guidewire at all times!).
  iii. Use Seldinger technique to dilate the skin and subcutaneous tissue, place the catheter over the wire, and remove the wire and ensure that it is complete (no fractures).
  iv. Place dressing and confirm catheter positioning via radiography.

e. Complications
  i. Insertion
    a) Injury to nearby nerves, arteries, veins, soft tissue
    b) Air embolus, tamponade, catheter misplacement
    c) Greatly reduced by appropriate patient positioning and use of ultrasound guidance[3]
  ii. Catheter dysfunction
    a) Early: Improper tip positioning, kinks, thrombosis
    b) Late: Fibrin sheath formation, tip migration, luminal thrombosis
  iii. Infection
    a) There is 2 times greater relative risk of fatal infection and 5 times greater relative risk of nonfatal infection compared with **arteriovenous fistula** (AVF).[4]
    b) Exit-site infections usually respond to antibiotics alone.
    c) Infections involving the cuff/tunnel or with systemic symptoms require catheter exchange/removal in addition to IV antibiotics (typically with vancomycin and gentamycin).
  iv. Central vein stenosis
    a) May result in loss of permanent access options in ipsilateral extremity.
    b) Incidence varies (5%-50%) based on site, type, and duration of access.
    c) Usually requires repeated interventions with angioplasty and stents, eventually leads to total occlusion.
    d) Catheter retention/removal depends on adequacy of catheter function and availability of other access sites; alternative access will ultimately be required.
  v. Mortality
    a) There is 53% and 38% higher relative risk of all-cause mortality compared with AVF and AVG (**arteriovenous graft**), respectively.[4]

2. **Arteriovenous access** (AVA) planning
   a. Permanent connection between artery and vein for HD
   b. Patient evaluation, planning, and maturation of new autogenous access requires ~6 months.
   c. Examination
      i. Arterial (inflow)
         a) Palpate pulses, and if nonpalpable, obtain arterial Doppler and/or duplex studies.
         b) Cuff pressures bilaterally: >20 mm Hg difference suspicious for proximal stenosis.
         c) **Allen test:** Assess integrity of palmar arches and palmar perfusion dominance (radial vs ulnar arteries).
      ii. Venous (outflow)
         a) Clinic evaluation using dilation techniques (e.g., tourniquets)
         b) Presence of visible/palpable upper arm/chest wall collateral veins may indicate upstream stenosis/occlusion.
   d. Ultrasound imaging
      i. **Vein mapping:** Cross-sectional measurements of several prominent arm veins recorded at intervals down the arm.
      ii. **Color Doppler-duplex ultrasound scanning** (CDDUS) should always be performed for both functional and structural evaluation of peripheral arteries and veins.
      iii. Intraoperative ultrasound imaging is essential in determining favorable fistula/graft targets as veins previously deemed unsuitable may dilate to appropriate size once limb is anesthetized.[5]
   e. Additional imaging
      i. Indicated when concern for central lesions such as arterial stenosis/atherosclerotic narrowing or central vein stenosis
      ii. **CT angiography** and/or **contrast angiography** can be performed.
         a) Angiography can be performed in conjunction with treatment (e.g., dilation, stenting).
         b) When using iodinated contrast, risk of contrast-induced nephropathy for either modality
         c) Angiography can be performed with carbon dioxide contrast when iodinated contrast will not be tolerated (requires a specialized injection system).
   f. Day-of-surgery laboratory tests: Hemoglobin, serum potassium, and glucose (goal to avoid procedural/anesthesia-related complications)
   g. AVA creation generally performed on an outpatient basis, using conscious sedation, local anesthetics/regional blocks
3. **AVF**
   a. Benefits: Superior longevity, patency, and resistance to infections compared with catheter and AVGs.
   b. Pitfalls: Requires maturation of the **needle-access segment** (NAS; vein dilation to appropriate size for needle access) over 4 weeks to

4 months, potential need for additional procedures to assist maturation (~40%) or due to maturation failure (6%-54%).[4,6]

c. Principles
   i. Nondominant limb preferred.
   ii. Distal over proximal: Lower risk of ischemic complications as well as keep proximal veins for potential future use.
   iii. Multiple established upper-limb locations (**Figure 38.2**) where anatomy may lend itself to direct arteriovenous anastomosis.
   iv. Artery with >2 mm diameter adequate for inflow.
   v. The mature NAS should be ≥6 mm in diameter and <5 mm deep to the skin and have ≥10 cm straight segment.
   vi. End-to-side vein to artery anastomosis using conventional or **piggyback straight line onlay technique** (pSLOT).[7]

d. **Surgical approach: Radiocephalic (Brescia–Cimino) fistula creation**
   i. Use intraoperative ultrasound imaging to identify, mark, and assess the cephalic vein and radial artery.
   ii. Make a 2- to 3-cm incision that will allow exposure of both vessels.
   iii. Dissect the vein, mark it to prevent torsion/kinking. Ligate and divide the vein distally.
   iv. Swing the vein over the artery to locate the anastomosis site, control the artery proximally and distally with vessel loops/clamps, and make a longitudinal arteriotomy.
   v. Anastomosis with fine polypropylene/polytetrafluoroethylene (PTFE) sutures
      a) Conventional end-to-side: Spatulate the end of the vein.
      b) pSLOT: Close the end of the vein, make a short 4-mm anastomosis between the posterior vein and anterior artery.
   vi. Check for AVF thrill, palpate the distal arterial pulse to ensure presence.
   vii. Ensure hemostasis, close the skin and subcutaneous tissue in layers.

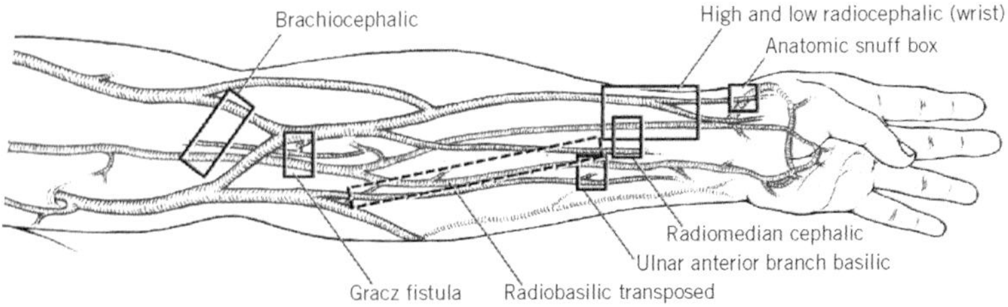

FIGURE 38.2 Possible sites of arteriovenous anastomosis in the upper extremity. *(From Shenoy S. Surgical anatomy of upper arm: what is needed for AVF planning. J Vasc Access. 2009;10(4):223-232. Copyright 2009, SAGE Publications. Reprinted by permission of SAGE Publications, Inc.)*

e. Postoperative evaluation
   i. Early assessment (7-10 days): Evaluate incision and fistula patency, detect any distal vascular insufficiency (ischemia/swelling)/neurologic deficit.
   ii. Maturation evaluation (4-6 weeks): Clinical assessment, CDDUS.
      a) Abnormalities are further evaluated with **fistulogram**.
f. Secondary surgical procedures may include
   i. Surgical superficialization required for NAS with adequate flows but too deep for easy cannulation.[8]
   ii. Ligate flow-diverting tributaries.

4. **AVG**
   a. Graft materials: PTFE, polyurethane, bovine artery/vein (xenograft), or cryopreserved human artery/vein (allograft)
   b. Benefits
      i. Rigid walls make graft cannulation easier than some AVFs.
      ii. No maturation needed.
   c. Pitfalls
      i. Prone to repeated thrombosis requiring significantly higher number of interventions than AVFs
      ii. Poor longevity relative to well-matured AVF
   d. Choice of vessels
      i. Artery: Proximal radial, brachial, or axillary
      ii. Vein: Deep veins of the upper arm (basilic, brachial, or axillary)
         a) Patients requiring AVG often lack sufficient superficial venous anatomy.
   e. Procedure considerations
      i. Prophylactic antibiotics (e.g., second-generation cephalosporin) are commonly administered immediately prior to surgery.
      ii. Two incisions (one over artery, one over vein) are made, and a tapered graft (4 mm arterial end diameter, to limit the inflow) is tunneled subcutaneously between the two and anastomosed at each end using fine monofilament suture.
   f. Postoperative use
      i. Conventional AVGs need good tissue incorporation prior to cannulation (3-6 weeks).
      ii. Newer composite graft materials permit early cannulation.

5. **AVA complications**
   a. Stenosis
      i. Responsible for over 90% of AVA dysfunctions.
      ii. Caused by venous neointimal hyperplasia in areas with higher hemodynamic stress (AVG graft-vein anastomosis, AVF juxta-anastomotic area).
      iii. Can lead to venous hypertension if central and/or late thrombosis.
      iv. Management: First line = **balloon angioplasty** (with or without thrombectomy as needed) and second-line = **surgical venoplasty/stenting**

b. Early thrombosis
  i. Due to technical error, inflammatory outflow narrowing, preexisting upstream vein occlusions, thrombophilia, hypotension
  ii. Often results in AVF loss
  iii. AVG salvage by thrombectomy and/or revision
c. Infection
  i. Cutaneous flora (commonly *Staphylococcus* species)
  ii. Can lead to skin ulceration, chronically infected aneurysm thrombi, and seeding of graft material.
  iii. Management depends on severity and presentation:
    a) Most AVF infections are treated with antibiotics.
    b) Most AVG infections require graft removal and AVA loss, although focal infections may be salvaged with resection of the infected portion and reconstruction with xenograft/allograft.
d. Aneurysms
  i. Defined as true dilations of the vein due to flow disruptions, repeated trauma, increased back-pressure from stenosis.
  ii. More common in AVF.
  iii. Skin overlying the aneurysm can thin and ulcerate risking rupture with life-threatening bleeding.
e. Pseudoaneurysms
  i. More common in AVG
  ii. High pressure in the graft leads to leaking of blood into subcutaneous tissue from needle holes.
f. Steal syndrome
  i. Increased blood flow in the AVA "steals" a fraction of blood from the distal circulation, usually well tolerated.
  ii. About 1% to 4% of patients have ischemic pain, worsening neuropathy, ulceration, or gangrene.[9]
  iii. Management depends on severity
    a) Mild symptoms (subjective coolness, paresthesia without sensory/motor loss) may be managed expectantly.
    b) Failure to improve or worsening symptoms
      1) Surgical banding can reduce access flow.
      2) If low AVA flow, enhance distal perfusion with
        - Proximalization of arteriovenous inflow: Use of a graft to maintain patency of the AVF from a proximal inflow source
        - **Distal revascularization interval ligation:** Ligation of the artery distal to the AVF inflow and revascularization of the distal arm with a bypass taken from a more proximal inflow source
    c) Severe ischemia with new-onset motor dysfunction/tissue-loss: Immediate AVA ligation

Key References

Citation	Summary
Lok CE, Huber TS, Lee T, et al. KDOQI Clinical practice guideline for vascular access: 2019 update. *Am J Kidney Dis.* 2020;75(4 suppl 2):S1-S164.	• Most recent update of the National Kidney Foundation's guidelines for hemodialysis vascular access. • Includes a summary of all guidelines, algorithms, and justification/description of supporting data.
Beathard GA, Lok CE, Glickman MH, et al. Definitions and end points for interventional studies for arteriovenous dialysis access. *Clin J Am Soc Nephrol.* 2018;13(3):501-512.	• Recommendations from the American Society of Nephrology on trial end points that would be useful in creating clinical practice guidelines, with the goal of facilitating design of future trials.
Shenoy S. Surgical anatomy of upper arm: what is needed for AVF planning. *J Vasc Access.* 2009;10(4):223-232.	• Overview of upper arm anatomy relevant to AVF creation, with recommendations for preoperative evaluation and systematic planning for multiple HD access sites that will likely be needed over the lifetime of a patient with ESKD.
Darcy M, Vachharajani N, Zhang T, et al. Long-term outcome of upper extremity arteriovenous fistula using pSLOT: single-center longitudinal follow-up using a protocol-based approach. *J Vasc Access.* 2017;18(6):515-521.	• Retrospective observational single-center cohort study of 342 patients, evaluating results of 372 AVF creations via pSLOT performed from 2008 to 2012. • Rate of primary patency (access patent without any intervention to improve/reestablish patency) at 1, 2, and 5 y was 42.8%, 31.6%, and 20.8%. • Rate of secondary patency (access patent but has required intervention) at 1, 2, and 5 y was 81.8%, 77.6%, and 71.7%.
Tan TW, Siracuse JJ, Brooke BS, et al. Comparison of one-stage and two-stage upper arm brachiobasilic arteriovenous fistula in the vascular quality initiative. *J Vasc Surg.* 2019;69(4):1187-1195.e2.	• VQI is the national US + Canada clinical database run by the Society of Vascular Surgery and spanning almost 1,000 centers. • This study was a retrospective multicenter observational cohort study of 2,648 patients who underwent either one- or two-stage creation of brachiobasilic arteriovenous fistula from 2010-2016. • Primary and secondary patency at 1 y were equivalent between groups on multivariate analysis accounting for history of previous access failure and preoperative diameter of the vessels used.

Citation	Summary
Wagner JK, Dillavou E, Nag U, et al. Immediate-access grafts provide comparable patency to standard grafts, with fewer reinterventions and catheter-related complications. J Vasc Surg. 2019;69(3):883-889.	• Immediate-access grafts (IAAVG) is an AVG in which the graft material somewhat seals around a puncture hole, allowing for immediate use of the AVG (as opposed to needing time after AVG implantation to allow for scar tissue formation for adequate hemostasis). • Retrospective two-center observational cohort study of 210 patients who underwent either SAVG or IAAVG creation. • Reported no instances of bleeding or infection attributable to early cannulation (within 10 d of placement), the majority of which was done in IAAVG grafts. • Primary and secondary patency equivalent between SAVG and IAAVG at 12 and 18 mo on univariate analysis.
Ryan SV, Calligaro KD, Scharff J, Dougherty MJ. Management of infected prosthetic dialysis arteriovenous grafts. *J Vasc Surg.* 2004;39(1):73-78.	• Retrospective observational single-center cohort study of 45 patients who underwent AVG creation between 1995 and 2002 and had subsequent AVG infection, who were treated with total graft excision (TGE), subtotal graft excision (SGE), or partial graft excision (PGE), with TGE and SGE requiring temporary dialysis catheter placement and PGE allowing for continued use of the original graft. • Hundred percent of TGE/SGE wounds healed by secondary intention, but (by definition) 100% lost use of the original graft. • Seventy-four percent of patients with PGE had graft patency and good wound healing, with failures (all due to poor wound healing) treated with TGE. • Concluded that PGE may be of use in select patients with highly localized infection of only a portion of graft.

CHAPTER 38: DIALYSIS ACCESS

Review Questions

1. At which stage of chronic kidney disease (CKD) should a patient be referred for surgical dialysis access?
2. What is the most common cause of arteriovenous graft (AVG) dysfunction?
3. What are five absolute contraindications to PD?
4. What is an acceptable initial empiric antibiotic regimen for peritonitis/sepsis in a patient on peritoneal dialysis (PD)?
5. What is the most common site of flow-limiting stenoses in arteriovenous fistulae (AVF)?
6. With symptomatic steal syndrome, what are indications for attempts at arteriovenous access (AVA) preservation vs ligation (loss)?
7. In what kind of AVA is aneurysm most common? Pseudoaneurysm?

REFERENCES

1. Johansen KL, Chertow GM, Gilbertson DT, et al. US renal data system 2021 annual data report: epidemiology of kidney disease in the United States. *Am J Kidney Dis*. 2022;79(4 suppl 1):A8-A12.
2. Li PKT, Szeto CC, Piraino B, et al. Peritoneal dialysis-related infections recommendations: 2010 update. *Perit Dial Int*. 2010;30(4):393-423.
3. Saugel B, Scheeren TWL, Teboul JL. Ultrasound-guided central venous catheter placement: a structured review and recommendations for clinical practice. *Crit Care*. 2017;21(1):225.
4. Ravani P, Palmer SC, Oliver MJ, et al. Associations between hemodialysis access type and clinical outcomes: a systematic review. *J Am Soc Nephrol*. 2013;24(3):465-473.
5. Hui SH, Folsom R, Killewich LA, Michalek JE, Davies MG, Pounds LL. A comparison of preoperative and intraoperative vein mapping sizes for arteriovenous fistula creation. *J Vasc Surg*. 2018;67(6):1813-1820.
6. Allon M, Robbin ML. Increasing arteriovenous fistulas in hemodialysis patients: problems and solutions. *Kidney Int*. 2002;62(4):1109-1124.
7. Bharat A, Jaenicke M, Shenoy S. A novel technique of vascular anastomosis to prevent juxta-anastomotic stenosis following arteriovenous fistula creation. *J Vasc Surg*. 2012;55(1):274-280.
8. Wilson SE. *Vascular Access: Principles and Practice*. 5th ed. Lippincott Williams and Wilkins; 2009.
9. Goff CD, Sato DT, Bloch PHS, et al. Steal syndrome complicating hemodialysis access procedures: can it Be predicted? *Ann Vasc Surg*. 2000;14(2):138-144.
10. Lok CE, Huber TS, Lee T, et al. KDOQI clinical practice guideline for vascular access: 2019 update. *Am J Kidney Dis*. 2020;75(4 suppl 2):S1-S164.
11. Beathard GA, Lok CE, Glickman MH, et al.. Definitions and end points for interventional studies for arteriovenous dialysis access. *Clin J Am Soc Nephrol*. 2018;13(3):501-512.
12. Shenoy S. Surgical anatomy of upper arm: what is needed for AVF planning. *J Vasc Access*. 2009;10(4):223-232.

13. Darcy M, Vachharajani N, Zhang T, et al. Long-term outcome of upper extremity arteriovenous fistula using pSLOT: single-center longitudinal follow-up using a protocol-based approach. *J Vasc Access*. 2017;18(6):515-521.

14. Tan TW, Siracuse JJ, Brooke BS, et al. Comparison of one-stage and two-stage upper arm brachiobasilic arteriovenous fistula in the vascular quality initiative. *J Vasc Surg*. 2019;69(4):1187-1195.e2.

15. Wagner JK, Dillavou E, Nag U, et al. Immediate-access grafts provide comparable patency to standard grafts, with fewer reinterventions and catheter-related complications. *J Vasc Surg*. 2019;69(3):883-889.

16. Ryan SV, Calligaro KD, Scharff J, Dougherty MJ. Management of infected prosthetic dialysis arteriovenous grafts. *J Vasc Surg*. 2004;39(1):73-78.

39 Pediatric Surgery

Cathleen M. Courtney and Brad W. Warner

I. FLUIDS AND NUTRITION IN CHILDREN

A. Fluid requirements

1. Normal daily fluid requirements of children are higher than those of adults due to greater insensible and urinary losses.
2. Infants have a particularly high body surface area-to-volume ratio and limited ability to concentrate urine due to immature renal function.
3. Total body water comprises a higher percentage of body weight in children (75% vs 60% in adults).
4. Postoperative fluid replacement can be calculated using the "4-2-1" rule and should be adjusted to support hemodynamic stability and urine output between 1 and 2 mL/kg/h (**Table 39.1**).
5. Total body weight is a surrogate for total blood volume (approximately 80 mL/kg).
6. Isotonic fluid boluses should be in a volume of 10 to 20 mL/kg.
7. Initial transfusion of packed red blood cells is typically 10 mL/kg.

B. Nutrition

1. Nutritional intake for infants and children must account for both growth and maintenance.
   a. Newborn enteral caloric requirements are 100 to 120 kcal/kg/d while parenteral are 90 to 100 kcal/kg/d.
   b. Daily caloric needs decrease throughout childhood to adult values of roughly 25 to 30 kcal/kg/d (**Table 39.2**).
   c. A newborn is expected to gain 15 to 30 g/d.
   d. Most enteral infant formulas and breast milk contain ~20 kcal/oz.
2. **Parenteral nutrition**. Several surgical conditions, particularly neonatal gastrointestinal anomalies, may require administration of total parenteral nutrition (TPN) (**Table 39.3**).

TABLE 39.1 Postoperative Fluid Replacement

Weight (kg)	Fluids (mL/kg/h)
0-10	+4
11-20	+2
>20	+1

TABLE 39.2 Daily Caloric Needs in Children

Age (y)	REE (kcal/kg/d)	Average (kcal/kg/d)
<36 wk	63	120
0-0.5	53	108
0.5-1	56	98
1-3	57	102
4-6	48	90
7-10	40	70
11-14	32	55
15-18	27	45

REE, resting energy expenditure.

TABLE 39.3 Components of Parenteral Nutrition and Titration in Neonates[a,b]

	Caloric Density (kcal/g)	Daily Calories (%)	Starting Value	Daily Titration	Goal
Carbohydrate	3.4	60	5.5 mg/kg/min	2-3 mg/kg/min	12-14 mg/kg/min
Fat	4	30	1 g/kg/d	1 g/kg/d	3 g/kg/d
Protein	9	10	2.5 g/kg/d	0.5–1 g/kg/d	Term infant: 3 g/kg/d Preterm infant: 3.4-4 g/kg/d

[a]Please note that starter TPN is indicated when neonates are <1,500 g or <32 wk. This helps promote an anabolic state after withdrawal of placental nutrients and protein and aids in glucose utilization, overall improving neurodevelopment.

[b]Addition of insulin is not routine in pediatric TPN infusions, as exogenous insulin-naive cells are particularly sensitive to its effects and risk hypoglycemia. However, blood glucose should be monitored to prevent seizures and impaired neurodevelopment from hypoglycemia and osmotic diuresis with possible resultant intraventricular hemorrhage in the setting of hyperglycemia.

II. NEONATAL SURGICAL CONDITIONS

A. Tracheoesophageal malformations

1. A spectrum of anomalies including isolated **esophageal atresia** (EA) or combined **tracheoesophageal fistula** (TEF) (**Figure 39.1**)
2. Incidence is 3 in 10,000 births
3. Slight male predominance
4. Diagnosis
   - a. Presentation: Neonatal patient with difficulty clearing secretions, regurgitation of saliva, or respiratory difficulty during feeds.
     - i. The classic finding is inability to pass an oro- or nasogastric tube.
   - b. Imaging
     - i. Radiography: Visualization of a coiled orogastric tube in the upper chest on plain radiograph implies EA (**Figure 39.2**), and presence of gas in the gastrointestinal (GI) tract confirms a distal communication between the respiratory and GI systems (TEF).
       - a) Plain imaging should be reviewed for aspiration.
     - ii. Contrast studies are rarely necessary to visualize the level of EA and/or TEF and are associated with risk for aspiration.
   - c. Up to two-thirds of patients with EA/TEF have associated anomalies, and workup for **VACTERL anomalies** (*V*ertebral, *A*norectal, *C*ardiac, *T*racheal, *E*sophageal, *R*enal, and *L*imb) should be completed.
   - d. Treatment
     - i. Decompression of the proximal esophageal pouch with oral or nasal tube
     - ii. A 30° elevation of the head of the bed to reduce the risk of aspiration
     - iii. Ventilation may prove challenging in the presence of a TEF.
       - a) Positive pressure can transmit through the TEF into the GI system, increasing abdominal distention and pressure.
       - b) Passage of an endotracheal tube beyond the fistula, right mainstem intubation, or high-frequency oscillatory ventilation may be necessary.
     - iv. Operative approach is determined by the side of the aortic arch (e.g., operative repair for infants with a right-sided aortic arch requires an alternative approach, often through the left chest).
     - v. **Surgical approach: Repair of tracheoesophageal fistula (normal left-sided aortic arch)**
       - a) Retropleural thoracotomy through the right fourth intercostal space
       - b) Identification and ligation of fistula (multiple options)
       - c) Mobilization of proximal esophageal stump
       - d) Tension-free primary hand-sewn anastomosis (unless a long-gap EA)
       - e) Placement of a chest tube and chest closure

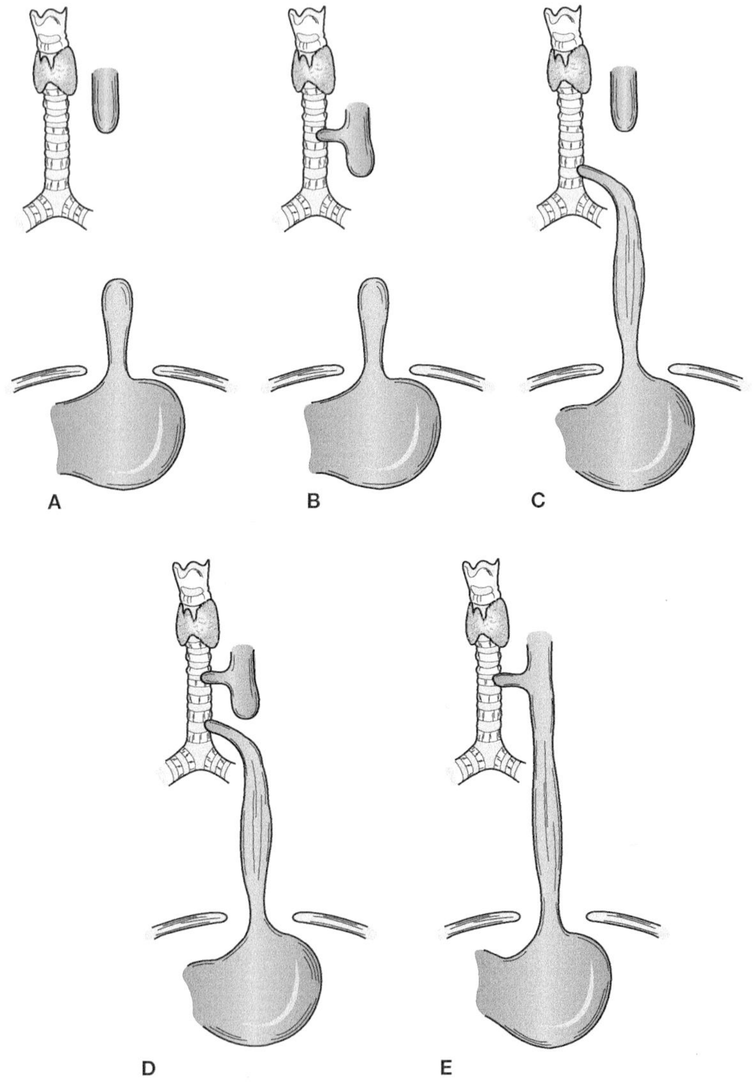

FIGURE 39.1 Variants of TEF. A, Pure esophageal atresia without fistula (5%-7% of cases). B, Proximal fistula and distal pouch (<1% of cases). C, Proximal pouch with distal fistula (85%-90% of cases). D, Atresia with proximal and distal fistulas (<1% of cases). E, Fistula without atresia ("H type") (2%-6% occurrence).

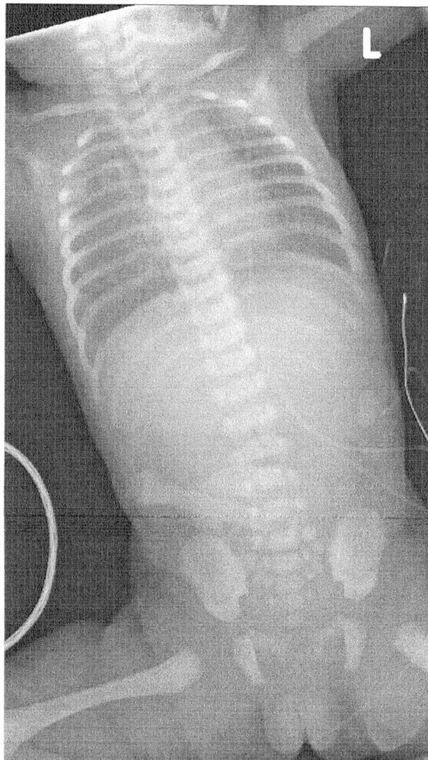

FIGURE 39.2 Radiographic findings of esophageal atresia. Note the orogastric tube ending in upper chest and the absence of bowel gas, suggesting pure esophageal atresia without any communication between the airway and gastrointestinal tract.

vi. A long-gap EA can be reconstructed with a variety of techniques including lengthening myotomy, colonic interposition, gastric pull-up, or delayed repair after a period of growth or traction (the **Foker process**).

vii. An isolated TEF without EA is often more proximal and can be approached via a cervical incision.

B. Congenital diaphragmatic hernia (CDH)

1. Incidence of 1 in every 3,000 live births
2. Equal male to female distribution
3. Result of incomplete diaphragm development at 8 weeks of gestation
   a. Abdominal contents herniate into the chest, resulting in lung compression and subsequent hypoplasia.
   b. The pulmonary vasculature develops increased tone in the muscular arterioles, which predisposes to pulmonary hypertension and vasospasm.

4. The majority (80%-90%) of hernias are posterolateral (**Bochdalek**), with the remainder presenting anteriorly (**Morgagni**).
5. Approximately 90% of hernias occur on the left.
6. Presentation
   a. Frequently diagnosed during routine prenatal screening ultrasound scans
      i. Prenatal diagnosis should lead to a multidisciplinary team of critical care neonatologists and surgeons available for respiratory management at the time of birth.
   b. For patients not diagnosed prenatally, presentation may include significant respiratory distress (tachypnea, cyanosis, retractions), asymmetric chest wall diameter, and a scaphoid abdomen as a result of abdominal contents herniating into the chest.
   c. Fewer than 20% of cases present >24 hours of life with respiratory distress, pneumonia, feeding intolerance, or intestinal obstructions.
   d. Major negative predictors of outcome include an intrathoracic liver, presence of major congenital heart disease, and other associated anomalies.
7. Diagnosis through imaging: Plain CXR demonstrating bowel gas patterns in the chest is sufficient for diagnosis (**Figure 39.3**).

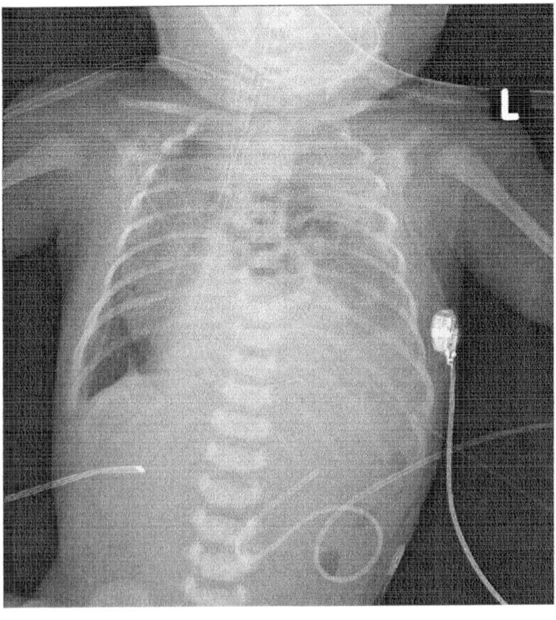

FIGURE 39.3 A case of congenital diaphragmatic hernia showing bowel filling the left chest.

8. Treatment
   a. Immediate postnatal care focuses on cardiopulmonary stabilization.
   b. Endotracheal intubation and oro- or nasogastric tube decompression to reduce gastric distension is often required.
   c. Management of pulmonary hypertension is key with avoidance of severe hypoxia, inhaled nitric oxide, prostacyclin, maintenance of systemic blood pressure.
   d. Ventilation with low positive-pressure, permissive hypercapnia, and stable hypoxemia (tolerance of preductal oxygen saturations >80%) minimizes barotrauma.
   e. About 20% to 40% of CDH neonates will require **extracorporeal membrane oxygenation**.
   f. Once the patient is stable on lower ventilator settings, operative fixation of the hernia should be undertaken.
   g. **Surgical approach: Repair of congenital diaphragmatic hernia**
      i. A subcostal abdominal incision or thoracotomy is made on the affected side (in smaller defects in which the liver is not above the diaphragm and patients are stable, thoracoscopic or laparoscopic approaches may be used).
      ii. Herniated abdominal contents are reduced into the abdomen.
      iii. The defect is repaired primarily and usually requires dissection of the posterior leaf away from the chest wall.
      iv. In larger defects a synthetic or biologic patch may be used.
      v. The abdominal or chest incisions are closed.
9. Outcomes
   a. Outcomes differ greatly between cases presenting with profound respiratory distress at birth compared with infants presenting >24 hours after birth.
   b. Overall survival rates are approximately 70%.
   c. Significant respiratory disease at birth can result in neurologic deficits, including developmental delay, gastroesophageal reflux, and seizures.
   d. Patients must be followed to observe for respiratory symptoms, gastroesophageal reflux, chronic lung disease, hernia recurrence, and the possibility of need for reoperation if a patch was used in the initial operation.

C. Abdominal wall defects
1. Neonatal development
   a. During normal embryologic development, the midgut herniates outward through the umbilical ring.
   b. By the 11th week of gestation, the midgut returns to the abdominal cavity and undergoes counterclockwise rotation and fixation, along with closure of the umbilical ring.
   c. **Omphalocele** is the failure of the abdominal contents to reduce back into the abdomen, resulting in a large hernia covered by a peritoneal sac.
   d. **Gastroschisis** is believed to be the result of an isolated intrauterine vascular insult resulting in an abdominal wall defect to the right of

the umbilical cord. The bowel herniates through the defect but is not covered by a sac.

e. Gastroschisis defects tend to be smaller than those of an omphalocele.
f. Omphalocele is typically associated with congenital anomalies (50% of cases have an associated genetic and/or cardiac anomaly) that often has a major impact on the prognosis of the infant.
g. There is a smaller incidence of associated anomalies with gastroschisis (10% rate of associated intestinal atresias).

2. Diagnosis: Often made at the time of prenatal ultrasound imaging after 13 weeks of gestation or by clinical examination at the time of birth.
3. Treatment
    a. Naso- or orogastric tube decompression
    b. Broad-spectrum prophylactic antibiotics
    c. Heat and fluid losses from exposed viscera should be corrected with IV fluids (IVFs) and warming while covering the exposed organs and lower body in a clear plastic bag.
    d. Do not cover the bowel with gauze and pour warm saline on the infant as the gauze prevents visualization of the bowel, and the warm saline ultimately drops to room temperature, cooling the infant.
    e. In gastroschisis, the bowel may be placed within a **Silastic silo** at the bedside, with gradual gravity-based reduction into the abdomen while monitoring for abdominal compartment syndrome and respiratory compromise.
    f. In omphalocele, the sac serves as sufficient coverage until operative closure is undertaken.
4. Operative repair
    a. Once the herniated abdominal contents can be reduced into the abdomen, the abdominal wall defect may be closed primarily.
    b. In some cases, the umbilical cord can be used to cover the defect thereby avoiding the need for operative closure.
        i. Usually results in umbilical hernia, which can be repaired later in life
        ii. Associated with a better cosmetic result
    c. In omphalocele, the sac is excised with care to ligate the umbilical vessels.
        i. Large omphalocele that cannot be closed primarily, sac is allowed to desiccate and ultimately separate, leaving an epithelialized covering over the bowel, then wrapping with elastic wraps followed by fascial closure is undertaken.
        ii. Fascial closure may require abdominal component separation, skin flaps, prosthetic or biologic patches, and/or tissue expanders to allow for closure.

D. Necrotizing enterocolitis

1. Etiology
    a. The most common neonatal gastrointestinal emergency.
    b. Acute inflammatory disease of the intestine associated with ulceration and necrosis of the gastrointestinal tract most frequently affecting the small bowel.

   c. Pathogenesis is believed to be multifactorial involving prematurity, an immature gut barrier defense, bacteria, enteral feeding, and hypoxia/ischemia or low-flow states.
   d. Incidence is 1 to 3 per 1,000 live births.
   e. Prematurity is the most prominent risk factor.
2. Diagnosis
   a. Requires a high clinical suspicion.
   b. Unusual within the first few days of life, but approximately 80% of cases occur within the first month of life.
   c. Presentation: Lethargy, irritability, abdominal distention, feeding intolerance, temperature instability, apneic, or bradycardic episodes or passage of bloody stools
      i. Advanced cases may show signs of peritonitis including erythema of the abdominal wall.
   d. Laboratory studies: Leukocytosis or leukopenia, metabolic acidosis, and thrombocytopenia.
   e. Imaging: Plain radiographs often reveal dilated loops of bowel with evidence of ischemia including **pneumatosis intestinalis** (**Figure 39.4**), **portal venous gas**, and/or pneumoperitoneum.
   f. Based on clinical examination and laboratory and imaging data, patients and their expectant management can be guided by **Bell staging**.[1]
3. Initial management
   a. If hemodynamically stable, then bowel rest, nasogastric decompression, parenteral nutrition, and broad-spectrum antibiotics.

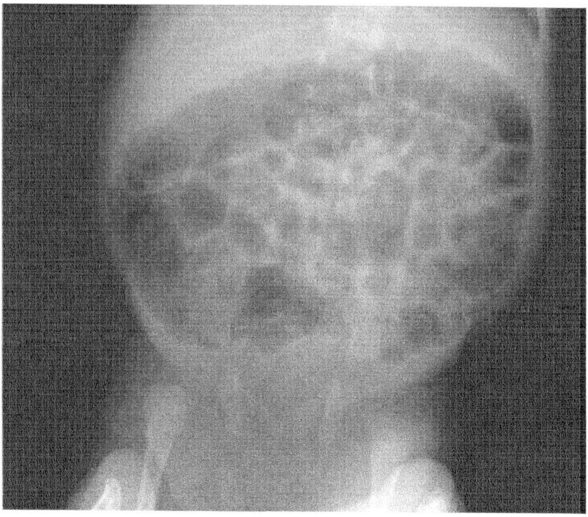

FIGURE 39.4 Radiographic findings of necrotizing enterocolitis. Pneumatosis intestinalis is visualized in the right upper quadrant.

b. Serial abdominal examinations, laboratory studies (complete blood count, blood gas) and plain radiographs are used to determine the success of nonoperative management (**Figure 39.5**).
c. Fifty percent of patients will improve with nonoperative management alone.

4. Operative management
   a. Indications
      i. Intestinal perforation (free air on abdominal radiograph)
      ii. Overall clinical deterioration
      iii. Abdominal wall cellulitis
      iv. Worsening acidosis
      v. Falling white blood cell or platelet count
      vi. Palpable abdominal mass
      vii. Persistent fixed loop on repeated abdominal radiographs
   b. Improvement of clinical status can be achieved with laparotomy, including resection of nonviable bowel and anastomoses or stomas as necessary, or with **peritoneal drainage**, a bedside procedure performed under local anesthesia that has shown outcomes comparable with laparotomy in select patients.

E. Meconium syndromes
1. Etiology: Associated with **cystic fibrosis** (CF) and **Hirschsprung disease**.
   a. Testing for these diseases is recommended even in the setting of simple and resolved meconium plugs.
   b. **Meconium ileus** may be the earliest manifestation of CF.
2. Diagnosis
   a. Unrecognized obstruction can progress to enterocolitis, sepsis, and perforation.
   b. Water-soluble contrast enemas can be both therapeutic and diagnostic.
   c. Imaging: Plain radiographs demonstrate dilated loops of small bowel filled with meconium with absent air–fluid levels.
   d. Treatment: Relief of the obstructed bowel, frequently in the distal ileum, may require laparotomy, in which case an enterotomy is made to remove and irrigate inspissated meconium using saline or *N*-acetylcysteine.

F. Malrotation
1. Etiology: Intestine fails to complete its normal 270° counterclockwise rotation around the superior mesenteric artery between the 4th and 10th weeks of gestation.
2. Presentation
   a. Bilious emesis and abdominal distention in the neonatal period
   b. Bilious emesis in a neonate should be considered a surgical emergency and mandates an emergent upper GI contrast study to rule out midgut volvulus.
   c. Intestinal rotation abnormalities may also present later in life with intermittent or chronic abdominal pain with or without bilious emesis.
   d. Mesenteric attachments (**Ladd's bands**) to the ileal-cecal region can result in mechanical obstruction (usually at the duodenum due to the attachments in the right upper quadrant to the colon).

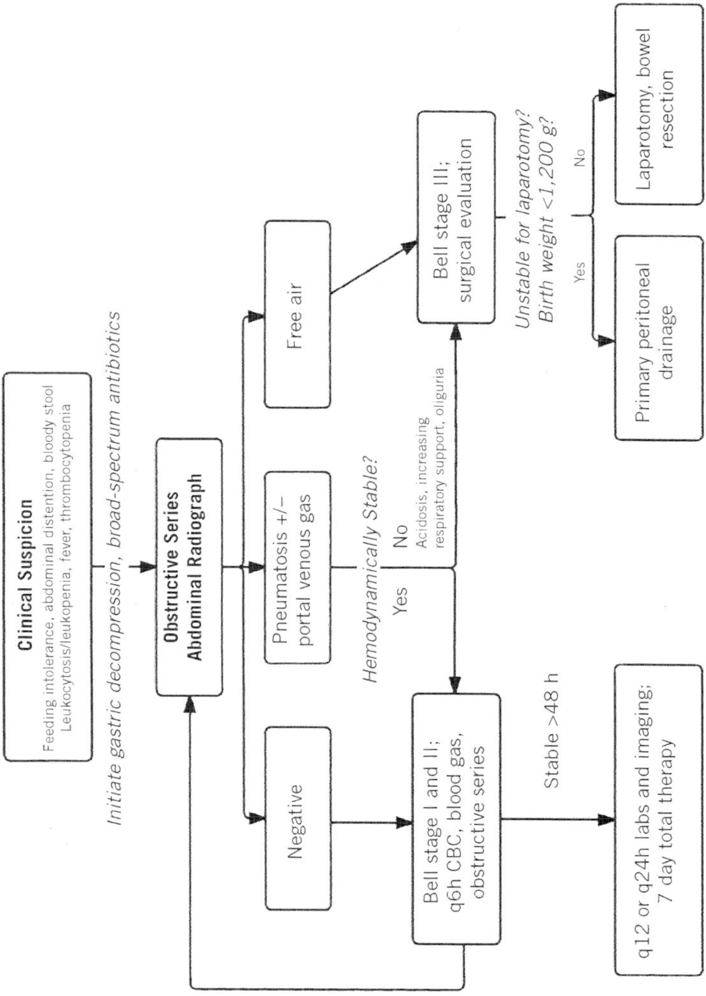

FIGURE 39.5 Algorithm for management of patients with suspected necrotizing enterocolitis.

e. Imaging
    i. Abdominal radiographs can show dilated or normal bowel patterns.
    ii. Upper GI contrast study is the test of choice and demonstrates failure of the duodenojejunal junction to cross midline with jejunum in the right hemiabdomen.
    iii. Volvulus may appear as a classic "bird's beak" or corkscrew appearance of the intestine.

3. **Surgical approach: Ladd procedure for correction of malrotation**
    a. Supraumbilical transverse incision
    b. Bowel is untwisted in a counterclockwise manner ("turn back the hands of time"), then resection of compromised bowel, if any.
    c. Division of Ladd's bands between the duodenum and colon, allowing for broadening of the mesenteric base.
    d. Appendectomy to prevent future diagnostic uncertainty since the cecum is in an aberrant location.
    e. The small bowel is placed in the right hemiabdomen and the colon is placed in the left hemiabdomen, and the abdomen is closed.

G. Jejunoileal intestinal atresia

1. Etiology is intrauterine vascular insult
2. Presentation
    a. Distal obstructive symptoms (failure to pass meconium) or proximal symptoms (feeding intolerance, bilious emesis)
    b. The most common location is the distal small bowel.
    c. Prenatal ultrasound may demonstrate polyhydramnios.
    d. Imaging
        i. Abdominal radiograph will show dilated proximal loops with absence of air distally.
        ii. Upper gastrointestinal contrast studies are helpful in identifying the suspected level of the atresia and ruling out volvulus.
3. Treatment
    a. Resection of atretic segment with care to preserve adequate small intestinal length and then reanastomosis.
    b. Stomas can be used if primary anastomosis is not technically feasible or high risk.

H. Duodenal atresia

1. Etiology
    a. Failure of recanalization of the duodenal lumen
    b. Much higher association with other conditions than jejunoileal atresias, including prematurity, Down syndrome, maternal polyhydramnios, malrotation, annular pancreas, and biliary atresia
2. Presentation: Plain radiographs demonstrate the "**double bubble**" sign caused by air within both the stomach and duodenum.
3. Treatment: Operative repair may be through duodenoduodenostomy with or without duodenoplasty to account for proximal dilatation of the bowel.

I. Anorectal malformations
   1. Anorectal malformations include a variety of congenital defects.
   2. Often associated with other congenital defects as part of the VACTERL syndromes.
   3. Lesions are characterized by their level—low or high—and that distinction determines whether or not repair can be done in the newborn period without the need for a colostomy.
   4. Low lesions are indicated by an anocutaneous fistula (meconium noted at the perineum) and are often amenable to perineal anoplasty in the newborn period.
   5. Management follows an algorithmic approach in the majority of cases (**Figure 39.6**).

J. Hirschsprung disease
   1. Etiology/epidemiology
      a. Due to absent ganglion cells in the **myenteric (Auerbach)** and **submucosal (Meissner) plexuses** starting in the rectum and extending proximally.
         i. Associated with nerve fiber hypertrophy and muscular spasm of the distal colon and internal anal sphincter resulting in a functional obstruction.
      b. Occurs in 1 of 5,000 live births.
      c. There is a predisposition for patients with affected family members as well as those with trisomy 21.
   2. Diagnosis
      a. Abdominal distention and failure to pass meconium within 24 hours.
      b. Older patients may present with chronic constipation, even in adulthood.
      c. Imaging
         i. Radiography demonstrates absence or paucity of air distal to the obstruction.
         ii. Contrast enema reveals a transition zone between proximally dilated and distally decompressed pathologically abnormal bowel (inversion of rectosigmoid ratio).
      d. *Rectal biopsy is required for pathologic confirmation of the diagnosis*, performed transanally with a suction device or linear full-thickness biopsy to assess for presence of ganglion cells.
   3. Treatment
      a. Preoperative decompression accomplished by saline colonic irrigations to evacuate impacted stool.
      b. Operative technique aimed at identifying the transition zone ("leveling") with serial biopsies, then bringing ganglionated bowel down to the anus while preserving sphincter function. Historically, two-stage procedures with stoma formation were utilized, now single-stage procedures are preferred.
         i. **Swenson procedure:** Aganglionic bowel is removed to the level of the internal sphincters, and a coloanal anastomosis is performed on the perineum.

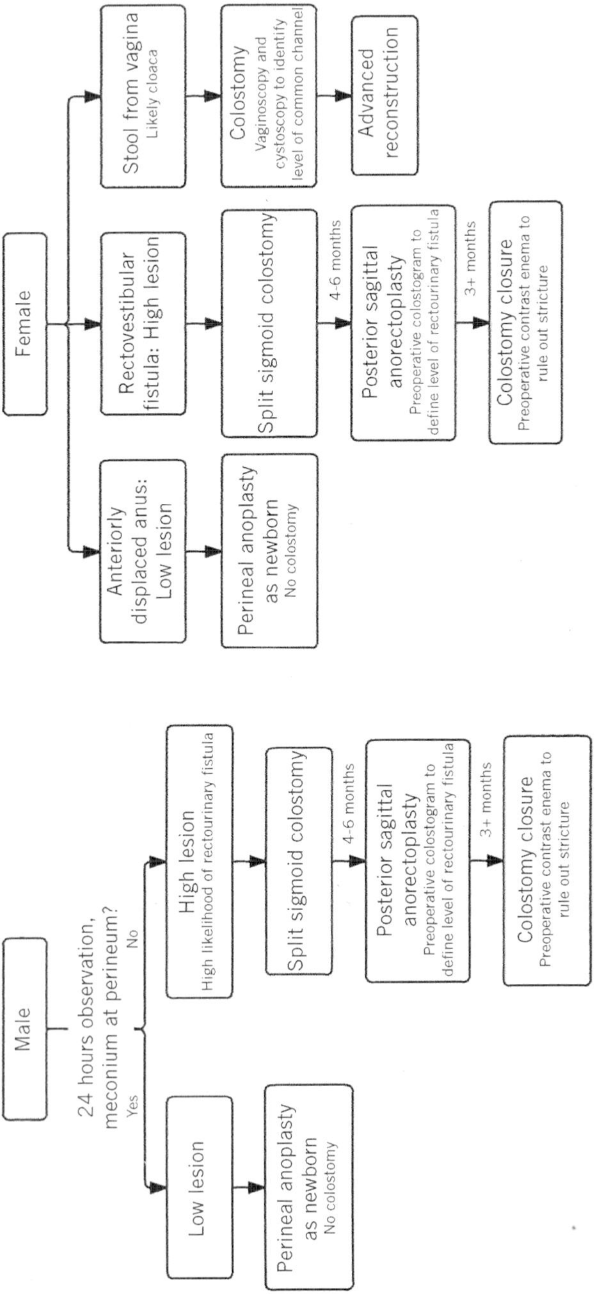

FIGURE 39.6 Algorithm for management of neonatal anorectal anomalies.

ii. **Duhamel procedure:** Aganglionic rectal stump is left in place, and the ganglionated, normal colon is pulled behind and anastomosed to this stump.
iii. **Soave procedure:** Endorectal mucosal dissection within the aganglionic distal rectum is performed, and normal colon is pulled through the remnant muscular cuff and a coloanal anastomosis performed, usually done by a combined abdominal/transanal approach or completely transanal approach with equivalent outcomes.

III. THORACIC PATHOLOGY

A. Congenital airway malformations

1. **Pulmonary sequestrations**
   a. Lung malformations with an aberrant blood supply and no bronchial communication.
   b. **Intralobar sequestrations** are contained within lung parenchyma.
      i. Commonly in medial and posterior segments of the lower lobe.
      ii. Two-thirds are left sided.
      iii. Eighty-five percent receive anomalous arterial supply from the infradiaphragmatic aorta via the inferior pulmonary ligament.
      iv. CT and MRI are useful studies to elucidate the vascular supply.
      v. Indications for surgery include risk of hemorrhage or infection.
   c. **Extralobar sequestrations** are surrounded by a separate pleural layer.
      i. Predominantly male disease (3:1).
      ii. Associated with other anomalies in 40% of cases, including CDH, chest wall deformities, and congenital heart disease.
      iii. Lower infection risk, allowing for a period of observation for asymptomatic patients.
2. **Congenital pulmonary airway malformations**
   a. Multicystic lesions of bronchial tissue with relatively little alveoli.
   b. Typically do not have normal bronchial communication.
   c. Classified by size
      i. Type I—macrocystic (>2 cm)
      ii. Type II—epithelial-lined cysts (<1 cm), frequently associated with CDH, cardiac malformations, or other anomalies
      iii. Type III—microcystic, have poor prognosis
   d. Pulmonary resection in the newborn period should be performed because of the potential for size increase, infection, or malignancy.
3. **Bronchogenic cysts**
   a. Lined by ciliated cuboidal or columnar epithelium and mucous glands
   b. Two-thirds of cysts are within lung parenchyma, and the remainder are within the mediastinum.
   c. Resected due to symptoms and concern for malignant potential
4. **Congenital lobar emphysema**
   a. Most commonly in the left upper lobe
   b. Due to overdistention of one or more lobes within a histologically normal lung due to abnormal cartilaginous support of the feeding bronchus

c. Bronchial collapse creates a one-way valve promoting air trapping.
d. Many patients are asymptomatic.
e. Respiratory distress with radiographic imaging mimicking tension pneumothorax may occur; thus, placement of a chest tube in these instances would be detrimental and emergent lobar resection may be needed.

B. Chest wall deformities

1. Classifications
   a. **Pectus carinatum**—abnormal protrusion of the chest wall and sternum
   b. **Pectus excavatum**—abnormal caved-in appearance of the chest wall
      i. Five times more common than carinatum
      ii. A 3:1 male to female ratio
2. Etiology: Both believed to be related to abnormal and asymmetric costal cartilage development.
3. Diagnosis
   a. CXR
   b. Examination for scoliosis, present in 15% of cases
   c. Evaluation for cardiorespiratory abnormalities
   d. Additional workup may require echocardiogram and ophthalmologic examination if concern for cardiac abnormalities or Marfan syndrome exists.
   e. Pulmonary function tests should be obtained if there is concern for the condition causing pulmonary impairment.
   f. CT scan allows evaluation of the **Haller index** (transverse chest diameter divided by the anterior–posterior diameter: Normal <2, mild 2-3.2, moderate 3.2-3.5, severe >3.5) to document severity of the defect, but has little bearing on operative consideration.
4. Treatment
   a. Surgery is largely cosmetic, as the condition becomes exaggerated physically and psychosocially in the pubescent years.
   b. Correction generally performed after 8 years of age to prevent restrictive chest wall deformities.
   c. Two standard techniques, **Ravitch** and **Nuss (minimally invasive)**, offer effective approaches; both require subsequent surgery to remove hardware.
   d. Carinatum defects are usually corrected with external brace therapy. Infrequently cartilage resection and sternal fixation are performed.

IV. ABDOMINAL PATHOLOGY

A. Hypertrophic pyloric stenosis (HPS)

1. The most common surgical cause of nonbilious vomiting
2. Occurs in 1 in 400 births
3. Occurs between 2 and 8 weeks of age
4. Male to female ratio of 4:1
5. Infants of Northern European descent are most affected.
6. Increased incidence for children of parents with HPS

7. Characterized by hypertrophy of the circular muscle of the pylorus resulting in gastric outlet obstruction
8. Presentation
   a. Projectile nonbilious emesis associated with feeding and persistent fussiness
   b. Pediatrician may initially diagnose a symptomatic child with more common diagnoses such as reflux or simple intolerance of particular formula.
9. Diagnosis
   a. Evaluation for dehydration (urine output) and electrolyte abnormalities
   b. **Hypokalemic, hypochloremic metabolic alkalosis** is the most common electrolyte abnormality due to hydrochloric acid loss from gastric secretions and potassium from the kidney in attempt to compensate for hypovolemia.
   c. Physical examination may reveal the "**olive sign**," the palpable pylorus to the right of and superior to the umbilicus.
   d. Imaging with abdominal ultrasound: Pyloric channel length >14 mm and single-wall muscular thickness of 4 mm or greater is diagnostic (these criteria have 99.5% sensitivity and 100% specificity for identifying HPS[2]).
10. Treatment
   a. Evaluation and treatment of dehydration and electrolyte abnormalities
   b. Nil per os to prevent further episodes of emesis
   c. IVF titrated to urine output >1 mL/kg/h; addition of potassium into fluids is withheld until urine output has been restored.
   d. Surgical timing is decided by the severity of electrolyte abnormalities, particularly HCO_3, which, if significantly elevated, results in compensatory respiratory acidosis that may result in apnea, a devastating consequence exaggerated by postanesthetic respiratory depression.
   e. **Operative treatment is pyloromyotomy.**
      i. Through open or laparoscopic approach, hypertrophied pylorus is identified.
      ii. A linear incision is made over the pylorus 2 mm proximal to the pyloroduodenal junction extending onto the antrum, and hypertrophied muscle fibers are split down to the mucosa.
      iii. Pylorus halves are tested for independent mobility.
      iv. Mucosa is inspected for perforation; the abdomen is closed.
   f. Postoperative feeding typically starts with an electrolyte solution with gradual advancement over the first 24 hours postoperatively to formula or breast milk volumes that are appropriate for age.
   g. Vomiting is a common postoperative issue, but, rarely, may be an indicator of incomplete myotomy.
   h. Complications include perforation of the mucosa, which is generally identified intraoperatively and treated by mucosal repair and nasogastric drainage.

B. Intussusception

1. Invagination or telescoping of the proximal intestine into distal bowel
2. Most common in infants 3 months to 3 years of age, and frequently originates at the ileocecal junction
3. Pathologic or anatomic lead point is often not present, although may be found in up to 20% of patients requiring surgery.[3]
    a. Most frequently Meckel diverticulum (remnant of the omphalomesenteric duct), intestinal polyp, or tumor
4. Presentation
    a. "Attacks" of a few minutes with periods of intense crying and leg retraction in infants
    b. Recent gastrointestinal or upper respiratory illness is common.
    c. Obstruction may result in ischemia, which produces stool with a mix of blood and mucus (i.e., "**currant jelly**" stools).
5. Diagnosis
    a. Abdominal radiographs show abnormal gas patterns concerning for a mass with subsequent paucity of gas in the right lower abdomen, sufficient for diagnosis in up to 50% of cases.
    b. Ultrasound may identify a "**target**" lesion representing a transverse view of the intussuscepted layers of bowel.
6. Treatment
    a. Contrast or air enema
        i. Successful in 80% of cases
        ii. Recurrence rate is approximately 10% within the first 24 hours.
        iii. Management of first recurrence is usually again attempted nonoperatively.
        iv. Failure and a second recurrence are indications for operation, as is peritonitis or concern for bowel ischemia at any stage of presentation.
    b. **Operative management of intussusception via open or laparoscopic approach**
        i. The abdomen is entered through open midline or transverse incision or can be performed laparoscopically.
        ii. The bowel is inspected for signs of ischemia or for evidence of a pathologic lead point.
        iii. If no ischemia or pathologic lead point is identified, an attempt is made at manual reduction by retrograde milking of the intussuscepted segment.
        iv. If manual reduction is unsuccessful, bowel ischemia is present, or a pathologic lead point is found, a segmental bowel resection with reanastomosis is performed.
        v. Abdomen is closed.
    c. With the open approach, reduction is achieved with retrograde (distal to proximal) squeezing or milking of the intussusceptum (portion intussuscepted) until reduced.
    d. With laparoscopy, the affected bowel is pulled in opposing directions to reduce the intussusception.
    e. Lymphoid tissue is often noted to be hypertrophic, but it is unclear if this is causative or reactive.
    f. Incidental appendectomy may also be performed.

C. Hepatobiliary

1. **Jaundice**
    a. Transient jaundice may be a normal physiologic condition of the newborn.
    b. Any infant with direct, conjugated hyperbilirubinemia (>2 mg/dL) beyond 2 weeks of age should undergo further workup.
    c. Unconjugated hyperbilirubinemia is often caused by physiologic jaundice of the newborn, hemolytic conditions, or breast milk jaundice.
    d. Conjugated hyperbilirubinemia may be caused by hepatitis or biliary obstruction.
2. **Choledochal cysts**
    a. A spectrum of abnormalities characterized by cystic dilatation of the biliary system.
    b. Fifty percent of affected children present within the first 10 years of life.
    c. Presentation: Jaundice, abdominal pain, and right upper quadrant mass.
    d. Diagnosis: Right upper quadrant ultrasound imaging, demonstrating biliary dilatation.
    e. Treatment
        i. Operation generally indicated for resolution of symptoms and potential for malignant degeneration.
        ii. Procedure is specific to the type of cyst (see Chapter 18).
3. **Biliary atresia**
    a. Progressive obliteration of extrahepatic bile ducts.
    b. No identified causative factor in the majority of cases, although genetic factors may play a causative role in a small subgroup of infants.
    c. Incidence 1 in 15,000 births
    d. Presentation: Jaundice, acholic stools, dark urine, and/or hepatomegaly
    e. Diagnosis
        i. Right upper quadrant ultrasound imaging demonstrating shrunken or absent gallbladder and incomplete or nonvisualized extrahepatic bile ducts.
        ii. Percutaneous liver biopsy is performed to confirm the diagnosis (bile duct plugs, biliary epithelial proliferation).
        iii. **Technetium-99m hepatobiliary iminodiacetic acid scan** aids in differentiating liver parenchymal disease and biliary obstructive disease.
            a) In biliary atresia, the liver takes up the tracer molecule but does not excrete into the extrahepatic biliary system or duodenum.
        iv. Cholangiography may be performed.
    f. Treatment
        i. **Kasai hepatoportoenterostomy:** Distal bile duct and gallbladder remnant are excised and a Roux-en-Y limb of jejunum is anastomosed to the divided portal plate (the scarred remnant of the biliary tract).

ii. Best outcomes if surgical correction takes place within the first 60 days of life with 30% requiring no further surgical intervention.[3]
iii. The remainder of patients inevitably progress to fibrosis, portal hypertension, and cholestasis and will require liver transplantation.
iv. Older patients or those with significant fibrosis at initial presentation may require immediate transplantation.

V. HEAD AND NECK MASSES

A. Branchial cleft cyst

1. Head and neck structures are embryologically derived from six branchial arches and the corresponding external clefts and internal pouches.
2. Congenital cysts, sinuses, or fistulae result from failure of appropriate migration or regression.
3. Branchial remnants are present at birth but may not become clinically evident until later in life.
4. In children, fistulas are more common than external sinuses or cysts.
5. Presentation: Visible or palpable lesions (see below), mucoid drainage, or development of infected cystic masses.
6. **First branchial remnants**
   a. Located in front or back of the ear or in the upper neck (mandibular region)
   b. May involve the parotid gland, facial nerve, or external auditory canal
7. **Second branchial cleft remnants**
   a. Most common
   b. Located along the anterior border of the sternocleidomastoid muscle
   c. May ascend along the carotid sheath
   d. Fistula may course up to the tonsillar fossa.
8. **Third branchial cleft remnants**
   a. Usually no associated sinuses or fistulae
   b. Often contain cartilage
   c. Located in the suprasternal notch or clavicular region
   d. Present as a firm mass or as a subcutaneous abscess

B. Thyroglossal duct cysts

1. Common in the midline of the neck located along the normal course of thyroid migration from foramen cecum to the anatomically normal site of the pyramidal lobe of the thyroid
2. Present in preschool-aged children
3. Represent incomplete thyroid gland formation
4. Frequently involves tongue or hyoid bone
5. Indications for operation
   a. Increasing size
   b. Infection or risk for infection
   c. Carcinoma risk (1% to 2%)
6. Diagnosis: Neck ultrasound imaging to identify involved structures including the site of normal thyroid tissue

7. Treatment is **Sistrunk procedure**—excision of the central portion of the hyoid bone in addition to the cyst in continuity with its tract

C. Lymphatic malformation (previously referred to as cystic hygroma)

1. Results from abnormal development of a lymphatic network that fails to drain into the venous system.
2. Seventy-five percent involve the lymphatic jugular sacks, presenting as a posterior neck mass.
3. The majority of lymphatic malformations present at birth (50%-65%), with most becoming apparent by the second year of life.
4. Diagnosis: MRI needed to determine extent of the lesion and neurovascular involvement.
5. Indications for operation
   a. Cosmetic
   b. Expansion that threatens compression of the airway
   c. Infection
   d. Pain
6. Treatment
   a. Complete surgical excision is preferred with caution to spare neurovascular structures. A subtotal resection is therefore often performed.
   b. Alternatively, malformations can be treated by sclerosing agent injection (bleomycin, tetracycline, hypertonic saline) for those that comprise large cysts (macrocystic).
   c. Postoperative complications: Recurrence, lymphatic leak, infection, and neurovascular injury

VI. TUMORS AND NEOPLASMS

A. Neuroblastoma

1. The most common solid tumor of childhood (6%-10% of all childhood cancers)
2. Approximately 600 to 700 new cases are diagnosed each year, with median age of diagnosis of 19 months with 90% diagnosed before age 10 years.
3. Neural crest origin and are thus found along the sympathetic nervous system, 75% in the abdomen or pelvis and half within the adrenal medulla
4. Median age of diagnosis of 2 years
5. Only 25% of patients present with isolated disease, often found incidentally; the remainder present with metastatic disease (most commonly to bone and lung) and have a poor prognosis
6. Young patients with early disease and favorable pathology have >90% survival, while older patients with unfavorable pathology or metastatic disease can have survival rates as low as 10%.
7. Diagnosis
   a. Evaluation for hypertension
   b. Urine testing for catecholamine metabolites
   c. CT or MRI to evaluate for vascular invasion or metastasis

d. Radiolabeled metaiodobenzylguanidine can be used to identify metastatic disease.
e. Bone marrow aspirate and biopsy are necessary for staging.
f. Staging and survival are determined by disease burden and genetic markers including N-*myc* overexpression and chromosomal deletions, which portend a worse prognosis.

8. Treatment
 a. Operation is first line for patients with low-risk, resectable, nonmetastatic disease.
 b. For patients with high-risk disease, multimodal treatment with chemotherapy, surgery, and radiotherapy is required to attempt to achieve disease control.

B. Wilms tumor
1. Six percent of all malignancies in children
2. The most common renal malignancy in children
3. Approximately 500 cases are diagnosed annually in the US
4. Average age of diagnosis of 3 or 4 years
5. No gender predominance
6. Most cases are sporadic, although heritable forms exist (**Beckwith–Wiedemann syndrome**).
7. Five percent of cases are bilateral.
8. Presentation: Incidental abdominal masses, possible hypertension, or hematuria
9. Diagnosis/staging
 a. Ultrasound imaging is used to confirm renal origin and evaluate for intravascular extension.
 b. CT or MRI may assist in differentiating Wilms tumor from neuroblastoma.
 c. Urine catecholamines
 d. CT chest is needed for complete staging.
10. Treatment
 a. Surgical intervention requires radial nephroureterectomy and lymph node sampling; intraoperative spillage of tumor contents must be carefully avoided, as it upstages the patient's disease (**Table 39.4**).
 b. For higher-risk disease, adjuvant chemotherapy can be added.
 c. Patients with bilateral renal involvement will require preoperative chemotherapy and parenchymal sparing resection.
 d. For resectable disease, combination surgery and chemotherapy result in cure rate >90%.

C. Teratomas
1. Tumors containing tissue from more than one of the **embryonic germ cell layers** (endoderm, ectoderm, mesoderm)
2. A frequent presentation in the neonatal period is sacrococcygeal teratoma
 a. Female to male ratio of 4:1
 b. Ultrasound and rectal examination are performed to rule out pelvic or presacral extension.
 c. The majority are benign and are removed with the sacrum to prevent recurrence.

TABLE 39.4 Wilms Tumor Staging System

Stage	Characteristics
I	Tumor confined to the kidney and completely excised intact
II	Tumor extends through the renal capsule into adjacent tissues (fat, vessels, etc.), but all affected tissue is completely excised intact. Stage II also includes cases in which the kidney is biopsied preoperatively or localized spillage occurs during resection
III	Tumor without hematogenous or extra-abdominal spread. Includes cases of positive lymph nodes, positive resection margins, or peritoneal implants
IV	Hematogenous metastases
V	Bilateral renal involvement

D. Soft tissue sarcomas

1. Account for 6% of childhood malignancies, most commonly rhabdomyosarcomas.
2. Wide local excision depending on the anatomic location with or without chemotherapy and lymph node sampling should be performed.
3. Additional information is located in Chapter 28.

VII. PEDIATRIC GENERAL SURGICAL CONDITIONS

A. Appendicitis

1. One of the most common pediatric surgical conditions
2. Presentation
   a. Abdominal pain followed by nausea
   b. Tenderness at **McBurney point** (one-third the distance between the right anterior iliac spine and umbilicus) and obturator, iliopsoas, or **Rovsing** signs (palpation of the left lower quadrant causes pain in the right lower quadrant) may be present on examination depending on location of the appendix.
   c. Scoring systems incorporating history, physical, and laboratory values such as the **Alvarado score**[4] can aid in risk stratification but are not frequently used in clinical practice.
3. Diagnosis
   a. Ultrasound is the first imaging modality of choice.
   b. CT can be used for patients in whom signs of advanced illness exist or ultrasound imaging was unsuccessful in identifying the appendix.
   c. Treatment
      i. Antibiotics
      ii. Laparoscopic appendectomy (see Chapter 22)
      iii. Some institutions are beginning to utilize nonoperative management.

B. Inguinal hernias
1. Affect approximately 1% to 5% of children
2. Predominance in males (8:1)
3. Increased rate in premature infants (7%-30%)
4. Bilateral hernias are present in 10% to 40% and occur more frequently in premature infants and girls.
5. Nearly all pediatric inguinal hernias are **indirect**; as such, the use of mesh is rare in the pediatric age group.
6. Due to an increased risk of recurrence and postanesthesia apnea in premature patients, neonatal inguinal hernias are frequently repaired prior to the patient leaving the hospital or at 50 weeks post conception.
7. Repair is recommended at approximately 6 months of age for infants who are asymptomatic or 24 to 48 hours after manual reduction for incarcerated hernias.
8. Surgical repair
   a. High ligation and excision of the processus vaginalis is performed.
   b. Plication or reconstruction of the floor of the inguinal canal may be necessary when the inguinal floor is particularly weak or the inguinal ring is very large.
   c. Mesh is generally not used in pediatric hernia repair.
   d. Teenagers near full growth potential may require a more traditional hernia repair, although this is decided on a case-by-case basis (see Chapter 25).

C. Umbilical hernia
1. Due to a persistence of the umbilical ring
2. Generally close spontaneously by age 4 to 5 years.
3. If the hernia has not closed by age 5 years or is large (>2 cm), or if the patient has had a history of bowel incarceration, operative primary closure is recommended.
4. Generally primary repair without mesh placement is preferred in the pediatric patient population.

D. Trauma—considerations in children
1. See additional information in Chapters 5 to 9.
2. Imaging
   a. Limiting radiation exposure and unnecessary testing is important in children. However, the inability to obtain reliable examinations in this population, particularly in trauma settings, complicates the decision to obtain imaging.
   b. Diffuse abdominal pain, a seatbelt sign, or distracting injuries can be indications for CT scan.
   c. In addition, elevated serum glutamic-oxaloacetic transaminase or serum glutamic-pyruvic transaminase levels higher than 200 or 100 IU/L, respectively, are accepted thresholds for obtaining a CT scan in the setting of blunt trauma.

3. Treatment of injury: Indications for exploratory laparoscopy or laparotomy are similar to adults and include hemodynamic instability with visible or suspected organ or vascular injury, penetrating abdominal injury, imaging findings consistent with bowel injury, or the presence of pelvic free fluid after blunt trauma without solid organ injury, suggestive of small bowel injury.
4. **Nonoperative management of isolated solid organ injury**
   a. Blunt injury to the liver and spleen is attempted to be managed nonoperatively in the pediatric population regardless of grading of injury by CT scan (see additional information regarding splenic and liver injury grading in Chapter 8) with close monitoring of hemodynamics and evidence of recurrent bleeding.
   b. Hemodynamic instability despite appropriate resuscitation with significant liver or splenic injury, as in adults, is an indication to proceed to the operating room for exploratory laparotomy and hemorrhage control.
   c. For patients with ongoing bleeding who are hemodynamically stable, angioembolization can be attempted for hemorrhage control to avoid the need for surgical intervention.
   d. Length of stay, need for intensive care unit admission, and activity restrictions are guided by the severity of solid organ injury.
   e. Regardless of the injury grade, and in the absence of specific indications, follow-up imaging either at the time of discharge or prior to resumption of normal activities is not indicated.

Key References

Citation	Summary
Blakely ML, Tyson JE, Lally KP, et al. Initial laparotomy versus peritoneal drainage in extremely low birthweight infants with surgical necrotizing enterocolitis or isolated intestinal perforation: a multicenter randomized clinical trial. *Ann Surg.* 2021;274(4):e370-e380.	• In extremely low-birthweight infants with necrotizing enterocolitis or isolated intestinal perforation, there is no difference in the rates of death or neurodevelopmental impairment (NDI) at 18-22 mo corrected age when compared in overall treatment groups of initial laparotomy vs initial peritoneal drainage. Preoperative diagnosis (NEC vs IP) is an effect modifier, and our data suggest that initial laparotomy is more likely than initial drainage to reduce death or NDI among infants with a preoperative diagnosis of NEC.

Citation	Summary
Minneci PC, Hade EM, Lawrence AE, et al. Association of nonoperative management using antibiotic therapy vs laparoscopic appendectomy with treatment success and disability days in children with uncomplicated appendicitis. *JAMA*. 2020;324(6):581-593.	• Among children with uncomplicated appendicitis, an initial nonoperative management strategy with antibiotics alone had a success rate of 67.1% and, compared with urgent surgery, was associated with statistically significantly fewer disability days at 1 y. However, there was substantial loss to follow-up, the comparison with the prespecified threshold for an acceptable success rate of nonoperative management was not statistically significant, and the hypothesized difference in disability days was not met.
Deprest JA, Nicolaides KH, Benachi A, et al. Randomized trial of fetal surgery for severe left diaphragmatic hernia. *N Engl J Med*. 2021;385(2):107-118.	• Fetal intervention for congenital diaphragmatic hernia consists of balloon occlusion of the fetal trachea to stimulate lung growth. This trial demonstrated that only those fetuses with isolated left-sided severe anomalies (<25% predicted fetal lung volume) with intervention at 27-29 wk of gestation resulted in a significant survival benefit over expectant care. Tracheal occlusion was associated with increased risk for prelabor rupture of membranes and preterm birth. In an accompanying article, tracheal occlusion did not improve survival in infants with mild or moderate diaphragmatic hernias (greater than 25% predicted lung volume).
Kelly RE, Goretsky MJ, Obermeyer R, et al. Twenty-one years of experience with minimally invasive repair of pectus excavatum by the Nuss procedure in 1215 patients. *Ann Surg*. 2010;252(6):1072-1081.	• This retrospective review studied the outcomes of 1215 patients undergoing a minimally invasive repair of pectus excavatum and demonstrated over 95% of patients had good to excellent anatomic result.

CHAPTER 39: PEDIATRIC SURGERY

Review Questions

1. What is the imaging modality of choice used to diagnose malrotation with intestinal volvulus of an infant?
2. What acid–base abnormality is expected in pyloric stenosis?
3. What is the most common solid tumor of childhood?

4. Ganglion cells are lacking in which plexuses in Hirschsprung's disease?
5. What is the most common type of tracheoesophageal fistula?
6. What is the initial transfusion volume of packed red blood cells in pediatric patients?
7. Where is the most common location for a 2nd branchial cleft remnant?
8. What are the two most important factors contributing to the pathogenesis of necrotizing enterocolitis?
9. What is the standard management of pectus carinatum?

REFERENCES

1. Hällström M, Koivisto AM, Janas M, Tammela O. Laboratory parameters predictive of developing necrotizing enterocolitis in infants born before 33 weeks of gestation. *J Pediatr Surg*. 2006;41(4):792-798.
2. Aspelund G, Langer JC. Current management of hypertrophic pyloric stenosis. *Semin Pediatr Surg*. 2007;16(1):27-33.
3. Shteyer E, Ramm GA, Xu C, White FV, Shepherd RW. Outcome after portoenterostomy in biliary atresia: pivotal role of degree of liver fibrosis and intensity of stellate cell activation. *J Pediatr Gastroenterol Nutr*. 2006;42(1):93-99.
4. Alvarado A. A practical score for the early diagnosis of acute appendicitis. *Ann Emerg Med*. 1986;15(5):557-564.
5. Blakely ML, Tyson JE, Lally KP, et al. Initial laparotomy versus peritoneal drainage in extremely low birthweight infants with surgical necrotizing enterocolitis or isolated intestinal perforation: a multicenter randomized clinical trial. *Ann Surg*. 2021;274(4):e370-e380.
6. Minneci PC, Hade EM, Lawrence AE, et al. Association of nonoperative management using antibiotic therapy vs laparoscopic appendectomy with treatment success and disability days in children with uncomplicated appendicitis. *JAMA*. 2020;324(6):581-593.
7. Deprest JA, Nicolaides KH, Benachi A, et al. Randomized trial of fetal surgery for severe left diaphragmatic hernia. *N Engl J Med*. 2021;385(2):107-118.
8. Kelly RE, Goretsky MJ, Obermeyer R, et al. Twenty-one years of experience with minimally invasive repair of pectus excavatum by the Nuss procedure in 1215 patients. *Ann Surg*. 2010;252(6):1072-1081.

40 Subspecialty Surgery for the General Surgeon

OBSTETRICS AND GYNECOLOGY FOR THE GENERAL SURGEON

James Doss and Andrea R. Hagemann

I. OBSTETRIC AND GYNECOLOGIC DISORDERS

A. Vaginal bleeding (**Figure 40.1**, **Table 40.1**)

1. Assessment
   - **a.** Take thorough history including pattern and intensity of bleeding and date of last menstrual period.
   - **b.** Physical examination including vital signs to assess stability, as well as speculum and bimanual pelvic examination.
   - **c.** Obtain urine β-human chorionic gonadotropin (β-hCG), complete blood count (CBC), coagulation studies, blood type.

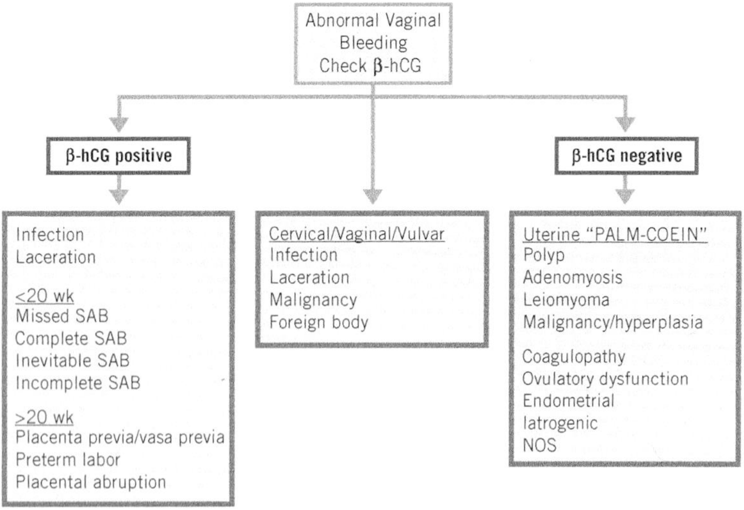

FIGURE 40.1 Management of vaginal bleeding. NOS, not otherwise specified; SAB, spontaneous abortion.

TABLE 40.1 Nonobstetric Causes of Vaginal Bleeding

Differential Diagnosis	Laboratory Data	Signs and Symptoms	Treatment
Menses	CBC count, urine hCG	Cyclic bleeding every 21-35 d	Iron therapy if indicated, consideration of hormonal regulation to control heavy or painful menses
Abnormal uterine bleeding	CBC count, urine hCG, endometrial biopsy if >45 y old, or any age with risk factors (see endometrial cancer section)	Noncyclic bleeding; may have associated dysmenorrhea, fatigue, or dizziness	Hormonal therapy if patient is hemodynamically stable; if unstable, transfuse as needed, IV estrogen or high-dose OCPs
Gonorrhea/*Chlamydia* cervicitis	Cervical culture, wet prep	Purulent vaginal discharge, possible spotting	Doxycycline 100 mg bid ×7 (or azithromycin 1 g ×1 in 2nd-3rd trimester) and ceftriaxone 500 mg ×1 (1 g if > 150 kg)
Trichomonas vaginitis	Wet prep	Yellow-green frothy vaginal discharge, possible spotting	Metronidazole 500 mg bid × 7 d; tinidazole 2 g × 1 (defer breastfeeding 12-24 h with metronidazole, 72 h with tinidazole)
Sexual trauma	Rape kit Sexual assault evidence collection kit (a.k.a. "rape kit")	Vaginal bleeding and/or discharge	Emergency contraception (copper/hormonal IUD, ulipristal acetate, levonorgestrel), prophylactic treatment for STDs; if laceration, pack vagina, possible surgical repair

CBC, complete blood cell; hCG, human chorionic gonadotropin; IUD, intrauterine device; OCP, oral contraceptive pill; STD, sexually transmitted disease.

   d. Pelvic/transvaginal ultrasound imaging
      i. Intrauterine gestation typically seen with β-hCG > 3,500 mIU/mL
      ii. Cardiac activity seen with β-hCG > 10,000 mIU/mL
2. **Nonobstetric etiologies of vaginal bleeding** (see **Figure 40.1** and **Table 40.1**)
3. **Obstetric etiologies of vaginal bleeding**
   a. *First trimester:* Spontaneous abortions (SAB), postcoital bleeding, ectopic pregnancy, lower genital tract lesions/lacerations, expulsion of molar pregnancy
   b. *Second/third trimester:* Placenta previa, placental abruption, vasa previa, preterm labor, lower genital tract lesions/lacerations
   c. Terminology
      i. **Threatened abortion:** Any vaginal bleeding <20 weeks of gestation without expulsion of products of contraception (POCs); cervix closed
      ii. **Missed abortion:** Nonviable gestation <20 weeks with retention of POCs; cervix closed
      iii. **Inevitable abortion:** Cervical dilation with or without ruptured membranes
      iv. **Incomplete abortion:** Partial passage of POCs; cervix open
      v. **Complete abortion:** Expulsion of all POCs; cervix closed
      vi. **Septic abortion:** Retained infected POC
      vii. **Ectopic pregnancy:** Pregnancy located outside the uterus, most often within the fallopian tube. Transvaginal ultrasound imaging with adnexal mass with or without pelvic free fluid
4. Treatment
   a. **Threatened abortion**
      i. **Viable:** Expectant management
      ii. **Indeterminate viability:** Repeat ultrasound imaging in 7 days, repeat β-hCG in 48 hours.
   b. **Missed/inevitable/incomplete abortion:** Expectant management, surgical management (**dilation and curettage** [D&C], manual vacuum aspiration), or medical therapy.
      i. After medical therapy, follow-up within 1 to 2 weeks to confirm completion.
      ii. Give bleeding (soaking one pad/h) and infection precautions (temperature of 101 °F, symptoms of septic abortion).
   c. **Complete abortion:** If hemodynamically stable, expectant management, but if unstable, D&C
   d. **Ectopic pregnancy:** Medical therapy with methotrexate is indicated in appropriate clinical circumstances,[1] but in the setting of hemodynamic instability or rupture, surgical management with salpingostomy or, more commonly, salpingectomy.
   e. **RhoGAM (50 μg intramuscular)** to any pregnant patient with vaginal bleeding who is Rh-negative with negative antibody screen

f. Risks and complications of D&C
   i. Ultrasound imaging guidance is recommended to prevent **uterine perforation**.
      a) Perform laparoscopy/cystoscopy if concerned for bowel/bladder injury.
      b) Manage expectantly if hemodynamically stable and no injury to surrounding organs.
   ii. **Endometritis**
      a) If unrelated to gonorrhea/chlamydia, doxycycline 100 mg bid × 7 days
      b) If high level of suspicion for gonorrhea/chlamydia infection, use pelvic inflammatory disease treatment regimen.

B. Evaluation of acute abdominal/pelvic pain
1. **Ovarian torsion**
   a. Epidemiology: Primarily reproductive age women, but can occur across age spectrum
   b. Presentation: Unilateral or diffuse abdominal/pelvic pain (out of proportion to examination), palpable adnexal mass, nausea, vomiting, fever
   c. Diagnosis: Primarily clinical diagnosis aided by leukocytosis and elevated lactate, and can confirm on transvaginal ultrasound imaging with edematous enlarged ovary with string of pearls and lack of Doppler flow.
   d. Management: Diagnostic laparoscopy with detorsion to preserve ovarian function, drainage or cystectomy if cyst present, or oophorectomy if ovarian tissue is diffusely necrotic
   e. A ruptured ovarian cyst will have similar presentation, with pelvic free fluid observed on imaging, proceed with symptomatic management. Diagnostic laparoscopy should be considered in setting of hemorrhagic cyst/**tubo-ovarian abscess (TOA)** rupture and hemodynamic instability.
2. **Pelvic inflammatory disease**
   a. Epidemiology: Majority reproductive age women
   b. Presentation: Abdominal/pelvic pain, fever, nausea, vomiting, diarrhea, dysmenorrhea, dyspareunia, abnormal vaginal discharge
   c. Diagnosis: Uterine, adnexal, or cervical motion tenderness, purulent cervical discharge, cervical friability, leukocytes on wet mount, elevated inflammatory markers (C-reactive protein, erythrocyte sedimentation rate)
      i. With diffuse abdominal pain and peritonitis, TOA can be evaluated by transvaginal ultrasound imaging.
   d. Management: IV to PO antibiotics, drainage of TOA
3. **Ectopic pregnancy** (see above)
   a. Imaging considerations
      i. With positive β-hCG and abdominal pain, transvaginal ultrasound imaging should be performed to assess the causes listed above.

ii. In pregnancy, MRI or nongynecologic ultrasound imaging is preferred to limit radiation exposure to fetus, but CT imaging can be performed as clinically indicated or if other imaging modalities are not readily available.

II. NONOBSTETRIC SURGERY IN THE PREGNANT PATIENT

A. Timing and risks

1. If nonemergent and unable to defer to postpartum, it is safest to proceed with surgery in the second trimester.
2. The risk of pregnancy interruption (any trimester) from nonobstetric surgery is approximately 3% to 11%.
3. Pregnancy is not a contraindication to indicated/emergent surgery.[2]

B. Perioperative considerations in the pregnant patient

1. Increased risk for aspiration results from upward displacement of the stomach and the inhibitory effects of progesterone on gastrointestinal motility (typically after 18 weeks gestation).
   a. Nonparticulate antacids and an H2-antagonist (metoclopramide) should be given prior to induction of anesthesia.[3]
2. Increased risk for difficult airway due to laryngeal and upper airway edema, always considered American Society of Anesthesiologists (ASA) classification II.
3. **Vena cava compression** necessitates maintaining left lateral positioning in third trimester to decrease inferior vena cava (IVC) compression and maintain adequate venous return/maternal circulation and placental blood supply.
4. Avoid maternal hypoxia (goal > 95% SpO_2), which can cause vasoconstriction, decreased uterine artery perfusion, and inadequate blood flow to the fetus.
5. **Fetal monitoring**
   a. If previable (<23 weeks, <400 g), perform portable Doppler assessment ("Doptones") pre- and postoperatively.
   b. If viable, perform intraoperative continuous fetal and uterine contraction monitoring and perform an emergent cesarean section if needed.
   c. If intraoperative continuous monitoring is not feasible, monitor fetal heart rate and uterine contractions pre- and postoperatively.
6. **Antenatal steroids** are recommended prior to any operation if gestational age is 23 to 34 weeks (betamethasone 12 mg IM q24h × two doses) to decrease neonatal morbidity and mortality due to prematurity.
7. **Maternal hematologic changes:** Pregnancy is a hypercoagulable state with increased hepatic production of coagulation factors, decreased fibrinolysis (in second/third trimesters), and venous stasis, so it is recommended to employ both mechanical and pharmacologic venous thromboembolism (VTE) prophylaxis if possible.
8. **Laparoscopy in pregnancy**
   a. Based on the SAGES Guidelines for laparoscopic surgery during pregnancy laparoscopy is safe and has similar advantages as in nonpregnant patients.[4]

b. Initial trocar placement can be accomplished by Hasson, Veress, or optical trocar techniques (adjusted for fundal height) and/or ultrasound imaging–guided left upper quadrant/subcostal entry as after ~16 weeks of gestation the uterus becomes an extrapelvic organ.
c. Carbon dioxide pneumoperitoneum up to 15 mm Hg is safe and unlikely to result in fetal hypoxia or acidosis, with intraoperative monitoring via capnography.
d. Avoid cervical or uterine manipulation.

III. GYNECOLOGIC SURGICAL ANATOMY

A. Uterus and cervix
1. The primary blood supply to the uterus and cervix comes from the uterine branch of the hypogastric artery; after passing through the cardinal ligament the uterine artery has ascending and descending branches (**Figure 40.2**).
2. The ureter travels through the cardinal ligament under the uterine artery and vein within the ureteric tunnel.

B. Ovary
1. The ovary receives its primary blood supply from the gonadal arteries, which branch off the aorta.
2. The left ovarian vein drains into the left renal vein, and the right ovarian vein empties into the vena cava.
3. The gonadal vessels travel retroperitoneally within the infundibulopelvic ligament. The infundibulopelvic ligament and gonadal vessels pass over the ureter approximately at the bifurcation of the iliac vessels as the ureter crosses the pelvic brim and descends into the pelvis.
4. The ovary attaches to the uterus via the utero-ovarian ligament.

C. Bladder: To safely perform a hysterectomy, the bladder must be dissected off the uterus and cervix by incising the vesicouterine peritoneum down to the pubocervical fascia and opening the vesicovaginal space.

D. Rectum: The rectovaginal septum can be developed by incising the posterior uterus just caudad to the attachment of the uterosacral ligament.

E. Pelvic avascular spaces: Developing the avascular spaces allows for identification of the major vessels and ureter, palpation of the parametrial tissue (an important step in evaluation of pelvic masses and gynecologic malignancies), and separation of pelvic organs.
1. **Prevesical (space of Retzius):** Lies between the posterior pubic bone and anterior wall of the bladder
2. **Vesicovaginal space:** Lies between anterior vagina and posterior bladder, laterally defined by bladder pillars
3. **Paravesical space:** Bordered by bladder pillars medially and pelvic sidewall/obturator internus laterally
4. **Pararectal space:** Identified between the ureter and the hypogastric artery
5. **Rectovaginal space:** Potential space between the rectum and vagina, laterally defined by the rectal pillars/uterosacral ligaments

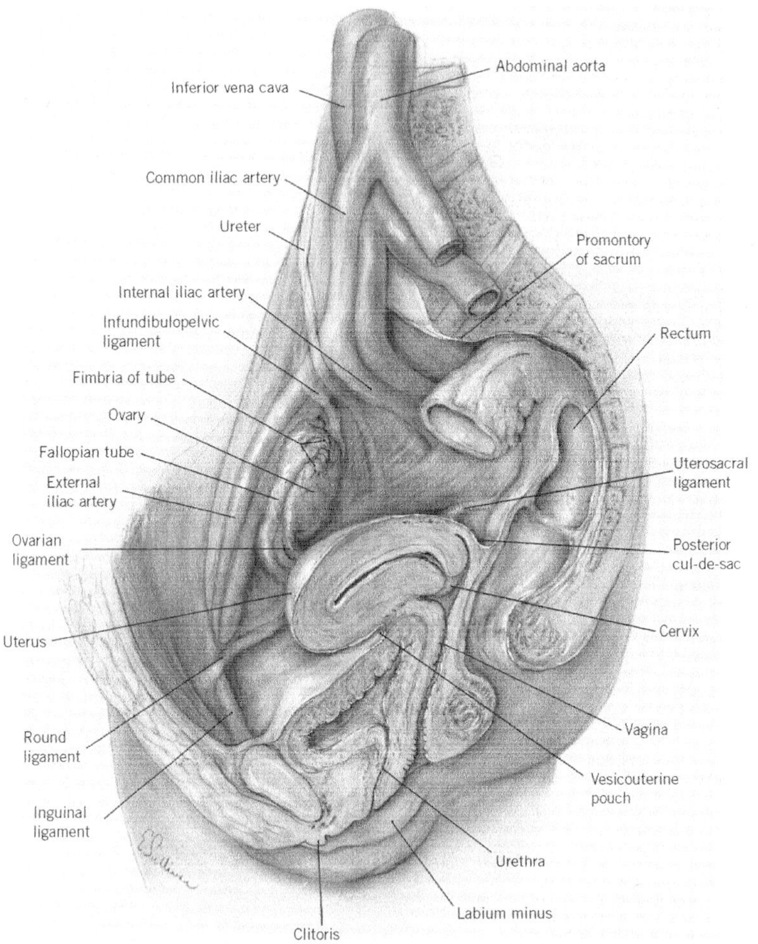

FIGURE 40.2 Pelvic viscera. *(Reprinted with permission from Rock JA, Jones HW, eds. Te Linde's Operative Gynecology. 10th ed. Wolters Kluwer Health/Lippincott Williams & Wilkins; 2008.)*

IV. GYNECOLOGIC MALIGNANCIES

A. Over 115,100 new cases of gynecologic malignancy were diagnosed in the US in 2022.[5]

B. If a gynecologic malignancy is suspected, all effort should be made to obtain an intraoperative consultation with a gynecologic oncologist.

C. Vulvar carcinoma

1. Epidemiology

   a. Mean age at diagnosis is 65 years, associated with **human papillomavirus (HPV)** in 60% of cases.

b. Other risk factors: Cigarette smoking, vulvar and cervical dysplasia, vulvar dystrophy, and immunodeficiency

2. Presentation and clinical features
   a. The most common symptom is itching, but lesions can be painful or asymptomatic.
   b. Vulvar examination typically shows an ulcerated, hyper- or hypopigmented, and/or exophytic lesion, most often on the skin of the labia.
3. Standard of care
   a. Vulvar cancer is staged using both clinical, radiographic, and surgical assessment to determine size of the lesion and regional/distant metastasis.
   b. Treatment options include radical vulvectomy and adjuvant radiation with or without chemotherapy.[6]
4. **What to do if a lesion is identified pre- or intraoperatively:** A punch biopsy should be taken, usually 4 mm in diameter and 1.5 mm deep.

D. Cervical carcinoma

1. Epidemiology
   a. Mean age of diagnosis is 50 years, with HPV detected in >99% of cases.
   b. Other risk factors: Cigarette smoking, immunosuppression, history of multiple sexual partners, early onset of sexual activity, history of sexually transmitted infections (STIs), limited prior screening, and vulvar/vaginal dysplasia.
2. Prevention
   a. Cervical cancer screening with **Papanicolaou (Pap)** testing and HPV testing to include Pap test every 3 years or cytology combined with HPV (co-testing) every 5 years, recommended for patients starting at age 21 to 25 years until age 65 years.
   b. Vaccines for multiple HPV genotypes are available (Gardasil, Gardasil 9, and Cervarix).
3. Presentation and clinical features
   a. Irregular or postcoital vaginal bleeding and malodorous, watery discharge are the most common symptoms.
   b. Advanced-stage disease may present with leg pain or edema, flank pain, renal failure, vesico/rectovaginal fistula formation, or rectal bleeding from a pelvic mass.
4. Standard of care
   a. Cervical cancer stage is summarized using the American Joint Committee on Cancer (AJCC) **TNM staging system** (*AJCC Cancer Staging System*: Cervix Uteri, 9th ed.) based on tumor extent of invasion and size, number and extent of lymph node metastases, and presence of distant metastases[7]
   b. Early-stage cervical cancers can often be cured by surgical management alone.
   c. For patients with early-stage disease desiring fertility, a loop electrosurgical excision procedure or cone biopsy with negative margins or a radical cervicectomy (also known as trachelectomy) and pelvic lymphadenectomy may be recommended.
   d. Locally advanced cervical cancers should be treated with radiation and cisplatin.

e. Cervical cancers with distant spread can be treated with combination taxane and platinum chemotherapy with anti-VEGF therapy.
f. **Pelvic exenteration** with removal of the bladder and rectum is reserved for recurrent cervical cancer localized to the pelvis.[8]

5. **What to do if suspected pre- or intraoperatively**
a. Perform a speculum examination and biopsy of malignant-appearing cervical tissue with Tischler forceps.
b. Hemostasis can be obtained using silver nitrate sticks and applying ferric subsulfate (**Monsel's solution**).

6. Uncontrolled vaginal bleeding due to cervical cancer
a. Place a tight vaginal packing and a transurethral Foley catheter.
b. Acetone-soaked gauze is the most effective packing for vessel sclerosis and control of hemorrhage from necrotic tumor.
c. If ineffective at controlling bleeding, interventional radiology (IR) embolization may be necessary.
d. Prompt consultation with radiation oncology is also indicated once a biopsy has confirmed invasive cancer.

E. Endometrial cancer

1. Epidemiology
a. The most common gynecologic cancer in the US with 65,950 new cases and 12,550 deaths in 2022; mean age of diagnosis is 63 years.
b. Risk factors: Excess/unopposed estrogen (obesity, medication, anovulation, estrogen-producing tumors, early menarche, late menopause), age, hereditary predisposition (such as Lynch syndrome).

2. Presentation and clinical features
a. The most common symptom is abnormal vaginal bleeding, often postmenopausal.
b. Workup should include a transvaginal ultrasound imaging and endometrial sample by in-office biopsy or D&C under anesthesia.
c. Paps with atypical glandular cells or endometrial cells in a patient over the age of 40 years should prompt endometrial assessment with biopsy or D&C.

3. Standard of care
a. Endometrial cancers are staged surgically by laparoscopic or robot-assisted hysterectomy, bilateral salpingo-oophorectomy with or without sentinel, or full pelvic lymphadenectomy.
b. Omental biopsy should be performed for high-grade cancers.
c. Adjuvant or postoperative treatment recommendations based on endometrial cancer stage as summarized by the AJCC **TNM staging system** (Chapter 53: Corpus uteri; *AJCC Cancer Staging Manual*, 8th ed.) based on tumor extent of invasion and size, number and extent of lymph node metastases, and presence of distant metastases.[9]

4. **What to do if suspected pre- or intraoperatively**
a. If suspected preoperatively, biopsy with curette or biopsy Pipelle.
b. If suspected intraoperatively because of uterine surface disease, biopsy and send for frozen pathology, and if positive for adenocarcinoma of Müllerian origin, consult a gynecologic oncologist, if available.
c. If consult is unavailable, if hemorrhage is occurring, and if within the scope of your practice, consider proceeding with

total abdominal or robotic-assisted hysterectomy, bilateral salpingo-oophorectomy.

i. If outside of your scope of practice or without available gynecologic consultation with current hemorrhage, uterine artery embolization with IR or tranexamic acid or acetone-soaked vaginal packing can be used.

F. Ovarian carcinoma

1. Epidemiology
   a. Deadliest gynecologic malignancy in the US with 19,880 new cases and 12,810 deaths in 2022 with mean age at diagnosis 63 years but can occur earlier in women with hereditary predisposition.
   b. Risk factors: Age, hereditary predisposition (such as *BRCA1* or *BRCA2* mutations), early menarche, late menopause, nulliparity, endometriosis, infertility.
2. Presentation and clinical features
   a. Early-stage disease is generally asymptomatic, and no good screening tests exist.
   b. Symptomatic patients experience pelvic pain or pressure, nausea, early satiety, weight loss, and bloating with increasing tumor burden.[10]
   c. Workup of a pelvic mass can differ by age but should include **CA-125**, pelvic ultrasound imaging, and referral to a gynecologist or gynecologic oncologist if cancer is highly suspected.
3. Standard of care
   a. Ovarian cancer is surgically staged with total abdominal hysterectomy, bilateral salpingo-oophorectomy, bilateral pelvic and para-aortic lymphadenectomy, peritoneal biopsies, and omental biopsy.
   b. If bulky disease is identified outside of the pelvis, the goal of the surgery is maximal cytoreduction of all gross disease.
   c. Adjuvant treatment recommendations based on ovarian cancer stage as summarized by the AJCC **TNM staging system** (Chapter 55: Ovary, Fallopian Tube, and Primary Peritoneal Carcinoma; *AJCC Cancer Staging Manual*, 8th ed.) based on tumor extent of invasion and size, number and extent of lymph node metastases, and presence of distant metastases.[9]
4. **What to do if suspected pre- or intraoperatively**
   a. If suspected preoperatively, obtain pelvic ultrasound imaging, serum CA-125 and and carcinoembryonic antigen (CEA).
   b. If ultrasound imaging is suspicious, a CT scan of the chest/abdomen/pelvis is indicated for staging.
   c. Consult a gynecologic oncologist if possible, and do not proceed with nonemergent operation until consultation is complete if suspicion for ovarian malignancy is high.
   d. If detected intraoperatively, obtain pelvic/peritoneal washings and biopsies of any extraovarian disease, and obtain an intraoperative gynecologic oncology consult.
   e. If consult is unavailable, bilateral salpingo-oophorectomy in a postmenopausal patient with or without hysterectomy is reasonable if within the operating surgeon's scope of practice.
   f. An isolated ovarian mass without signs of extraovarian spread should not be drained or biopsied, as this risks upstaging of a potential cancer.

OTOLARYNGOLOGY FOR THE GENERAL SURGEON

Theresa Tharakan and Nyssa Farrell

V. THE NECK

A. Anatomy
   1. The cervical fascia provides planes for passage of infection, hemorrhage, and surgical dissection (**Figure 40.3**).
   2. The lymphatic system of the neck helps predict spread of head and neck malignancy to lymph nodes and determine the extent of lymphadenectomy necessary during a neck dissection (**Figure 40.4**).

B. Neck masses
   1. **Adult neck masses** are presumed malignant; see workup algorithm in **Figure 40.5**.
   2. **Pediatric neck masses**
      a. Usually inflammatory or congenital
      b. Children often have palpable lymph nodes, but large/persistent neck masses should undergo workup (**Figure 40.6**).

C. Infectious disorders of the neck
   1. **Bacterial lymphadenitis**
      a. Etiology due to *Staphylococcus aureus* or group A streptococcal (GAS) infections in 40% to 80% of pediatric cases
      b. Presents as tender lymphadenopathy, fevers.
      c. Diagnosis/testing includes CBC, erythrocyte sedimentation rate, and C-reactive protein to inform illness severity and ultrasound imaging or CT to confirm diagnosis.
      d. Treatment is IV antibiotics and incision and drainage (I&D) of any abscesses.
      e. Outcomes/complications include abscess formation, progressive cellulitis, and sepsis.
   2. **Acute mononucleosis**
      a. Epidemiology/etiology due to **Epstein–Barr virus** (EBV) with peak incidence in 15 to 24 year olds.
      b. Presents with lymphadenopathy, fevers, tonsillitis, fatigue, hepatosplenomegaly.
      c. Diagnosis is confirmed with Monospot or EBV antibody test.
      d. Treatment is supportive, and avoiding contact sports in setting of hepatosplenomegaly.
      e. Complications: Splenic rupture
   3. **Deep neck space infections**
      a. Etiology from odontogenic or tonsillar infections, trauma, or instrumentation
      b. Present with fevers, tender neck swelling, local symptoms
      c. Diagnosis/testing is CT.

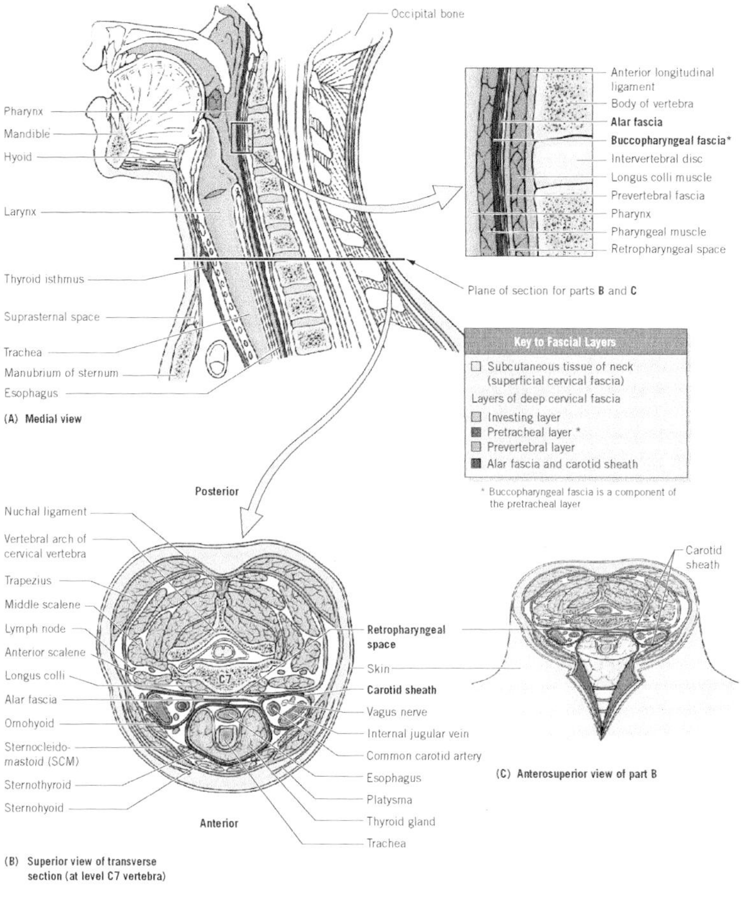

FIGURE 40.3 Fascial layers of the neck. A, Medial view. B, Superior view of transverse section (at level C7 vertebra). C, Anterosuperior view of (B). *(Reprinted with permission from Moore KL, Dalley AF, Agur AMR. Clinically Oriented Anatomy. 6th ed. Wolters Kluwer Health/Lippincott Williams & Wilkins; 2010.)*

d. Treatment is IV antibiotics and I&D of any abscesses.

e. Outcomes/complications

  i. Sepsis

  ii. Airway obstruction

  iii. Parapharyngeal, retropharyngeal, or prevertebral space infections can extend to the "danger space" bound by alar fascia and prevertebral fascia that extends from skull base to mediastinum, causing risk of mediastinitis.

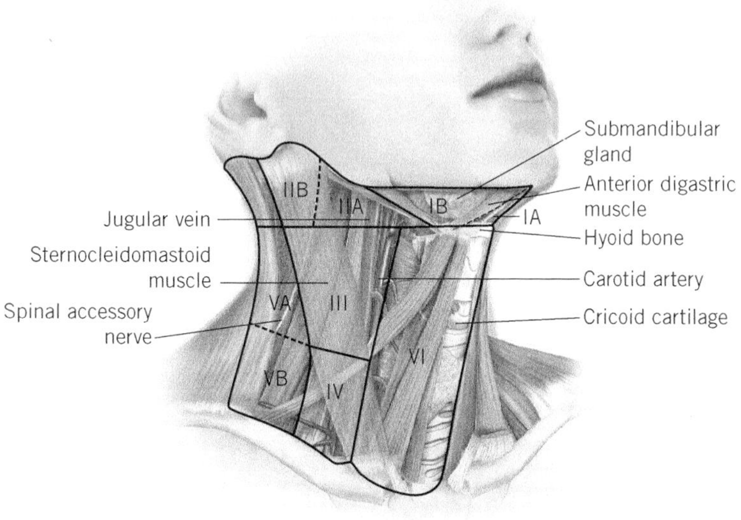

FIGURE 40.4 Neck node levels. IA, submental; IB, submandibular; II, upper jugular; III, middle jugular; IV, lower jugular; V, posterior triangle; VI, anterior compartment. *(Reprinted with permission from Mulholland MW, Hawn MT, Hughes SJ, et al., eds. Operative Techniques in Surgery. Wolters Kluwer Health; 2015.)*

f. Special cases
   i. **Necrotizing fasciitis:** Rapidly progressive infection of the skin and soft tissues of the neck
      a) Epidemiology/etiology
         1) Annual incidence 0.4/100,000
         2) Risk factors: Immunocompromise (e.g., diabetes, HIV)
         3) Mixed aerobic (predominantly GAS, *Staph*, gram-negative rods) and anaerobic spread from odontogenic infection, trauma, pharyngitis
      b) Present as painful swelling, crepitus, odynophagia
      c) Diagnosis/testing
         1) CT shows gas in deep neck spaces crossing fascial planes.
         2) Immediate surgical exploration if high clinical suspicion
         3) Laboratory Risk Indicator for Necrotizing Fasciitis (LRINEC) score > 6 is an adjunct tool for clinically indeterminate cases (sensitivity 75%, specificity 85%).[11]
      d) Treatment
         1) Serial surgical debridement

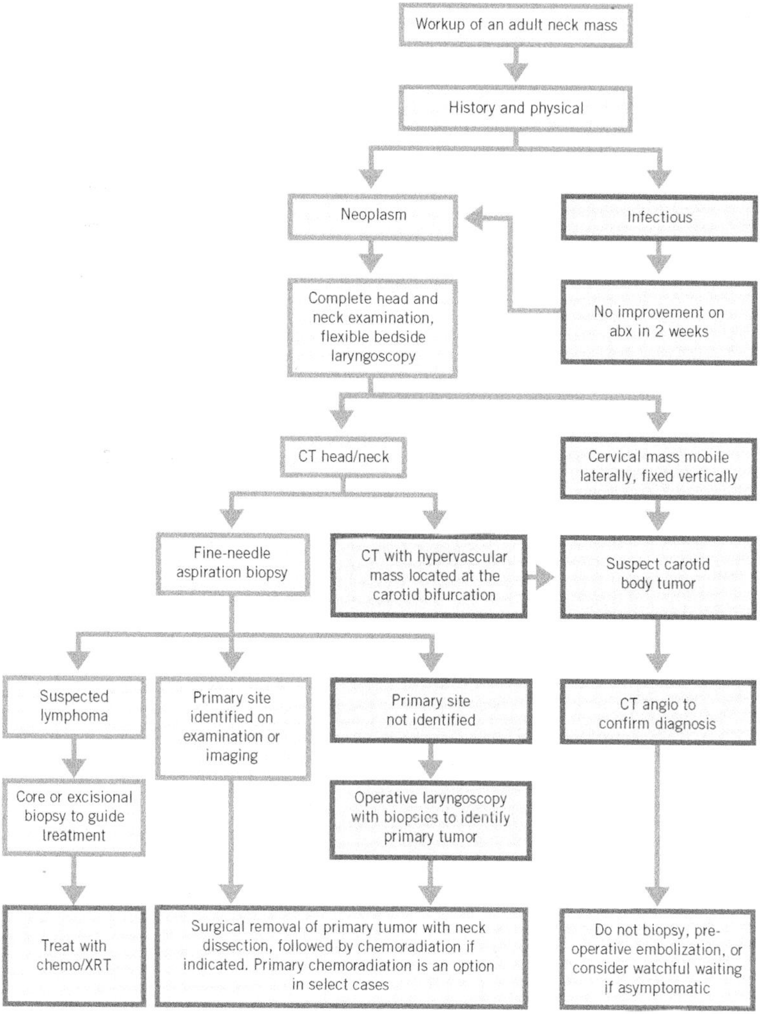

FIGURE 40.5 Workup of adult neck mass. XRT, radiation therapy.

2) IV antibiotics, ideally culture directed
3) Control of underlying comorbidities

e) Complications
1) Sepsis, multiorgan failure
2) Airway and vascular compromise
3) Mortality >20%

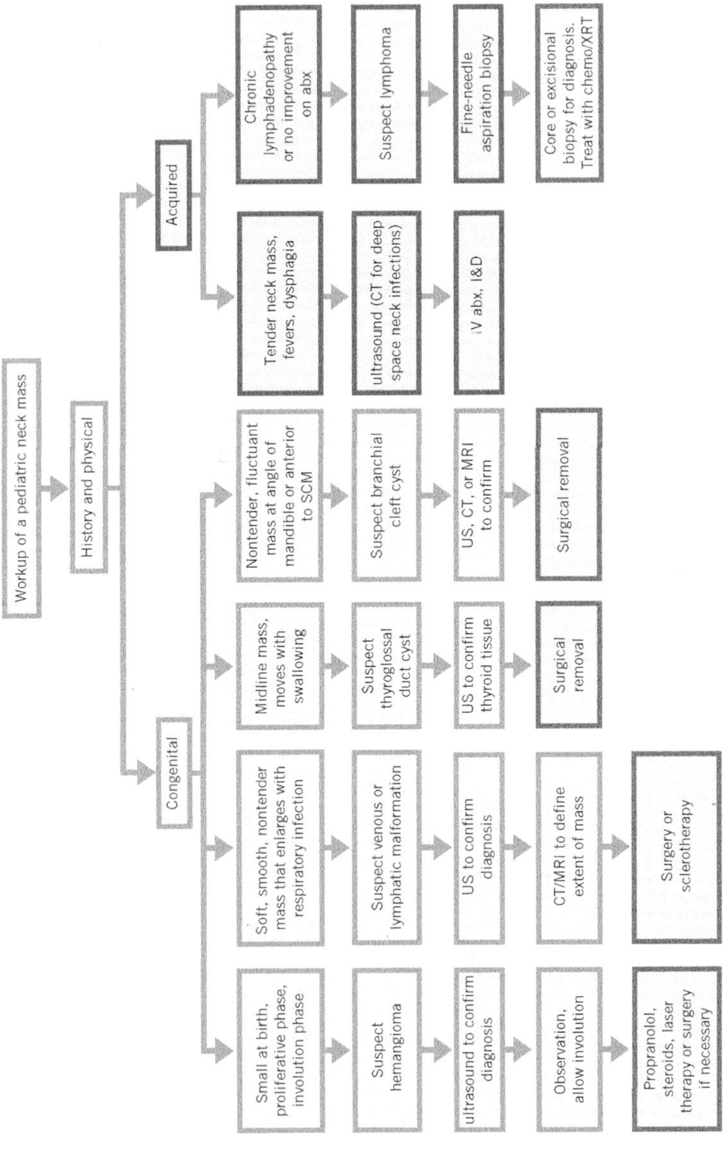

FIGURE 40.6 Workup of pediatric neck mass. SCM, sternocleidomastoid; XRT, radiation therapy.

ii. **Ludwig angina:** Bilateral cellulitis of submandibular and submental regions
  a) Etiology is odontogenic infection in majority of cases.
  b) Presents with floor of mouth elevation, tongue swelling, submandibular induration, rapidly progressive airway obstruction.
  c) Diagnosis/testing: CT
  d) Treatment
    1) Airway management (awake fiberoptic intubation or tracheostomy, if necessary)
    2) IV antibiotics and I&D of any abscesses
  e) Complications include airway obstruction and sepsis.

D. Neoplasms

1. **Benign**
  a. **Paragangliomas**
    i. Epidemiology/etiology
      a) Arise from **neural crest cells**
      b) Familial in 20%
    ii. **Location/Presentation**
      a) Carotid body (60%)
      b) Jugulotympanic (35%)—pulsatile tinnitus, CN VII-XII palsies
      c) Glomus vagale (5%)—neck swelling, rare dysphonia
    iii. Testing
      a) Plasma and urine metanephrines to rule out secreting jugulotympanic tumors
      b) CT abdomen/pelvis to rule out concomitant pheochromocytoma
    iv. Treatment
      a) Observation if asymptomatic
      b) Surgical resection and/or radiation if large, growing, symptomatic
2. **Malignant**
  a. **Squamous cell carcinoma (SCC)** is the most common **head and neck cancer (HNC)** in adults and often metastasizes to the neck.
    i. Epidemiology/etiology
      a) Unknown primary in 1% to 3% of new SCC cases
      b) Risk factors: Tobacco/alcohol use, HPV genotypes 16/18
    ii. Presentation
      a) Lymphadenopathy, often fixed/immobile
      b) Symptomatic primary lesion (see **Table 40.2**)
    iii. Diagnosis
      a) Cytology
        1) Staining + p16 is associated with an oropharyngeal primary.
        2) Staining + EBV is associated with a nasopharyngeal primary.
      b) CT with or without MRI for local staging
      c) PET/CT

TABLE 40-2 Presentation of Primary Head and Neck Malignancies by Location

Location	Symptoms	Common Pathologies
Oral cavity	Leukoplakia, erythroplakia, visible mass, difficulty chewing, bleeding, pain	Squamous cell carcinoma (SCC)
Pharynx (nasopharynx, oropharynx, hypopharynx)	Dysphagia, odynophagia, upper airway obstruction, unilateral otalgia/hearing changes/tinnitus	SCC
Larynx	Hoarseness, dyspnea, stridor, dysphagia, odynophagia	SCC
Paranasal sinuses and nasal cavity	Nasal obstruction, epistaxis, persistent/recurrent sinus infections, headaches, intracranial or orbital invasion, smell changes, middle ear effusion	SCC (e.g., nasopharyngeal carcinoma) (50%-80% of sinonasal tumors) Adenocarcinoma (10%) Melanoma (5%) Less common: Adenoid cystic carcinoma, mucoepidermoid carcinoma, esthesioneuroblastoma, sinonasal undifferentiated carcinoma
Salivary glands	Neck/facial swelling, pain, facial nerve palsy, trismus	Mucoepidermoid carcinoma (15% of salivary gland malignancies) Adenoid cystic carcinoma (10%) Less common: adenocarcinoma, acinic cell carcinoma, primary SCC
Cutaneous	BCC: Indolent growth, pearly papule or erythematous/scaly plaque SCC: Ulcerating, friable, tender plaque Melanoma: Pigmented, asymmetric lesion with irregular borders	Basal cell carcinoma (BCC) (80% of skin cancers) SCC (10%-20%) Melanoma (5%)

1) May help identify the primary lesion if unknown.
2) Evaluates for distant/metastatic disease.

iv. Treatment
a) Complex, depending on location/extent of disease
b) Surgical primary resection with or without neck dissection for cervical metastases
c) Neck dissection complications: chyle leak, vessel injury (e.g., carotid artery, internal jugular vein), or temporary or permanent nerve injury to the marginal mandibular branch of CN VII; CN X, XI, and XII; cervical plexus rootlets; sympathetic trunk.
d) Radiation with or without chemotherapy (combined radiation and cisplatin has improved progression-free and overall survival compared with radiation alone for stage III or IV HNC).[12]

b. **Thyroid carcinoma** (see Chapter 30)

c. **Lymphoma**

i. Epidemiology
a) The most common HNC in children
b) US annual incidence (per million children)
1) Non-Hodgkin's: 30
2) Hodgkin's: 50
c) Presentation
1) Cervical lymphadenopathy
- Eighty percent of pediatric Hodgkin's cases
- About 5% to 10% of pediatric Non-Hodgkin's cases
2) Extranodal masses (e.g., tonsils, thyroid, salivary gland, nasal)
3) **B symptoms** (fevers, night sweats, weight loss)
d) Diagnosis is based on core or excisional biopsy with flow cytometry and immunophenotyping.
e) Treatment is chemotherapy and radiation.

E. The Larynx

1. Anatomy

a. Regions (see **Figure 40.7**)
i. Supraglottis: Epiglottis, arytenoid cartilages, false vocal cords/folds, and ventricles
ii. Glottis: True vocal cords
iii. Subglottis: Below true vocal cords to cricoid cartilage

b. **Recurrent laryngeal nerve**
i. Branch of CN X
ii. Provides sensory and motor innervation to vocal cords, laryngeal muscles, and laryngeal mucosa.
iii. Injury risk during thyroid/parathyroid surgery due to proximity to the posterior thyroid capsule (see **Figure 40.8**)

2. **Infectious/inflammatory disorders**

a. **Viral laryngotracheitis (croup)**
i. Epidemiology/etiology

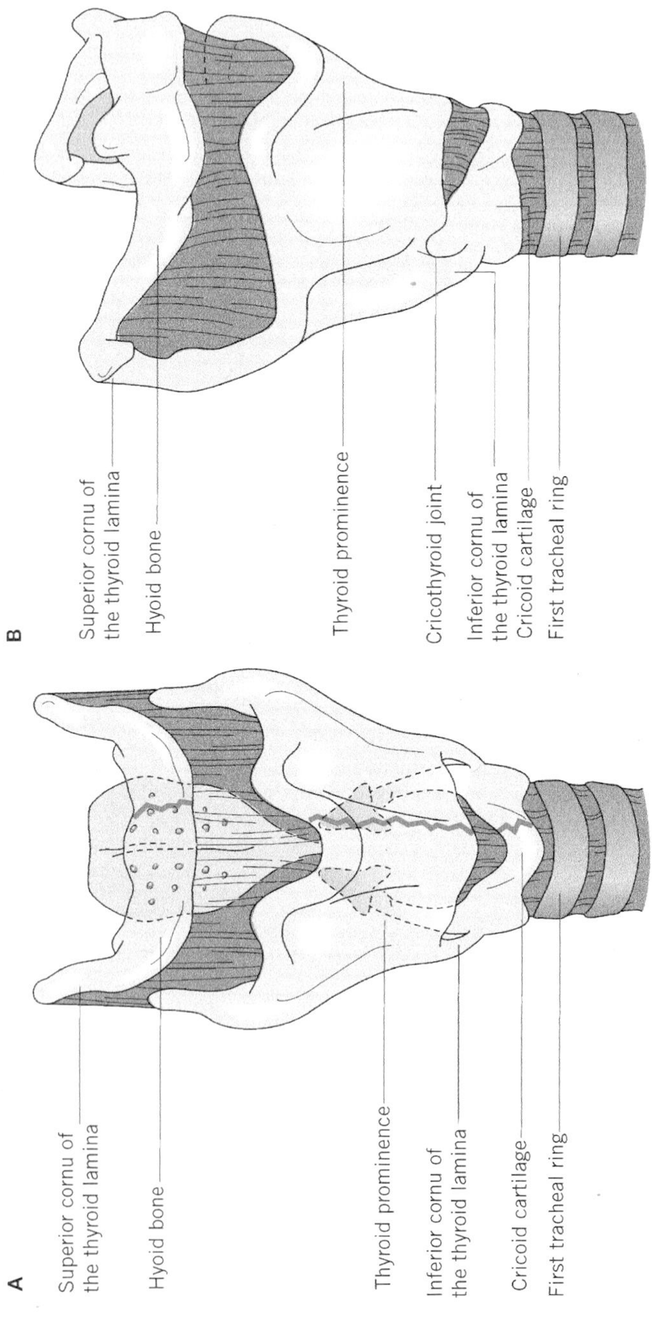

FIGURE 40.7 A and B, Anterior and lateral views, respectively, of the external larynx anatomy. *(Reprinted with permission from Mulholland MW, Lillemoe KD, Doherty GM, et al., eds. Greenfield's Surgery: Scientific Principles and Practice. 5th ed. Wolters Kluwer Health/Lippincott Williams & Wilkins; 2011.)*

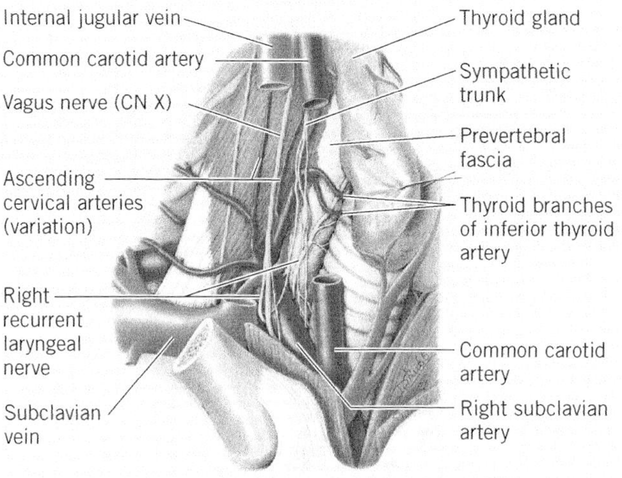

FIGURE 40.8 Injury to recurrent laryngeal nerves. *(Reprinted with permission from Moore KL, Dalley AF, Agur AMR. Clinically Oriented Anatomy. 8th ed. Wolters Kluwer; 2018. Figure B9.10.)*

- a) Affects 3% of children annually.
- b) Parainfluenza virus causes 75%.

- **ii.** Presents with barking cough, hoarseness, inspiratory stridor.
- **iii.** Diagnosis/testing
  - a) Clinical diagnosis
  - b) Lateral neck radiograph may show the **steeple sign** (subglottic edema).
- **iv.** Treatment
  - a) Airway management can include racemic epinephrine, heliox, and intubation.
  - b) Air humidification
  - c) Glucocorticoids
- **v.** Complications
  - a) Bacterial superinfection
  - b) Respiratory distress
  - c) Recurrence is suspicious for underlying airway abnormalities (subglottic stenosis, laryngomalacia, mass).

b. Epiglottitis

- **i.** Etiology/epidemiology
  - a) *Haemophilus influenzae* type B in 25%, streptococcal infections, trauma, caustic injury
  - b) Adults:children approximately 2:1
- **ii.** Presents with fever, muffled voice, drooling, stridor, tripod positioning.
- **iii.** Diagnosis: Laryngoscopy in stable patients

iv. Treatment: Airway management, IV antibiotics
v. Complications: Respiratory distress

3. **Neoplasms**
   a. **Benign**
      i. **Recurrent respiratory papillomatosis** is characterized by bulky papillomas on the laryngotracheobronchial tree.
      ii. Etiology: HPV 6, 11 at junctions of ciliated and squamous epithelium
      iii. Presentation: Hoarseness, airway obstruction
      iv. Treatment
         a) Repeated excision
         b) Avoid tracheostomy (resulting squamous metaplasia creates a site of extension).
   b. Complications
      i. Airway compromise
      ii. Hemorrhage
      iii. Scarring
      iv. Distal tracheal/pulmonary spread
   c. Malignant: Most commonly SCC (**Table 40.2**)
4. **Trauma/injury** (see Chapter 6)
5. **Management of upper airway obstruction**
   a. History: Dyspnea, voice changes, dysphagia
   b. Physical examination
      i. Inspection: Assess oxygenation, respiratory effort, tachypnea, positioning, drooling, craniofacial abnormalities
      ii. Auscultation
         a) High-pitched inspiratory stridor with supraglottic/glottic obstruction
         b) Expiratory stridor with tracheal/bronchial obstruction
         c) Assess for bilateral breath sounds.
      iii. Palpation: Neck masses, mobility
      iv. Airway visualization by fiberoptic nasolaryngoscopy in stable patients
   c. **Nonsurgical airway options**
      i. Bag-mask ventilation
      ii. Supraglottic airway device (e.g., laryngeal mask airway)
      iii. Intubation either transoral or awake transnasal fiberoptic
   d. **Emergent cricothyrotomy**
      i. Indication: Inability to ventilate and intubate
      ii. Convert to tracheostomy within 24 to 72 hours to decrease risk of subglottic stenosis.
   e. **Tracheostomy**
      i. Surgical options: Open (see Chapter 4) vs percutaneous approach
      ii. **Indication**
         a) Respiratory failure requiring prolonged ventilatory support (expected > 7 days)
         b) Upper airway obstruction (e.g., tumor, trauma, severe persistent obstructive sleep apnea)

iii. Complications
- **a)** Tracheitis, pneumonia
- **b)** **Mucous plugging**
  - **1)** Presents as tracheostomy obstruction.
  - **2)** Prevention: Humidification, gentle suctioning, secretion management
  - **3)** Treatment: Replace tube and/or inner cannula on a scheduled and as-needed basis. If unable to replace trach, can ventilate using endotracheal tube through tracheostomy defect or nasal/oral intubation if appropriate. May use flexible fiberoptic tracheoscopy to identify area of obstruction and manually debride plug or crusting.
- **c)** Bleeding
  - **1)** Local oozing (e.g., from thyroid edges, skin edges, suction trauma causing bleeding) can be managed with topical agents or sutures.
  - **2)** Tracheoinnominate fistula
    - Epidemiology: Rare (<1% tracheostomies)
    - Presents as brisk, life-threatening (due to exsanguination and/or loss of air exchange from blood in the airways) upper airway bleeding often preceded by **sentinel bleed**.
    - Diagnosis: If stable enough, CT angiography may show vessel extravasation or pseudoaneurysm.
    - Treatment
      - Inflate cuffed endotracheal tube in the stoma.
      - Place direct pressure on the artery with a finger against the sternum through the tracheostomy defect.
      - Emergent endovascular or open surgical repair
- **d)** **False passage**
  - **1)** Risk factors: Percutaneous tracheostomy placement, morbid obesity, and/or new tracheostomy site
  - **2)** Presents as airway obstruction, inability to pass flexible suction through distal tube, and/or crepitus.
  - **3)** Treatment
    - Direct visualization while replacing tube
    - Place over flexible laryngoscope, suction catheter, or bougie.
    - Intubate and proceed with replacement in the operating room (OR).
- **e)** **Pneumothorax**
  - **1)** Etiology
    - Tracheal injury
    - Paratracheal false passage of tracheostomy tube
  - **2)** Presents as respiratory decompensation, hypotension, loss of breath sounds, pneumothorax noted on post-placement CXR.
  - **3)** Treatment (see Chapter 31)

- Thoracostomy/chest tube based on size and symptomatology

f) **Tracheal stenosis**
   1) Etiology due to prolonged tracheostomy placement
   2) Prevention
      - Minimize trauma to the tracheal wall (e.g., gentle suctioning, low cuff pressures).
      - In children, decreased incidence with vertical tracheostomy incisions
   3) Treatment: If severe, may require repeat operative dilation or tracheal resection.

iv. **Total laryngectomy**
   a) Removal of entire larynx for laryngeal cancer
   b) Trachea sewn directly to neck skin
   c) These patients can never be intubated orally.

VI. ORAL CAVITY AND PHARYNX

A. Anatomy
   1. Oral cavity boundaries (**Figure 40.9**)
      a. Anterior: Vermillion border of lips
      b. Posterior: Circumvallate papillae, junction of hard and soft palate
   2. The pharynx is divided into the nasopharynx, oropharynx, and hypopharynx (**Figure 40.10**).

B. Malignancy: Most commonly SCC (**Table 40.2**).

C. Trauma (see Chapter 6)

VII. THE SALIVARY GLANDS

A. Anatomy
   1. **Parotid gland**
      a. Lies over the masseter muscle
      b. Divided into superficial and deep lobes by CN VII
      c. CN IX provides parasympathetic innervation
   2. **Submandibular gland**
      a. Inferomedial to mandible
      b. Chorda tympani (CN VII) provides secretomotor innervation.
   3. **Sublingual gland**
      a. Beneath the floor of mouth mucosa
      b. Chorda tympani provides secretomotor innervation.
   4. Many **minor salivary glands** in the mucosa of the oral cavity, oropharynx, and nasopharynx

B. Inflammatory diseases
   1. **Acute sialadenitis**
      a. Etiology
         i. Salivary stasis with stagnation of oral bacteria
         ii. Risk factors: Dehydration, deconditioning, radiation, immunocompromise, sialolithiasis

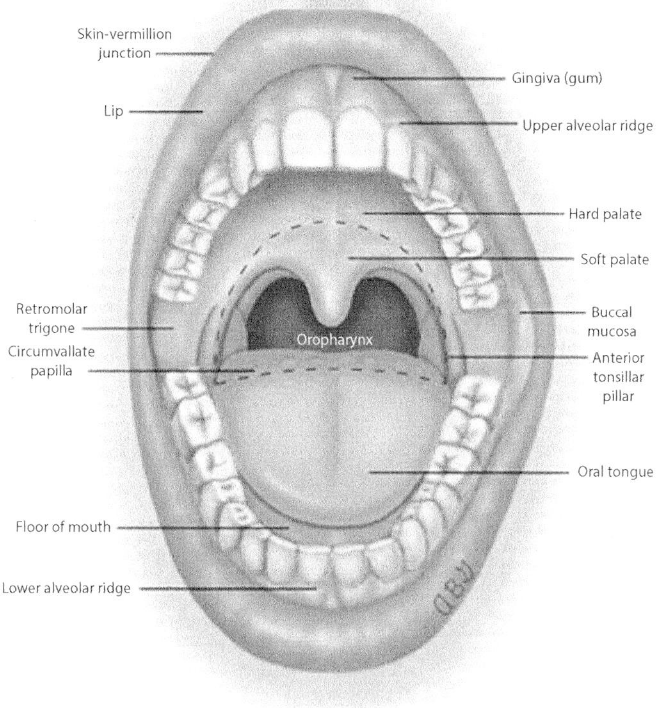

FIGURE 40.9 Oral cavity anatomy. *(Reproduced with permission from Lodi G. Oral lesions. In: UpToDate, Post TW (ed.), UpToDate. Accessed November 1, 2022. Copyright 2022, UpToDate, Inc. and its affiliates and/or licensors. All rights reserved.)*

b. Presentation
   i. Tender swelling
   ii. Worse with eating
   iii. Purulence expressed from the **parotid duct (Stensen's duct)** or **submandibular duct (Wharton's duct)**
c. Diagnosis is clinical with cultures as needed.
d. Treatment is antibiotics as well as hydration, warm compresses, massage, and/or sialogogues to stimulate saliva flow.

C. Neoplasms
1. Epidemiology
   a. Incidence 2,000 to 2,500 cases/y in the US.
   b. Seventy percent of parotid neoplasms are benign.

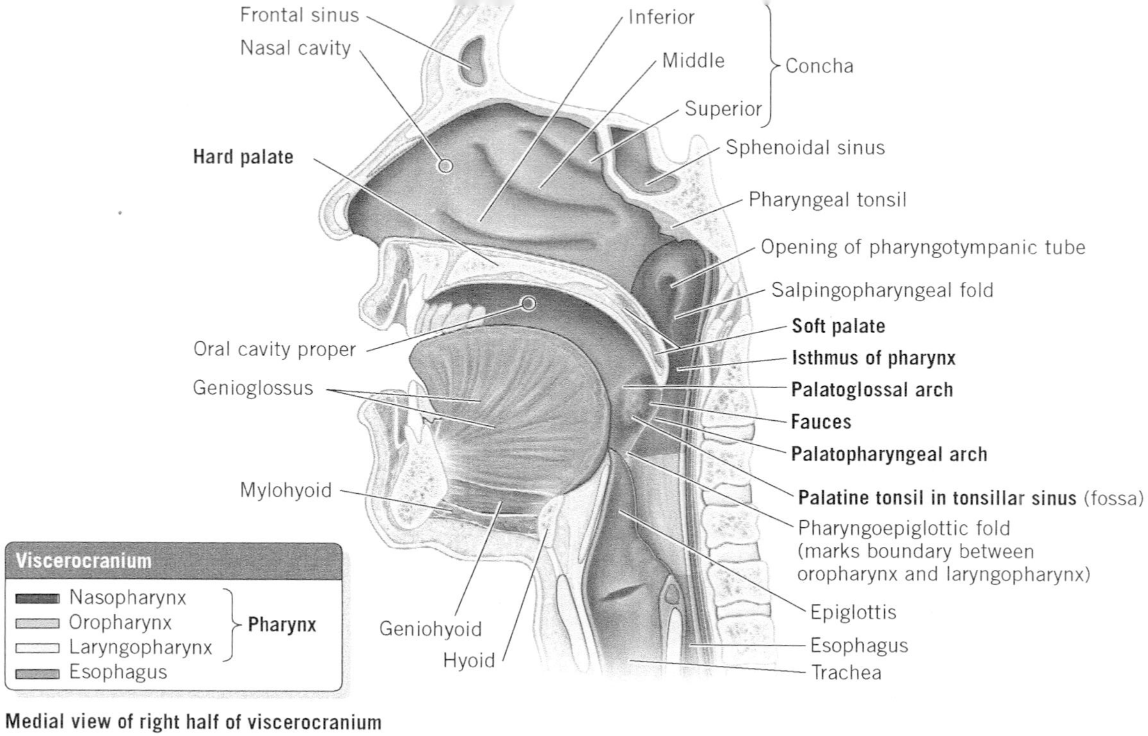

FIGURE 40.10 Median section of oral cavity and pharynx. *(Reprinted with permission from Moore KL, Dalley AF, Agur AMR. Clinically Oriented Anatomy. 8th ed. Wolters Kluwer; 2018. Figure 8.83.)*

c. Fifty percent of neoplasms of the submandibular gland are malignant.
d. Primary sublingual tumors are rare.

2. **Benign**
   a. Etiology
      i. Most common: **Pleomorphic adenoma** (50%-75%)
      ii. Second most common: **Warthin tumor** (5%-15%)
   b. Present as painless, slow growing masses, usually within the parotid gland.
   c. Diagnosis/testing
      i. Fine needle aspiration (FNA) biopsy
      ii. CT for surgical planning
   d. Treatment: Parotidectomy with facial nerve preservation.
3. **Malignant**
   a. Etiology and presentation **Table 40.2**
   b. Diagnosis/testing
      i. FNA
      ii. CT for surgical planning
   c. Treatment: Parotidectomy, with possible facial nerve sacrifice, possible neck dissection, possible adjuvant radiation

VIII. THE EAR AND TEMPORAL BONE

A. Anatomy
   1. The **temporal bone** lies on the lateral aspect of the head, posterior to the mandible and anterior to the occiput, and contains important vessels including the internal carotid artery, jugular vein, and sigmoid sinus.
   2. The external, middle, and inner ear are depicted in **Figure 40.11**.
   3. The **facial nerve** (**CN VII,** which innervates the facial musculature, stapedius muscle, taste to the anterior tongue via the chorda tympani, and the parotid gland) travels through the temporal bone where it is vulnerable to trauma.

B. Trauma (see Chapter 6)

IX. THE NOSE AND PARANASAL SINUSES

A. Anatomy
   1. The nose and septum are composed of bone superiorly/posteriorly and cartilage anteriorly.
   2. The **turbinates** are mucosa-covered bony prominences from the lateral nasal cavity that humidify, warm, and filter air.
   3. The **nasopharynx** contains the eustachian tube orifices laterally and the adenoid pad centrally, which involutes in late childhood.
   4. The **paranasal sinuses** are pneumatized cavities lined with respiratory epithelium and named for their surrounding bone (frontal, sphenoid, ethmoid, or maxillary). They reduce the weight of the skull, contribute to voice resonance, and cushion the cranial contents against trauma.

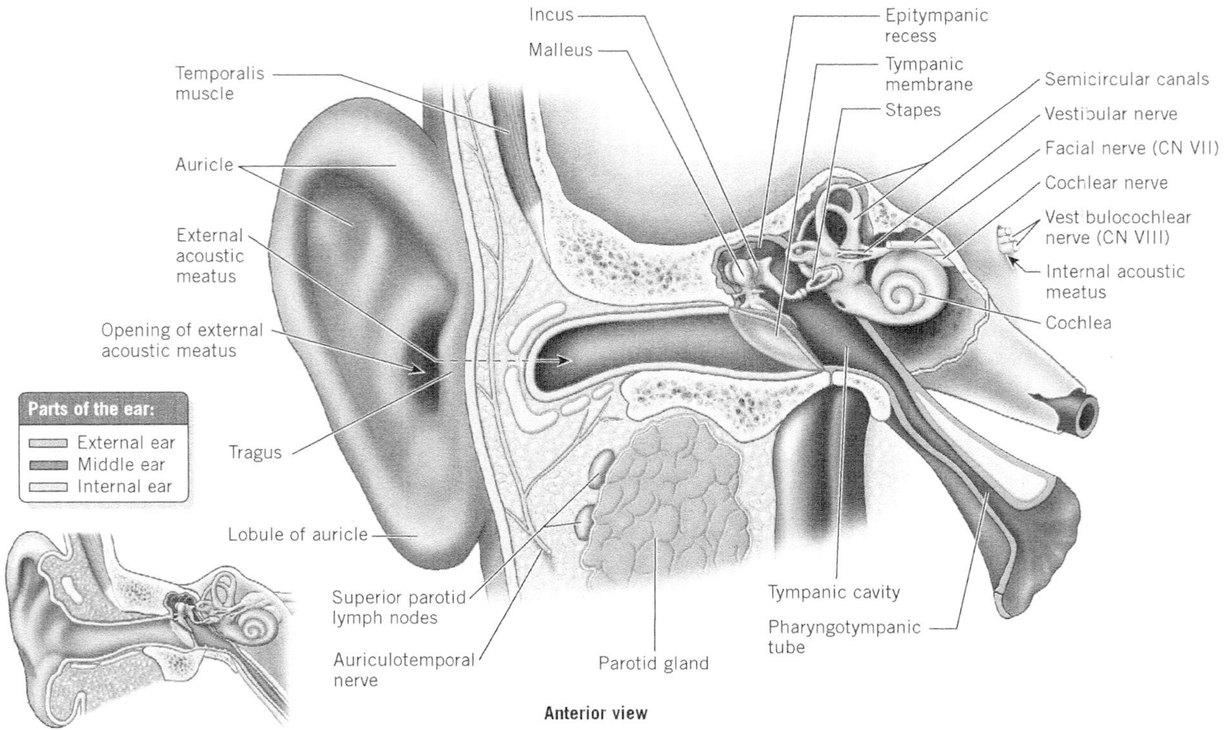

FIGURE 40.11 External, middle, and inner ear anatomy. *(Reprinted with permission from Moore KL, Dalley AF, Agur AMR. Clinically Oriented Anatomy. 8th ed. Wolters Kluwer; 2018. Figure 8.109.)*

PLASTIC AND RECONSTRUCTIVE SURGERY FOR GENERAL SURGEONS

Damini Tandon and Shoichiro Tanaka

X. TECHNIQUES AND PRINCIPLES

A. Reconstructive elevator defines a systematic reconstructive approach that starts with considering solutions in increasing complexity.
   1. **Secondary intention healing** allows wound to heal with time through maintaining clean, protected wound with dressings; contraindications include exposed critical structures, aesthetically sensitive areas.
   2. **Negative-pressure wound therapy (NPWT)** can accelerate secondary healing if wound is free of infection/malignancy.
   3. **Primary closure** best with minimized tension to prevent tissue ischemia, dehiscence, scarring, and displacement of adjacent structures.
   4. **Skin grafting** requires a vascularized wound bed, and exposed critical structures, infected/irradiated wounds will not support graft survival, although NPWT can promote granulation and create a graftable wound.
   5. **Tissue expansion** involves stretching existing tissue to cover a defect.
   6. **Local tissue transfer** involves moving healthy tissue into the wound bed while leaving it attached to its blood supply.
   7. **Free tissue transfer** involves distant movement of healthy tissue requiring division of vascular pedicle and anastomosis to donor vessels.

B. Graft types
   1. **Skin grafts (Figure 40.12)**

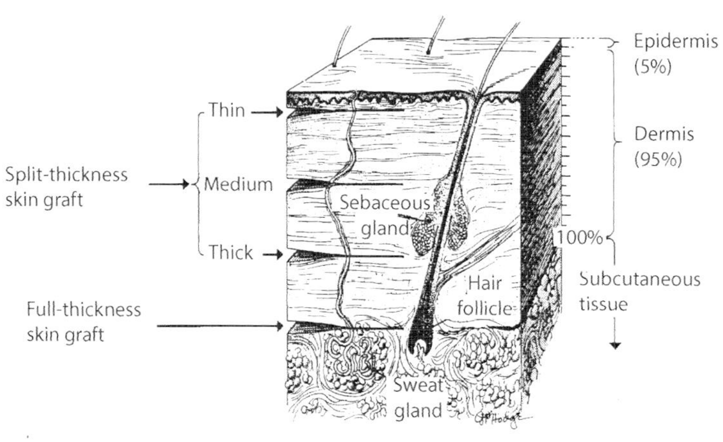

FIGURE 40.12 Skin graft thickness. *(Reprinted with permission from Thorne CH, Chung KC, Gosain AK, et al., eds. Grabb and Smith's Plastic Surgery. 7th ed. Wolters Kluwer Health/Lippincott Williams & Wilkins; 2014.)*

a. **Split-thickness skin grafts (STSGs)** include epidermis and portion of dermis.
   i. Contracture: 20% primary, 40% secondary
   ii. Donor sites: Thigh, buttock
   iii. Mesh (1.5:1) to increase surface area and fluid egress
   iv. Relative contraindications: Joint surface, aesthetically demanding location
b. **Full-thickness grafts** include epidermis and dermis.
   i. Contracture: >40% primary, ~0% secondary
   ii. Donors: Groin, postauricular, supraclavicular
c. Skin graft healing (**Table 40.3**)
   i. 6 weeks: 90% of maximum tensile strength
   ii. Can fail due to hematoma, seroma, infection, or shearing.

2. Other grafts: Tendon, bone, cartilage, fat, nerve

C. Flap types
1. Definition: Flap is tissue that is transferred to another site with intact blood supply.
2. Classification by blood supply
   a. **Random pattern flaps** (**Figure 40.13A**) are used to cover adjacent defects with blood supply from dermal/subdermal plexus (3:1 length-to-width ratio).
      i. **Rotation flaps** (**Figure 40.14**) and **transposition flaps** (**Figure 40.15**) rotate about a pivot point.
      ii. **Advancement flaps** bring skin into defect without rotation (e.g., **V-Y advancement**, **Figure 40.16**).
   b. **Axial pattern flaps** contain a longitudinal, named arteriovenous system (**Figure 40.13B**).
3. Specialized flaps: See **Table 40.4**.

D. Tissue expansion uses an inflatable silicone balloon to expand surrounding tissue with serial expansions using saline beginning 2 to 4 weeks after expander placement.
1. Indications: Burn alopecia, congenital nevi, postmastectomy breast reconstruction.
2. Advantages: Like replaces like.
3. Disadvantages: Staged, visible deformity during expansion, multiple visits, infection/extrusion risk

TABLE 40-3 Stages of Skin Graft Healing

Days	Stage	Description
1-2	Imbibition	Diffusion of nutrients from the wound bed
3-5	Inosculation	Graft and wound bed capillaries align
5	Revascularization	Graft revascularized by capillary ingrowth
4-7	Adherence	Graft anchored by collagen, earliest possible time for bolster removal

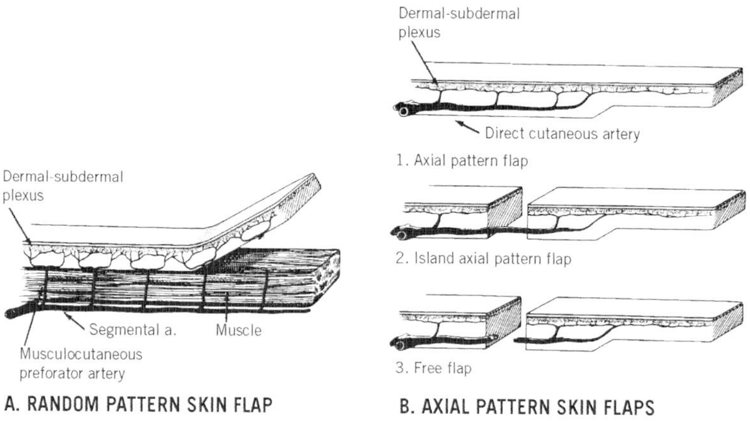

FIGURE 40.13 A, Random pattern skins flap are supplied by the dermal/subdermal plexus. B, Axial pattern skin flaps are supplied by a longitudinal, named septocutaneous artery in various forms, including: 1. In a *peninsular axial flap*, the skin and vessels are moved together. 2. In an *island axial flap* skin is divided from surrounding tissue but maintained on its vascular pedicle. 3. In an *axial free flap* the vascular pedicle is isolated, divided, and anastomosed at a new site. *(Reprinted with permission from Thorne CH, Chung KC, Gosain AK, et al., eds. Grabb and Smith's Plastic Surgery. 7th ed. Wolters Kluwer Health/Lippincott Williams & Wilkins; 2014.)*

XI. ACUTE INJURIES

A. Facial trauma

1. Assessment

a. C-spine: Ten percent of patients with facial trauma have associated C-spine injury.

b. Examination

i. Oral: Assess malocclusion, trismus, loose teeth (aspiration risk).

ii. Facial nerve: Assess branches, noting paresis or asymmetry (**Table 40.5**).

a) Injuries lateral to the pupil should be explored/repaired within 72 hours; but if more medial, manage expectantly.

iii. Ocular: Assess eye/extraocular movements.

a) Limited upgaze in orbital fracture may indicate muscle entrapment (needs urgent operation).

b) **Orbital compartment syndrome** with proptosis, vision loss, and severe eye pain from retrobulbar hematoma requires emergent lateral cantholysis.

iv. Nasal: Assess for septal hematoma using otoscope; drain acutely to prevent deformity.

2. Imaging: Maxillofacial CT to characterize facial fractures.

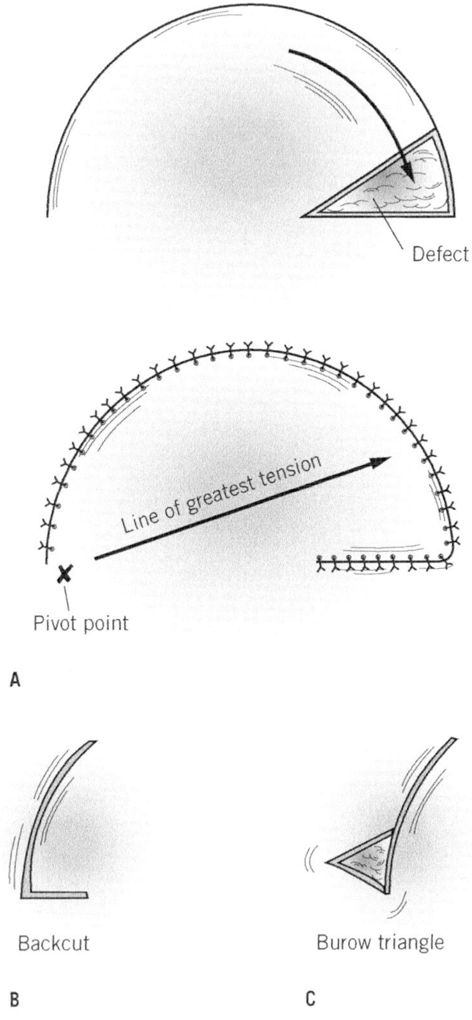

FIGURE 40.14 Rotation flap. A, The edge of the flap is four to five times the length of the base of the defect triangle. B and C, A back cut or Burow triangle can be useful if the flap is under tension.

3. Nasal hemorrhage usually ceases with packing, but if refractory, likely an external carotid branch requiring embolization.
4. Laceration: Close in layers and align anatomic structures after local block/irrigation.
5. Repair fractures electively within 1 to 2 weeks unless airway compromise and/or muscle entrapment (**Table 40.6**).

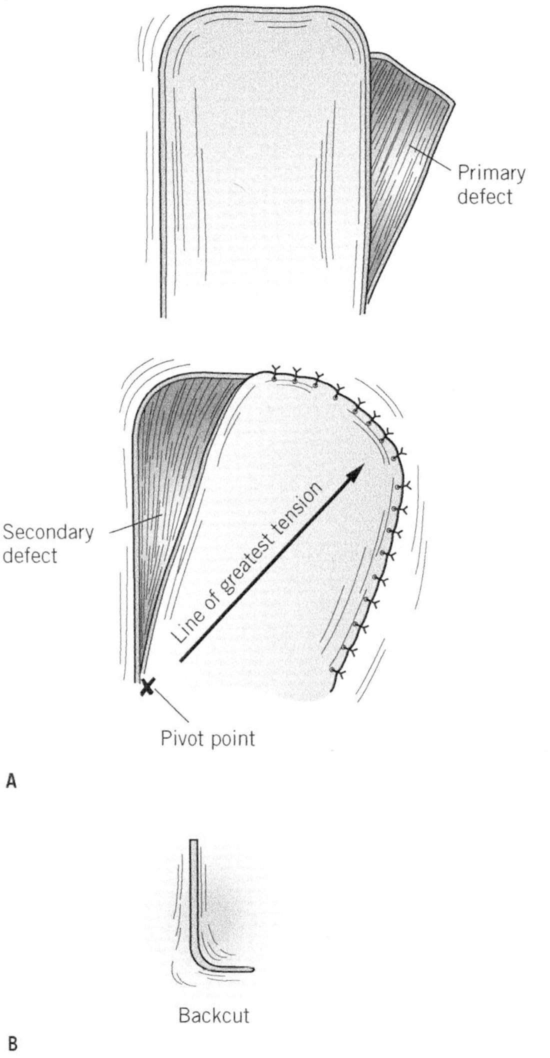

FIGURE 40.15 A, Transposition flap (more complex rotation flap that creates a defect that must be closed). The secondary defect is typically covered with a skin graft. B, A back cut may be added to reduce tension at the pivot point.

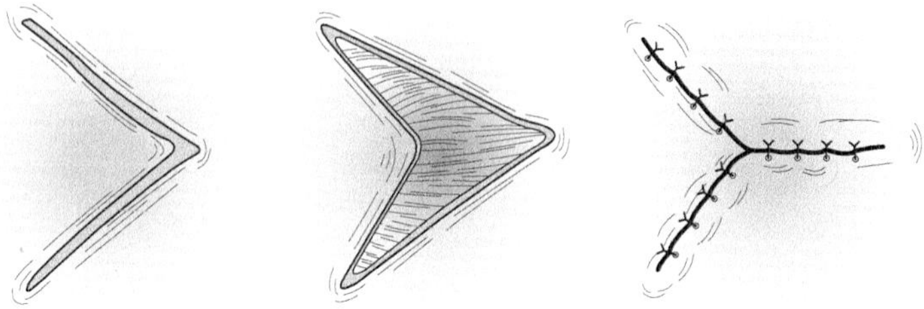

FIGURE 40.16 V-Y advancement. The skin to the sides of the V is advanced.

TABLE 40-4 Specialized Flaps

Type	Common Examples	Notes
Fascial flap	Temporoparietal flap	Used for thin vascularized coverage
Fasciocutaneous flap	Radial forearm flap Anterolateral thigh flap Lateral arm flap Groin flap	
Muscle flap Groin coverage Chest coverage	Sartorius muscle flap Rectus femoris muscle flap Gracilis muscle flap Pectoralis major muscle flap Rectus abdominus muscle flap Latissimus dorsi muscle flap	Used for robust vascularized coverage to obliterate dead space or provide bulk
Musculocutaneous flap Chest coverage Perineal coverage	Thoracodorsal artery perforator flap Vertical rectus abdominus muscle flap	
Vascularized bone flap	Fibular bone flap Scapular bone flap Iliac crest bone flap Intercostal bone flap	Used for bony defects > 6 cm
Functional muscle flap	Gracilis free functional muscle flap Latissimus free functional muscle flap	Transferred with dominant nerve to retain muscle function after location change

TABLE 40.5 Facial Nerve Testing

Branch	Test
Temporal	Brow raise
Zygomatic	Squeeze eyes shut
Buccal	Puff out cheeks
Marginal mandibular	Smile and grimace to depress lower lip
Cervical	Flex platysma

B. Hand trauma

1. Assessment

a. History: Handedness, occupation, hobbies

b. Vascular/perfusion: Color, temperature, capillary refill, and pulses (palpation/Doppler)

i. Allen test to assess for intact palmar arch, radial/ulnar artery transection/occlusion.

ii. Control hemorrhage with pressure; reserve tourniquets for life-threatening exsanguination and place as distally as possible.

c. Examination: Test sensation and motion in ulnar/radial/median distributions (**Table 40.7**).

d. Imaging: Obtain three-view radiographs including joint above and below injury to look for fractures, dislocations, and foreign bodies.

e. Laceration: Close primarily after local block/irrigation, and evert **glabrous skin** to prevent inclusion cysts.

2. Fractures (see Chapter 9)

TABLE 40.6 Indications for Facial Fracture Fixation

Fracture	Indication
Mandible	Malocclusion, trismus
Orbital	Persistent diplopia, enophthalmos, extraocular muscle entrapment, hypoglobus
Midface	Cosmetic deformity, malocclusion/trismus
Nasal bone	Cosmetic deformity, airway obstruction

TABLE 40.7 Unambiguous Tests of Hand Nerve Function

Test	Radial Nerve	Median Nerve	Ulnar Nerve
Sensory	Dorsum first web	Index fingertip	Small fingertip
Extrinsic motor	Extend wrist	FDP index	FDP small
Intrinsic motor	None	Abduct thumb perpendicular to palm	Cross long finger over index (interossei)

FDP, flexor digitorum profundus.

3. **Tendon injuries**
   a. **Flexor tendons** are lacerated during everyday activities (see **tendon zones, Figure 40.17**).
      i. Acute management: Irrigate/close wound, place extension-blocking splint to minimize retraction of tendon ends.
      ii. Definitive repair within 10 days to avoid tendon grafting; zone II-IV injuries have worse prognosis.
   b. **Extensor tendon injuries** result from lacerations and closed axial loading of digits.
      i. Acute management: Irrigate/close wound, place flexion-blocking splint to minimize retraction of tendon ends; can repair acutely, unlike flexors.
      ii. Treat **Mallet finger** (terminal tendon rupture) with distal interphalangeal (DIP) joint extension splinting for 6 weeks.
4. **Infections (Figure 40.18)**
   a. Hand infections result from penetrating trauma (**Table 40.8**).
      i. Management: I&D of purulence, regular irrigation/dressing changes, and splinting/elevation
      ii. Preprocedure radiographs to assess for foreign bodies (e.g., needles).
5. Surgical emergencies
   a. **Compartment syndrome:** Increased pressure within the osseofascial space leading to decreased perfusion pressure, tissue ischemia, and necrosis if left untreated (see Chapter 9).
   b. **Flexor tenosynovitis:** Infection in flexor tendon sheath after volar injury.
      i. **Kanavel signs (Table 40.9)**
      ii. Urgent OR for I&D, IV antibiotics.
   c. **Palmar abscess** requires I&D of involved palmar fascial spaces.
   d. **Necrotizing infections** threaten limb and life and require aggressive, repeated OR debridement, broad-spectrum IV antibiotics, and resuscitation.

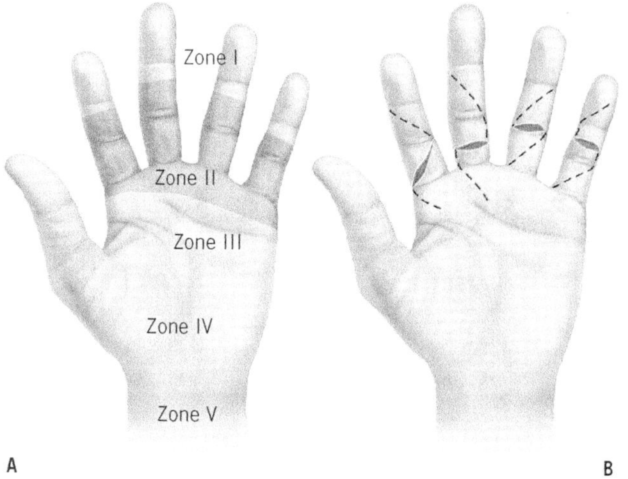

FIGURE 40.17 Zones of flexor tendon injury. A, Zone I, at the DIP level, distal to the FDS insertion. Zone II, from proximal A1 pulley (MCP joint) to FDS insertion. Injuries in this zone may affect both FDS and FDP. Zone III, from distal transverse carpal ligament (carpal tunnel) to A1 pulley. Look for associated palmar arch or median/ulnar nerve injury. Zone IV, within the carpal tunnel, look for median nerve injury. Zone V, proximal to the carpal tunnel. In general, flexor tendons repaired in zones I, III, IV, and V have a better prognosis than those in zone II, known as "no man's land." B, Brunner zigzag extensions to optimize exposure of the proximal and distal ends of the flexor tendon. DIP, distal interphalangeal; FDP, flexor digitorum profundus; FDS, flexor digitorum superficialis; MCP, metacarpophalangeal. *(Reprinted with permission from Thorne CH, Chung KC, Gosain AK, et al., eds. Grabb and Smith's Plastic Surgery. 7th ed. Wolters Kluwer Health/Lippincott Williams & Wilkins; 2014.)*

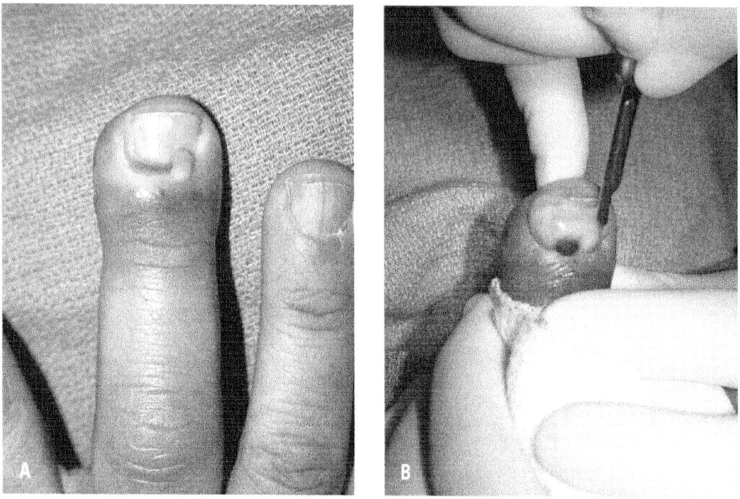

FIGURE 40.18 Acute paronychia. A, As seen in the emergency room. B, Incision is made through the most fluctuant region. *(Reprinted with permission from Thorne CH, Chung KC, Gosain AK, et al., eds. Grabb and Smith's Plastic Surgery. 7th ed. Wolters Kluwer Health/Lippincott Williams & Wilkins; 2014.)*

TABLE 40.8 Hand Infections

Type	Treatment
Paronychia: Infection of lateral nail fold (Figure 44.18)	• I&D with or without nail removal
Felon: Infection of finger pulp	• I&D requiring division of involved septae
Cellulitis: Presents with soft tissue erythema, induration, and warmth	• Antibiotics with or without I&D if abscess develops
Animal bites	• Irrigated for decontamination and removal of foreign bodies (e.g., teeth) • Infection prophylaxis with PO antibiotics • IV antibiotics for established infection
Human bites/fight bites	• Urgently operative for exploration and debridement when over MCP (75% have a bone, tendon, or cartilage injury) • Treated with IV antibiotics and multiple washouts

I&D, incision and drainage.

XII. GENERAL RECONSTRUCTION

A. Scalp
   1. Scalp layers (**Figure 40.19**)
   2. Lacerations
      a. Assess for associated skull, C-spine, or intracranial injuries.
      b. Rich blood supply can lead to significant blood loss, and hemostasis can be achieved with layered closure.
      c. Stapling the hair-bearing scalp reduces trauma to hair follicles.

TABLE 40.9 Kanavel Signs for Clinical Diagnosis of Flexor Tenosynovitis

Finger held in flexion
Fusiform swelling of the finger
Tenderness along the flexor tendon sheath
Pain with passive extension of finger

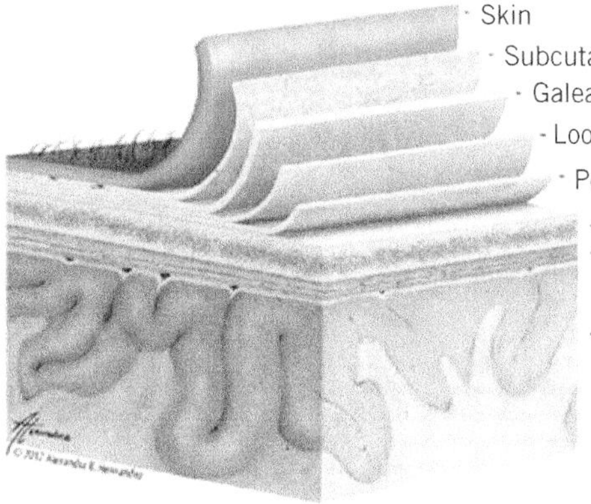

FIGURE 40.19 Scalp layers from superficial to deep are A, **S**kin, B, sub**C**utaneous tissue, C, **G**alea, D, loose **A**reolar tissue, E, **P**ericranium. These layers spell out the acronym **SCALP**. *(Reprinted with permission from Sokoya M, Inman J, Ducic Y. Scalp and Forehead Reconstruction. Semin Plast Surg. 2018;32(2):90-94. Copyright 2018, Georg Thieme Verlag KG.)*

3. **Partial-thickness scalp loss** occurs at the subaponeurotic layer, large avulsions can be skin grafted, and tissue expansion can be used for the hair-bearing scalp.
4. **Full-thickness scalp loss** can occur from trauma or tumor extirpation, with reconstruction dependent on defect size (**Table 40.10**).

B. Trunk
1. **Breast reconstruction**
   a. **Postmastectomy reconstruction** aims to recreate a breast mound with or without **nipple–areola complex** (NAC) (**Figure 40.20**).
      i. **Autologous reconstruction** uses the patient's own tissue (**Table 40.11**).
         a) Advantages: Natural, fewer visits/radiation complications
         b) Disadvantages: Longer procedure/recovery, donor-site morbidity

TABLE 40.10 Scalp Reconstruction of Full-Thickness Defects

Defect Size	Options
Small (<3 cm)	Primary closure after undermining
Medium (3-10 cm)	Skin graft or skin substitute (e.g., integra) Local scalp flap with skin graft of donor site Tissue expansion for hair-bearing scalp
Large (>10 cm)	Free tissue transfer (e.g., latissimus dorsi flap, omentum flap)

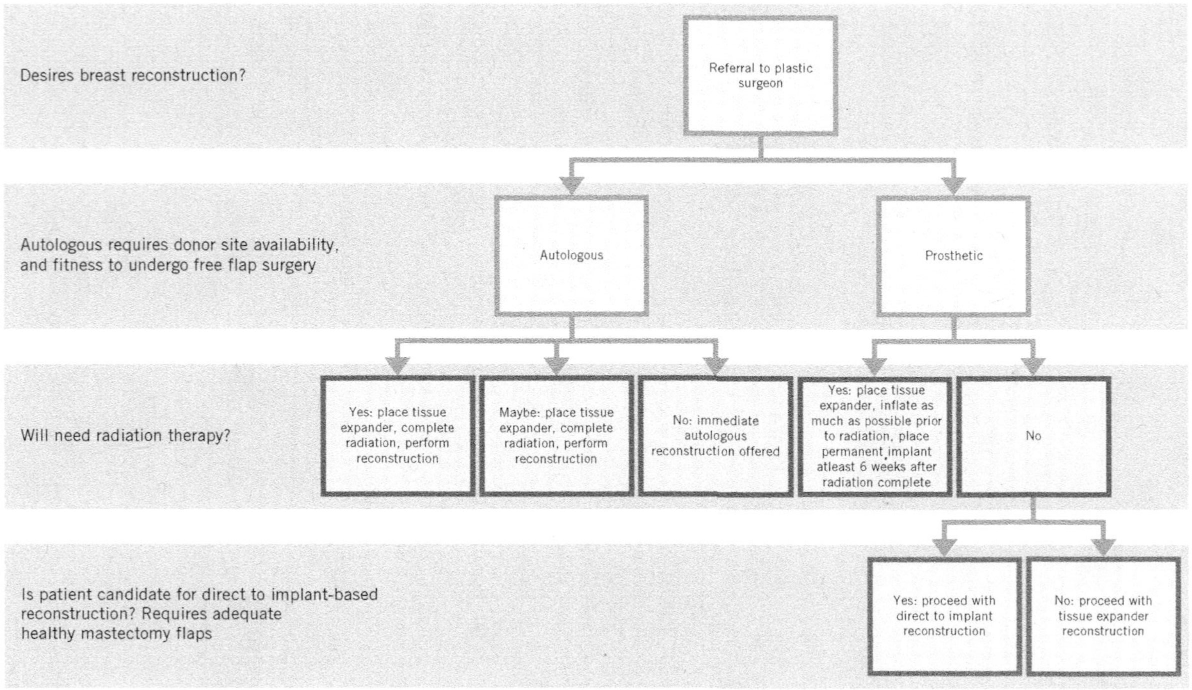

FIGURE 40.20 Breast reconstruction algorithm.

TABLE 40.11 Autologous Breast Reconstruction Options

Flap Type	Options
Pedicled	Transverse rectus abdominis myofascial (TRAM) flap Latissimus dorsi myocutaneous flap
Free	Deep inferior epigastric perforator (DIEP) abdominal flap Transverse upper gracilis (TUG) thigh flap

ii. **Implant-based reconstruction** is more common.
   a) A **tissue expander** is placed at the time of mastectomy and replaced with a permanent implant after expansions achieve desired size.
   b) Advantages: Shorter procedure/recovery, fewer scars.
   c) Disadvantages: Implant rupture/infection/contracture, less natural, possible need for replacement.

b. **Breast implant–associated anaplastic large cell lymphoma** is rare lymphoma associated with capsule formation around textured implants.
   i. Presents as late seroma, and diagnosis is confirmed by aspiration cytology.
   ii. Treatment includes complete capsulectomy/implant removal with or without systemic treatment.
   iii. Lifetime risk: 1:1,000 to 1:30,000 after textured implants.

c. Radiation increases wound healing complications, tissue fibrosis, infection, and implant contracture, but timing reconstruction around radiation can reduce complications (**Figure 40.20**).

d. Prophylactic contralateral mastectomy is controversial; bilateral reconstruction has better symmetry but greater risk of complications.

e. **NAC reconstruction** is done via local flaps with areolar tattoo or 3D tattoo alone.

f. **Symmetry procedures** include contralateral reduction or mastopexy, fat grafting, inframammary fold (IMF) modification, or flap revision/liposuction.

g. **Reconstruction after breast conservation therapy** is complicated by radiation, include:
   i. Ipsilateral volume replacement with fat grafting or local tissue rearrangement
   ii. Contralateral reduction or mastopexy

2. **Chest wall reconstruction**
   a. Goals
      i. Restoration of chest wall integrity
      ii. Dead space obliteration
      iii. Durable, well-vascularized coverage

b. Preoperative assessment
   i. Evaluate for available vascular pedicles (e.g., prior bypass with internal mammary artery precludes using ipsilateral rectus abdominis flap or pectoralis turnover flap).
   ii. Defect must be clear of neoplasm, radiation damage, and infected tissue/hardware; NPWT can bridge to definitive coverage.
   iii. Wound location determines flap options, and flaps should cover wound without tension (**Figure 40.21**).
   iv. Skeletal stabilization (autologous or prosthetic) is required if missing more than four rib segments or 5 cm of chest wall.

3. **Abdominal wall reconstruction**
   a. Goals: Recreate competent abdominal wall.
   b. **Primary fascial closure** can be assisted by **component separation** (lateral release of external oblique fascia, **Figure 40.22**).
   c. Mesh (synthetic or biologic) can strengthen fascial closure or provide closure when component separation is inadequate (see Chapter 25).
   d. Skin coverage: STSGs can be used over vascularized tissue, while advancement flaps should be used over mesh.
   e. Challenging cases may require locoregional myofascial/myocutaneous flaps (e.g., anterolateral thigh flap, tensor fascia lata [TFL], rectus femoris).

4. **Pressure sores**
   a. Etiology/staging (see Chapter 11)
   b. Management
      i. Stage I-II ulcers: Wound care
      ii. Stage III-IV ulcers: Consider coverage once wound is free of infection/devitalized tissue, osteomyelitis has been treated, and nutrition is optimized.
   c. **Diverting colostomy** is controversial; laparoscopic colostomy reduces recurrence in select patients.[13]
   d. Common flaps: Gluteus maximus, TFL, hamstring, or gracilis-based rotation/advancement flaps.

C. Lower extremity
   1. Soft tissue defects from trauma, tumor, or ulceration require multidisciplinary care (e.g., orthopedic/vascular/plastic surgery).
   2. Thigh soft tissue defects are usually closed by primary closure, skin grafts, or local flaps.
   3. Open tibia fractures frequently involve degloving of anterior tibial surface, described using **Gustilo classification** (**Table 40.12**); fractures in distal tibia watershed zone have high infection/nonunion risk.
   4. Large bony defects can be reconstructed with endoprosthesis, nonvascular bone graft, vascularized bone flap, or distraction osteogenesis.
   5. Foot wound coverage is based on surface involved and addressing wound etiology (e.g., arterial insufficiency) prior to coverage.
      a. **Plantar surface:** Durable sensate coverage using dermal substitutes, rotation of instep tissue, or free flap.

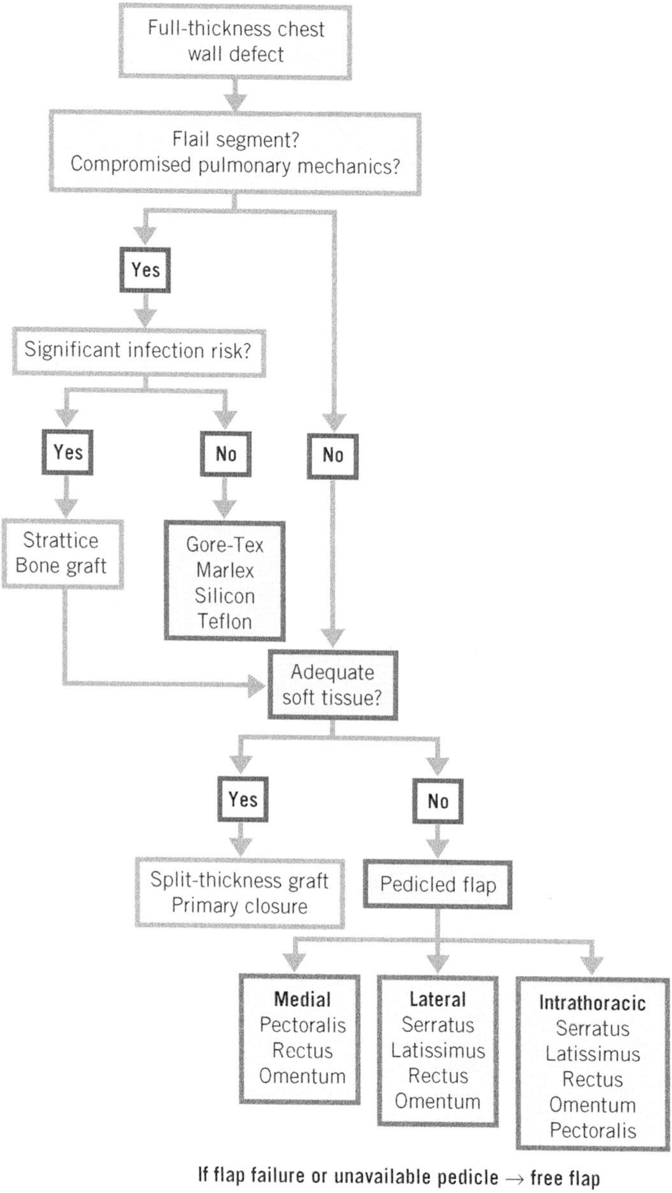

FIGURE 40.21 Chest wall reconstruction algorithm.

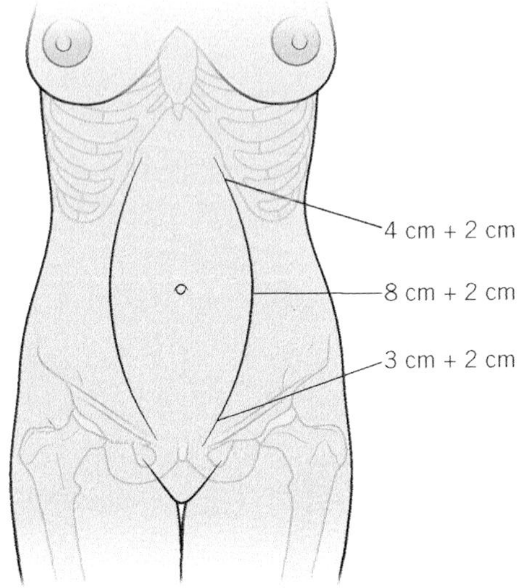

FIGURE 40.22 Maximal unilateral rectus complex mobility in the upper, middle, and lower thirds of the abdomen using component separation. Rectus muscle separation from the posterior sheath can gain an additional 2 cm. The anterior sheath of one or both muscles can also be incised to provide additional fascia for closure. *(Reprinted from Neligan PC, Buck DW II, eds. Abdominal wall reconstruction. In: Core Procedures in Plastic Surgery. 2nd ed. Elsevier; 2020:277-290. Copyright 2020, Elsevier. With permission.)*

b. **Dorsal foot:** Thin pliable coverage for standard footwear use with skin grafting (paratenon present) or dermal substitute/fascial free flaps + skin graft.

D. Peripheral nerve

1. Assessment requires clinical motor and sensory evaluation with or without electrodiagnostic studies (EDX).
   a. Motor evaluation is standardized (**Table 40.13**).
   b. Nerve injuries are classified by severity (**Table 40.14**).
2. Acute management
   a. **Sharp transection:** Repair nerve within 72 hours, and if tension-free primary repair is not possible, use nerve graft.
   b. **Closed injury:** Usually first- or second-degree injury, so full recovery can be expected without operation (e.g., post-op deficit at nonsurgical site secondary to positioning); but if no improvement by

TABLE 40.12 Gustilo Open Fracture Classification

Classification	Characteristics
I	Clean wound <1 cm long
II	Laceration >1 cm long with extensive soft tissue damage
III	Extensive soft tissue laceration, damage, or loss; open segmental fracture; or traumatic amputation
IIIa	Adequate periosteal cover of the bone despite extensive soft tissue damage; high-energy trauma with small wound or crushing component
IIIb[a]	Extensive soft tissue loss with periosteal stripping and bone exposure requiring soft tissue flap closure; usually associated with massive contamination
IIIc[a]	Vascular injury requiring repair

[a]Types IIIb and IIIc frequently require flap coverage using pedicled gastrocnemius or soleus flap, or a free flap for more distal wounds.

Adapted with permission from Gustilo RB, Anderson JT. Prevention of infection in the treatment of one thousand and twenty-five open fractures of long bones: retrospective and prospective analyses. *J Bone Joint Surg Am.* 1976;58(4):453-458. Copyright 1976, by The Journal of Bone and Joint Surgery, Inc.

6 weeks, obtain EDX, and if no improvement by 3 months, repeat EDX and refer to nerve surgeon.

c. Treat **nerve deficit from compartment syndrome** with emergent fasciotomy, expect rapid functional improvement if decompressed within 6 hours.

TABLE 40.13 Classification of Motor Function

Grade	Motor Function
M0	No contraction
M1	Perceptible contraction in proximal muscles
M2	Perceptible contraction in proximal and distal muscles
M3	All important muscles powerful enough to act against gravity
M4	Muscles act against strong resistance; some independent movement possible
M5	Normal strength and function

Adapted with permission of Georg Thieme Verlag KG from Mackinnon SE, Dellon AL. *Surgery of the Peripheral Nerve.* Thieme; 1988:118; permission conveyed through Copyright Clearance Center, Inc.

TABLE 40.14 Classification of Nerve Injuries

Sunderland[a]	Seddon[b]	Structure Injured	Prognosis
First degree	Neurapraxia	Schwann cell (demyelination)	Complete recovery within 3 mo
Second degree	Axonotmesis	Axon (Wallerian degeneration)	Complete recovery, regeneration 1 mm/d
Third degree		Endoneurium	Incomplete recovery
Fourth degree		Perineurium	No recovery
Fifth degree	Neurotmesis	Epineurium	No recovery
Sixth degree		Mixed injury, neuroma in continuity[c]	Unpredictable recovery

[a]Sunderland S. A classification of peripheral nerve injuries producing loss of function. *Brain.* 1951;74:491.

[b]Seddon HJ. Three types of nerve injury. *Brain.* 1943;66:237.

[c]Mackinnon SE. New direction in peripheral nerve surgery. *Ann Plast Surg.* 1989;22(3):257-273.

XIII. AESTHETIC SURGERY

A. Augmentation mammoplasty
   1. **Implants**
      a. Types: Saline or silicone (smooth)
      b. Placement: Subglandular, submuscular, or dual plane
      c. Monitoring
         i. Cancer screening (see Chapter 27) using **standard mammography plus Eklund views**
         ii. Saline **implant rupture** presents as a deflated breast.
         iii. Silicone implants must be monitored by MRI or ultrasound imaging, with initial study 5 to 6 years after placement and every 2 to 3 years thereafter.
   2. **Fat transfer** can fill the upper pole following implant placement.

B. Reduction mammoplasty
   1. High patient satisfaction from improvement in symptoms
   2. Indications: Neck pain, IMF rashes/infections, shoulder grooving, functional limitations to exercise
   3. Goal: Reduction of breast tissue volume/skin excess while maintaining blood supply to NAC, which can be removed and grafted.

C. Abdominoplasty
   1. Goal: Removal of redundant abdominal skin/fat by elevating large subcutaneous flaps from umbilicus to xiphoid and transposing umbilicus (with or without rectus plication)
   2. High VTE risk, so patients discharged on deep vein thrombosis prophylaxis

D. Postbariatric body contouring
  1. Includes liposuction, abdominoplasty, upper body/lower body lift, back/thigh lift, brachioplasty.
  2. Timing: Weight stability for 3 to 6 months (~12-18 months after a bariatric operation) as lower body mass index equates to lower complications and better cosmesis
  3. Nutrition optimization: Recommend pre-op iron, vitamin B_{12}, calcium, folate, and albumin testing.

UROLOGY FOR THE GENERAL SURGEON

Nicholas A. Pickersgill and Eric H. Kim

XIV. HEMATURIA

A. Etiology: Malignancy, urinary tract infection (UTI), stones, **benign prostatic hyperplasia** (BPH), recent trauma, instrumentation, gynecologic sources

B. Presentation
  1. **Gross hematuria** is visible blood in the urine while **microscopic hematuria** is defined as ≥3 red blood cells per high-power field.
  2. Often painless
  3. Severe gross hematuria may present with urinary retention due to blood clot retention.

C. Diagnosis
  1. Laboratory studies: Urinalysis (UA), urine culture
  2. Imaging/invasive studies
     a. Upper urinary tract imaging is required.
        i. CT or magnetic resonance (MR) urogram
        ii. Renal ultrasound imaging with retrograde pyelograms if end-stage renal disease or history of renal transplant to evaluate the native kidneys and ureters
        iii. For microscopic hematuria, renal ultrasound imaging alone is sufficient in low-risk patients.
     b. Cystoscopy

D. Nonoperative treatment
  1. Clot retention requires urgent urologic consultation and a three-way large-bore (22 or 24 Fr) catheter for irrigation.
  2. **Continuous bladder irrigation** may be required for persistent bleeding once all bladder clots have been aspirated; used with caution in patients with recent urologic reconstruction due to risk of perforation.

E. Operative treatment
  1. Persistent lower tract bleeding may require cystoscopy, clot evacuation, and/or fulguration.
  2. Persistent, severe upper tract bleeding may require surgery or angiography with or without selective angioembolization.

XV. DISEASES OF THE KIDNEY: SOLID AND CYSTIC RENAL MASSES

A. Epidemiology/etiology
   1. Eighty percent of solid renal masses are malignant.
   2. **Renal cell carcinoma** (RCC) is the most common solid renal mass.
   3. Other etiologies: Urothelial carcinoma, oncocytoma, angiomyolipoma, metastatic tumors
   4. Renal cysts are mostly benign and occur in approximately 50% of people >50 year old.

B. Presentation
   1. Mostly incidentally diagnosed
   2. Classic triad of flank pain, hematuria, and flank mass is uncommon (<10%).
   3. Paraneoplastic syndromes occur in 10% to 40% of RCC.
   4. Incidence of metastatic disease at presentation is approximately 20% to 30%.

C. Diagnosis
   1. Imaging/invasive studies
      a. Renal protocol CT or MRI with renal cysts risk-stratified; see **Table 40.15**.[14]
      b. CXR or chest CT for staging
      c. Bone scan if elevated alkaline phosphatase or bone-related complaints
      d. Head CT/MRI if neurologic symptoms
      e. Percutaneous biopsy is increasingly used but not routinely necessary; diagnostic accuracy is >90% with a complication rate <5%.[15]
   2. Laboratory studies
      a. CBC, renal function panel (RFP), liver function tests, UA
      b. Lactate dehydrogenase (LDH) may be prognostic in metastatic disease.
   3. RCC staged using the AJCC **TNM staging system** (Chapter 60: Kidney; *AJCC Cancer Staging Manual*, 8th ed.) based on tumor size and depth of invasion, presence of lymph node metastases, and presence of distant metastases[9]

D. Nonoperative treatment
   1. Active surveillance with imaging every 6 to 12 months for small or complex cystic masses
   2. Metastatic RCC: Targeted systemic therapy with *immune checkpoint inhibitors*, *tyrosine kinase inhibitors*, or mTOR inhibitors[16]

E. Operative treatment
   1. Options include ablation, nephron-sparing partial nephrectomy, and radical nephrectomy depending on tumor stage.
   2. Metastatic RCC: Cytoreductive therapy in select patients[17]

XVI. DISEASES OF THE URETER

A. Hydronephrosis
   1. Definition/etiology
      a. Hydronephrosis refers to renal collecting system dilation.

TABLE 40.15 Bosniak Classification System of Renal Cystic Masses, Version 2019

Bosniak Category	Characteristics	Risk of Malignancy (%)	Management
I	Simple cyst; thin (≤2 mm) wall; no septa or calcifications; wall may enhance	0	No follow-up
II	Thin (≤2 mm) wall that may enhance; few septa; may have calcification; homogenous; nonenhancing; can have high attenuation	5-18.5[a]	No follow-up
IIF	Minimally thickened (3 mm) enhancing wall, or smooth minimal thickening of septa, or many smooth thin enhancing septa	15-25	Surveillance imaging at 6 and 12 mo, then annually for 5 y
III	One or more enhancing thick (≥4 mm) or enhancing irregular walls or septa	33+	Surveillance, resection, or ablation
IV	Contains one or more enhancing nodule(s)	92.5	Surveillance, resection, or ablation

[a]There are limited data on category II cysts as most studies combine II and IIF cysts. Category II cysts (excluding IIF) are thought to be essentially benign.

Adapted from Silverman SG, Pedrosa I, Ellis JH, et al. Bosniak classification of cystic renal masses, version 2019: an update proposal and needs assessment. *Radiology.* 2019;292(2):475-488.

- **b.** Commonly caused by ureteral obstruction.
  - **i. Intrinsic:** Stones, ureteropelvic junction obstruction, stricture, or tumor
  - **ii. Extrinsic:** Compression from abdominal/pelvic masses, crossing blood vessels, pregnancy, or retroperitoneal fibrosis
- **c.** Nonobstructive etiologies: Urinary reflux from the bladder, excessive hydration, or prominent extrarenal pelvis.
- **d.** Bilateral hydronephrosis with a distended bladder may be due to **bladder outlet obstruction** (e.g., BPH).

2. Presentation

- **a.** Flank pain/renal colic
- **b.** Elevated serum creatinine
- **c.** Can be asymptomatic

3. Diagnosis
    a. Laboratory studies: UA, urine culture, RFP
    b. Imaging/invasive studies
        i. Anatomic studies such as noncontrast CT/ultrasound imaging are best if urolithiasis is suspected.
        ii. Functional studies provide information on renal function and urine flow.
            a) CT/MR urogram
            b) **Diuretic renal scintigraphy** (**furosemide renal scan**) measures urine flow and relative function of each kidney.
        iii. **Retrograde pyelogram** can determine the location of obstruction.
4. Nonoperative treatment
    a. Observation if asymptomatic, nonobstructive, and the affected kidney demonstrates stable or absent function.
5. Operative treatment
    a. **Ureteral stent** or **percutaneous nephrostomy tube**
    b. Long-term management (e.g., chronic indwelling ureteral stent or nephrostomy tube, endoureterotomy, ureteral reconstruction) is dependent on the etiology.

B. Urolithiasis (urinary tract calculi)
1. Epidemiology/etiology
    a. Most common in fourth and sixth decades of life, although incidence in pediatric populations is rising.
    b. Male predominance
    c. Modifiable risk factors: Low fluid intake and diets high in animal protein, sodium, or oxalate
    d. Other risk factors: Obesity, diabetes, inflammatory bowel disease (IBD), gout, hyperparathyroidism, and type I renal tubular acidosis, medications, high doses of vitamins C/D.[18]
2. Presentation
    a. Acute onset of severe flank pain often associated with nausea/vomiting
    b. May present with hematuria.
    c. Obstruction in the setting of UTI can quickly progress to sepsis and become life threatening.
3. Diagnosis
    a. Laboratory studies: UA, urine culture, RFP, CBC.
    b. Imaging/invasive studies
        i. Noncontrast CT preferred.
        ii. Renal ultrasound imaging may not accurately determine stone size and location.
4. Nonoperative treatment
    a. **Medical expulsive therapy:** >70% of stones <5 mm and ~40% of stones 5 to 10 mm will pass spontaneously, may take up to 4 weeks.[19]
    b. Narcotics and daily α-blocker therapy (e.g., tamsulosin)
    c. Urine should be strained.

5. Operative treatment
   a. Urgent ureteral stent or percutaneous nephrostomy tube placement for concomitant infection, acute renal failure, solitary kidney, bilateral obstruction, or intractable pain.
   b. Definitive surgical options include **shock wave lithotripsy**, **ureteroscopy with or without laser lithotripsy**, or **percutaneous nephrolithotomy**.

C. Ureteropelvic junction obstruction
1. Epidemiology/etiology
   a. **Congenital:** Intrinsic (e.g., scarring, ureteral valves, aperistaltic proximal ureter) or extrinsic (e.g., crossing vessel, high ureteral insertion), typically presents in childhood.
   b. **Acquired:** Trauma, ureteral instrumentation, failed prior reconstruction (e.g., endopyelotomy or pyeloplasty).
2. Presentation
   a. Intermittent flank pain
   b. Nausea/vomiting
   c. Pyelonephritis
   d. **Dietl's crisis:** Worsening of flank pain after aggressive hydration or diuresis
3. Diagnosis
   a. Laboratory studies: UA, urine culture, RFP.
   b. Imaging/invasive studies
      i. CT/MR urogram can assess location and cause of obstruction.
      ii. Diuretic renal scintigraphy confirms functional obstruction and assesses differential function.
4. Nonoperative treatment
   a. Observation if mild/absent symptoms and stable renal function.
5. Operative treatment
   a. **Pyeloplasty** or **endopyelotomy**.

XVII. DISEASES OF THE URINARY BLADDER

A. Bladder cancer
1. Epidemiology/etiology
   a. **Urothelial carcinoma** (>90% of bladder cancers in the US); SCC and adenocarcinoma are rare.
   b. Risk factors: Smoking, textile dyes, cyclophosphamide, chronic indwelling catheters, chronic parasitic infection (*Schistosoma haematobium*), radiation.
2. Presentation
   a. Hematuria is the most common presenting symptom.
   b. Irritative voiding symptoms may be present.
3. Diagnosis
   a. Imaging/invasive studies
      i. Diagnosis established via **transurethral resection of bladder tumor(s) (TURBT)** or cystoscopic biopsy

ii. CT/MR urogram to assess for concomitant upper tract urothelial carcinoma (<5% of cases); if unable, or history of renal transplant, renal ultrasound imaging or noncontrast CT/MRI with bilateral retrograde pyelograms is sufficient.

b. Bladder cancer staged by AJCC **TNM staging system** (Chapter 62: Urinary bladder; *AJCC Cancer Staging Manual*, 8th ed.) based on tumor depth of invasion, level of lymph node metastases, and presence of distant metastases.[9]

4. Treatment

a. **Non–muscle invasive bladder cancer**

i. TURBT is both diagnostic and therapeutic.

ii. Intravesical **bacillus Calmette–Guérin** or chemotherapy decreases the risk of recurrence.[20]

iii. Recurrent tumors are treated with TURBT and intravesical therapy.

b. **Muscle-invasive bladder cancer**

i. Cisplatin-based neoadjuvant chemotherapy, radical cystectomy (RC), bilateral pelvic lymph node dissection, and urinary diversion (**Table 40.16**)

ii. Locally advanced disease: Adjuvant chemotherapy or immunotherapy

iii. **Trimodal therapy** with TURBT, chemotherapy, and radiation may be utilized for patients who are unfit for RC or desire bladder preservation.[21]

XVIII. DISEASES OF THE PROSTATE

A. Prostate cancer

1. Epidemiology

a. The most common malignancy and second leading cause of cancer death in men in the US; mean age at diagnosis in 60s.

b. Risk factors: African American race, family history of prostate cancer, genetic mutations (e.g., *BRCA*), advanced age.

TABLE 40.16 Common Types of Urinary Diversion

Type	Name	Outlet
Noncontinent	Ileal conduit	Abdominal stoma empties into urostomy bag continuously
Continent	Indiana/Miami pouch	Continent catheterizable channel made of the ileocecal valve and terminal ileum
	Neobladder	Orthotopic anastomosis to the native urethra

2. Presentation is rarely symptomatic until locally advanced or metastatic.
3. Diagnosis
   a. Laboratory studies
      i. Screening consists of measurement of **serum prostate-specific antigen (PSA)**.
         a) PSA screening has garnered controversy.[22,23]
         b) American Urological Association guidelines (2022) and US Preventive Services Task Force recommendations (2018) recommend shared decision making and annual screening between ages 55 to 70 years for men at average risk, while men with risk factors should begin screening at age 45 years.[24]
4. Digital rectal examination (DRE) and other biomarkers are not independently sufficient for screening.
   a. Imaging/invasive studies
5. **Transrectal ultrasonography with needle biopsy** if PSA > 4 ng/mL.
6. **Multiparametric prostate MRI-targeted biopsy** improves accuracy.[25]
7. Staging imaging consists of **prostate-specific membrane antigen PET scan** or abdomen/pelvis CT/MRI and Tc^{99} bone scan for patients with high-risk disease.
8. Prostate cancer staging based on AJCC **TNM staging system** (Chapter 58: Prostate; *AJCC Cancer Staging Manual*, 8th ed.) based on extent of prostate involved with tumor or extraprostatic invasion, presence of lymph node metastases, and presence of distant metastases.[9]
9. Treatment
   a. Localized disease: Active surveillance (low- or intermediate-risk disease), radical prostatectomy, radiation therapy
   b. Recurrent or metastatic disease: **Androgen deprivation therapy**, testosterone suppression, and/or chemotherapy

B. BPH
1. Epidemiology/etiology
   a. Affects ~70% of men in their sixties and ~80% of men 70 years or older.
2. Presentation
   a. **Lower urinary tract symptoms (LUTSs):** Weak stream, frequency/urgency, incontinence, nocturia
   b. Severe BPH may cause hematuria, UTI, bladder stones, renal failure, urinary retention.
3. Diagnosis
   a. Studies
      i. UA, urine culture
      ii. Examination, DRE
      iii. **Urodynamic studies**
4. Nonoperative treatment
   a. Observation if minimally symptomatic or asymptomatic
   b. **Selective α-blockers** (e.g., tamsulosin) or **5α-reductase inhibitors** (e.g., finasteride) and combination therapy for moderate to severe BPH
   c. Catheterization for patients in urinary retention, monitor for **postobstructive diuresis**

5. Operative treatment
   a. Indicated in patients who have failed medical therapy or have severe symptoms
   b. **Transurethral resection of the prostate**, alternatives include prostatic urethral lift, water vapor thermal therapy, photoselective vaporization, laser enucleation, simple prostatectomy.[26]

C. Acute bacterial prostatitis
   1. Etiology
      a. Typically caused by gram-negative bacteria.
      b. Other forms of prostatitis include chronic bacterial prostatitis, chronic pelvic pain syndrome, nonbacterial prostatitis.
   2. Presentation
      a. Fevers, malaise, perineal/pelvic pain, voiding complaints
   3. Diagnosis
      a. Laboratory studies: UA, urine culture, CBC
      b. Examination: DRE reveals tender, boggy, enlarged prostate.
   4. Nonoperative treatment: Antibiotics for 4 to 6 weeks; if no improvement, pelvic CT to rule out abscess
   5. Operative treatment: Prostatic abscess is managed via transurethral resection.

XIX. DISEASES OF THE PENIS

A. Priapism
   1. Etiology
      a. Medications, blood dyscrasia, malignant infiltration, trauma/iatrogenic
   2. Diagnosis
      a. Rigid, tender corpora cavernosa with soft glans is indicative of **ischemic priapism**.
      b. Cavernosal blood gas can distinguish ischemic vs. nonischemic priapism (ischemic blood gas values: $pO_2 < 30$ mm Hg, $pCO_2 > 60$ mm Hg, pH < 7.25).
   3. Treatment
      a. Urologic emergency
      b. Corporal irrigation and aspiration via a 14- to 18-gauge needle
      c. Intracorporal injection of phenylephrine (100-500 μg/mL)
      d. **Cavernosal venous shunting** if above methods fail
      e. If no prospect of regaining erectile function, a penile prosthesis may be placed in the future.

B. Paraphimosis
   1. Etiology: May occur following Foley catheter placement if foreskin is not reduced
   2. Presentation: Urologic emergency in which the foreskin becomes constricted proximal to the glans, resulting in penile edema, pain, and potentially necrosis
   3. Treatment: Immediate manual reduction; if unsuccessful, urgent urology consult

C. Phimosis
  1. Etiology: Inability to fully retract foreskin
  2. Presentation: Mostly asymptomatic but can result in glans/foreskin infections or urinary retention (rare)
  3. Treatment is circumcision if symptomatic

XX. DISEASES OF THE SCROTUM AND TESTICLES

A. Testicular torsion
  1. Epidemiology/etiology
    a. Urologic emergency caused by rotation of the testicle on its vascular pedicle resulting in ischemia
    b. Most common in males 12 to 18 years of age but can occur at any age.
    c. Risk factors: **Bell-clapper deformity**, **cryptorchidism**
  2. Presentation: Acute onset of severe testicular pain and swelling often associated with abdominal pain, nausea/vomiting
  3. Diagnosis
    a. Examination: Tender, swollen testicle that may be high-riding with a transverse lie, and cremasteric reflex is often absent.
    b. Doppler ultrasound imaging can confirm or exclude the diagnosis; however, diagnosis is clinical, and treatment should not be delayed for imaging.
  4. Treatment
    a. Emergent scrotal exploration and bilateral orchiopexy
    b. Manual detorsion may be attempted; however, bilateral orchiopexy is still necessary to prevent future episodes of torsion.
    c. **Orchiectomy** if the testicle is nonviable.

B. Torsion of testicular/epididymal appendage (appendix testis)
  1. Presentation: Gradual onset of mild to moderate testicular pain.
  2. Diagnosis
    a. Examination: Tenderness in the superior testicle and/or epididymis with a normal lie
    b. Palpable nodule visible through the scrotal skin may be present (**"blue dot" sign**).
    c. Diagnosis can be confirmed with scrotal ultrasound imaging.
  3. Treatment: NSAIDs, light physical activity, and scrotal support until resolution over 7 to 14 days.

C. Acute epididymitis, orchitis, and epididymo-orchitis
  1. Etiology
    a. Inflammation of the testis most commonly caused by STI in men <35 years of age and *E. coli* in older men
    b. Other causes: Viral infection, autoimmune disease
  2. Presentation: Unilateral testicular pain and swelling, sometimes associated with dysuria, urethral discharge, or LUTS
  3. Diagnosis
    a. Examination: Painful, indurated epididymis and/or testis
    b. UA, urine culture, CBC, STI testing
    c. Ultrasound imaging can evaluate for scrotal abscess and assess testicular perfusion.

4. Treatment
   a. If low risk for STI, treat empirically with oral fluoroquinolone, although broad-spectrum antibiotics may be required for severe cases.
   b. If STI suspected, treat empirically.
   c. NSAIDs

D. Fournier's gangrene
1. Definition/etiology
   a. **Necrotizing fasciitis** involving the subcutaneous tissue of the genitals and perineum
   b. Surgical emergency with 20% to 30% mortality rate.
   c. Risk factors: Obesity, diabetes, alcoholism, immunodeficiency.
2. Presentation
   a. Painful swelling and induration of the genitalia and/or perineum, often associated with foul odor.
   b. Fever or sepsis may be present.
3. Diagnosis
   a. **Examination:** Painful edema and erythema of the perineum (and scrotum or penis in men); may feature necrosis, crepitus, and malodor.
   b. CBC, electrolytes, UA, urine and blood cultures.
   c. CT can evaluate for extent of infection and presence of subcutaneous gas but should never delay surgical intervention.
4. Treatment
   a. Broad-spectrum antibiotics with aerobic, anaerobic, gram-positive and negative coverage should be started immediately.
   b. Emergent wide surgical debridement (multiple may be necessary); orchiectomy is rarely indicated.

E. Nonacute scrotal masses
1. **Hydrocele**
   a. Etiology
      i. Fluid collections around the testicle that **transilluminate**
      ii. May be reactive due to infection or trauma.
   b. Presentation: Mostly asymptomatic, but larger hydroceles can cause scrotal swelling or discomfort
   c. Diagnosis
      i. Examination: Scrotal swelling without tenderness, testis is frequently nonpalpable in larger hydroceles.
      ii. Scrotal ultrasound imaging
   d. Treatment
      i. Supportive care; hydrocelectomy if symptomatic
2. **Varicocele**
   a. Etiology
      i. Abnormally dilated testicular veins
      ii. More commonly left-sided, and unilateral right-sided hydroceles are rare and may be caused by retroperitoneal masses (e.g., kidney tumor).
   b. Presentation is mostly asymptomatic, but clinical manifestations can include inguinal or scrotal pain, infertility, testicular atrophy.

c. Diagnosis
   i. Examination: "Bag of worms" above testis that enlarges with Valsalva or standing
   ii. Retroperitoneal imaging for unilateral right-sided varicoceles.
d. Treatment
   i. The **most common surgically correctable cause of male infertility**; nevertheless, most men with varicoceles remain fertile, asymptomatic, and never require treatment.
   ii. Varicocele repair results in improved semen quality in approximately 70% of patients.

3. **Testicular tumors**
   a. Epidemiology
      i. The most common solid tumor in males aged 15 to 35 years.
      ii. Most common histologies are **seminoma and nonseminomatous germ cell tumors** (NSGCTs).
      iii. Risk factors: Cryptorchidism, HIV, intratubular germ cell neoplasia, gonadal dysgenesis.
   b. Presentation: Testicular mass, usually asymptomatic.
   c. Diagnosis
      i. Scrotal ultrasound imaging.
      ii. Serum tumor markers: α-Fetoprotein, β-hCG, and LDH.
      iii. Radiographic staging CXR and CT/MRI of the abdomen/pelvis. Testicular cancer is staged using the AJCC **TNM staging system** (Chapter 59: Testis; *AJCC Cancer Staging Manual*, 8th ed.) based on tumor invasion, level and size of lymph node metastases, and presence and extent of distant metastases.[9]
   d. Treatment
      i. Radical inguinal orchiectomy is initial management.
      ii. Postorchiectomy management is stage-dependent.
         a) **Seminoma:** Surveillance, chemotherapy, or radiation.
         b) **NSGCT:** Surveillance, chemotherapy, or **retroperitoneal lymph node dissection** (RPLND).
      iii. RPLND and/or chemotherapy may be used for advanced or recurrent disease.

XXI. GENITOURINARY TRAUMA

A. Renal, ureteral, and bladder trauma (see Chapter 8)

B. Urethral injury
   1. Etiology
      a. **Anterior urethral injuries** involve the bulbous and penile urethra in males and distal one-third of the urethra in females.
      b. **Posterior urethral injuries** involve the prostatic and membranous urethra in males and proximal two-thirds of the urethra in females.
   2. Presentation
      a. Blood at the urethral meatus, genital or perineal hematoma ("butterfly" pattern in anterior injury), penile fracture, high-riding prostate, pelvic fracture, or difficulty voiding/urinary retention.

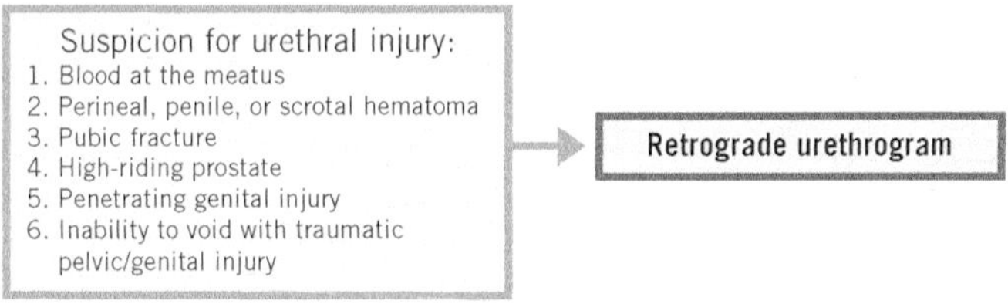
Suspicion for urethral injury:
1. Blood at the meatus
2. Perineal, penile, or scrotal hematoma
3. Pubic fracture
4. High-riding prostate
5. Penetrating genital injury
6. Inability to void with traumatic pelvic/genital injury
Retrograde urethrogram

FIGURE 40.23 Workup for suspected urethral injury. *(Adapted from Wieder JA. Pocket Guide to Urology. 5th ed. J Wieder Medical; 2014. Used with permission.)*

3. Diagnosis/evaluation: See **Figure 40.23**.
4. Treatment
   a. Urologic consultation for catheterization; if unsuccessful, **suprapubic catheter placement**
   b. **Anterior:** Endoscopic primary realignment with delayed urethroplasty in males.
   c. **Posterior:** Surgical repair not recommended in the acute setting.
   d. Immediate surgical repair if penetrating injury

C. Penile fracture
1. Etiology: Tear of the *tunica albuginea* from excessive bending of the erect penis, typically during intercourse
2. Presentation
   a. "Pop" with rapid detumescence and penoscrotal swelling.
   b. Difficulty voiding or blood at the meatus indicates concomitant urethral injury (10%-20% of cases)
3. Diagnosis
   a. Examination: Edema and ecchymosis/hematoma of the penis (**"eggplant deformity"**) and/or perineum
   b. Penile MRI/ultrasound imaging if presentation is unclear.
4. Treatment: Early surgical exploration (<48 hours) with tunica albuginea repair.

D. Scrotal trauma
1. Diagnosis: Ultrasound imaging diagnoses testicular injury with 100% sensitivity/93.5% specificity.[27]
2. Treatment
   a. Scrotal exploration if penetrating scrotal trauma or concern for testicular rupture
   b. Testicular rupture: Hematoma evacuation, debridement of necrotic tubules, and tunica albuginea closure; orchiectomy is rarely indicated.

Key References

Citation	Summary
Pearl JP, Price RR, Tonkin AE, Richardson WS, Stefanidis D. SAGES guidelines for the use of laparoscopy during pregnancy. *Surg Endosc*. 2017;31(10):3767-3782.	• Recommendations and guidelines from Society of American Gastrointestinal Endoscopic Surgeons regarding the (nonobstetric) surgical treatment of pregnant patients, focusing on laparoscopy.
Kim DH, Kim SW, Hwang SH. Application of the laboratory risk indicator for necrotizing fasciitis score to the head and neck: a systematic review and meta-analysis. *ANZ J Surg*. 2022;92(7-8):1631-1637.	• Systematic review of seven cohort studies using the Laboratory Risk Indicator for Necrotizing Fasciitis (LRINEC) score in cervical necrotizing fasciitis. In this study, a cutoff of 6 had 75% sensitivity and 85% specificity, making it a useful clinical adjunct tool in diagnosing head and neck necrotizing infections.
Schroder FH, Hugosson J, Roobol MJ, et al. Screening and prostate-cancer mortality in a randomized European study. *N Engl J Med*. 2009;360(13):1320-1328.	• Randomized controlled study in which over 160,000 men were randomized to screening with prostate-specific antigen (PSA) every 4 y or no screening. Approximately 80% of the screening group was screened at least once. Prostate cancer incidence was 8% in the screening group and 5% in the control group, while the death rate ratio was 0.80. There might be overdiagnosis with PSA screening, but the study is limited by noncompliance in the screening group. Screening in select patients based on first PSA or greater screening intervals might result in greater mortality reductions.

CHAPTER 40: SUBSPECIALTY SURGERY FOR THE GENERAL SURGEON

Review Questions

1. What is the most appropriate next step in an asymptomatic 52-year-old woman with a suspected adnexal mass on clinical examination?
2. A 23-year-old female at 32 weeks' gestation is diagnosed with ruptured appendicitis and requires laparoscopic appendectomy. What changes to the standards of care must be considered?
3. A 62-year-old postmenopausal female presents with intermittent vaginal bleeding for the past 3 months, with unintentional weight loss. What is your initial evaluation?

4. What types of airway management can be initiated in a patient with history of total laryngectomy in respiratory distress?
5. What is the most likely diagnosis for a 5-year-old, otherwise healthy male with a nontender midline mass that moves vertically with swallowing?
6. A 12-year-old female presents with bulky persistent cervical lymph nodes, despite a 2-week course of antibiotics. FNA is suspicious for lymphoma. What is the next best step in management?
7. What are the three stages of skin graft healing?
8. What are Kanavel's signs and what are they used for?
9. How soon should you explore and repair a sharp facial/hand nerve injury?
10. What is the appropriate management for an obstructing ureteral stone with urinary tract infection or sepsis?
11. What is the appropriate management for Fournier's gangrene?
12. What is the recommended age range for PSA screening in men at average risk for prostate cancer?

REFERENCES

1. American College of Obstetricians and Gynecologists' Committee on Practice Bulletins—Gynecology. ACOG practice bulletin No. 193: tubal ectopic pregnancy. *Obstet Gynecol.* 2018;131(3):e91-e103.
2. ACOG Committee Opinion No. 775: nonobstetric surgery during pregnancy. *Obstet Gynecol.* 2019;133(4):e285-e286.
3. Vasco Ramirez M, Valencia GCM. Anesthesia for nonobstetric surgery in pregnancy. *Clin Obstet Gynecol.* 2020;63(2):351-363.
4. Pearl JP, Price RR, Tonkin AE, Richardson WS, Stefanidis D. SAGES guidelines for the use of laparoscopy during pregnancy. *Surg Endosc.* 2017;31(10):3767-3782.
5. Siegel RL, Miller KD, Fuchs HE, Jemal A. Cancer statistics, 2022. *CA Cancer J Clin.* 2022;72(1):7-33.
6. Olawaiye AB, Cuello MA, Rogers LJ. Cancer of the vulva: 2021 update. *Int J Gynaecol Obstet.* 2021;155(suppl 1):7-18.
7. Olawaiye AB, Mutch DG, Bhosale P, et al. *AJCC Cancer Staging System: Cervix Uteri.* 9th ed. American College of Surgeons; 2020.
8. Cohen PA, Jhingran A, Oaknin A, Denny L. Cervical cancer. *Lancet.* 2019;393(10167):169-182.
9. Amin MB, ed. *AJCC Cancer Staging Manual.* 8th ed. Springer; 2017.
10. Goff BA, Matthews B, Andrilla CH, et al. How are symptoms of ovarian cancer managed? A study of primary care physicians. *Cancer.* 2011;117(19):4414-4423.
11. Kim DH, Kim SW, Hwang SH. Application of the laboratory risk indicator for necrotizing fasciitis score to the head and neck: a systematic review and meta-analysis. *ANZ J Surg.* 2022;92(7-8):1631-1637.
12. Bernier J, Domenge C, Ozsahin M, et al. Postoperative irradiation with or without concomitant chemotherapy for locally advanced head and neck cancer. *N Engl J Med.* 2004;350(19):1945-1952.

13. de la Fuente SG, Levin LS, Reynolds JD, et al. Elective stoma construction improves outcomes in medically intractable pressure ulcers. *Dis Colon Rectum*. 2003;46(11):1525-1530.
14. Silverman SG, Pedrosa I, Ellis JH, et al. Bosniak classification of cystic renal masses, version 2019: an update proposal and needs assessment. *Radiology*. 2019;292(2):475-488.
15. Lane BR, Samplaski MK, Herts BR, Zhou M, Novick AC, Campbell SC. Renal mass biopsy: a renaissance? *J Urol*. 2008;179(1):20-27.
16. Wallis CJD, Klaassen Z, Bhindi B, et al. First-line systemic therapy for metastatic renal cell carcinoma: a systematic review and network meta-analysis. *Eur Urol*. 2018;74(3):309-321.
17. Mejean A, Ravaud A, Thezenas S, et al. Sunitinib alone or after nephrectomy in metastatic renal-cell carcinoma. *N Engl J Med*. 2018;379(5):417-427.
18. Daudon M, Estépa L, Viard JP, Joly D, Jungers P. Urinary stones in HIV-1-positive patients treated with indinavir. *Lancet*. 1997;349(9061):1294-1295.
19. Preminger GM, Tiselius HG, Assimos DG, et al. 2007 guideline for the management of ureteral calculi. *J Urol*. 2007;52(6):1610-1631.
20. Chang SS, Boorjian SA, Chou R, et al. Diagnosis and treatment of non-muscle invasive bladder cancer: AUA/SUO guideline. *J Urol*. 2016;196(4):1021-1029.
21. Seisen T, Sun M, Lipsitz SR, et al. Comparative effectiveness of trimodal therapy versus radical cystectomy for localized muscle-invasive urothelial carcinoma of the bladder. *Eur Urol*. 2017;72(4):483-487.
22. Andriole GL, Crawford ED, Grubb RL III, et al. Mortality results from a randomized prostate-cancer screening trial. *N Engl J Med*. 2009;360(13):1310-1319.
23. Schroder FH, Hugosson J, Roobol MJ, et al. Screening and prostate-cancer mortality in a randomized European study. *N Engl J Med*. 2009;360(13):1320-1328.
24. Carter HB, Albertsen PC, Barry MJ, et al. Early detection of prostate cancer: AUA Guideline. *J Urol*. 2013;190(2):419-426.
25. Kasivisvanathan V, Rannikko AS, Borghi M, et al. MRI-targeted or standard biopsy for prostate-cancer diagnosis. *N Engl J Med*. 2018;378(19):1767-1777.
26. Lerner LB, McVary KT, Barry MJ, et al. Management of lower urinary tract symptoms attributed to benign prostatic hyperplasia: AUA GUIDELINE PART I-initial work-up and medical management. *J Urol*. 2021;206(4):806-817.
27. Buckley JC, McAninch JW. Use of ultrasonography for the diagnosis of testicular injuries in blunt scrotal trauma. *J Urol*. 2006;175(1):175-178.

41 Biostatistics and Study Design

Sydney C. Beache and Graham A. Colditz

I. INTRODUCTION

Evidence-based medicine aims to use information from the existing and ever-expanding body of published research to inform clinical practice. Whether contributing to the literature via the conduct and publication of original research, critically evaluating existing data to incorporate changes into day-to-day healthcare delivery, or evaluating practice patterns to improve patient outcomes at a systems level, a basic knowledge of biostatistics is essential for the general surgeon.

II. STUDY DESIGN

Study design can be stratified into three categories based on the aims of inquiry: **observational, descriptive, and experimental** (**Figure 41.1**).

A. Observational studies

1. Participants are not assigned to treatment or control groups, instead inferences are made by surveillance of a group of participants.
2. Observational studies **determine associations** between exposures and outcomes but **cannot establish causation**.
3. **Case–control study**
   - a. Study design where **participants are selected based on the presence or absence of the outcome of interest** to determine the relationship of exposure to outcome (i.e., a group of individuals with the disease [cases] are compared with a group of individuals without the disease [controls]).
     - i. For example, a group of women with breast cancer are compared with a group of women without breast cancer and their rates of exposure to second hand smoke are compared.
   - b. Evaluation of exposures in both cases and controls is conducted to determine systematic differences between groups, and selected controls should be similar to cases except for presence of disease and should originate from a similar population.
   - c. Can be a quick and relatively inexpensive first step in evaluating the association of an exposure with a disease.
   - d. Useful for investigation of rare diseases or diseases with long induction periods.
   - e. Can also be used to sample cases and controls from a larger randomized trial or cohort study in which biomarkers or other laboratory measures are being considered for additional analysis (**Figure 41.2**).

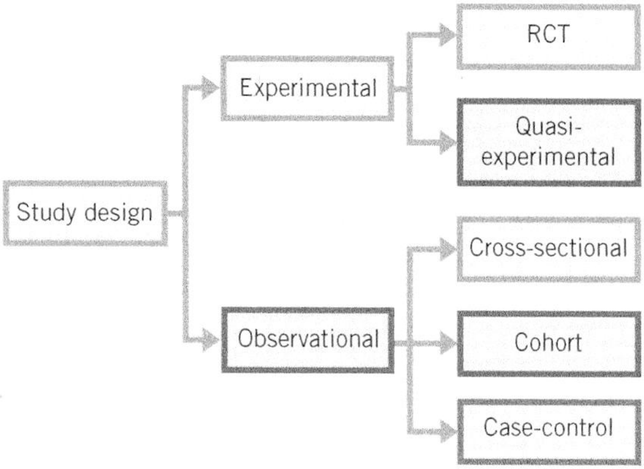

FIGURE 41.1 Summary of study designs.

4. **Cohort study**
   a. Can be retrospective or prospective (**Figure 41.3**) studies in which **individuals are divided into groups based on exposure** and followed over time to document incidence of disease or the development of the outcome of interest.
      i. For example, a group of individuals receives a new type of vaccine to prevent flu infection and is compared with a group of individuals who did not receive the vaccine, and both groups are monitored for incidence of flu infection.
   b. Individuals in the unexposed group should be similar to those in the exposed group in all manners except exposure status, and thus cohort studies require that the study population be followed for a period of time in order to evaluate whether the outcome has developed.
   c. Cohort studies are limited by several factors:
      i. **The age effect:** Differential risk in disease occurrence associated with aging
      ii. **The cohort effect:** Group-level variations in health status associated with a common societal or environmental exposure among individuals born during a certain period

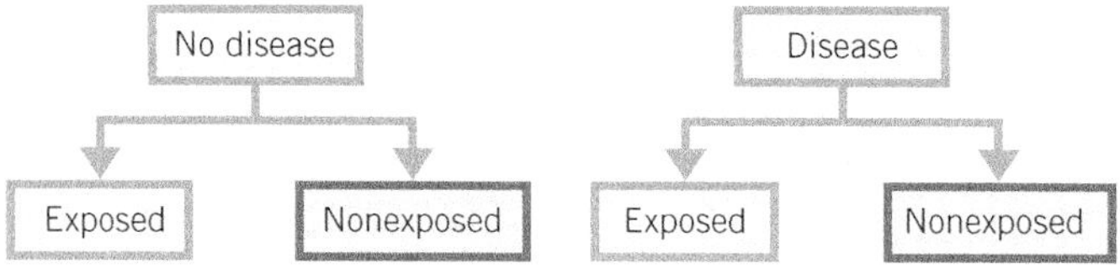

FIGURE 41.2 Design of a case–control study.

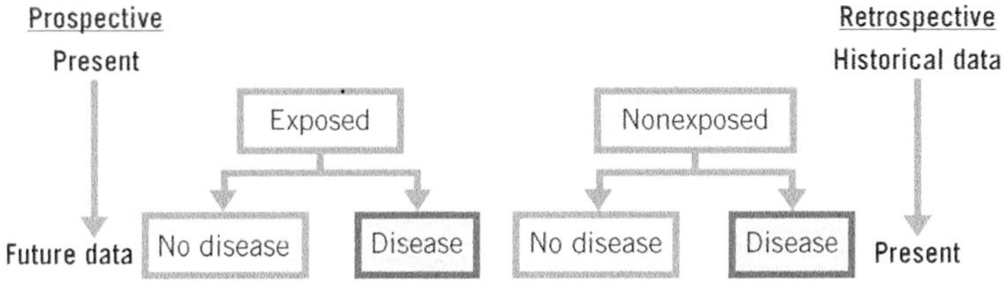

FIGURE 41.3 Design of prospective and retrospective cohort studies.

iii. **The period effect:** Group-level changes in health outcomes because of an event that affects all individuals in a particular period (e.g., breast cancer incidence increasing with the advent of screening mammography).

d. In a **prospective cohort design**, the study population is identified at the outset of the study, data are collected, and participants are followed for a sufficient time for the outcome of interest to develop in a portion of the population.

i. This study design is useful for investigating the effects of **rare exposures**; however, it is not ideal for projects studying rare outcomes, as a large number of patients must be enrolled and followed for a prolonged period of time for the specified outcome to occur.

e. In a **retrospective cohort design**, historical data are assembled and used to compare an outcome of interest in exposed and nonexposed individuals.

i. This methodology allows for quicker completion of studies but is limited by the post hoc definition of exposure and by having to rely on the quality of the historical record.

B. Descriptive studies

1. Helpful for **hypothesis-generating** purposes but are limited due to lack of a comparison group and cannot generate statistical associations.

2. **Cross-sectional study**

a. Provides information from a single period of observation when **exposure and outcomes are measured simultaneously** in a defined study population.

i. For example, the entire population of patients who receive care at a clinic are surveyed to determine their current activity levels and the rates of hypertension.

b. Low cost, and a large volume of information can be obtained quickly.

c. Useful for describing populations, identifying risk factors, quantifying the magnitude of health problems, and generating hypotheses about exposures and disease outcomes.

d. **Ecological study:** Compare the relationship between exposure and outcome at the population level, where the unit of analysis is a group with a shared characteristic (e.g., socioeconomic status, geography, ethnicity).

e. **Case report/case series:** Describes the experience of a patient (report) or small group of patients (series) and documents the natural course of a disease, associated treatment, and outcome.
   i. Typically used to document rare disease processes.
   ii. Including all cases in a defined period is necessary to reduce bias given the small sample size.

C. Experimental studies

1. Properly crafted, experimental studies **can establish a causal relationship** between exposure and outcome by assigning participants to treatment and nontreatment groups and observing a specified effect.
2. **Randomized controlled trial (RCT)**
   a. Patients are randomly assigned to intervention and control groups or "arms." Considered the **gold standard** for clinical research in that causality can be determined via an appropriately designed RCT.
      i. **Randomization** is a key element in this study design as this facilitates unbiased distribution to the study arms of both known/measured and unknown/unmeasured participant covariates that may bias an observer's interpretation of the relationship between the intervention being studied and the outcome to be observed.
      ii. **Blinding** is the concealment of participant allocation to treatment and control groups and can be utilized by researchers with respect to investigators and participants.
         a) From the trial participant perspective, blinding means participants do not know if they are in the treatment or control group.
         b) Investigators can also be blinded so they are not aware of patient assignment.
         c) When neither investigators nor participants are informed of participants' allocation status, an experiment is considered **double blinded**.
      iii. For example, patients with metastatic melanoma are randomized to receive standard chemotherapy or to receive standard chemotherapy with the addition of a new immunotherapeutic, but neither the patients nor the researchers know who is receiving the new drug, and all patients are monitored for disease progression and overall survival.
   b. **Pragmatic trial**
      i. Designed for the primary purpose of performing **comparative effectiveness research** between interventions as they are experienced in the "real world."
      ii. Developed in response to the fact that RCTs may be limited in their generalizability and face challenges in recruiting a diverse, representative population due to strict inclusion/exclusion criteria and testing under artificial conditions.
      iii. According to one commonly cited definition by Califf and Sugarman,[1] pragmatic trials share three common traits:

a) The intention to inform decision makers from multiple backgrounds (patients, clinicians, policy makers) rather than characterize a biologic or social mechanism
b) Enrollment of patients who are representative of the populations and settings for whom the study in question is relevant
c) Streamlined study procedures and data collection to increase the chances of performing an adequately powered study that can inform clinical/policy decisions or measure an expansive range of outcomes

iv. Pragmatic clinical trials have several advantages:
a) Maximize external validity and generalizability.
b) Generally easier to obtain sufficient power due to less restrictive inclusion criteria.

v. However, given these characteristics, analysis may be more complicated due to influence of more **confounding factors** compared with RCTs.

vi. Agencies tasked with promoting patient-centered comparative effectiveness research, including the National Institutes of Health and the Patient-Centered Outcomes Research Institute, have given increased attention and funding to pragmatic trials.

vii. Designed in 2013, **Pragmatic Explanatory Continuum Indicator Summary** (PRECIS-2) is a tool that evaluates pragmatic trials in nine domains (eligibility criteria, recruitment, setting, organization, flexibility delivery, flexibility adherence, follow-up, primary outcome, primary analysis) to determine whether a study design replicates ideal conditions (explanatory) or real-world conditions (pragmatic).[2]

D. Systematic reviews and meta-analysis (SRMA)

1. Methods to critically appraise the published literature and develop a consensus on a particular clinical question, the two terms are often used interchangeably, but they are distinct entities.
2. A **systematic review** is a literature review conducted by establishing a clear clinical question, completing an exhaustive search of published data, identifying relevant studies, and analyzing the data to draw more reliable conclusions that minimize bias.
   a. Analysis is largely qualitative but may have quantitative components.
   b. A **Cochrane review** is a type of systematic review conducted in a systematic way according to a specific published method (https://www.cochranelibrary.com/).
3. A **scoping review** is a literature review aimed at identifying the scope of the current literature on a particular topic and determining knowledge gaps.
   a. Scoping reviews do not aim to produce an answer to a specific question, and thus assessments of methodological limitations or risk of bias are not performed.
4. A **meta-analysis** is a quantitative statistical analysis of results synthesized from a literature search of published data.

a. If individual patient data are abstracted from these results, they can be analyzed in a pooled analysis that summarizes the effect of a therapy or intervention.
b. This analysis reduces heterogeneity among studies by using a more uniform classification of participant covariates.
5. The **Preferred Reporting Items for Systematic Reviews and Meta-Analyses** (PRISMA) is a checklist used to guide reporting in SRMAs to ensure quality and reproducibility of methodology and results.[3]

III. DATA SOURCES

A. When designing a study, appropriate selection of a data source entails selecting a population relevant to your research question.
B. Databases can help researchers answer clinical questions in a cost-conscious manner that minimizes risk or ethical concerns to the cohort under study.
C. Population health data sources
1. The **Healthcare Cost and Utilization Project** (HCUP) collects data from insurance claims to provide insight into health outcomes, healthcare utilization, quality, and cost for adults and children in the ambulatory, emergency, and inpatient settings (HCUP Overview. Healthcare Cost and Utilization Project (HCUP). February 2022. Agency for Healthcare Research and Quality, Rockville, MD [https://www.hcup-us.ahrq.gov]).
2. National health surveys sponsored by the Centers for Disease Control and Prevention (e.g., The Behavioral Risk Factor Surveillance System [https://www.cdc.gov/brfss/index.html], National Health Interview Survey [https://www.cdc.gov/nchs/nhis/index.htm], National Health and Nutrition Examination Survey [https://www.cdc.gov/nchs/nhanes/index.htm]) represent additional sources of longitudinal data on the health status of adults and children in the US.
D. Surgical outcomes data sources
1. There are specialized databases that use hospital data to monitor outcomes for surgical patients (e.g., American College of Surgeons National Surgical Quality Improvement Program [https://www.facs.org/quality-programs/data-and-registries/acs-nsqip/]) and oncology patients (e.g., National Cancer Database [https://www.facs.org/quality-programs/cancer-programs/national-cancer-database/] and Surveillance, Epidemiology, and End Results Program [https://seer.cancer.gov/]).
2. These databases are advantageous given large sample sizes and diverse cohorts that allow for high-quality analyses, but they are limited by lack of clinical context.

IV. DATA ANALYSIS

A. Basic statistical principles
1. **The null hypothesis (H_0)** is the premise that there is *no* difference between control and treatment groups.
2. **The alternative hypothesis (H_a)** is the premise that there *is* a difference between the control and treatment groups.

3. A ***P*-value (*P*)** is defined as the probability of obtaining a study's results, or more extreme results, if H_0 is true.
   a. A large (high) *P*-value means there is a high probability the data are compatible with the null hypothesis, and therefore H_0 is not rejected.
   b. A small (low) *P*-value indicates the data are not compatible with the null hypothesis, and therefore there is sufficient evidence to reject H_0.
   c. In the typical clinical study, authors refer to a finding as statistically significant when $P < .05$.
4. A **confidence interval (CI)** is a measure of uncertainty in how sample data estimate a population parameter, expressed as a lower limit (A) and an upper limit (B) bounded by parentheses (A,B).
   a. When the *P*-value is set at 0.05, the CI is 95%, indicating that, if a study were repeated, there is 95% confidence that the population parameter would fall between sample estimates of A and B.

B. Measures of effect
1. **Prevalence** is the proportion of individuals in each population with a specific disease process or risk factor at a particular point in time.
2. **Incidence** is the number of new cases developing in a population over a discrete period of time.
3. Absolute measures
   a. **Absolute risk (AR):** The number of events (people with disease) divided by the number of event-free people in that group.
      i. AR is a measure of **cumulative incidence.**
      ii. Absolute risk, exposed (AR_e): The AR in a group that is exposed to a risk factor
      iii. Absolute risk, nonexposed (AR_0): The AR in a group that is not exposed to a risk factor
   b. **Absolute risk reduction (ARR).** $AR_e - AR_0$. The excess risk (or disease burden) associated with exposure to a risk factor, also known as the **risk difference.**
   c. **Number needed to treat/number needed to harm (NNT/NNH)** is calculated as 1/ARR, and this represents the number of people who would need to receive a particular treatment for one person to benefit (NNT) or be harmed (NNH) by that treatment.
   d. **Relative risk (RR)** is a **measure of association for cohort studies** and is calculated by evaluating the incidence of a disease in those who were exposed to a certain risk factor and comparing it with the incidence of that disease in those who were not exposed.
      i. **Interpreting RR**
         a) If RR = 1, the risk of developing the outcome is the same for individuals with and without the risk factor (i.e., exposed and unexposed individuals have the same outcome).
         b) If RR > 1, the risk of developing the outcome is greater among the exposed individuals.
         c) If RR < 1, the risk of developing the outcome is less in the exposed group.

e. **Odds ratio (OR)** is a **measure of association for case–control studies** and is calculated by comparing odds of an event (disease) in people with exposure to a risk factor with the odds of the event-free group (no disease) in people with this same exposure.
   i. This is comparable with a **hazard ratio (HR)** in a survival analysis.
   ii. In general, it is inappropriate to use ORs interchangeably with RRs; however, in cases where the disease is very rare, an OR can approximate the RR.
   iii. **Interpreting OR**
      a) If OR = 1, there is no difference in the odds of developing an outcome between the exposed and unexposed individuals.
      b) If OR > 1, there are greater odds of developing the outcome among exposed individuals.
      c) If OR < 1, there are lower odds of developing the outcome among the exposed individuals.

f. **Using contingency tables (2 × 2 tables) to calculate RR, OR, and ARR**
   i. A contingency table organizes data according to outcome and exposure status (**Table 41.1**).
   ii. Calculating RR
      a) RR = Incidence among exposed group/Incidence among nonexposed group
   iii. Calculating OR
      a) OR = Odds a case was exposed/Odds a control was exposed
   iv. Calculating ARR
      a) ARR = incidence among unexposed – incidence among exposed

$$RR = \frac{\frac{a}{(a+b)}}{\frac{c}{(c+d)}}$$

$$OR = \frac{a/b}{c/d} = \frac{ad}{cb}$$

$$ARR = \frac{c}{c+d} - \frac{a}{a+b}$$

TABLE 41.1 Sample 2 × 2 Table

	Outcome (Disease)	No Outcome (No Disease)
Exposed	A	B
Unexposed	C	D

C. Evaluating screening and diagnostic tests
   1. Sensitivity and specificity evaluate the accuracy of a screening or diagnostic tool from the perspective of the disease status.
   2. The predictive value of a tool describes its performance from the perspective of the test result (**Table 41.2**).
   3. **Sensitivity (true-positive rate)** is the ability of a test to correctly identify those with disease, the probability of having a positive test result provided that the disease is present.
      a. A high sensitivity means there will be a low "false-negative" rate.
   4. **Specificity (true-negative rate)** is the ability of a test to correctly identify individuals without disease, the probability of having a negative test result if the disease is not present.
      a. A high specificity means there will be a low "false-positive" rate.
   5. **Positive predictive value (PPV)** is the proportion of true-positive results among all positive test results, the probability of having the disease given a positive test result.
   6. **Negative predictive value (NPV)** is the proportion of true-negative results among all negative results, the probability of being disease-free given a negative test result.
   7. The predictive value of a test is related to the prevalence of a disease: As disease prevalence decreases, the PPV decreases and the NPV increases.
   8. Sensitivity and specificity are not affected by disease prevalence.

D. Commonly used statistical tests and analytic approaches
   1. **Statistical tests for continuous response variables**
      a. **T-tests** allow for comparison of a continuous, normally distributed response variable between two groups.
         i. An **unpaired t-test** compares two independent groups (e.g., compare hospital lengths of stay after laparoscopic vs open colectomy).
         ii. A **paired t-test** allows for comparison of variables, usually for the same subject before and after an intervention (e.g., compare the effect of an educational program on weight loss in patients undergoing bariatric surgery by measuring their weights before and after the intervention).

TABLE 41.2 Calculating Sensitivity, Specificity, PPV, and NPV Using a 2 × 2 Table

	Disease Present	Disease Absent	
Positive test	True positive (A)	False positive (B)	PPV = A/(A + B)
Negative test	False negative (C)	True negative (D)	NPV = D/(C + D)
	Sensitivity = A/(A + C)	Specificity = D/(B + D)	

NPV, negative predictive value; PPV, positive predictive value.

b. **Analysis of variance (ANOVA)** allows for comparison of continuous, normally distributed continuous variables of interest between more than two groups (e.g., compare hospital lengths of stay after laparoscopic vs open vs robotic colectomy).
c. **Linear regression** can be used to measure the relationship between one or more continuous predictor variables on a continuous response variable (e.g., evaluate body mass index and age's effects on weight loss in patients undergoing bariatric surgery).

2. **Statistical tests for categorical response variables**
   a. **Chi-square statistic** is used to compare categorical response variables across two groups from a contingency table that can be constructed based on frequencies of these variables, used to assess observed vs expected results in a large sample size (e.g., compare frequencies of operative management vs observation for small bowel obstruction in patients with malignancy compared with patients obstructed from nonmalignant causes).
      i. When there are small frequencies within the contingency table (i.e., small sample size), the **Fisher's exact test** may be a more appropriate test of association.
   b. **Logistic regression** can be used to measure the probability of a categorical response variable given one or more predictor variables (e.g., examine the effects of operative time and total bilirubin on major postoperative bleeding following hepatectomy).
3. **Statistical tests for time-to-event data**
   a. **The Kaplan–Meier (K-M)** method is a log-rank test used for survival analysis that compares differences in times-to-event between groups (e.g., evaluate the effect of imatinib [a tyrosine kinase inhibitor] on survival of unresectable and metastatic gastrointestinal stromal tumors).
      i. "Time-to-event" is the duration of time between entry into a study or diagnosis of disease and a specified endpoint.
      ii. Endpoints can include death, disease recurrence, or when patients are censored (i.e., the time-to-event is unknown either because the patient is lost to follow-up or the study ends before the patient experiences the event).
   b. **Cox proportional hazards regression** allows for the comparison of the effect of one or more covariates on survival in a given population (i.e., multivariable analysis, in contrast to K-M plots that are not controlled for multiple covariates), and it assumes the relationships between the covariates and the effects of the covariates upon survival do not vary over time.

V. ASSESSING STUDY QUALITY

A. Internal validity
1. A **type I error** (α) is also known as a "false positive."
   a. Occurs when the null hypothesis (H_0) is true but is incorrectly rejected.

b. Type I error is closely related to the *P*-value: The lower the *P*-value the lower the likelihood of a type I error to occur.

2. A **type II error** (β) is known as a "false negative."
   a. Occurs when the H_0 is false but is incorrectly accepted.
   b. In other words, a difference between the experimental and control groups is not detected, even though the difference actually exists.
3. **Power** is defined as the probability of rejecting a H_0 that is false (i.e., it is the ability of a statistical test to correctly detect a difference between the experimental and control groups).
   a. Power is closely related to sample size and the magnitude of the effect being studied.
   b. Researchers typically deem power of 80% or greater as acceptable.
   c. Power is expressed as $1 - \beta$ (i.e., correctly rejecting H_0) (**Table 41.3**).
4. **Bias** is the existence of a spurious difference between groups that affects the observed causal relationship between exposure and outcome.
   a. **Internal validity** may be compromised by biases that arise due to errors in study design.
   b. **Selection bias** occurs when there are systematic differences in participants' and nonparticipants' covariates or when the selected study population is not representative of the general population.
      i. **The "Healthy Worker" effect** is a type of selection bias that occurs within the context of cohort studies (e.g., if workers from an occupational cohort are chosen and their death rates are compared with those of the general population, the occupational cohort represents a population that is healthy enough to work and, thus, are not representative of the general population).
   c. **Measurement or misclassification bias** occurs when there is an error in how the exposure status of participants or the recording of outcomes is coded; this type of error may be introduced through variation in laboratory assays or recall of exposure in epidemiologic studies, for example.
      i. This type of bias is called **nondifferential** if it affects both comparison groups and **differential** if it only affects one comparison group.

TABLE 41.3 Assessing Internal Validity: Power and Error

		Null Hypothesis	
		True	False
Decision	Accept	Correct decision $1-\alpha$	Type II error (β)
	Reject	Type I error (α)	Correct decision Power = $1-\beta$

d. **Immortal time** bias refers to a period of time during the study in which an outcome cannot or should not be able to occur, therefore leading to bias in evaluating outcomes (e.g., a measured event occurs after a patient is entered in a trial but before they receive the intervention being studied).
e. **Recall bias** is an error that results from the incomplete or inaccurate recall of past events by participants in a way that is systematically different between participants in different arms of a study.
f. **Interviewer bias** occurs when interviewers are not blinded to exposure or disease status and structure questions in a way that is influenced by the participant's status.
g. **Hawthorne effect** describes participants' tendency to alter their behavior because they are aware of being observed.
h. **Lead-time bias** describes an apparent increase in survival due to differential (earlier) dates of diagnosis.
i. **Will Rogers phenomenon** references a satirical quotation from comedian Will Rogers in the 1930s describing US migration during the Great Depression. This phenomenon describes an event that leads to stage migration, which leads to apparent increases in survival, for example.
j. **External validity** refers to the ability to generalize the results of a study to the greater population.
   i. To improve the external validity, the study population must be similar to the reference population from which the study population was extracted.
   ii. More extensive reporting of patient selection processes, study participants' demographic information, and providers' professional and personal characteristics assist with the extrapolation of study conclusions to other clinical settings and patient populations.
k. **Confounding variables**
   i. Data are often subject to confounding variables (i.e., extraneous factor that is associated with both the predictor and the response variable) that affect our ability to determine associations between predictor and response variables.
   ii. There are several methods available to control for confounding variables, including stratification, matching, propensity scores, and use of multivariable regression models.

VI. CLINICAL PRACTICE GUIDELINES

With the wealth of published data, evaluating the integrity of research findings and determining best practices to implement can be challenging for the clinician.

A. Researchers have developed a hierarchical grading system to assess the quality of data and clinical recommendations, and while there are many published grading systems, the US Preventive Services Task Force has developed one of the most widely accepted systems (see **Tables 41.4** and **41.5**).

TABLE 41.4 USPSTF Quality of Data Classification

Level of Evidence	Source of Evidence
I	Evidence from systematic review of randomized controlled trials
IIa	Evidence from controlled trials without randomization
IIb	Evidence from cohort or case–control studies
IIc	Evidence from multiple time series or historic controls
III	Expert opinion based on clinical experience

USPSTF, US Preventive Services Task Force.

TABLE 41.5 USPSTF Clinical Practice Recommendations

Grade of Evidence	Recommendations for Practice
A	High certainty that the net benefit is substantial. Offer or provide this service.
B	High certainty that the net benefit is moderate to substantial. Offer or provide this service.
C	Moderate certainty that the net benefit is small. Provide this service based on individual patient preference and professional judgment.
D	Moderate to high certainty that this service has no benefit or the harms outweigh the benefit. Discourage use of this service.
I	Insufficient evidence to assess benefits and harms of service.

USPSTF, US Preventive Services Task Force.

These systems for synthesis of evidence have now been more formally accepted by many professional societies. The Institute of Medicine has published a set of guiding principles addressing the methods for developing these types of practice guidelines in order to bring a more consistent approach to their development across the overlapping sectors in healthcare delivery.

Key References

Citation	Summary
Mahmood SS, Levy D, Vasan RS, Wang TJ. The Framingham Heart Study and the epidemiology of cardiovascular disease: a historical perspective. *Lancet.* 2014;383(9921):999-1008.	• Established in 1948, The Framingham Heart Study is a renowned cohort study that aimed to determine risk factors for cardiovascular disease among a cohort of men and women in Framingham, Massachusetts.
Doll R, Hill AB. Smoking and carcinoma of the lung; preliminary report. *Br Med J.* 1950;2(4682):739-748.	• This classic case–control study published by Richard Doll and Bradford Hill in 1950 uncovered an association between smoking and lung cancer.
Colditz, G., Hankinson, S. The Nurses' Health Study: lifestyle and health among women. *Nat Rev Cancer.* 2005;5:388-396.	• The Nurses' Health Study was the first large cohort study of women examining exposures associated with cancer and other chronic conditions.

CHAPTER 41: BIOSTATISTICS AND STUDY DESIGN

Review Questions

1. What statistical analytic method would be most appropriate to retrospectively investigate the impact of sodium bicarbonate preprocedural hydration versus placebo on the rates of contrast-induced nephropathy?
2. What statistical analytic method would be most appropriate to investigate the role of alvimopan, a peripherally acting μ-opioid antagonist, on the number of days until return of bowel function following open colectomy?
3. As the prevalence of a disease increases, what happens to the:
   a. **Positive predictive value?**
   b. **Negative predictive value?**
   c. **Sensitivity?**
   d. **Specificity?**
4. Statins, or hydroxymethyl glutaryl coenzyme A reductase inhibitors, are commonly prescribed medications that confer powerful preventive benefits against cardiovascular disease. Consider a hypothetical cohort study of 3,000 patients investigating the effect of atorvastatin therapy on developing a cerebrovascular accident (CVA): in this study, 1,000 individuals were treated with atorvastatin therapy and 2,000 individuals did not receive therapy. This cohort was followed for 15 years. At the study endpoint, 100 individuals in the atorvastatin cohort developed a CVA. One-fourth of patients who did not receive statin therapy developed a CVA.

a. **Create a 2x2 contingency table describing the study outcome.**

	CVA	No CVA
Atorvastatin therapy		
No atorvastatin therapy		

b. **What is the relative risk of CVA in the atorvastatin group vs. no therapy group?**
c. **What is the absolute risk reduction of CVA associated with atorvastatin therapy?**
d. **How many people would need to receive atorvastatin therapy for one person to benefit from its CVA protective effects?**

REFERENCES

1. Califf RM, Sugarman J. Exploring the ethical and regulatory issues in pragmatic clinical trials. *Clin Trials*. 2015;12(5):436-441.
2. Loudon K, Treweek S, Sullivan F, Donnan P, Thorpe KE, Zwarenstein M. The PRECIS-2 tool: designing trials that are fit for purpose. *BMJ*. 2015;350:h2147.
3. Page MJ, McKenzie JE, Bossuyt PM, et al. The PRISMA 2020 statement: an updated guideline for reporting systematic reviews. *BMJ*. 2021;372:n71.

42 Patient Safety and Quality Improvement

Britta J. Han and Shaina Eckhouse

I. PATIENT SAFETY AND QUALITY IMPROVEMENT:

A. Modern era traced to two Institute of Medicine reports
   1. *To Err Is Human: Building a Safer Health System* (safety).[1]
   2. *Crossing the Quality Chasm: A New Health System for the 21st Century* (quality improvement).[2]

B. Definitions
   1. **Patient safety (PS):** The focus on increasing freedom from accidental injury in health care by "designing safety into the system" to reduce preventable harm and by shifting blame away from the individual.
   2. **Quality improvement (QI):** The focus on developing safe, effective, and patient-centered heath care delivery systems by tracking quality measures.

C. Why does patient safety and quality improvement (PSQI) matter?
   1. Estimated 180,000 to 195,000 annual deaths due to medical error in Medicare beneficiaries alone; extrapolating to all US hospital admissions translates to 400,000 deaths per year.[3]
   2. Economic impact and cost of preventable medical errors estimated as high as $1 trillion and $980 billion, respectively.[4-7]

II. PATIENT SAFETY

A. Key vocabulary
   1. **Safety:** Freedom from accidental injury
   2. **Error:** Failure to complete an action or meet an aim[8]
      a. **Error of execution:** Failure of a planned action to be completed as intended
      b. **Error of planning:** Failure to use the correct plan to achieve an aim or goal
      c. **Error of commission:** Doing the wrong thing
      d. **Error of omission:** Not doing the right thing; difficult to detect, but may be more common than error of commission
   3. **Adverse event (AE):** An injury resulting from a medical intervention, specifically not due to the underlying condition of the patient.
   4. **Near miss:** An error that is caught before an AE or harm occurs.
   5. **High-reliability organization:** Organization operating in a complex, high-hazard domain for extended periods that experiences fewer accidents or failures than expected due to specific organization characteristics.

B. Strong culture of PS: Requires dynamic factors that build on the values, attitudes, perceptions, and behaviors of healthcare providers to encourage commitment to PS.[9]

1. Organizational approach
   a. "Just culture" organization
      i. Focuses on **systems approach** that acknowledges inevitability of human error, works to create systems that minimize AEs by placing barriers and safeguards.[10]
      ii. Prioritizes **human factors engineering** to design systems and environments that account for human strengths and weaknesses.
   b. **Hospital-wide mindset** promotes multidisciplinary focus on PSQI efforts and reminds all practitioners and staff to be "hospital-level," not just "department-level," team members and also empowers individuals, regardless of level, to "**stop the line**" and report behaviors or other concerns related to PS.
   c. Organizations must also support providers in addition to patients and families after an AE.
      i. **Second victim effect:** When providers involved in errors experience increased anxiety over future errors, poor sleep, reduced job satisfaction, and increased job-related stress.[11] While patients and families often receive support after an AE, healthcare providers are often neglected.
2. Consistent, systematic approach to analyzing AEs as they occur.
   a. **Swiss cheese model of accident causation (Figure 42.1):** Systems approach that views AEs to be the result of small, multiple system failures.

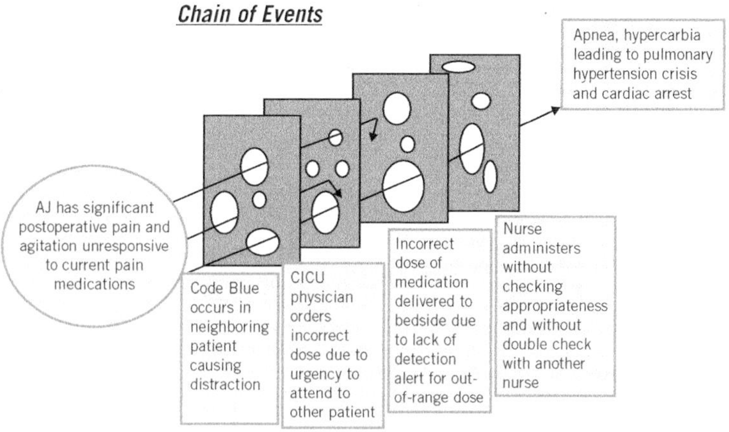

FIGURE 42.1 Accident trajectory passing through corresponding holes in layers of defenses and safeguards (Swiss cheese model). *(Reprinted with permission from Lee A, Samora J, Bartman T, Davis JT, Brilli RJ. Safety and quality in the heart center. In: Shaddy RE, Penny DJ, Feltes TF, Cetta F, Mital S, eds. Moss & Adams' Heart Disease in Infants, Children, and Adolescents Including the Fetus and Young Adult. 10th ed. Wolters Kluwer; 2022:1750-1763. Figure 78.2.)*

i. Many potential sources of error ("holes"), but the holes in a single "slice" are not sufficient for a serious error or AE due to safeguards and barriers in place.

ii. When multiple holes over many slices line up, a trajectory of "accident opportunity" is present, may result in AE.

iii. The holes comprise **active failures** and **latent conditions** (**Table 42.1**).

a) Active failures: Unsafe actions by people who are directly in contact with patients.

b) Latent conditions: Existing structures that, under the right circumstances, can lead to errors.

c) Identification of active failures and latent conditions is the first step to analyzing AEs and errors, which will ultimately determine any need to change a system(s).

b. **Root cause analyses:** Used to review AEs and near misses retrospectively and systematically.

i. Map out actions and processes that led to an identified outcome, help determine the key contributors that resulted in the outcome.

ii. Strategies are developed to address the key contributors and prevent future harm/recurrence.

iii. To visually map out the actions and processes, a **Fishbone diagram,** or **Ishikawa diagram**, is created asking "five whys" (**Figure 42.2**).

3. **Reliable, safe, and easy-to-use reporting systems** create cultural norms that promote safety, facilitate reporting and recording errors and near misses.

TABLE 42.1 Examples of Active Failures vs Latent Conditions

Active Failures Actions by Humans	Latent Conditions Inherently Systemic—"Accidents Waiting to Happen"
- Incorrectly programming infusion dosing on pump	- Multiple types of infusion pumps being provided on the hospital floor
- Ordering the wrong medication dose for a patient	- A medical chart lacking a system to notify providers when multiple patients have the same last name
- Mislabeling of specimens	- When order medications, no notifications about drug interactions are provided to the order provider
- Marking the wrong laterality for surgery	- Faulty equipment
- Failure to check whether equipment is working appropriately	- No clear systematic method for communication between team members or sign-out between team members
- Not signing out patients to team or between teams	
- Forgetting tasks related to patient care	- Lack of a standardized checklist to ensure certain tasks are completed

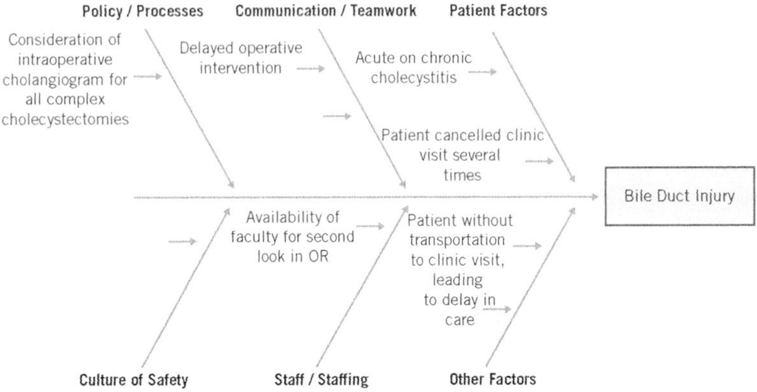

FIGURE 42.2 **Fishbone, or Ishikawa, diagram** is a method that maps out factors, actions, and processes that may have contributed to the outcome listed in the pink box, in this example a bile duct injury to discuss during Morbidity and Mortality conference. The diagram can include both factors that exacerbated the adverse outcome and factors that went well despite the outcome.

4. **Consistent and systematic methods to improve and reinforce clear communication between team members**, examples include the following:
   a. Checklists create reliable "closed-loop" written communication opportunities to increase standardization and reduce complications. Formatted checklists, such as I-PASS (Illness severity, Patient summary, Action list, Situational awareness/contingency planning, Synthesis by receiver) and SBAR (Situation, Background, Assessment, Recommendation), are established written hand-off methods.
   b. The surgical time-out is a verbal and written standardized hand-off method.
   c. Teams should eliminate unnecessary patient hand-offs and standardize timing of verbal communication.
   d. Morbidity and Mortality is a recurring conference to discuss adverse events and QI initiatives.

III. QUALITY IMPROVEMENT

A challenge to improve quality of healthcare through a drastic redesign of care coordination was proposed in *Crossing the Quality Chasm: A New Health System for the 21st Century*, highlighting six key aims in QI: **Care should be safe, effective, patient-/person-centered, timely, efficient, and equitable.**[2]

A. Identifying areas for QI
   1. Can feel daunting, but QI is a daily component of surgery (e.g., QI initiatives can be generated from morbidity and mortality conferences;

daily workflows, including intentional and unintentional, can adversely impact PS or quality of care).

2. Department and/or institutional PSQI representatives can offer guidance and access to learning more about QI through certification programs and/or PSQI committees as well as mentors involved in PSQI research.

B. Models of tracking and improving quality outcomes
 1. "Model for Improvement" (**Figure 42.3**) asks three key questions to address a problem.
  a. What are we trying to accomplish?
   i. Identify an aim to address the problem.
   ii. Effective aims must be **SMART: Specific, Measurable, Achievable, Realistic, and Time bound.**[12]
  b. How will we know that any change is an improvement?
   i. Monitoring a system change is imperative to understanding whether a SMART aim is achieving the desired result.

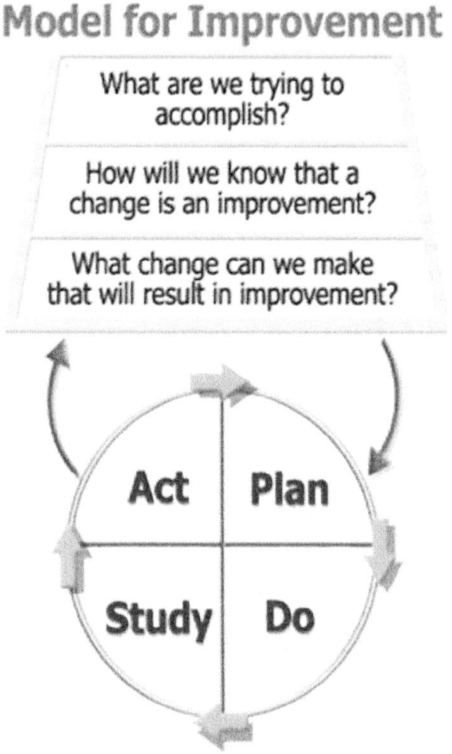

FIGURE 42.3 Model for improvement. *(Reprinted with permission from Associates in Process Improvement. Available at https://www.apiweb.org.)*

ii. Some outcomes may lead to new problems in other parts of the system, defined as a **"balancing measure."**[12] Thus, monitoring the desired outcome and balancing measure ensures the QI initiative solves the correct problem.

c. What change can we make that will result in the desired improvement?

i. Once specific, small changes are identified, the **PDSA cycle (Plan, Do, Study, Act)** can be used iteratively to track change implementation and outcomes.

ii. These small changes can subsequently be implemented on a larger scale through repeated PDSA cycles.

iii. Tracking for compliance through auditing and feedback can reinforce changes and improvements made from those changes.

2. **Lean** framework: Iterative process that focuses on creating and optimizing value and reducing nonvalue items (e.g., wasting time, resources).

a. Core principles: Defining value from the key players' perspectives (e.g., patients and staff), empowering employees (work should not be punitive), creating standard work, continuously identifying and removing waste, and creating a system that naturally maintains improvement.[13]

3. **Six Sigma** framework: Aims to improve quality by removing causes of errors and focusing on reducing the variability in the healthcare provided to patients.[14]

a. Five key elements ("DMAIC"): Define (definition of the problem), Measure (measurement of current state), Analyze (characterize the root of the problem), Improve (develop and test an intervention), Control (implement the changes).

C. Determining how to measure QI: Quality measures are defined as tools to track or quantify a health care outcome or event.

1. **Outcome measures** track how a specific practice or healthcare system impacts patient well-being.

a. Can be defined by variety of items such as 30-day mortality, 30-day readmission rates, specific postoperative complications, discharge disposition, and self-reported postoperative pain.

b. **Patient-reported outcomes** (PROs) are becoming a widely used outcome measure.

i. Some are tied to specific reimbursement incentives or penalties through the Centers for Medicare and Medicaid Services.

ii. PROs can both be tied to objective postoperative outcomes and be used to track postoperative recovery.

2. **Process measures** track how well the steps of an implemented process are being followed and how well each step is performing (e.g., time to intervention, time to complete an intervention, or percentage of individuals adhering to a protocol).

3. **Balancing measures** track unintended consequences of an implemented change and whether these consequences cause problems in another metric not being measured (e.g., whether decreased length of hospital stay results in increased readmissions or emergency room visits).

IV. VISUALIZING QI

Collecting and tracking data through quality measures that determines whether an initiative is leading to intended outcomes that can motivate/reinforce the changes made.

A. Pareto chart: A cause-analysis tool represented as a bar graph where the bars represent frequency or cost, and the graph is arranged with the tallest bar on the left and shortest on the right.
   1. Helps to visualize significant key causes, obstacles, or problems in a process being studied (e.g., determine what key factor may hinder nurses from mobilizing their patients after an operation [**Figure 42.4**]).

B. Run chart: A line graph that allows for identification of trends or patterns in a process over time.
   1. Useful tool at the beginning of a QI project because it can demonstrate key information about a preexisting process before changes are implemented.
   2. Often precedes a **control chart** (below) and can help create **control limits** to understand expected process variation.
   3. Cannot demonstrate how a process changes over time or whether the process remains stable.

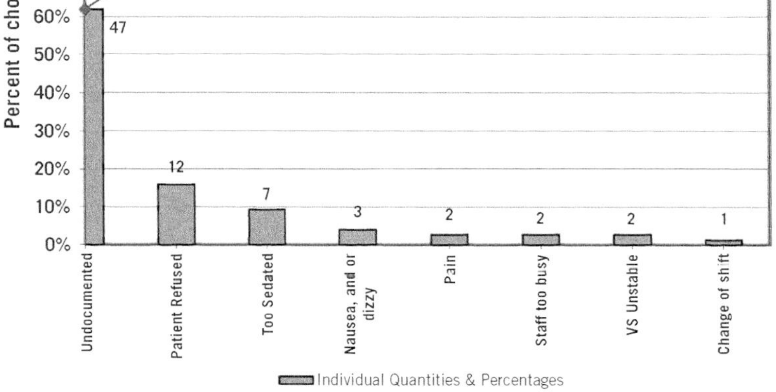

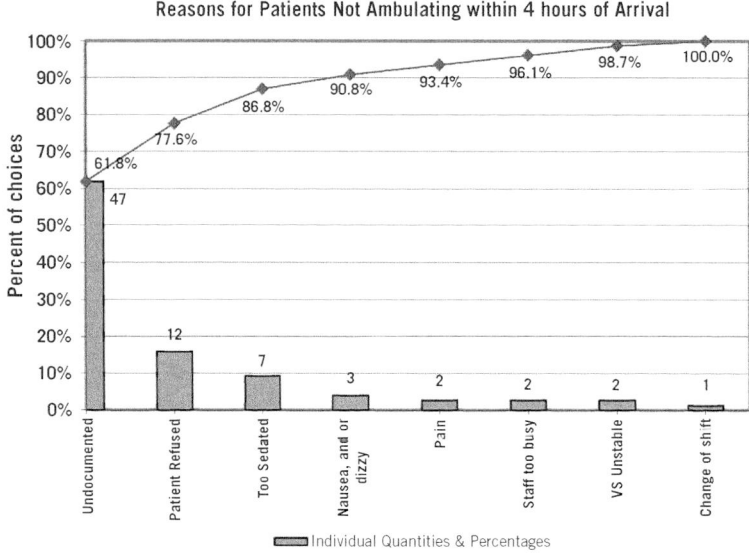

FIGURE 42.4 **Pareto chart** example of the reasons patients are not ambulating within 4 hours of arriving to the hospital ward following minimally invasive surgeries, including bariatric, foregut, and hernia surgeries, performed by Washington University surgeons at Barnes Jewish Hospital (*unpublished data*). The number of responses for a specific answer, depicted by the bar graph, is listed in descending order. The line graph represents the cumulative total. VS, vital signs.

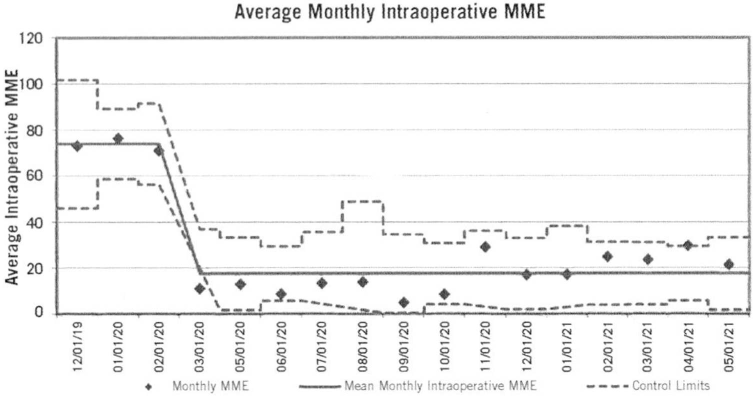

FIGURE 42.5 **Control chart** with **control limits** example demonstrates longitudinal data of average morphine milligram equivalents (MME) per month given intraoperatively to patients undergoing bariatric surgery while creating and implementing a reduced narcotic patient protocol perioperatively. The narcotic free protocol was implemented 03/2021, which is where the reduction in MMEs is noted by the change in the central line for the means (*unpublished data*).

C. Control chart: A line graph used to study how a process changes over time and whether the process is stable.
   1. Data are plotted over time with **control limits** determined from historical data (upper control limit line, lower control limit line, central line for the average).
   2. Can determine whether a process variation is consistent or unpredictable.
   3. Patterns can be analyzed when special causes (nonroutine events) or common causes occur over a period of time.
   4. As problems to a process are identified, control chart can identify how addressing problems can change a process (**Figure 42.5**).

Key References

Citation	Summary
Kohn LT, Corrigan JM, Donaldson MS (eds). *To Err Is Human: Building a Safer Health System.* National Academies Press; 2000.	• Landmark report from the Institute of Medicine highlighting nearly 98,000 people die a year due to preventable medical errors.
Institute of Medicine (US) Committee on Quality of Health Care in America. *Crossing the Quality Chasm: A New Health System for the 21st Century.* National Academies Press (US); 2001.	• An urgent call for closing the quality gap in the American healthcare system.

Citation	Summary
Mason SE, Nicolay CR, Darzi A. The use of lean and six sigma methodologies in surgery: a systematic review. *Surgeon.* 2015;13(2):91-100.	• A systematic review of the use and utility of Lean and Six Sigma methodologies in surgery.
Boysen PG. Just culture: a foundation for balanced accountability and patient safety. *Ochsner J.* 2013;13(3):400-406.	• Description of the framework of a just culture in healthcare.

CHAPTER 42: PSQI

Review Questions

1. What does *safety* mean in the context of patient safety and quality improvement?
2. What are the six key aims of quality improvement in the context of patient safety and quality improvement?
3. What is an *adverse event?*
4. What is a *near miss?*
5. What is the definition of a *just culture?*
6. What is the difference between *error of commission* and *error of omission?*
7. What is *Root Cause Analysis (RCA)* used for in the context of patient safety and quality improvement?
8. What are the components of a SMART aim?
9. What does a *run chart* allow you to identify or monitor?

REFERENCES

1. Institute of Medicine. Committee on quality of health care in America. In: Donaldson MS, Corrigan JM, Kohn LT, eds. *To Err Is Human: Building a Safer Health System.* National Academies Press; 2000.
2. Institute of Medicine. Committee on quality of health care in America. In: Baker A, ed. *Crossing the Quality Chasm: A New Health System for the 21st Century.* vol. 323. 2001.
3. Makary MA, Daniel M. Medical error-the third leading cause of death in the US. *BMJ.* 2016;353:i2139.
4. Ottosen MJ, Sedlock EW, Aigbe AO, Bell SK, Gallagher TH, Thomas EJ. Long-term impacts faced by patients and families after harmful healthcare events. *J Patient Saf.* 2021;17(8):e1145-e1151.
5. Sokol-Hessner L, Folcarelli PH, Sands KE. Emotional harm from disrespect: the neglected preventable harm. *BMJ Qual Saf.* 2015;24(9):550-553.
6. Gandhi TK, Feeley D, Schummers D. Zero harm in health care: how a comprehensive systems-focused approach can help to prevent all types of harm in health care. *NEJM Catalyst.* 2020;1(2):20200219.
7. Andel C, Davidow SL, Hollander M, Moreno DA. The economics of health care quality and medical errors. *J Health Care Finance.* 2012;39(1):39-50.

8. Reason J. *Human Error*. Cambridge university press; 1990.
9. Pronovost PJ, Berenholtz SM, Goeschel CA, et al. Creating high reliability in health care organizations. *Health Serv Res*. 2006;41(4 pt 2):1599-1617.
10. Boysen PG. Just culture: a foundation for balanced accountability and patient safety. *Ochsner J*. 2013;13(3):400-406.
11. Waterman AD, Garbutt J, Hazel E, et al. The emotional impact of medical errors on practicing physicians in the United States and Canada. *Jt Comm J Qual Patient Saf*. 2007;33(8):467-476.
12. Doran GT. There's a SMART way to write management's goals and objectives. *Manag Rev*. 1981;70(11):35-36.
13. Ojo B, Feldman R, Rampersad S. Lean methodology in quality improvement. *Paediatr Anaesth*. 2022;32(11):1209-1215.
14. Shah NK, Emerick TD. Lean six sigma methodology and the future of quality improvement education in anesthesiology. *Anesth Analg*. 2021;133(3):811-815.

Answer Key

Chapter 1

1. "Geriatric syndromes," although these not only impact elderly patients but can also affect younger ones depending on their functional status.
2. There are a number of scales, including single-item assessments such as a timed walking test, and surveys such as the Clinical Frailty Scale, the Frail scale, the Frailty Index and the Comprehensive Geriatric Assessment. One scale or assessment has not demonstrated superiority over others in terms of their prognostic ability.
3. Pacemakers should be turned to their uninhibited mode, and bipolar cautery should be used if possible. Internal defibrillators should be turned off intraoperatively.
4. About 6 to 12 months. This should be considered when timing elective operations.
5. Ideally by postoperative day 1, unless there is an operative indication for longer use (e.g., low pelvic dissection), oliguria, and/or concern for urinary tract injury.
6. Wound and tissue flap necrosis, anastomotic leak, and surgical site infections are some of the short-term complications associated with smoking. Long-term complications related to smoking include increased risk for hernias and delayed fistula and bone healing.
7. Prehabilitation has gained popularity as a means of optimizing patients preoperatively. Typically, prehabilitation programs have mental, physical, and nutritional components, in addition to weight loss in the setting of obesity, glucose control in the setting of diabetes, smoking cessation, and correction of malnutrition, if present. The exact benefits of prehabilitation continue to be investigated.

Chapter 2

1. 4 mg/kg × 60 kg = 240 mg > 240 mg/10 mg/mL = 24 mL
2. Enteric gram-negative bacilli, anaerobes, enterococci
3. Class III/Contaminated
4. No (see "Common Intraoperative Problems")
5. Direct vessel ligation with a clip, suture, or tie (see "Hemostasis techniques")
6. Cryoprecipitate
7. 1:1:1

Chapter 3

1. Naloxone 40 µg IV with repeat dosing at 2- to 5-minute intervals until patient is responsive
2. Oral fidaxomicin
3. Necrotizing fasciitis and urgent operative debridement
4. Atelectasis; incentive spirometry, ambulation, pain control
5. Tachycardia and oliguria
6. Urgent DC cardioversion
7. 4 days
8. Bivalirudin

Chapter 4

1. Significant hypotension due to myocardial depression, vasodilation, and increased venous capacitance, respiratory depression, and bradycardia
2. Hypovolemic/hemorrhagic, distributive, obstructive, cardiogenic
3. Auscultation, return of end-tidal CO_2, and imaging with CXR
4. Wound complication from leaking, perforation, dislodgement
5. Sepsis includes life-threatening organ dysfunction
6. Conventional glucose targets (110-180 mg/dL)
7. H2 blocker

Chapter 5

1. Airway, breathing, circulation, disability, and exposure/environment
2. Hypotension, tracheal deviation to the contralateral side, decreased breath sounds, distended neck veins
3. In the midaxillary line at the level of the nipple or inframammary fold (around the 4th intercostal space)
4. Can diagnose on echocardiogram, which will show pericardial effusion and decreased cardiac function. Treat with pericardial window to evaluate for blood. If blood is detected, may need to perform median sternotomy to identify and treat cardiac injury.
5. Vital signs (heart rate, blood pressure), signs of peripheral perfusion (capillary refill, skin turgor, temperature), mental status, urine output
6. Urethral injury. Blood at the urethral meatus, unable to palpate prostate
7. Motor, verbal, and eye opening

Chapter 6

1. Arterial hemorrhage from neck/nose/mouth, cervical bruit in patient <50 years old, expanding cervical hematoma, focal neurologic defect: TIA, hemiparesis, vertebrobasilar symptoms, Horner syndrome, Neurologic deficit inconsistent with head CT, ischemic stroke on CT or MRI
2. Yes
3. Yes
4. Epidural hematoma
5. Epidural—biconvex hyperdensities that typically respect the suture lines

   Subdural—hyperdense crescents representing blood interspersed between the brain surface and dura
6. Zone 1—Median sternotomy with possible extension along sternocleidomastoid or supraclavicular incision

   Zone 2—Transverse cervical collar incision or anterior sternocleidomastoid incision

   Zone 3—Preferably endovascular, difficult to control operatively, need to dislocate mandible

Chapter 7

1. Decompression of the right chest via finger thoracostomy or needle decompression, based on proceduralist skill level
2. Patient stability, initial output >1.5 L or continued output of >200 mL/h for 4 hours
3. Salvageable postinjury cardiac arrest:

   a. Penetrating thoracic trauma and <15 minutes prehospital CPR
   b. Penetrating nonthoracic trauma and <5 minutes prehospital CPR
   c. Blun t trauma and <10 minutes prehospital CPR

   Persistent and severe postinjury hypotension (systolic blood pressure <60 mm Hg) due to:
   a. Cardiac tamponade
   b. Hemorrhage (intra-abdominal, intrathoracic, extremity, cervical)
   c. Air embolism
4. ECG with or without troponin I
5. Water-soluble (Gastrografin) contrast esophagram
6. Obstructive shock
7. Hypotension, diminished heart sounds, distended neck veins; suggestive of cardiac tamponade

Chapter 8

1. Hemodynamically stable, awake, and unimpaired patients without abdominal complaints with or without CT imaging
2. Blunt trauma patients with hypotension
3. A single dose of broad-spectrum antibiotics with both aerobic and anerobic coverage. Redosing or increasing dose if more than 10 units of blood has been transfused
4. *Streptococcus pneumoniae*, *Haemophilus influenzae*, and *Neisseria meningitidis*
5. Determining presence and location of ductal involvement
6. Long-term nasogastric decompression and parenteral nutrition with repeat imaging at 2 weeks
7. CT with intravenous contrast with delayed images
8. All central hematomas (zone I), flank hematomas that are rapidly expanding or pulsatile, central pelvic hematomas (zone III) if suspected iliac artery injury
9. Greater than 20 weeks gestation or unknown gestational age

Chapter 9

1. Intravenous antibiotics
2. Anterior, lateral, superficial posterior, deep posterior

   Medial incision—superficial and deep posterior, and lateral incision—anterior and lateral
3. Femoral shaft fractures, distal femur fractures, unstable complex fractures

Chapter 10

1. *S. aureus.* Gram-positive organisms are most commonly isolated early in hospitalization; however, gram-negative organisms become more common after hospital day 5. *Pseudomonas aeruginosa* is the most common gram-negative organism.
2. Sepsis. Factors affecting mortality include extremes of age, comorbidities, TBSA (total body surface area), and presence of inhalational injury.
3. Securing the airway. Burn patients should be assessed per ATLS guidelines.
4. With suspicion of sepsis or spreading wound infection. Prophylactic antibiotics are not recommended for burn patients and may contribute to antimicrobial resistance.

5. Cyanide and carbon monoxide toxicity. Continued O_2 therapy is the treatment of CO toxicity, although hyperbaric O_2 proves the fastest resolution. Cyanide toxicity is treated with hydroxycobalamin, the highly active form of vitamin B12. Cyanocobalamin and sodium thiosulfate are also treatment options.
6. Thirty-six percent. Note that tools to approximate TBSA are subjective with variability among providers. Resuscitation efforts based on TBSA are useful in initiation of resuscitation; however, ongoing fluid requirements are based on clinical parameters (e.g., urine output, blood pressure).
7. Superficial partial thickness. Burn injury may manifest with varying depths even within bordered segments.

Chapter 11

1. Never; maximum strength achieved is 80% of uninjured tissue.
2. Lifestyle modifications, topical washes, topical clindamycin, oral antibiotics, spironolactone, adalimumab
3. 10^6
4. Primary intention—closure by direct approximation of skin edges
   Secondary intention—closure by granulation, epithelialization, and contraction
5. Keeps wounds clean, increases angiogenesis, decreases edema, increases granulation tissue growth
6. Macrophages
7. Stage I: nonblanchable erythema
   Stage II: partial-thickness skin loss
   Stage III: full-thickness skin loss, subcutaneous fat exposed
   Stage IV: full-thickness skin loss, muscle/tendon/bone exposed
   Unstageable: eschar covering wound

Chapter 12

1. Sudden, severe pain
2. Free intraperitoneal air seen under the diaphragm on upright radiograph
3. Intermittent, cramping abdominal pain
4. Smoking, alcohol consumption, chronic use of NSAIDs or steroids
5. Right upper quadrant, epigastric, or occasionally left upper quadrant
6. Hypokalemic, hypochloremic metabolic alkalosis

Chapter 13

1. Asymptomatic type I hernias
2. A collis gastroplasty can be performed
3. Toupet fundoplication
4. Progressive dysphagia beginning with solids and progressing to liquids
5. Diffuse esophageal spasm
6. Enucleated from the esophageal muscular wall without entering the mucosa
7. Esophagogastroduodenoscopy

Chapter 14

1. Left and right gastric arteries and left and right gastroepiploic arteries
2. Duodenal—95%
3. Submucosa—collagen-rich layer of connective tissue
4. Idiopathic
5. Gastric
6. Lymphadenectomy is not indicated for GIST
7. Intermediate- or high-risk disease (>5 cm tumor or >10 mitoses)

Chapter 15

1. Failed medical weight loss, BMI > 40, BMI > 35 with obesity-related comorbidities
2. Diabetes, hypertension, obstructive sleep apnea
3. Sleeve gastrectomy
4. Transverse mesocolon, jejunojejunostomy, Petersen's space
5. Leak and small bowel obstruction
6. Smoking, NSAIDs, steroids

Chapter 16

1. Nonoperative management (with bowel rest, nasogastric tube decompression, intravenous fluid hydration, correction of electrolyte abnormalities, and serial abdominal examinations)
2. Small bowel follow through (SBFT) or "small bowel challenge" with water-soluble contrast
3. Parenteral nutrition (TPN), assuming enteral nutrition distal to the fistula is not possible

4. FRIENDS: **F**oreign body, **R**adiation, **I**nflammation or **I**nfection, **E**pithelialization, **N**eoplasm and/or lack of **N**utrition, **D**istal obstruction, or **S**teroids
5. Tyrosine kinase inhibitor
6. Magnetic resonance enterography (MRE)
7. Stricturoplasty

Chapter 17

1. Hyperenhancement relative to the background liver on the arterial phase with contrast washout (hypoenhancement) relative to the background liver in portal venous or delayed phases
2. Antibiotics and percutaneous drainage
3. Hepatic adenoma

Chapter 18

1. Inspiratory arrest during deep palpation of the RUQ
2. Gallbladder wall thickening (>5 mm)
   Pericholecystic fluid
   + Sonographic Murphy's sign (tenderness with compression of the gallbladder by the ultrasound probe)
   Gallstones or sludge in the gallbladder
3. Fever, jaundice, RUQ pain
4. Charcot's triad + hypotension and altered mental status
5. Two and only two structures entering the gallbladder
   The bottom one-third of the gallbladder is dissected off the liver bed
   The hepatocystic triangle is cleared of fat and fibrous tissue
6. Transcystic or transcholedochal

Chapter 19

1. Zollinger–Ellison
2. Lateral pancreatojejunostomy (Puestow)
3. Supportive care (volume resuscitation, nutrition, analgesics)
4. Standard oncologic resection (pancreaticoduodenectomy or distal pancreatectomy)
5. Pancreaticojejunostomy, gastrojejunostomy, Hepaticojejunostomy
6. During the same hospitalization

Chapter 20

1. Extramedullary hematopoiesis
2. Right upper quadrant ultrasound imaging
3. Extremities, ears, and nose where temperatures are below body temperature
4. Symptomatic splenomegaly or treatment-limiting hypersplenism
5. Splenosis
6. CT with intravenous contrast
7. *Strep. pneumoniae, H. influenzae type B, Neisseria meningitidis*

Chapter 21

1. HLA-A, -B, and -DR (HLA-C, -DP, -DQ are not as important)
2. Hyperacute, accelerated, acute cellular, and chronic rejection
3. Corticosteroids: e.g., prednisone, methylprednisolone/Solu-Medrol

   Antiproliferative agents/antimetabolites: e.g., azathioprine/Imdur, mycophenolic acid/CellCept/Myfortic

   Calcineurin inhibitors: e.g., cyclosporin/CsA/Sandimmune/Neoral/Gengraf, tacrolimus/FK506/Prograf

   mTOR inhibitors: e.g., sirolimus/Rapamune, everolimus/Zortress

   Costimulation blockade: e.g., belatacept/Nulojix

   Antithymocyte antibodies: Thymoglobulin, basiliximab/Simulect
4. Bacterial infections: e.g., urinary tract infection, pneumonia

   Viral infections: e.g., CMV, EBV, HSV, BK virus

   Fungal infections: e.g., candidiasis (oral, esophageal, disseminated)

   Malignancies: squamous cell, basal cell, Kaposi sarcoma, lymphomas, hepatobiliary carcinomas, cervical carcinoma
5. Waiting time, pediatric status, being a prior living donor, distance from donor hospital and survival benefit, KDPI (kidney donor profile index)
6. MELD (model for end-stage liver disease) score: bilirubin, serum creatinine, INR, and for patients with MELD < 11, sodium
7. Living, donation after brain death (DBD), donation after cardiac death (DCD) donors
8. Lymphocele: ultrasound imaging, CT

   Renal artery and/or vein thrombosis: Doppler ultrasound, technetium-99m renal scan

   Urine leak: technetium-99m renal scan

   Rejection: renal biopsy

9. Primary nonfunction: retransplant
   Hepatic artery thrombosis: retransplant
   Portal vein stenosis or thrombosis: thrombectomy, possible retransplant
   Biliary stricture: percutaneous or endoscopic dilation, possible surgical revision
10. Simultaneous kidney-pancreas (SKP), pancreas after kidney (PAK), pancreas alone transplantation (PAT)

Chapter 22

1. True, it has all layers of the bowel wall, unlike false diverticula.
2. Ultrasound imaging followed by MRI if nondiagnostic
3. True, so appendectomy is recommended with the presence of a fecalith.
4. Appendectomy, including laparoscopic approaches (see chapter 40)
5. Neuroendocrine tumor (NET)
6. No additional therapy warranted after appendectomy for appendiceal NET < 1 cm.
7. Formal right hemicolectomy is warranted.

Chapter 23

1. Neostigmine can cause significant bradycardia and bronchospasm and should only be administered in a monitored setting; it is contraindicated in patients with significant cardiac disease or asthma.
2. Initial management involves endoscopic decompression and placement of a rectal tube, followed by elective sigmoidectomy due to the high recurrence rate.
3. Hinchey III (purulent peritonitis) and Hinchey IV (feculent peritonitis) require surgical intervention in addition to bowel rest and intravenous antibiotics.
4. Crohn's disease can be characterized by some or all of the following, including the presence of perianal disease, "skip lesions," ileal inflammation on colonoscopy, and the presence of upper gastrointestinal and/or small bowel (SB) involvement on endoscopy or imaging. Ulcerative colitis does not involve the SB, extends continuously from the rectum proximally, and is not associated with perianal disease.
5. In the emergent/urgent setting, the operation of choice is total abdominal colectomy with end ileostomy. Electively, surgical therapy involves total proctocolectomy with ileal pouch–anal anastomosis

(IPAA) in three, two, or just one stage depending on patient factors and eligibility.

6. Flexible sigmoidoscopy. The presence of full-thickness or severe necrosis on endoscopy is an indication for laparotomy with emergent resection and diversion. (CT scan is helpful, but endoscopy gives a better assessment of mucosal status.)
7. Adjuvant therapy should be considered in this patient because, although the patient has a stage II colon cancer, there was inadequate lymph node harvest (<12).
8. Chest/abdomen/pelvic CT to assess for metastatic disease and pelvic MRI to assess the local tumor stage (EUS [endorectal ultrasound imaging] can be considered if MRI is unavailable).

Chapter 24

1. Grade III internal hemorrhoids, can offer excisional hemorrhoidectomy or THD (transanal hemorrhoidal dearterialization).
2. Anal pain, followed by urinary retention
3. Medical treatment including fiber supplementation, stool softeners/laxatives, sitz baths, topical anesthetics (e.g., lidocaine), nonnarcotic pain medications, and topical nifedipine or nitroglycerin ointment
4. Anorectal examination with cytology with or without anoscopy
5. Chemoradiation (mitomycin/5-FU + radiotherapy)
6. Delorme procedure if short segment versus Altemeier procedure
7. Draining seton placement
8. Endoanal ultrasound imaging

Chapter 25

1. Indirect inguinal hernia
2. Inguinal ligament, rectus muscle, inferior epigastric vessels
3. Obturator hernia
4. McVay repair
5. Inferomedial to the internal ring or inferior to the iliopubic tract because of the risk of injury to the external iliac vessels ("triangle of doom") and ilioinguinal, genitofemoral, lateral femoral cutaneous, and femoral nerves ("triangle of pain")
6. Obesity, smoking, poor glycemic control, malnutrition
7. 5 cm

Chapter 26

1. Inability to tolerate general anesthesia; hemodynamic instability; uncorrected coagulopathy; no available experienced laparoscopic surgeons or staff
2. Reduces afferent arterial renal flow, leading to decreased glomerular filtration rate and elevated renal venous pressure
3. Increased intra-abdominal pressure leads to increased systemic vascular resistance secondary to compression of venous and arterial structures.

   Decreased flow leads to renin–angiotensin–aldosterone axis activation.

   Compression of the inferior vena cava leads to reduced preload and lower cardiac output.
4. 38 cm
5. Presence of peritonitis or suspected colorectal perforation, severe acute diverticulitis, and fulminant colitis
6. 6 minutes

Chapter 27

1. Superiorly, the clavicle; inferiorly, the inframammary fold; medially, the lateral edge of the sternum; and laterally, the anterior border of the latissimus dorsi
2. Superiorly, the axillary vein, outer border of the first rib, and edge of the clavicle; laterally, the latissimus dorsi muscle; medially, the serratus anterior muscle; posteriorly, the subscapularis and teres major muscles; and anteriorly, the pectoralis major and minor muscles
3. All women beginning at age 50 years per the USPTF, while the American College of Obstetricians and Gynecologists (ACOG) and the American Cancer Society (ACS) recommend annual screening mammography for women starting at 45 years and older.
4. Reduces the risk for local disease recurrence
5. Neoadjuvant chemotherapy and/or neoadjuvant hormonal therapy should be administered to all patients with primary tumors measuring >2 cm, node-positive disease at presentation, triple-negative breast cancer, or *HER2*-positive disease.
6. A modified radical mastectomy involves a total mastectomy and axillary lymph node dissection.
7. Seldomly performed, a radical mastectomy (or Halstead mastectomy) involves total mastectomy, complete axillary lymph node dissection, removal of the pectoralis major and minor muscles, and removal of all overlying skin.

Chapter 28

1. WLE (wide local excision) with 1-cm margins, consider SLNB (sentinel lymph node biopsy)
2. Punch biopsy or resection, suspect BCC (basal cell cancer)
3. Squamous skin cancer
4. WLE with 2-cm margins and SLNB
5. Excisional biopsy or deep shave biopsy including the entire depth of the lesion
6. Lipoma
7. Combination immunotherapy with anti-PD-1/CTLA-4 antibodies is indicated. Other immunotherapeutics can be considered in the setting of a clinical trial. Metastasectomy can be discussed in a multidisciplinary setting.
8. CNBx (core needle biopsy)
9. Histologic grade
10. WLE (sparing critical structures), always with adjuvant radiotherapy
11. Management should include en bloc resection of the tumor with the right kidney, if the patient is eligible.

Chapter 29

1. The left renal vein
2. Neural crest
3. Nonfunctioning cortical adenoma
4. Plasma fractionated metanephrines or urine catecholamines/metanephrines, overnight low-dose dexamethasone suppression test, and (if hypertensive) aldosterone and plasma renin activity
5. Functional, size >4 to 5 cm, or imaging characteristics suspicious for malignancy
6. ACTH-secreting pituitary adenoma (also known as Cushing disease)
7. Adrenal vein sampling
8. α-Adrenergic blocker
9. Mitotane
10. *MENIN, RET, RET*

Chapter 30

1. All glands are supported by the inferior thyroid artery.
2. Infusion of normal saline
3. 50%
4. Thyroid ultrasound imaging
5. Follicular and papillary thyroid carcinoma
6. Pheochromocytoma (and genetic testing should also be considered)
7. Hashimoto's thyroiditis

Chapter 31

1. The descending thoracic aorta
2. Type II pneumocytes
3. Talc (talcum, hydrated magnesium silicate)
4. Open or VATS (video-assisted thoracoscopic surgery) decortication
5. People aged 50 to 80 years with at least a 20-pack-year smoking history who currently smoke or quit within the past 15 years
6. Mesothelioma
7. Thymoma, teratoma/germ cell tumor, lymphoma, thyroid tumor
8. Chronic obstructive pulmonary disease (COPD), idiopathic pulmonary fibrosis (IPF), cystic fibrosis (CF), alpha-1-antitrypsin deficiency, pulmonary arterial hypertension (PAH)

Chapter 32

1. The left internal mammary artery (LIMA)
2. Age, life expectancy, ability to take warfarin (bleeding issues, adherence, health literacy, care access, expected future fertility)
3. Intra-aortic balloon pump (IABP), Impella heart pump, venoarterial extracorporeal membrane oxygenation (VA ECMO)
4. Left ventricular assist device (LVAD), heart transplant
5. Arrhythmia, bleeding, cardiac tamponade, myocardial ischemia, postoperative myocardial stunning, hypovolemia. Remember that ventricular arrhythmias should be treated as ischemia until proven otherwise.
6. Aortic insufficiency, aortic dissection, severe peripheral vascular disease (unless central cannulation for VA ECMO is used)
7. Mechanical complications of myocardial infarction (papillary muscle rupture, ventricular septal defect, ventricular rupture)

Chapter 33

1. Where the artery runs over the medial half of the femoral head
2. Catheters are defined by their *outer* diameter while sheaths are defined by their *inner* diameter.
3. 1 Fr = 0.33 mm
4. Endothelial injury
5. Blunt dehiscence of lesion, fracture and separation of media from intima, and stretching of media and adventitia
6. To mechanically remove/reduce heavy plaque burden, prepare a vessel for balloon angioplasty and/or stenting, and for use instead of stenting when stents are contraindicated in the anatomical location of the lesion (e.g., behind the knee)

Chapter 34

1. Antiplatelet therapy (aspirin and/or Plavix), antihypertensive therapy, good blood sugar control for patients with diabetes (HgbA1C < 7), smoking cessation, and statin therapy
2. Within 2 to 14 days
3. With >70% carotid artery stenosis
4. Vagus and hypoglossal nerves
5. Cerebral hyperperfusion syndrome, severe headache
6. Transcarotid artery revascularization with flow reversal (TCAR) and transfemoral stenting with distal embolic protection (TF-CAS)
7. Stump pressure (threshold <40 mm Hg), somatosensory evoked potentials, transcranial doppler, or cerebral oximetry
8. A1C < 7; LDL < 70 mg/dL or 50% reduction from baseline

Chapter 35

1. Cigarette smoking
2. Individuals meeting the following criteria should be screened: 65 to 75 year olds with history of tobacco use and/or with first-degree relatives with AAA (abdominal aortic aneurysm); >75 year olds in good health.
3. 5.0 to 5.4 cm in females, ≥5.5 cm in males; increase of >0.5 cm over 6 months or >1 cm over a year
4. AAA and femoral artery aneurysm
5. Improved 30-day/in-hospital mortality after EVAR (endovascular aortic aneurysm repair)

6. When they lead to expansion of the aneurysm sac and/or if they are type I, III, or V
7. (1) Goal is 90 minutes or less from door to intervention; (2) patients should be managed with permissive hypotensive resuscitation, as aggressive fluid/blood resuscitation can worsen hemorrhage; (3) if patient will require general anesthesia, induction should be delayed until patient is in the OR and surgeons are ready to begin intervention.
8. Preoperative planning with established protocols consisting of multimodal therapies for spinal protection
9. A—involves the proximal ascending aorta with or without the arch; B—descending aorta only (distal to the left subclavian)
10. (1) Revascularization of the ischemic territory; (2) assessment of bowel viability; (3) temporary abdominal closure and second-look operations for patients with questionable bowel or requiring bowel resection

Chapter 36

1. Risk factor modification and structured exercise
2. Perform four-compartment calf fasciotomies on that side
3. Knee reduction and repeat perfusion evaluation, with pulse examination, ABI (ankle brachial index), and CTA (CT angiography)
4. >6 hours
5. Proximal and distal vascular control
6. IIb—emergent revascularization

   III—amputation
7. Deep posterior compartment
8. Rest pain, nonhealing wounds, tissue loss
9. Claudication < 0.8; rest pain < 0.4
10. Smoking cessation, weight management, exercise program, diabetes management, hypertension management, high-intensity statin, dual antiplatelet therapy

Chapter 37

1. Outpatient venous duplex
2. Start the patient on anticoagulation. There is no role for an IVC (inferior vena cava) filter in a patient who can tolerate anticoagulation.

3. There is no role for prophylactic IVC filter placement. The patient should be placed on appropriate DVT (deep venous thrombosis) prophylaxis postoperatively.
4. Serial ultrasound imaging of the deep veins, starting at 1 week or sooner if the patient develops symptoms. You do not need to start anticoagulation at this time.
5. IVC filter removal
6. Outpatient DOAC (direct oral anticoagulants) for 3 months with reevaluation at that time
7. Prescribe the patient compression stockings to be worn during waking hours for her chronic venous insufficiency.

Chapter 38

1. CKD stage 4
2. Stenosis. Endothelial cell injury leads to smooth muscle proliferation and neointimal hyperplasia, which causes graft stenosis.
3. Intra-abdominal infection, inflammatory bowel disease (IBD), severe/refractory psychiatric disorders, unstable housing conditions, late pregnancy (3rd trimester)
4. Intraperitoneal cefazolin and gentamicin
5. The juxta-anastomotic area
6. Improving distal perfusion while preserving access can be performed via proximalization of arteriovenous inflow (PAI) or distal revascularization interval ligation (DRIL) procedures in the setting of worsening or nonimproving symptoms. If symptoms progress to new-onset motor dysfunction or tissue loss, arteriovenous access (AVA) must be ligated immediately.
7. Aneurysm—AVF (arteriovenous fistula); pseudoaneurysm—AVG (arteriovenous graft)

Chapter 39

1. Upper GI contrast study
2. Metabolic alkalosis with associated hypochloremia and hypokalemia
3. Neuroblastoma
4. Myenteric–Auerbach and submucosal Meissner plexuses
5. Type C: where the upper portion of the esophagus ends in a blind pouch and the lower portion is connected to the trachea by a tracheoesophageal fistula
6. 10 mL/kg

7. Along the anterior border of the sternocleidomastoid
8. Prematurity and enteral feeding
9. External brace therapy

Chapter 40

1. Workup with imaging (pelvic/transvaginal ultrasound and/or CT abdomen/pelvis), serum CA-125/CEA levels, and referral to gynecologist.
2. Left lateral tilt positioning to prevent IVC (inferior vena cava) compression, laparoscopic port site location adjustments, awareness of increased aspiration risk, ASA II airway, increased thromboembolism risk, need for intraoperative external fetal monitoring.
3. A speculum examination to view the cervix, consider cervical or endometrial biopsies based on examination findings.
4. Tracheostomy collar or intubation through cervical stoma. Patients with a history of total laryngectomy have their trachea sewn directly to the skin, so they cannot be intubated orally/nasally.
5. Thyroglossal duct cyst. Ultrasound imaging should be performed to evaluate for the presence of normal thyroid tissue outside the cyst before surgical excision (Figure 40.4).
6. Tissue samples from core or excisional biopsy are necessary for flow cytometry, immunophenotyping, and architectural pattern, which are used for subclassification of lymphoma to direct further management.
7. Imbibition, inosculation, revascularization (Table 40.7)
8. (a) Finger held in flexion, (b) pain with palpation of flexor tendon sheath, (c) fusiform swelling of finger, and (d) pain with passive extension of finger. Used for clinical diagnosis of flexor tenosynovitis, which requires urgent operation for finger I&D.
9. Within 72 hours, otherwise neurotransmitters will be depleted and the distal end cannot be stimulated intraoperatively.
10. Urine culture, antibiotics, urgent Urology consult for ureteral stent placement
11. Intravenous antibiotics, immediate surgical exploration and debridement
12. 55 to 69 years old

Chapter 41

1. Chi-square test, which would compare the frequency of a categorical response variable (contrast-induced nephropathy) in two groups (with or without sodium bicarbonate)
2. (Unpaired) t-test that would compare the effect of an intervention (opioid antagonist) on a continuous, normally distributed variable (days until return of bowel function) in two groups
3. (a) Increases; (b) Decreases; (c) Unchanged; (d) Unchanged

4a.

	CVA	No CVA
Atorvastatin therapy	100	900
No atorvastatin therapy	500	1,500

4b. RR = (1/1,000)/(500/2,000) = 0.4, or 40%

4c. ARR = (500/2,000) – (100/1,000) = 0.15, or 15%

4d. This is the number needed to treat (NNT). Recall, NNT = 1/ARR, so 1/0.15 = 6.67, or 7 people

Chapter 42

1. Freedom from accidental injury
2. Safety, effectiveness, patient (person) centered, timeliness, efficiency, equity
3. An injury to the patient that results from a medical intervention and is not specifically due to a patient's underlying condition
4. It is an error that is caught before an AE (adverse event) or harm occurred.
5. Focus on systems-based errors rather than individual-based errors.
6. "Error of commission" is when someone actively does the wrong thing, whereas "error of omission" is failing to do the right thing. Error of omission can be difficult to detect because no action may occur, but the lack of action itself can result in an error.
7. It is a retrospective and systematic approach to analyzing adverse events and near misses. RCAs (root cause analyses) can map out actions and processes that lead to an identified outcome of interest (for example, an AE).
8. Specific, Measurable, Achievable, Realistic, and Time-bound (SMART)
9. A run chart collects data over time and allows you to identify or monitor trends or patterns in a process.

Index

Note: Page numbers followed by "f" indicate figures and "t" indicate tables.

A

AAAs. *See* Abdominal aortic aneurysms (AAAs)
AAS. *See* Acute aortic syndrome (AAS)
ABCDE mnemonic of melanoma, 551, 552f
Abdomen/gastrointestinal tract
- critical care, 104–106

Abdominal access, in laparoscopic procedure
- abdominal wall hemorrhage, 521
- closed technique, 519
- complications of, 521
- open technique, 519–521
- physiologic effects of, 521–522
- port removal and closure, 521
- trocar insertion, 521

Abdominal aorta, 702–704, 705f
Abdominal aortic aneurysms (AAAs)
- clinical presentation, 708
- diagnosis, 708
- elective management, 708–715, 709f, 711f–712f
- epidemiology, 706–707
- late graft-specific complications, 717–719, 718f
- pathophysiology/etiology, 707–708
- postoperative period after, complications in, 716–717
- screening recommendations, 706–707
- urgent/emergent management, 715–716

Abdominal genitourinary injuries, 170–171
Abdominal pain, 317, 825–826
Abdominal pathology. *See also* Pediatric surgery
- hepatobiliary, 813–814
- hypertrophic pyloric stenosis (HPS), 810–811
- intussusception, 812

Abdominal plain films, 303
Abdominal transplantation
- deceased donor procurement operation, 423
- immunosuppression, 414–417, 414t–415t, 416f, 418–419
- organ allocation, 419–421
- organ donation, 421–422
- organ preservation, 423
- organ transplantation
  - kidney transplantation, 423–426
  - liver transplant, 427–430
  - lung and heart transplant, 432
  - pancreas transplant, 430–432
  - small intestine transplant, 432
- physiologic immunity
  - adaptive immune system, 412–413
  - innate immune system, 412
- transplant immunology, 413
- transplant rejection, 413

Abdominal trauma
- anatomy, 163
- imaging modalities in, 163
- injury classification, 163, 164f, 164t
- solid organ injuries
  - abdominal genitourinary injuries, 170–171
  - common bile duct injuries, 167
  - diaphragmatic injuries, 164–166
  - duodenal injuries, 169–170
  - gallbladder injuries, 167
  - gastric injuries, 169
  - hepatic injuries, 166–167
  - intestinal injuries, 170
  - pancreatic injuries, 169
  - pregnancy, 172
  - splenic injuries, 167–169, 168f
  - vascular injuries, 171–172
- trauma laparotomy, 163–164
- trauma resuscitation management, 163

Abdominal wall
- defects, 801–802
- hemorrhage, 521
- reconstruction, 862, 864f

Abdominal wall hernia
- etiology of, 508–510
- incidence of, 508–510
- operative approach
  - laparoscopic repairs, 514
  - open repairs, 511–514
  - open *vs.* minimally invasive approach, 514
- treatment and operative management
  - mesh choice, 510–511, 512t–513t
  - patient and hernia factors, 510, 511t
  - prosthetic mesh in, 510

Abdominoplasty, 866–867
Above-knee amputation, 755
Abscesses/cystic disease
 amebic abscesses, 336
 echinococcal cysts, 336
 intrahepatic biliary cysts, 336–337
 pyogenic abscesses, 335–336
Abscopal effects, 560
Absolute risk (AR), 888
Absolute risk reduction (ARR), 888
Acalculous cholecystitis, 349
ACC. *See* Adrenocortical carcinoma (ACC)
Acetabular fractures, 189
Acetylcholine, 270
Achalasia, 255–256
Achilles tendon ruptures, 191
Acid–base disorders, 103
Acquired disorders, 394–400
Acquired strictures, 257–258
Acromioclavicular dislocations, 187
ACR Thyroid Imaging, Reporting and Data System (TI-RADS), 608, 609f
Actinic keratosis, 564
Active external warming, 205
Active internal rewarming, 205
Acute abdomen. *See* Acute abdominal pain
Acute abdominal pain
 epigastric pain, 233
 etiologies
  infectious colitis, 245–247
  ischemic colitis, 245–247
  mesenteric ischemic, 243–244
  rectus sheath hematoma, 240, 243
  small bowel obstruction (SBO), 244–245, 247
 evaluation
  differential diagnosis, 240, 241t–242t
  laboratory evaluation, 238–239
  medications, 234–235
  physical examination, 235–238
  present illness, history of, 234
  radiographic evaluation, 239–240
 parietal pain, 233
 periumbilical pain, 233
 referred pain, 233
 suprapubic pain, 233
 visceral pain, 233, 234f
Acute adrenal insufficiency, 587–588
Acute aortic syndrome (AAS)
 clinical management, 724–726
 clinical presentation, 724
 diagnosis, 724
 epidemiology, 723
 pathophysiology and classification, 723, 724f–725f
Acute arterial occlusion of extremity
 clinical management, 743–746
 clinical presentation, 740–741
 complications, 746–747, 748f
 diagnosis, 741–743, 742t
 etiology, 740
Acute bacterial prostatitis, 874
Acute calculous cholecystitis, 346–349
Acute cholangitis, 350–351
Acute idiopathic thrombocytopenic purpura (ITP), 399
Acute kidney injury, 103–104
Acute mesenteric ischemia (AMI), 726–727
Acute myeloid leukemia, 395
Acute pancreatitis
 complications of, 379
 diagnosis, 376–378, 376t
 etiology, 376
 treatment, 378
Acute paronychia, 857f
Acute respiratory distress syndrome (ARDS), 57, 95–96
Acute sialadenitis, 844–845
Acute subdural hematomas, 134
Acute suppurative thyroiditis, 617
Acute wounds
 hidradenitis suppurativa (HS), 212–213, 213t, 214t
 necrotizing soft tissue infections (NSTIs), 213–216, 216f
Adaptive immune system, 412–413
Adenocarcinoma, 634
Adenomas, 458
Adjunctive therapies, 203
Adjuvant chemoradiotherapy, 277
Adrenal cortex, 573
Adrenalectomy, 582, 588–590, 590f–592f
Adrenal gland, diseases of
 acute adrenal insufficiency, 587–588
 adrenalectomy, 588–590, 590f–592f
 adrenal incidentaloma, 575–578, 576f, 577t
 adrenocortical carcinoma (ACC), 585–586, 586f
 anatomy, 573, 574f
 Cushing syndrome, 578–581, 579f
 embryology, 573
 histology, 573–575
 hypercortisolism, 578–581, 579f
 miscellaneous nonfunctional adrenal masses, 586–587
 paraganglioma, 582–585
 pheochromocytoma, 582–585
 physiology, 573–575
 primary hyperaldosteronism, 581–582

Adrenal incidentaloma, 575–578, 576f, 577t
Adrenal medulla, 573, 575
Adrenal metastases, 587
Adrenal myelolipoma, 587
Adrenal vein sampling (AVS), 582
α-Adrenergic blockade, 583
β-Adrenergic blockade, 584
Adrenocortical carcinoma (ACC), 585–586, 586f
Adrenocortical insufficiency, 587
Adrenocorticotropic hormone (ACTH), 575
Advanced/metastatic disease, 277
Advancement flaps, 850, 854f
Adverse event (AE), 897
Aenocarcinoma, 441
Aesthetic surgery, 866–867
Airway injuries, 204–205
Aldosterone, 573
  adrenal adenoma, 581
  adrenal carcinoma, 581
Allen test, 661, 787, 855
ALND. *See* Axillary lymph node dissection (ALND)
Altered mental status (AMS), 44
Alternative hypothesis (H_a), 887
Alvarado score, 817
Alveolar epithelium, 625
Amaurosis fugax, 692
Ambulatory phlebectomy, 768
Amebic abscesses, 336
American College of Cardiology (ACC), 658
American Gastroenterological Association (AGA), 318
American Heart Association (AHA), 658
American Joint Committee on Cancer (AJCC) system, 539
AMI. *See* Acute mesenteric ischemia (AMI)
Amputation, 744, 754–755
Amyand hernia, 501
Amylase, 271
Anal canal anatomy, 475, 476f
Anal fissure
  etiology, 485
  evaluation, 486
  symptoms, 486
  treatment, 486–487
Anal intraepithelial neoplasia (AIN), 494, 495f
Anal manometry, 445
  incontinence, 479
Anal neoplasia
  anal intraepithelial neoplasia (AIN), 494, 495f
  basal cell carcinoma (BCC), 495
  melanoma, 496
  Paget disease, 495
  primary anal adenocarcinoma, 495–496
  squamous cell carcinoma (SCC), 494–495
Anal seepage, 477
Anal sphincter
  external, 475
  internal, 475
  mechanism, 475–476
Anal stenosis, 487
Analysis of variance (ANOVA), 891
Anaplastic carcinoma, 610
Anastomotic leaks, 294
Anesthesia, 14–20, 16t, 20t
  common anesthetic agents, 15–16, 17–20
  conscious sedation, 15
  general, 14–15
  local anesthetic systemic toxicity, 16
  monitored anesthesia care (MAC), 15
  neuroaxial blockade, 16–17
  postoperative management problems, 43–44
  regional/local anesthetic, 15
  types of, 14–15
Angina pectoris, 657
Angioplasty, 4
Angiosarcoma, 545
Ankle-brachial index (ABI), 741
  chronic arterial and athero-occlusive disease, 750
Ankle fractures, 191
Anlotinib, 566
Annular pancreas, 364
Annuloplasty, 665
Anoderm, 475
Anorectal abscess, 488f
  cryptoglandular, 487–488, 489t
  fistula-in-ano, 488–491, 490f–491f
Anorectal disease
  abnormal rectal fixation
    external/full-thickness rectal prolapse, 482
    internal intussusception, 480, 480f, 481t
  anatomy, 475, 476f
  histology, 475
  incontinence
    etiologies of, 476
    evaluation of, 477, 478t
    symptoms of, 477
    treatment of, 479
  obstructive defection, 479
  physiology, 475–476, 477f

Anorectal malformations, 807, 808f
Anorectal melanoma, 496
Anorectal testing modalities, endoscopic and physiologic, 477, 478t
Anorectum, infectious pathology of
 anorectal abscess, 487–491
 condyloma acuminatum, 493–494
 hidradenitis suppurativa, 493
 necrotizing anorectal infection, 491
 pilonidal cyst, 491–493
 pruritus ani, 493
Ansa cervicalis, 688
Antenatal steroids, 826
Anterior tibial artery (AT), 733
Antibiotic prophylaxis, 24t, 75t–77t
Antibiotics, 5
Antidiuretic hormone (ADH), 538
Antiplatelet therapy, perioperative use of, 55
Antiproliferative agents/antimetabolites, 416
Antiseptic agents, 25
Antithymocyte antibodies, 417, 418f
Aorta, 702, 703f
Aortic arch, 702
Aortic insufficiency (AI), 661–662
Aortic stenosis (AS), 661
Aortic valve disease, 650
 aortic insufficiency (AI), 661–662
 aortic stenosis (AS), 661
 surgical aortic valve replacement (SAVR), 662
 transcatheter aortic valve replacement (TAVR), 662
Aortobifemoral bypass grafting, 752
Aortography, 708
Aortoiliac disease, 752–753
Aortoiliac endarterectomy, 753
Apendiceal mucinous neoplasms, 440–441
Appendiceal neoplasms
 adenocarcinoma, 441
 appendiceal mucinous neoplasms, 440–441
 appendiceal tumors, 440t
 neuroendocrine tumor (NET), 439–440
Appendicitis, 817
Appendix
 anatomy, 435
 appendicitis
  children, 439
  diagnosis, 435–436
  epidemiology/etiology, 435
  pregnancy, 438–439
  presentation, 435
  treatment, 436–441, 437f
Arrhythmias, 657, 672
Arterial blood gas (ABG), 5, 625
Arterial insufficiency ulcers, 750
Arterial pressure monitoring, 85
Arteriovenous access (AVA)
 complications
  aneurysms, 790
  early thrombosis, 790
  infection, 790
  pseudoaneurysms, 790
  steal syndrome, 790
  stenosis, 789
 planning, 787
Arteriovenous fistula (AVF), 787–789, 788f
Arteriovenous graft (AVG), 789
Associating liver partition and portal vein ligation for staged hepatectomy (ALPPS), 343
Asthma, 56–57
Asymptomatic cholelithiasis, 346
Atelectasis, 55–56, 521
Atherosclerosis, 737–739
Atrial fibrillation, 54–55, 667, 740
ATTRACT trial, 771
Atypical lobular hyperplasia (ALH), 538
Augmentation mammoplasty, 866
Autoimmune diffuse toxic goiter (Graves' disease)
 classification, 615
 clinical presentation/symptoms, 615
 diagnosis/testing, 615
 epidemiology, 615
 etiology, 615
 nonoperative treatment, 615–616
 operative treatment, 616
 outcomes/complications, 616
Axilla
 defined, 527
 lymphatic structures, 529
 sensory and motor nerves, 529, 530t
Axillary lymph node dissection (ALND), 529, 529t, 544–545
Axillobifemoral bypass, 752–753
Azygous vein, 620

B

Balancing measure, 902
Bariatric surgery techniques, 290t
 biliopancreatic diversion with duodenal switch (BPD-DS), 292–293, 292f
 gastric band surgery, 289

long-term surveillance, 297
postoperative issues and complications, 294–297, 295f, 296f
postoperative management, 293
Roux-en-Y gastric bypass (RYGB), 291–292, 291f
sleeve gastrectomy, 289–291, 290f
Baroreceptor, 688
Barrett esophagus, 261–264, 263f
Basal cell carcinoma (BCC), 495
diagnosis, 560
epidemiology, 560
etiology, 560
treatment, 560–561, 561t
Bassini repair, 503
Bedside pleurodesis, 627
Bell staging, 803
Below-knee amputation (BKA), 755
Benign breast conditions
cysts, 535
fibroadenoma, 535–536
fibrocystic breast change (FBC), 535
mastalgia, 536
nipple discharge
benign intraductal papilloma, 537
galactorrhea, 537
lactation, 536
pathologic, 537
Benign esophageal neoplasms, 264
Benign intraductal papilloma, 537
Benign liver tumors
focal nodular hyperplasia (FNH), 333–334
hemangioma, 333
hepatic adenoma, 334–335
Benign prostatic hyperplasia (BPH), 873–874
Benign skin lesions
actinic keratosis, 564
congenital nevi, 564
dysplastic nevi, 564
seborrheic keratoses, 563
Benign soft tissue lesions
cutaneous cysts, 567
ganglion cysts, 568
lipomas, 568
neurofibromas, 567–568
Beta-blockade, perioperative, 4
Bethesda System for Reporting Thyroid Cytopathology, 606, 606t
Bianchi, 312
Bile duct injury, 353
Biliary atresia, 813–814
Biliary neoplasms
cholangiocarcinoma, 356–358
gallbladder cancer, 353–356
Biliary operations
cholecystectomy, 358–359
common bile duct exploration (CBDE), 359–360
Biliary strictures, 351–352
Biliary tree
benign biliary obstruction
acalculous cholecystitis, 349
acute calculous cholecystitis, 346–349
acute cholangitis, 350–351
asymptomatic cholelithiasis, 346
choledocholithiasis, 349–350
symptomatic cholelithiasis, 346
bile duct injury, 353
biliary neoplasms
cholangiocarcinoma, 356–358
gallbladder cancer, 353–356
biliary operations
cholecystectomy, 358–359
common bile duct exploration (CBDE), 359–360
biliary strictures, 351–352
choledochal cyst, 352–353
Biliopancreatic diversion with duodenal switch (BPD-DS), 292–293, 292f
Biological/physiologic age, 3
Biostatistics, for general surgeon
clinical practice guidelines, 893, 894t
data analysis
measures of effect, 888–889, 889t
screening and diagnostic tests, 890, 890t
statistical principles, 887–888
statistical tests and analytic approaches, 890–891
data sources, 887
study design, 883f
case–control study, 882, 883f
cohort study, 883–884, 884f
cross-sectional study, 884–885
experimental studies, 885–886
observational studies, 882–884
pragmatic trial, 885–886
randomized controlled trial (RCT), 885–886
systematic reviews and meta-analysis (SRMA), 886–887
study quality, 891–893, 892t
Bipolar instruments, 523

BI-RADS. *See* Breast Imaging Reporting and Data System (BI-RADS)
Bladder, 827
  cancer, 871
Blood glucose, 25
Blood urea nitrogen (BUN), 6
Blue toe syndrome, 741
Blunt cardiac injury, 149
Blunt cerebrovascular injury (BCVI)
  diagnosis, 141
  grading system, 143t
  management, 141
  risk factors, 143t
  signs/symptoms, 143t
Bosniak classification system, 868, 869t
Botulinum toxin injections, 486
Bowel obstruction, postoperative management, 67
Brachiocephalic trunk, 688
Branchial cleft cyst, 814
BRCA1, 532
BRCA2, 532
Breast
  anatomy of, 528f
    axillary, 527–529, 529t–530t
    boundaries and attachments, 527
    lymphatic, 527
    neurovascular, 527
  cancer risk
    hereditary, 532
    risk factors, 531t
  conditions during pregnancy, 546–547
    cancer, 547
    nipple discharge, 547
  infarcts, 547
Breast biopsy
  core needle biopsy, 534
  excisional biopsy, 534
  fine-needle aspiration biopsy (FNAB), 534
  stereotactic core biopsy, 535
Breast conservation therapy (BCT), 541
Breast diseases
  clinical assessment
    of cancer risks, 529–532, 531t
    patient history, 529
    physical examination, 532
    in supine position, 532
    in upright position, 532
  gynecomastia, 538
  high-risk/premalignant conditions, 538–539
  infections
    granulomatous mastitis, 537–538
    lactational mastitis, 537
    nonpuerperal abscesses, 538
  invasive breast cancer, 541–543
  malignancy of
    ductal carcinoma in situ (DCIS), 540–541, 541f
    epidemiology, 539
    staging, 539
    tumor biomarkers and prognostic factors, 540
Breast imaging
  Breast Imaging Reporting and Data System (BI-RADS), 533t
    benign mammographic findings, 532
    cysts, 532
    malignant mammographic findings, 532
    screening, in high-risk patients, 533
  diagnostic mammograms, 533–534
  magnetic resonance imaging (MRI), 534
  screening mammograms, 532
  ultrasound, 534
Bromocriptine, 536, 593
Bronchial system, 620
Bronchiolitis obliterans syndrome (BOS), 645
Bronchodilators, 6
Bronchogenic cysts, 809
Bronchopleural fistula, 640
Brooke ileostomy, 320, 320f–322f, 445
Budesonide, 455
Bundles of His, 650
Burns
  chemical injuries, 205
  cold injuries, 205–206
  electrical injuries, 205
  evaluation, 195f
  excision, 201–202
  infection, 203–204, 204t
    burn sepsis, 203–204
    burn wound infection, 203
  inhalation injuries, 204–205
  local wound care
    debridement, 199, 201
    dressings, 199
    irrigation, 199
    ointments, 199, 201
  long-term care, 206
  management
    associated injuries, treatment of, 199
    continuous pulse oximetry, 199
    diagnostic testing, 199
    foley catheter, 199
    naso- and orogastric tubes, 199

pain control and sedation, 198–199
tetanus prophylaxis, 199
management of, 195f
nutrition, 203
operative management
burn excision, 201–202
escharotomy, 201
wound coverage, 202–203, 202t
primary survey
airway, 194
breathing, 194
circulation, 194
disability, 196
exposure, 196
resuscitation
fluids, 198
oxygen, 198
secondary survey
burn center referrals, 198
depth, 196–197, 196t
total body surface area (TBSA) estimation, 197, 197f
sepsis, 203–204
topical antimicrobial agents for, 200t
wound infection, 203
Butyrate, 444
Bypass *versus* Angioplasty in Severe Ischemia of the Leg (BASIL) trial, 752

C

Calcaneus fractures, 191
Calcineurin inhibitors, 416–417
Calcitonin, 593, 598
Calcium channel blockers, 486, 583
Canadian C-Spine criteria, 141, 142f
Capillary perfusion pressure, 746
Carbon monoxide poisoning, 205
Carcinoembryonic antigen (CEA), 464
Carcinoid syndrome, 316
Cardiac arrest, 656
Cardiac catheterization, 652–654
Cardiac index (CI), 669
Cardiac injury
blunt, 149
diagnosis/testing, 150–152
outcomes/complications, 152
penetrating, 149–150
treatment, 152
Cardiac risk index, 9
Cardiac surgery
anatomy, 650, 651f–652f
aortic valve disease
aortic insufficiency (AI), 661–662
aortic stenosis (AS), 661
surgical aortic valve replacement (SAVR), 662
transcatheter aortic valve replacement (TAVR), 662
cardiopulmonary bypass (CPB)
benefits, 655
drawbacks, 655–656, 656f
coronary artery disease
acute complications, 657–658
angina pectoris, 657
chronic complications, 658
myocardial infarction (MI), 657
operative management, 658–661
mitral valve disease, 663–664
postoperative management and complications, 669–673, 670t, 671f
preoperative evaluation
assessment tools, 651
cardiac catheterization, 652–654
chest X ray (CXR), 652, 654f
computed tomography (CT), 652, 654f
echocardiography, 654–655
history/physical examination, 652, 653t
viability studies, 655
Cardiac tamponade, 670
Cardiogenic shock, 124
Cardioplegia, 655
Cardiopulmonary bypass (CPB), 721
benefits, 655
drawbacks, 655–656, 656f
Cardiovascular disease
cardiac risk indices/calculators, 4
functional status assessment, 3
mortality rate of, 3, 4
preoperative management
angioplasty/stenting, patients with, 4–5
internal defibrillators, patients with, 4
patients with pacemakers, 4
perioperative beta-blockade, 4
preoperative testing, 4
risk factors for, 4
Carotid artery, 688, 689f
Carotid duplex ultrasonography, 693
Carotid endarterectomy (CEA), 695
Carotid flow reversal, 697, 697f
Carotid sinus/bulb, 688
Carotid–subclavian bypass, 756
Case–control study, 882, 883f
Catheter-based angiography, 693
Catheter-directed thrombolysis, 771
Catheter-related bloodstream infections, 82
Caustic ingestion, 260–261

C cells, 599
CDH. *See* Congenital diaphragmatic hernia (CDH)
CEA. *See* Carotid endarterectomy (CEA)
CEAP classification, 765, 766t–767t
Cecal bascule, 447
Cecal volvulus, 447–448
Cecopexy, 447
Cellulitis, 777
Central venous pressure (CVP) monitoring, 85
Cerebral contusions, 134
Cerebral hyperperfusion syndrome, 696
Cerebral perfusion, preservation of, 136
Cerebrovascular disease
  anatomy, 688–689
  stroke and extracranial carotid artery atherosclerosis
    clinical presentation, 692
    diagnosis, 693
    epidemiology, 690
    nonoperative management, 693, 694t
    operative management, 693–698, 697f
    pathophysiology, 692
Cervical carcinoma, 829–830
Cervical spine, 140–141, 142f
Cervix, 827, 828f
Chamberlain procedure, 637
Chest trauma
  anatomy, 148–149
  cardiac injury
    blunt, 149
    diagnosis/testing, 150–152
    outcomes/complications, 152
    penetrating, 149–150
    treatment, 152
  chest wall injuries
    classification, 152–153
    diagnosis/testing, 153
    epidemiology, 152–153
    etiology, 152–153
    outcomes/complications, 156
    treatment, 153–156
  diaphragm injuries
    classification, 152–153
    diagnosis/testing, 153
    epidemiology, 152–153
    etiology, 152–153
    outcomes/complications, 156
    treatment, 153–156
  esophageal injury
    classification, 157
    diagnosis/testing, 157
    epidemiology, 157
    etiology, 157
    outcomes/complications, 157–159
    treatment, 157
  initial workup, 148
  lung injury
    classification, 159
    diagnosis/testing, 159
    epidemiology, 159
    etiology, 159
    outcomes/complications, 159
    treatment, 159, 160f
  physiology, 149
  pleural injuries
    classification, 152–153
    diagnosis/testing, 153
    epidemiology, 152–153
    etiology, 152–153
    outcomes/complications, 156
    treatment, 153–156
  thoracic injuries, 148
  tracheobronchial injury
    classification, 159
    diagnosis/testing, 159
    epidemiology, 159
    etiology, 159
    outcomes/complications, 159
    treatment, 159, 160f
Chest wall deformities, 810
Chest wall injuries
  classification, 152–153
  diagnosis/testing, 153
  epidemiology, 152–153
  etiology, 152–153
  outcomes/complications, 156
  treatment, 153–156
Chest X ray (CXR), 5, 625
  cardiac surgery, 652, 654f
  thoracic aortic aneurysms (TAAs), 720
Chi-square statistic, 891
Cholangiocarcinoma, 340, 356–358
Cholecystectomy, 358–359
Choledochal cyst, 352–353
Choledochal cysts, 813
Choledocholithiasis, 349–350
Chordae tendinae, 663
Chromaffin cells, 582
Chronic arterial and athero-occlusive disease
  clinical presentation, 749
  diagnosis, 750–751
  distribution, 747–749
  nonoperative management, 751
  operative management, 751–757, 753f

Chronic idiopathic thrombocytopenic purpura (ITP), 399
Chronic kidney disease (CKD)
  epidemiology, 782, 782t
  planning for/initiation of, 782–783
Chronic limb-threatening ischemia (CLTI), 749
Chronic lung allograft dysfunction (CLAD), 645
Chronic lymphocytic leukemia (CLL), 398
Chronic mesenteric ischemia, 727
Chronic myeloid leukemia (CML), 395–396
Chronic pancreatitis
  complications, 383–384
  diagnosis, 380–381
  etiology, 380
  treatment, 381–383
Chronic vascular rejection, 669
Chronic venous insufficiency (CVI)
  epidemiology, 764
  imaging, 765
  nomenclature, 765, 766t–767t
  nonoperative management, 765–768
  operative management, 768
  pathophysiology, 764–765
  physical examination, 765, 767f
  symptoms, 765
Chronological age, 3
Chvostek sign, 603
Cilostazol, 751
CKD. *See* Chronic kidney disease (CKD)
Clagett window, 632
Clavicle fractures, 184
Clopidogrel, 751
Cloquet's node, 558
Clostridioides difficile, 456
Clostridioides difficile infection (CDI), 81–82
Coagulopathy, 136–137
Cobblestoning, 317
Colitides
  Crohn's disease (CD), 454–455
  indeterminate colitis, 455
  infectious colitis, 456–457
  ischemic colitis, 455–456
  neutropenic enterocolitis, 457
  radiation proctocolitis, 456
  ulcerative colitis, 453–454
Colitis
  infectious, 245–247
  ischemic, 245–247
Colocutaneous fistulas, 450
Coloenteric fistulas, 450
Colon
  cancer, 461–466, 462t–463t
  colonic pseudo-obstruction, 446
  diverticular disease, 448–450, 449t
  functional constipation, 444–446
  lower gastrointestinal bleeding, 450–452, 452f
  neoplastic disease
    adenomas, 458
    colorectal neoplasms, 457
    malignant polyps, 458–461, 460t
    nonadenomatous polyps, 457–458
  normal physiology, 444
  volvulus, 446–448, 447f
Colonic pseudo-obstruction, 446
Colonoscopy, 445, 451, 517, 524–525
Color Doppler-duplex ultrasound scanning (CDDUS), 787
Colorectal cancer (CRC), 337
  adjuvant chemotherapy, 465
  clinical presentation, 461
  diagnosis and staging, 461–464
  hereditary, 462t–463t
  screening recommendations, 457, 459t, 461, 462t–463t
  surgical treatment, 464–465
Colostomy, 470–471
  abnormal rectal fixation, 480
  incontinence, 479
Colovesical fistulas, 450
Common bile duct exploration (CBDE), 359–360
Common bile duct injuries, 167
Common carotid artery (CCA), 688
Common femoral artery (CFA), 680, 680f, 733
Compartment syndrome, 205, 746, 856
Complete abortion, 824
Complete bowel rest, 308
Completion lymph node dissection (CLND), 557
Compression therapy, 765
Computed tomography (CT)
  appendicitis, 817
  cardiac surgery, 652, 654f
  cecal volvulus, 447
  colorectal cancer, 464
  Crohn's disease (CD), 454
  cryptoglandular abscess, 487
  fistula-in-ano, 489
  galactorrhea, 537
  hyperparathyroidism (HPT), 600
  inguinal hernia, 501
  lung cancer, 635
  lymphedema, 776
  melanoma, 554
  neutropenic enterocolitis, 457

Computed tomography (CT) (*continued*)
sigmoid volvulus, 446
soft tissue masses, 564
Spigelian hernias, 510
squamous cell carcinoma (SCC), 494
Computed tomography angiography (CTA), 451, 693
abdominal aortic aneurysms (AAAs), 708
acute aortic syndrome (AAS), 724
acute arterial occlusion of extremity, 741
chronic arterial and athero-occlusive disease, 750
chronic mesenteric ischemia, 727
thoracic aortic aneurysms (TAAs), 720
Condyloma acuminatum, 493–494
Confidence interval (CI), 888
Confounding variables, 893
Congenital airway malformations
bronchogenic cysts, 809
congenital lobar emphysema, 809–810
extralobar sequestrations, 809
intralobar sequestrations, 809
pulmonary sequestrations, 809
Congenital diaphragmatic hernia (CDH), 799–801, 800f
Congenital disorders, 391–394
Congenital lobar emphysema, 809–810
Congenital nevi, 564
Congenital primary lymphedema, 775
Congenital pulmonary airway malformations, 809
Congenital webs, 257
Congestive heart failure (CHF), 658
exacerbation, 54
Conn syndrome, 581
Continence, 476
Contrast-enhanced digital mammography, 533
Contrast-enhanced spiral chest computed tomography, 773
Control chart, 904, 904f
Cooper ligament repair (McVay), 507
Core needle biopsy, 534
Coronary artery anatomy, 650, 651f
Coronary artery bypass grafting (CABG), 650, 660
Coronary artery disease
acute complications, 657–658
angina pectoris, 657
chronic complications, 658
myocardial infarction (MI), 657
operative management, 658–661
Coronary artery vasculopathy, 669
Coronary sinus, 650
Cortical-sparing adrenalectomy, 585
Corticotropin-releasing hormone (CRH), 573
Cortisol, 573
Costimulation blockade, 417
Cox–Maze IV procedure (CMP-IV), 667
Cox proportional hazards regression, 891
CPB. *See* Cardiopulmonary bypass (CPB)
Cricothyroidotomy, 633
Critical care
abdomen and gastrointestinal tract, 104–106
acid–base disorders, 103
acute kidney injury, 103–104
cardiovascular, 96–97
circulatory failure, 97–102
electrolyte abnormalities, 102–103
endocrine dysfunction, 107–108
glycemic control, 107–108
hematology, 108
infection, 106–107
medications, 108, 109t–110t
monitoring
arterial pressure monitoring, 85
central venous pressure (CVP) monitoring, 85
neurologic monitoring, 86
noninvasive cardiac output (CO) monitoring, 86
pulmonary artery (PA) catheters, 85–86
respiratory monitoring, 86
temperature monitoring, 85
neurologic, 87–89, 88t
obstructive shock, 102
renal failure, 103–104
respiratory failure
acute respiratory distress syndrome (ARDS), 95–96
diagnosis, 89–90
inadequate gas exchange, 89
mechanical ventilation, 90–95, 94f
treatment, 90
shock, 101–102
specific therapy, 101–102
Crohn's colitis (CC), 454
Crohn's disease (CD), 454–455
Cross-sectional study, 884–885
Cryopreservation, of parathyroid glands, 602
Cryptoglandular abscess, 487–488, 489t
Cumulative incidence, 888
Curettage with electrodesiccation (CED), 560
Cushing syndrome, 578–581, 579f

Cutaneous cysts, 567
CVI. *See* Chronic venous insufficiency (CVI)
Cystic disease, 400–401
  intraductal papillary mucinous neoplasm (IPMN), 373, 374t
  mucinous cystic neoplasm (MCN), 374
  pancreatic pseudocyst, 371–373
  serous cystadenoma (SCA), 374–376
Cystic fibrosis (CF), 804
Cysts, breast, 535

D

Danazol, 536
Da Vinci Surgical System, 522
DeBakey classification system, of aortic dissection, 723, 724f
Decision-making capacity, 2
Deep venous thrombosis (DVT), 68–69, 70t, 71t–72t, 764
  diagnosis, 769–772
  management, 769–772
Defecation, 476, 477f
Defecography, 445
  abnormal rectal fixation, 480
Delirium, 44–46
Deoxygenated systemic venous blood, 650
Dermatofibrosarcoma protuberans, 566
Descending thoracic aorta, 702, 704f
Desmoid tumor, 567
Destination therapy, 667
Dexmedetomidine, 18
Diabetes mellitus (DM), 287
  preoperative assessment and care, 7
Dialysis, 6
  chronic kidney disease (CKD), 782–783, 782t
  hemodialysis (HD), 785–790, 785f, 788f
  peritoneal dialysis (PD), 783–785, 783t
Diaphragmatic injuries, 164–166
  classification, 152–153
  diagnosis/testing, 153
  epidemiology, 152–153
  etiology, 152–153
  outcomes/complications, 156
  treatment, 153–156
Diarrhea, 312, 317
Diet-controlled diabetes mellitus, 7
Diffuse esophageal spasm, 257
Diffuse-types of cancers, 274–275
Digital rectal examination (DRE), 444
Digital subtraction arteriography, 750
Disseminated intravascular coagulopathy (DIC), 33
  postoperative management problems, 68
Distal femur fractures, 190
Distal humerus fractures, 187
Distal radius fractures, 188
Distal tumors, 276
Diverticular disease
  complications
    diverticulitis, 448–450, 449t
    fistulization, 450
  general considerations, 448
Diverticulectomy, simple, 305
Diverticulitis
  complicated, 448
  Hinchey classification of, 448, 449t
  uncomplicated, 448
Doppler waveforms, 750
Doxazosin, 583
Dual antiplatelet therapy, 751
Ductal carcinoma in situ (DCIS), 540–541, 541f
Duhamel procedure, 809
Dumping syndrome, 294–297
Duodenal atresia, 806
Duodenal injuries, 169–170
Duplex scanning, 765
Dysplastic nevi, 564
Dyssynergic defection, 479

E

Ear anatomy, 847, 848f
Ebstein anomaly, 665
Echinococcal cysts, 336
Echocardiography, 654–655
Ectopic Cushing syndrome, 634
Ectopic pregnancy, 824–826
EGD. *See* Esophagogastroduodenoscopy (EGD)
Elastic band ligation, 483
Elbow dislocations, 187–188
Electrolyte abnormalities, 59, 61t–63t, 102–103
Electrosurgery, 27–29, 523
Embolization, 740
Emergent situations, 2
Empyema
  classification, 631
  clinical presentation/symptoms, 631
  complications, 632
  diagnosis/testing, 631–632
  epidemiology, 631
  etiology, 631
  nonoperative management, 632
  operative management, 632

End ileostomy (EI), 322–325, 445
Endobronchial ultrasound (EBUS), 637
Endocrine dysfunction, 107–108
Endometrial cancer, 830–831
Endometriosis, 312
Endometritis, 825
Endoscopic mucosal resection, 276
Endoscopic surgery, 517
Endoscopy, 451
Endovascular access, 678–681, 679t, 680f
Endovascular aortic aneurysm repair (EVAR), 709
Endovascular basics
  access, 678–681, 679t, 680f
  treating lesion, 681, 685t
  vascular lesion, 681, 682t–684t
Endovascular mechanical thrombectomy, 771
Endovenous techniques, 768
End-stage kidney disease (ESKD), 782
Enhanced recovery after surgery (ERAS), 293
Enteral feeding, 308
Enteral nutrition, 310
Epidural anesthesia, 17
Epidural hematomas (EDHs), 133
Epigastric hernias, 509
Epigastric pain, 233
Epiglottitis, 841–842
Ergonomics, 23
Eribulin, 566
Escharotomy, 201
Esophageal atresia (EA), 797
Esophageal carcinoma, 264–266
Esophageal diverticula, 258–259
Esophageal injury
  classification, 157
  diagnosis/testing, 157
  epidemiology, 157
  etiology, 157
  outcomes/complications, 157–159
  treatment, 157
Esophageal perforation, 259–260
Esophageal strictures
  acquired strictures, 257–258
  congenital webs, 257
  evaluation, 258
  symptoms, 258
  treatment, 258
Esophageal tumors
  Barrett esophagus, 261–264, 263f
  benign esophageal neoplasms, 264
  esophageal carcinoma, 264–266
Esophagogastroduodenoscopy (EGD), 451, 517, 524
Esophagus
  disorders of
    achalasia, 255–256
    diffuse esophageal spasm, 257
    gastroesophageal reflux (GERD), 252–255
    hiatal hernia, 250–252
    nutcracker/jackhammer esophagus, 257
    progressive systemic sclerosis, 257
    secondary dysmotility, 257
  esophageal diverticula, 258–259
  esophageal strictures
    acquired strictures, 257–258
    congenital webs, 257
    evaluation, 258
    symptoms, 258
    treatment, 258
  esophageal tumors
    Barrett esophagus, 261–264, 263f
    benign esophageal neoplasms, 264
    esophageal carcinoma, 264–266
  traumatic injury
    caustic ingestion, 260–261
    esophageal perforation, 259–260
Etomidate, 18
*Euro*SCORE II, 651
Excisional biopsy, 534
Excisional hemorrhoidectomy, 484–485
Exophthalmos, 616
External carotid artery (ECA), 688
External hemorrhoids, 483
External iliac artery (EIA), 733
External iliac vein, 733
Extracorporeal membrane oxygenation (ECMO), 668
Extracranial carotid artery atherosclerosis
  clinical presentation, 692
  diagnosis, 693
  epidemiology, 690
  nonoperative management, 693, 694t
  operative management, 693–698, 697f
  pathophysiology, 692
Extraintestinal manifestations, 317
Extrapleural pneumonectomy (EPP), 641
Extremity trauma
  common orthopedic implants, 178f, 179
  common orthopedic terms, 176, 177f–178f
  distal tibia and ankle
    Achilles tendon ruptures, 191
    ankle fractures, 191
    pilon fractures, 191

foot
calcaneus fractures, 191
Lisfranc injuries, 191–192
metatarsal fractures, 192
talus fractures, 191
toe fractures, 192
forearm, wrist, and hand
distal radius fractures, 188
metacarpal and phalangeal fractures, 188
radial and ulnar shaft fractures, 188
scaphoid fractures, 188
hip and femur
femoral shaft fractures, 189–190
hip dislocations, 189
hip fractures, 189
initial assessment, 179, 180t
knee and tibia
distal femur fractures, 190
knee dislocations, 190
patellar fractures, 190
tibial plateau fractures, 190
tibial shaft fractures, 190–191
management, 179, 180t
orthopedic injuries, 181t–183t
pelvic fractures
acetabular fractures, 189
pelvic ring disruption, 188–189
pubic rami fractures, 189
sacral fractures, 189
Young–Burgess classification, 188
peripheral nerve examination, 180t
shoulder
acromioclavicular dislocations, 187
clavicle fractures, 184
dislocations (glenohumeral), 184–187
proximal humerus fractures, 184
scapula fractures, 184
sternoclavicular (SC) dislocations, 187
upper arm and elbow
distal humerus fractures, 187
elbow dislocations, 187–188
humeral shaft fractures, 187
radial head fractures, 187
Extubation, 38–39
Exudative pleural effusions, 628
Ex vivo lung perfusion (EVLP), 644–645

F

Facial injuries, 133, 134t
Facial trauma, 851–855, 855t
Familial atypical multiple-mole melanoma syndrome, 553
Familial hypocalciuric hypercalcemia (FHH), 600
Felty syndrome, 403
Femoral hernias
anatomy of, 507
clinical presentation, 507
incidence of, 507
treatment
femoral approach, 508
inguinal approach, 507
preperitoneal approach, 507–508
Femoral shaft fractures, 189–190
Femoral thromboembolectomy, 743–744
Femorofemoral bypass, 753
Fentanyl, 18
FES. *See* Fundamentals of Endoscopic Surgery (FES)
Fever, postoperative management, 73–74
Fiberoptic bronchoscopy, 638
Fibroadenomas, 535–536, 547
Fibrocystic breast change (FBC), 535
Fibromas, 312
Fine-needle aspiration (FNA)
hyperparathyroidism (HPT), 600
thyroid nodules, 606, 606t, 607f
Fine-needle aspiration biopsy (FNAB), 534, 551
Fisher's exact test, 891
Fistula-in-ano, 488–491, 490f–491f, 492t
Fistulas
anatomic considerations, 305, 306t
defined, 305
diagnosis, 306–307
etiology, 305, 307t
nonoperative treatment, 307–309
operative management, 309, 309t
pathophysiology, 306
Fistulization, 450
Fistulogram, 789
Fistulography, 306
Flail chest, 121
Flexible endoscopy, 517
Flexor tendon injury, zones of, 857f
Flexor tenosynovitis, 856, 858t
FLS. *See* Fundamentals of Laparoscopic Surgery (FLS)
Fluid requirements, of children, 795, 795t
Focal nodular hyperplasia (FNH), 333–334
Focused Assessment Sonography in Trauma (FAST) examination, 128, 129f
Fogarty (balloon) catheter, 744
Foker process, 799

Follicular cells, 599
Follicular thyroid cancer (FTC), 610
Fournier gangrene, 491, 876. *See also* Necrotizing anorectal infection
Frailty, 3
Frostbite, 205–206
Functional capacity, 3
Functional recovery, 137–138
Functional status assessment, 3
Fundamentals of Endoscopic Surgery (FES), 523
Fundamentals of Laparoscopic Surgery (FLS), 522–523
Fundamental Use of Surgical Energy (FUSE), 523
Fusiform aneurysms, 708–710

G

68-Ga DOTATATE positron emission tomography, 583
Gaiter distribution, 765
Galactorrhea, 537
Gallbladder
  cancer, 353–356
  injuries, 167
Gallstone
  formation, 294
  ileus, 303
Ganglion cysts, 568
Gastrectomy, 276
Gastric adenocarcinoma, 274–277
  classification, 274–277
  epidemiology/etiology, 274
Gastric band surgery, 289
Gastric injuries, 169
Gastrin, 270
Gastrinomas, 593
Gastroesophageal reflux (GERD), 252–255
Gastrointestinal considerations
  postoperative management problems
    bowel obstruction, 67
    nausea, 60–66
    paralytic ileus, 66–67
    vomiting, 60–66
Gastrointestinal stromal tumors (GISTs), 279–280
Gastrointestinal tract, 104–106
Gastroparesis, 272–274
  classification, 272
  diagnosis/testing, 273
  epidemiology, 272
  etiology, 272
  nonoperative treatment, 273
  operative treatment, 273–274
  presentation/symptoms, 273
Gastroschisis, 801–802
Gastroscopes, 517
Genitourinary infections, 8
Genitourinary trauma, 877–878, 878f
Geriatric syndromes, 2–3
Germ cell tumors, 642–643
3.5-Gland parathyroidectomy, 593, 602
Glasgow Coma Scale (GCS), 132
Gleevec. *See* Imatinib
Glenohumeral dislocations, 184–187
Global Limb Anatomic Staging System (GLASS), 751
Glucocorticoid-suppressible aldosteronism, 581
Glucose-6-phosphate dehydrogenase (G6PD) deficiency, 394
Glycemic control, 107–108
Gonadorelin, 536
Goodsall's rule, 489, 491f
Granulomas, 317
Granulomatous mastitis, 537–538
Graves' disease (autoimmune diffuse toxic goiter)
  classification, 615
  clinical presentation/symptoms, 615
  diagnosis/testing, 615
  epidemiology, 615
  etiology, 615
  nonoperative treatment, 615–616
  operative treatment, 616
  outcomes/complications, 616
Greater saphenous vein (GSV), 733, 761
Gustilo classification, 862, 865t
Gynecologic malignancies
  cervical carcinoma, 829–830
  endometrial cancer, 830–831
  ovarian carcinoma, 831–832
  vulvar carcinoma, 828–829
Gynecologic surgical anatomy, 827, 828f
Gynecomastia, 538

H

Hairy cell leukemia, 398–399
Haller index, 810
Hamartomatous polyps, 458
Handoff, 39
Hand trauma, 855–858, 856t, 858t
Hartmann procedure, 447
Hashimoto thyroiditis, 611, 616
Hasson cannula, 519
Hasson technique, 519–521

Hawthorne effect, 893
Hazard ratio (HR), 889
HD. *See* Hemodialysis (HD)
Headache, 17
Head injuries
  management of, 136–138
  radiographic evaluation, 133, 134t
  types of
    acute subdural hematomas, 134
    cerebral contusions, 134
    chronic SDHs, 134
    epidural hematomas (EDHs), 133
    intraparenchymal hemorrhages, 135
    skull and facial fractures, 136
Head/neck masses. *See also* Pediatric surgery
  branchial cleft cyst, 814
  lymphatic malformation, 815
  thyroglossal duct cysts, 814–815
Healthcare Cost and Utilization Project (HCUP), 887
Health care power of attorney (HCPOA), 2
Healthy Worker effect, 892
Heart failure, surgical treatment of
  epidemiology, 667
  heart transplantation, 669
  mechanical circulatory support (MCS), 667–669
Heart transplantation, 432, 667, 669
Hedgehog pathway inhibitors, 561
Helicobacter pylori, 289
Hemangioma, 333
Hematochezia, 451
Hematologic diseases
  acquired disorders, 394–400
  congenital disorders, 391–394
Hematuria, 867
Hemiazygous vein, 620
Hemodialysis (HD)
  physiology, 785
  vascular access, types of, 785f
    arteriovenous access (AVA), 787, 789–790
    arteriovenous fistula (AVF), 787–789, 788f
    arteriovenous graft (AVG), 789
    catheters, 785–786
Hemoglobinopathies, 391–392
Hemolytic anemias, 392–394
Hemophilia, 32
Hemorrhage, 521, 614
Hemorrhagic shock, 121–124, 122t
Hemorrhoids
  classification of, 483f
  etiology, 482
  evaluation, 482–483
  symptoms, 482
  treatment, 483f
    nonoperative, 483–484
    operative procedures for, 484–485, 484t
Hemostasis, 680
  coagulation, inherited and acquired disorders of, 31–33
  inherited and acquired disorders, 31–33
  lab assessment of, 35
  mechanisms, 30–31
  techniques, 33–34
  thrombus formation, 30–31
Hemothorax, 120
Heparin-induced thrombocytopenia (HIT), 32–33
  postoperative management problems, 67–68
Heparinize, 678
Hepatectomy, 341–342
Hepatic adenoma, 334–335
Hepatic injuries, 166–167
Hepatic transection, 342
Hepatic venous pressure gradient, 332
Hepatocellular carcinoma (HCC), 338–339, 339f
Hereditary breast cancer, 532
Hereditary elliptocytosis, 393
Hereditary endocrine tumor syndromes
  multiple endocrine neoplasia type 1 (MEN-1), 592–593, 592t
  multiple endocrine neoplasia type 2 (MEN-2), 593–594
Hereditary spherocytosis, 392–393
Hernias. *See also specific types*
  abdominal wall, 508–514
  femoral, 507–508
  inguinal, 499–507
Hesselbach triangle, 500
Hiatal hernia, 250–252
Hidradenitis suppurativa, 493
High spinal blockade, 17
Hinchey classification, complicated diverticulitis, 448, 449t
Hip
  disarticulation, 755
  dislocations, 189
  fractures, 189
Hirschsprung disease, 804, 807–809
Histamine, 270
Hodgkin lymphoma, 397

Hollenhorst plaques, 692
Horner syndrome, 634
Howship–Romberg sign, 510
HPT. *See* Hyperparathyroidism (HPT)
Human epidermal growth factor receptor 2 (HER2)/neu, 540
Human papillomavirus (HPV), 828
Humeral shaft fractures, 187
Hydrogen cyanide poisoning, 205
Hydronephrosis, 868–870
Hypercortisolism, 578–581, 579f
Hyperparathyroidism (HPT), 592–593
  clinical outcomes, 602
  clinical presentation/symptoms, 600
  complications, 602–603
  diagnosis/testing, 600
  nerve injury and hemorrhage, 603
  nonoperative treatment, 600–601
  operative treatment, 601–602, 601t
  persistent disease/missed glands, 603
  primary, 599
  secondary, 599–600
  tertiary, 600
Hyperpigmentation, 765
Hyperplastic polyps, 457–458
Hypertension, 53
Hyperthyroidism, 599
Hypertrophic cardiomyopathy, 666–667
Hypertrophic pyloric stenosis (HPS), 810–811
Hypocalcemia, 602–603, 614
Hypoglossal nerve, 688
Hypotension, 17
  postoperative management problems, 52–53
  preoperative assessment and care, 17
Hypothermia, 205, 206t
Hypothyroidism, 599

I

Idiopathic hyperaldosteronism, 581
Ileocolectomy, 447
Ileorectal anastomosis (IRA), 445
Ileostomy closure, 322, 323f–324f
Ileus, 301
Imatinib, 280
Imiquimod, 494
Immortal time bias, 893
Immune checkpoint proteins, 558
Immune-mediated hemolytic anemias, 394–395
Immunosuppression, 416f
  antiproliferative agents/antimetabolites, 416
  antithymocyte antibodies, 417, 418f
  calcineurin inhibitors, 416–417
  classes of, 414, 416f
  complications of, 418–419
  corticosteroids, 416
  costimulation blockade, 417
  dosing and indications for, 414t–415t
  mTOR inhibitors, 417
Incarcerated inguinal hernias, 501
Incomplete abortion, 824
Indeterminate colitis, 455
Inevitable abortion, 824
Infarction, 301
Infectious colitis, 245–247, 456–457
Infectious complications
  assessment, 8
  morbidity and mortality, 7
  patient-specific risk factors, 8
  procedure-specific risk factors, 8
  prophylaxis, 8
Infective endocarditis, 665–666
Inferior glands, 597
Inferior mesenteric artery (IMA), 704
Inferior vena cava (IVC), 771
  compression, 826
  placement, 771–772
  removal, 772
Inflammatory bowel disease (IBD), 452
  Crohn's disease (CD), 454–455
  indeterminate colitis, 455
  ulcerative colitis (UC), 453–454
Inguinal hernia, 818
  anatomy of, 499–501, 500f
  classification of, 499
  diagnosis of
    clinical presentation, 501
    physical examination, 501
    radiographic evaluation, 501
  incidence of, 499
  terminology, 499–501
  treatment
    laparoscopic/minimally invasive inguinal hernia repair, 504–507, 504f–505f
    open tension-free repairs (with mesh), 503–504
    preoperative evaluation and preparation, 501–502
    primary tissue repairs (without mesh), 502–503
    reduction, 502
    surgical, 502, 502f

Initial trauma evaluation
  primary survey, 132
  secondary survey, 132–133
Innate immune system, 412
Innominate artery, 688
Insufflation, 518–519
Insulin-dependent diabetic patients, 7
Intermittent pneumatic compression, 775
Internal hemorrhoids, 483
Interstitial cells of Cajal, 279
Interviewer bias, 893
Intestinal injuries, 170
Intestinal-type cancers, 274
Intra-abdominal abscess, 80
Intra-aortic balloon pump (IABP), 657, 667–668
Intracranial hypertension, 137t
Intracranial injuries, 126
Intrahepatic biliary cysts, 336–337
Intralesional therapy, 560
In-transit metastases, 555
Intraoperative considerations
  anesthesia, 14–20, 16t, 20t
  electrosurgery, 27–29
  ergonomics, 23
  extubation, 38–39
  handoff, 39
  hemostasis, 30–35, 34t
  intraoperative monitoring, 29–30
  operating room, culture of safety in, 13
  operation, 25–27, 26f–27f
  patient positioning, 20–23, 22t
  preparation and draping, 23–25
  timeout, surgical, 13, 14t
  transfusion, 35–38, 35f, 37t
Intraoperative monitoring, 29–30
Intraparenchymal hemorrhages, 135
Intravascular volume expansion, 7
Intravascular volume status, 6
Intussusception, 812
  internal, 480, 480f, 481t
Invasive breast cancer
  breast conservation therapy (BCT), 542
  histologies, 541
  locally advanced breast cancer (LABC), 546
  modified radical mastectomy (MRM), 543
  radical (Halsted) mastectomy, 543
  surgical options, for early-stage, 541
Invasive monitoring, 129
Irritable bowel syndrome, 444
Irubin, international normalized ratio (INR), 332
Ischemic cardiomyopathy, 658
Ischemic colitis, 245–247, 455–456
Isolated limb infusion (ILI), 560
Isolated limb perfusion (ILP), 560
Isolated small-bowel transplants, 312

J
Jaundice, 813
Jejunoileal intestinal atresia, 806
Juxtacarotid structures
  nerves, 688–689, 691f
  veins, 688, 690f

K
Kaplan–Meier (K-M) method, 891
Kasai hepatoportoenterostomy, 813–814
Ketamine, 18–19
Kidney
  diseases of, 868
  transplantation, 423–426
Kinase inhibitors, 558–559
Knee dislocations, 190
Kocher incision, 601
Kono-S anastomosis, 326, 326f

L
Lactate dehydrogenase, 554
Lactation, 536
Lactational mastitis, 537
Ladd's bands, 804
Lambert–Eaton syndrome, 635
Laparoscopic adrenalectomy, 588
Laparoscopic appendectomy, 438
Laparoscopic gastric resections, 276
Laparoscopic inguinal hernia repair, 504–507, 504f–505f
Laparoscopic sigmoid colectomy, 449–450
Laparoscopic surgery
  abdominal access, 519–521
  equipment and troubleshooting
    imaging system, 519, 520f
    insufflation, 518–519
    room setup and positioning, 518
  limitations, 518
  patient selection, 518
  physiologic effects of
    cardiovascular, 521
    neurologic, 522
    pulmonary, 521
    renal, 522
  port removal and closure, 521
  principles, 517–518
Laparoscopic transabdominal left adrenalectomy, 589

Laparoscopic transabdominal right adrenalectomy, 588–589, 590f–591f
Laparoscopy
  in pregnancy, 826–827
  Spigelian hernias, 510
Laparotomy, 447
Larynx
  anatomy, 839, 840f–841f
  infectious/inflammatory disorders, 839–842
  neoplasms, 842
  trauma/injury, 842
  upper airway obstruction, management
    emergent cricothyrotomy, 842
    nonsurgical airway options, 842
    physical examination, 842
    tracheal stenosis, 844
    tracheostomy, 842–844
Lateral internal sphincterotomy (LIS), 486–487
Lauren Classification system, 274
Lead-time bias, 893
Lean framework, 902
Left anterior descending artery (LAD), 650
Left brachiocephalic vein, 702
Left circumflex artery (LCx), 650
Left internal mammary artery (LIMA), 659
Left-sided heart (atriofemoral) bypass, 722
Left vagus nerve, 702, 704f
Leonardo vein, 761
Leriche syndrome, 749
Leser–Trélat sign, 563
LGIB. *See* Lower gastrointestinal bleeding (LGIB)
Lichtenstein repair, 503–504
Ligamentum arteriosum, 722
Light's criteria, 628
Linear regression, 891
Lipodermatosclerosis, 765
Lipomas, 568
Liposarcoma, 565
Lisfranc injuries, 191–192
Littré hernia, 305, 500
Liver
  abscesses and cystic disease
    amebic abscesses, 336
    echinococcal cysts, 336
    intrahepatic biliary cysts, 336–337
    pyogenic abscesses, 335–336
  anatomic features, 330
  associating liver partition and portal vein ligation for staged hepatectomy (ALPPS), 343
  benign liver tumors
    focal nodular hyperplasia (FNH), 333–334
    hemangioma, 333
    hepatic adenoma, 334–335
  disease, 32
  inflow
    arterial, 330
    venous, 330
  malignant liver tumors
    cholangiocarcinoma, 340
    hepatocellular carcinoma (HCC), 338–339, 339f
  metastatic disease
    colorectal cancer (CRC), 337
    neuroendocrine tumors, 338
  outflow
    biliary, 330
    venous, 330
  physiology, 331–333
    bile, 331
    bilirubin, 331
    laboratory testing, 331
    liver failure and cirrhosis, 331–332
  portal vein embolization, 342
  segmental and surgical anatomy, 330
  specific resections
    complications, 342
    hepatectomy, 341–342
    hepatic transection, 342
    segmental resections, 341
    wedge resections, 340
  transplant, 427–430
  two-stage hepatectomy, 343
Liver function tests (LFTs), 539
Lobular carcinoma in situ (LCIS), 535, 539
Locally advanced breast cancer (LABC)
  inflammatory, 546, 546f
Logistic regression, 891
Loop ileostomy closure, 322, 323f–324f
Low-dose unfractionated heparin (LDUH), 774
Lower extremity, vascular anatomy of, 734f–739f
Lower gastrointestinal bleeding (LGIB)
  causes of, 450
  computed tomography angiogram, 451
  endoscopy in, 451
  management, 450–451
  massive, 450–451
  mesenteric angiography in, 452
  nuclear scan in, 451, 452f

Low-molecular-weight heparin (LMWH), 774
Ludwig angina, 837
Lumbar hernia, 510
Lung
 abscess, 632
 anatomy, 620, 621f–623f
 injury
  classification, 159
  diagnosis/testing, 159
  epidemiology, 159
  etiology, 159
  outcomes/complications, 159
  treatment, 159, 160f
 neuroendocrine tumor, 634
 transplantation, 432
  donor selection, 643, 644t
  ex vivo lung perfusion (EVLP), 644–645
  indications, 643
  outcomes and complications, 645
  surgical approach, 643–644
Lung cancer
 clinical presentation, 634–635, 635f–636f
 complications after lung resection, 639–640
 diagnosis
  computed tomography (CT), 635
  positron emission tomography (PET), 637
  tissue biopsy, 637
 epidemiology, 633
 etiology, 633
 management by stage, 638
 nonoperative management, 638–639
 operative management, 639
 pathology, 633–634
 screening, 633
 staging, 637–638
 surveillance, 640
Lymphangitis, 777
Lymphatic malformation, 815
Lymphedema, 545, 558
 classification, 775–776
 differential diagnosis, 776
 epidemiology, 775
 imaging, 776
 nonoperative management, 776–777
 operative management, 777
 pathophysiology, 775–776
 physical examination, 776
 symptoms, 776
Lymphomas, 469–470, 643, 839
Lymphoproliferative disorders, 397–399
Lymphoscintigraphy, 775–776

M

Magnetic resonance angiography (MRA), 693
 abdominal aortic aneurysms (AAAs), 708
 acute aortic syndrome (AAS), 724
 chronic arterial and athero-occlusive disease, 750–751
 thoracic aortic aneurysms (TAAs), 720
Magnetic resonance imaging (MRI)
 abdominal aortic aneurysms (AAAs), 708
 breast, 534
 colorectal cancer, 464
 Crohn's disease (CD), 454
 galactorrhea, 537
 lymphedema, 776
 melanoma, 554
 rectal cancer, 466, 467f
 soft tissue masses, 564
Major adverse cardiac events (MACE), 4
Major (oblique) fissure, 620
Malignant liver tumors
 cholangiocarcinoma, 340
 hepatocellular carcinoma (HCC), 338–339, 339f
Malignant polyps, of colon and rectum
 Haggitt classification, 458, 460t
 Kudo classification, 458, 460t
Malnutrition, 9
Malrotation, 804–806
Mammoplasty
 augmentation, 866
 reduction, 866
Marfan syndrome, 720
Marjolin ulcers, 562
Massive hemoptysis, 632–633
Mastalgia, 536
Mastectomy
 modified radical mastectomy (MRM), 543
 nipple-sparing, 542
 radical (Halsted), 543
 skin-sparing, 542
Mastitis
 granulomatous, 537–538
 lactational, 537
McVay repair, 503
Mechanical circulatory support (MCS), 667–669
Mechanical ventilation, 90–95, 94f

Meckel's diverticulum
  diagnosis, 305
  management, 303–305
  treatment, 305
Meconium ileus, 804
Meconium syndromes, 804
Median sternotomy, 659–660
Mediastinal anatomy, 620–621
Mediastinoscopy, 637
Mediastinum, tumors of
  anterior mediastinal masses, 642–643
  clinical presentation, 642
  differential diagnosis of, 641, 641t
  epidemiology, 641–642
  etiology, 641–642
  middle mediastinal masses, 643
  posterior mediastinal masses, 643
  radiographic evaluation, 642
Medullary thyroid cancer (MTC), 610
Melanoma
  ABCDEs of, 551, 552f
  anorectal, 496
  cutaneous, 555, 555f
  diagnosis, 553–554
  epidemiology, 551–553
  etiology, 551–553
  imaging and laboratory studies, 554
  perioperative systemic therapy
    immunotherapy, 558
    kinase inhibitors, 558–559
  regional therapies for, 560
  risk factors, 553–554, 554t
  rule of two's and three's for, 554, 554t
  staging, 554–555
  treatment
    completion lymph node dissection (CLND), 557
    melanoma excision, complications of, 558
    metastases, resection of, 558
    neoadjuvant, 559, 559f
    sentinel lymph node biopsy (SLNB), 557
    sentinel nodes, detection of, 557
    surgical management, 555, 556f
    therapeutic lymph node dissection (TLND), 557–558
    wide local excision (WLE), 555–557
Melena, 451
MelMarT trial, 555
MEN-2A, 594
MEN-2B, 594
Merkel cell carcinoma, 563
Merkel cell polyoma virus (MCPyV), 563
Mesenteric angiography, 452
Mesenteric ischemia, 243–244, 726–727
Mesenteric whirl, 446
Mesh plug, 504
Mesothelioma, 640–641
Meta-analysis, 886–887
Metacarpal/phalangeal fractures, 188
Metastatic disease
  colorectal cancer (CRC), 337
  neuroendocrine tumors, 338
Metatarsal fractures, 192
Methimazole, 616
Metronidazole, 457
Miami criterion, 601
Microbiota, intraluminal, 444
Micronutrient supplementation, 203
Microporous polytetrafluoroethylene (PTFE) mesh, 511
Midazolam, 18
Midbody tumors, 276
Middle mediastinal masses, 643
Mild autonomous cortisol secretion (MACS), 578
Minimally invasive approach
  endoscopic surgery, 517
  flexible endoscopy, 517
  inguinal hernia repair, 504–507, 504f–505f
  laparoscopic surgery, 517–522
  parathyroidectomy, 601
  robotic surgery, 522
  splenectomy, 404
Minor (horizontal) fissure, 620
Missed abortion, 824
Mitotane, 585
Mitral regurgitation (MR), 658, 663–664
  primary, 664
  secondary, 664
Mitral stenosis (MS), 663
Mixed venous oxygen saturation, 669
Model for end-stage liver disease (MELD), 332
Modified radical mastectomy (MRM), 543
Mohs micrographic surgery, 560
Mondor disease, 536
Monoclonal antibodies, 558
Monopolar instruments, 523
MRA. *See* Magnetic resonance angiography (MRA)
Multiple endocrine neoplasia type 1 (MEN-1), 592–593, 592t

Multiple endocrine neoplasia type 2 (MEN-2), 593–594
Multivisceral transplantations, 312
Musculoskeletal disorders (MSDs), 23
Myasthenia gravis (MG), 642
Myelofibrosis, 396–397
Myeloproliferative/myelodysplastic disorders, 395–397
Myocardial infarction (MI), 657
Myocardial ischemia, 670
Myocardial revascularization, 658
Myocardial stunning, 669
Myxofibrosarcoma, 566

N

Nasopharynx, 847
Nausea, postoperative management, 60–66
Neck
  anatomy, 832, 833f–834f
  cervical spine injuries, 138–141, 139f
    penetrating, 138–140, 139f
    radiographic evaluation, 140–141
  infectious disorders of
    acute mononucleosis, 832
    bacterial lymphadenitis, 832
    deep neck space infections, 832–837
  larynx
    anatomy, 839, 840f–841f
    infectious/inflammatory disorders, 839–842
    neoplasms, 842
    trauma/injury, 842
    upper airway obstruction, 842–844
  masses, 832, 835f–836f
  neoplasms
    benign, 837
    malignant, 837–839, 838t
Necrotizing enterocolitis, 802–804, 803f, 805f
Necrotizing fasciitis, 834
Necrotizing infections, 858
Necrotizing soft tissue infections (NSTI), 74–80
Needle-access segment (NAS), 787
Needle thoracostomy, 626–627
Negative predictive value (NPV), 890
Negative pressure wound therapy (NPWT), 223, 228–229, 228f, 849
Neonatal surgical conditions. *See also* Pediatric surgery
  abdominal wall defects, 801–802
  anorectal malformations, 807, 808f
  congenital diaphragmatic hernia (CDH), 799–801, 800f
  duodenal atresia, 806
  Hirschsprung disease, 807–809
  jejunoileal intestinal atresia, 806
  malrotation, 804–806
  meconium syndromes, 804
  necrotizing enterocolitis, 802–804, 803f, 805f
  tracheoesophageal malformations, 797–799, 798f–799f
Neoplasms, 401–402, 815–817. *See also* Tumors
  benign tumors, 312
  biliary, 353–358
  larynx
    benign, 842
    complications, 842
    malignant, 842
  malignant tumors, 312, 316
  metastatic disease, 316
  neck
    benign, 837
    malignant, 837–839, 838t
  salivary glands, 845–847
  spleen, 401–402
Neostigmine, 446
Nerve injury, 615
Neuroendocrine tumor (NET), 338, 439–440, 470
Neurofibromas, 312, 567–568
Neurofibromatosis type 1, 567
Neurogenic shock, 125
Neurologic considerations
  postoperative management problems
    altered mental status (AMS), 44
    anesthesia, delayed emergence from, 43–44
    delirium, 44–46
    seizures, 46–47
    withdrawal, 47–48
Neurologic monitoring, 86
Neuromuscular blockade, reversal of, 38–39
Neuropathic ulcers, 750
Neutropenic enterocolitis, 457
Nipple discharge
  benign intraductal papilloma, 537
  galactorrhea, 537
  lactation, 536
  pathologic, 537
Nipple-sparing mastectomy, 542
Nitrates, 486
Nonacute scrotal masses, 876–877

Nonadenomatous polyps, 457–458
Nonfunctional adrenocortical adenoma, 586–587
Non-Hodgkin lymphoma (NHL), 397
Noninvasive cardiac output (CO) monitoring, 86
Nonmelanoma skin cancers
basal cell carcinoma (BCC), 560–561
Merkel cell carcinoma, 563
squamous cell carcinoma (SCC), 561–563
Nonobstetric surgery, in pregnant patient, 826–827
Nonopiate adjuncts, 50, 50t
Nonpuerperal abscesses, 538
Nonseminomatous germ cell tumors, 643
Non–small cell lung carcinoma (NSCLC), 634
Nonsteroidal anti-inflammatory drugs (NSAIDs)
desmoid tumor, 567
thyroiditis, 617
Normetanephrines, 575
Nose/paranasal sinuses, 847
Null hypothesis (H_0), 887
Number needed to treat/number needed to harm (NNT/NNH), 888
Nutcracker/jackhammer esophagus, 257
Nutrition, 59–60, 64t–66t
Nutritional deficiencies, 297
Nutrition, in children, 795, 796t

O

Obesity
bariatric surgery techniques, 290t
biliopancreatic diversion with duodenal switch (BPD-DS), 292–293, 292f
gastric band surgery, 289
long-term surveillance, 297
postoperative issues and complications, 294–297, 295f, 296f
postoperative management, 293
Roux-en-Y gastric bypass (RYGB), 291–292, 291f
sleeve gastrectomy, 289–291, 290f
classification, 285t
comorbidities, 286t
definition, 285
epidemiology, 285
nonsurgical management of, 285, 286f
preoperative assessment and care, 9
preoperative evaluation/optimization, 288–289
treatment, 285, 286f
weight loss surgery, 287t
Obstetric/gynecologic disorders, 822–826, 822f, 823t
gynecologic malignancies
cervical carcinoma, 829–830
endometrial cancer, 830–831
ovarian carcinoma, 831–832
vulvar carcinoma, 828–829
gynecologic surgical anatomy, 827, 828f
nonobstetric surgery, in pregnant patient, 826–827
Obstipation, 301
Obstruction
complete, 301
partial, 301
Obstructive defection disorders, 479
Obstructive shock, 102
Obturator hernias, 510
Odds ratio (OR), 889
Ogilvie syndrome, 446
Ohm's law, 523
Olaratumab, 566
Omphalocele, 801
Oncotype Dx, 540
Open appendectomy, 438
Open splenectomy, 404
Open tension-free repairs (with mesh), 503–504
Open wound care options, 223
Operation
closure considerations, 25
skin closure, 27
steps in, 25, 26f
Opiates, 48–50
Oral cavity, 844, 845f–846f
Oral hypoglycemic agents, 7
Orbital compartment syndrome, 851
Organ allocation, 419–421
Organ donation, 421–422
Organ preservation, 423
Organ transplantation
kidney transplantation, 423–426
liver transplant, 427–430
lung and heart transplant, 432
pancreas transplant, 430–432
small intestine transplant, 432
Orthopedic injuries, 181t–183t
Ovarian carcinoma, 831–832
Ovarian torsion, 825
Ovary, 827
Oxygenated pulmonary venous blood, 650
Oxygenation, 621–622
Oxyphil cells, 599

P

Pacemakers, patients with, preoperative management, 4
PAD. *See* Peripheral arterial disease (PAD)
Paget disease, 495
  nipple, 547
Paired t-test, 890
Pancoast tumor, 634
Pancreas
  acute pancreatitis
    complications of, 379
    diagnosis, 376–378, 376t
    etiology, 376
    treatment, 378
  anatomy, 362, 362f
  blood supply, 362–363
  chronic pancreatitis
    complications, 383–384
    diagnosis, 380–381
    etiology, 380
    treatment, 381–383
  cystic disease
    intraductal papillary mucinous neoplasm (IPMN), 373, 374t
    mucinous cystic neoplasm (MCN), 374
    pancreatic pseudocyst, 371–373
    serous cystadenoma (SCA), 374–376
  divisum, 363–364
  embryology
    annular pancreas, 364
    pancreas divisum, 363–364
  pancreatic ductal adenocarcinoma
    complications, 368
    diagnosis, 364–365
    epidemiology, 364
    etiology, 364
    treatment, 366–368, 366f
  pancreatic neuroendocrine tumors (pNETs)
    diagnosis, 368–370
    etiology, 368, 369t
    treatment, 370
  pseduotumors, 370
  rare neoplasms, 370
  transplant, 430–432
Pancreatic ductal adenocarcinoma
  complications, 368
  diagnosis, 364–365
  epidemiology, 364
  etiology, 364
  treatment, 366–368, 366f
Pancreatic injuries, 169
Pancreatic islet cell tumors, 593
Pancreatic neuroendocrine tumors (pNETs)
  diagnosis, 368–370
  etiology, 368, 369t
  treatment, 370
Papanicolaou (Pap) testing, 829
Papillary muscle rupture, 658
Papillary thyroid cancer (PTC), 610
Paragangliomas, 573, 582–585, 837
Paralytic ileus, 303
  postoperative management, 66–67
Paranasal sinuses, 847
Paraneoplastic syndromes, 634–635
Paraphimosis, 874
Pararectal space, 827
Parathyroid autotransplantation, 602
Parathyroid cancer
  classification, 603
  clinical presentation/symptoms, 603–604
  diagnosis/testing, 604
  epidemiology, 603
  etiology, 603
  nonoperative treatment, 604
  operative treatment, 604
  outcomes/complications, 604
Parathyroid glands
  anatomy, 597, 598f
  histology, 599
  physiology, 598
Parathyroid hormone (PTH), 598
Paravesical space, 827
Parenteral nutrition, 795, 796t
Pareto chart, 903, 903f
Parietal pain, 233
Partial mastectomy, 541
Passive rewarming, 205
Patellar fractures, 190
Patient positioning, 22 (table)
Patient-reported outcomes (PROs), 902
Patient safety (PS), 897
  consistent and systematic methods, 900
  organizational approach, 898
  reliable, safe, and easy-to-use reporting systems, 899
  systematic approach, 898–899, 898f, 899t, 900f
  vocabulary, 897
Pazopanib, 566
PD. *See* Peritoneal dialysis (PD)
Pediatric general surgical conditions
  appendicitis, 817
  inguinal hernias, 818
  trauma, 818–819
  umbilical hernia, 818

Pediatric surgery
  abdominal pathology
    hepatobiliary, 813–814
    hypertrophic pyloric stenosis (HPS), 810–811
    intussusception, 812
  fluid requirements, 795, 795t
  general surgical conditions
    appendicitis, 817
    inguinal hernias, 818
    trauma, 818–819
    umbilical hernia, 818
  head/neck masses
    branchial cleft cyst, 814
    lymphatic malformation, 815
    thyroglossal duct cysts, 814–815
  neonatal surgical conditions
    abdominal wall defects, 801–802
    anorectal malformations, 807, 808f
    congenital diaphragmatic hernia (CDH), 799–801, 800f
    duodenal atresia, 806
    Hirschsprung disease, 807–809
    jejunoileal intestinal atresia, 806
    malrotation, 804–806
    meconium syndromes, 804
    necrotizing enterocolitis, 802–804, 803f, 805f
    tracheoesophageal malformations, 797–799, 798f–799f
  nutrition, 795, 796t
  thoracic pathology
    chest wall deformities, 810
    congenital airway malformations, 809–810
  tumors/neoplasms
    neuroblastoma, 815–816
    soft tissue sarcomas, 817
    teratomas, 816
    Wilms tumor, 816, 817t
Pelvic avascular spaces, 827
Pelvic fractures
  acetabular fractures, 189
  pelvic ring disruption, 188–189
  pubic rami fractures, 189
  sacral fractures, 189
  Young–Burgess classification, 188
Pelvic inflammatory disease, 825
Pelvic pain, 825–826
Pelvic ring disruption, 188–189
Penetrating aortic ulcer (PAU), 723
Penile fracture, 878
Penis, diseases of, 874–875
Pepsin, 271
Peptic ulcer disease, 280–281
Percutaneous catheter, 627
Percutaneous retrograde common femoral artery access, 681
Perforated appendicitis, 438
Perianal fistula, 488
PeriOperative ISchemic Evaluation (POISE) trial, 4
Perioperative systemic chemotherapy, 277
Peripheral arterial disease (PAD)
  acute arterial occlusion of extremity
    clinical management, 743–746
    clinical presentation, 740–741
    complications, 746–747, 748f
    diagnosis, 741–743, 742t
    etiology, 740
  chronic arterial and athero-occlusive disease
    clinical presentation, 749
    diagnosis, 750–751
    distribution, 747–749
    nonoperative management, 751
    operative management, 751–757, 753f
  epidemiology, 736
  pathophysiology/etiology, 736–740
Peripheral nerve, 864–865, 865t–866t
Peritoneal dialysis (PD)
  catheter placement, 783–784
  complications, 784–785
  indications/contraindications, 783, 783t
  physiology, 783
Peritonitis, 447
Periumbilical pain, 233
Pharmacomechanical thrombectomy, 744
Pharynx, 844, 846f
Pheochromocytoma, 573, 611
  diagnosis, 583, 584f
  epidemiology, 582–583
  etiology, 582–583
  treatment, 583–585
Phimosis, 874–875
Phlebitis, 769
Phlegmasia alba dolens, 769
Phlegmasia cerulea dolens, 769–770
Phospholipase C, 270
Phyllodes tumors, 548
Pilon fractures, 191
Pilonidal cyst
  diagnosis, 492
  etiology, 491–492
  treatment, 493
Pituitary tumors, 593

Plasma aldosterone concentration (PAC), 581
Plasma metanephrines, 575
Plasma renin activity (PRA), 581
Plastic/reconstructive surgery
  acute injuries
    facial trauma, 851–855, 855t
    hand trauma, 855–858, 856t, 858t
  aesthetic surgery, 866–867
  lower extremity, 862–864, 865t
  peripheral nerve, 864–865, 865t–866t
  scalp, 858–859, 859f, 859t
  techniques and principles
    flap types, 850, 850t, 851f–854f, 854t
    graft types, 849–850, 849f
    reconstructive elevator, 849
    tissue expansion, 850–851
  trunk
    abdominal wall reconstruction, 862, 864f
    breast reconstruction, 859–861, 860f, 861t
    chest wall reconstruction, 861–862, 863f
    pressure sores, 862
Platelet disorders, 399–400
Pleural effusion, 629f
  classification, 628
  clinical presentation, 629
  diagnosis/testing, 629
  epidemiology, 628
  etiology, 628
  nonoperative management, 629–631, 630f
  operative management, 631
Pleural injuries
  classification, 152–153
  diagnosis/testing, 153
  epidemiology, 152–153
  etiology, 152–153
  outcomes/complications, 156
  treatment, 153–156
Pleura, tumors of, 640–641
Pleurodesis, 628
Pneumatic compression devices, 767–768
Pneumatosis intestinalis, 303, 803, 803f
Pneumonia (PNA), 9, 57, 80–81, 156, 265, 418, 628
Pneumothorax, 56, 120, 843–844
  clinical presentation, 625
  diagnosis/testing, 625
  etiology, 625
  nonoperative management, 626–627
  operative management, 627–628
  subtype definitions, 625, 626f
Podofilox, 494
Polycythemia vera (PCV), 396
Polyps, colon, 457–460
Popliteal fossa, 733
Portal vein embolization, 342
Positive predictive value (PPV), 890
Positron emission tomography (PET), 464
  lung cancer, 637
  melanoma, 554
  soft tissue masses, 564
Postbariatric body contouring, 867
Posterior descending artery (PDA), 650
Posterior mediastinal masses, 643
Posterior tibial artery (PT), 733
Posterolateral thoracotomy with decortication, 632
Postoperative management problems
  cardiovascular considerations
    antiplatelet therapy, perioperative use of, 55
    atrial fibrillation, 54–55
    congestive heart failure exacerbation, 54
    hypertension, 53
    hypotension, 52–53
    myocardial ischemia (MI), 53–54
  gastrointestinal considerations
    bowel obstruction, 67
    nausea, 60–66
    paralytic ileus, 66–67
    vomiting, 60–66
  hematologic considerations
    deep vein thrombosis (DVT), 68–69, 70t, 71t–72t
    disseminated intravascular coagulopathy (DIC), 68
    heparin-induced thrombocytopenia (HIT), 67–68
    pulmonary embolism (PE), 69–73
  infectious considerations
    antibiotic prophylaxis, 75t–79t
    catheter-related bloodstream infections, 82
    Clostridioides difficile infection (CDI), 81–82
    fever, 73–74
    intra-abdominal abscess, 80
    necrotizing soft tissue infections (NSTI), 74–80
    pneumonia (PNA), 80–81
    surgical site infections (SSIs), 74
    urinary tract infection (UTI), 80

Postoperative management problems (*continued*)
neurologic considerations
altered mental status (AMS), 44
anesthesia, delayed emergence from, 43–44
delirium, 44–46
seizures, 46–47
withdrawal, 47–48
pain control
nonopiate adjuncts, 50, 50t
opiates, 48–50
regional and local anesthesia, 51
pulmonary considerations
acute respiratory distress syndrome, 57
asthma, 56–57
atelectasis, 55–56
pneumothorax, 56
postoperative pneumonia, 57
pulmonary effusion, 56
pulmonary embolism, 57
respiratory support, 57
renal considerations
electrolyte abnormalities, 59
nutrition, 59–60
renal failure, 57
renal insufficiency, 57
urinary retention, 57–59
Postoperative pneumonia. *See* Pneumonia (PNA)
Postpartum thyroiditis, 616
Precedex. *See* Dexmedetomidine
Predicted postoperative DLCO (ppoDLCO), 625
Preferred Reporting Items for Systematic Reviews and MetaAnalyses (PRISMA), 887
Pregnancy, 172
breast conditions, 546–547
Prehabilitation, 9
Preoperative assessment and care
goals, 1–2
specific considerations
cardiovascular disease, 4–5
diabetes mellitus, 7
infectious complications, 7–8
pulmonary disease, 5–6
renal disease, 6–7
surgical patient, 1–2
Preoperative pulmonary function testing, 5
Prevesical (space of Retzius), 827
Priapism, 874
Primary anal adenocarcinoma, 495–496
Primary graft dysfunction (PGD), 645
Primary hyperaldosteronism
clinical presentation, 581
diagnosis, 581–582
epidemiology, 581
etiology, 581
subtypes of, 581
treatment, 582
Primary hyperparathyroidism (HPT), 599, 601t
Primary intention, 223
Primary lymphedema, 775
Primary survey
adjuncts to, 127–129
airway, 118, 119f
breathing, 120–121
circulation, 121–125
disability, 125–126
exposure, 127
Primary thyroid lymphoma, 610–611
Proctoscopy, abnormal rectal fixation, 480
Progressive systemic sclerosis, 257
Prolonged ileus, 310
Prophylactic thyroidectomy, 593
Propofol, 18
Propylthiouracil, 616
Prostate cancer, 872–873
Prostate, diseases of, 872–874
Prosthetic valve selection, 666
Proximal humerus fractures, 184
Proximal tumors, 276
Pruritus ani, 493
Pseduotumors, 370
Pseudomembranous colitis, 456–457
Pseudomonas species, 767
PTH. *See* Parathyroid hormone (PTH)
Pubertal hypertrophy, 538
Pubic rami fractures, 189
Puborectalis, 475
Pulmonary angiography, 773
Pulmonary artery (PA) catheters, 85–86
Pulmonary disease
postoperative management problems
acute respiratory distress syndrome, 57
asthma, 56–57
atelectasis, 55–56
pneumothorax, 56
postoperative pneumonia. *See* Pneumonia (PNA)
pulmonary effusion, 56
pulmonary embolism, 57
respiratory support, 57

preoperative assessment
antibiotics, 5
bronchodilators, 6
diagnostic evaluation, 5
history, 5
physical examination, 5
prophylaxis and management, 5
smoking cessation, 6
Pulmonary effusion, 56
Pulmonary embolism (PE), 57
diagnosis, 772–774
management, 772–774
massive, 773
postoperative management, 69–73
submassive, 773
Pulmonary function tests, 622, 624f
Pulmonary insufficiency, 665
Pulmonary stenosis, 665
Pulmonary system, 620
P-value *(P)*, 888
Pyogenic abscesses, 335–336
Pyruvate kinase deficiency, 393

Q

Quality improvement (QI), 897
identifying areas for, 900–901
measure, 902
tracking and improving quality outcomes, 901–902
visualizing, 903–904, 903f–904f

R

Radial head fractures, 187
Radial/ulnar shaft fractures, 188
Radiation proctocolitis, 456
Radical (Halsted) mastectomy, 543
Radioactive iodine (RAI) ablation, 608
Radiocephalic (Brescia–Cimino) fistula creation, 788–789
Radiocontrast dye administration, 7
Radiofrequency ablation, 608
Radionucleotide ventilation and perfusion lung imaging (V/Q scan), 773
Randomized controlled trial (RCT), 710, 885–886
Random pattern flaps, 850, 851f
Rapid sequence intubation, 19
Recall bias, 893
Rectal cancer
diagnosis and staging, 466
endorectal ultrasound, 466
neoadjuvant chemoradiation, 466
obstructing, 469
pelvic magnetic resonance imaging, 466, 467f
recurrence, 469
surgical approach, 468–469
Rectocele, 479
Rectovaginal space, 827
Rectum, 827
Rectus sheath hematoma, 240, 243
Recurrent laryngeal nerve (RLN), 597, 688
Red blood cell (RBC), 35
Referred pain, 233
Regional and local anesthesia, 51
Riedel thyroiditis, 616–617
Relative risk (RR), 888
Renal cell carcinoma (RCC), 868
Renal disease
postoperative management problems
electrolyte abnormalities, 59, 61t–63t
nutrition, 59–60, 64t–66t
renal failure, 57
renal insufficiency, 57
urinary retention, 57–59
preoperative assessment and care
diagnostic testing, 6
history, 6
perioperative management, 6
physical examination, 6
prevention, 7
risk factors, 6
Renal failure, 57, 103–104
Renal insufficiency, 57
Renin–angiotensin pathway, 573
Respiratory epithelium, 625
Respiratory failure
acute respiratory distress syndrome (ARDS), 95–96
diagnosis, 89–90
inadequate gas exchange, 89
mechanical ventilation, 90–95, 94f
treatment, 90
Respiratory infections, 8
Respiratory monitoring, 86
Respiratory rate, 622
Respiratory system, 620
Resuscitative thoracotomy, 123
RET proto-oncogene, 593, 611
Retroperitoneal endoscopic adrenalectomy, 590, 591f–592f
Retroperitoneal hematomas, management of, 173
Retrorectal tumors, 470
Rhabdomyolysis, 747

RhoGAM (50 μg intramuscular), 824
Richter hernia, 500
Right coronary artery (RCA), 650
Rivaroxaban, 751
Robotic splenectomy, 407
Robotic surgery, 521
Rome criteria, 444
Root cause analyses, 899
Rotational thromboelastometry (ROTEM), 35
Rotation flaps, 850, 852f
Roux-en-Y gastric bypass (RYGB), 291–292, 291f
Run chart, 903
Rutherford classification, 741, 742t

S

Saccular aneurysms, 708, 709f
Sacral fractures, 189
SAGES. *See* Society of American Gastrointestinal and Endoscopic Surgeons (SAGES)
Salivary glands
  anatomy, 844
  inflammatory diseases, 844–845
  neoplasms, 845–847
Saphenous vein grafts (SVGs), 660
Sappey plexus, 527
Satellite lesions, 555
SBO. *See* Small bowel obstruction (SBO)
SBS. *See* Short-bowel syndrome (SBS)
Scalp, 858–859, 859f, 859t
Scaphoid fractures, 188
Scapula fractures, 184
Schwann cell nerve sheath tumors, 567
Sclerotherapy, 768
Scrotal trauma, 878
Scrotum, diseases of, 875–877
Seborrheic keratoses, 563
Secondary dysmotility, 257
Secondary hyperparathyroidism (HPT), 599–600
Secondary intention, 223
  healing, 849
Secondary lymphedema, 775–776
Segmental resections, 341
Segmental small-bowel resection, 305
Seizures, 46–47
Seminomas, 643
Senescent gynecomastia, 538
Sensitivity (true-positive rate), 890
Sentinel lymph node biopsy (SLNB), 541, 543–544, 557
Sepsis control, 308
Septal ablation, 667
Septal myectomy, 667
Serial transverse enteroplasty procedure, 312
Serrated polyps, 458
Shock, 101–102
Short-bowel syndrome (SBS)
  acute phase management, 310
  defined, 309–310
  etiology, 310
  pathophysiology, 310
Short-chain fatty acids, 444
Shouldice repair, 503
Shunting, 696
Sickle cell disease (SCD), 391
Sigmoidoscopy, 445
  abnormal rectal fixation, 480
Sigmoid volvulus
  diagnosis, 446, 447f
  treatment, 446–447
Simple Endoscopic Score for Crohn's Disease (SES-CD), 317
Simple pneumothorax, 625, 626f
Single-photon emission computed tomography (SPECT)
  hyperparathyroidism (HPT), 600
Sinoatrial node, 650
Sinuses of Valsalva, 650
Sistrunk procedure, 815
Six sigma framework, 902
Skin and soft-tissue tumors
  benign skin lesions
    actinic keratosis, 564
    congenital nevi, 564
    dysplastic nevi, 564
    seborrheic keratoses, 563
  benign soft tissue lesions
    cutaneous cysts, 567
    ganglion cysts, 568
    lipomas, 568
    neurofibromas, 567–568
  melanoma, 551–560
  nonmelanoma skin cancers
    basal cell carcinoma (BCC), 560–561
    Merkel cell carcinoma, 563
    squamous cell carcinoma (SCC), 561–563
  skin lesions, 551, 552f–553f
  soft tissue masses, 564–565
  soft tissue sarcoma, 565–567
Skin grafting, 203
Skin graft thickness, 849, 849f
Skin punch biopsy, 534
Skin-sparing mastectomy, 542
Skip lesions, 317
Skull/facial fractures, 136
Sleeve gastrectomy, 289–291, 290f

Sliding hernia, 500
Small bowel obstruction (SBO), 244–245, 247, 294, 502
  definition, 301
  diagnosis, 302–303
  etiology, 301, 302t
  management, 303, 304f
  presentation, 301
Small bowel resection/ileocolic resection, 318
Small cell lung carcinoma (SCLC), 633–634
Small intestinal resection/ileocolic resection, 318
Small intestine (SI)
  Crohn's disease (CD)
    clinical presentation, 316–317
    defined, 316
    diagnosis, 317–318
    etiology/bowel involvement, 316
    prognosis, 326
    treatment, 318–326, 319t, 320f–326f
  fistulas
    anatomic considerations, 305, 306t
    defined, 305
    diagnosis, 306–307
    etiology, 305, 307t
    nonoperative treatment, 307–309
    operative management, 309, 309t
    pathophysiology, 306
  Meckel's diverticulum
    diagnosis, 305
    management, 303–305
    treatment, 305
  neoplasms
    benign tumors, 312
    malignant tumors, 312–316
    metastatic disease, 316
  short-bowel syndrome (SBS)
    acute phase management, 310
    defined, 309–310
    etiology, 310
    maintenance phase management, 310–312
    operative management, 312
    pathophysiology, 310
Small intestine transplant, 432
SMART objectives, 901
Smoking, 289
  cessation, 6
  preoperative assessment and care, 8
Soave procedure, 809
Society of American Gastrointestinal and Endoscopic Surgeons (SAGES), 522–523
Society of Thoracic Surgeons Risk Score, 651
Soft tissue sarcoma
  classification/staging, 565–566
  diagnosis, 565
  epidemiology, 565
  etiology, 565
  sarcoma-like tumors, 566–567
  treatment, 566
Solid/cystic renal masses, 868, 869t
Solid organ injuries
  abdominal genitourinary injuries, 170–171
  common bile duct injuries, 167
  diaphragmatic injuries, 164–166
  duodenal injuries, 169–170
  gallbladder injuries, 167
  gastric injuries, 169
  hepatic injuries, 166–167
  intestinal injuries, 170
  pancreatic injuries, 169
  pregnancy, 172
  splenic injuries, 167–169, 168f
  vascular injuries, 171–172
Solitary pulmonary nodules, 635
Solitary rectal ulcer, 480
Somatostatin, 270
Sonidegib, 561
Specificity (true-negative rate), 890
Spigelian hernias, 509–510
Spinal cord
  injuries, 126–127
  ischemia, 721
Spinal injuries
  neck and cervical, 138–141, 139f
  thoracolumbar
    diagnostic imaging, 141–143
    types of, 143–144
Spitz nevi, 564
Spleen
  abnormal development/anatomy, 389
  anatomy, 389, 390f
  cystic disease, 400–401
  hematologic diseases
    acquired disorders, 394–400
    congenital disorders, 391–394
  neoplasm, 401–402
  physiology, 390–391
  postoperative considerations
    early complications, 407
    late complications, 407–409
  preoperative considerations, 403–404
  splenectomy, 404–407, 405t–407t
  splenic abscess, 400
  surgical management
    Felty syndrome, 403
    splenic artery aneurysm, 402–403
    trauma, 402
  vascular supply, 389–390

Splenectomy, 404–407, 405t–407t
Splenic abscess, 400
Splenic artery aneurysm, 402–403
Splenic flexure volvulus, 448
Splenic injuries, 167–169, 168f
Split-thickness skin grafts (STSGs), 850
Squamous cell carcinoma (SCC), 494–495, 561–563, 837
- risk factors for, 562t

STAMPEDE trial, 287
Stanford classification system, of aortic dissection, 723, 724f
Staphylococcus aureus, 537
Steal syndrome, 790
Steatorrhea, 317
Stenting, coronary, 4
Stereotactic body radiation therapy (SBRT), 638–639
Stereotactic core biopsy, 535
Sternoclavicular (SC) dislocations, 187
Stomach
- anatomy, 269, 270f
- gastric adenocarcinoma, 274–277
- gastric blood supply, 271f
- gastrointestinal stromal tumors, 279–280
- gastroparesis, 272–274
- histology, 272
- peptic ulcer disease, 280–281
- physiology, 269–272
- upper gastrointestinal (GI) bleeding, 277–279

Strangulated hernias, 501
Strangulation, small bowel obstruction (SBO), 301
Streptococcus pyogenes, 767
Stricturoplasty, 325, 325f, 455
Stroke
- clinical presentation, 692
- diagnosis, 693
- epidemiology, 690
- nonoperative management, 693, 694t
- operative management, 693–698, 697f
- pathophysiology, 692

ST-segment elevation myocardial infarction (STEMI), 659
Subacute (de Quervain) thyroiditis, 617
Subclavian artery transposition, 756
Subclavian–subclavian bypass, 756
Subcutaneous vein dilation, 765
Submucosal tumor, gastrointestinal stromal tumors, 279
Superficial femoral artery (SFA), 733
Superior glands, parathyroid, 597
Superior laryngeal nerve (SLN), 597, 688
Superior mesenteric artery (SMA), 704
Superior sulcus tumors, 637
Superior vena cava syndrome, 634
Suprapubic pain, 233
Surgical aortic valve replacement (SAVR), 662
Surgical site infection (SSI), 8, 23–24, 23–25
- postoperative management problems, 74
- preparation and draping, 23–24

Surgical stabilization of rib fractures (SSRF), 155, 155f
Suspensory ligaments (Cooper's ligaments), 527
Swedish Obese Subjects (SOS), 285
Swenson procedure, 807
Swiss cheese model of accident causation, 898–899, 898f
Symptomatic cholelithiasis, 346
Systematic reviews and meta-analysis (SRMA), 886–887

T

T_3. *See* Triiodothyronine (T_3)
T_4. *See* Thyroxine (T_4)
TAC. *See* Total abdominal colectomy (TAC)
Talc, 628
Talimogene laherparepvec (T-VEC), 560
Talus fractures, 191
Tamoxifen, 536
Technetium-99m hepatobiliary iminodiacetic acid scan, 813
Technetium-99m sestamibi scintigraphy, 600
Technetium-99m tagged red blood cell scan, 451, 452f
Temperature monitoring, 85
Temperature regulation, 25
Temporal bone, 847
Tension pneumothorax, 625
Teratomas, 642
Terminal ileum, 316
Tertiary hyperparathyroidism (HPT), 600
Tertiary intention, 223
Testicles, diseases of, 875–877
Testicular torsion, 875
Tetralogy of Fallot, 665
Thalassemia, 391–392
Therapeutic lymph node dissection (TLND), 557–558
Thionamides, 608
Thoracentesis, 629, 630f
Thoracic aortic aneurysms (TAAs)
- classification, 719
- clinical management, 720–722

clinical presentation, 719–720
complications, 722–723
diagnosis, 720
epidemiology, 719
pathophysiology, 719
Thoracic emergencies, 632–633
Thoracic endovascular aortic repair (TEVAR), 721
Thoracic lymph node stations, 620, 623f
Thoracic pathology. *See also* Pediatric surgery
chest wall deformities, 810
congenital airway malformations, 809–810
Thoracoabdominal vascular disease
abdominal aortic aneurysms (AAAs)
clinical presentation, 708
diagnosis, 708
elective management, 708–715, 709f, 711f–712f
epidemiology, 706–707
late graft-specific complications, 717–719, 718f
pathophysiology/etiology, 707–708
postoperative period after, complications in, 716–717
screening recommendations, 706–707
urgent/emergent management, 715–716
acute aortic syndrome (AAS)
clinical management, 724–726
clinical presentation, 724
diagnosis, 724
epidemiology, 723
pathophysiology and classification, 723, 724f–725f
anatomy, 702–706, 703f–705f
histology, 702–706, 706f
mesenteric ischemia, 726–727
thoracic aortic aneurysms (TAAs)
classification, 719
clinical management, 720–722
clinical presentation, 719–720
complications, 722–723
diagnosis, 720
epidemiology, 719
pathophysiology, 719
Thoracoscopic decortication, 632
Threatened abortion, 824
Thromboelastography (TEG), 35
Thromboembolism, 21t
Thrombolysis, 774
Thrombosed hemorrhoid excision, 485
Thrombotic thrombocytopenic purpura, 399–400
Thymomas, 642
Thymus, 597
Thyroglossal duct cysts, 597, 814–815
Thyroid cancer, 612t
classification, 610–611
clinical presentation/symptoms, 611
diagnosis/testing, 611
epidemiology, 610–611
etiology, 610–611
outcomes/complications, 614–615
treatment, 611–614
Thyroid carcinoma, 839
Thyroid gland
anatomy, 597, 598f
histology, 599
physiology, 598–599
Thyroid hormone synthesis, 599
Thyroiditis
classification, 616–617
diagnosis/testing, 617
epidemiology, 616–617
etiology, 616–617
nonoperative treatment, 617
operative treatment, 617
outcomes/complications, 617
Thyroid nodules
classification, 604–605
clinical presentation/symptoms, 605
diagnosis/testing
fine-needle aspiration (FNA), 606, 606t, 607f
imaging, 608, 609f
laboratory studies, 605–606
molecular testing, 606
epidemiology, 604–605
etiology, 604–605
evaluation algorithm, 605, 605f
nonoperative treatment, 608
operative treatment, 608–610
outcomes/complications, 610
Thyroid-stimulating hormone (TSH), 598
Thyrotoxicosis, 608
Thyrotropin-releasing hormone, 598
Thyroxine (T_4), 599
Tibial plateau fractures, 190
Tibial shaft fractures, 190–191
Tibioperoneal (TP) trunk, 733
Tidal volume, 622
Tissue biopsy, cholangiocarcinoma, 637

TNF-α inhibitors, 455
Toe fractures, 192
Total abdominal colectomy (TAC), 445
Totally extraperitoneal (TEP) repair, 505–506, 505f
Total (simple) mastectomy, 541
Total neoadjuvant therapy (TNT), 466
Total parenteral nutrition (TPN), 308, 795, 796t
Trabectedin, 566
Tracheal stenosis, 844
Tracheobronchial disruption, 121
Tracheobronchial injury
  classification, 159
  diagnosis/testing, 159
  epidemiology, 159
  etiology, 159
  outcomes/complications, 159
  treatment, 159, 160f
Tracheoesophageal fistula (TEF), 797, 798f
Tracheoesophageal malformations, 797–799, 798f–799f
Tracheostomy, 842–844
Transabdominal preperitoneal (TAPP) repair, 505
Transanal hemorrhoidal dearterialization, 485
Transcarotid artery revascularization (TCAR), 697–698
Transcatheter aortic valve replacement (TAVR), 662
Transcatheter (transfemoral) mitral valve therapies, 664
Transesophageal echocardiogram (TEE), 655
Transfemoral carotid artery stenting (TF-CAS), 696
Transfusion
  blood components, 36, 37t
  preparation, 35–36
  risks, 36–38
Transient ischemic attack (TIA), 692
Transmetatarsal amputation, 755
Transmural inflammation, 317
Transposition flaps, 850, 853f
Transsphenoidal hypophysectomy, 593
Transthoracic echocardiogram (TTE), 654
Transudative pleural effusions, 628
Transverse volvulus, 448
Trauma, 402, 818–819
  laparotomy, 163–164
Trauma resuscitation
  Advanced Trauma Life Support (ATLS), 115, 125t
  epidemiology, 115
  management, 163
  prehospital care, 115–117
  primary survey
    adjuncts to, 127–129
    airway, 118, 119f
    breathing, 120–121
    circulation, 121–125
    disability, 125–126
    exposure, 127
  secondary survey, 129
Traumatic acute arterial ischemia, 741–743
Traumatic injury
  caustic ingestion, 260–261
  esophageal perforation, 259–260
Triangle of Koch, 650, 652f
Triangulation, principle of, 518
Trichloroacetic acid, 494
Tricuspid regurgitation (TR), 665
Tricuspid stenosis (TS), 664–665
Triiodothyronine (T_3), 599
Triple-negative breast cancer, 540
Trousseau's sign, 603
Trunk
  abdominal wall reconstruction, 862, 864f
  breast reconstruction, 859–861, 860f, 861t
  chest wall reconstruction, 861–862, 863f
  pressure sores, 862
T-tests, 890
Tube thoracostomy, 629–631, 630f
Tube thoracostomy placement, 120
Tubular adenomas, 458
Tubulovillous adenomas, 458
Tumors
  benign liver tumors, 333–335
  biomarkers and prognostic factors, 540
  colorectal tumors, 469-470
  esophageal, 261–266
  gastrointestinal stromal tumors, 279–280
  malignant liver tumors, 338–340
  of mediastinum
    anterior mediastinal masses, 642–643
    clinical presentation, 642
    differential diagnosis of, 641, 641t
    epidemiology, 641–642
    etiology, 641–642
    middle mediastinal masses, 643
    posterior mediastinal masses, 643
    radiographic evaluation, 642
  and neoplasms. *See* Neoplasms
  pancreatic neuroendocrine tumors, 368–370

pseduotumors, 370
of pleura, 640–641
Turbinates, 847
Two-stage hepatectomy, 343
Type I pneumocytes, 625
Type II pneumocytes, 625

U

Ulcerative colitis, 453–454
Ulcers, 765
Ultrasonic energy devices, 523
Ultrasonography
abdominal aortic aneurysms (AAAs), 708
appendicitis, 817
hemodialysis (HD), 787
hyperparathyroidism (HPT), 600
inguinal hernia, 501
Spigelian hernias, 510
Umbilical hernia, 509, 818
Undifferentiated pleomorphic sarcoma, 565
Undifferentiated thyroid carcinoma, 610
Unna boots, 767
Unpaired t-test, 890
Unstable angina, 657
Upper endoscopy, pH monitoring, 289
Upper gastrointestinal (GI) bleeding
classification, 277–278
diagnosis/testing, 278
epidemiology, 277–278
etiology, 277–278
nonoperative treatment, 278
operative treatment, 279
presentation/symptoms, 278
Uremia, 32
Ureter, diseases of
hydronephrosis, 868–870
ureteropelvic junction obstruction, 871
urolithiasis, 870–871
Ureteropelvic junction obstruction, 871
Urethral injury, 877–878, 878f
Urinary bladder, diseases of, 871–872, 872t
Urinary retention, 17, 57–59
Urinary tract infection (UTI), 80
Urolithiasis, 870–871
Urologic surgery
genitourinary trauma, 877–878, 878f
hematuria, 867
kidney, diseases of, 868, 869t
penis, diseases of, 874–875
prostate, diseases of, 872–874
scrotum, diseases of, 875–877
testicles, diseases of, 875–877
ureter, diseases of
hydronephrosis, 868–870
ureteropelvic junction obstruction, 871
urolithiasis, 870–871
urinary bladder, diseases of, 871–872, 872t
Urothelial carcinoma, 871
Uterus, 827, 828f

V

VACTERL syndromes, 807
Vaginal bleeding
clinical assessment, 822–824
management of, 822, 822f
nonobstetric causes of, 822, 823t
obstetric etiologies of, 824
treatment, 824–825
Vagus nerve, 688
Valvular disease, 666
Vancomycin, 457
Varicose veins, 764–765
Vascular injuries, 171–172
Vascular smooth muscle cells (VSMCs), 707
Vein mapping, 787
Venous and lymphatic disease
anatomy, 761–764, 762f–763f
chronic venous insufficiency (CVI)
epidemiology, 764
imaging, 765
nomenclature, 765, 766t–767t
nonoperative management, 765–768
operative management, 768
pathophysiology, 764–765
physical examination, 765, 767f
symptoms, 765
lymphedema
classification, 775–776
differential diagnosis, 776
epidemiology, 775
imaging, 776
nonoperative management, 776–777
operative management, 777
pathophysiology, 775–776
physical examination, 776
symptoms, 776
venous thromboembolism (VTE)
deep venous thrombosis diagnosis and management, 769–772
epidemiology, 768–769
pathophysiology, 769
prevention, in surgical patients, 774–775
pulmonary embolism diagnosis and management, 772–774

Venous claudication, 765
Venous ulcer
  lower extremity distribution of, 765, 767f
  management, 765
Ventilation, 622
Ventral mesh rectopexy, 480
Ventricular assist devices (VADs), 668
Ventricular septal defect (VSD), 650, 657–658
Veress needle, 519
Vesicovaginal space, 827
Video-assisted thoracoscopic surgery (VATS), 156, 627–628
Villous adenomas, 458
Visceral pain, 233, 234f
Vismodegib, 561
Vitamin D, 598
Vitamin K
  antagonists, 770
  deficiency, 32
Volvulus
  cecal, 447–448
  sigmoid, 446–447, 447f
  splenic flexure, 448
  transverse, 448
Vomiting, postoperative management, 60–66
Von Willebrand disease (vWD), 31–32
VTE. *See* Venous thromboembolism (VTE)
Vulvar carcinoma, 828–829

W

Waterhouse–Friderichsen syndrome, 587
Wedge resections, 340, 628
Weight loss, 317
  surgery, 287t
Weiss criteria, 586
Wide local excision (WLE), 555–557
Will Rogers phenomenon, 893
Withdrawal, postoperative management problems, 47–48
Wound care
  acute wound healing, 209–212
    special categories of, 212–216
  chronic wounds, 218–223
    healing, 216–218
  negative pressure wound therapy, 223–229, 224t–227t, 228f
  wound closure, 223
Wound closure, 223
Wound healing
  acute, 209–212
  chronic
    chronic leg ulcers, 219–220
    diabetic foot ulcers, 218–219, 219f
    physiology of, 216–218, 217t
    pressure injuries, 220–223, 220t, 221f
  early
    hemostasis, 209
    inflammatory phase, 209
    intermediate wound healing, 211
  intermediate
    angiogenesis, 211
    epithelialization, 211
    fibroblasts, 211
  late, 211
    collagen, 211
    wound contraction, 211
  medications, 211–212
  scars, 212

X

X-ray
  inguinal hernia, 501
  chest X ray (CXR). *See* Chest X ray (CXR)
  orthopedic injuries, 181t–183t

Y

Young–Burgess classification, 188

Z

Zollinger–Ellison syndrome, 593
Zona fasciculata, 573
Zona glomerulosa, 573
Zona reticularis, 575